MEDIAN HEIGHTS AND [illegible]E

Category	Age (years) or Condition	Weight (kg)	Weight (lb)	Height (cm)	Height (in)	REE* (kcal/day)	Average Energy Allowance (kcal)[b†] Multiples of REE	Per kg	Per day[‡]
Infants	0.0–0.5	6	13	60	24	320		108	650
	0.5–1.0	9	20	71	28	500		98	850
Children	1–3	13	29	90	35	740		102	1300
	4–6	20	44	112	44	950		90	1800
	7–10	28	62	132	52	1130		70	2000
Men	11–14	45	99	157	62	1440	1.70	55	2500
	15–18	66	145	176	69	1760	1.67	45	3000
	19–24	72	160	177	70	1780	1.67	40	2900
	25–50	79	174	176	70	1800	1.60	37	2900
	51+	77	170	173	68	1530	1.50	30	2300
Women	11–14	46	101	157	62	1310	1.67	47	2200
	15–18	55	120	163	64	1370	1.60	40	2200
	19–24	58	128	164	65	1350	1.60	38	2200
	25–50	63	138	163	64	1380	1.55	36	2200
	51+	65	143	160	63	1280	1.50	30	1900
Pregnant	1st trimester								+0
	2nd trimester								+300
	3rd trimester								+300
Lactating	1st 6 months								+500
	2nd 6 months								+500

*Calculation based on FAO equations, then rounded.
†In the range of light to moderate activity, the coefficient of variation is ±20%.
‡Figure is rounded.
From National Research Council. Recommended Dietary Allowances. 10th ed. Washington, DC, National Academy Press, 1989.

ESTIMATED SODIUM, CHLORIDE, AND POTASSIUM MINIMUM REQUIREMENTS OF HEALTHY PERSONS[a]

Age	Weight (kg)[a]	Sodium (mg)[a,b]	Chloride (mg)[a,b]	Potassium (mg)[c]
Months				
0–5	4.5	120	180	500
6–11	8.9	200	300	700
Years				
1	11.0	225	350	1000
2–5	16.0	300	500	1400
6–9	25.0	400	600	1600
10–18	50.0	500	750	2000
>18[d]	70.0	500	750	2000

[a]No allowance has been included for large, prolonged losses from the skin through sweat.
[b]There is no evidence that higher intakes confer any health benefit.
[c]Desirable intakes of potassium may considerably exceed these values (~3500 mg for adults—see text).
[d]No allowance included for growth. Values for those below 18 years assume a growth rate at the 50th percentile reported by the National Center for Health Statistics (Hamill et al., 1979) and averaged for males and females. See text for information on pregnancy and lactation.

Applied Nutrition and Diet Therapy for Nurses

SECOND EDITION

Applied Nutrition and Diet Therapy for Nurses

SECOND EDITION

Judi Ratliff Davis
M.S., C.N.S.D., R.D., L.D.

Kim Sherer
R.N., M.N.

Photography for chapter openers courtesy of

Doug A. Davis

W.B. SAUNDERS COMPANY
A Division of Harcourt Brace & Company
Philadelphia London Toronto Montreal Sydney Tokyo

W.B. Saunders Company
A Division of
Harcourt Brace & Company
The Curtis Center
Independence Square West
Philadelphia, Pennsylvania 19106

Library of Congress Cataloging-in-Publication Data

Davis, Judi.
Applied nutrition and diet therapy for nurses / Judi Davis, Kim Sherer.—2nd ed.
p. cm.
Rev. ed. of: Applied nutrition and diet therapy / Grace Burtis, Judi Davis, Sandra Martin. 1988.
Includes bibliographical references and index.
ISBN 0-7216-6785-6
1. Diet therapy. 2. Nutrition. 3. Nursing. I. Sherer, Kim. II. Burtis, Grace. Applied nutrition and diet therapy. III. Title.
[DNLM: 1. Diet Therapy—nurses' instruction. 2. Nutrition—nurses' instruction. WB 400 D262a]
RM216.B96 1993
615.8'54—dc20
DNLM/DLC 92-49079

APPLIED NUTRITION AND DIET THERAPY
FOR NURSES, 2nd Edition ISBN 0-7216-6785-6

Printed in the United States of America.

Last digit is the print number: 9 8 7 6 5 4 3 2

Dedication

To instructors and students who

struggle to squeeze the study of nutrition

into the ever-expanding nursing curriculum

About the Authors

Judi Ratliff Davis, M.S., C.N.S.D., R.D., L.D., received her B.S. from the University of Texas at Austin and her M.S. in nutrition from Texas Woman's University in Denton and completed a dietetic internship at Indiana University Medical Center in Indianapolis. She has had a variety of experiences in the field of nutrition, including teaching, clinical dietitian, and consultant. She has taught various nutrition and food service courses at Tarrant County Junior College in Fort Worth, Texas. She has served as a clinical dietitian at Rehabilitation Hospital of North Texas, Arlington, Texas; Fort Worth State School, Fort Worth, Texas; Rex Hospital in Raleigh, North Carolina; and Baptist Memorial Hospital in San Antonio, Texas. She has also worked as a nutrition consultant for nursing homes and mental health facilities in western Virginia, San Antonio, and the Dallas–Fort Worth area; for the Greenhouse, a health spa in Arlington, Texas; and for the Sugar Association.

Kim Sherer, R.N., M.N., obtained her B.S. in nursing at Oklahoma University Health Science Center in Oklahoma City and her M.N. at Wichita State University. She has worked as staff nurse, charge nurse, and House Supervisor at Stillwater Medical Center in Stillwater, Oklahoma. In addition to teaching nursing students at Northern Oklahoma College in Tonkawa, Oklahoma, she is currently the Chair of the Nursing Division.

Preface

The study of nutrition can be an interesting and rewarding subject for nursing students, not only for client education, but also for their own health. This book is designed to show nursing students how to apply sound nutrition principles in assessing, diagnosing, planning, implementing, and evaluating total care of clients and to help the student contribute to the nutritional well-being of clients. A holistic approach to dietary management of a disease by the entire health care team is especially appropriate to coordinate totally integrated client care.

Since the subject of nutrition is a top priority in today's society, the public faces the challenge of understanding nutritional information. As key members on the health care team, nurses are expected to discuss sound nutritional practices knowledgeably and authoritatively with their clients or the general public.

Nutritional information in this book is compiled clearly and concisely to provide an understanding of the therapeutic value of foods in the normal diet. Using the *Behavioral Objectives* as a guide, both the student and the instructor know the important information to be gained from each chapter. The *Chapter Outline* lists specific subjects to be covered. Questions in the margins and *Student Readiness* at the end of each chapter help students determine their comprehension of the subject. *Test Your NQ* (nutrition quotient) is a brief true-false pretest to stimulate interest in the reading assignment. Answers are located in Appendix G. Learning is also challenged by *Case Studies* in many chapters. Throughout the text, nutrition is integrated into the nursing process. In basic nutrition chapters, *Nursing Applications* provide practical information about how this information can affect the client's care or nutritional status; tips for *Client Education* help the student realize what the client should know or be taught. In therapeutic chapters, *Nursing Applications* provide specific information established during an *assessment* (physical, dietary, and laboratory), *interventions* or factors that need to be considered in caring for the client, some suggestions for *evaluation* of nursing care of the client's nutritional status, and information for *Client Education.* The *Nursing Process in Action* in each chapter describes a situation and is followed by the five-step nursing process care plan so students can see how to "pull it all together." *Nutrition Update*, presented in some chapters, provides state-of-the-art information on emerging issues in nutrition. An institutional-type menu introduced in Chapter 12 is used as a basis for therapeutic menus so students can realize types of changes in food choices necessary to meet dietary restrictions.

Section I deals with basic principles of nutrition. An understanding of basic nutrition facts is required for the student to evaluate the flood of new information available, to make wise judgments about eating habits, and to counsel clients about dietary changed needed. Nutrient deficiencies and excesses are addressed in sections entitled *Hyper- and Hypo-*, terms that are more familiar to nursing students and are more congruent with real-life occurrences. This unit contains sections on how a vegetarian can obtain an adequate balance of nutrients, food fads and misinformation, sugar and fat substitutes, carbohydrate loading for trained athletes, and many other relevant topics.

Section II, "Orientation to Clinical Nutrition," helps the student apply basic nutrition principles while providing care to clients in a community or hospital setting. Alternate methods of feeding, or using tube feedings or intravenous feedings, may be encountered in the clinical or home setting. Since the nurse is usually the health care team member most closely associated with intravenous and tube feedings, a thorough discussion of this subject is presented.

Problems specifically involved in application of basic nutrition principles through the life span and with ethnic groups are presented in Section III so the nurse can recognize other dietary habits and incorporate any necessary modifications with sensitivity and respect. Changes in nutritional requirements and eating patterns affected by various stages of life are discussed. Breast-feeding has been covered extensively to enable students to encourage this practice. Other subjects include premenstrual syndrome (PMS), hyperactivity, and Alzheimer's disease.

Nutrition support for vulnerable populations is discussed in Section IV. A nutritional assessment is a basic essential for the nutritional well-being of all clients; this involves performing a physical assessment, evaluating dietary intake/history, and monitoring pertinent laboratory values. Many conditions and their outcomes are improved by encouraging clients to eat well or to make minor changes in food choices to improve their health.

Dietary modifications essential to treat diseases are described in Section V. Pathophysiology is limited to indications for diet therapy; principles for the dietary treatment are emphasized. Pertinent nursing applications are cited. Integrated into the discussions are related laboratory findings and drug–nutrient interactions.

The Appendix contains information for completing assignments and reference material. Food composition tables include the nutritive values of food from three sources: (1) the latest USDA Handbooks 8–1 through 8–21, (2) items from fast-food restaurants, and (3) supplementary and tube feedings. Tables that are important in nutritional assessments are included.

The nurse has considerable influence on the client's food acceptance. With a better understanding of the importance of diet, the entire health care team can complement each other and provide optimal care for the client. While specific amounts of nutrients are mentioned, much of this information is presented not so nurses can prescribe special diets, but so they can recognize usual therapeutic measures for specific conditions and call any discrepancies to the attention of the physician or dietitian. This will also enable them to explain the reason for various treatments to the client.

Acknowledgments

Because of the diversity of subjects presented in a general nutrition textbook, a compilation of the work of many people, whether direct or indirect, is necessary to present up-to-date information. Whether the aid was in the area of a research study or verbal or written communications, each person's help and support is truly appreciated.

For consultation in specific areas, our gratitude is extended to Sherrill Burgdorf, Speech-Language Pathologist at Rehabilitation Hospital of North Texas (dysphagia); Aisha Faulkner, Food Service Director with American Restaurant Association (cultural and religious influences); Helene Silver, Registered, Licensed Dietitian with Harris Methodist Hospital in Fort Worth (renal and religious influences); Marsha McCleskey, R.D., L.D., nutrition consultant (diabetes and nutrition computer expertise); Diane Wade, R.N., Nutrition Support Nurse (nutrition support); Bobbi Emmons, R.N., M.S.N., Nursing Sophomore faculty (nutritional nursing process) at Northern Oklahoma College; numerous local hospital pharmacists, including Jon Albrecht, R.Ph, BCNSP, for their help with drug usage and spelling; and pharmaceutical sales representatives, Patti Walsh, R.D., L.D., Catherine Chairez, R.D., L.D. (Mead Johnson), Wanda Pittard, R.D., L.D., Hadley Hoff, R.D., L.D. (Ross Laboratories), and Cindy McLaughlin, M.S., R.D., L.D. (Sandoz).

Many thanks to Texas College of Osteopathic Medicine for their superb collection of medical journals and monographs and especially for the use of the Mini-MEDLINE, which was invaluable in accessing the latest medical research.

We would especially like to extend appreciation to Lisa Kight, Stephanie Hoover Davis, and Judi's daughter, Debbie Davis, who performed superbly at secretarial tasks and computer input. We are greatly indebted to Frank Davis for keeping the computer functioning and always forcing us to update the computer to "speed up" this time-consuming process. Thanks to Doug A. Davis for his creative ideas for chapter theme photography and Tamara Timmons for many of the drawings. Besides those listed, there are countless other friends and relatives to whom we wish to express our gratitude for encouragement and support.

Objective critiques from reviewers are invaluable to a good publication. We do appreciate the insight, perspective, words of encouragement, and valuable ideas of these reviewers. The authors and publishers thank the following reviewers for their many helpful suggestions: Colleen H. Duggan, M.S.N., R.N., Johnson County Community College, Overland Park, Kansas; Dana L. Griffith, R.D., C.N.S.D. and Irene Muth, R.D., C.N.S.D., Temple University Hospital, Philadelphia; Donna S. Bacon, M.S., R.D./L.D., formerly at University of Oklahoma Health Sciences Center, Oklahoma City; Eileen Monahan Chopnick, M.B.A., R.D., Widener University School of Nursing, Chester, Pennsylvania; Betty Joan Sims Marsh, M.S.N., R.N., Central Florida Community College, Ocala; Alan M. Levine, Ph.D., R.D., Marywood College, Scranton, Pennsylvania; Barbara A. Troy, M.S., R.D., Marquette University College of Nursing, Milwaukee; and Julia Boyd Swarner, Ph.D., M.P.H., R.D., Joni

J. Pagenkemper, M.S., R.D., and Kenneth Iber Burke, Ph.D., R.D., Loma Linda University, Loma Linda, California.

We also wish to thank the many persons at W. B. Saunders Company who worked so tirelessly in the various phases of planning and producing this book. We are especially grateful to Daniel T. Ruth, nursing editor, for his helpful ideas and insistence that this edition be geared specifically to the nurse's needs. We also appreciate the input, assistance, and encouragement of Ilze Rader, Ellen Thomas, Mary Anne Folcher, and Linda R. Garber whenever it was needed.

Contents

SECTION

I

Orientation to Basic Nutrition

This section will cover all the basic nutrients essential for good health, what foods contain these essential elements, and what happens if you eat too much or too little of them. In other words, it prepares you to provide optimal nutritional care for yourself and your clients so you can assess nutrient intake and suggest ways to improve food choices. You will learn there is no one perfect food, but it is the overall food choices that affect one's health.

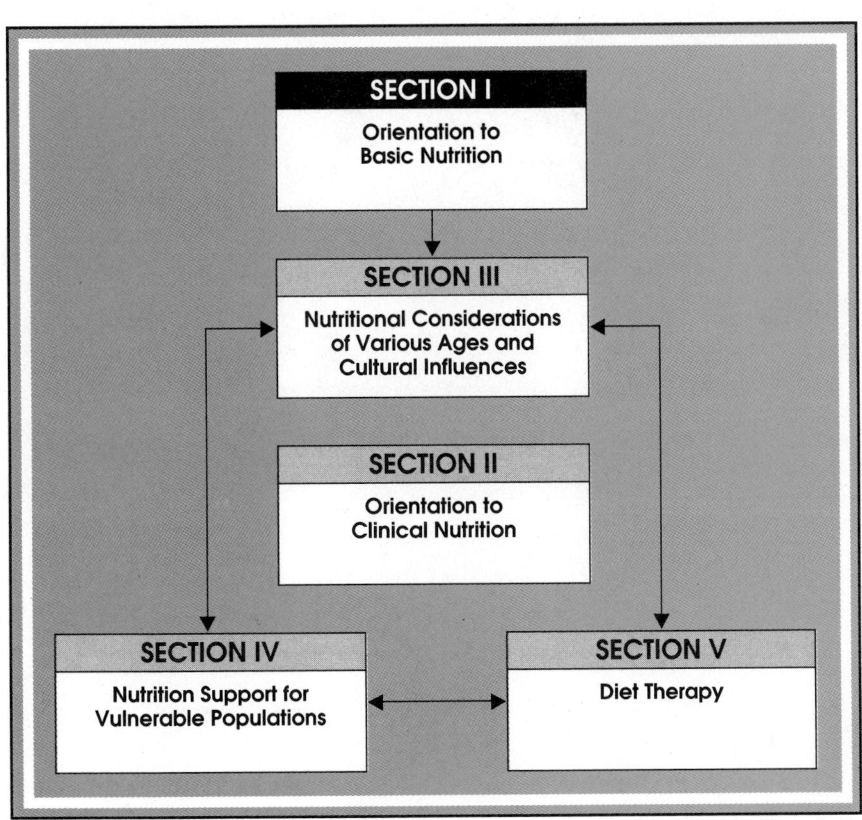

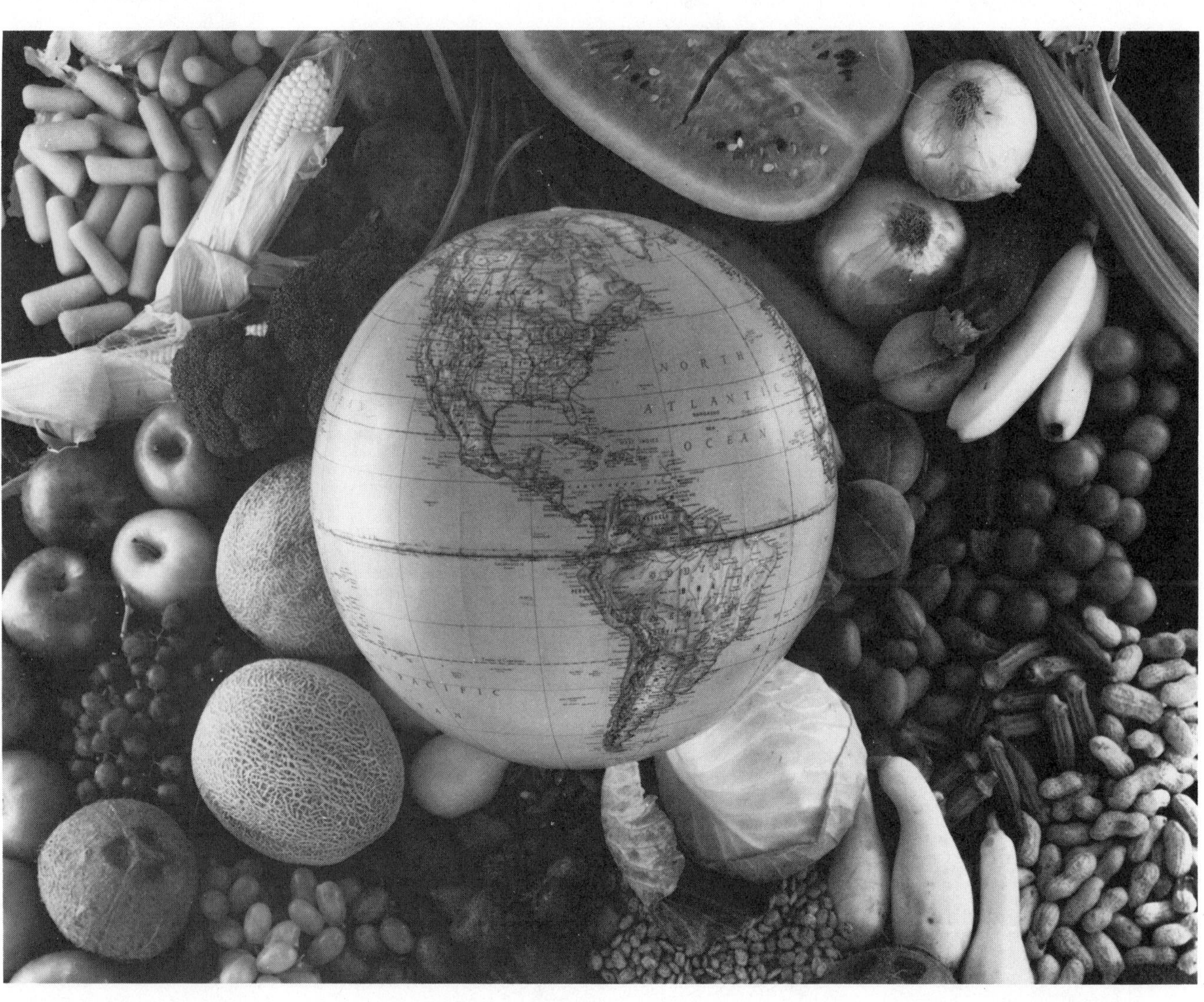
NORTH
OCEAN
PACIFIC

CHAPTER 1

World of Nutrition

OUTLINE

I. NUTRITION IN NURSING CARE
II. BASIC NUTRITION
III. PHYSIOLOGICAL FUNCTIONS OF NUTRIENTS
Nursing Applications
IV. BASIC CONCEPTS OF NUTRITION
V. NUTRITIONAL CONCERNS
Nursing Applications
VI. FOOD INFORMATION SYSTEMS
VII. RECOMMENDED DIETARY ALLOWANCES (RDAs)
Nursing Applications
VIII. FOOD GUIDE PYRAMID
A. Vegetables and Fruits
B. Breads, Cereals, Rice, and Pasta
C. Milk, Yogurt, and Cheese
D. Meats, Poultry, Fish, Dry Beans and Peas, Eggs, and Nuts
E. Other Foods
Nursing Applications
IX. DIETARY GUIDELINES FOR AMERICANS
A. Eat a Variety of Foods
B. Maintain Healthy Weight
C. Choose a Diet Low in Fat, Saturated Fat, and Cholesterol
D. Choose a Diet with Plenty of Vegetables, Fruits, and Grain Products
E. Use Sugars Only in Moderation
F. Use Salt and Sodium Only in Moderation
G. If You Drink Alcoholic Beverages, Do So in Moderation
H. Summation of the Dietary Guidelines
Nursing Applications
X. NUTRITION LABELING
Nursing Applications
XI. FOOD FADS AND MISINFORMATION
A. Evaluating Health Foods
B. Detecting Fraudulent Claims
C. Evaluating Scientific Information
D. The Role of Nurses
Nursing Applications

OBJECTIVES

THE STUDENT WILL BE ABLE TO:

- List the general physiological functions of the 6 nutrient classifications of foods.
- Assess factors that influence food habits.
- Name the basic food groups.
- State the number of servings needed from each of the food groups.
- Identify significant nutrient contributions of each food group.
- State the US Dietary Guidelines and their purpose.
- Identify dietary selections in each food group that significantly affect intake of kilocalories, fats, salt, and sugar.
- Assess dietary intake of a client, using the US Dietary Guidelines and the food guide pyramid.
- Explain the different purposes of the RDA, basic food groups, and the US RDIs.
- List reasons why health quackery can be dangerous.
- Identify common themes of health quackery and why they are contrary to scientific information.
- Analyze health information for its scientific validity.
- Apply basic nutritional concepts to help clients with nutritional disorders.
- Identify client educational principles for basic nutrition.

TEST YOUR NQ (True/False)

1. Milk is a perfect food.
2. Fad diets have magical healing qualities.
3. Water is the most important nutrient.
4. RDAs are required daily allowances essential for all clients to be healthy.
5. Americans consume 20 times more sodium than their bodies need.
6. Two to 4 servings are needed from the fruit and vegetable group.
7. The Dietary Guidelines were written for healthy Americans to help reduce chronic diseases.
8. Organic foods are more nutritious.
9. Alcohol is nutritionally inadequate.
10. The only nutrients that provide energy are carbohydrates, fats, and protein.

Nutrition involves the integration of physiological and biochemical reactions within the body as well as psychological and social factors that enter into the frequent decisions concerning food choices. Freedom of choice and variety in consumption are important components of individual and social life. Thus, to provide effective nursing care for a client's nutritional status, nurses must consider all these aspects.

To help you master nutritional care in a systematic process, this book is divided into 5 sections. Section I, "Orientation to Basic Nutrition," discusses the basic nutritional principles. Understanding "normal" nutrition is essential in caring for healthy as well as ill clients. An awareness of nutrient requirements and nutrient content of foods prepares you to assess adequacy of food choices and to make suggestions for needed changes. Additionally, this first chapter will give you the knowledge to make healthy food choices for yourself and your immediate family.

Once you have a grasp of normal nutrition, Section II, "Orientation to Clinical Nutrition," will show you how to apply these nutrition principles while providing care for all types of clients whether they are in the community or hospital setting. Various methods of providing nutrition to these clients will be presented. Section III, "Nutritional Considerations of Various Ages and Cultural Influences," discusses how nutritional requirements and eating patterns are affected during various stages of life. Although the same basic nutrients are essential for everyone, amounts are affected by a client's stage of life. The types of foods chosen to meet nutrient requirements are influenced by various ages, cultures, and lifestyles. These factors must be addressed to provide high-quality nutritional care.

Certain groups of the population are at greater risk of developing or experiencing nutritional problems. Nutrition support for these vulnerable populations will be discussed in Section IV. Section V, Diet Therapy, involves nutritional care for illnesses or disease states that may require dietary modifications. Some conditions or diseases alter the body's physiological needs or utilization of specific nutrients; in spite of this, adequate provision of other nutrients must be maintained.

As you will learn during your study, modifying nutrient intake may become complicated because each food contributes an assortment of nutrients. For example, milk not only provides calcium but also protein, lactose, and riboflavin; it may also be a source of saturated fats.

It is our hope that this book will equip you to meet the nutritional needs of your clients better. As summarized in the section opener, section I provides the basic essentials; section II builds on the foundation to help you provide nutritional care in various settings and presents basic skills for subsequent sections; section III streamlines information from previous sections to help you individualize nutritional care based on age and culture. Sections IV and V are interrelated because they both provide information on nutrition support to help you care for different conditions and actual disease processes.

NUTRITION IN NURSING CARE

A knowledge of basic nutrition principles will assist you to care for a client's nutritional concerns in the following ways:

1. **Assessing** a client's nutritional status.
2. Analyzing data gathered in the assessment to make appropriate nutritional nursing diagnosis. In nutrition, the 2 main nursing diagnoses used are "altered nutrition: less than body requirements" or "altered nutrition: more than body requirements." Other commonly used diagnoses for nutrition are "knowledge deficit" (specify particular area), "altered health maintenance," "feeding self-care deficit," and "impaired swallowing."
3. Planning realistic dietary goals for and with the client; goals are client centered and measurable. These goals also relate to the first part of a diagnosis, i.e., less or more than body requirements. Thus, depending on the diagnosis, a dietary goal could be "client will gain/lose 1 to 2 lbs in 1 week until desired weight is reached."
4. **Implementing** therapeutic nutritional **interventions** and understanding rationale for treatment.
5. **Evaluating** whether nutritional care was effective or not.

Assess—gather data about food intake by interviewing the client and family and reading the chart.

Implement—actual carrying out of interventions.

Interventions—measures a nurse performs to and/or with a client, such as monitoring intake and output or serving the food tray.

Evaluate—determine if goals were achieved or not. If goals were not achieved, revisions must be made, i.e., reassess the situation, make new nursing diagnosis or goals or try other interventions and reevaluate.

TABLE 1–1

GENERAL FUNCTIONS OF NUTRIENT CLASSES

Physiological Function	Nutrients
Furnish energy	Carbohydrates Fats Proteins
Build and maintain body tissues	Proteins Minerals Water
Regulate body processes	Proteins Minerals Vitamins Water

BASIC NUTRITION

Nutrition—the process by which living things utilize food for energy, growth and development, and maintenance.

Food—the substance taken into the body to provide nutrients.

Nutrients—biochemical substances that are required by the body and must be consumed in adequate amounts.

Nutrition involves eating foods to provide nutrients the body is unable to synthesize. Nutrition involves not only digesting **food** to make **nutrients** available, but also absorbing and delivering nutrients to the cells where they are utilized and eliminating waste products. Foods differ in the amount of nutrients they furnish. Any individual food can be compatible with good nutrition but should be evaluated in context of the client's physiological needs, the food's nutrient content, and other food choices.

PHYSIOLOGICAL FUNCTIONS OF NUTRIENTS

How is nutrition different from nutrients?

Why are foods eaten?

What are the 6 classes of nutrients?

Physiologically, foods eaten are used for energy, tissue building, and obtainment or production of numerous regulatory substances. The 6 classes of nutrients obtained from foods include (1) water, (2) proteins, (3) carbohydrates, (4) fats, (5) minerals, and (6) vitamins. Table 1–1 shows basic functions of the major nutrients; however, nutrients function interdependently, interacting in complex metabolic reactions.

NURSING APPLICATIONS

1. Assess client's physiological needs, food choices, and nutrient content of the foods consumed to determine adequacy of nutrition and nutrients.
2. Because nutrients work interdependently, a lack or excess in one can interfere with or prevent the use of another. Evaluate client's intake of the 6 classes of nutrients to determine adequacy or excessive intake. Ask client to record or list food intake for 24 hours so you can assess the nutrient intake.

Client Education

- No single food contains all the essential nutrients in the amounts needed for optimum health.
- Nutrition can either improve or adversely affect health.

BASIC CONCEPTS OF NUTRITION

The essential nutrients are needed throughout life; only the amounts of nutrients change. Nutrient requirements change according to the client's utilization of foods eaten, stage of growth and development, sex, body size, weight, physical activity, and state of health.

Some nutrients can be converted by the body to meet its physiological needs. Nonessential nutrients can be utilized by the body but either are not required or can be synthesized from dietary precursors. One example is cholesterol. Water is the most important nutrient. Following water, the nutrient of highest priority is **energy,** which must be supplied from foods or can be supplied from limited quantities stored in the body. The human body has adaptive mechanisms that allow clients to tolerate modest ranges in nutrient intakes. For instance, metabolic rate usually decreases as a result of decreased kilocaloric intake.

Energy—measured in kilocalories and provided by the basic nutrients: carbohydrate, fat, and protein.

Increasing the variety of foods in the diet reduces the probability of developing isolated nutrient deficiencies, nutrient excesses, and toxicities caused by nonnutritive components or contaminants in any particular food. When the intake of any single nutrient is changed, the amounts of other nutrients in the diet are also altered. For instance, because red meats and eggs are excellent sources of iron, decreasing cholesterol intake by limiting these foods reduces dietary iron. The premise of nutritional nursing care is that, in any cultural circumstance or for any personal taste or preference, good nutrition is possible.

What affects client's nutrient requirements? What nutrients supply energy? Why is a variety of foods important?

NUTRITIONAL CONCERNS

The Senate Select Committee on Nutrition and Human Needs originally published *Dietary Goals for the United States* in 1977 to promote healthy food choices. This was followed by *The Surgeon General's Report on Nutrition and Health* (USDHHS, 1988) confirming that 5 of the top 10 leading causes of death (coronary heart disease, certain types of cancer, stroke, diabetes mellitus, and atherosclerosis) have been associated with diet.

Both of these reports had similar conclusions. The US food supply provides adequate quantities of nutrients to protect healthy Americans from deficiency diseases.

What diseases have been associated with diet?

NURSING APPLICATIONS

1. Assess client's growth and development, sex, body size, weight, physical activity, and state of health to determine nutrient requirements. If there is an alteration in any of these, changes in nutrient requirements occur.
2. To provide good nutritional care, consider cultural influences and personal preferences when planning interventions.
3. Nurses must have a basic understanding of nutrient components in foods to suggest alternate food choices that provide the needed nutrients for clients who avoid or dislike a particular food. Additionally, this information may help nurses prevent a client from omitting needed nutrients inadvertently.
4. If the client has any of the diseases listed under "Nutritional Concerns," evaluate food or nutrient choices thoroughly. Asking the client to list typical intake for 24 hours will help in this effort.

Client Education

- It is the whole balance of the diet that matters, and the best balance incorporates a variety of foods.
- Unrestrained habits, especially overconsumption of certain dietary components, may contribute to the development of many diseases; i.e., saturated fat intake predisposes clients to atherosclerosis.

FOOD INFORMATION SYSTEMS

RDAs—identify nutritional needs in terms of specific amounts of essential nutrients that adequately meet the known nutrient needs of practically all healthy clients.

Since clients eat foods, nutrient requirements and information must be interpreted into the "food" language clients understand. The **Recommended Dietary Allowances (RDAs)** attempt to establish needed nutrients and amounts required at various stages of life. Food grouping systems are tools used to translate technical nutritional needs into practical guidelines for food selections. Several guidelines that facilitate appropriate food choices are discussed here, including the basic food groups, Dietary Guidelines for Americans, and nutrition labeling.

RECOMMENDED DIETARY ALLOWANCES (RDAs)

The RDAs are published by the government but are established by competent scientists and nutritionists who base their recommendations on evidence from epidemiological, physiological, clinical, and biochemical studies to ensure optimal physiological functioning.

Not all essential nutrients are addressed in the RDA table. Specifically, water, carbohydrates, essential fatty acids, and many trace elements are not included. The assumption is that a varied diet providing recommended amounts of the listed nutrients will also furnish sufficient amounts of the omitted nutrients. The RDAs include an **Estimated Safe and Adequate Daily Dietary Intake (ESADDI)** for 2 vitamins and 5 minerals.

ESADDI—estimated allowances established for nutrients in which data were sufficient to establish a range of requirements but insufficient for a specific RDA.

How are the RDAs established? Why are all nutrients not addressed in the RDA table?

RDAs are used most frequently as a measurement by professionals who assess the nutrition status of the American population; establish guidelines for feedings in institutions; and set standards for the use of food stamps, school lunch programs, and other forms of food assistance. Unfortunately, there are no sure guidelines for establishing at what point diets become inadequate. The government generally considers a diet adequate that provides two-thirds of the RDAs, whereas less than that is considered poor.

NURSING APPLICATION

1. Use of RDAs as an assessment guide is for healthy clients only.

Client Education

- The RDAs are intended as general guidelines rather than as specific requirements.

FOOD GUIDE PYRAMID

The food guide pyramid (Fig. 1–1) that replaces the basic four food groups can be adapted and modified imaginatively to meet the needs of clients and families with different levels of income, cultural patterns, and lifestyles. Broad families of foods with similar kinds of nutrients are grouped together, as shown in Table 1–2.

Vegetables and Fruits

The food guide pyramid separates fruits and vegetables into 2 groups, recommending 3 to 5 servings of vegetables and 2 to 4 servings of fruits daily. According

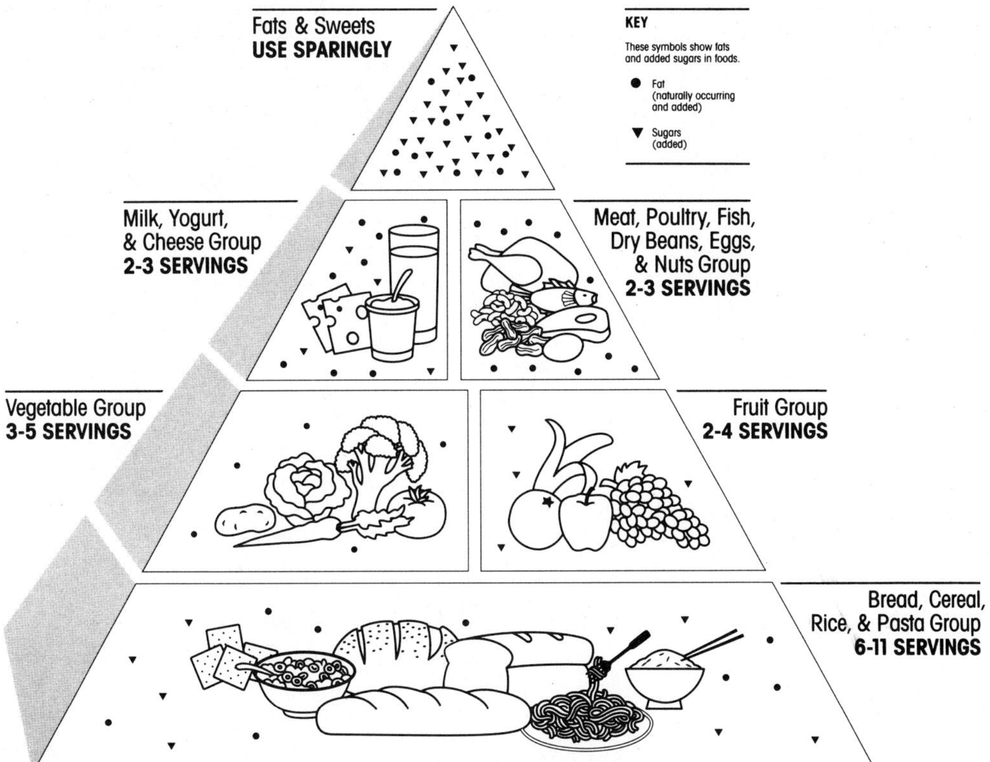

Figure 1–1 The food guide pyramid is a general guide of what to eat each day. It is not a rigid prescription, but will help you choose healthful foods. The pyramid presents a variety of foods to provide the nutrients you need and at the same time obtain the right amount of kilocalories to maintain a healthy weight. The food groups in the lower 3 sections are emphasized because of their contribution to nutrient requirements. (From U.S. Department of Agriculture and the U.S. Department of Health and Human Services, Washington, D.C., 1992. Home and Garden Bull. No. 252.)

the second National Health and Nutrition Examination Survey, 1976–1980, 45% of the American population consumed no fruits or juice and 22% consumed no vegetables in an entire day (Patterson et al, 1990). Vegetables and fruits in season (at their peak of production and lowest in price) are the most flavorful and highest in nutrient value in most cases. Although foods in both of these groups are valuable for their contribution of fiber and vitamins C and A, individual foods vary widely in their vitamin C and A content. Note that vitamin C is provided only by fruits and vegetables. A good source of vitamin C should be eaten daily. Vitamin A–rich foods should be chosen 3 to 4 times a week (Table 1–3). Dark green vegetables also contribute calcium, iron, magnesium, riboflavin, and folate. Because of their high water and high fiber content, most fruits and vegetables are relatively low in kilocalories.

Consumption of fruits and vegetables has been gradually increasing. Clients have the opportunity to purchase items such a kiwi fruit, papaya, Chinese cabbage, and snow peas that they had never heard of 10 years ago. Additionally, more clients are choosing fruits as snacks. They are concerned about consuming a well-balanced diet, with fewer kilocalories, and getting their money's worth (Segal, 1988).

How many servings are recommended for vegetables and for fruits? How often should a food source of vitamin C and vitamin A be eaten?

Breads, Cereals, Rice, and Pasta

Enrichment—the process of restoring nutrients removed from food during processing.

All whole-grain, refined and enriched, or fortified-grain products are included in this group. **Enriched** products have had iron, thiamin, riboflavin, and niacin re-

TABLE 1–2

THE FOOD GROUPS AND PRINCIPAL NUTRIENT CONTRIBUTION TO THE DIET

	Vegetable	Fruit	Meat	Milk	Grain
Recommended Number of Servings	3–5	2–4	2–3	Child, 2–9 yr, 2–3 Child, 9–12 yr, 3 or more Teenager, 4 or more Adult, 2 or more Pregnancy, 4 or more Lactation, 4 or more	6–11
Serving Sizes	½ cup chopped raw or cooked; 1 cup raw leafy greens	1 medium sized; or ½ of large fruit; ¼ cup dried fruit; ¾ cup juice; ½ cup canned fruit	2½ to 3 oz of cooked lean meat, poultry, or fish; ½ cup cooked dried beans, 1 egg, or 2 tbsp peanut butter is equivalent to 1 oz lean meat	1 cup milk or yogurt 1½ oz cheese 2 cups cottage cheese 2 oz processed cheese	1 slice bread; 1 oz dry cereal; ½ cup cooked cereal, pasta, rice
Protein			X	X	X
Vitamin A	X	X			
Vitamin D				X	
Vitamin E	X				
Vitamin C	X	X			
Thiamin			X		X
Riboflavin				X	
Niacin			X		X
Vitamin B_6			X	X	
Folacin	X	X			
Vitamin B_{12}			X	X	
Calcium				X	
Phosphorus			X	X	
Magnesium	X	X		X	
Iron			X		X
Zinc			X		
Fiber	X	X			X

TABLE 1–3

CONTRIBUTIONS OF SELECTED FRUITS AND VEGETABLES TO A HEALTHY DIET

	Vitamin A	Vitamin C	Fiber	Cruciferous Vegetable
Acorn Squash	X			
Apple			X	
Apricot	X		X	
Avocado	X		X	
Banana			X	
Bell Pepper		XX		
Broccoli	X	XX	X	X
Brussels Sprouts		XX	X	X
Cabbage		X	X	X
Cantaloupe	X	XX	X	
Carrot	X		X	
Cauliflower		X	X	X
Celery			X	
Collard Greens	X	X		
Grapefruit		X	X	
Iceberg Lettuce			X	
Kale	X	X		X
Kiwi Fruit		X	X	
Kohlrabi				X
Orange		XX	X	
Papaya	X	X	X	
Peach	X		X	
Prune			X	
Spinach	X		X	
Strawberry		XX	X	
Sweet Potato	X		X	
Swiss Chard	X			X
Tomato		X	X	

XX, Excellent source of Vitamin C. X, Good source of Vitamin C.

TABLE 1–4 **COMPARISON OF NUTRIENT VALUES OF SELECTED WHOLE-GRAIN AND ENRICHED PRODUCTS**

Types of Bread	Protein (gm)	Total Dietary Fiber (gm)	Thiamin (mg)	Riboflavin (mg)	Niacin (mg)	Vitamin B_6 (mg)	Folacin (mcg)	Pantothenic Acid (mcg)	Iron (mg)	Zinc (mg)	Calcium (mg)	Phosphorus (mg)	Magnesium (mg)
Whole wheat	2	2.8	0.09	0.05	1	0.05	14	0.18	0.9	0.42	18	65	23
Rye	2	1.6	0.10	0.08	0.8	0.02	10	0.11	0.7	0.32	20	36	6
Enriched white	2	0.4	0.11	0.07	0.9	0.08	8	0.10	0.7	0.14	29	25	5

Nutrient data from Nutritionist III software, Version 7.0, N-Squared Computing, Salem, Oregon.

Fortification—the process of adding nutrients not present in the natural product or higher than in the original product.

What is the difference between enriched and fortified?

placed approximately to their original levels. Enrichment is federally controlled by the Food and Drug Administration (FDA), which establishes the quantity of nutrients that can be added. Whole-grain products contribute more fiber, magnesium, and folacin than do enriched products (Table 1–4). A variety of grain products should be selected, such as wheat, rice, oats, and corn. Most processed breakfast cereals are **fortified** at nutrient levels higher than those occurring naturally in the grain.

Milk, Yogurt, and Cheese

The milk group excludes high-fat dairy products such as butter and cream because they are not high in calcium, riboflavin, and protein. Fortified milk products are important sources of vitamin D; however, many milk substitutes (cheese, yogurt, and ice cream) are not fortified with vitamin D (unless made with fortified milk). Use of low-fat milk products can decrease kilocalorie content significantly. Serving recommendations for this group are based on calcium requirements for various stages of life (Table 1–2).

Meats, Poultry, Fish, Dry Beans and Peas, Eggs, and Nuts

This group is an important source of protein and iron. Choices within this group should include a variety because each food has distinct nutritional advantages. Various meat choices are outstanding for their individual contributions (Table 1–5).

Other Foods

Foods not contained in the previously discussed groups might well be called "accessory foods." These kilocalorie-dense foods are high in fats, sugar, or alcohol,

TABLE 1–5

OUTSTANDING CONTRIBUTIONS OF VARIOUS PROTEIN FOODS

Protein Food	Nutrient
Lean red meats	Iron B vitamins Zinc
Pork	Thiamin
Liver and egg yolks	Vitamin A Iron
Dry peas and beans, soybeans, and nuts	Magnesium Fiber

providing mainly energy and few other nutrients. These foods contribute to palatability and make some nutritious foods more desirable. For instance, some clients may dislike milk but enjoy pudding or custard. In addition to providing a prolonged feeling of satiety, some fats and oils are a good source of vitamin A and E.

In general, the amounts of these foods to include in the diet depend on the amounts of energy needed. When only the specified amounts of foods from the basic food groups are consumed, the kilocaloric intake ranges from about 1400 to 1600 kcal—far below the energy needs of a teenager.

What are some examples of other foods? How much of these foods should be consumed?

NURSING APPLICATION

- Assess client's intake of food groups to determine nutrient adequacy or inadequacy. (If a client dislikes fruits and vegetables, vitamin A and C deficiencies may develop; if milk and other milk products are eliminated, calcium deficiencies may develop).

Client Education

- Within each food group, foods can vary widely in the number of kilocalories furnished.
- Milk products are poor sources of iron and vitamin C.
- Foods in the bread-cereal group are economical as well as nutritious; they may be staple items for lower socioeconomic groups.
- Cholesterol occurs naturally in all foods of animal origin.
- Foods not classified in the basic food groups, i.e., sugars, fats, and alcohol, are intended to complement, not replace, foods from the other groups.

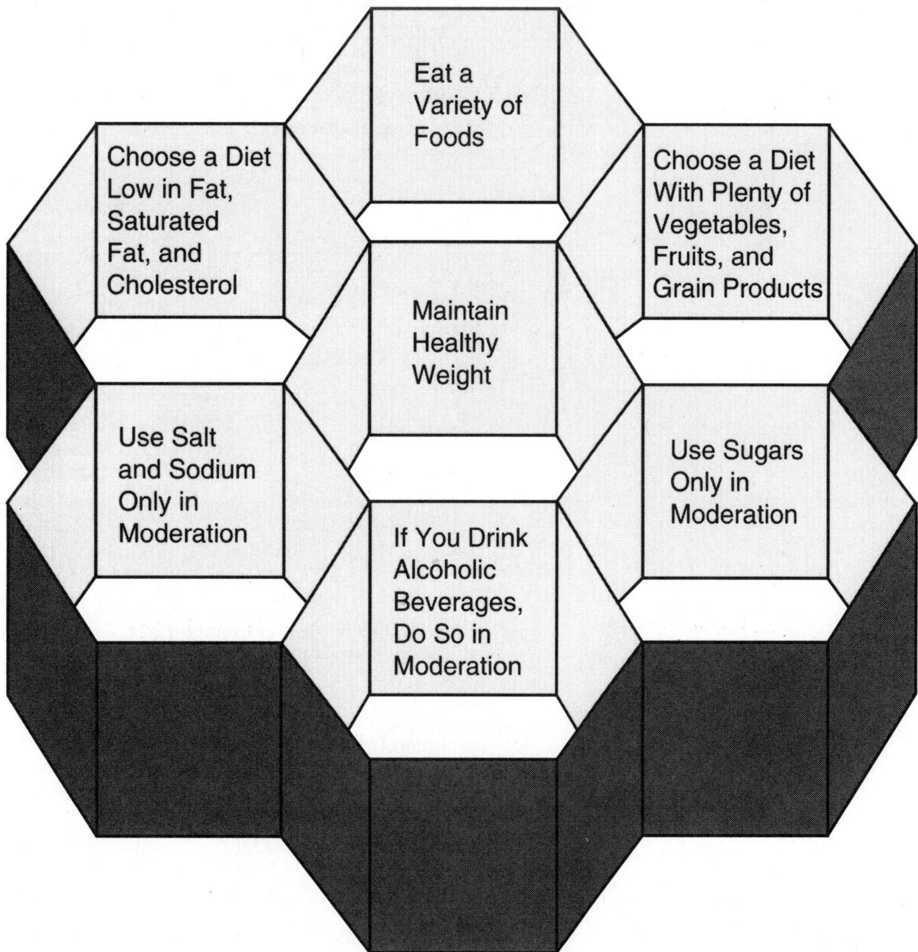

Figure 1–2 Seven guidelines that should be used together to choose a healthful and enjoyable diet. (From U.S. Department of Agriculture, U.S. Department of Health and Human Services. *Nutrition and Your Health: Dietary Guidelines for Americans.* 3rd ed. Home and Garden Bull. No. 232. Washington, D.C., Government Printing Office, 1990.)

DIETARY GUIDELINES FOR AMERICANS

Based on recommendations made from goals established in 1977, the US Department of Agriculture (USDA) and the former US Department of Health, Education, and Welfare (USDHEW) established the Dietary Guidelines for Americans, which were updated in 1990 (Fig. 1–2). The Dietary Guidelines are intended for healthy Americans and clients at risk of developing chronic diseases (family history of obesity, high blood pressure, or elevated cholesterol levels) who want to avoid nutritional deficiencies and reduce risks of some these diseases (Fig. 1–3). The 7 guidelines are discussed separately, indicating how they relate to nursing practice.

Eat a Variety of Foods

No healthy client with a broad range of likes and who regularly eats a wide variety of fruits, vegetables, milk, cereals, and small amounts of animal protein at each meal will be in any danger of developing nutritional deficiencies. This goal can be met by emphasizing variety from each of the basic food groups previously discussed.

Maintain Healthy Weight

Obesity involves clients of all ages and economic groups. The probability of developing hypertension, coronary heart disease, gallbladder disease, diabetes, and problems associated with osteoarthritis is increased with obesity. Obesity indicates that kilocaloric intake has exceeded output. Energy balance is most difficult to achieve with today's sedentary lifestyles and jobs, which are low in energy expenditure.

Being underweight also has risks. Numerous health problems are associated with anorexia, and underweight increases risk of osteoporosis in women.

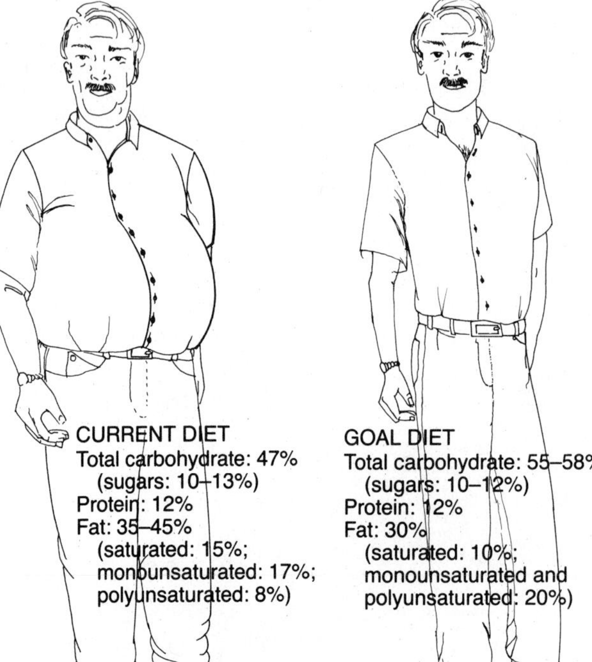

Figure 1–3 Comparison of current eating patterns versus recommendations from the Dietary Guidelines for Americans. (Data based on Raper N. Nutrient content of the U.S. food supply. *Food Rev* 1991 Jul/Sep; 14(4):13–18; Glinsman WH, et al. Evaluation of health aspects of sugars contained in carbohydrate sweeteners. U.S. Food and Drug Administration, 1986; *Dietary Goals for the United States.* 2nd ed. Washington, D.C., Senate Committee on Nutrition and Human Needs, 1977.)

TABLE 1–6

IMPLEMENTING THE FAT AND CHOLESTEROL GUIDELINE

Cooking with Fats and Oils
Check labels on foods to determine the amount of fat and saturated fat in a serving
Choose liquid vegetable oils most often because they are lower in saturated fat. Reduce saturated fats such as butter, lard, and palm and coconut oil
Limit foods with hidden fats such as chips, doughnuts, cookies, snack crackers, cakes, fried foods, and some processed and convenience foods
Use fats and oils sparingly in cooking (roast, bake, grill, or broil when possible). Baste meats with broth or stock
Use nonstick cookware and an aerosol cooking spray
Use small amounts of salad dressings and spreads, such as butter, margarine, gravy, and mayonnaise
Use the paste method for making gravy or sauces. Add flour or cornstarch to cold liquids slowly and blend well
Season with herbs, lemon juice, or stock rather than lard, bacon, or ham
Skim fat from homemade soups or stews by chilling and removing the fat layer that rises to the top
Use fat-free or low-fat salad dressings
Use jam, jelly, or marmalade spread instead of butter or margarine
Rely on mustard and salad greens to add moisture to sandwiches rather than fat-laden spreads
Substitute plain low-fat yogurt for mayonnaise or sour cream
Limit fruits and vegetables that contain high levels of fat: olives, avocados, and coconuts
Meat, Poultry, Fish, Dry Beans, and Eggs
Have 2 or 3 servings of meat, poultry, or fish, with a daily total of about 6 oz
Choose a vegetarian entree (dry beans and peas) at least once a week
Include all types of meat. Consumer demand has resulted in livestock producers breeding animals to produce leaner beef and pork
Trim visible fat from meat; take skin off poultry before eating
Choose a beef grade "select" because it contains fewer kilocalories as a result of less fat marbling. The fat content of the meat is also due to the type of cut, Leaner cuts include flank steak, sirloin, or tenderloin, loin pork chops, 85% lean ground beef
Marinate leaner cuts of meat in lemon juice, flavored vinegars, or fruit juices
Use low-fat ground turkey or extra lean ground beef for casseroles, spaghetti, and chili
Moderate the use of egg yolks (maximum 4 egg yolks weekly) and organ meats
Limit organ meats such as liver, brains, and kidney
Choose tuna packed in water not in oil
Milk and Milk Products
Choose skim or low-fat milk and fat-free or low-fat yogurt and cottage cheese most of the time. Look for the words "1% fat," "99% fat-free" or "skimmed"
Choose cheeses with 6 gm or less of fat/oz (90% of the kilocalories in cream cheese are from fat)

Moderation of kilocalorie intake is the key to maintaining ideal weight; it may be the most important dietary goal for clients. All food groups should be included, using more servings of lower kilocalorie foods. When the energy requirement is low, consumption of foods not included in the food groups (sugar, alcohol, and fats) should especially be reduced because these foods provide kilocalories but few other nutrients. Weight control is further discussed in Chapter 19.

What are some complications of overweight and underweight? What is the key to maintaining ideal body weight?

Choose a Diet Low in Fat, Saturated Fat, and Cholesterol

High blood cholesterol levels denote an increased risk of coronary heart disease. In some clients, excessive kilocaloric intake can also increase blood cholesterol.

The guidelines recommend that everyone over 20 years of age have their cholesterol level checked, preferably by a physician. Clients falling into high-risk categories should be given a therapeutic diet and encouraged to achieve or maintain desirable weight.

Although cholesterol and saturated fats are not essential nutrients, cholesterol-rich foods are a good source of iron, which is a difficult nutrient to obtain in adequate amounts from the food supply. In addition, liver and eggs are economical for clients on a low budget.

The biggest change in dietary habits is reflected by the fact that consumption of fat increased about 6% between 1976 and 1988 (Raper, 1991). Fortunately, the kinds of fats have changed. A larger percentage of the fat intake is from vegetable products, especially margarine, vegetable shortenings, and other consumable oils. The proportion of fat from animal sources has markedly declined from 65% to 53% between 1968 and 1988 (Raper, 1991). By decreasing the total amount of fat ingested and continuing to use more polyunsaturated fats, this goal can be met and practiced by healthy clients with no adverse effects (Table 1–6).

To help reduce fat consumption, food manufacturers have developed fat substitutes to decrease the fat content of foods. The potential for fat substitutes is promising by promoting reduced kilocalories from fats consumed in dessert and snack foods. But they are not a panacea against obesity, cancer, or heart disease. Fat substitutes will not compensate for poor dietary choices or replace the benefits of a diet rich in whole grains, fresh fruits, and vegetables. Further discussion of various fat substitutes is found in Chapter 5.

What is the benefit of reducing fat and cholesterol intake?

Choose a Diet with Plenty of Vegetables, Fruits, and Grain Products

Starches are also known as complex carbohydrates.

Unrefined—generally indicates foods that are as close to the form in which they naturally occur as possible, i.e., whole grains or whole legumes as opposed to refined flours, cereals, and meat substitutes.

Grain products and many vegetables and fruits are emphasized especially for their **complex carbohydrates** and dietary fiber. Foods rich in complex carbohydrates and fiber are listed in Table 1–7. Dietary fiber is important for healthy bowel functioning and can reduce symptoms of chronic constipation, diverticular disease, and hemorrhoids. **Unrefined** complex starches contain significant amounts of fiber as well as vitamins and minerals, especially zinc, vitamin B_6, and folacin.

To accomplish this goal for increasing intake of grain products requires educational efforts to change food habits with different emphases in menu planning. Clients have avoided complex carbohydrates with the misconception that they are fattening. Owing to their low fat content, they are relatively low in kilocalories. A

TABLE 1–7

NATURAL FOOD SOURCES OF COMPLEX CARBOHYDRATES AND FIBER

Good Sources of Complex Carbohydrates
Breads, both whole-grain and enriched
Breakfast cereals, cooked or ready-to-eat (enriched or fortified)
Flours, whole-grain and enriched
Pastas such as noodles, macaroni, and spaghetti
Rice, whole-grain or white
Legumes such as dried beans, peas, and lentils
Starchy vegetables such as English peas, potatoes, lima beans, corn
Good Sources of Fiber
Whole-grain breads and other bakery products
Whole-grain cereals, cooked and ready-to-eat
Legumes such as dried beans, peas, and lentils
Fruits, especially with skins (figs, pears, apricots, nectarines, raisins, blueberries) and edible seeds (blackberries, raspberries, strawberries)
Vegetables, especially sweet potato, carrots, mushrooms, raw onions, pumpkin, spinach, turnip greens, kale, Brussels sprouts, parsnips, peas, beets, okra, and broccoli
Nuts and seeds

TABLE 1–8

IMPLEMENTING THE GUIDELINE FOR INCREASING FIBER

Include 2–4 servings of fruits and 3–5 servings of vegetables daily
Use breads and cereals in which the first listing in the ingredient list is "whole wheat" or "whole grain"
Choose cereals with at least 2 gm fiber but no more than 2 gm fat/serving
Add a little bran or wheat germ to recipes, even casseroles, main dishes, pancakes, and cooked cereal
Eat bagels and English muffins, which are good low-fat choices
Prepare raw vegetables to eat with low-fat dip as appetizers
Serve baked potatoes topped with steamed vegetables (broccoli, cauliflower, carrots)
Add vegetables (mushrooms, peppers, onions, tomatoes) to an omelet or scrambled eggs
Drink tomato juice
Add leafy greens, tomato, and sprouts to sandwiches
Add raw vegetables to brown bag lunches: zucchini, carrots, or celery sticks
Snack on fresh fruits and vegetables and plain popcorn instead of fried chips and cookies

diet high in complex carbohydrates may be more slimming than a diet of comparable kilocalories high in fat (Lissner et al, 1989; McCargar et al, 1989; Schutz et al, 1989; Tremblay et al, 1989). Foods containing complex carbohydrates are usually eaten with added fats or sugars. For example, sugar is usually added to cereal, and margarine is added to bread or potatoes.

Foods rich in vitamins A and C may help lower the risk for cancers of the larynx, esophagus, and lungs (Block, 1991; Garewal, 1991; Stahelin, 1991; Ziegler, 1991). **Cruciferous** vegetables help reduce cancer susceptibility (Butrum et al, 1988). Good sources of vitamin A and C and cruciferous vegetables are listed in Table 1–3. Tips for implementing this guideline are presented in Table 1–8.

Cruciferous—a botanical family of plants including cabbage and mustard.

What are the benefits of increasing complex carbohydrate and fiber and vitamins A and C?

Use Sugars Only in Moderation

Refined sugar contains kilocalories and no other nutrients. This guideline was not meant to decrease the intake of natural sugars found in fruits, vegetables, and milk. The only health risk associated with sugar is tooth decay; however, many other factors are involved in the formation of caries. Routine oral hygiene and use of a fluoride toothpaste and/or fluoridated water are more important factors in healthy teeth.

Many forms of sugar can be added to foods by a client or a manufacturer: table sugar, brown sugar, raw sugar, glucose (dextrose), fructose, maltose, lactose, honey, syrup, corn sweetener, high-fructose corn syrup, molasses, and fruit juice concentrate. Therefore, client teaching concerning labeling is essential.

Many other sweeteners are now on the market as substitutes for sucrose. Several, including fructose, sorbitol, mannitol, and xylitol, contain the same number of kilocalories as table sugar. "Dietetic" products containing these sweeteners can mislead clients to believe they contain no kilocalories. Based on the prevalence of obesity, it is doubtful whether these products have actually helped curtail either sugar or kilocaloric consumption. These will be discussed further in Chapter 4.

What forms of sugar may be added to foods by clients or manufacturers? Which sweeteners contain the same number of kilocalories as sugar?

Use Salt and Sodium Only in Moderation

The average amount of salt intake in the US is about 10 gm daily, which is approximately 20 times more than the body's requirement. It is especially important to identify clients with a family history of hypertension or who are salt-sensitive. A low-salt intake begun at an early age may possibly protect against development of hypertension. The preferred amount of salt is dependent on the level of salt consumption; this preference can be lowered after reducing sodium intake for a while.

TABLE 1–9

IMPLEMENTING THE GUIDELINE FOR SALT INTAKE

Compare sodium content of products by reading nutrition labels. Try the lower sodium versions of canned soups, salad dressings, sauces, and other processed foods
Minimize intake of foods with a large amount of sodium added during food processing—bacon, cured meats, luncheon meats, sausage, sauerkraut, olives, and pickles
Learn to enjoy other seasonings or the natural flavors of foods; try seasonings such as lemon, garlic, or ginger
Use little or no salt at the table. Salt gives a sharper taste when on food rather than in food, so if you can go easy on the shaker, it is best to add salt after food is prepared
Cook with only small amounts of added salt

Table 1–9 presents some suggestions to help lower salt intake. The sodium content of many fast foods is significant (a cheeseburger and french fries may contain more than 1300 mg). Additionally, many food manufacturers have reduced the sodium content of their products or offer a reduced-sodium line.

If You Drink Alcoholic Beverages, Do So in Moderation

Moderation of alcohol consumption is classified as 1 drink a day for women and no more than 2 drinks a day for men.

Alcohol is high in kilocalories and contains few if any nutrients. Alcohol may be retained in the blood for 3 to 5 hours; this poses a risk to clients who engage in activities that require attention or skill, especially driving. Heavy drinking by pregnant women has been associated with birth defects. Many medications may be adversely affected (decreased benefits or increased toxicity) by alcohol.

Summation of the Dietary Guidelines

These goals work in conjunction with the basic food groups to help clarify some points lacking in the food groups relating to optimal health, as shown in Table 1–10. All of these guidelines support healthy eating habits to improve the health and quality of life (Fig. 1–4). Although the initial guidelines were controversial, other health and governmental organizations, such as the National Cancer Institute and American Heart Association, have also issued guidelines regarding nutrition and health advice to reduce risk of nutrition-related diseases in the US. Although each organization differed in their target population, the overall message is consistent with the Dietary Guidelines for Americans (Table 1–11).

NURSING APPLICATIONS

1. These guidelines do not necessarily apply to clients who require special diets or to those with conditions that interfere with normal nutrition or to children under 2 years of age.
2. Assess client's intake of the food groups; weight; blood pressure; and family history of hypertension, cardiovascular disease (strokes, heart attacks), and cancer.
3. Encourage foods listed in Tables 1–3 and 1–7.
4. Follow suggestions listed in Table 1–9.
5. Evaluate client's knowledge of foods low or high in fat, saturated fats, and cholesterol. A quick check is to have the client verbalize 1 or 2 foods that are high in these nutrients followed by 1 or 2 foods that can be substituted that are low in fat, saturated fats, and cholesterol. If the client is unable to do this, determine if he or she knows where to find this information. If not, provide booklet or information sheet.

Client Education

- Eat a variety of foods, but consume salt, sugar, alcohol, and fat in moderation.
- Describe advantages of diets high in grains, fruits, and vegetables.
- Dietetic and sugar-free foods may not be low in kilocalories; this is dependent on other ingredients in the food.
- Instruct the client not to use these guidelines if he or she has been told to follow a special diet or is ill.
- Instruct the client to consult a physician, nurse, or dietitian before radically modifying his or her diet.
- Encourage the use of polyunsaturated fat.
- Explain that 1 tsp salt = 5 gm salt or 2000 mg (2 gm) sodium.
- Encourage women who are pregnant or trying to conceive to abstain from alcohol.

NUTRITION LABELING

To help clients make informed decisions about food choices in the supermarket, the government has established a standard guideline for nutritional information on food labels. Nutrition labels on product packaging help nurses and clients to be aware of the nutrients in a food and to compare the nutritional values of various products. Based on a law passed in November 1990 (FDA, 1990), nutrition labels have had a complete overhaul in 1993 that will be fully implemented in May, 1994. This is a concerted effort of both the USDA and the FDA to improve the health and well-being of the American people by enhancing nutrition knowledge. The new label requires that all foods, including fresh produce, meat, and fish, provide nutritional information based on the nutrients provided in a single serving. Serving portions are based on the reference amount normally consumed by an average person. The number of servings in a container is expressed to the nearest whole number. For foods that are not packaged, the information is displayed at the point of purchase (e.g., counter card, sign, booklet).

Nutrients provided on the label include total kilocalories; total kilocalories from fats; total fat and saturated fat (gm); cholesterol (gm); total carbohydrates, complex carbohydrates, and sugars (gm); dietary fiber (gm); protein (gm); sodium (mg); and vitamins and minerals (vitamins A and C, calcium, iron). Labeling of the following nutrients is voluntary: kilocalories from saturated fat, amounts (gm) of polyunsaturated and monosaturated fats, other carbohydrates, sugar alcohol, soluble and insoluble fiber, potassium, and other vitamins (thiamin, riboflavin, niacin).

To make labels less confusing to consumers, the term *Daily Value* is used and reflects two new sets of dietary standards—**Reference daily intakes (RDIs)** and **daily reference values** (DRVs). RDIs are the basis for the percentage of daily values for protein, vitamins, and minerals. The RDIs are different from the RDAs previously discussed and should not be confused with them. The 5 sets of RDIs are designed for special foods for infants, children under 4, pregnant women, lactating women, and adults and children over 4 years of age (see Appendix B-1).*

RDIs, a new term for US RDA, are based on a population-adjusted average of all the age/sex groups of RDA values excluding those for pregnant and lactating women.

DRVs represent the energy-producing nutrients (based on an intake of 2000 kcal/day) and saturated fat, cholesterol, sodium, and fiber (Table 1–12). DRVs for

Text continued on page 25

Daily Reference Values (DRVs) are based on desirable levels of nutrients considered important for health: total fat, saturated fatty acids, protein, cholesterol, carbohydrate, fiber, and sodium.

* The RDI will replace the US RDAs. At the time of publication, the new values for the RDIs are not available. Therefore, the US RDA values are provided in Appendix B-1, but this text will use the term RDIs.

SAMPLE MENU BASED ON U.S. DIETARY GUIDELINES

Sample Menu

Breakfast
1 cup orange juice
1 bagel with 1 oz cream cheese and 1 packet raisins
1 cup 1% milk
coffee with creamer

Lunch
tuna salad sandwich (1 oz tuna with 2 tbsp mayonnaise, 2 slices tomato, lettuce slices on 2 slices whole wheat bread)
1 apple
1 cup 1% milk

Dinner
2 oz lean roast beef with 1/4 cup gravy
1/2 cup brown rice
1/2 cup corn
1/2 cup three bean salad
2 whole wheat rolls
1 tbsp light tub margarine
1/2 cup strawberries
iced tea

Evening Snack
12 oz diet cola beverage
1 oz dry roasted nuts

Nutrient	RDA: female-19 to 24 years	Actual	% RDA
Kilocalories	================	1969 kcal	90
Protein	=================*==============	82 gm	177
Carbohydrate	=================	264 gm	96
Fat	=================*	75 gm	102
Saturated fat	==============	20 gm	81
Monounsaturated fat	================	23 gm	93
Polyunsaturated fat	===============	21 gm	86
Linoleic fatty acid	=================*==================	16 gm	334
Cholesterol	========	125 mg	42
Fiber-dietary	=================*======	30 gm	135
Vitamin A	=============	583 RE	73
Thiamin	=================*=======	1.6 mg	141
Riboflavin	=================*======	1.8 mg	137
Niacin	=================*=====	20 mg	131
Vitamin B6	===============	1.4 mg	86
Folate	=================*==========	286 mcg	159
Vitamin B12	=================*==================	4.3 mcg	214
Pantothenic acid	==============	4.5 mg	82
Biotin	============	43 mcg	66
Vitamin C	=================*==================	168 mg	280
Vitamin D	==========	5.4 mcg	54
Vitamin K	=================*==================	169 mcg	282
Sodium	=================*	2441 mg	102
Potassium	=================*==========	3186 mg	159
Calcium	==============	952 mg	79
Phosphorus	=================*=====	1526 mg	127
Magnesium	=================*========	412 mg	147
Iron	==============	12 mg	82
Zinc	================	12 mg	94
	^0 ^50 ^100 ^150 ^200		

Carbohydrate, Protein, and Fat Distribution

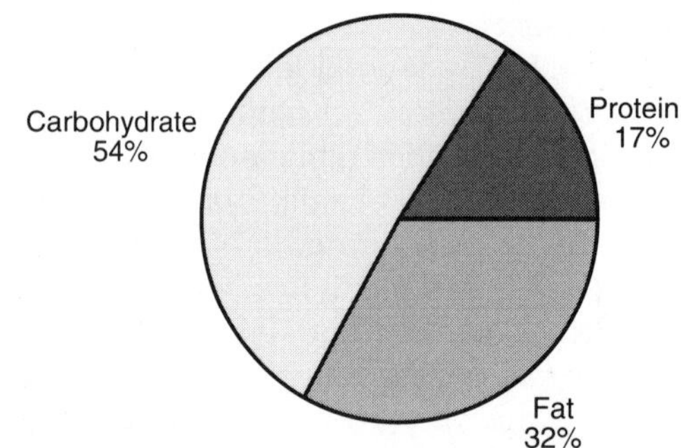

Figure 1–4 Sample menu based on the U.S. Dietary Guidelines. RDA, recommended dietary allowances; RE, retinol equivalents.

TABLE 1–10

SUMMARY OF FOODS HIGH IN CHOLESTEROL, FAT, SALT, AND SUGAR

	Bread/Cereal Group	Fruit/Vegetable Group	Milk/Dairy Group	Meat/Protein Group
High in Cholesterol			Butter and cream	Egg yolks, shrimp, organ meats, bacon, salt pork, and animal products
High in Salt	Pretzels, salted crackers, highly seasoned rice, and pasta mixtures	Pickled vegetables (pickles and sauerkraut), regular canned vegetables, vegetable juices with added salt	Buttermilk	Canned fish and meats, chipped beef, and textured vegetable protein analogs
High in Salt and Fat	Salted snacks and chips	Potato chips, frozen vegetables in sauce, and olives	Natural cheeses, especially blue, Camembert, processed cheese, and cheese foods	Canned, dried, salted, cured meats or fish such as bacon, salt pork, ham, corned beef, sausage, frankfurters, luncheon meat, and corned beef
High in Fat		French fries, fried vegetables, and avocados	Cream cheese, sour cream, whole milk, butter, cream, and whole milk yogurt	Duck, goose, nuts, brisket, oily fish (mackeral), and fish packed in oil
High in Sugar and Fat	Commercial granola, doughnuts, and pastries		Sweetened condensed milk; ice cream; malts and shakes; chocolate milk; whole-milk; fruit-flavored yogurt	
High in Sugar	Presweetened breakfast cereals	Fruits canned or frozen in heavy syrup, juices with added sugar, and maraschino cherries	Ice milk	
Reduced in Fiber; Low in Salt, Fat, and Sugar	Refined grains, especially white rice, degerminated cornmeal or flour, and white flour	Fruit juices and peeled fruits and vegetables		

Other foods or accessory foods provide kilocalories and flavor but few nutrients. These foods should not replace foods in the food groups but can be used to enhance a diet

Use Moderation When Selecting These Foods:

Fats: Gravy, mayonnaise, cream and cream sauces, chocolate, coconut, solid shortening, most nondairy creamers

Condiments (most are high in salt): Barbecue sauce, catsup, horseradish, mustard, olives, pickles, soy sauce, taco sauce

TABLE 1–11

DIETARY GUIDANCE FOR THE HEALTHY US POPULATION

Title and Organization	Type of Guidance (General or Specific)	Achieve and Maintain Desirable Body Weight	Fats (%kcal)			Cholesterol, Limit or Reduce	Carbohydrates			Sodium, Limit or Reduce	Alcohol in Moderation if at All
			Total, Limit or Reduce	*Saturated, Reduce*	*Polyunsaturated, Limit or Reduce*		*Complex, Increase*	*Fiber, Increase*	*Refined Sugar, Limit or Reduce*		
Nutrition and Your Health; Dietary Guidelines for Americans, 1990 (1)	General	Yes	< 30%	< 10%	*	Avoid too much	Choose a diet with plenty of vegetables, fruits, and grain products		Use in moderation	Use in moderation	Not to exceed 1–2 oz of ethanol/day
The Healthy American Diet, American Heart Association, 1988 (2)	General	Yes	30% or less	< 10% of kilocalories	< 10% of kilocalories	< 300 mg/day	Yes	*Yes	*	< 3 gm/day	< 1–2 oz/day
American Cancer Society Dietary Guidelines, American Cancer Society, 1990 (3)	Cancer	Yes. Avoid obesity	Yes. To 30% or less	*	*	*	*	Eat more high-fiber foods such as whole-grain cereals, vegetables, and fruits	*	Limit consumption of salt-cured, smoked, and nitrite-cured foods	Yes

* No specific dietary advice given.

(1) From US Department of Agriculture, US Department of Health and Human Services. *Nutrition and Your Health; Dietary Guidelines for Americans.* 3rd ed. Government Printing Office, Washington, DC, 1990.

(2) American Heart Association. Dietary guidelines for healthy American adults. *Circulation* 1988; 77(3):721A–724A.

(3) Nixon DW. Nutrition and cancer: American Cancer Society guidelines, programs and initiatives. *CA* 1990; 40(2):71–75.

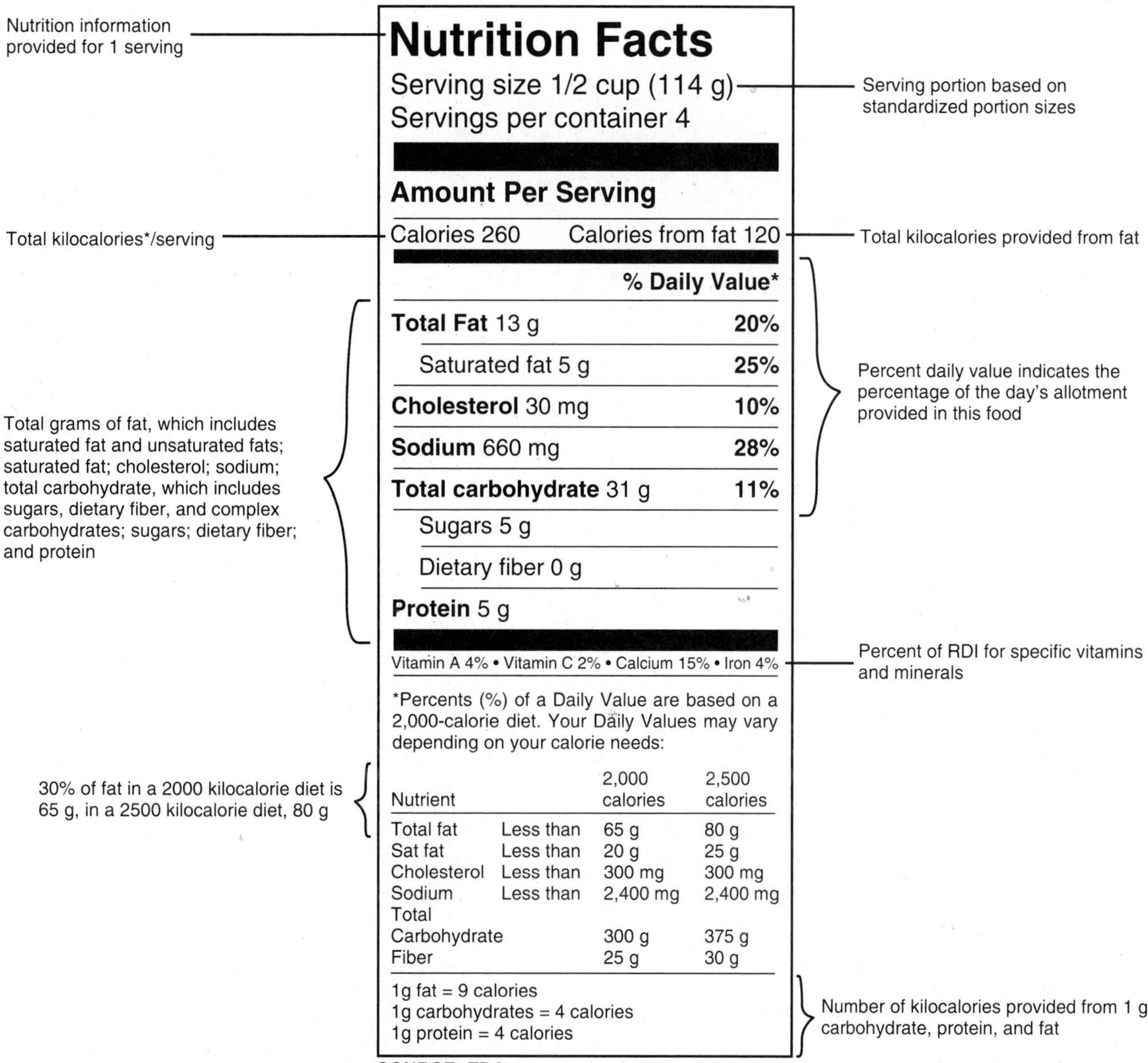

Nutrition information provided for 1 serving
Nutrition Facts
Serving size 1/2 cup (114 g)
Servings per container 4
Serving portion based on standardized portion sizes
Amount Per Serving
Total kilocalories*/serving
Calories 260
Calories from fat 120
Total kilocalories provided from fat
% Daily Value*
Total Fat 13 g 20%
Saturated fat 5 g 25%
Cholesterol 30 mg 10%
Sodium 660 mg 28%
Total carbohydrate 31 g 11%
Sugars 5 g
Dietary fiber 0 g
Protein 5 g
Percent daily value indicates the percentage of the day's allotment provided in this food
Total grams of fat, which includes saturated fat and unsaturated fats; saturated fat; cholesterol; sodium; total carbohydrate, which includes sugars, dietary fiber, and complex carbohydrates; sugars; dietary fiber; and protein
Vitamin A 4% • Vitamin C 2% • Calcium 15% • Iron 4%
Percent of RDI for specific vitamins and minerals
*Percents (%) of a Daily Value are based on a 2,000-calorie diet. Your Daily Values may vary depending on your calorie needs:
30% of fat in a 2000 kilocalorie diet is 65 g, in a 2500 kilocalorie diet, 80 g
Nutrient | | 2,000 calories | 2,500 calories
Total fat | Less than | 65 g | 80 g
Sat fat | Less than | 20 g | 25 g
Cholesterol | Less than | 300 mg | 300 mg
Sodium | Less than | 2,400 mg | 2,400 mg
Total Carbohydrate | | 300 g | 375 g
Fiber | | 25 g | 30 g
1g fat = 9 calories
1g carbohydrates = 4 calories
1g protein = 4 calories
Number of kilocalories provided from 1 g carbohydrate, protein, and fat
SOURCE: FDA

*Total kilocalories needed per day depends on the client's age, body size, and activity level. Average range is 1600–2500 kilocalories.

Example of the new food label that is required by 1994.

Figure 1–5 Explanation of nutritional information on food labels. DRVs, Daily reference values; RDI; reference daily intakes.

TABLE 1–12

DAILY REFERENCE VALUES*

	% of kilocalories†	Highest Desirable Amount
Protein	10‡	
Carbohydrate	60	
Fat	30	<65 gm
Saturated fat	10	<20 gm
Cholesterol		<300 mg
Sodium		<2400 mg
Fiber	11.5 gm/1000 kcal	

* Daily reference values (DRV) are not seen on the nutrient label. The term daily value, which appears on the label for ease of understanding, reflects the DRV and the RDI standards.
† Based on a reference intake of 2000 kcal/day.
‡ Protein amount is for adults and children over age 4 only.

TABLE 1–13

DEFINITIONS OF NUTRITION LABELING TERMS

	Free*	Low*	Reduced† or Less‡	Other
Synonyms	No, zero, without, trivial source of, negligible source of, dietarily insignificant source of	Little, few, small amounts of, low source of, low in	Reduced, reduced in, fewer, less, lower, lower in	
Generalized Meaning	Contains no or "physiologically inconsequential" amounts of one or more of the following: kilocalories, sugars, fat, saturated fat, cholesterol, or sodium; or no added sugar, salt, or fat.	Appropriate for foods that could be eaten frequently without exceeding dietary guidelines for one or more of the following: kilocalories, fat, saturated fat, cholesterol, sodium.	Nutritionally altered product that contains ≤25% of a nutrient or of kilocalories than the regular or reference product	
Kilocalories	≤5 kilocalories/serving	≤40 kilocalories/serving	≥25% fewer kilocalories/serving	"Light": ≥33.3% reduction of kilocalories/serving

TABLE 1–13

DEFINITIONS OF NUTRITION LABELING TERMS *Continued*

	Free*	Low*	Reduced† or Less‡	Other
Sugars§	≤0.5 gm/serving‖		≥25% less sugar/serving	
Sodium	≤5 mg/serving	≤140 mg/serving	≥25% less sodium/serving	Very low sodium: ≤35 mg/serving Light: ≥50% reduction of sodium/serving
Fat	≤0.5 gm/serving	≤3 gm/serving	≥25% less fat/serving	"Light'" ≥50% reduction of fat/serving
Saturated Fatty Acids¶	≤0.5 gm/serving	≤1 gm/serving	≥25% less saturated fat/serving	
Cholesterol	≤2 mg/serving	≤20 mg/serving	≥25% less cholesterol/serving	

* A claim for a food being "free" or "low" implies that the food differs from other foods of the same type. These foods have been specially processed, altered, formulated, or reformulated to decrease the amount of the nutrient in the food.
† The term "reduced" cannot be made if the reference food already meets the requirement for a "low" claim.
‡ Whether the food is altered or not, product contains 25% less than the regular or reference product.
§ Sugars are defined as the sum of all free monosaccharides and disaccharides (glucose, fructose, lactose, sucrose).
‖ If sugar-free or sugarless terms are used, must note whether the food is "low kilocalorie" or "kilocalorie reduced" or "not a reduced kilocalorie food" or "not for weight control."
¶ If claims are made with respect to the level of saturated fat, the level of total fat and cholesterol in the food must be disclosed unless the food contains ≤2 mg of cholesterol/serving and ≥3 gm total fat/serving, in which case the cholesterol or fat content, respectively, can be omitted.
Data from *FDA Backgrounder:* The New Food Label. Washington, D.C., Dec.; 1992 and *Fed. Register* 58: Jan; 1993.

fat, saturated fat, cholesterol, and sodium represent the highest limit considered desirable. The sample nutrition label provided in Figure 1–5 explains the type of information displayed.

A label cannot carry an explicit or implied nutrient content claim unless it uses terms that have been defined, such as "free," "low," "more," or "reduced." Tables 1–13 and 1–14 define the established terms and will be helpful to you as reference tools. Only health claims that are supported by substantial scientific evidence and authorized by the FDA can be used. If the product meets specified guidelines, health claims may be made for the following nutrient-disease relationships: sodium and hypertension, calcium and osteoporosis, lipids and cancer, lipids and cardiovascular disease, fiber and heart disease, fiber and cancer, and fruits and vegetables and cancer.

What are the RDIs and DRVs?

TABLE 1–14

NUTRIENT CONTENT DESCRIPTORS

Expressed Nutrient Claim

Any direct statement about the level or range of a nutrient in the food.

Implied Nutrient Claim

Describes the product in a manner that suggests a nutrient is absent or present in a certain amount or suggests the food may be useful in maintaining healthy dietary practices and is made in association with an explicit claim or statement about a nutrient. These misleading claims are prohibited. For example, a product that contains oat fiber must contain enough oat bran to meet the definition for "good source" of fiber to claim "made with oat bran."

Table continued on following page

TABLE 1–14

NUTRIENT CONTENT DESCRIPTORS
Continued

Substitute Food

Can be used interchangeably with another food that (1) has similar performance characteristics, (2) is not nutritionally inferior to the reference food (unless labeled "imitation"), and (3) complies with compositional requirements set by FDA.

High

Contains 20% or more of the daily value per serving for particular nutrient.

Good Source

Contains 10–19% of the daily value per serving for particular nutrient.

Relative Claims

These statements compare the level of a nutrient in the product with the level of a nutrient in a reference food. Relative claims include "light," "reduced," "less," "fewer," and "more." Relative claims cannot be made for a product if the nutrient content of the reference food meets the requirement for "low." "Less," "fewer," and "more" can be compared with a dissimilar food within a product category that can generally be substituted for the product in the diet (potato chips as reference for pretzels) or a similar food (potato chips as reference for potato chips). For "light," "reduced," "added," "fortified," and "enriched" claims, the reference food must be a similar food. To bear a relative claim, the amount of the nutrient in that food must be compared with the amount of that nutrient in an appropriate reference food, and the label must indicate the following: (1) identify the reference food; (2) state the percentage (or fraction) of the amount the nutrient in the reference food has been modified (⅓ fewer kilocalories than ____); (3) provide quantitative comparison of the amount of nutrient in the product with the amount in the reference food; (4) provide information immediately adjacent to the most prominent claim.

More

Natural or added content of a nutrient is at least 10% of the daily value more than the reference food; applies to "fortified" and "enriched" foods.

Fresh

Indicates a food is raw or unprocessed (raw, never been frozen or heated, and contains no preservatives). Low levels of irradiation are allowed. "fresh frozen," "frozen fresh," and "freshly frozen" can be used for foods that are quickly frozen while still fresh. Blanching is allowed. Exceptions to the use of fresh include "fresh," as used in "fresh milk" or "freshly baked bread."

Percent Fat Free

The product must be a low-fat or a fat-free product. The claim must also reflect the amount of fat in 100 gm of the food.

Lean and Extra Lean

Describes fat content of meat and seafood products. *Lean*—$\leq$10 gm fat, $\geq$4 gm saturated fat, and $\leq$95 mg cholesterol per serving and per 100 gm. *Extra lean*—$\leq$5 gm fat, $\leq$2 gm saturated fat, and $\leq$95 mg cholesterol/serving and per 100 gm.

Meals and Main Dishes

Must meet same requirements as those for individual foods. *Low kilocalorie*—contains $<$120 kcal. Low sodium—contains $<$20 mg cholesterol/100 gm and no more than 2 gm saturated fat. *Light*—can be low fat, or low kilocalorie, or sodium content of low kilocalorie, low-fat food has been decreased by 50%.

Healthy

Describes a food that is low in fat and saturated fat and contains $\leq$480 mg sodium and $\leq$60 mg cholesterol per serving. (This is a proposed FDA term with a final ruling expected in 1993.)

Data from *FDA Backgrounder:* The New Food Label. Washington, D.C., Dec; 1992 and *Fed Register* 58: Jan; 1993.

NURSING APPLICATIONS

1. Nurses must make sure they have the correct set of RDIs that correlate with client's age or grouping, i.e., when talking to pregnant women, use the RDI for pregnancy.
2. The acronyms RDI and DRV are not on the label; however, nurses need to be aware of the basis for the daily values.

Client Education

- Read labels carefully. Ingredients are listed in order of quantity (by weight). Choose products that have less fat or oils or in which fats are listed last.
- The RDIs are a useful tool to compare nutrient values of foods and to learn valuable sources of nutrients. Review a label together with the client and/or family.
- Fortified foods and supplements should not be purchased to attempt to meet 100% of the RDIs because this may be more than is needed, especially for young children.
- The DRVs on nutrition labels help in comparing processed foods for their fat, saturated fats, cholesterol, carbohydrate, sodium, and fiber content. Using a nutrient label, review the information presented and discuss how the information can be used to compare various products that are available.

FOOD FADS AND MISINFORMATION

Nutrition is a popular subject to clients, but even with all the current knowledge, it is no easier to educate today than it was 50 years ago:

> More food notions flourish in the United States than in any other civilized country on earth, and most of them are wrong. They thrive in the minds of the same people who talk about their operations; and like all mythology, they are a blend of fear, coincidence, and advertising (Anonymous, 1938).

As the client's interest in nutrition increases, myths surrounding nutrition continue to confuse. Purveyors of nutritional misinformation capitalize on clients' fears and hopes by exaggerating and oversimplifying health virtues or curative properties of foods. Too few clients understand the effects of various nutrients on the body and how the body uses these nutrients, thereby opening the door to food faddism or nutrition quackery.

A **food fad** may be based on a food fact or fallacy. Clients often begin a diet or believe claims for specific foods or supplements on the basis of something they read or hear without investigating its validity or effectiveness. Although some fads are physically harmless, they may create an economic hardship for clients with limited income because the foods or supplements may be expensive. Still others are nutritionally inadequate and could lead to serious deficiencies. A fad is frequently harmful because a client substitutes this therapy for the advice of a physician, thereby delaying medical treatment.

Food fad—a catchall term covering all aspects of nutrition nonsense, characterized by exaggerated beliefs about the value of nutrition in health and disease.

Food quackery claims or promises may be due to ignorance, delusion, misconception, or intent to deceive. At a National Health Conference in 1988, quackery was estimated to cost Americans between $10 billion and $40 billion yearly (Grigg, 1988).

Food quackery—the promotion of nutrition-related products or services having questionable safety and/or effectiveness for the claims made.

The unknowns of medicine and disagreement among reputable scientists re-

TABLE 1–15

FEDERAL LAWS TO PROTECT CONSUMERS

Laws	Enforcing Agency
Federal Food, Drug, and Cosmetic Act (1938)	Food and Drug Administration (FDA)
Truth in Advertising Act (1938)	Federal Trade Commission (FTC)
Mail Fraud and False Representation Statutes (1948)	US Postal Service

garding interpretation of research findings foster nutritional misinformation. Given the right circumstances, such as confronting a chronic or incurable disease, potentially everyone is capable of exchanging sound judgment and common sense for miraculous cures.

How do unscrupulous health promoters get away with their lies and fake products? Strict laws protect against false advertising and mislabeling, as outlined in Table 1–15, but health food ripoff or food terrorism thrives. The government actively pursues health swindlers, but enforcing agencies lack adequate staff and resources needed to handle all the problems reported.

The First Amendment to the US Constitution protects free speech and a free press; this also protects a person's right to dispense false, misleading, or deceptive health claims. If a food product makes false or misleading claims on the label, the FDA can take action because of mislabeling. For many years, health-related claims on a food product were prohibited by the FDA. In November 1990, new legislation was passed allowing health claims on food labels if (1) it is well documented that a particular nutrient can reduce risk and (2) the benefits of this nutrient are not offset by another ingredient present (FDA, 1990). (For instance, a high-fiber cereal that is high in fat could not be touted as being beneficial for health owing to its fat content.) Implementation of these new regulations should be completed by mid-1993.

What is the difference between food fads and food quackery?

The Federal Trade Commission can take action if false claims are made in advertising, so claims made on labels or in promotions are not usually false. However, products can be legally promoted in books and magazine articles and on radio and television talk shows owing to protection from the First Amendment.

Evaluating Health Foods

Organically grown—foods generally defined as being grown without synthetic pesticides or fertilizers.

Organically processed—foods that have not been treated with additives, preservatives, hormones, antibiotics, dyes, or waxes.

Organically grown and **organically processed** foods have become increasingly popular because of concerns about the effect of chemicals on health and the environment. Legal standards have been established by 26 states for organic food; the federal government is in the process of developing standards that should be implemented by late 1993 (Lynch, 1991a). Products sold both in health food and in grocery stores labeled as health foods or organic foods imply that all other foods are unhealthy or are not as beneficial to health. Terms are frequently used to imply a meaning different from the officially accepted one, thus misleading clients. Standardization of terminology is essential to assure consumers that what they are buying meets their personal definitions and that all products have been produced according to the regulations.

Numerous studies and reputable scientists have concluded that there are no demonstrable nutritional benefits from the consumption of "health" instead of conventional foods; yet health food sales continue to soar, with annual sales in excess of $1 billion. Consumers choose organic foods for many different reasons, such as environmental food safety or sensory concerns (Lynch, 1991a). Many are truly concerned about the uses of pesticides. Information about reduced use of pesticides on fresh fruits increases client acceptance of fruit that is imperfect in appearance (Lynch, 1991b).

What is the difference between organically grown and organically processed?

Detecting Fraudulent Claims

Evaluating nutritional information for quackery can be a tedious chore. Nurses and clients should begin by checking a person's credentials. The information should be objective, based on scientifically well-designed studies. Well-documented information written by reliable professionals is usually reported in scientific journals. The questions in Table 1–16 help to evaluate oral or written claims. If the answer to several of these questions is yes, stop and investigate further.

Evaluating Scientific Information

In addition to evaluating information for its nutritional validity, even scientific data need evaluation before recommendations are made based on the conclusions. Both the strengths and the weaknesses of a study design should be considered. A scientific study incorporates certain information that should be evaluated for its relevance to the acceptance of the hypothesis. Table 1–17 provides tips in evaluating research studies with an intelligent skepticism.

The Role of Nurses

What role can the nurse play in combating nutrition fads and misinformation? Natalie Van Cleve stated in 1938, when times were different but widespread misinformation on diet was just as prevalent as today:

It is the duty of all professions active in the field of food and nutrition to co-

TABLE 1–16

SCRUTINIZING FOR FRAUDULENT INFORMATION

Is the information based mainly on testimonials and case histories?
Is the medical profession or a government agency prosecuting him or her because it does not accept the superior discovery?
Are the claims extravagant or emotionally appealing, such as promises of youth, beauty, glamor, long life, or cure of disease?
Are superlatives such as "amazing," and "exclusive" used frequently to describe the product?
Are most diseases caused by a bad or faulty diet?
Does the product contain "biologically active" ingredients?
Is there danger of being poisoned by food additives and preservatives?
Are "natural" vitamins better than "synthetic" ones?
Will the cure be quick, dramatic, or miraculous?
Is the product good for a wide variety of ailments?
Is the product or service being offered a "secret remedy" or a "recent discovery" not available from other resources?
Is the remedy being sold door-to-door, by a self-styled "health advisor," or promoted by public lecture series or in a popular magazine?
Are self-diagnosis and treatment being promoted?
Does the product claim to be approved by the FDA?
Can the treatment be obtained only across the border or ocean?

FDA, Food and Drug Administration.

TABLE 1–17

EVALUATING SCIENTIFIC RESEARCH INFORMATION

A well-written research paper probably contains reliable information of scientific value if the author has:

- Summarized and referenced other studies on the subject
- Stated the hypothesis and purpose
- Clearly outlined and described the procedures used
- Presented data in a clear, concise, and systematic format
- Provided tables and figures to show results
- Discussed relationship of data to that done by others along with reasons for discrepancies
- Supported conclusions by the results presented

Some questions that the reader must consider to evaluate a study's relevancy include:

- What are the author's qualifications?
- Was it based on human or animal studies?
- Was this an appropriate sampling of the population?
- How many subjects were involved?
- Was there a control to determine effects of the change?
- How many factors in the study were changed, altered, or affected?
- Did the change affect anything else in the lifestyle that may have affected the outcome?
- Can the outcome of this study be duplicated by others?
- Is the length of time for the study long enough to allow the body to adapt to the change (as has been found with triglycerides)?

operate in clarifying any misconceptions of the laity. If the nurse does not know her vitamins, the patients will find a radio announcer who does.

Physicians, nurses, and even dietitians have sometimes promoted nutritional misinformation by failing to apply their knowledge, misunderstanding how nutrients are used, or searching for fame and fortune. The nurse is in a unique position to understand the causes of food faddism and to recognize their dangers. Understanding clients and their love of "miracle" answers should help in recognizing the appeal of such misinformation. A scientific background permits assessment of the potential effects or uselessness of food faddism. Nurses can provide clients with a clear understanding of the true essence of nutritional science—the process of nourishing or being nourished—rather than the polypharmacy of supernutrition and organic foods.

How can nurses help clarify misconceptions about food?

NURSING APPLICATIONS

1. Assess client's use of food fads, economic level, educational level, and nutrient adequacy of any fad diet practiced.
2. If a client restricts food choices because of a food fad or beliefs in organic food, ensuring nutrient adequacy is more difficult (Spillman et al, 1990). Therefore, a thorough assessment and evaluation by the nurse and/or a dietitian are needed.
3. Clarify for clients any misinformation about the use of organic foods, but respect their beliefs and help them obtain economical products that are acceptable for them.
4. Help clients choose a variety of foods to ensure a balanced intake and lessen contamination from any one source.
5. Provide clients with positive advice based on a broad knowledge and understanding of nutritional concepts and current research findings.
6. Answer any questions about any therapies, products, or treatments clients may be contemplating.
7. Speak out to protect the public from misinformation.

8. Do not offer proposals or remedies unless they have been demonstrated to be safe and effective.
9. If a client is using or contemplating a food fad or diet you are unfamiliar with, do not hesitate to consult a registered dietitian, home economist, or a nutrition professor.

Client Education

- Populations that consume large amounts of fruits and vegetables, even with the use of fertilizers and pesticides, have a lower rate of cancer (Tribole, 1989).
- Organic foods cost more money but are not more nutritious or significantly different in taste.
- Organic produce will not look as attractive and unblemished as traditionally grown produce; organically processed foods will have a shorter shelf life than products containing preservatives (Spillman et al, 1990).
- Wash produce thoroughly. Some fruits can be scrubbed with a brush under running water.
- In addition to the government health agencies already mentioned, numerous health and professional organizations listed in Appendix E-1 provide health information. Other organizations such as the Better Business Bureau may also be helpful.

SUMMARY

Nutrition not only involves eating, but also includes why clients make food choices, what happens to those foods in the body, and how the food affects a client's state of health. Certain basic concepts are fundamental for nurses to be able to learn, understand, and evaluate nutritional information and care.

To make planning a well-balanced diet easier, guidelines have been formulated. RDAs indicate desirable levels of nutrient intake that are formulated for determining the adequacy of diets for different groups of clients. The dietary guidelines can be used to help interpret the basic food groups about items that are of concern to improve quality of life and to encourage moderation in food consumption. Nutrition labels on processed foods can help a client make wise food choices based on the product's nutrient content.

Misinformation regarding nutrition is abundant. Health professionals are qualified to fight this ever-increasing problem by using their scientific knowledge and staying current with new information.

NURSING PROCESS IN ACTION

A young healthy mother comes to the clinic with her 18-month-old son seeking information about ways to improve or maintain optimal nutrition for herself and her family. She wants to keep current on the dietary guidelines and labeling changes. She is a little unsure about the RDAs and RDIs.

 ### Nutritional Assessment

- Willingness to seek nutritional information.
- Desire for increased control of nutritional health habits.
- Knowledge of community resources.

- Cultural or religious influences.
- Knowledge regarding the dietary guidelines, labeling, RDAs, RDIs, food groups, desired weight.
- Definition of optimal nutrition.

Dietary Nursing Diagnosis

Health seeking behaviors related to lack of knowledge concerning optimal nutrition and current standards.

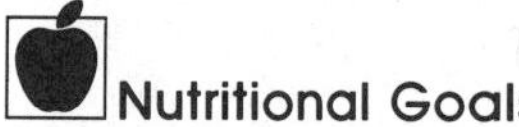

Nutritional Goals

Client verbalizes correct information concerning the US guidelines, labeling, RDAs, and RDIs.

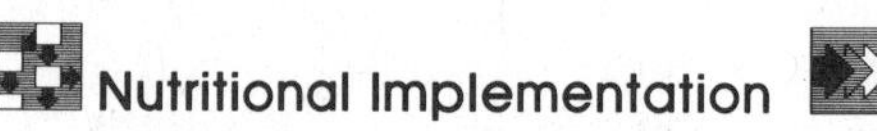

Nutritional Implementation

Intervention: Encourage a variety of food intake, using the basic food groups.

Rationale: It is the whole balance of diet that matters, and the best balance incorporates variety to prevent nutritional deficiencies.

Intervention: (1) Monitor weight of client and child; (2) compare findings to height-weight chart; (3) stress importance of maintaining ideal body weight; (4) determine kilocaloric intake.

Rationale: Monitoring weight will determine if overweight, ideal, or underweight. Overweight and underweight increase health risks. Moderation of kilocaloric intake is the key to maintaining ideal weight.

Intervention: (1) Check cholesterol level if not recently done; (2) emphasize a decreased intake of fats, saturated fats, and cholesterol by trimming excess fat, eating smaller servings of meat (about the size of a fist or a deck of cards); (3) encourage use of polyunsaturated fats.

Rationale: By decreasing fats, saturated fats, and cholesterol, one can decrease the risk of heart disease.

Intervention: (1) Stress importance of vegetables, fruits, and grains; (2) explain that complex carbohydrates are not fattening; (3) encourage selection of foods from Table 1–3; (4) use guidelines in Table 1–8.

Rationale: Dietary fiber is important for healthy bowel functioning and can reduce symptoms of chronic constipation, diverticular disease, and hemorrhoids and decrease the incidence of obesity, cancer, and diabetes.

Intervention: (1) Explain how to read labels for sugar. Most names end in "ose"; (2) emphasize moderation of sugar intake; (3) explain that dietetic and sugar-free labeling do not necessarily mean low in kilocalories.

Rationale: Refined sugar contains kilocalories and no other nutrients but is acceptable when used in items that contain appreciable amounts of other nutrients; i.e., a pudding would provide more nutrients than a congealed dessert or carbonated beverages.

Intervention: (1) Stress using sodium and salt in moderation; (2) follow suggestions in Table 1–9; (3) emphasize that no salt added does not mean low in sodium; (4) help client change mg of sodium to gm, i.e., 355 mg salt is the same as 0.355 gm of sodium (always move the decimal 3 places to the left).

Rationale: Good habits that do not foster a high level of salt preference are recommended and may protect against development of hypertension.

Intervention: Emphasize that any alcohol intake should be in moderation (1 drink/day), if at all.

Rationale: Alcohol is high in kilocalories and contains few if any nutrients.

Intervention: (1) Explain RDAs and RDIs; (2) go over recommendations with client; (3) stress that they are only guidelines and not absolutes; (4) explain that they should not be used to determine child's intake, unless the RDI for children is used.

Rationale: RDAs identify nutritional needs in terms of specific amounts of essential nutrients that adequately meet the known nutrient needs of most healthy individuals. RDIs help determine the nutrient content (protein, vitamins, and minerals) of certain food products. Food labels use RDIs for people above 4 years of age unless the food is intended for a specific population (e.g., baby foods).

Intervention: (1) Actually review an entire label with the mother to help her understand how to use it; (2) determine serving size; (3) determine gm of carbohydrates; (4) determine the percentage of fat by multiplying the gm of fat by 9 and compare this number to the total kilocalories (if amount is more than 30%, limit consumption); (5) look at cholesterol level; (6) find sodium level (if above 400 mg, use in moderation).

Rationale: Knowledge increases compliance and allows client to make informed choices regarding food selections.

Intervention: Refer to county extension agencies.

Rationale: These agencies provide practical guidelines via newsletters, workshops, and written materials for healthy clients who want to improve health.

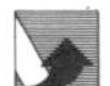

Evaluation

To determine effectiveness of care, have client read labels and choose the best buy for the nutrient content. Have client state the 7 basic guidelines for nutrition and include that this is not an accurate guide for her son. Client verbalizes the definitions of RDA and RDI and how these can help her with planning meals, but they are not absolutes and they do not apply to her son. Additionally, client will be able to plan a menu using foods recommended and state how to obtain or use community information or support.

STUDENT READINESS

1. A client asks you the difference between food and nutrition. What would you say?
2. Compare the cost of 3 foods from a health food store with the cost of similar items in a supermarket. Which is more economical?
3. Locate an advertisement in a popular magazine or newspaper for a health food product and list the merits of the product stated in the ad. Then list information about the product that might have been omitted or should be questioned.
4. Discuss current food fads and how they may have adverse effects.
5. A client wants to know the functions of foods in the body. List the nutrients necessary for each of the functions.
6. Distinguish between recommendations and requirements.
7. Keep a record of all the foods you eat for 24 hours. Was it adequate, as evaluated by the basic food groups? How does it measure up to the US Dietary Guidelines?
8. Collect nutrient labels for 3 similar products. Compare the nutrient values to determine which is a better source of nutrients. Which is a better buy for the amount of nutrients it contains?
9. List the US Dietary Guidelines. List your favorite food items from each category and the frequency of consumption. Are foods listed as "high" (see Table 1–10) consumed in moderation? If not, what are some foods that you can substitute for them?
10. A client states, "I want to follow the cure-all diet because my favorite actor swears by it." How would you respond?

REFERENCES

Anonymous, cited by Wilder RM. Fads, fancies, and fallacies in adult diets. *Sigma Xi Q* 1938; 26:73.

Block G. Vitamin C and cancer prevention: The epidemologic evidence. *Am J Clin Nutr* 1991 Jan; 53(Suppl 1):270S–282S.

Butrum RR, et al. NCI dietary guidelines: Rationale. *Am J Clin Nutr* 1988 Sept; 48(Suppl 3):888–895.

Food and Drug Administration (FDA), DHHS. *Fed Register* 55:5176, 1990.

Garewal HS. Potential role of beta carotene in prevention of oral cancer. *Am J Clin Nutr* 1991 Jan; 53(Suppl 1):294S–297S.

Grigg W. Quackery: It costs more than money. *FDA Consumer* 1988; July-Aug; 22(6):30–32.

Lissner L, et al. Dietary fat and the regulation of energy intake in human subjects. *Am J Clin Nutr* 1989 Dec; 46(6):886–892.

Lynch L. Congress mandates national organic food standards. *Food Rev* 1991a Jan-Mar; 14(1):12–15.

Lynch L. Consumers choose lower pesticide use over picture-perfect produce. *Food Rev* 1991b Jan-Mar; 14(1):9–11.

McCargar LJ, et al. Dietary carbohydrate-to-fat ratio: Influence on whole-body nitrogen retention, substrate utilization, and hormone response in healthy male subjects. *Am J Clin Nutr* 1989 June; 49(6):1169–1178.

Patterson BH, et al. Fruit and vegetables in the American diet: Data from the NHANES II survey. *Am J Public Health* 1990 Dec; 80(12):1443–1449.

Raper N. Nutrient content of the U.S. food supply. *Food Rev* 1991 July/Sept; 14(4):13–18.

Schutz Y, et al. Failure of dietary fat intake to promote fat oxidation: A factor favoring the development of obesity. *Am J Clin Nutr* 1989 Aug; 50(2):307–314.

Segal M. Fruit—something good that's not illegal, immoral, or fattening. *FDA Consumer* 1988 May; 22(4):10–12.

Select Committee on Nutrition and Human Needs, United States Senate. *Dietary Goals for the United States.* Washington, D.C., Government Printing Office, 1977.

Spillman M, et al. Organic foods: Are they better? *J Am Diet Assoc* 1990 Mar; 90(3):367–370.

Stahelin HB, et al. Beta carotene and cancer prevention: The Basel study. *Am J Clin Nutr* 1991 Jan; 53(Suppl 1):265S-269S.

Tremblay A, et al. Impact of dietary fat content and fat oxidation on energy intake in humans. *Am J Clin Nutr* 1989 May; 49(5):799–805.

Tribole E. In search of meaning. *Food Management* 1989 Sept; 24(9):53.

US Department of Agriculture, US Department of Health and Human Services. *Nutrition and Your Health: Dietary Guidelines for Americans.* 3rd ed. Home and Garden Bull. No. 232. Washington, D.C., Government Printing Office, 1990.

US Department of Health and Human Services, (USDHHS), Public Health Service. *The Surgeon General's Report on Nutrition and Health.* (PHS) 88–50210. Washington, D.C., Government Printing Office, 1988.

Van Cleve N. Food: Facts, fad, and fancy. *Am J Nurs* 1938 Mar; 38(3):285.

Ziegler PG. Vegetables, fruits and carotenoids and the risk of cancer. *Am J Clin Nutr* 1991 Jan; 53(Suppl 1):251S-259S.

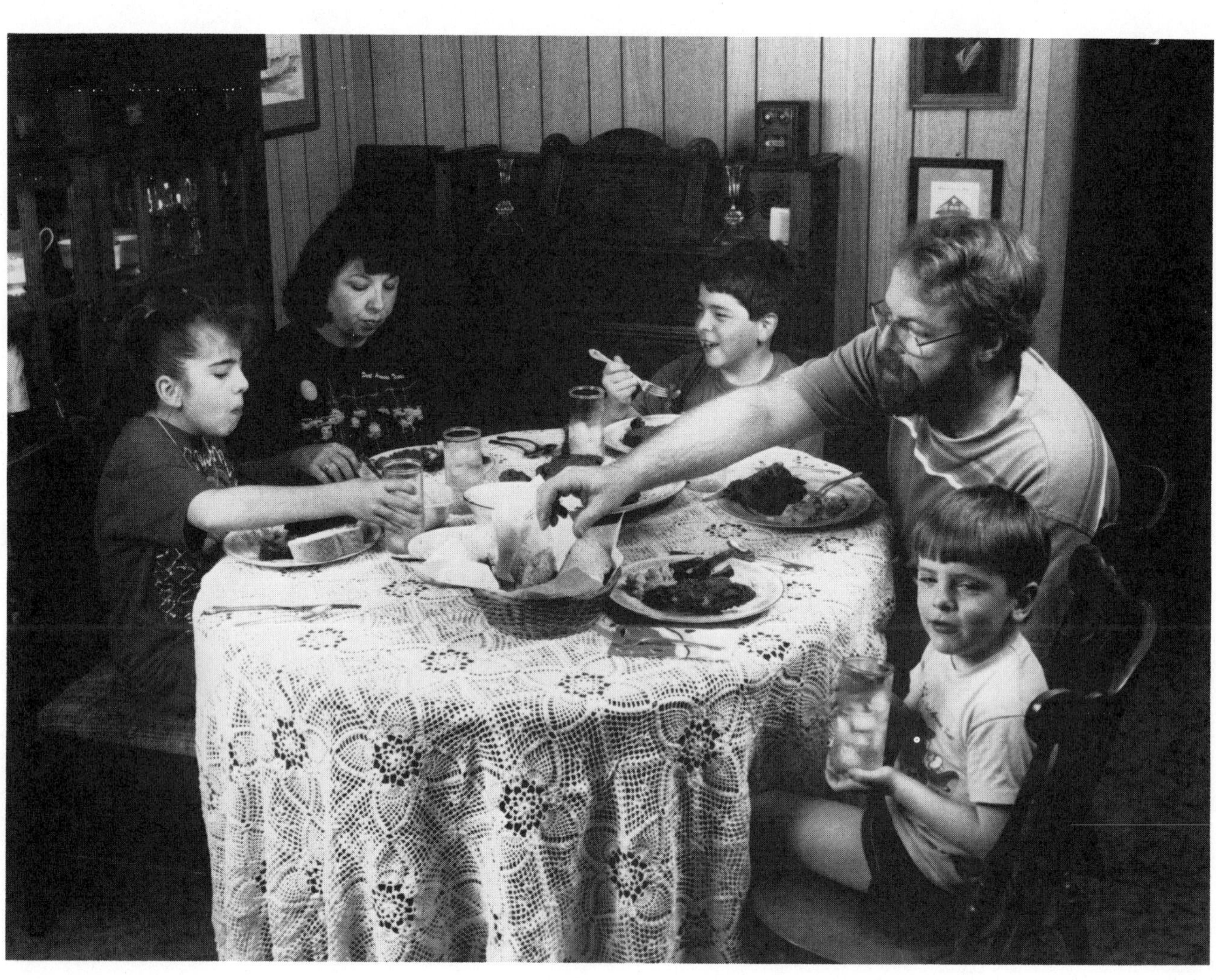

CHAPTER 2

Digestion and Metabolism

OUTLINE

I. PHYSIOLOGY OF THE GASTROINTESTINAL TRACT
II. CHEMICAL ACTION
III. MECHANICAL ACTION
   Nursing Applications
IV. MOUTH
   A. Taste and Smell
   B. Teeth
   C. Saliva
   Nursing Applications
V. ESOPHAGUS
VI. GASTRIC DIGESTION
   Nursing Applications
VII. GASTRIC ABSORPTION
VIII. SMALL INTESTINE
   A. Digestion
   Nursing Applications
   B. Absorption of Nutrients
      1. Absorption into Portal Circulation
      2. Absorption of Fat-Soluble Nutrients
   Nursing Applications
   C. Absorption of Drugs
   D. Drug and Nutrient Absorption
      1. Decreased Absorption of Nutrients
      2. Adsorption of Bile Salts
      3. Damage of Intestinal Mucosa
      4. Decreased Gastrointestinal Transit Time
      5. Increased Absorption
   Nursing Applications
   E. Effect of Foods on Drug Absorption
   Nursing Applications
IX. LARGE INTESTINE
   A. Functions
   B. Undigested Residues
   C. Microflora
   D. Peristalsis
   Nursing Applications

OBJECTIVES

THE STUDENT WILL BE ABLE TO:

- Discuss factors that influence ingestion.
- Describe general functions of each digestive organ.
- Identify chemical secretions necessary for digestion of energy nutrients and in what part of the gastrointestinal tract they are located.
- Name the energy nutrients and their end products of digestion that can be absorbed.
- Explain the role of gastrointestinal motility in the digestion and absorption process.
- State the purpose of the Krebs or tricarboxylic acid (TCA) cycle in metabolism.
- Identify ways drugs can potentially affect nutritional status.
- State why the time of drug administration is important.
- Discuss how nutrients and non-nutritive substances can alter drug metabolism and absorption.
- Identify client education aspects for digestion and metabolism.
- Apply nursing principles for digestion and metabolism.

TEST YOUR NQ (True/False)

1. The alimentary tract is about 30 feet long.
2. The hydrolysis of carbohydrate yields fatty acid and glycerol.
3. Most absorption occurs in the stomach.
4. Fat-soluble nutrients always enter the portal circulation.
5. Laxatives increase the amount of time for nutrient absorption.
6. Lactose is the name of an enzyme.
7. Enteric-coated drugs are designed to be released in the small intestine.
8. Villi are located in the large intestine.
9. Anabolism means to build or synthesize more complex compounds.
10. Caffeine can increase gastric secretions.

Foods are composed of large chemical molecules that cannot be used unless they are broken down to an absorbable form. The digestive system is designed to (1) ingest foods; (2) digest or break down complex molecules into simple, soluble materials that can be absorbed; and (3) eliminate unused residues. Only the 3 energy nutrients must be digested for absorption. Most vitamins, minerals, and water can be absorbed as eaten.

Name the 3 functions of the digestive system.

The gastrointestinal (GI) tract is also used to deliver necessary oral medications. Drugs, like foods, are complex chemical substances. Medications can frequently affect or be affected by foods, thereby modifying either food or drug absorption, metabolism, or excretion. Nurses need to become familiar with the processes of digestion and metabolism because these are disrupted in any GI disturbance and some metabolic disorders.

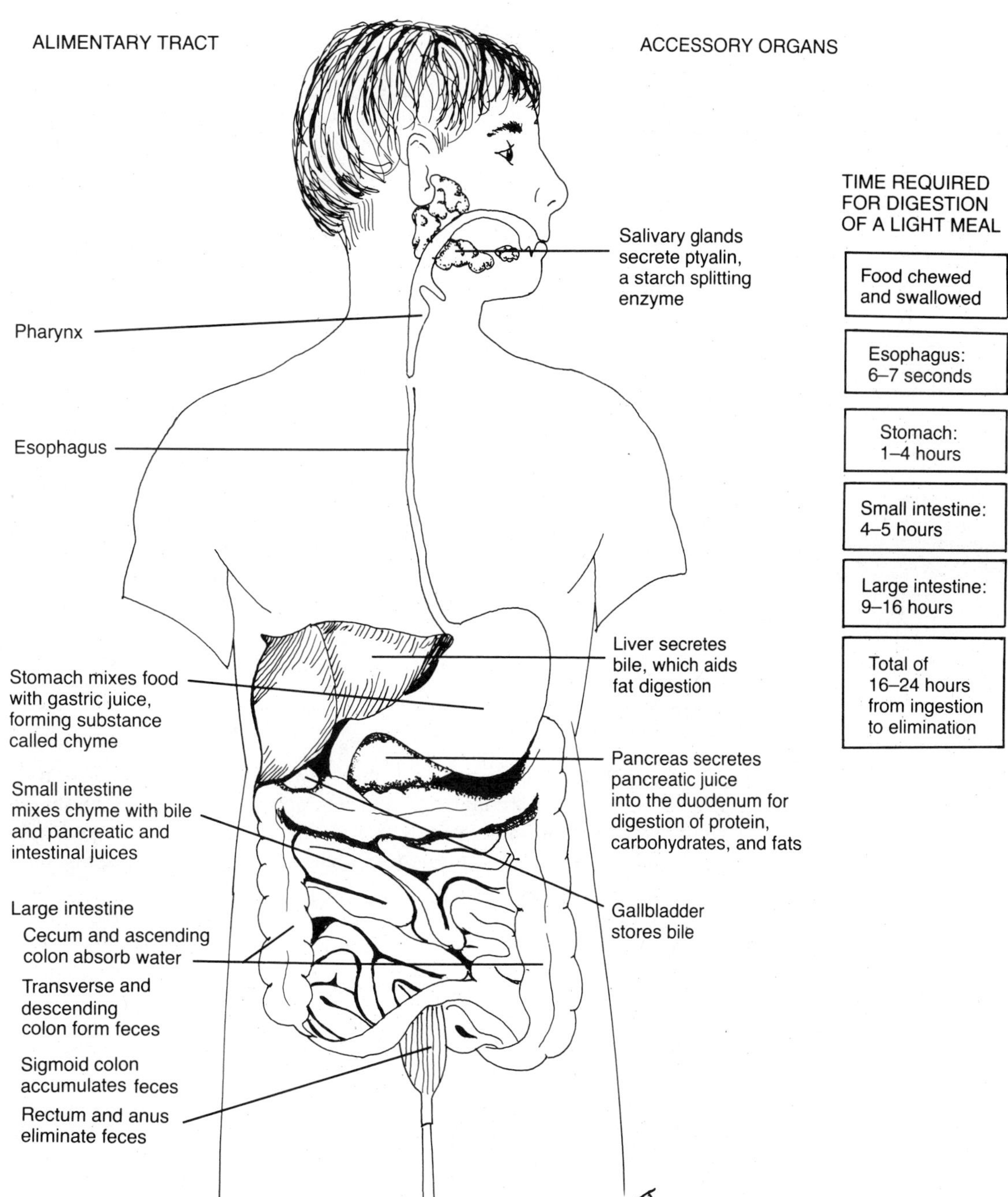

Figure 2–1 The digestive process.

PHYSIOLOGY OF THE GASTROINTESTINAL TRACT

The digestive system includes the alimentary canal and several accessory organs (Fig. 2–1). The alimentary canal is a tubular structure, extending from the mouth to the anus, with a length of about 30 feet (5 times the height of an average man). It includes the mouth, pharynx, esophagus, stomach, **small intestine,** and **large intestine.** The accessory organs include the salivary glands, liver, gallbladder, and pancreas. Digestion involves 2 basic types of action on the food: (1) **Mechanical** activities and (2) **chemical** activities.

Small intestine includes the duodenum, jejunum, and ileum; large intestine includes the cecum, colon, and rectum.

Mechanical actions include chewing and peristalsis, which break up and mix foods, permitting better blending with the chemicals; chemical actions involve digestive juices that reduce foodstuffs to absorbable molecules.

CHEMICAL ACTION

The process of digesting energy nutrients involves **hydrolysis.** The following are basic hydrolysis reactions in food digestion:

Hydrolysis is the splitting of a large molecule into smaller ones that are water-soluble and can be used by the cells; the reaction requires water.

$$\text{Protein} + H_2O \longrightarrow \text{amino acids}$$

$$\text{Fat} + H_2O \longrightarrow \text{fatty acids} + \text{glycerol}$$

$$\text{Carbohydrate} + H_2O \longrightarrow \text{monosaccharides}$$

Enzymes are complex protein agents that enable metabolic reactions to proceed at a faster rate without being consumed themselves.

These reactions are dependent on **enzymes.** In the hydrolysis of protein, the substrate for the enzyme is protein, and the amino acids are the product. The enzyme forms a temporary chemical compound with the substrate. When the reaction is completed, the complex separates, releasing the new chemical compound and the enzyme.

What substances occur when protein, fat, and carbohydrate are hydrolyzed? What is the function of enzymes, and how are they usually named?

Because the enzyme is reused, only small amounts are needed. Enzymes function somewhat like keys in that they are very specific and will function on only 1 substrate, similar to a key fitting a particular lock (Fig. 2–2). The name for some enzymes is derived from the name of the substrate, with the suffix "-ase", i.e., lactase is the enzyme produced to catalyze the breakdown of lactose.

MECHANICAL ACTION

Peristalsis is the involuntary rhythmic waves of contraction traveling the whole length of the alimentary tract.

The wall of the alimentary canal is the same from the esophagus to the rectum (Fig. 2–3). A circular layer of muscles encircles the tube, allowing the diameter of the tube to expand and contract. Food particles are therefore broken up and mixed by the churning action. The outer fibers of the muscular coat (longitudinal muscle) run lengthwise and are responsible for **peristalsis.**

Valves, also called sphincter muscles, are door-like mechanisms between the digestive segments.

Valves are designed to (1) retain food in that segment until the work of the mechanical actions and digestive juices has been completed, (2) allow measured

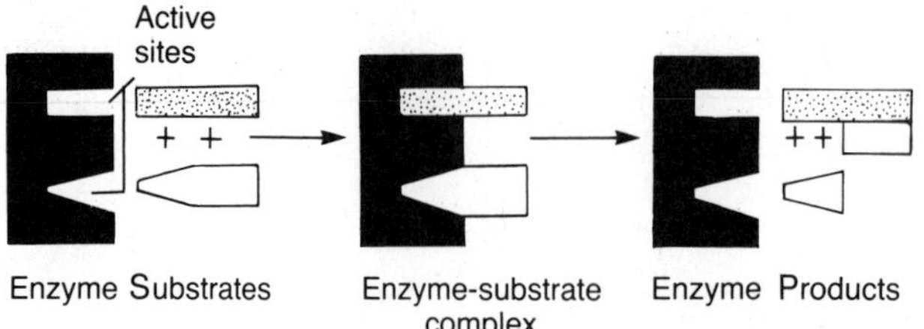

Figure 2–2 Lock-and-key mechanism of enzyme action. Like keys, substrates fit in the active sites of the enzyme. Following the reaction, the products separate and the unchanged enzyme is available to catalyze production of additional products.

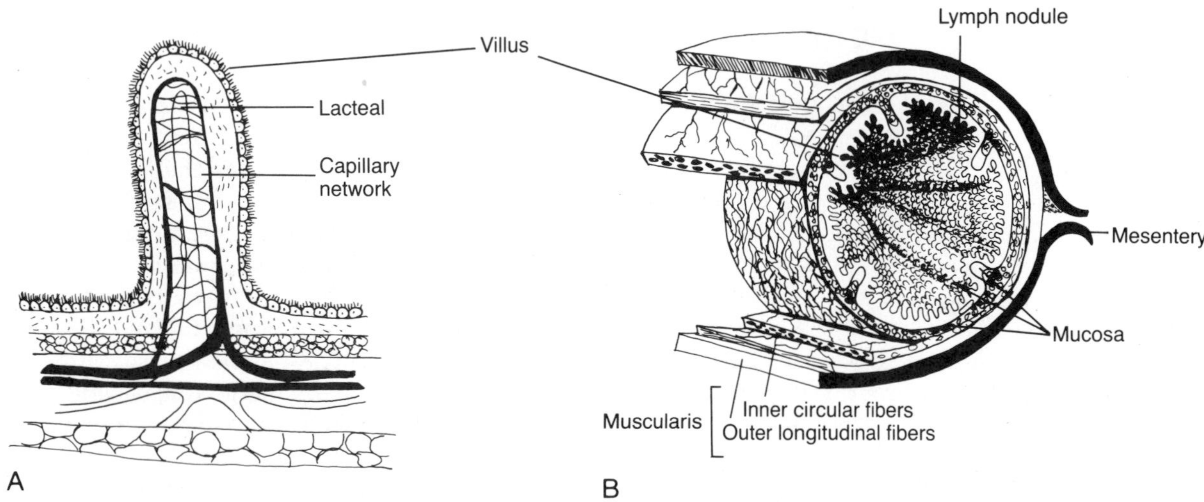

Figure 2–3 *A*, Villus, the absorptive organ of the small intestine. *B*, Layers composing the intestinal wall.

amounts of food to pass into the next segment, and (3) prevent food from "backing up" into the preceding area. The regulation of these valves is complex, involving muscular function and different pressures on each side of the valve.

NURSING APPLICATIONS

1. GI function can be assessed by auscultation. Gurgling, caused by air and fluid in the normal abdomen, indicates peristalsis.
2. Assess bowel sounds because if the alimentary tract is not functioning properly, the body may not be provided adequate amounts of nutrients. The client may be prone to deficiencies, poor healing, or impactions.
3. Loss of motility in the stomach and small intestine results in impaired stomach and intestinal emptying. This allows excessive growth of bacteria, which may injure the surface of the intestine, cause diarrhea, and interfere with nutrient absorption. Closely monitor clients who are not eating or who are immobile because they may be prone to these disorders.

Food–drug interactions have the potential to cause nutritional problems or erratic drug responses. Therefore, knowledge of the drugs given and how they interact with food is necessary. For example, giving milk with tetracycline decreases the amount of tetracycline available to the body.

Client Education

- Taking over-the-counter (OTC) enzyme tablets may not be beneficial because they are digested as any other protein. Prescription pancreatic enzymes are effective because of a special enteric coating that prevents the enzyme from exposure to gastric juices. Lactase, a nonprescription enzyme, is also effective because it is either added to or taken with lactose-containing foods so the lactase converts lactose into glucose and galactose before the gastric juices affect the enzyme (lactase).
- Digestion involves 2 types of action: Mechanical and chemical. Both must be functioning properly for digestion to occur.

MOUTH

Taste and Smell

Generally, food choices are influenced by the 3 senses of sight, smell, and taste. Taste is the first determinant of food choices in the US (Hess, 1991). The presentation of food, its color or aroma, may be the basis for acceptance or rejection.

Taste buds are the receptors for the sense of taste.

Olfactory nerves are the receptors for smell.

The mouth plays an important role in the digestive system, not only because it is the "port of entry," but also because of the presence of **taste buds.** Food stimulates the taste buds, and aromas stimulate the **olfactory nerves.** Satisfaction derived from food determines its acceptability. The basic taste sensations of sweet, sour, salty, and bitter are located on different parts of the tongue (Fig. 2–4). These 4 basic tastes reflect specific constituents of food. In general, taste and smell are essential for influencing the intake to meet physiological needs.

Foods are sometimes judged to be harmful or spoiled because of their odors, so the sense of smell may be a protective mechanism. On the other hand, clients with a cold usually lose their appetite because of a decreased sense of smell, which causes decreased palatability and enjoyment. Taste disorders are often the result of problems in smell rather than taste. Taste and smell abnormalities must always be considered in nutritional care of clients.

Anosmia—loss of smell. Hypogeusia—loss of taste. Hypergeusia—heightened taste acuity.

How do taste and smell affect food intake?

Certain diseases and medicines may produce **anosmia, hypogeusia,** or **hypergeusia** (Table 2–1). Drug-induced loss of taste acuity also results in anorexia. Taste and smell disorders, whether caused by disease states or drugs, are not mere inconveniences or neurotic symptoms. They affect food choices and dietary habits and can result in deterioration of a client's general condition or nutritional status. Because taste stimulants affect salivary and pancreatic flow, gastric contractions, and intestinal motility, taste disorders can also affect digestion.

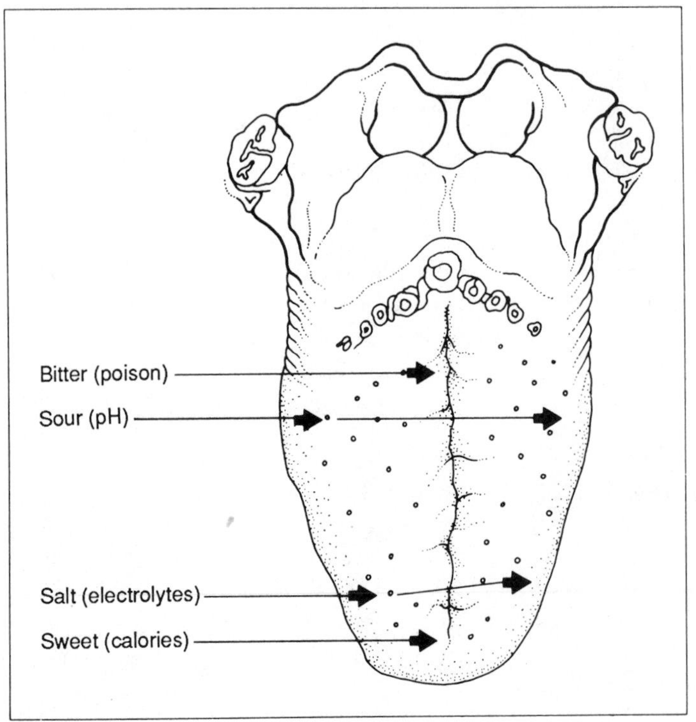

Figure 2–4 Regions of taste on the tongue.

TABLE 2–1

SOME FACTORS AFFECTING TASTE AND SMELL

Factor	Taste	Smell
Disorders		
Damage to chorda tympani	Absent/diminished	
Familial dysautonomia	Absent/diminished	
Head trauma	Absent/diminished	Absent/diminished
Cancer	Absent/diminished (sweet) Heightened (bitter)	
Chronic renal failure	Absent/diminished/distorted (sweet, salt, sour)	Absent/diminished
Cirrhosis	Absent/diminished	Absent/diminished
Niacin deficiency	Absent/diminished/distorted	
Thermal burn	Absent/diminished distorted	
Vitamin B_{12} deficiency		Absent/diminished
Zinc deficiency	Absent/diminished	
Adrenal cortical insufficiency	Increased detection but decreased recognition	
Multiple sclerosis	Absent/diminished/distorted	Absent/diminished
Cushing's syndrome	Absent/diminished	Absent/diminished
Hypothyroidism	Absent/diminished/distorted	Absent/diminished/distorted
Diabetes mellitus	Absent/diminished (sweet)	Absent/diminished
Allergic rhinitis, nasal polyps, sinusitis, bronchial asthma		Absent/diminished
Radiation therapy	Absent/diminished/distorted	
Cystic fibrosis	Individual variation, frequently increased	Individual variation, frequently increased
Hypertension	Absent/diminished (salt)	
Drugs		
Dimercaprol, fluorouracil, lincomycin, griseofulvin	Altered/distorted	
Phenformin, lithium, metronidazole, disulfiram, sulfonylureas, streptomycin	Metallic taste	
Metaproterenol, potassium iodide, chloral hydrate	Bad taste	
Amphetamines	Increased sensitivity (bitter)	
Furosemide	Peculiar sweet taste	
D-Penicillamine, clofibrate, cholestyramine, phenytoin, methylthiouracil, methimazole	Diminished	
Bromide–containing medications	Salty, bitter taste	

Data from Schiffman S. Taste and smell in disease. *N Engl J Med* 1983; 308(21):1275.

TABLE 2–2

DIGESTIVE FUNCTIONS OF SALIVA

Saliva Component	Classification	Function
Mucin	Glycoprotein	Lubricates food for easier passage
Amylase	Enzyme	Begins hydrolysis of starch to maltose
Lysozyme	Enzyme	Kills some ingested bacteria
Lingual lipase	Enzyme	Begins digestion of fats

Teeth

How do teeth aid digestion?

Another important role of the mouth in food digestion is the mechanical action of teeth. Chewing reduces the size of food particles. Digestion of food is facilitated by increasing its surface area.

Saliva

Some chemical action begins with secretions in the mouth. Saliva, secreted by the salivary glands, is mixed with food particles. Thus, moistened foods are more easily manipulated and prepared for swallowing. The functions of the different constituents in saliva are shown in Table 2–2.

List the functions of saliva.

Because food is normally in the mouth only briefly, salivary amylase just initiates starch digestion. If a carbohydrate food, such as a cracker, is chewed and held in the mouth for a few seconds, it will begin to taste sweet, denoting the fact that some starch is being hydrolyzed to maltose.

NURSING APPLICATIONS

1. Clients commonly complain about the "taste" or "flavor" of food when in fact olfactory as well as gustatory (taste) sensations are impaired (Mattes et al, 1990). Assess weight and adequacy of intake.
2. Assess for nutritional deficiencies because they can cause taste abnormalities (zinc, copper, nickel, niacin, and vitamin A).
3. Upper respiratory infections, nasal and/or sinus disease, or head trauma may cause olfactory disorders. Hypogeusia and hypergeusia arise from head trauma, numerous medications, oral diseases, and radiation. Assess these clients for appetite, increased use of spices (especially salt and sugar), and development of food cravings and/or dislikes.
4. Toddlers have the largest number of taste buds (and a higher degree of taste sensitivity), resulting in an aversion for highly seasoned foods. Thus, bland food is more appealing to these youngsters.
5. The number of taste buds declines in later life, explaining the fact that elderly adults have a diminished taste sensitivity. The elderly may inadvertently use too much sodium for seasoning. If cardiac problems are present, this can complicate matters. Other spices should be offered.
6. Clients who have difficulty chewing are likely to develop decreased taste acuity; therefore, monitor food intake.
7. Edentulous clients or those with ill-fitting dentures should be monitored because both quality and quantity of food intake may be compromised.

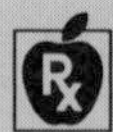 For clients unable to swallow whole tablets or capsules, particularly children or elderly individuals, use a liquid or suspension form of medication.

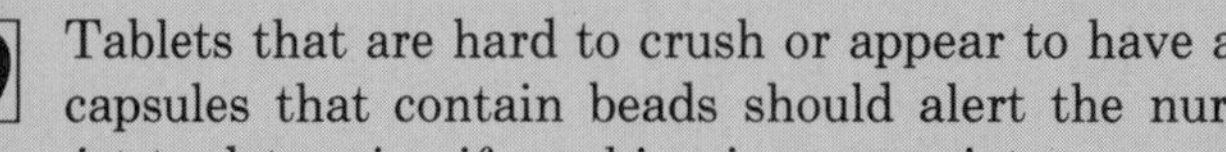 Tablets that are hard to crush or appear to have a special hard coating or capsules that contain beads should alert the nurse to consult the pharmacist to determine if crushing is appropriate.

Client Education

- Consider specific taste alterations to make food more acceptable to clients. Suggest additional sugar, salt, or spices as applicable.
- Most medications are not designed to be chewed, and their effectiveness is altered if they are not swallowed whole.

ESOPHAGUS

The swallowing reflex moves a **bolus** into the esophagus, which is transported to the stomach by peristalsis and gravity. The esophagus, a continuous tube about 10 inches long connecting the mouth with the stomach, penetrates the diaphragm through an opening called the esophageal hiatus. The **lower esophageal sphincter (LES)** relaxes to permit food to enter the stomach but contracts tightly to prevent the regurgitation or "backwashing" of the stomach contents.

Bolus is a mass of food that is swallowed and passed into the stomach.

LES is a group of very strong circular muscle fibers located just above the stomach.

GASTRIC DIGESTION

A bolus entering the stomach is mixed with gastric secretions by peristaltic contractions, producing chyme, a semifluid paste. Gastric secretions include mucus, hydrochloric acid (HCl), 2 enzymes, and a component called intrinsic factor. The low pH of the stomach contents (about 1.5 to 3.0) is beneficial for several reasons: (1) It kills or inhibits the growth of most food bacteria, (2) denatures proteins and makes them more easily hydrolyzed to amino acids, (3) activates gastric enzymes, (4) hydrolyzes some of the sugars, and (5) increases solubility and absorption of calcium and iron.

Two major enzymes are found in gastric juice—pepsin and lipase. Pepsin is capable of hydrolyzing large protein molecules to smaller fragments. Gastric lipase is involved in digestion of short-chain and medium-chain triglycerides (such as those found in butter fat). Mucus forms an alkaline coating on the lining of the stomach for protection against digestion of the stomach by pepsin. Intrinsic factor secreted in the stomach is essential for absorption of vitamin B_{12} in the small intestine.

Normal gastric secretion is regulated by nerve and hormonal stimuli. The senses that allow one to see, smell, and taste food stimulate the vagus nerve to increase gastric secretions. The vagus nerve also affects gastric secretions in response to emotions. Fear, sadness, pain, or depression are generally accompanied by decreased secretions; anger, stress, and hostility, by increased secretions.

In addition to foods, the stomach receives medication and other substances. Although most nutrients must be digested before absorption, most medications simply involve dissolving the dosage form in the stomach. Some medications are irritants to the stomach, making it subject to erosion, ulceration due to hypersecretion and intolerances. Most pass through the stomach unchanged.

The adult stomach has a capacity to hold 1 to 2 L and functions as a reservoir to hold an average meal from 3 to 4½ hours. The stomach empties at different rates depending on its size and composition of the chyme. Rate of passage through the stomach (fastest to slowest) is: liquids, carbohydrates, proteins, fats. When a mixture of foods is presented, however, this pattern is not as well defined. The smaller the stomach capacity, the more rapidly it will empty. (This is exemplified in the infant or person with a partial gastrectomy, who must be fed frequently.) Fats remain in the stomach longer. Chyme is released from the stomach through the pyloric sphincter in small amounts to allow for adequate digestion and absorption in the small intestine.

Why is the low pH of the stomach beneficial? What are the functions for pepsin, lipase, and intrinsic factor? What stimulates the vagus nerve? What inhibits the vagus nerve? What nutrient stays in the stomach longest?

NURSING APPLICATIONS

1. Peptic ulcers are usually due to the digestive action of pepsin, when the HCl somehow overwhelms the mucous protective coating of the stomach, which makes it vulnerable to the digestive action of pepsin.
2. Dietary constituents that increase HCl and pepsin secretions are proteins, calcium, caffeine, coffee, and alcohol. These may need to be limited in clients with ulcers or certain GI tract disorders. Consult with the dietitian as needed.
3. Because gravity facilitates the movement of food down the esophagus, clients who must remain horizontal have some difficulty swallowing and may have reflux of gastric contents after eating. If at all possible, raise head of bed or place the client in a chair during mealtime to avoid these discomforts. If this is not permissible, monitor for aspiration and heartburn. H_2 antagonists or antacids may be helpful.

Client Education

- Vomiting is one of the methods the body has of eliminating toxins from contaminated foods. Vomiting can also be stimulated by rapid changes in body motion or by drugs.
- Heartburn is a result of regurgitation of the stomach contents back into the esophagus. The acidic gastric secretions produce discomfort or pain, which may be relieved if the client remains in the upright position after eating.
- Eating in a relaxing atmosphere helps reduce gastric secretions.
- A stomachache may be the result of eating more than the stomach can comfortably hold or eating too rapidly.

GASTRIC ABSORPTION

Very little absorption takes place in the stomach because very few foods are completely hydrolyzed to nutrients the body can use at this stage. Nutrients that can be absorbed from the stomach include some water, alcohol, and a few water-soluble substances (sodium, potassium, amino acids, and glucose).

SMALL INTESTINE

Within the small intestine, most of the energy nutrients are completely hydrolyzed and absorbed. Most vitamins and minerals are also absorbed in the small intestine. The small intestine is specially designed to perform these tasks with juices from the intestine and the accessory organs and its complex structure along the lumen walls (Table 2–3). The small intestine is approximately 15 feet long, and foods are retained for 3 to 10 hours.

Digestion

Throughout the walls of the small intestine are villi, finger-like projections rising out of the mucosa into the intestinal lumen (see Fig. 2–3). These villi increase the surface area of the alimentary tract to about 3000 square feet. Each villus is

TABLE 2–3

DIGESTION IN THE GASTROINTESTINAL TRACT

Location	Secretion/Enzyme	Function	Nutrient Action
Mouth	Salivary amylase (ptyalin)		Hydrolyzes starch into disaccharides
Stomach	Hydrochloric acid	Antibacterial Activates pepsinogen, which is then called pepsin	Converts Fe^{3+} to Fe^{2+}
	Pepsin		Hydrolyzes proteins into polypeptides
	Gastric lipase		Hydrolyzes emulsified fats (butterfat) into glycerol and fatty acids
	Intrinsic factor	Combines with vitamin B_{12}	
	Mucin	Protects mucosa	
Small intestine:			
Pancreatic juices	Trypsinogen		
	Trypsin	Converts chymotrypsinogen to chymotrypsin	Hydrolyzes proteins and polypeptides into dipeptides
	Chymotrypsinogen	Is converted to chymotrypsin	
	Chymotrypsin		Hydrolyzes proteins and polypeptides into dipeptides
	Procarboxypeptidase		
	Carboxypeptidase		Hydrolyzes polypeptides and dipeptides into amino acids
	Pancreatic lipase (requires bile salts)		Hydrolyzes fats into glycerol, monoglycerides and diglycerides and fatty acids
	Pancreatic amylase		Hydrolyzes starch into maltose
	Phospholipase		Converts lecithin into lysolecithin
Intestinal juices (in microvilli)	Enterokinase	Activates trypsin, chymotrypsin, and carboxypeptidase	
	Aminopeptidase		Hydrolyzes polypeptides and dipeptides into amino acids
	Dipeptidases		Hydrolyzes dipeptides into amino acids
	Intestinal lipase		Hydrolyzes fats into glycerol and glycerides and fatty acids
	Sucrase		Hydrolyzes sucrose into glucose and fructose
	Maltase		Hydrolyzes maltose into glucose
	Lactase		Hydrolyzes lactose into glucose and galactose
	Lecithinase		Hydrolyzes lecithin into fatty acids and glycerol and phosphoric acid
	Bile	Accelerates action of pancreatic lipase Emulsifies fats Neutralizes chyme Stabilizes emulsions	
Large Intestine	Mucus	Protects mucosa	

also covered with a layer of epithelial cells containing microvilli that collectively form the brush border cells. This further increases the surface area. The pH change and motility in the small intestine inhibit bacterial growth.

Acidic chyme entering the intestine stimulates the hormones, secretin and pancreozymin, to release bicarbonate ions and pancreatic juices into the duodenum. Cholecystokinin, released in response to the presence of fat, stimulates the gallbladder to contract and release bile.

Pancreatic enzymes hydrolyze carbohydrates, protein, and fats.

Proteolytic enzymes function to hydrolyze proteins.

Emulsify means to break up fats into smaller particles by lowering the surface tension.

Pancreatic enzymes enter the duodenum through the pancreatic duct and function best in the neutralized chyme. The **proteolytic** enzymes are produced and stored in the pancreas in inactive form. Enterokinase, an intestinal enzyme, activates trypsinogen to its active form, precipitating a domino effect to activate the remaining proteolytic enzymes.

Approximately 1 L of bile is secreted daily by the liver. It is stored in the gallbladder, where reabsorption of water concentrates the bile. Bile salts have an **emulsifying** effect, allowing greater exposure to intestinal and pancreatic lipases.

Specific digestive enzymes located within the microvilli are responsible for completing the hydrolysis of carbohydrates, proteins, and fats. Not everything in foods can be completely digested. The human body does not have enzymes to digest cellulose, a carbohydrate found in plants.

Where are most nutrients absorbed? What nutrients are partially hydrolyzed by pancreatic secretions? What is the primary function of bile?

Other factors affecting digestion and absorption are as important to nutritional status as adequate intake: (1) the amount of the nutrient consumed; (2) the physiological need; (3) the condition of the digestive tract, such as the amount of secretions, motility, and absorptive surface; (4) the level of circulating hormones; (5) the presence of other nutrients or drugs ingested at the same time that enhance or interfere with absorption; and (6) the presence of adequate amounts of digestive enzymes.

NURSING APPLICATIONS

1. The 6 factors listed that affect digestion and absorption need to be assessed for each client.
2. The absence of bile leads to impaired digestion and absorption of fats and fat-soluble vitamins. Thus, monitor for fat and fat-soluble vitamin deficiencies.
3. An enzymatic deficiency in the GI tract results in some nutrients not being digested; therefore, they cannot be absorbed, and the client is at risk for deficiency. The most prevalent enzyme deficiency is lactase deficiency, discussed in Chapter 23.
4. If pancreatic juice is blocked from being released from the pancreas, it may accumulate and activate trypsinogen, which can digest portions of the pancreas (a condition called acute pancreatitis). Monitor for nausea, vomiting, and abdominal pain.

Client Education

- The rate of digestion is affected by how well the food is broken apart. If food is not chewed well, the food passes through the GI tract at a slower rate.
- In clients with gallbladder problems, eating a high-fat diet may cause distress.

Absorption of Nutrients

The small intestine is the principal site for nutrient absorption (Fig. 2–5). Only after the nutrient is absorbed into the intestinal mucosa is it considered to be "in" the body. As a general rule, absorption of nutrients by **passive diffusion** occurs in the duodenum, whereas absorption by **active transport** mechanisms is prevalent in the ileum. Approximately 80 to 90% of the water intake is absorbed in the small intestine by **osmosis.** Actually, water moves freely in both directions across the intestinal mucosa.

Absorbable nutrients pass through the microvilli and enter the portal circulation if they are water soluble or lymphatic circulation if they are fat soluble.

Passive diffusion is the passage of a permeable substance from more concentrated solution to an area of lower concentration.

Active transport occurs when absorption is from a region of low concentration to a higher concentration and requires a carrier and cellular energy.

Osmosis is the passage of water through a semipermeable membrane to equalize the osmotic pressure exerted by the ions in solutions.

How is food absorbed? How is water absorbed?

Absorption into Portal Circulation

Monosaccharides, amino acids, glycerol, water-soluble vitamins, minerals, and short-chain and medium-chain fatty acids are absorbed from the small intestine through the mucosa into the portal circulation. They are transported through the portal vein directly to the liver, where metabolism begins.

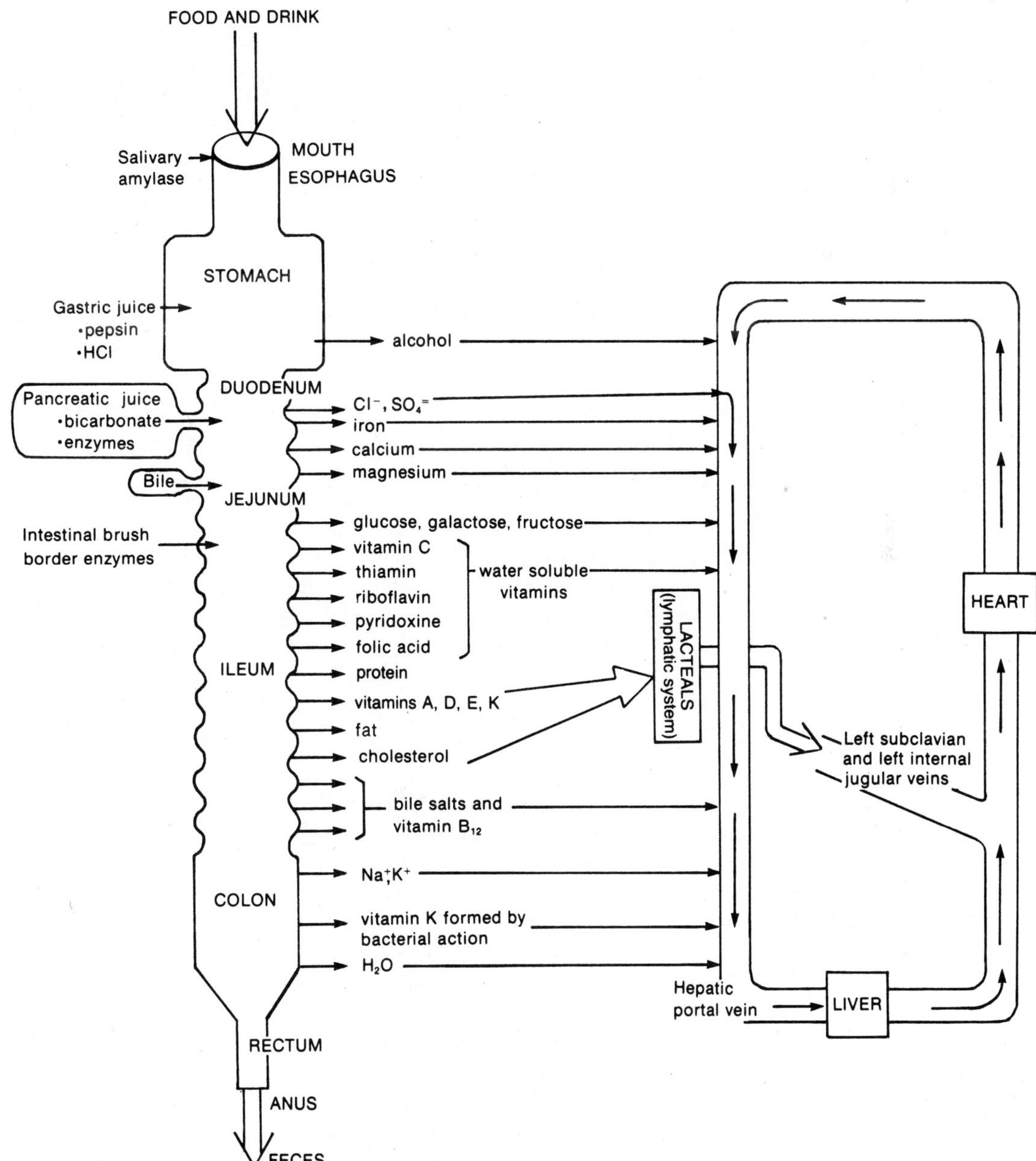

Figure 2–5 Sites of secretion and absorption in the gastrointestinal tract. (From Mahan LK, Arlin MT. *Krause's Food, Nutrition, and Diet Therapy.* 8th ed. Philadelphia, WB Saunders, 1992.)

Absorption of Fat-Soluble Nutrients

The absorption process for long-chain fatty acids is complex because the molecules are large and insoluble. Long-chain fatty acids are broken apart so they can pass through the intestinal wall into the lymphatic system, which transports them to the left subclavian and internal jugular veins. Absorption of the 4 fat-soluble vitamins—A, D, E, and K—is not as complex. Bile salts and lipases increase their water solubility so they are absorbed as a micellar complex along with other fats in the lymphatic system.

NURSING APPLICATIONS

1. Unless preventive care is taken, clients with partial or complete removal of the stomach, duodenum, jejunum, or ileum may develop deficiency symptoms when digestive secretions or absorptive areas are removed (see Fig. 2–5). Monitor weight closely and assess for possible complications (diarrhea, altered electrolytes).
2. If motility is increased, such as in diarrhea, nutrients are not exposed to digestive secretions and absorption surfaces long enough for maximum absorption. Severe or prolonged diarrhea may result in numerous deficiencies, the most rapid being a fluid deficit or dehydration.

Client Education

- Do not eliminate all dietary fat because it is necessary for absorption of fat-soluble vitamins.
- Most nutrients are absorbed in the small intestine.

Absorption of Drugs

Because both nutrients and drugs are blended in the GI tract before absorption, many different things can happen to the nutrient, the drug, or the GI tract that can affect absorption. Drugs are absorbed by passive diffusion. Weakly acidic drugs are absorbed in the stomach, but most drugs are absorbed in the small intestine.

Drug and Nutrient Absorption

The fact that a drug reduces nutrient absorption does not mean that a deficiency will occur. Medications that are generally of concern include those used for chronic diseases over an extended period of time.

The types of drugs that most frequently affect absorption of specific nutrients are laxatives, antacids, hypocholesterolemics, oral contraceptives, hypoglycemics, anticonvulsants, alcohol, and **cytotoxic** drugs (Table 2–4). Several conditions may result in drug-induced malabsorption of nutrients.

Cytotoxic drugs are tumor-inhibiting medications that are harmful to normal or body cells.

Decreased Absorption of Nutrients

A nutrient can bind with a medication; the decreased solubility prevents both from being absorbed. An example of this involves malabsorption of fat-soluble vitamins with concomitant mineral oil ingestion. Long-term antacid therapy and

TABLE 2–4

DRUGS AFFECTING NUTRIENT ABSORPTION

Drug	Nutrient Affected
Isoniazid (antitubercular), levodopa (Parkinson's disease)	Vitamin B_6, pyridoxine
Coumarin (anticoagulant)	Vitamin K
Primidone, phenobarbital, phenytoin (anticonvulsants)	Vitamin D, vitamin K, folate
Corticosteroids	Carbohydrates
Antacids	Phosphate, calcium, vitamin D
Antibiotics	Vitamin K

potassium chloride supplements neutralize the gastric HCl, thereby hindering absorption of the vitamins, folic acid and vitamin B_{12}, and the minerals, calcium and iron.

Adsorption of Bile Salts

Antilipemic medications **adsorb** bile salts. Not only is cholesterol excreted, but also fat-soluble vitamins are bound along with bile salts by the drug, resulting in their excretion.

Adsorb—attract and retain substances.

Damage of Intestinal Mucosa

Drugs can decrease the amount of enzymes available and thereby interfere with the transport system of nutrient absorption. For example, phenytoin (an anticonvulsant) and sulfasalazine (an anti-inflammatory) inhibit the complex enzyme system required for absorption of naturally occurring folate and vitamin B_{12}.

Decreased Gastrointestinal Transit Time

Laxatives decrease the amount of transit time and therefore decrease nutrient absorption in the intestinal tract. Peristaltic stimulants (containing bisacodyl or phenolphthalein) can interfere with the intestinal uptake of glucose, potassium, and calcium. Saline cathartics (milk of magnesia, magnesium sulfate, and sodium phosphate) are hypertonic, and water is osmotically attracted into the lumen. The increased volume causes the intestine to contract and expel the contents faster.

Increased Absorption

Few drugs enhance nutrient absorption. Increased absorption of cholesterol, however, has been documented with long-term use of the laxative docusate sodium. This is an undesirable effect.

What are some of the ways drugs affect the digestive process? Give examples.

NURSING APPLICATIONS

1. Although overuse of cathartics may decrease nutrient availability, nutritionally, they are not as hazardous as peristaltic stimulants. Thus, evaluation of clients' nutritional status is not as essential with other drugs.

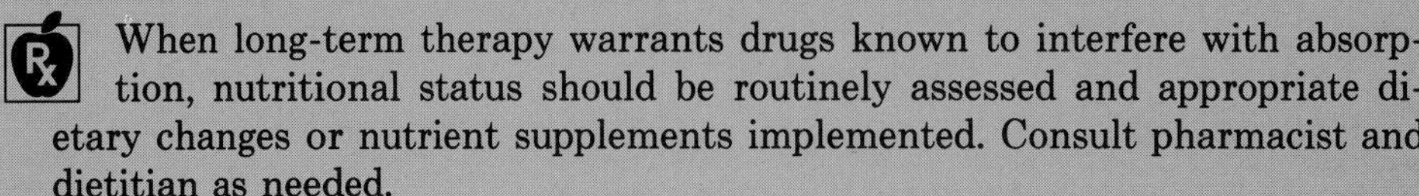

When long-term therapy warrants drugs known to interfere with absorption, nutritional status should be routinely assessed and appropriate dietary changes or nutrient supplements implemented. Consult pharmacist and dietitian as needed.

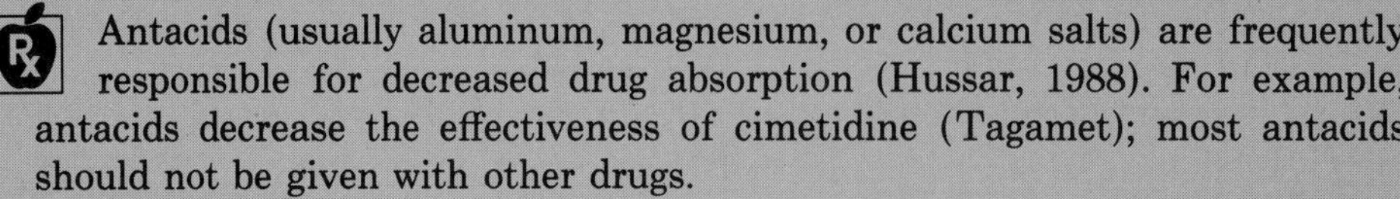

Antacids (usually aluminum, magnesium, or calcium salts) are frequently responsible for decreased drug absorption (Hussar, 1988). For example, antacids decrease the effectiveness of cimetidine (Tagamet); most antacids should not be given with other drugs.

Client Education

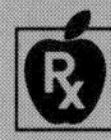

Vegetable bulk laxatives (e.g., psyllium [Konsyl, Metamucil]) are the least likely to cause nutrient malabsorption.

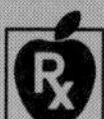

The use of mineral oil as a laxative is discouraged because it decreases the absorption of fat-soluble vitamins and the mineral, calcium.

Effect of Foods on Drug Absorption

Not only is nutrient absorption important, but also the absorption of a medication is necessary for it to have a therapeutic effect. Food intake as well as the composition of food may affect drug absorption. The time a drug is given in relation to food intake has clinical and economic implications. The established time of day for drug administration in health care institutions frequently conflicts with the optimal **bioavailability** of the drug. When food is in the digestive tract, studies show altered absorption response of 77 to 93% of drugs (Murray & Healy, 1991).

Bioavailability is the amount of nutrient available to the body following absorption.

In most cases, the absorption of drugs is delayed by concomitant food intake; this may or may not decrease the amount of drug absorption. Thus, other considerations determine whether to give the drug with food. If a rapid effect is necessary (such as with analgesics, hypnotics, or anti-infectives for acute infection), the drug is taken on an empty stomach (Appendix C-10).

In general, most drugs are water soluble. If taken with fatty food, absorption is significantly delayed. Some drugs should be taken with food to decrease GI distress or enhance their absorption. Because GI distress is a common side effect of many drugs, trade-offs must sometimes be made. These drugs may need to be taken with food, even if absorption is decreased. To assure client compliance, refined carbohydrates such as fruits or fruit juice or crackers are ideal foods to give when drugs cause GI distress. Tetracycline frequently causes GI upsets. However, when given with milk and milk products or supplements containing calcium, magnesium, iron and sodium bicarbonate, or aluminum (from certain antacids), both the ion and the tetracycline are excreted, thereby reducing effectiveness. The absorption, safety, and effectiveness of many drugs are enhanced by fluid intake, especially water (Appendix C-11).

As a general guideline, recommended timing for drug therapy is at least 1 hour before or 2 hours after a meal unless the medication causes GI disturbances when taken on an empty stomach (Murray & Healy, 1991). This timing enhances drug absorption and decreases interference with nutrient absorption. Various rationales are given in Table 2–5. Tables listing specific drugs and appropriate timing are found in Appendix C-10. Effects of specific drug–nutrient interactions will

TABLE 2–5

MEDICATION TIMING AND RATIONALE

Guidelines	Rationale
Take with food	Prolongs time in stomach
	Increases solubility
	Increases absorption due to increased blood flow
	Available nutrients increase absorption
	Prevents GI upsets
Give before meals	Decreases gastric acid secretion
	Decreases gut motility
	Decreases nausea
Give on empty stomach	Prevents decreased stomach acidity
	Decreases length of time in stomach
Give with large amounts of water	Decreases acid degradation in the stomach
	Enhances bioavailability
	Promotes dispersion and dissolution
	Enhances gastric emptying
	Promotes normal GI function
	Ensures excretion
Do not give with milk products	Enteric coating dissolves in basic medium
	Combines with alkaline medium

be discussed with the disease state with which the medications are used as a treatment.

Because the timing of drug administration is frequently the responsibility of the nursing staff, charts such as those provided in Appendices C-9–C-11 should be readily available at each nursing station; if the drug is not listed, a pharmacist should be consulted.

Explain how food can affect drug absorption. Why should some drugs be given with food? Name some foods that are least likely to interfere with drug absorption.

NURSING APPLICATIONS

1. Although aspirin is absorbed more rapidly from an empty stomach, the use of 1 to 3 gm aspirin tablets causes a 3 to 8 ml fecal blood loss (Allen, 1991). If aspirin is taken frequently on a routine basis, give with food; monitor red blood cell level or feces for occult blood.

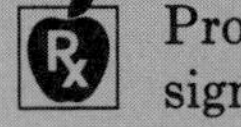
Provide enteric-coated drugs between meals. Enteric-coated drugs are designed to be released in the small intestine; foods in the stomach delay gastric-emptying time and interfere with their rate of absorption.

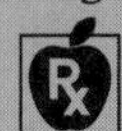
Alcohol and hot beverages can cause premature erosion of enteric-coated tablets. Thus, enteric-coated tablets should not be given with alcohol or hot beverages.

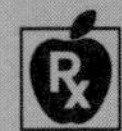
Antacids should not be given within 2 hours before or after drug administration.

Client Education

- Habitual users of aspirin may benefit by taking aspirin with food to minimize gastric irritation.

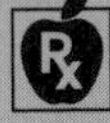
Drastic changes in dietary intake (such as a high-protein diet) can affect drug absorption, and clients should be advised to check with their physician before initiating radical dietary changes.

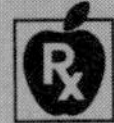
Clients should be taught optimal times to take medications in relation to meals for consistent and optimal absorption.

LARGE INTESTINE

Chyme remaining in the ileum is released through the ileocecal valve into the cecum in small amounts. Only about 1/20 of the ingested foods and digestive secretions arrives in the large intestine. For most adults, it takes between 1 and 3 days for foodstuffs to travel the full length of the gut.

Functions

The large intestine, so named because of its large diameter, has little or no digestive function. Its main functions are to reabsorb water and electrolytes (mainly sodium and potassium) and to form and store the residue (feces) until defecation. Chyme entering the large intestine with 500 to 1000 ml water is excreted as feces containing only 100 to 200 ml fluid (about 75% of the fecal weight). Essentially, all absorption occurs in the proximal half of the colon.

What is the main purpose of the colon?

The inner lining of the large intestine is relatively smooth, lacking the numerous villi found in the small intestine. The only important secretion is mucus, which protects the intestinal wall, aids in holding particles of fecal matter together, and helps to control the pH of the large intestine.

Undigested Residues

Residue is the total amount of fecal solids including undigested or unabsorbed food and metabolic (bile pigments) and bacterial products.

What is the benefit of residue? What can cause an increase in residue?

Fiber, obtained from fruits and vegetables or whole-grain products, results in increased **residue** and has a water-holding capacity, contributing to bulkier feces. Increased residue has a beneficial side effect of stimulating peristalsis, resulting in better muscle tone. Dietary fiber is undigestible and works as a laxative, but foods may contain other substances that increase fecal output. One example is prune juice, which yields no residue on chemical digestion but is classified as a high-residue food because it contains a laxative that indirectly increases the volume of the stool. Milk is fiber free and medium residue.

Microflora

Why are microflora important?

Decreased peristalsis and the neutral pH leads to proliferation of microflora in the colon. Some microflora can break down substances that human enzymes are unable to digest; others synthesize vitamins needed by humans. Vitamin K, vitamin B_{12}, biotin, thiamin, and riboflavin are produced in this manner. This source for obtaining vitamin K is especially important because the food supply normally contains insufficient amounts for adequate blood coagulation. The types of food and medications ingested influence the activity and relative numbers of bacteria. Bacterial activity produces various gases that contribute to flatus in the colon. Fecal odor is a result of the compounds produced by these bacteria.

Peristalsis

After chyme enters the large intestine, it takes about 18 hours to reach the distal colon. The purpose of peristalsis in the large intestine is to force the feces into the rectum. These large waves occur only 2 to 3 times daily.

NURSING APPLICATIONS

1. Bowel habits, stress, exercise, colonic anatomy, and diet (especially the amount of fiber) are assessed in each client because these important factors affect the GI transit rate.
2. Feces retained in the large intestine too long allows more reabsorption of water, and it becomes hard and dry, leading to constipation. Stress the importance of following the urge to defecate.
3. Know the difference between residue and fiber. Encourage constipated clients to consume foods high in fiber and/or residue.

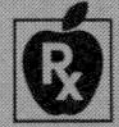 If the client is on long-term antibiotics, assess for bleeding problems because vitamin K production may be inhibited.

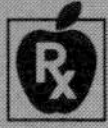 Antibiotic therapy normally kills the bacteria in the colon and inhibits bacterial production of vitamins. Assess clients for possible deficiencies of vitamin K, B_{12}, and biotin.

Client Education

- Constipation can be treated by increasing the fluid intake and/or by gradually increasing the nondigestible materials in the diet. Activity also affects GI motility. Active clients who routinely choose high-fiber foods and drink adequate amounts of liquids are less likely to become constipated than their sedentary counterparts.
- The frequency of bowel movements is an individual matter, and patterns can vary from after each meal to once every 2 days.

METABOLISM

In metabolic activity, the 2 major types of chemical reactions are **catabolism** and **anabolism.** Anabolic processes require energy. Examples of anabolism are building new muscle tissue, bone, or cellular secretions such as hormones.

Anabolism and catabolism are continuous reactions in the body. All cells in the epithelial lining of the GI mucosa are replaced about every 3 to 5 days. Despite this rapid turnover, catabolism is usually equal to anabolism in an adult. During certain stages of life, such as growth periods or pregnancy, more anabolism is occurring than catabolism. Conversely, when illness or stress occurs, excessive catabolism is evident.

Other phases of metabolism include delivery of nutrients to the cells where they are needed and wastes to sites where they can be excreted. The catabolic end products of carbohydrates, proteins, and fats are carbon dioxide, water, and energy. Nitrogen is an additional end product of protein.

Within the cell, the energy-yielding products of digestion—glucose, fatty acids, and amino acids—can be used via a common pathway to yield energy (Fig. 2-6). The energy-releasing process is performed in the mitochondria of cells. **Adenosine triphosphate (ATP)** moves out of the mitochondria and becomes a ready supply of cellular energy. Waste products—carbon dioxide and water—are removed from the body through the lungs and kidneys.

The Krebs cycle, which converts carbohydrates, proteins, and fats to a usable form of energy, requires many enzymes. For the activity of some of these enzymes, vitamins and/or minerals must be available. Some B vitamins function as **coenzymes** in the Krebs cycle. An enzyme may also require a **cofactor.**

Anabolism involves using glucose, amino acids, fatty acids, and glycerol to build the various substances that make up the body itself and the other substances nec-

Metabolism can be defined as the continuous processes whereby living organisms and cells convert nutrients into energy, body structure, and waste.

Catabolism—complex substances broken down into simpler substances.

Anabolism—absorbed nutrients are used to build or synthesize more complex compounds.

The major source of energy for the cell to transport ions, generate heat, synthesize chemical compounds, and contract muscles is stored in the form of ATP generated from the Krebs or tricarboxylic acid (TCA) cycle.

If the nonprotein enzyme portion is a vitamin, the structure is called a coenzyme; a mineral or electrolyte attached to an enzyme is called a cofactor.

Describe anabolism and catabolism. Give examples of each.

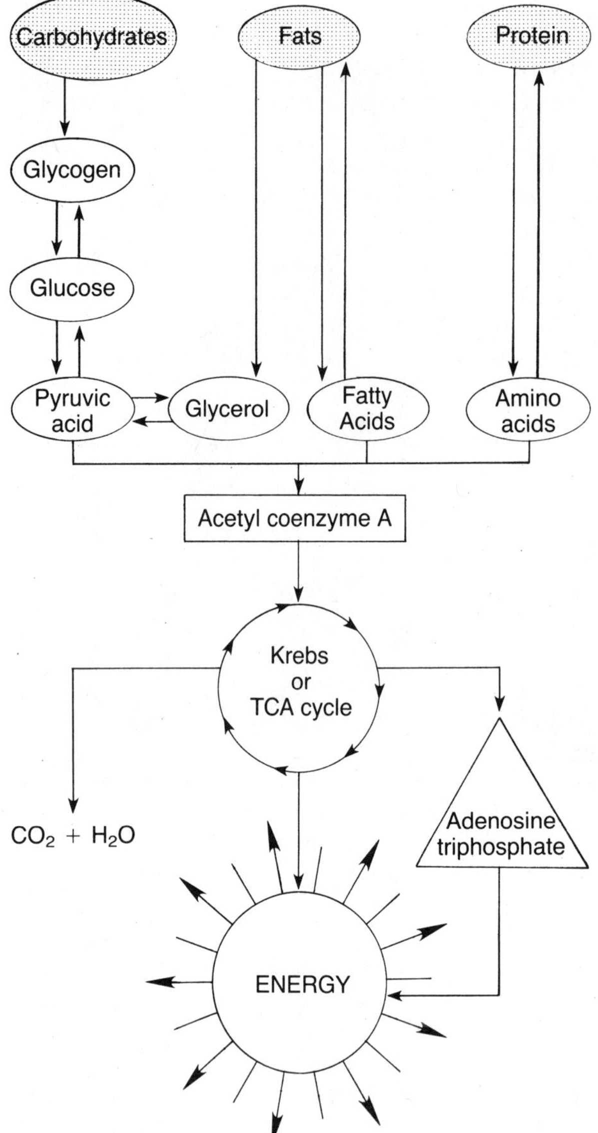

Figure 2–6 Central pathways of metabolism: How the body produces energy from the energy-containing nutrients using the Krebs or tricarboxylic acid (TCA) cycle.

essary for the body to function. All nutrients are intertwined in this process. Ordinarily, amino acids are used to build proteins; still, amino acids or fatty acids can be produced from glucose. To put it mildly, the body is a very complex system.

Role of the Liver

The major distributing organ of foodstuffs to the body is the liver, which regulates the kinds and quantities of nutrients in the blood stream. All monosaccharides are converted to glucose in the liver because glucose is the major energy supply for cells. Glucose is maintained in the blood stream at a certain level; the excess is stored as glycogen or fat. Glycogen can be broken down to glucose and released into the circulating blood as needed. Other end products of digestion may be oxidized to provide energy; converted to glucose, protein, fat, or other substances; or released to circulate at prescribed levels in the blood to be used by cells throughout the body.

Drug–Nutrient Interactions and Metabolism

In some instances, the therapeutic action of a drug directly interferes with the body's use of a particular nutrient in foods by competing with the nutrient at its site of action. This effect is more significant if the nutritional status is poor or if long-term intake of the drug is necessary. In these instances, drug–nutrient effects may precipitate clinical symptoms of nutrient deficiency.

Foods and the type of diet may also increase activity of drug-metabolizing enzymes, thereby enhancing drug metabolism. In general, a diet high in protein results in increased amounts of enzyme production. Other food components can also influence enzyme activity. The inclusion of cruciferous vegetables (e.g., cabbage, broccoli, and cauliflower) and charcoal-broiled foods increases the metabolism of drugs, especially theophylline, resulting in decreased effectiveness.

The metabolism of many drugs is reduced with marginal nutritional deficiencies (magnesium and vitamins A, E, and C), which may **potentiate** their actions. Other non-nutritive substances in foods, such as caffeine and alcohol, can alter metabolism to affect drugs or nutrients.

Potentiate—the action of 1 agent is enhanced by another so the combined effect is magnified.

Discuss how medications may affect nutritional status or vice versa.

NURSING APPLICATIONS

1. If liver function is compromised, monitor glucose levels closely to prevent complications precipitated by elevated or depressed blood glucose levels.
2. A nursing goal for nutrition is to promote anabolism.
3. Evaluate effectiveness of care in promoting anabolism by monitoring client's weight; intake of nutrients, food, and kilocalories; and adherence to prescribed diet.

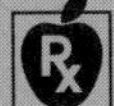

If client principally eats meats, drug dosage may need to be adjusted if desired effects are not noted. Therefore, inquire about dietary habits, and alert the physician if protein intake appears excessive.

Client Education

- The liver is a vital organ for metabolism of food and drugs.

Alcohol

Regardless of whether alcohol (ethanol) is considered a drug or a food, it does affect nutrient and drug metabolism. Alcohol is metabolized primarily by the liver. Large amounts of alcohol inhibit liver enzymes that metabolize drugs, whereas chronically large amounts of alcohol enhance the metabolism of many drugs. Nutritionally, alcohol enhances production of lipids and lipoproteins, decreases lipid oxidation, and interferes with carbohydrate metabolism. It may cause damage to the liver and interfere with the transport, activation, catabolism, and storage of almost every nutrient.

How does alcohol affect nutrient metabolism?

Caffeine

Although caffeine is a non-nutritive substance in food, it is probably the most widely used drug consumed in the US and Europe. It is frequently ingested in large enough quantities to alter metabolism. Caffeine, theophylline, and theobromine are all chemically similar compounds called methylated xanthine. They are found natu-

TABLE 2–6

XANTHINE CONTENT OF BEVERAGES

Beverage	Caffeine	Theophylline	Theobromine
Coffee (1 cup)	85 mg	—	—
Tea (1 cup)	50 mg	1 mg	—
Cocoa (1 cup)	5 mg	—	250 mg
Cola (12 oz)	40–50 mg	—	—

Data from Rall TW. Drugs used in the treatment of asthma. The methylxanthines, cromolyn sodium and other agents. *In* Gilman AG, et al, eds. *Goodman and Gilman's The Pharmacological Basis of Therapeutics.* 8th ed. New York, Pergamon Press, 1990, pp 618–637.

rally in coffee, tea, cocoa, and cola beverages (Table 2–6). These compounds affect body metabolism by:

1. Stimulating the central nervous system (more rapid thinking, reduced drowsiness and fatigue, keener appreciation of sensory stimuli, and decreased reaction time).
2. Stimulating the kidney and producing diuresis (especially theophylline).
3. Stimulating the cardiac muscle (especially theophylline).
4. Relaxing smooth muscles (especially the bronchial muscle).
5. Increasing gastric secretions.

There is no conclusive evidence that moderate amounts of caffeine are harmful to the average healthy client; however, its use should be minimized during pregnancy, even though its link to birth defects is inconclusive. Many drugs are affected by caffeine; it is definitely contraindicated when sedatives are given.

More than 1000 OTC drugs contain caffeine; it is most frequently found in weight-control remedies (e.g., Dexatrim), alertness or stay-awake tablets (e.g., Vivarin), headache and pain relief remedies (e.g., Excedrin), cold products (e.g., Triaminicin), and diuretics (e.g., Aqua-Ban).

NURSING APPLICATIONS

1. Vitamin and mineral requirements are higher in alcoholics than in nonalcoholics, so assess dietary intake and perform a thorough nutritional assessment.
2. Be aware of clients who are habitual users of alcohol, coffee, tea, and cola drinks. If the effectiveness of the prescribed drug is questionable, consult the physician, pharmacist, or dietitian.

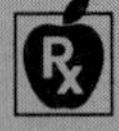

Alcohol potentiates the effect of many types of drugs, especially central depressants. Therefore, medications should not be given with alcohol.

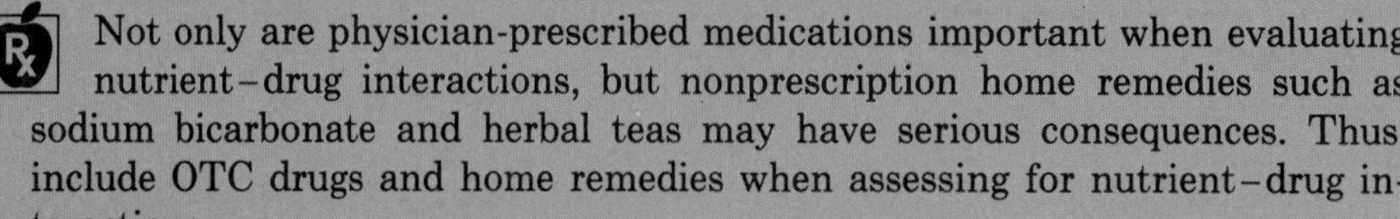

Not only are physician-prescribed medications important when evaluating nutrient–drug interactions, but nonprescription home remedies such as sodium bicarbonate and herbal teas may have serious consequences. Thus, include OTC drugs and home remedies when assessing for nutrient–drug interactions.

Client Education

- Alcohol and sedatives should not be taken together.
- The most common withdrawal symptom of caffeine is headache.

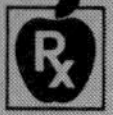

Clients on medications for long-term therapy should be advised to consult the physician or pharmacist before drastically altering their diet.

Kidney

The kidney performs an important metabolic task of removing waste products in the urine and, along with the liver, controls the amount of many nutrients in the circulating blood. Metabolic end products from the cells, unnecessary substances absorbed from the GI tract, potentially harmful compounds that have been detoxified by the liver, and drugs are all excreted by the kidney.

The kidneys accomplish this by a process of filtration and reabsorption. Glucose, amino acids, vitamins, and various mineral ions are reabsorbed or excreted by the kidney, depending on the body's need. In this way, kidneys help maintain nutrient balance within the body.

Hydration status can influence the therapeutic action of drugs and their retention in the body. The rate of urine elimination affects rate of drug excretion; urine elimination may be decreased in dehydrated or edematous clients, causing increased drug levels in the body.

Drugs may alter the kidney's ability to reabsorb a nutrient. Increased sodium excretion precipitated by diuretics is desirable; however, loss of other electrolytes, potassium, magnesium, and zinc is an undesirable side effect.

A number of foods can affect drug excretion by changing the pH of the urine. An alkaline urine decreases the excretion of some medicines, thereby increasing the duration of their action. For example, basic urinary pH increases tubular reabsorption of a weak-base drug. Toxic symptoms have been reported. The pH of the urine is alkalinized in clients taking antacids and some diuretics. Urinary pH may be altered to improve therapeutic efficacy. Vitamin C (approximately 2 to 3 gm) may be used to acidify the urine. It may accompany methenamine mandelate therapy to prevent alkalinization of the urine and to increase the therapeutic effectiveness of the drug.

Other routes of excretion of waste products are the bowel; the skin, which excretes water and electrolytes; and the lungs, which remove carbon dioxide and water.

NURSING APPLICATIONS

1. If the client is dehydrated or edematous, monitor for drug toxicity.
2. Thiazide diuretics can cause a loss of potassium. Monitor client for signs and symptoms of low potassium (weakness), and encourage high-potassium foods such as dried fruits and orange juice.

Client Education

- Kidneys help rid the body of waste products and drugs. Adequate fluid intake facilitates this process.
- If the kidneys are not working properly, drugs and nutrients may either be retained or lost. Both are undesirable.

NUTRITION UPDATE 2–1: PREVENTION OF NUTRIENT–DRUG PROBLEMS

Nutrient depletion occurs gradually, but when drugs are taken over a long period of time, malnutrition may result. Drug-induced nutritional deficiencies occur most frequently in clients with (1) multiple drug usage; (2) marginal nutritional status because of a poor diet, chronic disease, drug abuse, or physiological stress; or (3) impaired metabolic or excretory functions. Deficiencies have been identified in clients who abuse alcohol, drugs, or laxatives. Elderly clients are particularly at risk because of their need for many drugs combined with poor eating habits and a slow rate of drug metabolism.

Malnutrition caused by drug side effects or medication toxicities resulting from nutrient–drug interactions are largely preventable. Nurses need to be aware of circumstances that could lead to problems and carefully assess nutritional status, clinical signs, and laboratory reports of clients on long-term drug therapies. When an expected response to a planned therapeutic program does not occur, the possibility of interactions between the disease state, drugs, and food should be considered.

The requirements by the Joint Commission on Accreditation of Healthcare Organizations to provide clients with drug–nutrient information for medications to be taken at home is a positive step.

NURSING APPLICATIONS

1. Assess the elderly, chronically ill, health faddists, abusers of OTC drugs, and alcoholics because they are most at risk for nutrient–drug problems.
2. Assess elderly clients on numerous prescribed drugs and their attitudes about taking these medications. The probability of elderly clients correctly taking all the prescribed drugs decreases with the number of medications taken. Noncompliance is frequently associated with fear of side effects (Spagnoli et al, 1989).
3. Inquire about any OTC medications and offer advice regarding potential interactions.

Client Education

- Unless contraindicated, modification of the diet to include foods rich in the depleted vitamins and minerals is preferable to taking supplements.
- Advise clients to keep a list of the medications they take.
- When a client changes physicians, consults more than 1 physician, or relocates, provide a list of all medications and dosages to health care workers.
- Teach dosages, times, actions, and side effects of drugs ordered.

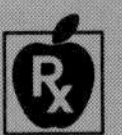
Supplemental vitamin and mineral mixtures can counter the effectiveness of certain drugs.

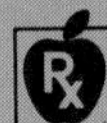
Provide clients with drug–nutrient information in written form.

SUMMARY

The process of furnishing nutrients for use by the body begins with the ingestion of foods, which can be physiologically affected by the senses of taste and smell. Intake can be affected by psychological status, food presentation, and medications. No matter how nutritious a food is, if it is not eaten, it cannot benefit the body, and nutritional status may be affected.

The GI tract is responsible for digesting the ingested foodstuffs into products the body can absorb and use. The liver, the gatekeeper of metabolism, receives all the nutrients and oversees the transport of nutrients to the cells where they are needed and waste products to the organs where they can be excreted (e.g., kidney or lungs).

Drug–nutrient interactions can alter therapeutic effectiveness of a drug or result in deterioration of nutritional status. Clinical deficiencies of nutrients occur most frequently during extended periods of drug usage, when multiple drugs are used, or when the diet is inadequate or marginal. Interrelationships among drugs, diets, and diseases have complex interactions that require careful attention of all health care professionals. A summary of nutrients detrimentally affected by drugs is shown in Appendix C-8.

NURSING PROCESS IN ACTION

A client taking theophylline smokes and consumes a low-carbohydrate, high-protein diet to lose weight. She still is having breathing problems and wants to stop taking theophylline because it does not appear to be working. She knows there is some connection between her diet and medication but does not really understand.

Nutritional Assessment

- Timing of theophylline medication and type of preparation (timed or immediate release).
- Food and nutrient intake.
- Concomitant intake of diet and medication.
- Willingness to learn and to change habits.

Dietary Nursing Diagnosis

Knowledge deficit of interaction between theophylline and diet related to (RT) lack of information and understanding.

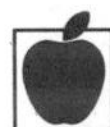

Nutritional Goals

Client will continue taking theophylline; consume a well-balanced diet; and state why a low-carbohydrate, high-protein diet is detrimental to the effectiveness of theophylline as well as the interaction between smoking and theophylline.

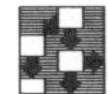

Nutritional Implementation

Intervention: (1) Monitor serum theophylline level. (2) Notify the laboratory to draw a sample 1 to 2 hours after administration of an immediate-release preparation and 4 hours after a sustained-release preparation, as ordered by physician.
Rationale: (1) For the medicine to be effective, the level must be 10 to 20 mcg/ml. Serum levels that are too high cause toxicity, and a depressed level results in a nontherapeutic response. (2) Blood must be drawn before dose is given to prevent a falsely elevated result.

Intervention: Discourage cigarette smoking.
Rationale: Smoking decreases theophylline effectiveness by increasing metabolism. These effects may last for 3 months to 2 years after smoking is discontinued (Karch & Boyd, 1989).

Intervention: (1) Discourage the low-carbohydrate, high-protein diet and excessive routine ingestion of charcoal-broiled beef, broccoli, and cauliflower. (2) Encourage use of a well-balanced diet.
Rationale: (1) These practices increase theophylline elimination, thereby decreasing its effectiveness. (2) Not only will this help theophylline work better, but overall health will also be enhanced.

Intervention: If theophylline is a timed-release capsule, teach the following: (1) Take on an empty stomach without food; (2) do not chew or crush the medication.

Rationale: Timed-release capsules have a special coating to prevent release of medication all at once; chewing or crushing causes this coating to be damaged, resulting in a possibility of overdose.

Intervention: Stress avoidance or use in moderation of coffee, tea, cocoa, cola beverages, or chocolate.

Rationale: These may increase the side effects of theophylline because these contain substances similar to theophylline that stimulate the CNS.

 Evaluation

The client should continue to take theophylline; consume a well-balanced diet; verbalize that a low-carbohydrate, high-protein diet causes theophylline not to work as well; and state that smoking also decreases the effectiveness of the medication. Other behaviors and observations include that the theophylline serum level is within 10 to 20 mcg; smoking is actually decreased; and excessive intake of coffee, tea, cocoa, chocolate, broccoli, and cauliflower are avoided.

STUDENT READINESS

1. Make a chart or diagram showing the GI secretions, where they are produced, and their digestive actions on the nutrients present in milk. Homogenized milk contains the following: lactose (a disaccharide), proteins, emulsified fats, calcium, riboflavin, and vitamins A and D. Where would the end products be absorbed?
2. Define metabolism, catabolism, anabolism, enzyme, and coenzyme.
3. A client has problems secreting too much HCl. What foods would you tell the client to avoid?
4. If kilocaloric intake were equal, which of the following breakfasts would probably delay the feeling of hunger the longest? (1) Dry cereal with skim milk, toast with jelly, and coffee with sugar. (2) Egg with ham, toast with butter, and coffee with cream.
5. What are the absorbable products resulting from the digestion of carbohydrates, proteins, and fats?
6. Within what section of the alimentary canal does most of the digestion and absorption take place?
7. A client asks why some drugs are given with food and others on an empty stomach. What would you say?
8. What vitamins are most frequently implicated in drug–nutrient interactions?
9. Discuss the commonplace use of antacids, laxatives, and analgesics. What are some dangers of these practices?

CASE STUDY

An 18-year-old high school student who has been placed on low-dosage tetracycline for acne is advised not to take the medication with dairy products. After several weeks of therapy, there is no appreciable improvement. When questioned further, she states that she never took the tetracycline with milk, but the capsule was taken each morning with her multivitamin-iron supplements.

a. Why was she advised not to take the medication with dairy products?
b. The nurse advised her to take the medication alone — not with the multivitamin and iron supplement. What is the rationale for this?
c. What OTC preparations should she avoid?

REFERENCES

Allen AM. *Powers and Moore's Food Medication Interactions.* 7th ed. Pottstown, PA, Food Medication Interactions, 1991.

Hess MA. President's page: Resetting the American table—creating a new alliance of taste and health. *J Am Diet Assoc* 1991 Feb; 91(2):228–230.

Hussar DA. Drug interactions in the older patient. *Geriatrics* 1988; 43(suppl):20–30.

Karch A, Boyd E. *Handbook of Drugs and the Nursing Process.* Philadelphia, JB Lippincott, 1989.

Mattes RD, et al. Dietary evaluation of patients with smell and/or taste disorders. *Am J Clin Nutr* 1990 Feb; 51(2):233–240.

Murray JJ, Healy DM. Drug-mineral interactions: A new responsibility for the hospital dietitian. *J Am Diet Assoc* 1991 Jan; 91(1):66–70.

Spagnoli A, et al. Drug compliance and unreported drugs in the elderly. *J Am Geriatr Soc* 1989 July; 37(7):619–624.

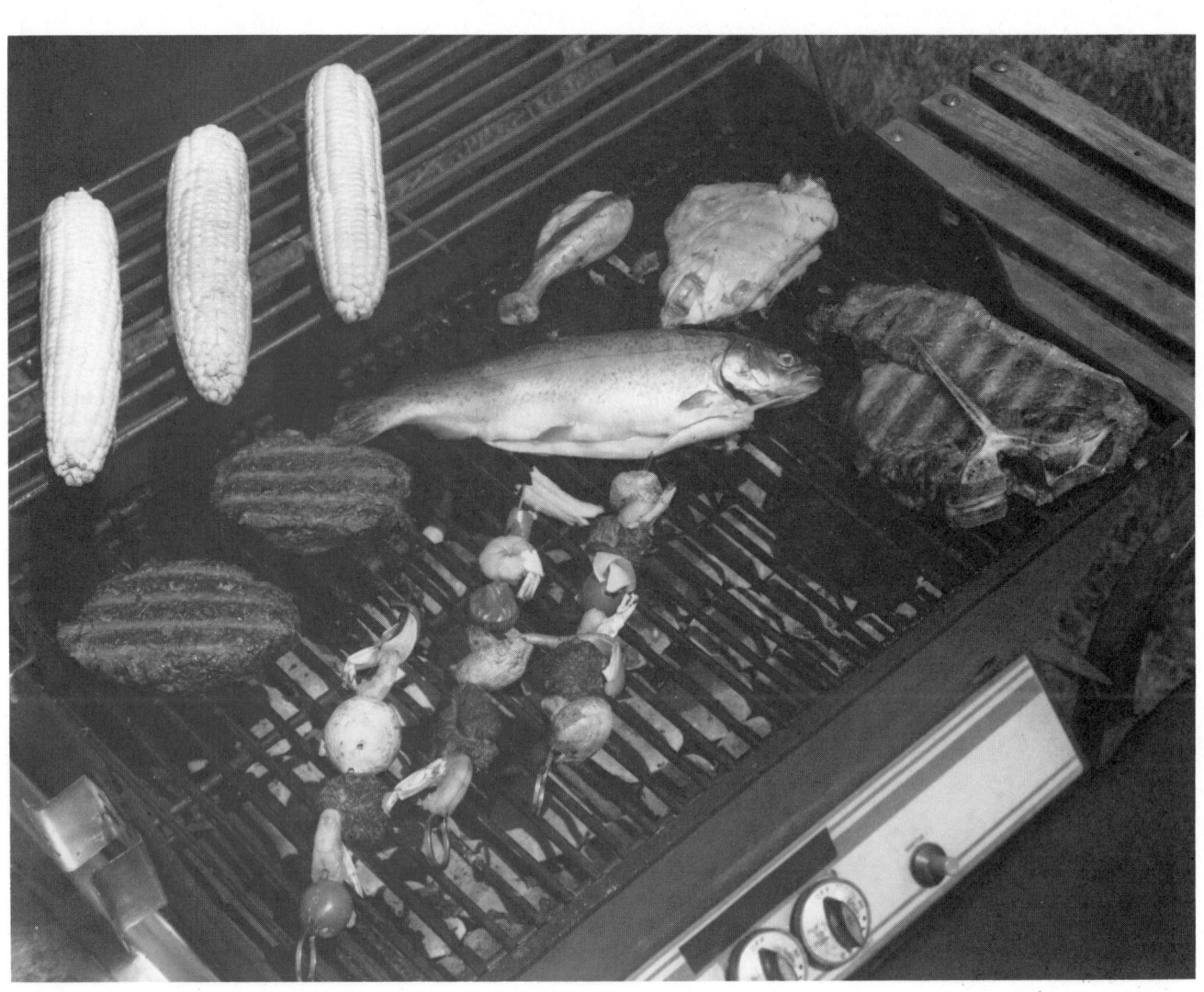

CHAPTER 3

Protein: The Cellular Foundation

OUTLINE

I. AMINO ACIDS
II. DENATURATION
III. CLASSIFICATION
NURSING APPLICATIONS
IV. DIGESTION
V. ABSORPTION
VI. METABOLISM
  A. Anabolism-Catabolism Balance
    1. Anabolism
    2. Catabolism
  Nursing Applications
VII. NITROGEN BALANCE AND BLOOD SERUM LEVELS
  A. Nitrogen Intake and Excretion
  B. Serum and Urine Nitrogen
  Nursing Applications
VIII. PHYSIOLOGICAL ROLES
IX. REQUIREMENTS
X. SOURCES
  A. Amino Acid Content of Foods
  Nursing Applications
XI. HYPER- AND HYPO- STATES
  A. Protein Deficiency
  B. Excessive Protein Intake
  Nursing Applications
XII. NUTRITION UPDATE 3–1: VEGETARIANISM
  A. Vegan or Strict Vegetarian Diet
  B. Lactovegetarian Diet
  C. Ovolactovegetarian Diet
  D. Ovovegetarian Diet
  E. Advantages and Problems
  Nursing Applications

OBJECTIVES

THE STUDENT WILL BE ABLE TO:

- Describe protein digestion.
- List the possible fates of amino acids.
- Classify foods as sources of high-quality or lower-quality proteins.
- Explain to clients how proteins can be used to complement one another.
- Explain the relationship between the nitrogenous substances in the body and protein nutriture.
- Plan menus to include the recommended protein level for a meat-containing diet and a vegetarian diet.
- Explain why various physiological states require different amounts of protein.
- State the problems associated with a protein deficiency or excess.
- Apply nursing principles to protein consumption, deficiency, or excess.
- Describe client education for protein intake to prevent protein deficiency and protein excess.

TEST YOUR NQ (True/False)

1. Eating a lot of foods high in DNA and RNA is the key to staying young.
2. Brown shell eggs are more nutritious than white shell eggs.
3. Gelatin is a good source of high-quality protein.
4. Elderly clients require less protein than younger clients.
5. Protein status of a client can be determined by serum and urine measurements containing nitrogen.
6. An increase in protein intake may lead to fat rather than muscle.
7. Amino acids are the building blocks of proteins.
8. Marasmus is a protein-deficiency disorder.
9. Lactovegetarians eat eggs and plant foods.
10. A biological value of 3.5 indicates a lower quality protein.

Until the middle of the nineteenth century, many scientists thought that life was made from one basic chemical—protein. Protein is present in each living cell, constituting almost half of the dry weight of a cell. Second to water, protein is the most plentiful substance in the body. Protein is considered the main ingredient by most Americans, who are frequently unable to plan a balanced meal without a meat entree, yet other essential nutrients frequently receive little or no attention.

AMINO ACIDS

Amino acids are basic building blocks for proteins.

All the billions of proteins associated with life are made from 22 different **amino acids.** They can be compared with letters of the alphabet used in different sequences and combinations to make billions of words. The general design of an amino acid is illustrated on the next page for better understanding. An amino acid contains a basic or amine grouping (—NH_2) and an acidic or carboxyl grouping (—COOH). The distinguishing feature of amino acids is the amine group, which is the body's source of nitrogen. The radical group shown is the part of the structure that varies to form 22 different amino acids.

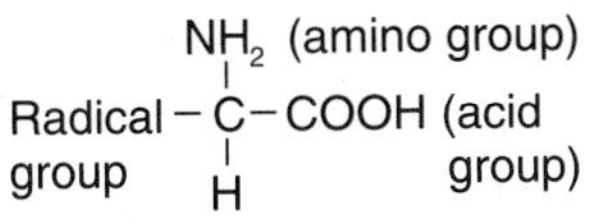

```
                 NH2 (amino group)
                  |
Radical      -   C  - COOH (acid
group             |          group)
                  H
```

Amino acids are able to combine with each other to make long chains. Two amino acids together form a dipeptide, as shown below. Several amino acids form a polypeptide. Foods and body proteins contain polypeptides. The number of amino acids in a protein varies greatly (from 100 to 300), but it is specific for that protein.

What is the relationship between amino acids and protein? Does the amine or radical group provide the body with nitrogen? What is the difference between a dipeptide and polypeptide?

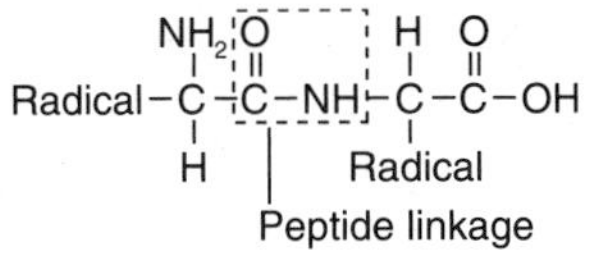

```
         NH2 O       H  O
          |  ||      |  ||
Radical - C - C - NH - C - C - OH
          |          |
          H          Radical
              |
       Peptide linkage
```

DENATURATION

Protein sensitivity to heat, surface action, and extremes in pH causes **denaturation.** Food preparation structurally alters protein molecules. For example, an egg white becomes white and fluffy when beaten; when subjected to heat, it becomes a solid or coagulates. When protein substances are subjected to the extremely acid medium in the stomach, they are denatured as the digestion process begins.

Denaturation is the result of change in the protein structure, causing alteration in its physical properties.

In most cases, digestibility and nutritional value are not unfavorably affected by cooking procedures. Proper cooking sometimes facilitates digestion and utilization. For example, cooking makes egg albumin more readily digestible, and cooking soybeans increases the amino acid bioavailability. On the other hand, processing affects proteins in cereal by binding lysine (an amino acid) so it is not usable by the body.

CLASSIFICATION

A very important classification of amino acids is whether they are **essential** amino acids (EAAs) or **nonessential** amino acids (NEAAs). The 9 EAAs are listed in Table 3–1. If any 1 of the EAAs is not present when the cell needs it for protein synthesis, the protein cannot be produced. The body is able to make adequate amounts of NEAAs if a sufficient amount of protein is available to furnish the nitrogen needed and enough kilocalories are present to spare the catabolism of amino acids.

EAAs are required in the diet.

NEAAs are essential for the body but are not required in the diet.

Tyrosine and cysteine are usually synthesized in adequate amounts from their **precursors,** phenylalanine and methionine, and are classified as semi-essential. Other amino acids may be conditionally essential in certain nutritional or disease states or in certain stages of development. Histidine, arginine, cysteine, tyrosine, and glutamine may be considered as conditionally EAAs for certain disease or stressed conditions (Lacey & Wilmore, 1990; Laidlaw & Kopple, 1987). Although the body is able to make glutamine, it is essential for growth of many rapidly dividing cells and a major energy source for intestinal cells.

Precursor is a substance from which another substance is formed.

TABLE 3–1

CLASSIFICATION OF AMINO ACIDS

Essential Amino Acids	Nonessential Amino Acids
Threonine	Glycine
Valine*	Alanine
Leucine*	Serine
Isoleucine*	Tyrosine†
Phenylalanine	Proline
Tryptophan	Histidine†
Methionine	Cysteine (cystine)†
Lysine	Arginine†
	Hydroxylysine
	Aspartic acid (asparagine)
	Glutamic acid (glutamine)†

* Branched-chain amino acid.
† These amino acids are semi-essential.

High-quality proteins are well balanced in their EAA content.

Biological value is a measure of how well the proteins from the food can be converted into body proteins.

Lower quality proteins, if fed as the only protein source, support life but not normal growth and are intermediate in biological value.

PER is a measurement to compare weight gain of an animal while eating a given amount of protein.

The amount of EAAs furnished by a food determines its ability to support growth, maintenance, and repair. Several methods of classification are used to evaluate a food's protein quality or its ability to support these functions. Foods that supply adequate amounts of the 9 EAAs to maintain nitrogen equilibrium and permit growth are known as **high-quality proteins** or proteins of high **biological value.** Biological values range from 1 to 100, with a higher score for proteins of higher quality. Foods of high biological value containing high-quality proteins are derived from animal sources—egg, dairy products, meat, fish, and poultry. One exception is gelatin, which contains no tryptophan.

Most protein-containing foods have all the EAAs present, although the quantity of 1 or more of the EAAs may be insufficient for optimum protein synthesis; these foods are sources of **lower quality proteins.** These include the proteins found in legumes, nuts, and grains. The amino acid in short supply relative to need is referred to as the limiting amino acid (Table 3–2).

Proteins that do not contain EAAs in adequate amounts to support life have a low biological value. Vegetable and some grain proteins fall into this category; they contain all the EAAs, but because 1 or more EAA is present in a very low ratio, the protein they furnish has a low biological value.

Another measurement of the protein quality of a food is the **protein efficiency ratio (PER).** This measurement is used for nutrition labeling on food packaging to show a comparable measurement of protein. For example, 1 gm of protein from cornmeal is not equal to 1 gm of protein from chicken. Foods of high

TABLE 3–2

AMINO ACID CONTENT OF SELECTED FOODS

Food	Limiting Amino Acids	High Amounts of Amino Acids
Corn	Lysine, threonine, tryptophan	
Cereal	Cystine, lysine, threonine	Methionine
Legumes	Cystine, methionine, tryptophan	Lysine, threonine
Whole grains	Threonine	Methionine, lysine
Nuts and soybeans	Methionine	Lysine, threonine
Sesame and sunflower seeds	Lysine	Cystine, methionine, tryptophan
Peanut	Methionine, lysine, threonine	
Green leafy vegetables	Methionine	
Gelatin	Methionine, lysine, tryptophan	
Yeast	Phenylalanine	Methionine, threonine

biological value receive a high score (above or equal to 2.5), whereas lower quality proteins score between 0.5 and 2.5.

What happens if an essential protein is not available? List the EAAs. Give an example of a semi-essential and conditionally essential protein. What is the difference between high-quality proteins and lower quality proteins? Give examples of each.

NURSING APPLICATIONS

1. Assess intake of amino acid supplements because toxicities and imbalances of amino acids are frequently produced when excesses of 1 amino acid are ingested (Darby, 1990).
2. If a client is taking tryptophan for insomnia, inquire about the dose. Daily intakes of 1.2 to 2.4 gm/day may result in muscular and abdominal pain, weakness, exertional dyspnea, mouth ulcers, and skin rash. These symptoms associated with tryptophan use may be related to contaminants in the tablets; nevertheless, the FDA has banned the use of tryptophan for insomnia.

Client Education

- Biological value and PER indicates how well the body uses the particular proteins. The higher the number, the higher the protein quality.
- Animal foods (except for gelatin) and fish are high-quality proteins.

DIGESTION

Endogenous sources of protein, including products of catabolism within the GI tract, are hydrolyzed and absorbed along with food proteins. The process of protein digestion is summarized in Table 3-3. The chemical process begins in the stomach. Hydrochloric acid activates the inactivated pepsinogen to pepsin. Pepsin is capable of digesting all types of proteins, even collagen (the connective tissue in meats), but owing to the length of time food is in the stomach, most proteins are hydrolyzed into **peptones** and polypeptides. In the small intestine, enzymes continue the process of hydrolyzing peptones and polypeptides into amino acids.

Endogenous indicates the substance is from within the body, such as protein available from degradation of blood or replaced cells.

Peptones—proteins partially broken down.

Describe digestion of proteins.

TABLE 3-3

PROTEIN DIGESTION

Location	Enzyme	Action
Stomach	Hydrochloric acid	Activates pepsinogen
	Pepsinogen	Activated to pepsin
	Pepsin	Hydrolyzes proteins into polypeptides
Small intestine	Trypsinogen*	Activated to trypsin by enterokinase
	Trypsin	Hydrolyzes proteins and polypeptides into dipeptides
	Chymotrypsinogen	Activated to chymotrypsin
	Chymotrypsin	Hydrolyzes proteins and polypeptides into dipeptides
	Procarboxypeptidase*	Converts trypsin to carboxypeptidase
	Carboxypeptidase	Hydrolyzes polypeptides and dipeptides into amino acids
Intestinal mucosa	Enterokinase	Activates trypsinogen
	Aminopeptidase	Hydrolyzes polypeptides and dipeptides into amino acids
	Dipeptidase	Hydrolyzes dipeptides into amino acids

* These enzymes are secreted by the pancreas.

ABSORPTION

Pinocytosis is the process of a cell engulfing the whole molecule before its hydrolysis.

A carrier picks up the particle outside the cell and releases it on the inside, then returns to pick up another particle.

Generally, all proteins are absorbed in the form of amino acids. Occasionally, however, a whole protein escapes digestion and is absorbed, probably by the process of **pinocytosis.** The digestion of amino acids is very slow, but absorption is rapid. Approximately 90 to 95% of the ingested proteins is converted to amino acids and usually absorbed in the proximal part of the intestine. Absorption by active transport requires energy and a **carrier.**

METABOLISM

Amino acids pass through the portal vein into the liver. The liver is an "aminostat," monitoring the intake and breakdown of all amino acids except the branched-chain amino acids, which are metabolized in the muscle. The liver allows individual amino acids to enter the general circulation at specific levels, so each amino acid is available as needed by the cells to synthesize each individual protein. Amino acids transported in the blood are rapidly removed for use by cells. If individual amino acids rise above the prescribed level in the blood, they are removed and oxidized for energy. Important aspects of protein metabolism are shown in Figure 3–1.

Protein metabolism is in a constant dynamic state with continuous catabolism and anabolism to replace worn-out proteins. Even during anabolic periods such as growth, muscle catabolism is elevated as the cell remodels itself.

A small reservoir of amino acids called the "amino acid metabolic pool" is available for anabolism and to maintain the dynamic state of equilibrium. This

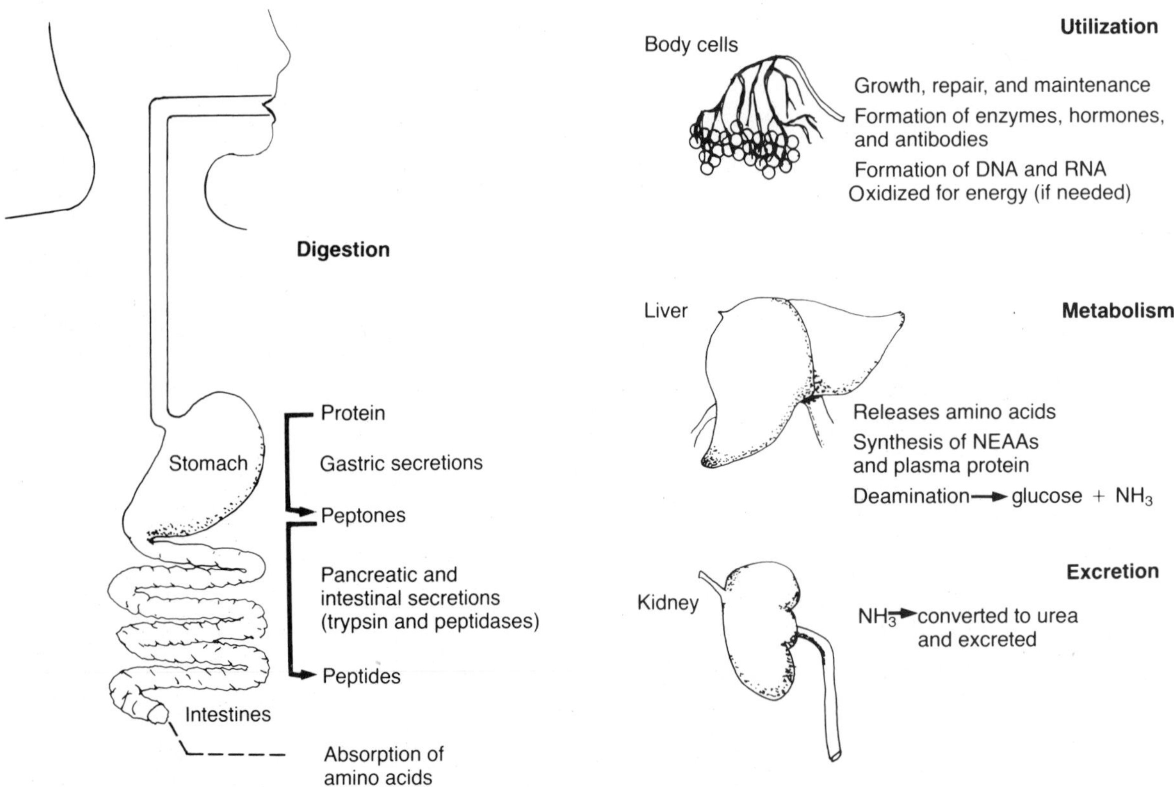

Figure 3–1 Body processes for protein. NEAAs, Nonessential amino acids.

TABLE 3–4

HORMONAL INFLUENCES IN PROTEIN METABOLISM

Hormone	Effect	Mechanism
Pituitary growth hormone	Anabolic	Stimulates extra tissue synthesis during infancy and childhood
Androgen and testosterone	Anabolic	Stimulate extra tissue synthesis during preadolescence and adolescence
Adrenocortical hormones	Catabolic	Stimulate increased nitrogen excretion
Insulin	Anabolic	Facilitates the entry of amino acids into the cells
Thyroid		
Normal amounts	Anabolic	Regulates basal metabolic rate
Excessive amounts	Catabolic	Increases basal metabolic rate
Glucagon	Catabolic	Stimulates gluconeogenesis and ketogenesis from proteins

Gluconeogenesis—production of glucose from non-carbohydrate sources such as amino acids and glycerol.
Ketogenesis—the production of ketones.

metabolic pool, containing about 70 gm of amino acids, could hardly be classified as a large storage of protein. Increasing muscle size is considered an increase in body mass, not protein storage. It is evident that to maintain a satisfactory protein status, a daily supply of EAAs is necessary.

Which amino acids are metabolized by muscle? Which organ metabolizes other amino acids? What helps maintain a satisfactory protein status?

Anabolism-Catabolism Balance

Anabolic and catabolic processes, which use amino acids from the metabolic pool and absorption, are controlled not only by the liver but also by hormones (Table 3–4).

Anabolism

In addition to the influence of hormones, anabolism is dependent on the presence of all EAAs simultaneously. It is not a stepwise process, in which a protein can be started and then completed by waiting until the needed amino acid appears. Protein synthesis is also affected by kilocaloric intake. If kilocaloric intake is inadequate, tissue proteins are used for energy, resulting in increased nitrogen excretion. In **transamination,** the amine group is transferred from an amino acid to a new carbon skeleton to form a new amino acid. This process requires the B vitamin, pyridoxine.

Transamination—production of NEAAs.

Proteins are synthesized by individual cells for their own use. Deoxyribonucleic acid (DNA), a **nucleic acid** present in the nucleus, controls protein synthesis. The messenger RNA (mRNA) copies the pattern from DNA in the nucleus and carries it to the **ribosomes** in the cytoplasm. Transfer RNAs (tRNAs) form a complex with each individual amino acid, directing it to its proper position in the chain. This RNA–amino acid complex moves to the mRNA, where enzymes are present to promote amino acid linkage (Fig. 3–2). On completion of synthesis, the protein is released from the ribosome to serve its specific function in the cell.

Nucleic acids, ribonucleic acid (RNA) and DNA, are present in every cell to form the genetic material of the cell and direct cellular protein synthesis.

Ribosomes present within the cell are responsible for protein synthesis.

What must be present for protein anabolism to occur? What is adequate kilocaloric intake necessary for anabolism? What are the purposes of DNA, mRNA, and tRNAs?

Catabolism

Amino acids are catabolized principally in the liver, but they are also catabolized to some extent in the kidney. **Deamination** of amino acids results in a carbon skeleton and ammonia. This process requires the B vitamins, pyridoxine and riboflavin.

Deamination is the catabolic processing of protein with the removal of the nitrogen grouping.

The carbon skeletons (keto acids) can be used to (1) make NEAAs, (2) produce

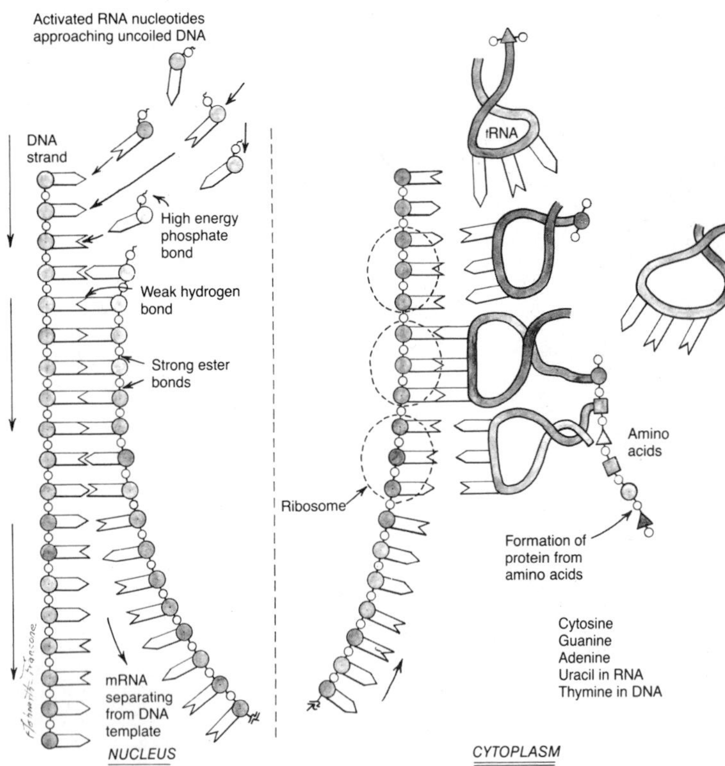

Figure 3–2 Protein synthesis. *A*, mRNA formation. The DNA strands separate in one area; a strand of RNA is built up as shown and then leaves the nucleus. *B*, The mRNA becomes associated with ribosomes. Then tRNA molecules are assembled on the mRNA strand in a sequence complementary to it. Each tRNA bears an amino acid. In this way, the amino acid sequence of the finished protein is determined. (From Jacob SW, Francone CA. *Elements of Anatomy and Physiology*. 2nd ed. Philadelphia, WB Saunders, 1989.)

energy via the Krebs cycle, or (3) be converted to fats and stored as fatty tissue. Thus, not all ingested protein is used to build muscle.

When amino acids are not needed for protein anabolism and energy is not needed, they are converted to fat and stored in the body. If kilocaloric intake is inadequate, proteins are used for energy rather than to build or repair lean body mass or produce essential protein-based compounds.

NURSING APPLICATIONS

1. Protein synthesis is sensitive to food intake and can be disrupted if intake is altered for any reason. Thus, assessment of intake is vital to detect possible protein deficiencies.
2. Determine a client's energy requirements and provide adequate amounts of both protein and energy so protein can be used for growth or healing, as needed. If energy is insufficient, healing is prolonged.
3. Even in extreme starvation, proteins can be digested as long as food can be swallowed, so maintaining some intake is helpful.
4. Protein pinocytosis may be an important factor in the development of immunity for infants and allergic reactions.
5. Evaluate intake of B vitamins. If deficient, protein metabolism is affected and the rate of healing is decreased.
6. Clients with compromised liver or renal functions may postpone progression of their condition by avoiding excessive amounts of protein.

Client Education

- Foods containing large amounts of DNA and RNA do not delay aging.
- A diet high in protein may be fattening because excess protein is stored as fat.
- Increasing protein intake does not necessarily increase muscle tissue and may lead to dehydration.

TABLE 3–5

NITROGEN BALANCE

N balance: body protein constant
N intake = N excretion
Positive N balance: increase in body protein
N intake > N excretion
Negative N balance: decrease in body protein
N excretion > N intake

Positive N Balance	Negative N Balance
Growth	Inadequate intake of protein (fasting, GI tract diseases)
Pregnancy	Inadequate kilocalorie intake
Convalescent periods	Illnesses, such as fevers, trauma, infections, or wasting diseases
Athletic training	Injury or immobilization
	Deficiency of EAAs
	Accelerated protein loss (albuminuria, protein-losing gastroenteropathy)
	Burns
	Increased secretion of thyroxine and glucocorticoids

NITROGEN BALANCE AND BLOOD SERUM LEVELS

Nitrogen balance refers to the balance of anabolic and catabolic reactions involving protein substances.

Because nitrogen is a unique characteristic of protein metabolism, measurements of nitrogen and nitrogenous constituents in the blood and urine assess protein equilibrium in the body. Although nitrogen balance means that the output is equal to input, excreted nitrogen atoms are usually not the same as those ingested. For a client to be in nitrogen equilibrium, not only must the diet contain required amounts of protein, but also kilocaloric intake must be adequate, or else protein will be used for energy. During certain stages of life, the body is in positive nitrogen balance, whereas other states indicate negative balance (Table 3–5).

Nitrogen Intake and Excretion

Nitrogen intake can be measured by the amount of protein ingested. The average nitrogen content of protein is 16%; each gram of nitrogen represents 6.25 gm of protein (Table 3–6). Nitrogen is excreted principally in the urine, but small amounts are lost in feces, sweat, vomitus, skin, menstrual fluid, and hair.

Serum and Urine Nitrogen

Protein status of a client is indicated by several blood serum and urine measurements containing nitrogen, which is the result of protein metabolism (Table 3–7). Urea is the major waste product of protein catabolism. Ammonia, a toxic

TABLE 3–6

PROTEIN-NITROGEN CONVERSIONS

To determine the amount of nitrogen (N) consumed from food, divide the gm of protein by 6.25
Example: 60 gm protein intake ÷ 6.25 = 9.6 gm N intake
To determine the amount of muscle wastage (gm of protein lost), add 4 (estimate of N lost in sweat, hair, skin and stool) to the 24 hour UUN
Example: 8 (UUN/24 hour) + 4 = 12 gm N output
Subtract the N output from N intake
Example: 9.6 gm N intake − 12 gm N output = −2.4 N loss
Based on an intake of 60 grams of protein and UUN/24 hours of 8, this client is in negative nitrogen balance, indicating protein intake needs to be increased

UUN, Urinary urea nitrogen.

TABLE 3–7

HEMATOLOGIC VALUES AND URINE MEASUREMENTS AFFECTED BY THE STATE OF NITROGEN

Test	Normal Values
Total protein	6–7.9 gm/dl
Albumin	3.5–4.5 gm/dl
Globulin	2.3–3.5 gm/dl
Serum transferrin	250–300 gm/dl
Urea nitrogen (BUN)	8–20 mg/dl
Creatinine (serum)	0.6–1.2 mg/dl
Creatinine clearance	
Males	1–2 gm/24 hr (95–135 ml/min)
Females	0.8–1.8 gm/24 hr (85–125 ml/min)
Urinary urea nitrogen (UUN)	6–17 gm/24 hr

substance, is transformed to urea in the liver and excreted by the kidneys. The levels of urea and ammonia vary directly with dietary protein levels. Thus, urinary urea nitrogen (UUN) reflects the rate of protein catabolism and adequacy of protein intake.

Creatinine and creatine are also end products of protein metabolism and are usually present in amounts proportional to the body's muscle mass. An increase of serum creatinine with an increase of blood urea nitrogen (BUN) is not indicative of dietary intake but rather kidney failure. Urinary creatinine, a waste product from creatine, is normally constant in any given client and indicates lean muscle mass. During kilocalorie deprivation or when inadequate amounts of EAAs are consumed, muscle is catabolized for fuel, and creatinine excretion falls. Serum creatine is used in diagnosing muscular disease.

What laboratory test can help determine protein status?

Plasma proteins are a source of protein available for the tissues. During slight protein deprivation, the body attempts to maintain a normal plasma protein level. This is accomplished by mobilizing protein from lean body mass. With continued protein deficit, serum protein levels decline. Serum albumin and transferrin are frequently used to assess protein status.

NURSING APPLICATIONS

1. In nutritional assessment of protein nutriture, blood and urine tests are beneficial and results must be monitored.
2. A diet containing large amounts of red meat can cause abnormally high levels of urinary creatinine, so if the level is high, inquire about the amount of red meat consumed.
3. The catabolization of amino acids results in the waste product urea. Therefore, a diet high in protein could make a falsely high reading. Evaluation of dietary protein is essential to determine if urea level is elevated because of diet or disease process.
4. Protein deprivation causing a decrease in albumin below 2.8 gm/dl or total serum protein below 5.2 gm/dl results in edema.

Client Education

- Some laboratory results may be affected by diet. Educate each client about foods to be eaten or omitted before tests, if applicable.

PHYSIOLOGICAL ROLES

Proteins perform many important physiological roles, but it is inaccurate to say that protein is more important than any other required nutrient, because other nutrients are required for the body to use available protein fully. These roles are described as they relate to nursing care.

Proteins are the principal source of nitrogen for the body. They are very large molecular structures, also containing the elements carbon, hydrogen, and oxygen and sometimes sulfur and phosphorus.

Proteins are essential for body functions; some of the more familiar roles are shown in Table 3-8. Actually, the functions of proteins fall into 8 categories.

1. Build new body tissues. Because protein is a constituent of all cells, it is necessary for anabolism. During periods of increased growth (infancy, childhood, adolescence, and pregnancy) as well as in periods of wound healing or recovery (illness, surgery, burns, or fever), protein needs are increased for building new tissues.
2. Repair body tissues. Owing to continuous catabolism in all body proteins, new ones must be resynthesized from amino acids. Therefore, assessment of both recent and usual protein intake is important.
3. Produce essential compounds. Amino acids or proteins are constituents of the regulatory enzymes and hormones and other body secretions. A low protein intake may affect all of these functions.
4. Regulate fluid balance. Protein dissolved in water forms a colloidal solution;

TABLE 3-8

CLASSIFICATION OF PROTEIN BY FUNCTION

Classification	Body Location	Example	Function
Structural proteins	Skin, cartilage, bone	Collagen	Principal substance in connective tissue
Contractile proteins	Skeletal muscle	Actin myosin	Muscle contraction
Antibodies	Blood plasma, spleen, lymphatic cells	Alpha globulins	Disease protection
Blood proteins	Blood plasma	Albumins	Control osmotic pressure of blood Maintain the buffering capacity of blood pH
	Blood	Fibrinogen	Blood clotting
	Blood	Hemoglobin	Transports oxygen from lungs to all parts of the body
Hormones	Endocrine or ductless glands (thyroid, pancreas, parathyroid, adrenals, pituitary)	Insulin	Regulates carbohydrate metabolism
		Growth hormone	Stimulates overall protein synthesis and growth
Enzymes	Throughout body—nearly 2000 different enzymes known; each highly specific in function		Biological catalysts; proteins that allow chemical reactions to proceed at their proper rate
	Stomach	Pepsin	Protein digestion
	Pancreas	Trypsin and chymotrypsin	Protein digestion
Nutrient proteins		Meat, fish, chicken, milk, cheese, eggs, peanut butter, nuts soybeans, tofu, dried peas and beans	Sources of amino acids required by humans and other animals
Viruses	Microscopic infective agents	Smallpox, measles	Cause disease
Nucleoproteins	Cell nucleus	DNA	Determines and transmits hereditary characteristics; carries genetic (hereditary) code

From Howard RB, Herbold NH. *Nutrition in Clinical Care.* 2nd ed. New York, McGraw-Hill, 1982.

in other words, it attracts water. Blood albumin (a protein) draws water from interstitial fluid or cells to maintain blood volume. During protein deficiency, a decreased amount of protein in the blood results in edema because of a loss of osmotic balance.

5. Regulate acid–base balance. Plasma proteins are buffers that react with either acidic or alkaline substances to maintain the correct blood pH (7.4).
6. Provide resistance to disease. Antibodies or immunoglobulins, the body's main protection from disease, are proteins. Thus, low protein levels may result in immunodeficiencies.
7. Provide transport mechanisms. Proteins enable insoluble lipid substances to be transported through the blood.
8. Provide energy. After the nitrogen grouping has been removed, the remaining carbon skeleton can be used for energy, furnishing 4 kcal/gm. Although this is not a main function for protein, it is used in this manner when (1) kilocaloric intake from carbohydrate and fat is inadequate, (2) protein intake exceeds requirements, and (3) the EAAs are not available for synthesis of proteins.

Name 4 roles of proteins.

REQUIREMENTS

Protein requirements are based on body size and rate of growth. (The body needs more protein during growth periods or for maintenance and repair of a larger body mass.) To a certain extent, the better the quality of protein, the less quantity is required. Protein requirements are based on the assumption that EAAs and kilocalories are provided in adequate amounts.

The RDAs for protein are proportionately higher for different ages and stages of life to adjust for increased anabolism. The requirement is based on the amount of nitrogen needed for nitrogen balance, allowing for amounts lost by the body through ordinary routes. Using data from many nitrogen balance studies, the National Research Council (1989) has determined that the minimum requirement of protein for adults is about 0.6 gm/kg. Using the 0.6 gm/kg, a client weighing 120 lbs (54.5 kg) would require 25.6 gm of protein. Because the RDAs provide a margin of safety, the National Research Council (1989) has established 0.8 gm/kg daily as the recommended allowance for all adults. With this standard, a client weighing 120 lbs (54.5 kg) requires 44 gm of protein.

When any condition of health or disease puts the body in negative nitrogen balance, an increased protein intake (above the RDAs) prevents excessive catabolism of tissue and plasma proteins. Although these disease states, or surgery, increase protein requirements, RDAs have not been established for these conditions. Supplementation with high quality proteins can help prevent protein malnutrition and shorten recovery periods. Individual laboratory studies that measure nitrogen intake and urinary excretion can be used to calculate the amount of protein needed to establish equilibrium.

Americans commonly ingest significantly more protein than is recommended. Ordinarily dietary protein is limited only in some physiological disease states affecting the liver and kidney. Because these organs are heavily involved in protein metabolism and the excretion of protein waste products (see Chapters 26 and 29, respectively), if they are diseased, excessive amounts of protein cannot be properly handled.

What are the minimum and recommended allowances for protein?

SOURCES

Foods with high protein content are readily available in the US. The average protein content of some foods is shown in Table 3–9. Most of the protein is furnished by the meat and milk food groups. As clients increase their intake from the

TABLE 3–9

PROTEIN CONTENT OF SELECTED FOODS

Food	Quantity	Amount Protein (gm)
Meats: chicken, beef, pork	3 oz	>20
Cottage cheese	½ cup	15
Thick milkshake	12 oz	12
2% protein fortified milk	8 oz	10
Instant nonfat dried milk	25 gm	9
Whole milk	8 oz	8
Cheddar cheese	1 oz	8
Peanut butter	2 tbsp	8
Cooked dried navy beans	½ cup	8
American processed cheese	1 oz	6
Eggs	1	6
Ice cream	1 cup	5
Macaroni	½ cup	4
Oatmeal	½ cup	3
Corn muffin	1	3
White bread	1 slice	2
White rice	½ cup	2
Vegetables	½ cup	1–2
Fruits	½ cup	0.1–1

Nutrient data from Nutritionist III Software, version 7.0. N-Squared Computing, Salem, OR.

cereal group, this group will contribute significantly more to the protein intake. The recommendation of an additional 12 to 19 gm protein during pregnancy or lactation can be met by increasing intake by 1 to 2 glasses of milk or by 1 to 2 oz of meat. Protein content of items from the sample menu displayed in Chapter 1, Figure 1–4 is shown in Figure 3–3.

Amino Acid Content of Foods

Table 3–10 lists the amounts of amino acids furnished by some high-quality and lower quality protein foods as compared with the requirements for adults. Despite the fact that amino acids are not limited in the food supply, some clients choose plant sources of protein for economic reasons or for philosophical, ecological, or religious convictions. EAAs can be provided by plants, but larger amounts of these foods must be consumed to match the protein obtained from animal sources.

EAAs that are low in grains are abundant in other plants such as legumes. As you can see in Table 3–2, beans are low in methionine and tryptophan, and corn is low in lysine and threonine. When both are eaten, as in pinto beans and cornbread, they are said to be complementary to each other. The deficiencies of one are offset by the adequacy of another. When a mixture of plant proteins is eaten throughout the day, the amino acids complement each other, and less volume is required. Additionally, small amounts of high-quality proteins can be combined with plant foods, such as in macaroni and cheese, to provide adequate amounts of EAAs.

Although it was previously thought that these complementary foods were necessary at the same meal, protein from a variety of foods is ordinarily consumed in excess of the RDA in the US. Protein from a single source is seldom consumed alone. Foods that are complementary to each other are usually combined without a lot of planning; i.e., beans are usually combined with rice, bread, or crackers (wheat) or tortillas or cornbread (corn).

PROTEIN CONTENT OF SAMPLE MENU AND MODIFICATIONS FOR OVOLACTOVEGETARIAN DIET

Sample Menu	Protein Content	Vegetarian Menu*	Protein Content
Breakfast			
Orange juice (1 cup)	1.7		1.7
Bagel (1)	6.0		6.0
Cream cheese (1 oz)	2.2		2.2
Raisins (1 packet)	0.5		0.5
1% Milk (1 cup)	8.0		8.0
Coffee	0		0
Creamer (1 tsp)	1.0		1.0
Lunch			
Tuna sandwich (1 oz)	7.6	Peanut butter (2 tbsp)	7.9
Mayonnaise (2 tbsp)	0.4	Jam (2 tbsp)	0
Tomato (2 slices)	0.6	Omit	
Lettuce slices	0.4	Omit	
Whole wheat bread (2 slices)	5.4		5.4
Apple (1)	0.3		0.3
1% Milk (1 cup)	8.0		8.0
Dinner			
Lean roast beef (2 oz)	15.5	Cheese-brown rice-broccoli	
Gravy (1/4 cup)	0.5	casserole (1 1/4 cup with	
Brown rice (1/2 cup)	2.8	2 oz cheese)	19.7
Corn (1/2 cup)	2.5		2.5
Three bean salad (1/2 cup)	2.8	Three bean salad (3/4 cup)	4.3
Whole wheat roll (2)	7.0		7.0
Margarine (1 tbsp)	0		0
Strawberries (1/2 cup)	0.5	Strawberries (1 cup)	1.0
Iced tea	0		
Evening Snack			
Diet cola (12 oz)	0.4		0.4
Dry roasted nuts (1 oz)	7.5		7.5
Totals	81.6		83.4

* Only items changed are listed; all others are the same.

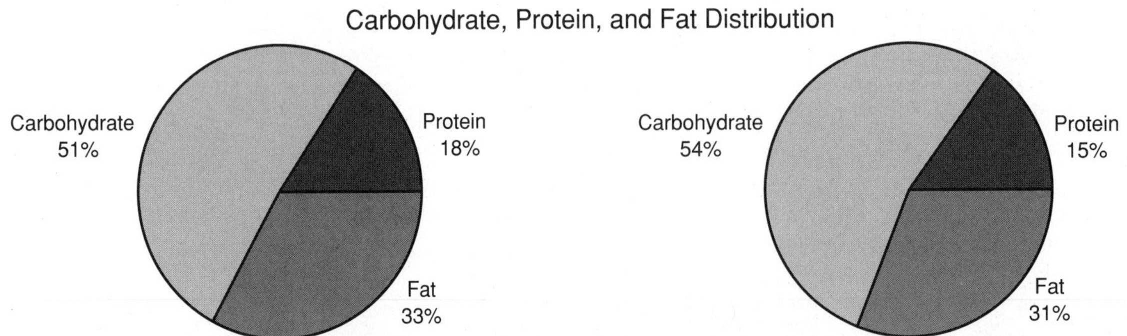

kcal, 1969; carbohydrate, 264 gm; protein, 82 gm; fat, 75 gm

kcal, 2179; carbohydrate, 311 gm; protein, 83 gm; fat, 79 gm

Figure 3–3 Protein content of sample menu and modifications for ovolactovegetarian diet. (Nutrient data from Nutritionist III Software, version 7.0. N-Squared Computing, Salem, OR.)

NURSING APPLICATIONS

1. Most Americans consume almost twice as much protein as recommended in the RDA. When assessment indicates the client normally consumes 1.5 gm/kg or more than the RDA for protein, this is considered a high-protein diet. Further increases would probably not be beneficial.
2. Nurses should assess the variety of protein sources when requirements are being met by plant sources.
3. The protein requirement of the elderly is at least equal to that of the young adult or may be increased, so monitor protein intake. Decreased protein intake is common as a result of ill-fitting dentures or loss of teeth, economic reasons, or poor access to the grocery store.
4. A lack of protein intake could cause any or all of the roles to be affected. Evaluate client's status in the 8 areas described under the discussion of Physiological Roles, especially if dietary intake appears inadequate.
5. One rule of thumb is that protein should never exceed 15 to 20% of kilocaloric intake. If protein intake appears excessive, determine kilocaloric and protein intake. The adequacy of intake can be established using either of the following 2 methods.

   Example: Client is consuming 2000 kcal, 115 gm protein.

   Recommended gm protein based on total energy intake:

   2000 kcal × 0.20 (% of total kcal) = 400 kcal from protein or less.
   400 kcal ÷ 4 (kcal/gm protein) = 100 gm protein recommended.
   Thus, the intake of 115 gm protein is more than the recommended amount.

   Actual intake based on the actual protein intake:

   115 (gm protein) × 4 (kcal/gm protein) = 460 kcal from protein.
   460 (kcal from protein) ÷ 2000 (total kcal intake) × 100 (%) = 23% of total kilocalories from protein.
   Because 20% is the upper limit, this client is consuming 3% more protein than is recommended.
6. Do not overemphasize protein foods to clients on restricted income (elderly, homeless, poverty). Too much emphasis on high-protein foods may result in inadequate amounts of other nutrients in the diet, especially when the food budget is low.
7. Healthy clients will be in nitrogen balance appropriate for their stage of life if their diet contains adequate kilocalories with the recommended number of servings from all the basic food groups. Evaluate food intake by gathering data from the client and comparing with basic food groups, stage of growth, RDA for kilocalories, and protein needed.

Client Education

- Increased muscular activity does not appear to elevate protein requirement except for a small increase for muscle development during conditioning.
- Protein requirements should be met by foods from several sources (even animal protein foods) because of other nutrients that accompany the protein. For example, pork is an excellent source of thiamin; red meats furnish a significant amount of iron. In contrast, too many eggs in the diet contribute excessive cholesterol.
- Protein sources are generally the most expensive foods. When clients have limited resources, counsel them to (1) eat protein in adequate but not excessive amounts, (2) use a variety of proteins of lower quality (these are less expensive), and (3) purchase less expensive kinds of protein foods (see Chapter 18).
- The color of the egg's shell is not related to its nutritional value. The breed of the hen determines the color.

TABLE 3–10

COMPARISON OF AMINO ACID CONTENT OF VARIOUS FOODS WITH REQUIREMENTS

Amino Acids	Hamburger	Egg	Dried Beans	Brown Rice	Peanuts	Broccoli	RDA for Adult Male
Isoleucine	1060	682	1216	120	1039	116	790
Leucine	1981	1068	1837	218	2010	139	1106
Lysine	2065	898	1589	98	1035	151	948
Methionine and cystine	813	680	428	45*	618	56	1027
Phenylalanine and tyrosine	1707	1174	2005	127*	2815	157	1106
Threonine	1036	600	926	98	775	97	553
Tryptophan	304.7	152	199	28	324	31	277
Valine	1198	762	1300	177	1211	137	790
Histidine	787	296	610	No data	780	53	790

* No data for cystine or tyrosine.
Nutrient data from Nutritionist III Software, version 7.0. N-Squared Computing, Salem, OR.

HYPER- AND HYPO- STATES

Protein Deficiency

Although protein supplies in the US are plentiful and drastic protein deficiency is uncommon, several groups of clients are susceptible to insufficient intakes: (1)

TABLE 3–11

CAUSES OF PROTEIN-ENERGY MALNUTRITION

- Impaired intake of dietary protein
  - Insufficient quantity or quality
  - Impaired intake due to systemic disease, e.g., cerebrovascular accident or chronic infections
  - Impaired intake due to localized GI disease, e.g., benign or malignant esophageal stricture
- Impaired digestion and/or absorption
  - Selective enzyme defect, e.g., enterokinase or trypsinogen deficiency
  - Generalized enzyme defect, e.g., pancreatic exocrine insufficiency
  - Impaired small intestinal assimilation, e.g., celiac sprue, short bowel syndrome
- Excessive enteric protein loss
  - Gastric or intestinal mucosal disease, e.g., Menetrier's disease, intestinal lymphangiectasia
  - Extraintestinal disease, e.g., constrictive pericarditis, thoracic or abdominal lymphatic blockade, i.e., lymphoma
- Disorders with multiple causes
  - Advanced malignancy
  - Chronic renal failure with uremia
  - Other chronic debilitating diseases

From Freeman HJ, et al. Protein digestion and absorption in man. Normal mechanisms and protein-energy malnutrition. *Am J Med* 1979 Dec; 67:1030.

elderly clients who are unable to prepare nutritious meals or are uninspired to eat, (2) low-income groups, (3) strict vegetarians, (4) those with a lack of education or who are unwilling to shop wisely, and (5) chronically ill and hospitalized clients.

Although protein-energy malnutrition (PEM) is uncommon in the US, given the above-mentioned conditions, malnutrition frequently lurks behind closed doors. Certain physiological conditions, listed in Table 3–11, may also precipitate PEM. An insufficient intake of protein as well as inadequate kilocalories causes negative nitrogen balance. Tissues are depleted of reserves, blood protein levels are lowered, and resistance to infections are lowered. Also, the ability to withstand the stresses of injury or surgery is lowered with increased recovery periods.

Because of insufficient quantity of high-quality proteins and kilocalories in other areas of the world, PEM is commonly seen. Kwashiorkor develops when young children receive adequate kilocalories but not enough high-quality protein (Fig. 3–4). It usually appears after the child has been weaned from breast milk. Marasmus is also seen in infants when there is a deficiency of both protein and kilocalories (see Chapter 18).

Kwashiorkor and marasmus are serious health problems that have received much attention by the United Nations and the World Health Organization. Supplementation has been made in the form of skim-milk powder, Incaparina (a food powder made from corn, cottonseed, and sorghum with mineral and vitamin supplements), and the addition of lysine to cereal products. However, most of these efforts to improve the status of world nutrition have not been well accepted for various reasons, and the protein-energy problems of the world still exist.

What clients are at risk for PEM?

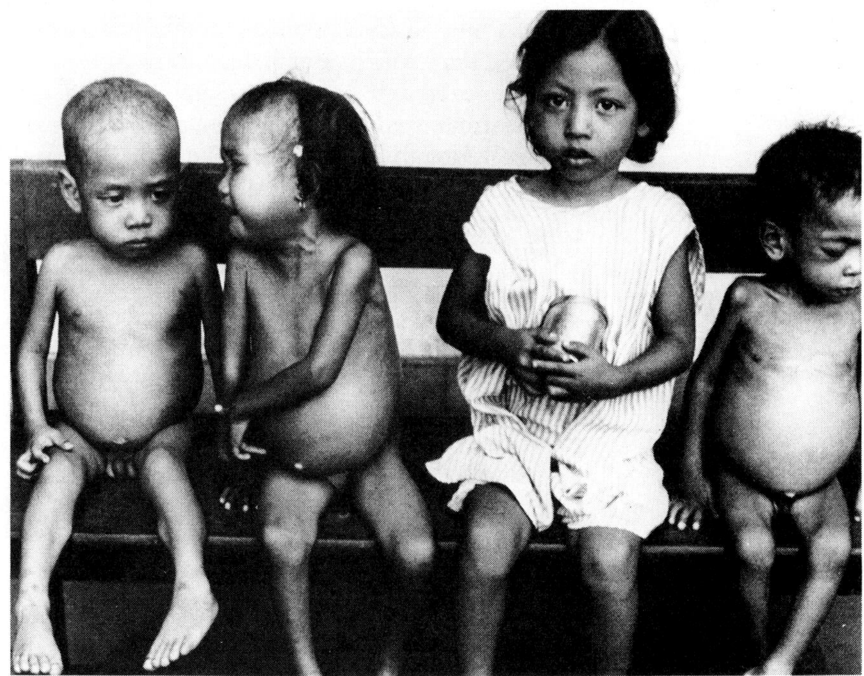

Figure 3–4 One child in this picture is healthy; the other three, all from the same community and of about the same age, are victims of the deficiency disease kwashiorkor. Note that the faces and abdomens of the two on the left look quite full, because of the accumulation of water as edema. The fact that the children are in reality pitifully thin is apparent from looking at the arms. (Courtesy of World Health Organization, photo by H. Omen.)

Excessive Protein Intake

An upper limit for safe levels of protein intake has not been determined. Most clients give proteins a high priority and believe there is no such thing as too much protein in the diet. Frequently, 150 to 200% of the RDA is eaten.

One concern regarding high-protein intake is its effect on calcium balance. The RDAs in the US for calcium are approximately double the allowances established for most other nations because of the large amounts of protein consumed. Studies indicate that high-protein foods with a high phosphorus content do not cause calcium loss in clients. On the other hand, phosphorus from carbonated beverages may have an undesirable effect on calcium balance when protein intake is high. (Spencer et al, 1988).

A concern especially in infant nutrition is fluid imbalances resulting from excessive protein intake. The metabolism of 100 kcal of protein requires 350 gm of water, compared with 50 gm of water for a similar amount of carbohydrates or fats. Therefore, water requirements are increased as well as the end products of protein metabolism in the blood stream.

NURSING APPLICATIONS

1. When assessing for marasmus or kwashiorkor, the main difference is edema. Edema is present in kwashiorkor, especially in the feet and legs, and absent in marasmus.
2. Assess client's financial status because poverty is a major cause of PEM.
3. To assess for inadequate protein: frequent or extended NPO (nothing by mouth) status (for diagnostic tests or surgical procedures), medications (some cause anorexia), food intake, skin (flaky and dry), nausea and vomiting, hair (dull, dry, brittle, breaks easily), and prolonged glucose intravenous (IV) feedings only. Laboratory findings of decreased albumin, protein, and urine creatinine indicate malnutrition.
4. With infants, monitor I&O (intake and output) and protein intake. If serum protein levels increase, make sure adequate fluids are provided for metabolism and excretion of proteins.
5. Treatment of malnutrition involves oral feedings and supplements, enteral tube feedings, and occasionally total parenteral nutrition.
6. Malnourished clients take longer to heal and regain strength and are at risk for infections and decubitus ulcers. Rest periods, hand washing, and turning are necessary nursing measures.
7. Too much protein can result in additional fat stores and obesity.

Client Education

- Suggest Meals on Wheels for elderly clients and refer them to the social worker.
- The protein content of the diet can be supplemented by adding dry skim milk powder to milk, soups, or mashed potatoes if the client is not lactose intolerant.
- Extremely high intake of protein is especially undesirable in infants.

NUTRITION UPDATE 3-1: VEGETARIANISM

Vegetarianism has become a way of life for many clients. Basically, a vegetarian diet consists of no meat, poultry, or fish. With some basic nutrition knowledge, it can provide a healthy, balanced diet. Four types of vegetarian diets differ in the types of foods included.

Vegan or Strict Vegetarian Diet

This diet contains only food from plants, including vegetables, fruits, and grains. No foods of animal origin are allowed (meat, milk, cheese, eggs, butter). This is the strictest type of diet and requires cautious planning to achieve combinations that provide the necessary amounts of amino acids. The use of complementary proteins can provide proper quantities of EAAs. By using a variety of principally unrefined foods and enough kilocalories to promote good health, the protein quality and quantity, in addition to other nutrients, may be adequate.

TABLE 3-12

VEGETARIAN FOOD GUIDE

Food Group	Standard Serving	Number of Servings (by Age)			
		1-3 Years	*4-6 Years*	*7-12 Years*	*Adult*
Milk and milk products*	1 cup	2-3	2-3	3-4	2-3
Vegetable protein foods					
1. Legumes	1 cup	¼	½	½	1†
Textured vegetable protein	20-30 gm, dry				
Meat analogs	2-3 oz				
2. Nuts and seeds	1½ tbsp	¼	½	¾	1
Peanut butter	4 tbsp				
Fruit and vegetables		3-4	4-5	5-7	5-9‡
Total daily	½ cup cooked 1 cup raw ½ cup juice				
Green leafy	daily	1	1	1	1
Vitamin C rich	daily	1	1	1	1
Breads and cereals§		4	4-5	9-11	6-11
Whole-wheat bread	1 slice				
Cooked cereal	½-¾ cup				
Other					
Eggs	1	1	1	1	3-4/week
Fats	1 tsp	1-3	2-3	2-3	3

Adapted from Vyhmeister IB, Register UD, Sonnenberg LM. Safe vegetarian diets for children. *Pediatr Clin North Am* 1977; 24(1):207.

* Soy milk fortified with vitamin B_{12} may be used if desired.

† To help meet the female adult requirement for iron, 2 cups legumes should be included.

‡ Include 1 cup dark greens to help meet the adult female iron requirement.

§ Include a variety of yeast-raised, whole-grain breads and a serving of whole-grain cereal. (Yeast breads contain more nutrients than quick breads when made with the same ingredients.)

TABLE 3–13

TIPS FOR PLANNING A VEGETARIAN DIET

Follow the vegetarian food guide (Table 3–12)
Use unrefined foods as much as possible, which, based on their kilocaloric contribution, provide a greater variety of nutrients. Substantially reduce high-kilocalorie, low–nutrient density foods
Replace meat with plant proteins from legumes, seeds, and nuts
Ensure that all the essential amino acids are present in adequate amounts. Suggestions are provided for combining complementary proteins in appropriate combinations
Grains and legumes: rice and beans, wheat-soy bread, corn-soy bread, cornbread and black-eyed peas, corn tortillas and beans, lentil soup and rye crackers, baked beans with brown bread, beans in a tostada, or brown rice and peas
Legumes and nuts/seeds: roasted soybean snacks with bean dip, raw peanuts and sunflower seeds, stir fry tofu with slivered almonds and broccoli, seed bread with split-pea soup
Grains and nuts/seeds: rice and sesame seeds, wheat germ and peanuts, rice and cashews, peanut butter on wheat bread, or noodles and cashews
Vegetables and legumes, grains or corn, or potatoes: dark green leafy vegetables with pinto beans; stir-fried vegetables with kidney beans; steamed broccoli and corn over brown rice; fresh lima beans and corn; corn and potato casserole; spinach-potato salad; or gumbo with okra, corn, and lima beans
Grains and milk products: cottage-cheese salad with sesame seeds and garbanzos, milk in legume soup, cheese sauce for beans, or vegetable quiche with peanut butter muffins
Commercially prepared plant protein products are not essential for adequate protein intake but may be used to replace the traditional entree
If milk/milk products are used, utilize low-fat or nonfat milk/milk products (low-fat cheese, ice cream, and yogurt)
Increase whole-grain breads and cereals to meet energy requirements
Use a variety of fruits and vegetables. Include a vitamin C–rich food at each meal
Tips for a vegan diet:
Provide adequate energy intake using whole-grain breads and cereals, legumes, nuts, and seeds
Use a variety of legumes and whole-grain products with some seeds and nuts
Because milk/milk products are eliminated, foods need to replace the nutrients contained in milk:
Use a fortified soybean milk drink
Incorporate a modest amount of nutritional yeast
Increase the use of green leafy vegetables
Increase the use of legumes, nuts, and dried fruits
Obtain vitamin D by exposure to the sunshine daily (20–30 min)
Use foods fortified with vitamin B_{12} or take a vitamin B_{12} supplement

Lactovegetarian Diet

In addition to foods from plants, dairy products are consumed. ("Lacto-" comes from the Latin word for milk, *lactis.*) Meat, poultry, fish, and eggs are excluded. Milk and cheese products complement plant products and enhance the amino acid content.

Ovolactovegetarian Diet

This vegetable diet is supplemented with milk, cheese, and eggs. ("Ovo-" comes from the Latin word for egg, *ovum.*) Only meat, poultry, and fish are excluded. If adequate quantities of eggs, milk, and milk products are consumed, all nutrients are likely to be provided in sufficient quantities (see Fig. 3–3). Strict supervision is not warranted unless serum cholesterol levels require dietary fat restrictions.

Ovovegetarian Diet

This diet consists of foods from plants with the addition of eggs. Meat, poultry, fish, and dairy products are excluded.

Advantages and Problems

Much can be said of the healthy aspects of the vegetarian diets. There is no reason why an adequate diet cannot be obtained (with the exception of the strict vegan diet). As shown in Table 3–12, the only food group changed is the protein or meat group. Various combinations of protein-containing foods are used to complement or supplement one another (Table 3–13).

As you will note from Table 3–2, methionine (a sulfur-containing amino acid) is limited in many of the vegetarian foods and is the most difficult to obtain. Cysteine (another sulfur-containing amino acid), which can be made from methionine in the body, is available from nuts and soybeans.

Some groups, especially the Seventh-Day Adventists, have supplemented protein intake with many textured vegetable protein (TVP) products. These are meat analogs produced from vegetable proteins, usually soybeans.

Because vitamin B_{12} is available only from meat and animal products, vitamin B_{12} supplements are necessary for vegans. It may take years to deplete an adult's body stores of vitamin B_{12} and to develop deficiency symptoms. In a group of strict vegans, 51% of the adults had low concentrations of serum vitamin B_{12}, which was inversely correlated with the duration of the diet (Miller et al, 1991). Unfortunately, anemia caused by vitamin B_{12} deficiency may result in serious and irreversible damage to the central nervous system before diagnosis (Dwyer, 1991).

Strict vegetarians and lactovegetarians are also at risk of iron deficiency. Iron-enriched foods or iron supplementation can be used. Iron supplementation is mandatory during pregnancy, early childhood, and adolescence, and after any major loss of blood. The use of eggs in the ovolactovegetarian diet increases iron intake. Because iron-deficiency anemia is not observed as frequently as predicted, it is thought that the increased consumption of vitamin C–containing foods may be responsible for enhancing iron absorption from plant sources.

Although calcium intake is low because of the lack of milk products in the vegan diet, the low intake of phosphorus and protein makes absorption of calcium from plant sources more efficient. Calcium supplementation, however, is recommended during pregnancy and lactation, when requirements are high.

Of primary concern is the lactating woman who strictly adheres to the vegan diet, thus affecting the nutritional quality of breast milk and increasing the chances that the infant may not thrive. Additionally, the weaned child is prone to protein deficiency; cases of PEM in vegans have been documented in the US. Soy-based milk products can be used to complement other plant proteins eaten. The use of peanut butter is also encouraged. Vegan-like diets pose special problems early in infancy and childhood with respect to sufficiency of energy, iron, and vitamin D, especially if the pregnancies are unplanned and unaccompanied by ongoing health supervision (Jacobs & Dwyer, 1988). An ovolactovegetarian diet, however, can promote growth in preadolescent children and compares favorably for most nutrients with a regular diet (O'Connell et al, 1989; Tayter & Stanek, 1989).

NURSING APPLICATIONS

1. When working with vegetarians, keep lines of communication open by respecting the client's decision, unless eating habits are clearly potentially harmful.
2. Benefits of the vegetarian diet include better weight control and less constipation, less diverticular disease, less colon cancer, lower incidence of gallstones, less breast cancer, lower blood pressure, less osteoporosis, and decreased rate of coronary artery disease (Allinger et al, 1989; Dwyer, 1988; Kowalski et al, 1987).
3. Minerals most likely to be inadequate in the vegetarian diet include calcium, iron, and zinc (see Chapter 9). A thorough assessment of these minerals is needed.
4. Suggest brewer's yeast, tempeh (fermented soy), or fortified breakfast cereals as sources of vitamin B_{12}. Direct vitamin supplementation may also be appropriate.
5. The protein in TVP products is of good quality. These products may also have a high sodium content so clients with hypertension need to be advised.
6. The limitations of the vegetarian diet should be recognized during periods of positive nitrogen balance (such as infancy or growth) or during periods of increased catabolism (such as stress, surgery, and illness) in which nitrogen requirements are increased. Strict monitoring of food intake is indicated in these instances. Refer the client to a dietitian.
7. Evaluate energy intake by recording foods eaten and totaling kilocaloric intake. Low-energy intake is a common problem of vegetarians. During pregnancy, this may result in inadequate weight gains. High-energy, nutrient-dense foods are recommended to increase energy intake. When energy intakes are adequate, protein intakes are usually satisfactory, especially among ovolactovegetarians.

Client Education

- Vegetarian diets (like nonvegetarian diets) have the potential to be either beneficial or detrimental to health.
- Nutrient needs of a vegetarian are the same as for any other client. The major difference is the protein source. The basic food groups can still be used for planning well-balanced menus, using combinations of foods allowed.
- A mixture of protein-containing foods throughout the day will provide enough EAAs (ADA, 1988).
- Encourage the consumption of whole-grain or unrefined grain products.
- Iron-rich vegetables accompanied by good sources of vitamin C are encouraged for optimum iron absorption.
- For clients on strict vegan diets, use foods fortified with vitamin B_{12}, such as soy milk and breakfast cereals.

SUMMARY

Proteins, made up of amino acids, are required in sufficient quantities for replacement of body tissues that are constantly in a dynamic state. Additional amounts are needed to support growth.

EAAs are not made in the body and must be provided by the diet. Animal proteins contain the EAAs in balanced proportions and are considered high quality. Plant foods contain protein; however, the amino acid content may not be in the proper proportions for human needs. They can be combined within the day's meals to complement one another to provide the required quantities of amino acids. Not only is this essential for all clients, but especially needs to be assessed in vegetarians.

Nurses need to know the requirements and sources for protein to teach clients effectively and monitor for excessive or deficient intakes of protein, which can lead to serious health problems.

NURSING PROCESS IN ACTION

A male client thinks he should eat as much protein as possible to build muscle. He is a college student and participates in intramural sports on the weekend but usually does not work out on weekdays. He believes that protein is the best food and the others are of "no value." His kilocaloric intake is 1800 kcal, and protein intake is 150 gm. He does not understand why everyone is so concerned about his intake because he wants to be sure protein is available for body building.

Nutritional Assessment

- Willingness to learn.
- Knowledge base of protein, carbohydrate, and fat principles of optimal nutrition.
- Cultural beliefs.
- Percent of kilocalories from protein (33%).
- Types of protein intake and total nutrient intake.
- Kidney functioning.
- Carbonated beverage intake.

Dietary Nursing Diagnosis

Altered health maintenance RT insufficient knowledge of protein and optimal nutrition.

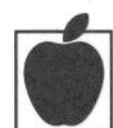

Nutritional Goals

Client will verbalize 3 principles concerning protein as well as the benefits from other nutrients. Client will consume 15 to 20% of total kilocalories from protein.

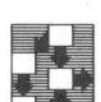

Nutritional Implementation

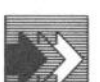

Intervention: Teach the (1) 8 functions or roles of protein; (2) difference between EAAs and NEAAs; (3) difference between high-quality and lower quality protein; and (4) interaction among carbohydrate, fats, and protein and recommended percentages of each.
Rationale: Knowledge corrects inaccurate information.

Intervention: Explain that protein may be fattening. High protein intake does not necessarily increase muscle tissue.
Rationale: Excess protein is stored as fat.

Intervention: Monitor serum urea, albumin, protein, and creatinine.
Rationale: With a diet high in protein, these readings may be falsely elevated.

Intervention: Monitor fluid intake.
Rationale: Metabolism of 100 kcal of protein requires 350 gm of water, compared with 50 gm of water for similar amounts of carbohydrate or fats.

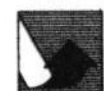 Evaluation

Client should state that he was mistaken about protein. To determine this, have client repeat 3 principles he remembers from teaching. He will be saying that 15 to 20% of the total kilocalories should come from protein, excessive protein is as bad as too little, and excessive protein does not necessarily turn into muscle but may increase fat deposits. The client will also state that he uses complementary proteins to provide adequate amounts of amino acids, which also provide other nutrients that are of "value." Additionally, all the above listed laboratory work should be within normal ranges.

STUDENT READINESS

1. Define amino acid, essential amino acid, nitrogen balance, and complementary proteins to a client.
2. Name the functions of proteins.
3. Using your desirable body weight, how many grams of protein should you consume?
4. Given a client weighing 150 lbs who has a kilocaloric intake of 2500 kcal, if the diet averages 15% protein, how many kilocalories are provided by protein? How many grams of protein is this? How does this fit into the RDA for this client?
5. What would you tell strict vegetarian parents about feeding their infant?
6. What are the effects of too much protein in the diet? Too little?
7. Explain the relationship between kilocalories and protein.
8. What are 2 methods of obtaining the EAAs from vegetarian foods? List 2 food combinations for each that would provide adequate amounts of EAAs.
9. If a client eats more protein than his or her body needs, what happens to the excess protein?
10. Evaluate the protein quality of the following meals: (1) cooked bulgur wheat with honey, oatmeal toast with margarine, fresh grapefruit, and herb tea; (2) peanut butter on whole-wheat bread, split-pea soup, a fresh peach, and soy milk; (3) lentils and rice, cooked Brussels sprouts, carrot-raisin salad, whole-wheat bread with margarine, an apple, and herb tea.

REFERENCES

Allinger UG, et al. Shift from a mixed to a lacto-vegetarian diet: Influence on acidic lipids in fecal water—a potential risk factor for colon cancer. *Am J Clin Nutr* 1989 Nov; 50(5):992–996.

American Dietetic Association (ADA). Position of the American Dietetic Association: Vegetarian diets—technical support paper. *J Am Diet Assoc* 1988 March; 88(3):352–355.

Darby WJ. The ban on tryptophan supplements. *Nutr Today* 1990 Jun; 25(3):5.

Dwyer JT. Nutritional consequences of vegetarianism. *Annual Rev Nutr* 1991; 11:61–92.

Dwyer JT. Health aspects of vegetarian diets. *Am J Clin Nutr* 1988 Sept; 48(suppl 3):712–738.

Jacobs C, Dwyer JT. Vegetarian children: Appropriate and inappropriate diets. *Am J Clin Nutr* 1988 Sept; 48(suppl): 811–818.

Kowalski R, et al. Congress investigates vegetarian nutrition. *Nutr Today* 1987 Aug; 22(4):30–33.

Lacey JM, Wilmore DW. Is glutamine a conditionally essential amino acid? *Nutr Rev* 1990 Aug; 48(8):297–306.

Laidlaw SA, Kopple JD. Newer concepts of the indispensable amino acids. *Am J Clin Nutr* 1987 Oct; 46(4):593–601.

Miller DR, et al. Vitamin B_{12} status in a macrobiotic community. *Am J Clin Nutr* 1991 Feb; 53(2):524–529.

National Research Council (NRC). *Recommended Dietary Allowances.* 10th ed. Washington, D.C., National Academy Press, 1989.

O'Connell JM, et al. Growth of vegetarian children: The farm study. *Pediatrics* 1989 Sept; 84(9):475–481.

Spencer H, et al. Do protein and phosphorus cause calcium loss? *J Nutr* 1988 June; 118(6):657–659.

Tayter M, Stanek KL. Anthropometric and dietary assessment of omnivore and lacto-ovo-vegetarian children. *J Am Diet Assoc* 1989 Nov; 89(11):1661–1663.

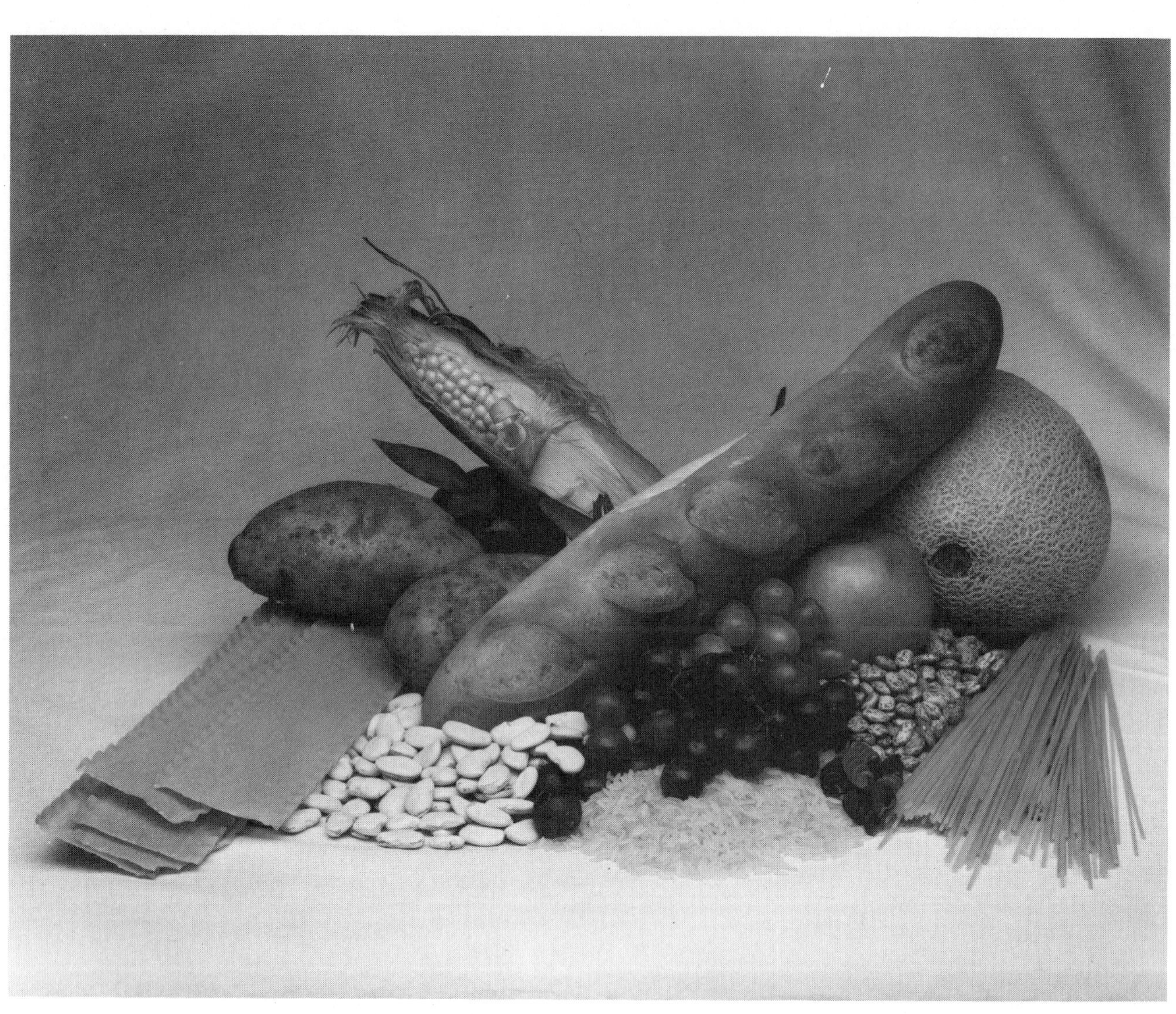

CHAPTER 4

Carbohydrate: The Efficient Fuel

OUTLINE

- I. CLASSIFICATION
  - A. Monosaccharides
    1. Glucose
    2. Fructose
    3. Galactose
    4. Sugar Alcohols
    5. Pentoses
    6. Other Sugars
  - B. Disaccharides
    1. Sucrose
    2. Lactose
    3. Maltose
  - *Nursing Applications*
  - C. Polysaccharides
    1. Starch
    2. Glucose Polymers
    3. Glycogen
    4. Structural Polysaccharides
    5. Cellulose
    6. Hemicellulose
    7. Pectin
    8. Lignin
    9. Gums, Mucilages, and Algal Polysaccharides
- II. DIGESTION AND ABSORPTION
  - *Nursing Applications*
- III. METABOLISM
- IV. PHYSIOLOGICAL ROLES
  - A. Energy
  - B. Lipogenesis
  - C. Conversion to Other Carbohydrates
  - D. Transamination
  - E. Normal Fat Metabolism
  - F. Protein Sparers
  - G. Intestinal Bacteria
  - H. Gastrointestinal Motility
  - I. Other Nutrients

OBJECTIVES

THE STUDENT WILL BE ABLE TO:

- Identify the major carbohydrates in foods and the body.
- Describe the digestion of carbohydrates in the stomach and small intestine.
- Identify normal body mechanisms that decrease and elevate blood glucose levels.
- List the ways glucose can be used by the body.
- State the functions of dietary carbohydrate.
- State why carbohydrate should be included in the diet.
- Identify dietary sources of lactose, other sugars, and starches.
- State the role and sources of dietary fiber.
- State the number of kilocalories provided per gram of carbohydrate.
- Apply nursing principles for carbohydrate ingestion, digestion, metabolism, and disturbances.
- Identify teaching interventions for carbohydrates.

TEST YOUR NQ (True/False)

1. Raw sugar is nutritionally superior to white sugar.
2. Fructose is the principal carbohydrate in honey.
3. Carbohydrate is the preferred nutrient for energy.
4. A blood glucose level of 150 mg/dl is called hypoglycemia.
5. Fiber tends to normalize intestinal transit time.
6. Carbohydrates are absorbed as monosaccharides.
7. Bananas and applesauce may help decrease diarrhea.
8. Glucose is the same as table sugar.
9. Sticky foods are more cariogenic than liquid foods.
10. Glycogen loading is not recommended for events lasting less than 90 minutes.

During the 1950s, carbohydrates acquired a bad reputation in the US. Statements have been made in best-selling books to the effect that we are the victims of "carbohydrate poisoning." Naturally, these unscientific rumors affected food patterns. After the government began advising Americans in late 1977 that risk for various chronic diseases could be reduced by eating foods containing more complex

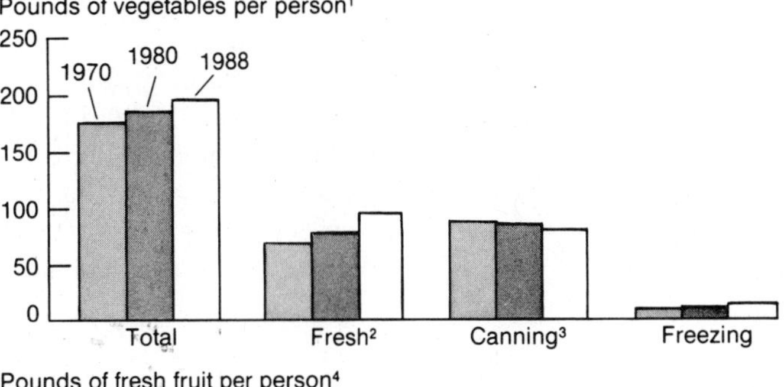

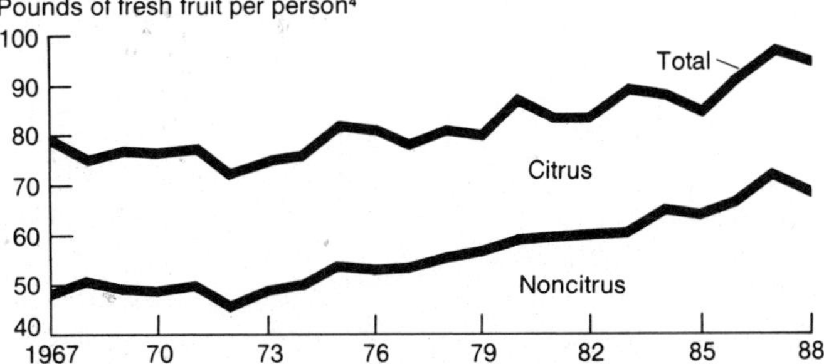

[1]Farm weight. [2]Asparagus, broccoli, carrots, cauliflower, celery, sweet corn, lettuce, onions, and tomatoes. [3]Tomato products are about 60 percent of the total. [4]Retail weight.

Figure 4–1 **The American diet includes more fresh fruits and vegetables. (From Putnam JJ. Food consumption. *Natl Food Rev* 1990 Jul-Sept; 13(3):1–9. (Original source: Putnam JJ. *Food Consumption, Prices, and Expenditures 1967–88.* U.S.D.A., E.R.S. Stat. Bull. No. 804. May 1990. Contact: Judith Jones Putnam (202) 786-1870.))**

carbohydrates (fruits, vegetables, grains, legumes, and cereal products), dietary patterns began to change. Between the 1970s and the early 1980s, vegetable and fruit consumption increased significantly (Fig. 4–1), and the intake of rice, pasta, and breakfast cereals increased 55% (Putnam, 1990), as shown in Figure 4–2. Clients are still consuming less dietary carbohydrate than is recommended (47% versus 58%) (Raper, 1991). Therefore, nurses need to become aware of ways to adjust carbohydrate consumption to help clients avoid health problems caused by too much or too little intake.

Carbohydrate has been the major source of energy for people since the dawn of

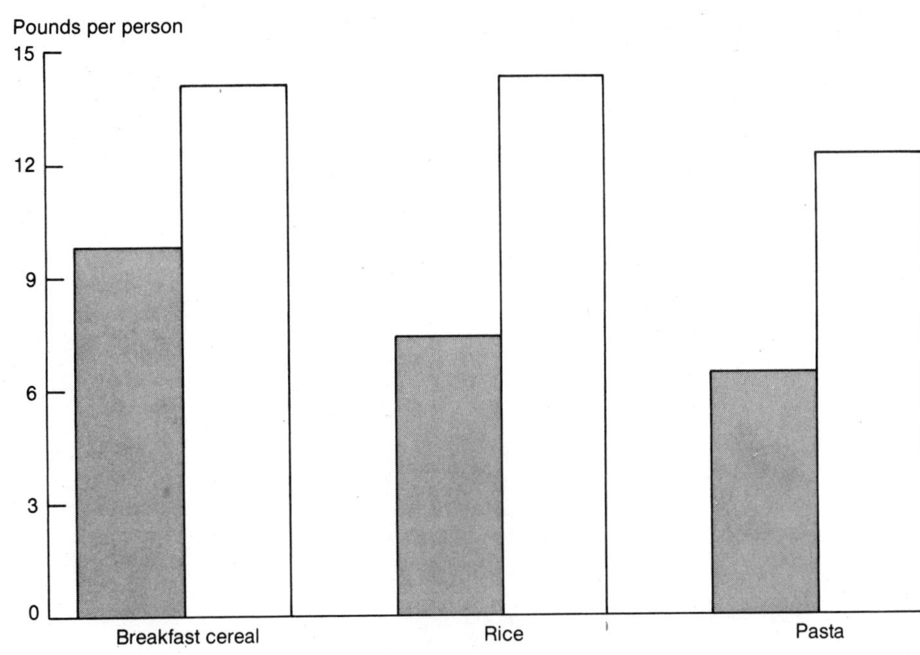

Figure 4–2 **Consumption of rice and pasta doubled between 1967 and 1988. (From Putnam JJ. Food consumption. *Natl Food Rev* 1990 Jul-Sept; 13(3):1–9. (Original source: Putnam JJ. *Food Consumption, Prices, and Expenditures 1967–88.* U.S.D.A., E.R.S. Stat. Bull. No. 804. May 1990. Contact: Judith Jones Putnam (202) 786-1870.))**

history. Worldwide, carbohydrates are the most important source of energy, furnishing up to 90% of the kilocalories for many African nations. Carbohydrates are the most economical form of energy. As you will learn in this chapter, and contrary to popular opinion, carbohydrates should not be considered as "fattening." Additionally, dietary carbohydrates add variety and palatability to the diet.

Carbohydrates are made by all plants from carbon, hydrogen, and oxygen. In the process of photosynthesis, the carbon is combined with a molecule of water, such as $C-H_2O$. As Deutsch (1976) stated, "A hydrated carbon is a carbohydrate."

CLASSIFICATION

Monosaccharides (simple sugars) contain 2 to 6 carbon atoms; disaccharides are double sugars, containing 12 carbon atoms; polysaccharides contain over 12 carbon atoms.

List the 3 classifications of carbohydrate.

Generally, the chemical structure is in these proportions: $C_n(H_2O)_n$. Hence, empiric formulas such as $C_6H_{12}O_6$ or $C_{12}H_{22}O_{11}$ could readily be identified as carbohydrates. The number of carbon atoms in the molecule is used to classify carbohydrates: **monosaccharides, disaccharides,** and **polysaccharides.**

Monosaccharides and disaccharides are sugars that contribute to the palatability of a food because of their sweetness. Temperature, pH, and the presence of other substances influence the sweetness of a food. Relative sweetness of sugars is measured by subjective sensory tasting; sucrose is used as the standard of comparison (Table 4–1).

Monosaccharides

The simplest carbohydrates are monosaccharides; they are absorbed without further digestion. The monosaccharides of greatest significance in foods and body metabolism are glucose, fructose, galactose, and mannose. Figure 4–3 identifies the slight differences between 3 of the 6-carbon sugars, as compared with glucose.

Glucose

Also called dextrose or corn sugar, glucose is naturally abundant in many fruits, such as grapes, oranges, and dates, and in some vegetables, including fresh corn and carrots. It is prepared commercially as corn syrup or by special processing of starch. Glucose is the principal product formed by the digestion of disaccharides and polysaccharides. It provides energy for the cells via the blood stream.

TABLE 4–1

RELATIVE SWEETNESS OF SUGARS AND SWEETENERS

Sugar and Principal Sources	Relative Sweetness (sucrose = 100)
Sugars and sugar alcohols	
Fructose (fruit, honey, carbonated beverages)	173
Invert sugar (honey)	130
Sucrose (table sugar)	100
Dextrose/glucose (corn syrup)	74
Sorbitol (dietetic candies, sugarless gum)	60
Mannitol (dietetic candies)	50
Lactose (milk)	16
Artificial sweetners	
Saccharin	300
Acesulfame K	200
Aspartame	180
Cyclamate	30

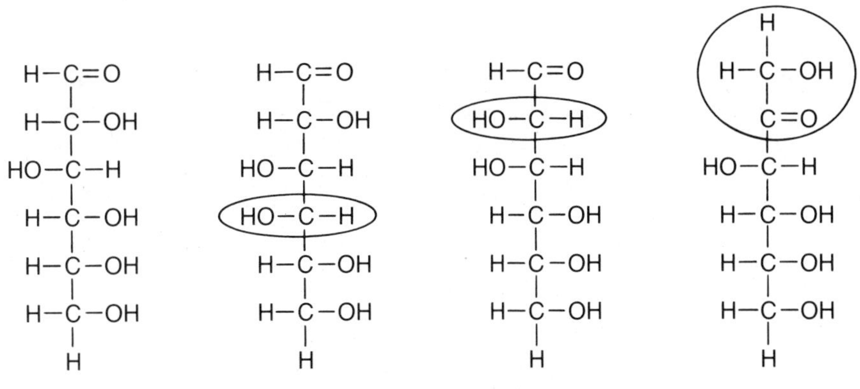

Glucose	Galactose	Mannose	Fructose
			H
H−C=O	H−C=O	H−C=O	H−C−OH
H−C−OH	H−C−OH	HO−C−H	C=O
HO−C−H	HO−C−H	HO−C−H	HO−C−H
H−C−OH	HO−C−H	H−C−OH	H−C−OH
H−C−OH	H−C−OH	H−C−OH	H−C−OH
H−C−OH	H−C−OH	H−C−OH	H−C−OH
H	H	H	H
Glucose ($C_6H_{12}O_6$)	Galactose ($C_6H_{12}O_6$)	Mannose ($C_6H_{12}O_6$)	Fructose ($C_6H_{12}O_6$)

Figure 4–3 The chemical structure of monosaccharides. Monosaccharides, or hexoses, are represented as straight chains called stick formulas. The chemical formula is the same, but the atoms are arranged differently, as shown by the encircled grouping.

Fructose

This sugar (also known as levulose) is found naturally in honey and fruits. It is the sweetest of the monosaccharides and is a product of the digestion of sucrose. Fructose can be manufactured from glucose.

Galactose

Another 6-carbon sugar is galactose, which is a product of lactose digestion (milk sugar). Although the primary source of galactose is milk, legumes also contain some galactose. Physiologically, it is a constituent of nerve tissue and produced from glucose during lactation in the synthesis of lactose.

Sugar Alcohols

Sugar alcohols, such as sorbitol, may appear naturally in foods or be added by a manufacturer. For a given quantity, it adds about the same amount of sweetness as glucose; it also furnishes the same amount of kilocalories (Beaugerie et al, 1990). The benefit of sorbitol is that it is absorbed and metabolized more slowly than sucrose.

Mannose is a 6-carbon sugar derived from some legumes. Mannitol, derived from mannose, is found in foods.

Xylitol is a sweetener with approximately the same perceived sweetness and kilocaloric value as sugar. It is found in fruits and vegetables (lettuce, carrots, and strawberries). Poor absorption of all the sugar alcohols causes a laxative effect.

Pentoses

Five-carbon sugars, called pentoses, include ribose, xylose, and arabinose. Ingested pentoses are not used but eliminated in the urine and feces. The body synthesizes pentose sugars from other carbohydrates, as needed by the cell. Physiologically, ribose is important as a constituent of RNA, DNA, and the B vitamin, riboflavin.

Other Sugars

Raffinose, a trisaccharide, and stachyose, a tetrasaccharide, cannot be hydrolyzed by humans. Their presence in dry beans may cause flatulence.

List sources for glucose, fructose, galactose, sugar alcohols, and pentoses. Which of these monosaccharides provide energy for the cell?

Disaccharides

Two simple sugars (monosaccharides) joined together are called a disaccharide.

Disaccharides are not important in human metabolism because they contribute to body function only after they have been digested. All are hydrolyzed during digestion to their constituent monosaccharides for absorption as shown:

Sucrose = glucose + fructose

Maltose = glucose + glucose

Lactose = glucose + galactose

Sucrose

Granulated table sugar is the most common form of sucrose. Commercially, sucrose is produced from sugar cane or sugar beets (not to be confused with red beets). It is also found in molasses, maple syrup, and maple sugar. Some fruits and vegetables (apricots, peaches, plums, raspberries, honeydew, cantaloupe, beets, carrots, parsnips, winter squash, peas, corn, and sweet potatoes) naturally contain large amounts of sucrose.

Lactose

The sugar found in milk is lactose. Lactose is unique to mammals, composing 4.5% of cow's milk and 7.5% of human milk. In the fermentation of milk, some of the lactose is converted to lactic acid, giving buttermilk and yogurt their characteristic flavors.

Maltose

List sources for sucrose, lactose, and maltose.

Also called malt sugar, maltose does not occur naturally. It is created in bread making and brewing and is present in beer, some processed cereals, and baby foods. It is also combined with dextrins in infant formulas.

NURSING APPLICATIONS

1. Assess dietary intake of clients with the genetic disorder galactosemia. Legumes may not be well tolerated because of their galactose content.
2. IV fluids are normally dextrose (glucose) solutions with some electrolytes added. Some kilocalories are provided, but the main purpose is to provide fluids.
3. Mannitol has been used as a diuretic agent to inhibit water reabsorption and maintain urine excretion in conditions such as cardiovascular operations and severe traumatic injury (Gilman et al, 1990). Closely monitor blood glucose levels of diabetic clients receiving this drug. Additionally, monitor I&O in all clients hourly.

Client Education

- Clients should limit their intake of hard candies containing sugar alcohols (mannitol, sorbitol) to 3 to 4 pieces throughout the day to prevent gastric cramping.
- Some sweeteners produced from corn, especially high-fructose corn syrup, may not be tolerated by persons allergic to the parent grain.
- Excessive consumption of sugar alcohols may have a laxative effect.

TABLE 4–2

SYNOPSIS OF FIBER

Type of Fiber	Major Food Sources	Physiological Mechanism	Clinical Implication
Insoluble fiber			
Noncarbohydrate			
Lignin	Fruits and mature vegetables; whole grains	Decreases free radicals in GI tract	Possibly anticarcinogen
Carbohydrate			May prevent:
Cellulose	Whole-wheat flour, bran, cabbage family, peas/beans, apples, root vegetables	Increases fecal bulk: Lowers GI transit time; Lowers intraluminal pressure	Constipation; Hemorrhoids; Diverticulosis
Hemicellulose	Bran, cereals, whole grains	Lowers GI exposure time to cancer-causing toxins	Colon cancer
		Decreases mineral absorption.	Potential for mineral deficiency
Soluble fiber			
Gums and mucilages	Oat products, dried beans, and legumes	Decreases rate for stomach emptying, delaying absorption of sugar	Increased satiety; Improved glycemic control
		Increases mouth to cecum transit time	Decreased serum lipids; Cholelithiasis
Pectin	Apples, citrus fruits, strawberries	Binds with bile acids, increasing their excretion	

Polysaccharides

Some **polysaccharides** have a role in energy storage and are digestible; the second group, largely indigestible by human intestinal enzymes, is called dietary fiber (Table 4–2).

Complex carbohydrates, also called polysaccharides, are composed of many (1500 or more) monosaccharides. The chains have different structures and can be branched or straight.

Starch

Most complex carbohydrates in the diet are in the form of starch from cereal grains, roots, vegetables, and legumes. The amount of starch present in a vegetable increases with its maturity. Freshly picked corn tastes much sweeter than after it has been picked for several days; i.e., simple sugars continue to develop into starch. The amount of starch in a fruit decreases as it ripens; i.e., the complex carbohydrates are broken down in the ripening process into simple sugars.

Starch granules are insoluble in cold water because of their cell wall, called cellulose. Cooking facilitates the digestive process by causing the granules to swell, rupturing the cell wall so digestive enzymes have access to the starch inside the cell. In cooking, this swelling is referred to as thickening. Industrially, food starch is modified by chemicals to produce a better thickening agent.

Name edible sources of starch.

Glucose Polymers

Industrially produced carbohydrate supplements are composed of glucose, maltose, and **dextrins.** They are used to increase kilocaloric intake when requirements are increased and/or inadequate amounts of kilocalories are consumed from regular foods. They are well suited for clear-liquid diets or protein-restricted, fat-restricted, or electrolyte-restricted diets. These products can be mixed easily with most foods

Dextrins are intermediate products of the digestive enzymes on the starch molecules.

When are glucose polymers used?

and beverages without making them excessively sweet. Glucose polymers have a relatively low osmolality and are absorbed as rapidly as glucose. The glucose provides 4 kcal/gm, similar to other carbohydrate products. These products include Polycose (Ross) and Moducal (Mead Johnson).

Glycogen

Glycogen is the carbohydrate storage form of energy for humans.

What does glycogen provide?

Stored in the muscle and liver, glycogen is readily available as a source of glucose and energy. Carbohydrates are frequently consumed in excess of immediate energy needs. Excess glucose is converted to glycogen until the limited glycogen storage capacity is filled; simultaneously, glucose is also being converted into fats and stored as adipose tissue.

The Structure of Glycogen*

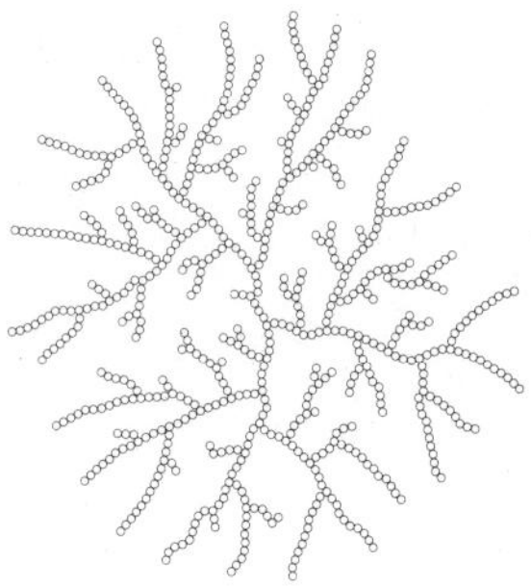

Structural Polysaccharides

Structural polysaccharides, or dietary fiber, are mixtures of several different types of polysaccharides and lignin.

Dietary constituents that contribute to dietary fiber cannot be digested by human GI enzymes. A large percentage, however, is digested in the large intestine by microflora, producing fatty acids and gas (Slavin, 1990). Each type exhibits different physiological roles (see Table 4–2), which are discussed later in the chapter.

Dietary fiber consists of the undigestible products that arrive in the large intestine.

Tables listing crude fiber content were determined by antiquated procedures that measured mainly cellulose and lignin fractions. These are being updated, reflecting higher **dietary fiber** amounts than crude fiber tables. For every gram of crude fiber, the food probably contains 2 or 3 gm of dietary fiber per serving.

What is the difference between dietary and crude fiber? Which more accurately reflects physiological function?

Cellulose

What is the function of cellulose?

The most plentiful polysaccharide found in plants is cellulose. Although it is not digested by human digestive enzymes, it serves as a substrate for microbial fermentation and has a hydrophilic ability to attract water, promoting efficient intestinal function.

Hemicellulose

Another important food fiber, hemicellulose, absorbs and retains water in the gut but has little effect on stool size. GI bacteria can digest much of the hemicellulose.

---

* From McGilvery RW. *Biochemistry: A Functional Approach.* 3rd ed. Philadelphia, WB Saunders, 1983.

Pectin

Pectins are nondigestible polysaccharides that form a gel with water. They are used in the preparation of fruit jams and jellies.

Lignin

Lignin is a woody substance, closely associated with cellulose in plants. Although it is the only noncarbohydrate fiber, it is grouped with the polysaccharides. Lignified fibers are less digestible by gut bacteria than other polysaccharides. Lignin combines with bile acids to prevent their absorption.

Gums, Mucilages, and Algal Polysaccharides

All these water-soluble polysaccharides are components of dietary fiber. These products are frequently used as additives, especially in milk products such as ice cream.

DIGESTION AND ABSORPTION

Ptyalin, or salivary amylase, begins the process of hydrolyzing starch to dextrins and maltose. Chyme enters the small intestine, where intestinal and pancreatic juices complete the digestion to monosaccharides. As disaccharides come into contact with the brush border cells, they are hydrolyzed by their enzymes into glucose, fructose, and galactose. Lactose is the slowest disaccharide to be hydrolyzed. Sucrase and, to a lesser extent, lactase activity is somewhat affected by levels of these sugars in the diet. In other words, if the intake of these sugars is routinely low, the amount of their respective enzymes will be decreased. A synopsis of carbohydrate digestion is shown in Table 4–3.

Absorption occurs mainly in the lower duodenum and jejunum, but studies indicate some starch may enter the large intestine undigested, contributing to fermentable carbohydrate and substrates available to microflora (Englyst & Cummings, 1985; 1986). Factors influencing the amount of time for carbohydrate digestion and absorption depend on how fast it is released into the small intestine and the mixture of foods already present in the intestine. The condition of the

TABLE 4–3

DIGESTION OF CARBOHYDRATE

	Secretion	Action/Products
Mouth	Ptyalin	Starch → maltose and dextrins
Stomach	Acid	Inhibits action of ptyalin; continues digestion of carbohydrates
Small intestine		
Pancreatic secretion	Amylase	Starch → dextrins and maltose
Intestinal secretions	Sucrase	Sucrose → glucose and fructose
	Lactase	Lactose → Glucose and galactose
	Maltase	Maltose → Glucose (2 molecules)

mucous membrane, hormones, and adequacy of vitamin intake also affect absorption rates.

NURSING APPLICATIONS

1. The desire for sweetness is not considered an acquired taste because newborn infants exhibit a preference for it. Judgment or criticism by the nurse is not beneficial in decreasing client's use of sugar, so be nonjudgmental.
2. If clients are on extremely restricted diets or need additional kilocalories, suggest glucose polymers to the physician.
3. Pancreatic amylase is present in sufficient quantities to hydrolyze starches even in clients with severe pancreatic disease. Starches are an important source of kilocalories for these clients and need to be offered.

Client Education

- Dietary fiber is more accurate than crude fiber amounts.
- Product labels list the amount of dietary fiber per serving.

METABOLISM

Glycogenesis is the process by which sugars, including fructose, galactose, sorbitol, and xylitol, are stored as glycogen.

Monosaccharides are transported through the portal vein to the liver for **glycogenesis.** Glucose is the most common circulating sugar in the blood; it is the main energy source for cells. The level of circulating glucose is closely monitored by

TABLE 4–4

GLYCEMIC INDEX OF FOODS

Food	Glycemic Index	Food	Glycemic Index
Grain and cereal products		Vegetables	
White bread	100	Baked potato	135
Whole-wheat bread	99	Instant potatoes	116
Brown rice	96	New potatoes	81
White rice	83	Yams	74
White spaghetti	66	Frozen peas	74
Whole-wheat spaghetti	61	Sweet potatoes	70
Rye bread	58	Dried legumes	
Breakfast cereals		Canned baked beans	60
Cornflakes	119	Kidney beans	54
Weetabix	109	Butter beans	52
Shredded Wheat	97	Chickpeas	49
All Bran	73	Lentils	43
Oatmeal	85	Soybeans	20
Fruits		Dairy products	
Raisins	93	Ice cream	52
Banana	79	Yogurt	52
Orange juice	67	Whole milk	49
Orange	66	Skim milk	46
Grapes	62	Sweeteners	
Apple	53	Maltose	152
Pear	47	Glucose	138
Peach	40	Honey	126
Grapefruit	36	Sucrose	86
Plum	34	Fructose	30

Adapted from Jenkins DJA, et al. The glycaemic response to carbohydrate foods. *Lancet* 1984; 2(August 18):388.

the liver, constantly maintained at a level between 70 and 110 mg/dl. After a meal, blood glucose levels peak in 30 to 60 minutes and return to normal within 3 hours in a normal individual.

This consistent blood glucose level is significant, indicating the necessity for a certain amount of sugar in the blood for normal functioning of body tissues. When the blood glucose level exceeds 160 to 180 mg/dl, some glucose will exceed the renal threshold, resulting in **glucosuria.** The blood glucose level is so closely regulated that glucosuria is infrequent. **Hyperglycemia** and **hypoglycemia** are serious conditions, and the precipitating cause should be identified. (Chapters 27 and 28 discuss these metabolic problems and appropriate therapeutic diets.)

The presence of glucose in the urine is called glucosuria.

A blood glucose level below 70 mg/dl is called hypoglycemia; a blood glucose level above 110 mg/dl is hyperglycemia.

In the past, it was assumed that all monosaccharides or disaccharides (sugars) produced a higher blood glucose response than starches. Dr. J. A. Jenkins and colleagues (1988) challenged this, comparing the glycemic response of individual foods with a white wheat bread. Sucrose has a glycemic effect similar to that of bread, potatoes, and rice (Bantle, 1989). In other words, differences in blood glucose response to different foods cannot be accurately predicted from the amount of simple sugars or complex carbohydrates (Jenkins et al, 1988), so foods have been classified by their glycemic index (Table 4–4). A food with a high glycemic index will cause the blood glucose to rise higher during a 2-hour period after ingestion than a food with a low glycemic index.

A complex hormonal system maintains a constant blood glucose level. The hormone that lowers the blood glucose level is insulin. Beta cells within the islets of Langerhans in the pancreas produce insulin. When hyperglycemia occurs, insulin is secreted to lower blood glucose levels. Conversely, hypoglycemia elicits the secretion of several hormones (thyroid hormone, epinephrine, glucagon, or growth hormone) to increase blood glucose levels. Blood glucose levels can be increased by **gluconeogenesis** and **glycogenolysis.**

Muscle tissue is also able to store carbohydrates as glycogen; however, muscles lack the enzymes necessary for glycogenolysis. Glycogen in muscle tissue is broken down to lactic acid, a process referred to as **glycolysis,** which also releases energy for the cells. Ordinarily, lactate is oxidized by oxygen (aerobically) to yield carbon dioxide, water, and energy (via the Krebs cycle), which is stored as adenosine triphosphate (ATP). Carbohydrate metabolism is summarized in Figure 4–4.

Noncarbohydrate sources, especially amino acids and glycerol (from fats), can be converted to glucose by a process called gluconeogenesis.

Glycogen broken down by the liver to glucose is referred to as glycogenolysis.

Glycolysis is an anaerobic (without oxygen) process involving the production of lactic acid or pyruvic acid from glucose or glycogen.

What hormones increase blood glucose levels? Which one decreases blood glucose? What happens when muscles break down glycogen?

PHYSIOLOGICAL ROLES

Energy

The principal role of the absorbed sugars is to provide energy for the body and heat to maintain body temperature. Glucose is the preferred source of energy for the brain and central nervous system, red blood cells, and the lens of the eye. Although many organs can use fats for energy, glucose is the preferred fuel. Each gram of carbohydrate, whether it was originally from a sugar or a starch, provides 4 kcal. Glycogen stores are a readily available source of glucose for the tissues.

Lipogenesis

The process of converting glucose to fats is called lipogenesis.

When large quantities of carbohydrates are eaten, glucose can be converted to triglycerides and stored as fat. Blood sugars ensure replenishing of glycogen stores;

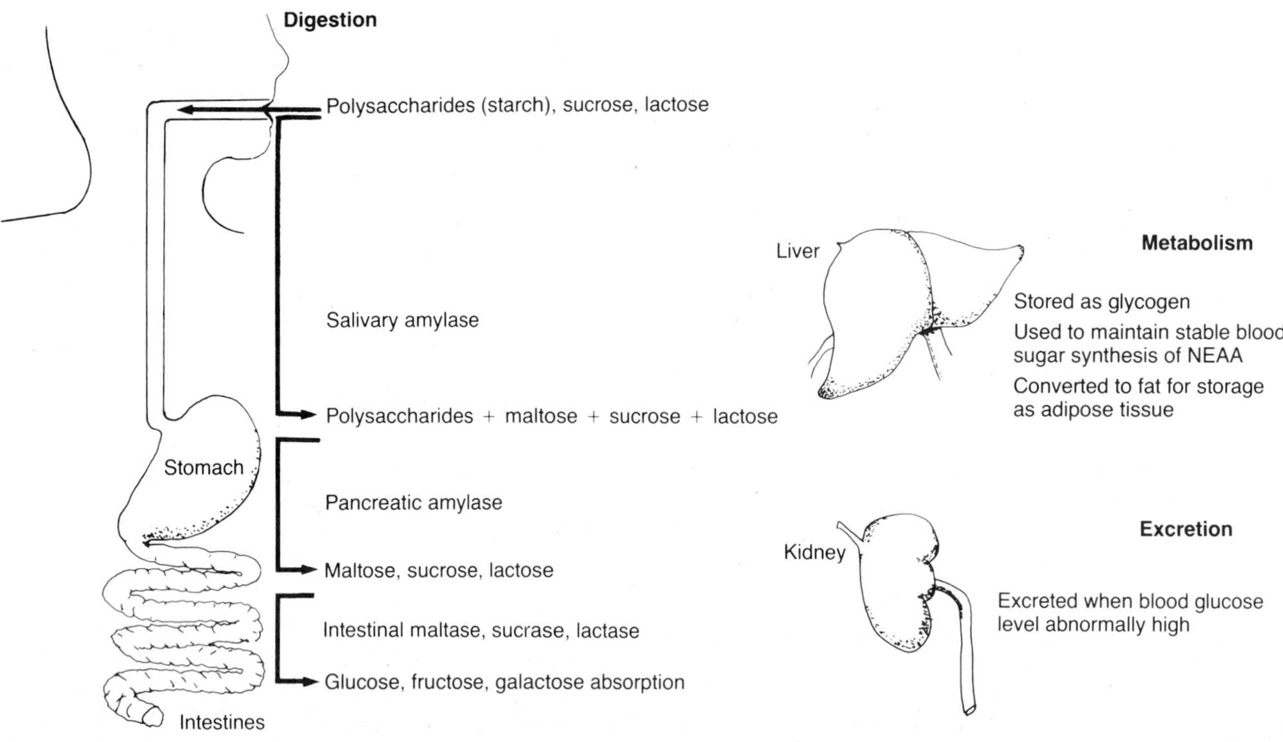

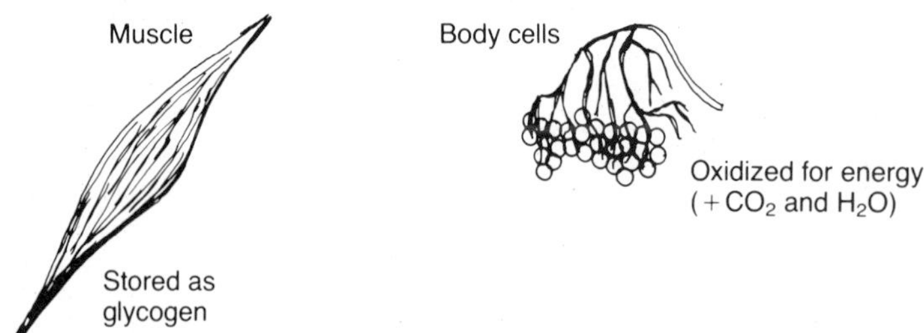

Figure 4–4 Body processes for carbohydrate. NEAA, Nonessential amino acid.

TABLE 4–5

SOME BODY COMPOUNDS CONTAINING CARBOHYDRATE

Compound	Function
Glucuronic acid	Combines with toxic chemicals and bacterial by-products in the liver, functioning as a detoxifying agent
Heparin	Prevents blood clotting
Chondroitin sulfates	Found in connective tissue, cartilage, and heart valves. Capable of binding water
Immunopolysaccharides	Part of infection-resistant mechanism
DNA and RNA	Compounds responsible for the genetic material and cell duplication
Galactolipins	Constituents of nervous tissue
Glycosides	Components of steroid and adrenal hormones
Keratan sulfate	In connective tissue
Hyaluronic acid	Component of intercellular material and synovial fluids. Can bind a large amount of water
Dermatan sulfate	Present in tissues rich in collagen, especially in the skin

however, excessive amounts result in less fat being oxidized and in carbohydrate being converted to fat and stored in fatty tissue.

Conversion to Other Carbohydrates

Monosaccharides are important constituents of many compounds that regulate metabolism (Table 4–5).

Transamination

The liver can use the carbon framework from the sugar molecule and the amine group contributed by the breakdown of an amino acid to produce NEAAs needed in the body.

Normal Fat Metabolism

Oxidation of fats requires the presence of some carbohydrates. When carbohydrate intake is low, the body relies on energy from fat intake or stores. Fats are metabolized faster than the body can oxidize them; the resulting intermediate products are called **ketone** bodies.

Ketones are normal products of lipid metabolism in the liver; they can be used by muscles for energy if adequate amounts of glucose are available. An accumulation of ketones, or incompletely oxidized fatty products, results in ketosis.

Protein Sparers

Carbohydrates, by furnishing energy in the diet, are said to be protein sparing. Energy is an essential physiological requirement. With insufficient carbohydrate intake, the body burns protein for fuel. With adequate carbohydrate intake, protein can be used to build and repair tissue.

Intestinal Bacteria

Lactose and dietary fiber remain in the GI tract longer than other nutrients. This encourages the growth of bacteria that synthesize certain vitamins (B complex and vitamin K).

Gastrointestinal Motility

The contribution of fiber in the GI tract has several functions (see Table 4–2). Dietary fiber **accelerates transit rate** in clients with slow transit time and decreases it in those with rapid transit time. Its ability to bind water in the intestine and increase bulk from nondigestible substances causes decreased length of time in the alimentary tract. Thus, an **increased transit time** allows tissues to be exposed to cancer-causing nitrogenous waste products for longer periods of time. An added benefit is stool softening, which helps prevent constipation.

Accelerated intestinal transit rate refers to faster movement through the GI tract, which alleviates or prevents constipation.

Increased transit time refers to food present in the GI tract for longer periods of time or a slower rate, which contributes to constipation.

TABLE 4–6

HIGH-FIBER DIET

Guidelines*

1. Assess current dietary fiber intake before initiating a fiber increase
2. Increase the consumption of high fiber foods gradually. Begin with 5–10 gm increments to avoid adverse side effects. A period of at least 6–8 weeks should be allowed for adaptation and preventing flatulence, abdominal cramping, and diarrhea/constipation (Flock et al, 1986)
3. Avoid large amounts of purified fiber such as lignin and bran because many minerals, especially calcium, iron and zinc, are bound by the fiber and possibly excreted
4. Substitute whole-wheat flour for some of the white flour in baked goods
5. Add bran, bran flakes, or oatmeal to mixed meat dishes, muffins, and pancake batter
6. Enjoy fresh fruits and vegetables in season, preferably unpeeled
7. Use whole-grain crackers
8. Incorporate beans into soups and casseroles
9. Use bran flakes for a crispy coating for meats or fish

Principles*

1. Fiber absorbs water in the intestines, so adequate fluids are important to keep the intestinal contents moving
2. Food rather than fiber supplements is the best way to increase both soluble and insoluble dietary fiber
3. Rice bran and corn bran may be just as effective in lowering serum cholesterol levels as oat bran (Hegsted et al, 1990; Earll et al, 1988)
4. Beans are an excellent source of soluble fiber and could be substituted for animal proteins
5. Insoluble fiber comes principally from whole-grain products; brown color is no guarantee of whole-grain content
6. Fiber normalizes bowel movements to 1 to 2 a day
7. In addition to oat bran, beans, barley, and psyllium also show cholesterol-reducing properties
8. The cholesterol-lowering properties of soluble dietary fiber are more effective when the diet is also low in fat
9. Cooking, freezing, and other preservation methods only slightly decrease fiber content
10. Unbuttered popcorn is a low-fat, high-fiber snack
11. Supplementation with concentrated or purified dietary fiber lacks the nutritional balance provided by a diet containing a variety of fruits, vegetables, whole-grain products, and legumes

Water-insoluble fibers affect the large bowel. Lignin, cellulose, and hemicellulose serve as substrates for microbial fermentation, producing fatty acids that can be used by colonic bacteria for growth. These fibers increase stool bulk, exercising the digestive tract muscles by increasing the radius of the colon and preventing the muscle from being chronically contracted. Therefore, muscle tone is maintained, colonic pressure is diminished, and the gut is able to resist bulging out into the pouches frequently seen in diverticulosis. Fiber accelerates intestinal transit rate, slows starch hydrolysis, and delays glucose absorption.

Water-soluble fibers such as pectins, gums, psyllium, mucilages, and algal polysaccharides influence the physiology of the upper GI tract. They are physiologically important for their gel-forming ability. Pectin increases the viscosity of chyme in the gut, thereby delaying gastric emptying and glucose absorption. These can also bind bile acids and are classified as being hypocholesteremic (Bell et al, 1991; Anderson et al, 1990; Kesaniemi et al, 1990). Another benefit is that fiber-rich foods are not kilocalorie-dense and may help a client to fill up on a fewer number of kilocalories (Anderson, 1986). Whether or not it plays a significant role in weight man-

TABLE 4–6

HIGH-FIBER DIET
Continued

Dietary Fiber Content of Sample Menu†

Sample Menu	***Dietary Fiber Content***
Breakfast	
Orange juice (1 cup)	0.5
Bagel (1)	1.2
Cream cheese (1 oz)	0
Raisins (1 packet)	0.7
1% Milk (1 cup)	0
Coffee	0
Creamer (1 tsp)	0
Lunch	
Sandwich: Tuna (1 oz)	0
Mayonnaise (2 tbsp)	0
Tomato (2 slices)	0.5
Lettuce slices	0.4
Whole-wheat bread (2 slices)	6.3
Apple (1)	3.0
1% Milk (1 cup)	0
Dinner	
Lean roast beef (2 oz)	0
Gravy (1/4 cup)	0
Brown rice (1/2 cup)	1.2
Corn (1/2 cup)	1.7
3-bean salad (1/2 cup)	6.1
Whole-wheat roll (2)	3.7
Margarine (1 tbsp)	0
Strawberries (1/2 cup)	1.9
Iced tea	0
Evening snack	
Diet cola (12 oz)	0
Dry roasted nuts (1 oz)	2.5
Totals	29.7‡

* Data from Earll L, et al. Feasibility and metabolic effects of a purified corn fiber food supplement. *J Am Diet Assoc* 1988 Aug; 88(9):950–952; Flock MH, et al. Practical aspects of implementing increased dietary fiber intake. *Am J Gastroenterol* 1986 Oct; 81(10):936–939; and Hegsted M, et al. Stabilized rice bran and oat bran lower cholesterol in humans. *FASEB* 1990; 4(3):A368.

† Nutrient data from Nutritionist III software, version 7.0. N-Squared Computing, Salem, OR.

‡ This menu could easily be increased by changing to 1 whole orange (3.1 gm fiber), increasing to 1 cup strawberries (additional 1.9 gm fiber), and/or increasing the amount of 3-bean salad.

agement has yet to be determined (Stevens, 1988). Guidelines for assisting clients in increasing dietary fiber are given in Table 4–6.

List 4 roles of carbohydrate.

Other Nutrients

Carbohydrates are normally accompanied by other nutrients. Starchy foods are especially important for their contribution of protein, minerals, and B vitamins. Whole-grain products are superior because of their fiber plus other nutrients (see Chapter 1, Table 1–10); enriched products should always be used as opposed to those processed but not enriched.

NURSING APPLICATIONS

1. Carbohydrate metabolism is dependent on an adequate supply of B vitamins and 2 minerals, phosphorus and magnesium. The amount of carbohydrate eaten affects these requirements. Usually adequate amounts of these nutrients accompany the increased carbohydrate intake, but this may not be true if refined sugars and breads are chosen predominantly. Assess dietary intake for adequacy of the B vitamins, phosphorus, and magnesium as well as carbohydrate intake (see Chapters 7 and 9).
2. The fasting blood glucose level is an indicator of overall glucose homeostasis and requires 8 hours of fasting before the test. The normal range for fasting blood glucose is 70 to 110 mg/dl. Monitor results.
3. Pain and emotional excitement (fear, anxiety, apprehension) accelerate hepatic glycogenolysis because of increased epinephrine and glucocorticoid secretion, so these may elevate blood glucose levels. Glucose levels may be elevated in clients scheduled for surgery because of stress, not a disease process.
4. A diet high in complex carbohydrates leads to a general increase in insulin's ability to promote glucose removal from plasma. In diabetic clients, this diet may be beneficial to lower the glucose level. However, medications should not be discontinued.
5. Blood glucose concentrations are increased only slightly when fructose, sorbitol, or xylitol is given because these sugars are absorbed more slowly; less insulin is required for their metabolism. Encourage diabetic clients to limit foods containing these sugars so blood glucose and total kilocaloric intake will not be adversely affected (with weight gain) and to avoid diarrhea.
6. Ketosis is associated with accelerated endogenous tissue breakdown, sodium excretion, and dehydration. It can be prevented with a minimum of 50 gm carbohydrate intake daily. Monitor carbohydrate intake for clients whose intake is poor and who are severely curtailing kilocalories.
7. Ketosis frequently occurs in clients with uncontrolled diabetes mellitus or in clients who are not eating (because of illness or dieting) because they are burning fat rather than carbohydrate. Therefore, monitor urine for ketones.
8. The best source of dietary fiber to relieve constipation is bran. However, clients with chronic constipation respond less well to bran treatment, and bran may be only partially effective in restoring normal transit time (Muller-Lissner, 1988). Therefore, evaluation of stools and use of other high-fiber foods is essential for individualizing care.

Rx Pectin is used in combination with an absorbent, kaolin, to treat diarrhea (Kaopectate).

Client Education

- Carbohydrates are not fattening.
- Fiber tends to normalize intestinal transit time.
- Enthusiastic clients who eat excessive amounts of bran (50 to 60 gm) gain no benefit from the surplus and expose themselves unnecessarily to known hazards, such as decreased mineral and vitamin absorption.
- Some vegetables and fruits (bananas, white potatoes, and apples) are high in pectins, which bind water. They are frequently used to check diarrhea but can also help relieve constipation by softening the stool.
- Even when reducing, it is important to consume as much carbohydrate as possible, especially vegetables, fruits, and whole-grain breads and cereals, to prevent ketosis and provide vital nutrients.
- Carbohydrates supply 4 kcal/gm and are a less concentrated source of energy than fats.

REQUIREMENTS

Since amino acids and a part of the fat molecule can be converted to glucose, a specific requirement for carbohydrate has not been established by the National Research Council. A reasonable proportion of the kilocaloric intake should consist of carbohydrates (minimum of 50 to 100 gm digestible carbohydrate) with the emphasis on complex carbohydrates to avoid ketosis, excessive breakdown of protein, loss of electrolytes, and involuntary dehydration.

Although dietary fiber is important, a specific RDA has not been made. Approximately 20 to 35 gm of dietary fiber daily has been suggested as an appropriate fiber intake (ADA, 1988; Butrum et al, 1988). Currently, about 13 gm dietary fiber is consumed daily in the US (Lanza et al, 1987).

Why should some carbohydrate be included in the diet? How much dietary fiber has been recommended?

SOURCES

Presently, the American diet furnishes about 45% of the kilocalories from carbohydrates, or almost 400 gm carbohydrate daily. Carbohydrates are furnished by the following food groups: milk, grain, and fruits and vegetables. The average sugar intake is about 11 to 13% of daily kilocaloric intake.

The only animal food supplying significant quantities of carbohydrate is milk and milk products, which furnish the disaccharide, lactose. In cheese-making, the lactose remains in the whey, which is removed as a by-product. Consequently, most cheeses contain only trace amounts of lactose.

Other sugars are furnished by table sugar, syrups, jellies, jams, and honey.

TABLE 4–7

SOURCES OF FIBER

	Insoluble Fiber	Soluble Fiber
Wheat bran	X	
Whole-wheat products	X	
Corn bran	X	
Oat bran	X	X
Whole-grain oats	X	X
Barley	X	X
Rice bran	X	
Brown rice	X	
Nuts	X	
Lentils	X	
Navy beans	X	X
Soy beans	X	X
Kidney beans	X	X
Bananas	X	
Apples	X	X
Cauliflower	X	
Potatoes	X	X
Citrus Fruits		X
Green beans and peas	X	
Broccoli	X	X
Carrots	X	X
Psyllium		X
Pectin		X
Carrageenan		X
Guar gum		X
Flax seed		X

Sugars are incorporated into many popular foods (e.g., candy, beverages, cakes and desserts, chewing gum, and ice cream), which accounts for their widespread acceptance. Approximately 20% of the kilocaloric intake is from refined sugars. Sugars, mainly glucose and fructose, are furnished in fruits and vegetables in varying amounts depending on their maturity (ripe bananas contain more simple sugars than green bananas) and their water content (spinach contains less carbohydrate than potatoes).

Complex carbohydrates or starches are furnished by grain products—wheat, corn, rice, oats, rye, barley, buckwheat, and millet. Some vegetables, especially root and seed varieties (potatoes, sweet potatoes, beets, carrots, peas, and winter squashes), also contain considerable amounts of starch. Dried beans and peas are excellent sources of complex carbohydrates.

Name sources for sugar, starches, and soluble and insoluble fiber.

Dietary fiber, especially hemicellulose, is furnished by whole-grain breads and cereals. Cellulose is found principally in the stems, roots, leaves, and seed coverings of plants; unpeeled fruits and leafy vegetables are good sources. Legumes are also a good source of dietary fiber. The pectin contributed by fruits and vegetables is an important source of fiber. Table 4–7 shows specific foods containing large amounts of soluble and/or insoluble fiber, and Table 4–6 indicates the fiber-containing foods provided in the sample menu.

NURSING APPLICATIONS

1. Offer high-fiber foods to clients. Fiber helps reduce constipation and diverticulosis and may help reduce some colon cancers.
2. A diet high in carbohydrate will maintain glycogen reserves, whereas a diet high in fat and low in carbohydrate and protein results in poor glycogen reserves. Because glycogen stores in the heart are critical for continuous functioning of heart muscles, the importance of carbohydrates should be emphasized.
3. Numerous studies indicate that carbohydrate-rich foods increase the synthesis and release of the brain neurotransmitter serotonin. Serotonin causes a calm, relaxing feeling, decreasing sensitivity to pain. Offering such foods to anxious or stressed clients may be beneficial.

Client Education

- Increased serotonin level curtails the need and desire for carbohydrate consumed at the following meal.
- Carbohydrate snacking seems to be related to a physiological need to increase the level of brain serotonin.
- Encourage clients to consume more complex carbohydrates and less refined sugar.
- A tablespoon of honey has more kilocalories than a tablespoon of sugar and only trace amounts of other nutrients.
- Inform clients on a weight reduction diet that a food label must indicate the total amount of carbohydrate (starch, sugar, and fiber) in a serving. Because fiber is not absorbed, it does not contribute any kilocalories. Hence, a product with 25 gm carbohydrate may have only 80 kcal if at least 5 gm of the carbohydrate are from fiber.
- The US FDA has labeled raw sugar as "unfit for direct use as food or as a food ingredient because of the impurities it ordinarily contains."
- Clients should be aware that sugar may be identified as any of the following on food labels: sucrose, fructose, corn sweetener, cane sugar, honey, molasses, high fructose corn syrup, raw sugar, and maple syrup. Clients trying to reduce concentrated sweets should avoid foods if the first ingredient is any of the above aforementioned.

HYPER- AND HYPO- STATES

Normal physiological conditions and disease states affect carbohydrate metabolism, which is reflected in serum glucose levels (hyperglycemia or hypoglycemia). Other factors that occur with too much or too little carbohydrate will be discussed.

Carbohydrate Excess

Soft drinks are increasingly being substituted for milk and coffee. Soft drink consumption reached 30.3 gallons per person in 1986 (Putnam, 1989). A diet high in sugar from too many pastries, candies, and soft drinks is less likely to be adequate in other nutrients.

On the other hand, sugar increases palatability and may induce clients to eat certain foods otherwise disliked. Combining sugar with other nutritious foods, as in milk used for pudding, may increase the variety of foods consumed and enjoyed.

Fiber Deficiency

Frequently, clients eliminate complex carbohydrates in the belief that they are fattening. This can result in an insufficient intake of B vitamins, iron, and fiber.

Dental Caries

Tooth decay is affected by many factors. Carbohydrates (including sugars and starches that are hydrolyzed by amylase) can be digested by bacteria in the mouth, leaving plaque and acids that lead to tooth decay. When a **cariogenic** food is eaten, the pH of the plaque is lowered by the bacterial fermentation of the carbohydrate. A pH below 5.5 will dissolve tooth enamel. Adequate amounts of saliva flow increase the clearance of the food and bacterial substrate from the mouth.

Cariogenic—conducive to the formation of dental cavities.

Bibby et al (1986) found that some foods high in sugar were removed quicker and did not lower the pH of plaque as much as starchy foods with less sugar. The less time the offending substance is exposed to the enamel, the less cariogenic. Sticky foods and those that remain in the mouth for a longer time are more cariogenic than liquid foods. Cough drops, raisins, and even peanut butter with crackers appear to be quite innocent, yet may cause extensive dental damage if proper cleaning does not follow and/or if they are eaten too often. Replacing potential cariogenic snacks with foods such as fresh fruits, vegetables, cottage cheese, cheese, yogurt, peanuts, or popcorn can decrease caries.

Why is sugar considered cariogenic? What are some options for preventing tooth decay?

Obesity

There is no evidence that carbohydrates or sugars are a cause of obesity. Excessive kilocaloric intake leads to obesity, whether from carbohydrates, proteins, fats, or alcohol. Although excessive kilocalories from sugar intake could lead to obesity, epidemiological studies and several individual studies have shown that obese clients actually consume less sugar than thin clients (Lewis et al, 1992).

NURSING APPLICATIONS

1. Scientific studies do not support the claim that sugars interfere with bioavailability of vitamins, minerals, or trace nutrients or the notion that dietary imbalances are preferentially caused by increased sugar consumption (Sugars Task Force, 1986). Thus, do not assume that just because a client is obese, increased sugar intake is the culprit. Perform a thorough nutritional assessment to help determine the cause.
2. Some foods, such as milk and aged cheese, actually protect the teeth by inhibiting acid production. If snacks are needed when oral hygiene cannot be performed, offer snacks consisting of milk or aged cheese or follow snack with these items.

Client Education

- Two tips to prevent dental caries include (1) always brush after eating and (2) offer sweets as part of the meal instead of as snacks.
- Using a straw may lessen contact with the teeth and reduce caries.
- Frequent snacks provide more opportunities for bacterial growth and increase the risk for development of caries.
- The use of wholesome, unprocessed grains, fruits and vegetables is to be encouraged.
- The amount of sugar in a food is unrelated to its caries potential; all carbohydrate foods are potentially cariogenic.
- Frequent exposure of the tooth surface to fluoride such as in drinking water, mouth rinses, and dentifrices is effective in controlling caries.

SUGAR SUBSTITUTES

The practice of flavoring foods without additional kilocalories is one of many approaches to the problems of excess kilocalorie intake and a sedentary life. The desire to decrease sugar consumption is being met through the widespread and increasing use of numerous sugar substitutes (Fig. 4–5). In the 1980s, consumption of

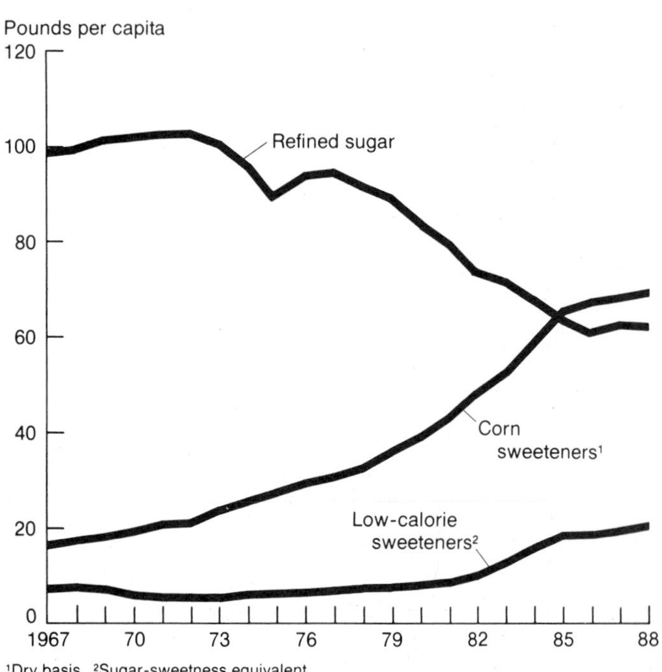

Figure 4–5 Total sweetener consumption is up, while low-kilocalorie sweeteners are becoming more popular. (From Putnam JJ. Food consumption. *Natl Food Rev* 1990 Jul-Sept; 13(3):1–9. (Original source: Putnam JJ. *Food Consumption, Prices, and Expenditures 1967–88.* U.S.D.A., E.R.S. Stat. Bull. No. 804. May 1990. Contact: Judith Jones Putnam (202) 786-1870.))

low kilocalorie sweeteners increased faster than kilocalorie sweeteners. Total use of kilocalorie sweeteners rose from 123 pounds per capita in 1970 to 133 lbs in 1988; low-kilocalorie sweeteners increased from 5.8 to 20.0 lbs per capita during the same time period (Putnam, 1991).

These products are used principally for their sweetening power, but they also make some foods more palatable. The large variety of sweeteners is desirable because each has certain advantages and limitations. Because each sweetener has different properties, the availability of various products helps satisfy flavor and texture requirement in foods and beverages. Taste buds may be fooled by artificial sweeteners, but they do not produce a prolonged feeling of satiety. Although saccharine consumption has been shown to increase hunger and food intake, the use of aspartame does not cause an increase in food intake (Canty & Chan, 1991; Rolls, 1991). Whether the use of these artificial sweeteners decreases the total kilocaloric intake depends on other food choices. Compensatory food choices such as using a diet carbonated beverage to permit a piece of cheesecake will be ineffective in weight control, whereas using a low-kilocalorie food to replace a high-kilocalorie food, watching other food intake, and engaging in some form of exercise may be beneficial.

Many clients question the safety of these products. All the products on the market have been extensively researched, and with the exception of aspartame, are safe for most clients if consumed in moderation. Information regarding sugar substitutes is summarized in Table 4–8.

NURSING APPLICATIONS

1. Sugar substitutes can reduce the kilocaloric content of a product and decrease cariogenicity of a product. Used in moderation, sugar substitutes are beneficial for many clients, especially diabetic clients.
2. Because aspartame contains phenylalanine, aspartame-containing products are labeled to warn clients with phenylketonuria. Advise clients with this disorder to avoid products containing aspartame.
3. A new sweetener called Acesulfame-K contains small amounts of potassium (the K stands for potassium). Clients with severe potassium restriction (renal conditions) should use Acesulfame-K in moderation.

Client Education

- Nonkilocalorie sweeteners do nothing to appease the appetite. Some studies have reported increases in hunger following use of artificial sweeteners, but others have found decreased or unchanged hunger (Canty & Chan, 1991; Rolls, 1991).
- Clients who need to rely on sugar substitutes to help with blood glucose control should use multiple types so that only small amounts of any one sweetener are consumed.
- When deciding whether young children should be given artificially sweetened foods, consider the child's body weight and limit to below recommended levels (500 mg/day for saccharin, 50 mg/kg body weight for aspartamine, and 15 mg/kg body weight for Acesulfame-K).
- During pregnancy, aspartame in limited amounts is the preferred sweetener because it is metabolized like other amino acids, whereas saccharin is known to cross the placenta (Bertorelli & Czarnowski-Hill, 1990).

NUTRITION UPDATE 4–1: GLYCOGEN LOADING

A high-carbohydrate diet to improve endurance capacity was recommended as long ago as 1940. Since the major source of energy for muscles and **anaerobic**-type activity is glycogen, a determinant for endurance in aerobic activity is the volume of

Anaerobic—without oxygen.

TABLE 4-8

LOW-KILOCALORIE SWEETENERS

	Saccharin	Aspartame	Cyclamate	Acesulfame K
Descriptions	Nonkilocaloric sweetener used commercially to sweeten foods and beverages since early 1900s	Nutritive sweetener made from 2 amino acids (L-phenylalanine and L-aspartic acid). Because of its intense sweetness, the small amounts ingested are considered virtually nonkilocaloric	Nonkilocaloric sweetener discovered in 1937; used widely during the 1960s in low-kilocalorie foods and beverages	Nonkilocaloric sweetener discovered in Germany; developed by the Hoechst Celanese Corp. White, odorless, crystalline sweetener; readily absorbed
Relative Sweetness	300 times sweeter than sucrose	180 times sweeter than sucrose	30 times sweeter than sucrose	200 times sweeter than sucrose
Metabolism	Not metabolized; excreted by the kidneys unchanged	Digested as a protein; the resulting amino acids are metabolized normally	Most people do not metabolize cyclamate	Not metabolized by the body; excreted by the kidneys unchanged
Assets	Stable shelf life; combines well with other sweeteners; synergistic effect when combined with aspartame and/or cyclamate	Sugar-like taste; enhances some flavors; synergistic effect when combined with saccharin and/or cyclamate; appropriate for many applications	Stable in heat and cold; good shelf life. Soluble in liquids. Has synergistic effect when combined with other low-kilocalorie sweeteners	Sweet taste is rapidly perceptible; good shelf life; relatively stable across temperature and pH ranges normally associated with food processing
Limitations	Slight aftertaste, which can be eliminated when blended with another low-kilocalorie sweetener	Unstable at prolonged high heat; not suitable for cooking or products that undergo heat sterilization. Can be added to heated recipes after cooking. Loses sweetness gradually depending on temperature and acidity. Restrict intake for clients with phenylketonuria	Least "sweetening power" of the commercially acceptable nonkilocaloric sweeteners	Some aftertaste noted at levels required to achieve adequate sweetness when used alone. When blended with other low-kilocalorie sweeteners, provides improved taste, economic, and stability advantages
Applications	Primarily in soft drinks, tabletop sweeteners, and other beverages and foods as well as cosmetics and pharmaceuticals	Wide variety of products, including tabletop sweeteners, soft drinks, cold breakfast cereals, chewing gum, dry beverage mixes, instant coffee and tea, gelatins, puddings, fillings, toppings, milk beverages, refrigerated or frozen beverages, gelatin desserts, breath mints, and multivitamin supplements	Before 1970, widely used as tabletop sweetener, in sugar-free beverages, and other low-kilocalorie foods, particularly with saccharin	Potentially useful for almost all applications including soft drinks and baked goods

muscle glycogen. Glycogen loading is commonly referred to as "carbohydrate loading." The purpose is to delay exhaustion by postponing the time at which glycogen depletion is reached.

Endurance activities for which this regimen may be effective include the marathon, cross-country skiing, distance cycling and swimming, and events that are intense for longer than 90 minutes. Because of numerous side effects of the classic glycogen-loading regimen, a modified technique leads to increasing muscle glycogen stores 2-fold to 3-fold. Normal glycogen storage is about 15 gm/kg body weight, and

TABLE 4-8

LOW-KILOCALORIE SWEETENERS *Continued*

	Saccharin	Aspartame	Cyclamate	Acesulfame K
Safety	Nearly a century of safe human use. Thirty human studies found no association between saccharin and bladder cancer. NCI concluded that there was "no evidence of increased risk with the long-term use of artificial sweeteners in any form or with use that began decades ago." FDA Commissioner has said that FDA has less concern about saccharin than in 1977, "The actual risk, if any, of saccharin to humans still appears to be slight." Research now demonstrates that saccharin is unlikely to cause cancer in humans; differences in rat urine and the type of saccharin used in rat studies cause the differences observed	Extensive animal and human studies provide strong evidence that aspartame is no more hazardous than normal dietary protein consumption. In 1986, the CDC found that the complaints "do not provide evidence of the existence of serious widespread, adverse health consequences." The majority of frequently reported symptoms were mild and uncommon in the general populace. In July, 1985, AMA's Council on Scientific Affairs concluded that consumption of aspartame is safe and "is not associated with serious adverse health effects"	Banned in the US in 1970. Current petition for reapproval in the US	Tested in approximately 90 studies. On approval, FDA said it "found that the safety studies did not show any toxic effects that could be attributed to the sweetener"
Status	A 1977 proposed ban on saccharin in the US was stayed by Congress pending further research. Congressional moratorium on saccharin ban has been extended 6 times; current moratorium is in effect until May 1, 1997. In 1991, FDA formally withdrew its 1977 proposal to ban saccharin use. It is used in more than 90 countries	Approved for use in more than 96 countries and is available in more than 5000 products worldwide	In June, 1985, NAS concluded, "the totality of the evidence from studies in animals does not indicate that cyclamate or its metabolites is carcinogenic by itself." Petitioned for reapproval pending. Approved for use in more than 50 countries worldwide	Approved by FDA in July, 1988, for use in dry beverage mixes, instant coffee and tea, dairy product analogs, and as table top sweetener. Approved for use in more than 50 countries. Petitions for use in confectionary, soft drinks, and baked goods are pending before FDA

Adapted from Sweetener Fact Sheets, Saccharin, May 1992; Aspartame, June 1991; Cyclamate, May 1989; Acesulfame K, April 1991. Calorie Control Council, 5775 Peachtree-Dunwoody Road, Suite 500-G, Atlanta, Georgia 30342. (NCI, National Cancer Institute; NAS, National Academy of Sciences.)

about 500 gm glycogen can be added to the normal glycogen stores before body fat significantly begins to increase (Acheson et al, 1988).

Carbohydrate loading begins a week before the event, with consumption of 300 to 350 gm of carbohydrate eaten in conjunction with the regular conditioning program. Three days before the competition, exercise is tapered to allow the muscles to rest; athletes gradually increase their carbohydrate, culminating in 525 to 550 gm carbohydrate daily (Kris-Etherton, 1989) (Table 4-9).

This technique is often used inappropriately, and adverse effects can occur

TABLE 4–9

HIGH CARBOHYDRATE DIET

Sample Menu	Carbohydrate Content	High-Carbohydrate Menu*	Carbohydrate Content
Breakfast			
Orange juice (1 cup)	27		27
Bagel (1)	31		31
Cream cheese (1 oz)	0.8		0.8
Raisins (1 packet)	11		11
1% Milk (1 cup)	12		12
Coffee	0.9		0.9
Creamer (1 tsp)	2.0		2.0
Lunch			
Sandwich: Tuna (1 oz)	0	2 sandwiches: Tuna (2 oz)	0
Mayonnaise (2 tbsp)	0.8	Mayonnaise (4 tbsp)	1.6
Tomato (2 slices)	2.6	Tomato (4 slices)	5.2
Lettuce leaves (2)	0.8	Lettuce leaves (4)	1.6
Whole wheat bread (2 slices)	25.4	Whole-wheat bread (4 slices)	50.8
Apple (1)	21.1		21.1
1% Milk (1 cup)	12		12
Dinner			
Lean roast beef (2 oz)	0		0
Gravy (1/4 cup)	4.1		4.1
Brown rice (1/2 cup)	28.6		28.6
Corn (1/2 cup)	16.8	Corn (3/4 cup)	25.3
Three bean salad (1/2 cup)	20.2		20.2
Whole wheat roll (2)	36.6		36.6
Margarine (1 tbsp)	0		0
Strawberries (1/2 cup)	5.3	Strawberries (1 cup)	10.6
Iced tea	0		0
Evening Snack			
Diet cola (12 oz)	0.4	Regular soft drink (12 oz)	38.4
Dry roasted nuts (1 oz)	5.4	Peanut butter (2 Tbsp)	6.6
		Crackers (8)	16.0
Totals	264 gm		363 gm

* Only items changed are listed; other items are the same.
Nutrient data from Nutritionist III software, version 7.0. N-Squared Computing, Salem, OR.

(Hopkins & Thompson, 1988). The athlete may gain 2 to 7 pounds (fluid) with carbohydrate loading, which makes the body sluggish. (However, this may help prevent dehydration). The extra glycogen and water stores may cause muscle stiffness and impair performance.

NURSING APPLICATIONS

1. This regimen is not advisable for anyone with heart disease, high blood lipids, or diabetes because of the stress it puts on the heart.
2. Carbohydrate supplementation during prolonged strenuous exercise (over 2 hours) has been shown to improve performance (Coggan & Coyle, 1989; Wheeler, 1989). This regimen is to be used only by athletes engaged in endurance events and should be used only 3 to 4 times a year. Athletes following this regimen are closely monitored for side effects.

Client Education

- Complex carbohydrates are advised to achieve more glycogen storage.
- Carbohydrate loading is not appropriate for events lasting less than 90 minutes because normal glycogen stores provide fuel for about 2 hours of moderate-intensity exercise.

SUMMARY

Carbohydrates include simple carbohydrates, or sugars, and polysaccharides (starches and dietary fiber). All dietary carbohydrates are broken down to monosaccharides in the GI tract. In the liver, most monosaccharides are converted to glucose, which is transported to and used by the cells. Carbohydrate is stored in small amounts in the body in the form of glycogen. This is used for cellular energy and to maintain blood glucose, which is essential for the central nervous system. Although no RDA has been established for carbohydrate or fiber, daily intake prevents ketosis and muscle wasting and promotes normal bowel functions.

NURSING PROCESS IN ACTION

A healthy client comes to the clinic seeking information on how to eat less refined sugar and consume more complex carbohydrate. He knows this regimen is being encouraged but is not sure about all the health reasons. Fiber intake is also important to him, but he does not know a lot about the types of food needed or the benefits.

 Nutritional Assessment

- Willingness/motivation to learn.
- Usual dietary habits; focus especially on carbohydrate.
- Basic knowledge of carbohydrate and carbohydrate principles.
- Usual food/nutrient intake.
- Financial status.
- Support persons, married, divorced, single.
- Use of community resources.
- Food shopping practices.

 Dietary Nursing Diagnosis

Health-seeking behavior RT lack of knowledge concerning carbohydrate and carbohydrate principles for optimal nutrition.

 Nutritional Goals

Client will consume a high fiber and complex carbohydrate food daily and state 3 principles concerning carbohydrate.

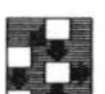 Nutritional Implementation 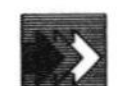

Intervention: Explain (1) that the main function of carbohydrate is to provide energy for the body, (2) that excessive amounts of carbohydrate in conjunction with excessive kilocalories are converted to triglycerides and stored as fat but that carbohydrates themselves do not cause obesity, and (3) roles of carbohydrate.
Rationale: Knowledge corrects misinformation.

Intervention: (1) Follow suggestions in Table 4–6. (2) Explain the importance of fiber. Recommend 20 to 35 gm of fiber daily, and help the client plan out a diet that will provide this amount, incorporating his food preferences.
Rationale: These will increase fiber in the diet. Fiber increases stool bulk, ex-

ercising the digestive tract muscles and thus preventing them from being chronically contracted. Therefore, muscle tone is maintained, colonic pressure is diminished, and the gut is able to resist bulging out into pouches. Additionally, fiber slows starch hydrolysis and delays glucose absorption.

Intervention: Explain sources of complex carbohydrates and fiber sources and provide the client with a list of these foods.
Rationale: These measures will help the client consume more complex carbohydrate and fiber by increasing knowledge and providing concrete information.

Intervention: (1) Teach about substituting artificial sweeteners for sugar. (2) Actually read a label with client to determine how to recognize sugars (usually end in "ose"). (3) Substitute fresh fruit for juices. (4) Avoid densely concentrated sugar in cola drinks, cookies, and pastries.
Rationale: He wanted to reduce refined sugar intake, and these measures will help meet this personal goal.

Intervention: Refer to dietitian and county extension agencies.
Rationale: These will provide expert knowledge and community resources for continued compliance.

Intervention: Review labeling—(1) high fiber just means that the food contains fiber (there is no set standard); (2) no sugar added means sugar was not added, but the product may naturally contain sugar; (3) sugar-free means the product contains no added sucrose but may have other sugars added such as sorbitol; (4) choose a product that has 5 gm or less of sucrose; (5) incorporate foods with 3 gm or more fiber per serving.
Rationale: If a client does not know how to read labels, unhealthy food choices may be selected inadvertently.

Evaluation

Client consumed a bran muffin or beans or other high-fiber foods daily and verbalized that carbohydrates provide energy and fiber, carbohydrate has several roles in maintaining gut functioning, and most sugars end in "-ose." Other indicators of success include reading a label correctly, reducing intake of refined sugars, and using the community resources.

STUDENT READINESS

1. Differentiate between the 3 classes of carbohydrates.
2. Trace the route of carbohydrate from ingestion to its metabolism, including the enzymes, the site of the activity, and the absorbable products.
3. What are the main sources of fiber in the American diet? What are the main sources of starch? List 3 of your favorite foods high in sugar.
4. Explain the functions of sugars and fiber in the diet in terms a client can understand.

CASE STUDY

Your client has been on a liquid diet for 3 days. She refuses to eat Jell-O and has taken very little bouillon. Today, the only intake she had was the following: 6 oz pineapple juice (26 gm carbohydrate), 4 oz cranberry juice (21 gm carbohydrate), 10 oz orange juice (36 gm carbohydrate), and 2 cups hot tea with 2 tsp sugar (8 gm carbohydrate).

a. How many kilocalories did she consume?

b. What is the carbohydrate circulating in her blood?
c. What is the normal range?
d. How is this maintained if too little carbohydrate is eaten?
e. How is this maintained if very large amounts are eaten?

REFERENCES

Acheson KJ, et al. Glycogen storage capacity and de novo lipogenesis during massive carbohydrate overfeeding in man. *Am J Clin Nutr* 1988 Aug; 48(2):240–247.

American Dietetic Association (ADA). Position paper: Health implications of dietary fiber. *J Am Diet Assoc* 1988 Feb; 88(2):216–221.

Anderson JW, et al. Serum lipid response of hypercholesterolemic men to single and divided doses of canned beans. *Am J Clin Nutr* 1990 June; 51(6):1013–1019.

Anderson JW. Fiber and health: An overview. *Am J Gastroenterol* 1986 Oct; 81(10):99–105.

Bantle JP. Clinical aspects of sucrose and fructose metabolism. *Diab Care* 1989 Jan; 12(1):56–61.

Beaugerie L, et al. Digestion and absorption in the human intestine of three sugar alcohols. *Gastroenterology* 1990 Sept; 99(3):717–723.

Bell LP, et al. Cholesterol-lowering effects of soluble-fiber cereals as a part of a prudent diet for patients with mild to moderate hypercholesterolemia. *Am J Clin Nutr* 1991 Dec; 52(6):1020–1026.

Bertorelli AM, Czarnowski-Hill JV. Review of present and future use of nonnutritive sweeteners. *Diab-Educator* 1990 Sept/Oct; 16(5):415–429.

Bibby BG, et al. Oral food clearance and the pH of plaque and saliva. *J Am Dental Assoc* 1986 March; 111(3):333–337.

Butrum RR, et al. NCI dietary guidelines: Rationale. *Am J Clin Nutr* 1988 Sept; 48(Suppl 3):888–895.

Canty DJ, Chan MM. Effects of consumption of caloric vs noncaloric sweet drinks on indices of hunger and food consumption in normal adults. *Am J Clin Nutr* 1991 May; 53(5):1159–1164.

Coggan AR, Coyle EF. Metabolism and performance following carbohydrate ingestion late in exercise. *Med Sci Sport Exerc* 1989 Feb; 21(1):59–65.

Deutsch RM. *Realities of Nutrition.* Palo Alto, CA, Bull Publishing Co., 1976.

Englyst HN, Cummings JH. Digestion of the carbohydrates of banana in the human small intestine. *Am J Clin Nutr* 1986 July; 44(1):42–50.

Englyst HN, Cummings JH. Digestion of the polysaccharides of some cereal foods in the human small intestine. *Am J Clin Nutr* 1985 Nov; 42(5):778–787.

Gilman AG, et al. Goodman and Gilman's *The Pharmacological Basis of Therapeutics.* 8th ed. New York, Pergamon Press, 1990.

Hopkins M, Thompson W. Specificity of sport and incorporation of a carbohydrate regime. *Ann Sports Med* 1988; 4(1):16–18.

Jenkins DJA, et al. Starchy foods and glycemic index. *Diab Care* 1988 Feb; 11(1):149–159.

Kesaniemi YA, et al. Low vs high dietary fiber and serum, biliary and fecal lipids in middle-aged men. *Am J Clin Nutr* 1990 June; 51(6):1007–1012.

Kris-Etherton PM. Nutrition and athletic performance. *Contemporary Nutrition* 1989; 14(8): 1–2.

Lanza E, et al. Dietary fiber intake in the United States population. *Am J Clin Nutr* 1987 Nov; 46(5):790–797.

Lewis CJ, et al. Nutrient intakes and body weights of persons consuming high and moderate levels of added sugars. *J Am Diet Assoc* 1992 June; 92(6):708–713.

Muller-Lissner SA. Effect of wheat bran on weight of stool and gastrointestinal transit time: A meter analysis. *Br Med J* 1988 Feb 27; 296(6622):615–617.

Putnam JJ. Food consumption, 1970–90. *Food Rev* 1991 July/Sept; 14(3):2–12.

Putnam JJ. Food consumption. *Nat Food Rev* 1990 July/Sept; 13(3):1–9.

Putnam JJ. Food consumption. *Nat Food Rev* 1989 Apr/June; 12(2):1–9.

Raper N. Nutrient content of the U.S. food supply. *Food Rev* 1991 July/Sept; 14(3):13–18.

Rolls BJ. Effects of intense sweeteners on hunger, food intake, and body weight: A review. *Am J Clin Nutr* 1991 Apr; 53(4):875–878.

Slavin JL. Dietary fiber: Mechanisms or magic on disease prevention. *Nutr Today* 1990 Nov/Dec; 25(6):6–10.

Stevens J. Does dietary fiber affect food intake and body weight? *J Am Diet Assoc* 1988 Aug; 88(8):934–945.

Sugars Task Force. Evaluation of health aspects of sugars contained in carbohydrate sweeteners. Washington, D.C., Division of Nutrition and Toxicology, Center for Food Safety and Applied Nutrition, FDA, 1986.

Wheeler KB. Sports nutrition for the primary care physician: The importance of carbohydrate. *Phys Sportsmed* 1989 May; 17:106–117.

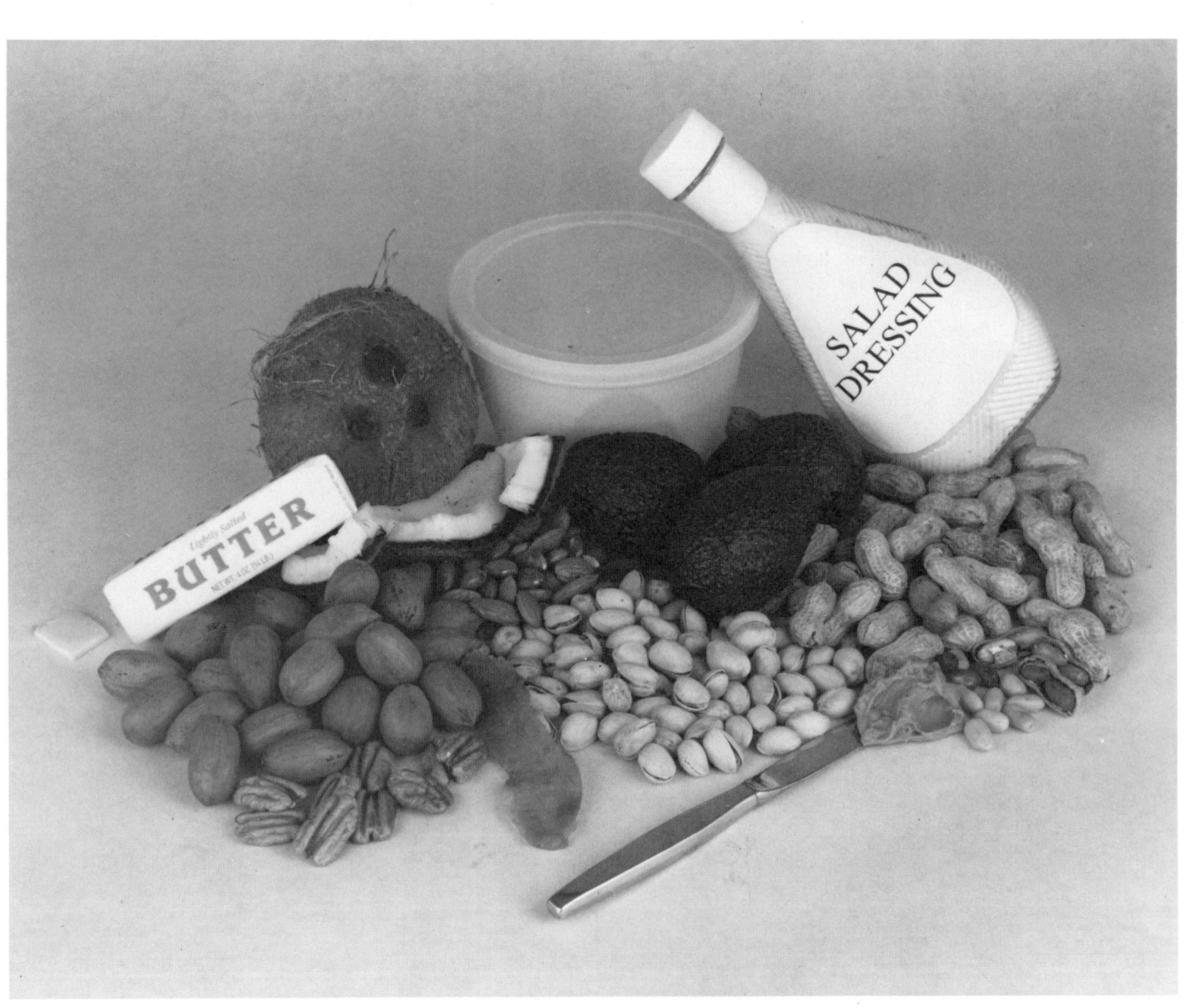
BUTTER
SALAD
DRESSING

Lipids: The Condensed Energy

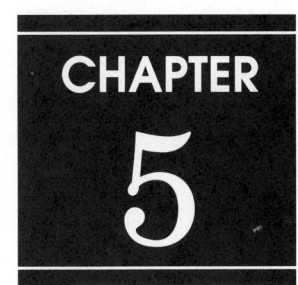

OUTLINE

I. CLASSIFICATION
  A. Chemical Structure
    1. Saturated Fatty Acids
    2. Monounsaturated Fatty Acids
    3. Polyunsaturated Fatty Acids
    4. P/S Ratio
  Nursing Applications
  B. Characteristics
    1. Chain Length versus Saturation
    2. Hydrogenation
    3. Rancidity
  C. Compound Lipids
    1. Phospholipids
    2. Lipoproteins
  D. Cholesterol
  E. Synthetic Fats
    1. Medium-Chain Triglycerides
    2. Structured Lipids
    3. Fat Substitutes
  Nursing Applications
II. DIGESTION
III. ABSORPTION
IV. DIGESTIBILITY
  Nursing Applications
V. FAT METABOLISM
VI. OXIDATION
VII. FAT SYNTHESIS
  Nursing Applications
VIII. PHYSIOLOGICAL ROLES
  A. Concentrated Energy
  B. Protein Sparers
  C. Satiety Value
  D. Palatability
  E. Complementary Relationships
  F. Fat Storage

OBJECTIVES

THE STUDENT WILL BE ABLE TO:

- Identify the basic structural units of dietary lipids.
- Describe how fatty acids affect the properties of fat.
- Identify the secretions and processes involved in triglyceride digestion and absorption.
- Name the essential fatty acid (EFA) and some of its functions.
- Describe the metabolism of fatty acids in cells.
- Describe the metabolic events leading to ketosis and the role of the diet.
- List the functions of fats in the body.
- List dietary sources for saturated and polyunsaturated fatty acids and cholesterol.
- Distinguish between chylomicrons and other lipoproteins.
- State the effect of polyunsaturated fatty acids on serum cholesterol.
- State the number of kilocalories provided per gram of fat.
- Describe nursing application principles for fat.
- Identify client teaching tips concerning fats.

TEST YOUR NQ (True/False)

1. Fried foods are not well digested.
2. Americans are being poisoned by manufacturers adding tropical oils to foods.
3. Products containing more polyunsaturated fatty acids than saturated fatty acids are healthier food choices than products containing a higher proportion of saturated fatty acids.
4. The fat content of the diet should be less than 30% of total kilocalories.
5. Bananas and avocados contain a lot of cholesterol.
6. Oils are less fattening than solid fats.
7. The liver is the principal regulator of fat metabolism.

TABLE 5-1

PERCENTAGE OF FAT IN FOODS

Percent Fat*	Food	Percent Fat*	Food
90-100	Salad and cooking oils and fats, lard	10-20	Broiled choice round steak, broiled veal chop, roast turkey, eggs, avocado, olives, chocolate cake with icing, french-fried potatoes, ice cream, apple pie
80-90	Butter, margarine		
70-80	Mayonnaise, pecans, macadamia nuts		
50-70	Walnuts, dried unsweetened coconut, meat, almonds, bacon, baking chocolate	1-10	Pork and beans, broiled cod, halibut, haddock, many other fish, broiled chicken, crabmeat, cottage cheese, beef liver, milk, creamed soups, sherbet, most breakfast cereals
30-50	Broiled choice T-bone and porterhouse steaks, spareribs, broiled pork chop, goose, cheddar and cream cheeses, potato chips, French dressing, chocolate candy	<1	Baked potato, most vegetables and fruits, egg whites, chicken consommé
20-30	Choice beef pot roast, broiled choice lamb chop, frankfurters, ground beef, chocolate chip cookies		

* Percent of fat by weight. This should not be confused with percent of kilocalories.
From FDA Consumer, *Primer on Three Nutrients*. HHS Publication No. (FDA) 81-2026, revised January 1981.

8. Food products labeled "no cholesterol" are low in fat.
9. Fats contain 9 kcal/gm.
10. Omega-3 fatty acids are polyunsaturated fatty acids.

Unsweetened coconut, mayonnaise, blue cheese salad dressing, almonds, pecans, sausage—what do all these things have in common? More than one-half of the kilocalories in each of these food items comes from fat, a vital constituent of our diet. The percentage of fat (by weight) in many foods is listed in Table 5-1.

Food supply trends indicate a fall in US fat intake; this preceded the decline in heart disease mortality (Stephen & Wald, 1990). Client concerns about healthy food choices explain these changes. Food manufacturers, producers, and grocers have responded by (1) trimming the fat from meats, (2) providing leaner cuts of beef and pork, (3) eliminating tropical oils from processed foods, and (4) manufacturing foods containing less fat. Even though prices for seafood and chicken rose faster than for beef and pork, consumers increased their consumption of fish and poultry and substituted lower fat milk (2%) for whole milk (Putnam, 1990).

CLASSIFICATION

Fats in the diet should actually be called lipids to include the structural and functional **lipids.** Lipids contain less oxygen in proportion to hydrogen and carbon than carbohydrates. Because of their structure, their metabolism uses more oxygen and releases more energy than either carbohydrates or amino acids.

Lipids contain the same 3 elements as carbohydrates: carbon, hydrogen, and oxygen.

The 2 classes of insoluble substances include (1) fats that occur both in foods and in the body (functional) and (2) structural or complex lipids that are produced

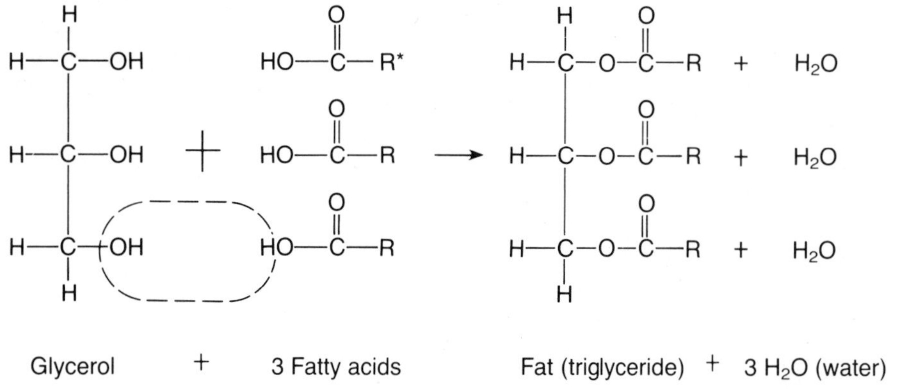

Glycerol + 3 Fatty acids → Fat (triglyceride) + 3 H_2O (water)

Figure 5–1 Chemical structure of a triglyceride. *Each of the fatty acids can be different: long or short, saturated or unsaturated.

What is another name for fat? Which fats are found in the diet; which are present in the body?

by the body for specific functions. Dietary fats usable by the body include triglycerides, fatty acids, phospholipids, and cholesterol. Lipids found solely in the body include lipoproteins and glycolipids.

A fatty acid is a chain of carbon atoms attached to hydrogen atoms with an acid grouping on the end.

Glycerol is the alcohol portion of a triglyceride to which the fatty acids attach.

Short-chain fatty acids contain 4 to 6 carbons; medium-chain fatty acids, 8 to 12 carbons; and long-chain fatty acids, more than 12 carbons.

Chemical Structure

Fats are composed of **fatty acids** and **glycerol,** as shown: monoglyceride = glycerol + 1 fatty acid, diglyceride = glycerol + 2 fatty acids, triglycerides = glycerol + 3 fatty acids. Triglycerides, or neutral fats, are the most common fat present in animal or protein foods (Fig. 5–1). Monoglycerides and diglycerides are found in the small intestine resulting from hydrolysis of triglycerides during digestion. **Medium-chain** and **short-chain fatty acids** are more readily digested and absorbed, but most foods (especially vegetable fats) contain predominantly **long-chain fatty acids** (16 to 18 carbon atoms).

Saturation of a fatty acid depends on the number of hydrogen atoms attached to the carbon. Saturated fatty acids contain only single bonds, with each carbon atom having 2 hydrogen atoms attached to it.

Name sources of saturated fatty acids.

Saturated Fatty Acids

Fatty acids are classified according to their degree of **saturation.** If each carbon atom has 2 hydrogen atoms attached, the fat is saturated (Fig. 5–2). Palmitic and stearic acids, the most prevalent saturated fatty acids, are found in animal fats, cheese, butter, coconut oil, and chocolate (Fig. 5–3).

Monounsaturated fats contain only 1 double bond.

What is the most abundant monounsaturated fatty acid, and what foods contain this monounsaturated fatty acid?

Monounsaturated Fatty Acids

When adjacent carbon atoms are joined by a double bond because 2 hydrogen atoms are lacking, the fatty acid is **monounsaturated.*** The most abundant monounsaturated fatty acid is oleic acid, which is found in olive, peanut, and canola oils (see Fig. 5–3).

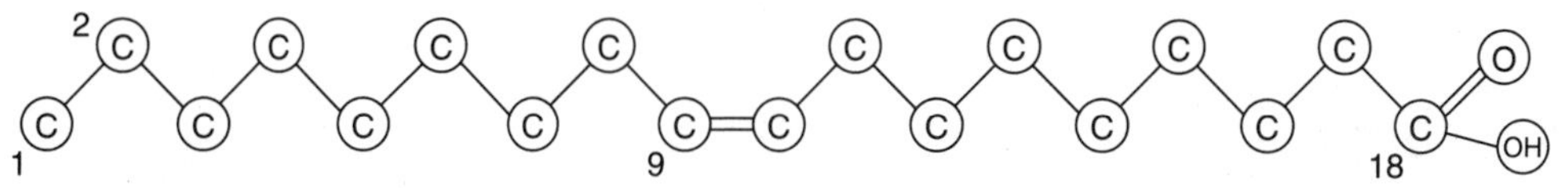

Oleic acid (18:1).

* Fatty acids are more clearly identified by numbers to indicate the position of any double bonds. The double bond can be designated in 2 ways. If the structure is numbered from the carboxyl group (C—OH), the symbol Δ is used. This text will be using the alternate system, whereby carbon atoms are numbered from the omega end, which is indicated by "n-" or "ω". (Omega, or ω, is the final letter in the Greek alphabet.)

```
    H H H H H H H H H H H H H H H H H O
    | | | | | | | | | | | | | | | | | ||
H—C—C—C—C—C—C—C—C—C—C—C—C—C—C—C—C—C—C—O—H
    | | | | | | | | | | | | | | | | |
    H H H H H H H H H H H H H H H H H
```

A

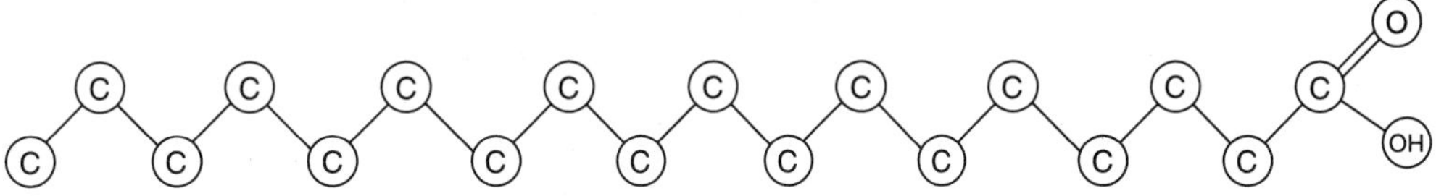

B

Figure 5–2 Structure of a fatty acid. Saturated fatty acid: stearic acid, an 18-carbon fatty acid (18:0). These numbers indicate the number of carbon atoms and how many double bonds are present. Thus stearic acid, a saturated fatty acid containing 18 carbon atoms and no double bonds, is labeled 18:0. *A*, Detailed structure. *B*, Simplified structure. Each of the C's at the corners of the zigzag lines represents a carbon atom with 2 atoms of hydrogen attached. The structure can rotate around single bonds and is constantly twisting and bending. A flat space with an extra line indicates a double bond, as will be seen in future examples.

COMPARISON OF DIETARY FATS

Dietary Fat	Cholesterol mg/Tbsp.	Saturated Fat	Polyunsaturated Fat	Other Fats	Monounsaturated Fat
Crisco Puritan® Oil (canola oil)	0	6%	31%	←1%	62%
Safflower Oil	0	9%	78%	←1%	12%
Crisco® Vegetable Oil	0	10%	51%		39%
Sunflower Oil	0	11%	69%		20%
Corn Oil	0	13%	62%		25%
Peanut Oil	0	13%	33%	5%	49%
Olive Oil	0	14%	9%		77%
Soybean Oil	0	15%	61%		24%
Margarine (fat)	0	18%	29%	5%	48%
Vegetable Shortening	0	26%	25%	6%	43%
Cottonseed Oil	0	27%	54%		19%
Chicken Fat	11	30%	22%	←1%	47%
Lard	12	41%	12%		47%
Animal Fat Shortening (precreamed)	9	43%	6%	←3%	48%
Beef Fat	14	51%	4%	←1%	44%
Palm Oil	0	51%	10%		39%
Butter (fat)	33	54%	4%	12%	30%
Coconut Oil	0	77%	←2%	15%	6%

The values shown for saturated and polyunsaturated fats are based on Federal Regulations, Title 21, Section 101.25(c)(2)(ii)(a&b). These state that: (a) saturated fat is the sum of lauric, myristic, palmitic and stearic acids, and (b) polyunsaturated fat is cis, cis-methylene-interrupted polyunsaturated fatty acids. "Other Fats" include saturated and polyunsaturated fatty acids that are outside of these definitions.

Provided as a Professional Service by Procter & Gamble© 1992 P&G

References:
Crisco Puritan Oil, Crisco Vegetable Oil, vegetable shortening, animal fat (precreamed) shortening; data on file, Procter & Gamble.
Margarine: Slover, H.T. et al, Lipids in Margarines and Margarine-Like Foods, Journal of the American Oil Chemists' Society, Vol. 62, 775-786, 1985.
All others: Reeves, J.B. and Weihrauch, J.L., Composition of Foods, Agriculture Handbook No. 8-4, Washington, D.C.: United States Department of Agriculture, 1979.

Figure 5–3 Comparison of dietary fats.

Polyunsaturated Fatty Acids

A polyunsaturated fatty acid (PUFA) has more than 2 double bonds.

When numerous carbons are connected by double bonds, the fatty acid is **polyunsaturated.** Linoleic, linolenic, and arachidonic acids are polyunsaturated. Linoleic acid is the most prevalent **PUFA** and is the predominant fatty acid in safflower, sunflower, corn, cottonseed, soybean, and sesame oils (see Fig. 5–3). These PUFAs are omega-6 fatty acids, having their first double bond on the sixth carbon from the omega (terminal) end.

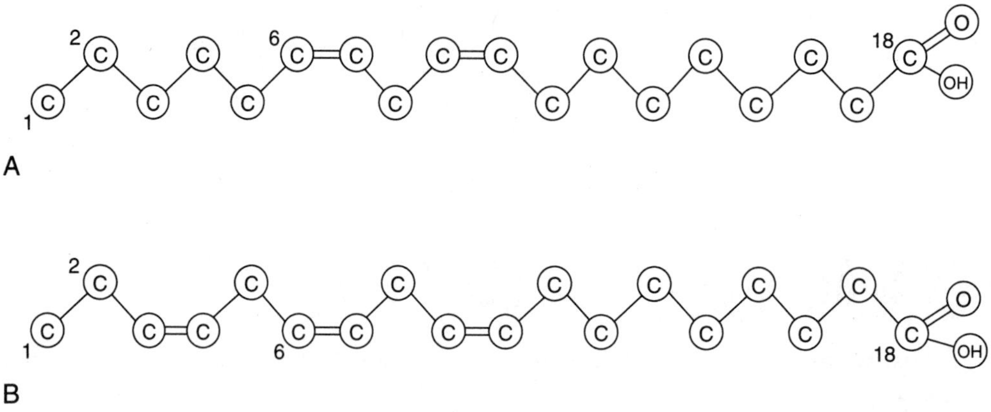

A

B

A, **Linoleic acid (18:2), an omega-6 fatty acid.** *B*, **Linolenic acid (18:3), an omega-6 fatty acid.**

Omega-3 fatty acids include eicosapentaenoic acid (EPA) and docosahexaenoic acid (DHA).

Give examples of PUFAs and where they are found.

Omega-3 is another class of PUFA. These fatty acids are unique in that the first double bond is located 3 carbons from the omega end of the molecule; hence they are called omega-3s or n-3s. Fish oils contain both omega-3 fatty acids, which appear to have many health benefits.

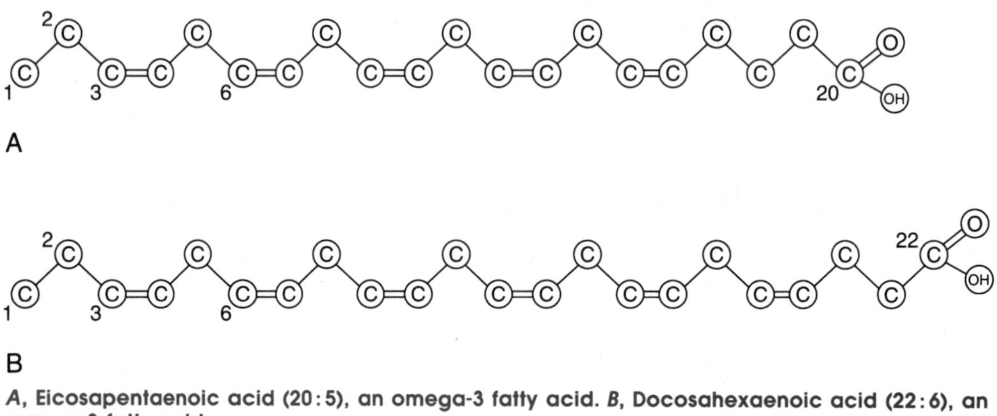

A

B

A, **Eicosapentaenoic acid (20:5), an omega-3 fatty acid.** *B*, **Docosahexaenoic acid (22:6), an omega-3 fatty acid.**

P/S Ratio

P/S ratio is the amount of PUFAs present as compared with the saturated fatty acid content.

If PUFAs exceed saturated fatty acids, the food is classified as polyunsaturated. No triglyceride occurring naturally is totally saturated or unsaturated.

A healthy diet is composed of more unsaturated fats (both monounsaturated and PUFA) than saturated fats. Nutrition labels indicated the grams of polyunsaturated and saturated fats so that the P/S ratio could be determined. New labels, however, only indicate the amount (in gm) of total fat and saturated fat.

NURSING APPLICATIONS

1. Foods having higher fat content are more kilocalorie-dense; ¼ cup of peanuts and 7 whole carrots have the same number of kilocalories (210). Carrots have only a trace of fat. Peanuts contain 18 gm of fat per ¼ cup. Therefore, knowledge of fat content of foods is necessary to assess for fat intake.
2. Because omega-3 fatty acids may be beneficial for health, determine the frequency of fish consumption. A higher intake may help clients recover faster.
3. Have client actually read a nutrition label to determine a good buy as well as a healthy choice for fat. A rule of thumb to remember is if fat content is greater than 3 gm/100 kcal, fat content is too high.

Client Education

- Tropical oils, including palm oil, palm kernel oil, and coconut oil, are saturated fats and undesirable in the diet.
- Total fat should be less than 30% of total caloric intake.
- Purchase processed foods that contain more polyunsaturated and monounsaturated fatty acids. If the food label contains only the required information (total fat and saturated fat content), subtract the gm saturated fat from the total fat.*

Characteristics

Carbon chain length and the degree of saturation determine various properties of fats, including flavor and melting point or hardness.

Chain Length versus Saturation

Saturated fatty acids are solid at room temperature, especially if most of the fatty acids contain more than 12 carbon atoms. Animal fats contain mostly saturated fats and are solids at room temperature. However, the chain length prevails over the effect of saturation. Short-chain fatty acids (12 carbon atoms or less), monounsaturated fatty acids, and PUFAs are liquids at room temperature and are called oils. Milk fat contains a large amount of short-chain saturated fatty acids.

Hydrogenation

Polyunsaturated vegetable oil can be converted to a saturated fat by a process called hydrogenation.

Hydrogen added to an unsaturated fat at the double bonds in the presence of a catalyst results in a saturated fat. This commercial process to produce solid margarine and vegetable shortening increases the proportion of saturated fatty acids. Hydrogenation can be controlled so that "tub" or "soft" margarine is available. These margarines usually contain "partially hydrogenated" vegetable oils.

During hydrogenation, the shape of the fatty acid is altered. PUFAs naturally occur in what is called the "cis" (i.e., on the same side) configuration; the carbon chain bends so hydrogens stick out on the same side of the molecule. During processing, the groups may rotate so they are on opposite sides of the bond, ion the "trans" position. In 1989, the National Academy of Sciences (NAS) (NRC, 1989a)

* Example: Product contains 8 gm fat and 3 gm saturated fat. Therefore, there are 5 gm monounsaturated and polyunsaturated fats (>3 gm saturated fat). This product is acceptable, but a similar product (if available) containing <3 gm saturated fat would be a wiser choice.

determined intake in the US to be about 6% of the total fat intake. Although NAS concluded that trans fatty acids do not appear to be harmful at current levels of consumption, the subject continues to be researched.

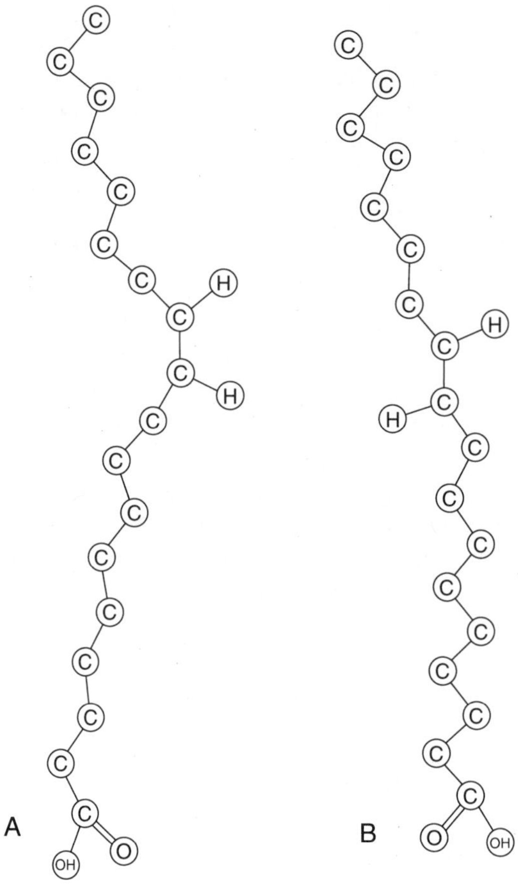

A, **Oleic acid: "cis" form (note the kink in the molecule).** *B*, **Elaidic acid: "trans" form.**

Rancidity

Fats become rancid when subjected to high temperatures and exposure to light, which cause oxidation and decomposition of fats.

Is hydrogenation nutritionally beneficial? How can rancidity of fats be prevented?

Fats with a high proportion of unsaturated fatty acids are more susceptible to **rancidity,** resulting in off flavors and odors. The decomposition results in peroxides that may be toxic in large amounts. Unpalatable flavors and odors, however, generally prevent clients from eating rancid fats.

Vitamin E, a fat-soluble vitamin, is an antioxidant and, to some degree, protects the oil. When used as an antioxidant, however, it is inactivated as a vitamin for the body. Antioxidants, for example butylated hydroxyanisole (BHA) and butylated hydroxytoluene (BHT), are added to commercially processed fats and oils to prevent their spoilage. They also help prevent vitamin E content from oxidation.

Compound Lipids

Glycerol and fatty acids combined with carbohydrate, phosphate, and/or nitrogenous compounds, are called compound lipids.

Compound lipids, such as phospholipids and lipoproteins, are found in foods and/or produced by the body.

Phospholipids

Phospholipids contain phosphorus and a nitrogenous base in addition to fatty acids and alcohol.

Fats from both plant and animal foods contain phospholipids. Commercially, phospholipids are used as additives in products to aid in emulsification.

Lipoproteins

The liver and intestinal mucosa produce **lipoproteins** to transport insoluble fats. Several types are present in the blood: high-density lipoproteins (HDL), low-density lipoproteins (LDL), very low-density lipoproteins (VLDL), and chylomicrons. Their role in heart disease is discussed in Chapter 24.

Lipoproteins contain triglycerides, phospholipids, and cholesterol combined with protein.

Give examples of compound lipids. Where are phospholipids found? What is the function of lipoproteins?

Cholesterol

Cholesterol is not a fat but a fat-like substance classified as a lipid. Cholesterol synthesis occurs predominantly in the liver and small intestine. Because the body can produce all the cholesterol it needs, cholesterol intake is not essential.

Cholesterol is a fat-related lipid with a complex ring structure called a sterol.

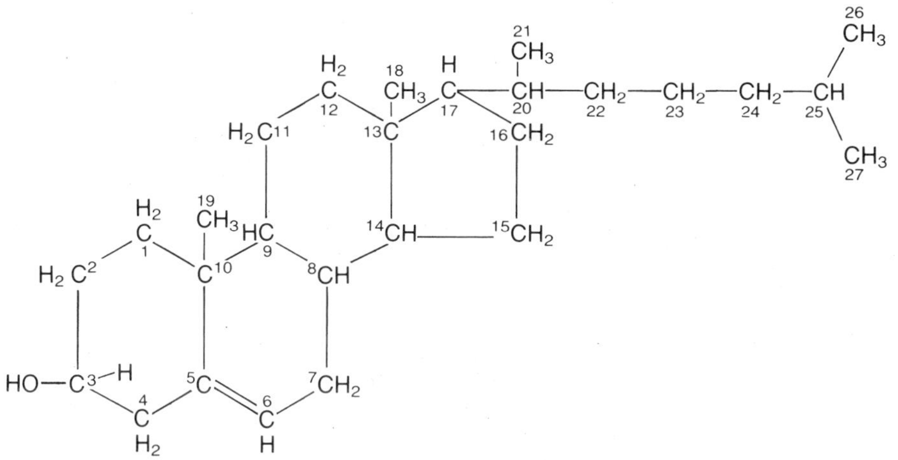

Cholesterol, $C_{27}H_{45}OH$.

Synthetic Fats

Medium-Chain Triglycerides

Medium-chain triglycerides (MCTs) are commercially produced for clients with fat malabsorption problems because of their ability to be easily absorbed. They can be purchased as an oil and are used in many infant and tube feeding formulas. The use of MCT oils can be beneficial by providing a concentrated source of kilocalories. Because they do not contain EFA, they cannot be used as the only source of fat.

MCTs contain 8 to 10 carbon atoms in each fatty acid.

Why are MCTs appropriate for clients with malabsorption?

Structured Lipids

Structured lipids are now used in some tube feeding formulas. These lipids are beneficial in providing readily available fuel and EFAs for various disease states.

Structured lipids combine specific fatty acids, including medium-chain fatty acids and long-chain fatty acids, from the omega-6 and omega-3 fatty acid families.

Fat Substitutes

As a result of growing concern over dietary fats, numerous foods are being manufactured containing less fat. Carbohydrate-based, protein-based, and lipid-based materials have been formulated that possess diverse sensory, functional, and physiological properties. Low-kilocalorie salad dressing, low-fat yogurt, and imitation margarine are all made by using modified starches and gums to reduce the oil or fat in the product.

Simplesse is a fat substitute containing only 1 to 2 kcal/gm made from egg white and milk protein. Fat content of a product can be reduced as much as 20 to 80% (ADA, 1988). Simplesse resembles fat by producing a creamy smooth feeling in the mouth like fats, but it coagulates and loses this creaminess at high temperatures. Thus, the use of this original product is limited to dairy products (such as ice cream and cream cheese) and oil-based products (such as salad dressings and margarine) that do not require heat in processing. A more versatile version of Simplesse has been introduced on the market that is a whey protein concentrate. It can be used in all food categories, including baked goods, cheese for hamburgers and pizza, soups, and sauces.

Trailblazer is another protein-based fat substitute similar to Simplesse. FDA clearance is expected in the near future.

Sucrose polyester is a synthetic fat that resembles conventional dietary fats and can be substituted in many foods. Olestra is the proposed name for sucrose polyester. Its status is pending FDA approval. Because it is not digested or absorbed, it contributes 0 kcal. It provides the taste, texture, and mouth feel of conventional fats. Olestra can be used to replace some of the fat in shortenings and oils and for deep fat frying (Morrison, 1990).

Already on the market is a reduced-kilocalorie fat, Caprenin, that resembles cocoa butter but contains only 5 kcal/gm. It has been approved for use in soft candy and confectionery coatings.

Needless to say, within the near future, countless other fat substitutes will be available. Because of the possible connection between excessive fat intake and chronic diseases, fat substitutes may be helpful in reducing fat consumption. By replacing fat with fat substitutes, some weight loss can be achieved (Kendall et al, 1991) or the total fat intake reduced (Rolls, 1991). An overall weight loss program, however, will still be needed to effect weight loss (Rolls, 1991). Fat substitutes appear to pose little risk to health, but data are sparse regarding possible benefits under conditions of normal consumer use (Mela, 1992).

NURSING APPLICATIONS

1. Assess use of fat substitutes.
2. A high serum level of HDLs is desirable to prevent heart disease, so monitor HDL levels in the blood.
3. MCT oil is used for clients with celiac disease and other GI conditions. If it is not being used and the client is underweight or losing weight, suggest a consultation with a dietitian or physician.
4. Evaluate dietary habits because clients may think fat substitutes will make a desirable change in health without considering other aspects of their diet.

Client Education

- Simplesse cannot be used for frying or baking and contains 1 to 2 kcal/gm. Other proposed fat substitutes may be used for frying.
- Clients allergic to egg or cow milk could be at risk for an allergic reaction to Simplesse.
- Intake of fat substitute products needs to be balanced with variety and moderation in food choices to achieve an overall healthy nutritious diet.

DIGESTION

Most fats in the diet are in the form of triglycerides. Of course, the first action on fats is the chewing process, which helps to break apart the fats physically and to warm them. Lingual lipase begins hydrolysis of triglycerides.

Gastric lipase is specific in hydrolysis of medium-chain and short-chain fatty acids. These fatty acids are then transported to the liver bound to albumin (Fig. 5–4). Gastric lipase plays a more important role in newborn infants and possibly in clients with cystic fibrosis as a result of low levels of pancreatic lipase and **bile salts.**

Bile salts emulsify and reduce surface tension of fats and thereby allow large insoluble molecules to be divided into smaller particles.

The presence of fat in chyme stimulates the release of cholecystokinin, which causes the gallbladder to contract and release its bile. Peristalsis facilitates the mixing and emulsification process by bile.

Describe digestion of fats.

Lipases in the pancreatic and intestinal secretions are able to hydrolyze triglycerides to fatty acids and glycerol.

ABSORPTION

As compared with medium-chain and short-chain fatty acids, which are water soluble, fatty acids with 12 or more carbon atoms are insoluble in water and must enter the blood stream via the lymphatic system. These large molecules can be ab-

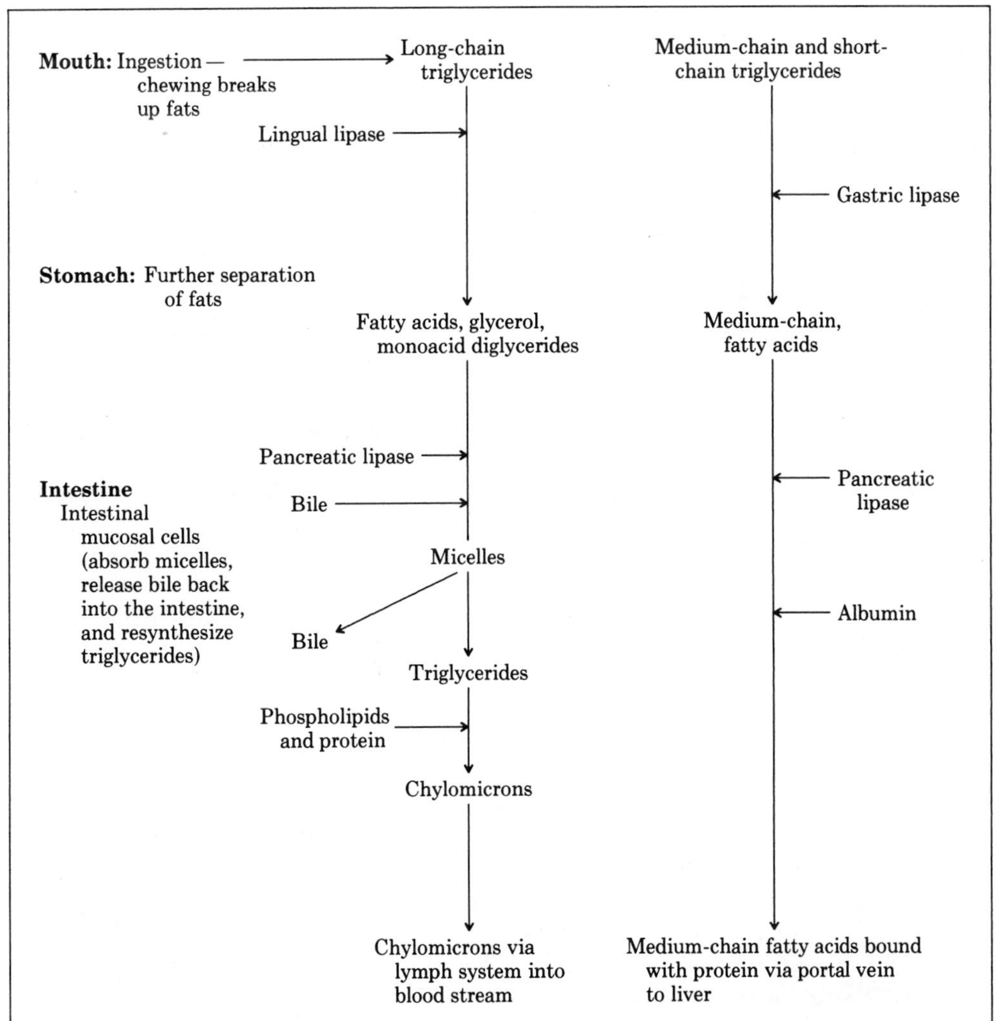

Figure 5–4 Digestion and absorption of fats.

sorbed by the intestinal villi. The mechanism for absorption of these fatty acids is a complicated procedure (see Fig. 5–4).

Micelles are bile salts complexed with fats for absorption.

1. Bile salts combine with products of fat digestion and disperse them into tiny units called **micelles.** These can pass through the intestinal membrane. Bile salts are separated from the fat products after they pass through the intestinal wall to be reused again.
2. In the intestinal mucosa, digestion of the monoglycerides and diglycerides may be completed by the action of intestinal lipase. All the available fatty acids and glycerol molecules are synthesized into new triglycerides.
3. In the final stage, the new triglyceride is enclosed with a protein coating. This lipoprotein complex, called a **chylomicron,** is produced in the intestinal mucosa. Chylomicrons are carried via the lymph system to enter the blood stream at the subclavian vein (see Fig. 5–4). They are then transported to the liver and adipose tissue for metabolism and storage.

Chylomicrons promote the absorption and transport of lipids from the GI tract.

Steatorrhea is a large amount of fat in the feces.

Describe the absorption of long-chain fatty acids.

When inadequate amounts of bile are available, **steatorrhea** occurs.

The amount of cholesterol absorbed is highly variable; generally about half of the dietary cholesterol is absorbed.

DIGESTIBILITY

Digestion of high-fat meals is slower than for other energy-containing nutrients, resulting in such phrases as "high satiety value" or "sticks to the ribs." The higher the fat content of a meal, the longer the food remains in the stomach. Nevertheless, about 95% of the ingested fats is absorbed. Soft fats that are liquids at body temperature (like margarine) are digested more quickly than hard fats, such as meat fats.

NURSING APPLICATIONS

1. In the geriatric client, assess serum cholesterol levels because aging changes lipid absorption and decreases uptake of cholesterol (Thomson, 1989).
2. Infants, young children, and some older clients may experience discomfort after high-fat meals. If this occurs, offer softer, emulsified fats (in milk and eggs) for better tolerance.
3. Foods fried in low temperatures absorb excessive amounts of fats, whereas those fried in very high temperatures result in decomposition of some fats, which can be irritating to the intestine. Therefore, monitor client's physical status after meals, especially with fried foods.
4. Lipid malabsorption occurs when bile salts and pancreatic lipase are not available or when mucosal cells are damaged (as in celiac disease), resulting in steatorrhea and loss of fat-soluble vitamins. Thus, monitor output (steatorrhea) and physical status for deficiencies in vitamins A, D, and K, and EFA (see Chapter 6).
5. In clients with fat malabsorption disorder, offer MCTs for effective digestion/absorption of the needed fats.

Client Education

- Although the digestion of fried foods takes longer, digestion is as complete as for other foods in most persons if the proper frying temperature is used.
- The use of mineral oil is not advisable because of its laxative effect, which reduces absorption of fat-soluble vitamins.

TABLE 5–2

HORMONAL ROLE IN FAT METABOLISM

Hormone	Effect	Action
Insulin		Activates lipoprotein lipase
Lack	Decreases lipogenesis; increases lipolysis	
Excess	Increases lipolysis; inhibits fat utilization	
Thyroxin	Increases lipolysis	Increases rate of energy metabolism
Glucocorticoids	Increase lipolysis	Increase fat-cell membrane permeability
Adrenocorticoids	Increase lipolysis	Stimulate secretion of glucocorticoids
Epinephrine and norepinephrine	Increase lipolysis	Increase release of free fatty acids from fat cells

FAT METABOLISM

The liver is the principal regulator of fat metabolism and lipoprotein synthesis. Hormones involved in carbohydrate metabolism also control fat metabolism (Table 5–2). In the liver, fatty acids can be hydrolyzed or modified by shortening, lengthening, or adding double bonds before their release into the circulation.

Cholesterol is produced, removed from the blood, and used to make bile acids by the liver. **Lipotropic substances** that prevent fatty liver include choline, vitamin B_{12}, and possibly inositol.

Lipotropic substances present in the liver prevent fat accumulation in the liver.

What organ is the principal regulator of fat metabolism?

Metabolism of chylomicrons in the liver results in triglycerides being transported to the tissues for energy or other uses or carried to adipose tissue to be stored. Serum triglycerides are the result of not only absorption from foods, but also the conversion of carbohydrates and proteins into fats (Fig. 5–5).

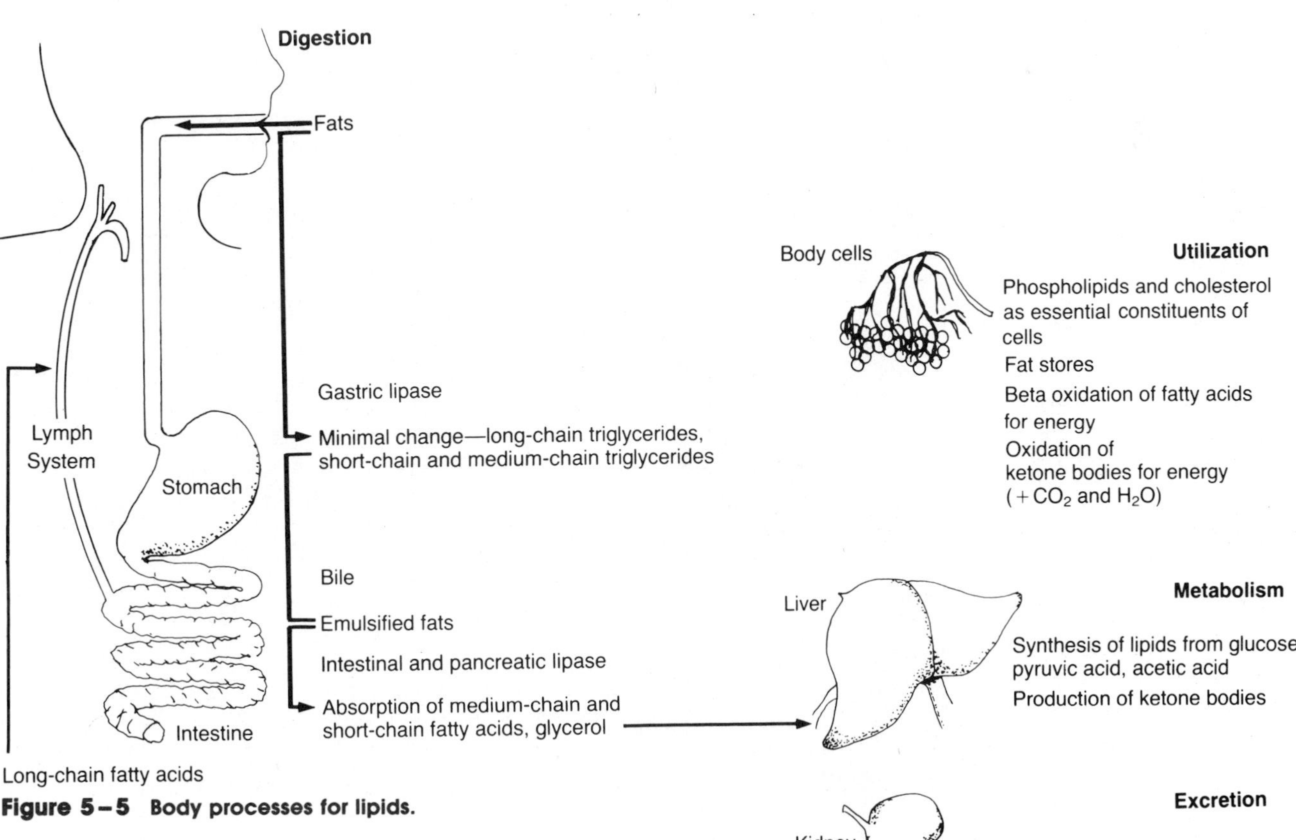

Figure 5–5 Body processes for lipids.

OXIDATION

Oxidation is the process of hydrolyzing triglycerides into 2-carbon entities to enter the Krebs cycle for energy production.

The oxidation of 1 lb of fat results in 3500 kcal released for energy. (This is more than most clients use in a 24-hour period).

When excessive amounts of fats are oxidized for energy, the liver is overwhelmed, and ketone bodies are formed. Ketone bodies are not oxidized in the liver but are carried to the skeletal and cardiac muscles, where they are rapidly metabolized under normal circumstances.

The capacity of the tissues to use ketone bodies may be exceeded when the glucose supply is reduced. Even during **ketosis,** some ketone bodies are being oxidized normally in the tissues.

Ketosis is accumulation of ketone bodies in the blood. Ketonuria is the excretion of ketones in the urine.

Hyperuricemia—elevated serum uric acid.

What occurs when large amounts of fats are oxidized for energy? What can ketosis cause?

Ketosis can be a dangerous condition for several reasons. These strong acids must be neutralized by bases to maintain the acid–base balance in the blood. Thus, they are generally carried through the blood and into the urine with sodium. If the amount of base available is inadequate, acidosis may result. In addition to the loss of sodium ions, large amounts of water are lost, which can lead to dehydration (or rapid weight loss for the dieter). Elevated blood ketones also promote **hyperuricemia.** When the blood glucose levels remain low for several days, the brain and nerve cells adapt to use ketones for some of their fuel requirements.

FAT SYNTHESIS

Lipogenesis is fat synthesis. Lipolysis is fat breakdown.

Triglycerides can be synthesized in the intestinal mucosa, in adipose tissue, and in the liver. **Lipogenesis** and **lipolysis** are continual processes, which are in equilibrium when the energy needs of the body are balanced.

NURSING APPLICATIONS

1. Cholesterol is present in the blood primarily in LDLs and HDLs. When monitoring serum cholesterol levels, be sure to check LDL and HDL levels.
2. Fatty livers can be the result of starvation, diabetes mellitus, deficiency of lipotropic substances, poisons, drugs, and excessive alcohol intake. Therefore, assess clients with fatty livers for these conditions.
3. Ketosis does not occur just because of rapid breakdown of adipose tissue but when accompanied by carbohydrate deprivation. Thus, be sure clients receive adequate carbohydrate intake.
4. Ketosis and ketonuria may occur in starvation or diabetes mellitus or on diets containing less than 50 gm of carbohydrate. If these conditions occur, check for ketones in the urine.
5. Because high ketone levels result in an unusual breath odor, similar to acetone or nail polish remover, smell the client's breath if ketosis is suspected.
6. Evaluate client's weight and use of diets because high ketone levels may be associated with starvation or high-protein, low-carbohydrate, low-kilocalorie diets. This results in decreased appetite and occasionally nausea, which can worsen the condition.

Client Education

- Serum cholesterol below 200 mg/dl is desirable.
- High-protein, low-carbohydrate diets have been promoted as an effective way of excreting kilocalories to lose weight through ketonuria. At most, however, about 20 gm/day of ketones may be excreted in the urine, or less than 100 kcal/day. This is an insignificant amount and not worth the risk involved.

PHYSIOLOGICAL ROLES

Concentrated Energy

Dietary fats are a concentrated source of energy, furnishing 9 kcal/gm. Foods high in fats are generally referred to as **"kilocalorie dense,"** which to a certain extent has its merits. The advantage of kilocalorie-dense foods is that it is not necessary to consume large volumes of food to furnish the energy requirements.

Kilocalorie-dense foods are usually high in fats (or fat and sugar) and low in other nutrients.

Protein Sparers

As an energy source, fats are also referred to as "protein sparing" because they allow protein to be used for important functions such as building and repairing tissues. Fats are also vitamin sparing when they are used for energy, as opposed to carbohydrates, which require thiamin and other B vitamins.

Satiety Value

Fats are important in the diet for their high **satiety** value. Because they depress gastric secretions and retard emptying of the stomach, they delay the rapid development of hunger.

Satiety is the state of being full; fats contribute to a feeling of fullness for a longer period of time than carbohydrates or protein.

Palatability

Fats contribute to palatability and flavor of foods. Their use in cooking improves texture.

Complementary Relationships

Fat-soluble vitamins and the EFAs are generally found in foods containing fat. The absorption of these vitamins is facilitated by the presence of fats in the GI tract.

Name 3 functions of fats.

Fat Storage

Adipose tissue has several roles: It provides a concentrated energy source, protects internal organs, and maintains body temperature.

Energy

Excess carbohydrates and protein are converted to fat and stored in adipose tissue. Fatty acids can be used as an energy source by all cells except erythrocytes (red blood cells) and those of the central nervous system. Clients have been known to survive total starvation for 30 to 40 days.

Protection of Organs

Fatty tissue surrounds vital organs and provides a cushion, thereby protecting them from traumatic injury and shock.

Insulation

The subcutaneous layer of fat functions as an insulator that preserves body heat and maintains body temperature. Excessive layers of fat can also deter heat loss during warm weather. Two types of fat are present in the body, white and brown. The fat in subcutaneous tissue, abdominal cavity, and intramuscular fat is known as white fat.

Describe how fat provides energy, protects organs, and insulates the body. What is the difference between white and brown fat?

Brown fat has a different role than energy storage. It is located particularly in the interscapular region and the back of the neck. Energy is not collected and stored as ATP but dissipates as heat to warm the body. The role of brown fat is unknown, but it may account for the variability in energy requirements of clients.

Essential Fatty Acids

Linoleic acid is considered an EFA because it must be supplied from dietary sources.

Linoleic acid (18-carbon chain with 2 double bonds) cannot be synthesized by the body. If linoleic acid is not furnished in the diet, deficiency symptoms result. Arachidonic (18-carbon chain with 4 double bonds) and linolenic (18-carbon chain with 3 double bonds) acids are also considered EFAs, but children and adults can produce them from sufficient quantities of linoleic acid. These EFAs are required for proper growth and healthy skin.

Phospholipids

Also called phosphatides, phospholipids are produced from EFAs. As key components of cellular membranes, they are the second most prevalent form of fat in the body. Phospholipids are a part of the lipoprotein molecule important in fat absorption and transport of fats in the blood.

Phospholipids include lecithin, cephalin, and sphingomyelins. Lecithin, the most widely distributed phospholipid, is a component of the erythrocyte plasma membrane and is present in all cells. Cephalin is present in thromboplastin, necessary for blood clotting. Sphingomyelins are important constituents of brain tissue and of the myelin sheath around nerve fibers.

Eicosanoids

The omega-3 fatty acids are found principally in fish. EPA and arachidonic acid are metabolized into eicosanoids. Eicosanoids are important physiologically in regulation of blood pressure, blood clotting, immune responses, GI secretions, cardiovascular function, and inflammatory reactions. The omega-3 fatty acids are discussed in further detail in Nutrition Update 5–1.

Which fatty acid cannot be produced by the body? What is the second most prevalent form of fat in the body? What are the functions of lecithin, cephalin, sphingomyelins, and eicosanoids?

Cholesterol

Although cholesterol is not a dietary essential, it has important functions as a constituent of brain and nervous tissues, a precursor of vitamin D and steroid hormones, a constituent of bile salts, and a structural component of cell membranes. It is transported in the blood via lipoproteins.

Glycolipids

Glycolipids are produced from fatty acids, carbohydrate, and nitrogen. Cerebrosides and gangliosides are included in this classification. Structurally they are components of brain and nerve tissue and certain cell membranes, where they function in cell permeability for fats.

Nursing Applications

1. Fat deficiency results in poor growth, dermatitis (Fig. 5–6), lowered resistance to infection, and poor reproductive capacity. Therefore, assess intake of fat through interviewing and monitoring intake.
2. If clients have a poor reserve of subcutaneous fat, monitor temperature closely. These clients are not able to regulate temperature as effectively as clients who have subcutaneous fat reserves.
3. Lecithin supplements lower serum cholesterol in some clients, but in other studies, lecithin lowers the blood cholesterol only transiently. Thus, close monitoring of serum cholesterol is needed.
4. Evaluate total fat intake. Clients need adequate amounts of fat to allow protein to perform its function (build and repair). If total energy intake is inadequate, healing is slower. Also, inadequate fat intake could lead to secondary deficiencies of the fat-soluble vitamins.

Client Education

- Serum cholesterol can be lowered by diets low in total fat and high in the EFAs or PUFAs.
- The consumption of soluble fibers may decrease serum cholesterol.
- The ratio of PUFAs to omega-3 fatty acids can affect platelet function and inflammatory responses and possibly influence disease conditions such as coronary heart disease and rheumatoid disease (Leaf & Weber, 1988).
- Fats act as a lubricant in the intestines, thereby decreasing constipation.
- The primary form of fat in the body is triglyceride, not cholesterol.

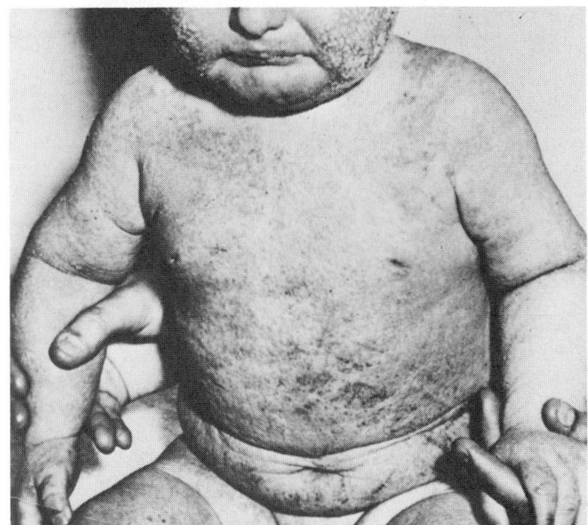

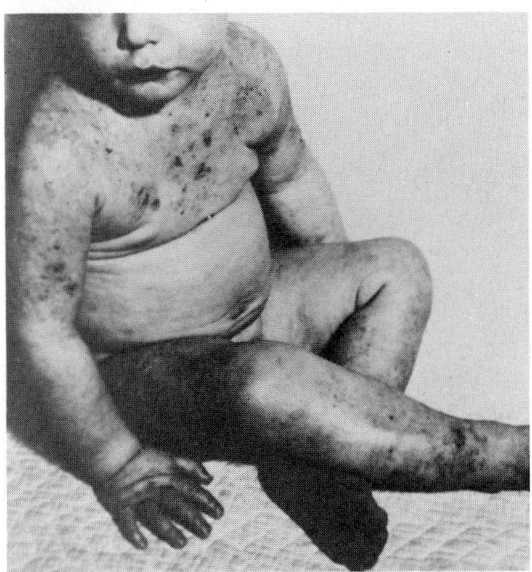

Figure 5–6 The first symptoms identified specifically as being due to essential fatty acid (EFA) deficiency were skin lesions in rats. Similar lesions were seen in infants given formulas devoid of EFAs. This research was carried out before the critical nature of EFAs was known. Ethical considerations would prohibit such research today. *A*, Six-month-old infant with very resistant eczema appearing at 2½ months of age. *B*, The same child 6 months later after a source of linoleic acid had been included in the diet. (Courtesy of the late Dr. A. E. Hansen.)

TABLE 5–3

CALCULATION OF DIETARY FAT*

(1) Determine kilocaloric level of the diet (the RDA on the inside cover can be used)
Example: Client needs 2000 kcal

(2) Multiply the kilocalories by 0.30 to determine the number of kilocalories of fat the diet can contain
Example: 2000 kcal × 0.30 (% of total kcal) = 600 kcal from fat

(3) Divide the answer by 9 to determine the grams of fat allowed daily
Example: 600 kcal from fat ÷ 9 kcal/gm fat = 66.6 gm fat

* Determination of the amount of fat a diet can contain to meet the Dietary Guidelines of 30% or less.

DIETARY REQUIREMENTS

Linoleic acid is the only dietary requirement for fat. The American Academy of Pediatrics (1985) recommends 2.7% of the kilocalories in infant formulas be EFAs. The requirement for adults is lower, about 3 to 6 gm/day (NRC, 1989a). When dietary intake is high, linoleic acid is stored in the tissues.

Human requirements for omega-3 fatty acids have long been disputed. Research by scientists at USDA Agriculture Research Service has determined that linolenic acid in soybean oil can rapidly be converted into omega-3 fatty acids (Anonymous, 1989). The conversion of linolenic acid to EPA and linoleic acid to arachidonic acid compete for the same enzyme. If intake of linoleic acid is substantially higher than intake of linolenic acid, the result is less EPA available (Nettleton, 1991). Omega-3 fatty acids may be shown to be essential as further studies examine their many and varied effects.

What are the requirements for linoleic acid and fat?

Currently, approximately 42% of the kilocalories in the typical American diet is from fat (Raper, 1991). As discussed in Chapter 1, numerous health organizations recommend total fat intake be limited to 30% of total kilocalories. To provide adequate amounts of fat-soluble vitamins and EFAs, a minimum of 15 to 25 gm fat is recommended. Determination of appropriate grams of dietary fat is shown in Table 5–3.

TABLE 5–4

FATS IN FOODS

Saturated

High fat content: Beef, lamb, luncheon meats (cold cuts, frankfurters, etc.), pork (including ham and salt pork), hard yellow cheeses, sweet cream, sour cream

Low fat content: Veal, organ meats, whole and part-skim milk, yogurt, cottage cheese

Monounsaturated

High fat content: Duck, goose, eggs

Low fat content: Chicken, turkey

Polyunsaturated

Low fat content: Fish, shellfish, salmon, tuna

Fats and Oils

Saturated: Butter, lard, coconut oil, palm oil, hydrogenated or "hardened" vegetable oils, regular margarine

Monounsaturated: Olive oil, peanut oil

Polyunsaturated: Safflower oil, corn oil, cottonseed oil, sesame oil, soybean oil, sunflower oil, salad dressings from these oils, special margarines listing liquid oil first

SOURCES

Foods high in saturated, monounsaturated, and polyunsaturated fatty acids are itemized in Table 5–4. The most important sources of saturated fats are the meat and milk groups; for monounsaturated fatty acids, the meat and grain groups; and for PUFAs, the grain group and additional fats and oils. Linoleic acid is highest in safflower, sunflower, and corn oil, with lesser amounts present in soybean and canola oil. Linolenic acid is present in linseed oil (not available in the US), canola oil, and soybean oil and in small amounts in green leafy vegetables, seaweed or plankton, and meat fats. EPA and DHA are found in fish.

Cholesterol is found only in animal products; it is not found in egg whites or plant foods. It is highest in egg yolk, liver, and other organ meats.

Food Choices

Percentage of fat by weight is widely used on food labels and advertising. Although this information is correct, it is misleading to the American public. The recommendation that fat intake should be limited to 30% refers to the percentage of fat based on the total kilocalories of the product. As shown in Table 5–5, the percentage of fat in milk by kilocalories is 49%, not 3.3% as the label normally indicates. Clients need to be aware of these differences to know that a label indicating "25% less fat" may still not be a desirable food choice.

Wide publicity about the benefits of a lower fat diet has resulted in some Americans changing their food habits without adequate information regarding fat content of foods and changes in food composition by the food industry. For most clients, a decrease in red meat consumption was probably desirable, but many have chosen to eliminate it from their diet altogether. In recent years, through improvements in breeding and feeding livestock, these products are lower in fat, kilocalories, and cholesterol, as shown in Figure 5–7. Other important nutrients are present in beef, pork, and lamb; moderate use of these products is encouraged. Loin (sirloin, tenderloin, center loin) and round cuts (top, bottom, eye, or tip) and lean or extra-lean ground beef contain the least amount of fat.

After consideration of total fat content of a product, the next priority is its saturated fat content. Figure 5–8 provides a general continuum of saturated and unsaturated fats.

What are food sources for saturated fatty acids, monounsaturated fatty acids, and PUFAs? What are food sources for linolenic acid, EPA, and cholesterol?

TABLE 5–5

ANALYSIS OF FAT CONTENT OF MILK

	Kilocalories (1 cup)	Total Fat (gm)	Percent of Fat by Weight	Percent of Fat by Kilocalories
Whole Milk	150	8.1	3.3	49
Low-fat Milk (2%)	120	4.7	2	35
Low-fat Milk (1%)	102	2.6	1	23
Skim Milk	86	0.4	<1	4

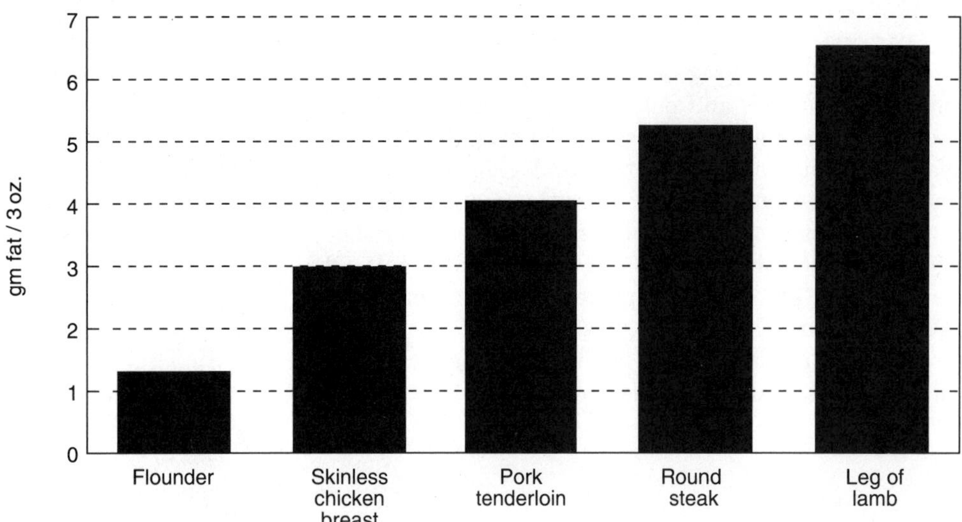

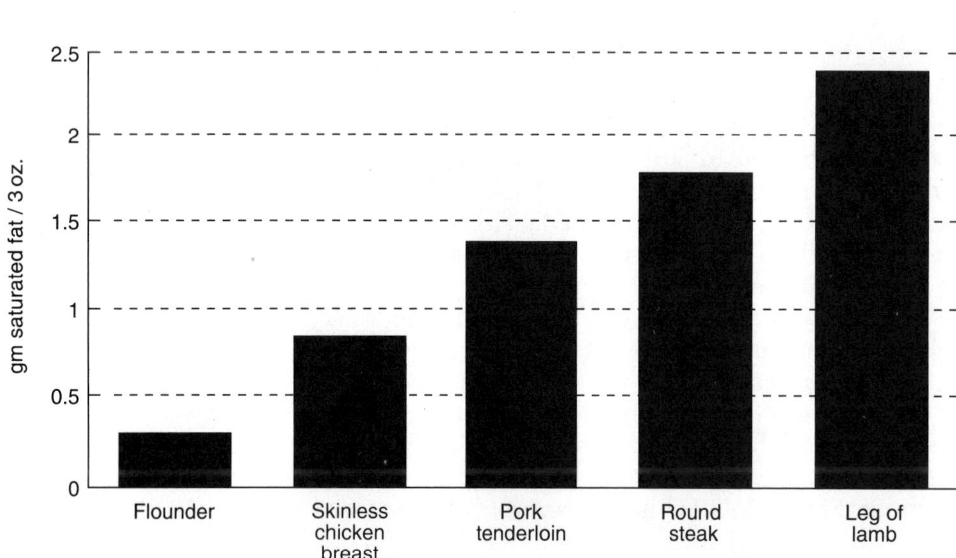

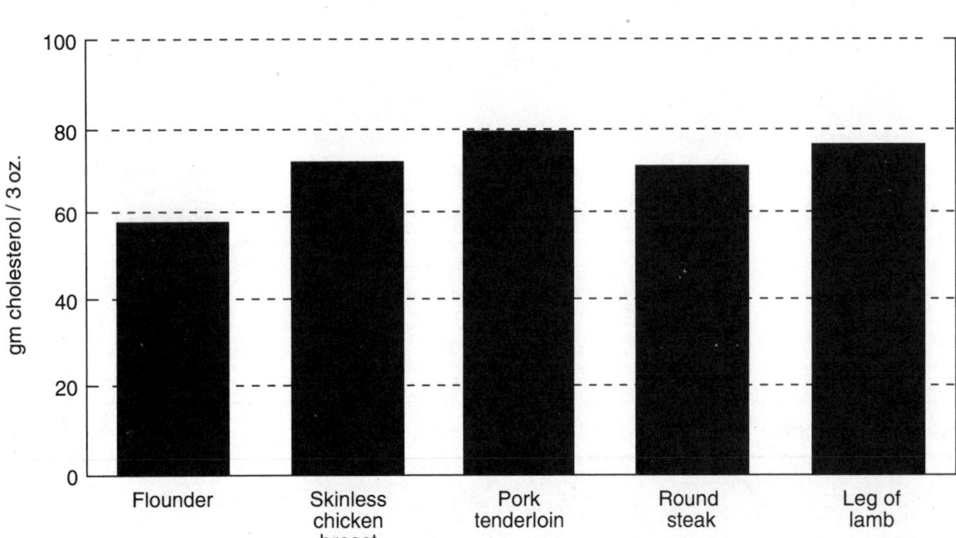

Figure 5–7 **Fat, saturated fat, and cholesterol content of meats (3 oz. cooked (baked/roasted) and trimmed).** ***A*****, Fat content comparison.** ***B*****, Saturated fat content comparison.** ***C*****, Cholesterol content comparison.**

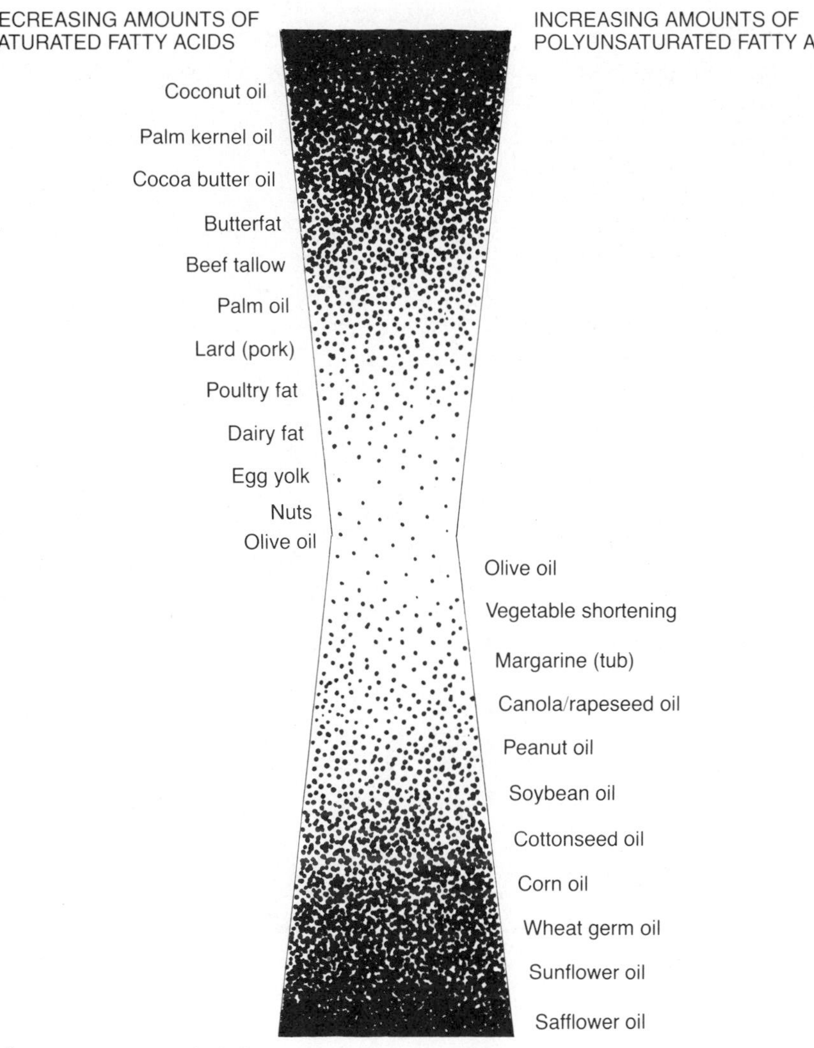

Figure 5–8 Continuum of fatty acid saturation.

Nursing Applications

1. Use Table 5–3 to assess fat recommendations.
2. Clients frequently consume more fat than they realize because of the "invisible" fats in the milk (including cheese) and meat groups. Therefore, interview clients to assess their intake of these foods.
3. Animal products contribute approximately 53% of total fat intake and contain principally saturated fatty acids (Raper, 1991). If mainly animal products are consumed, risk for cardiovascular disease may be increased because of the high intake of saturated fat. Monitor blood lipid levels.
4. To evaluate the client's knowledge of fat principles, have the client state the dietary requirements for linoleic acid and fat intake and foods high in saturated, monounsaturated, and polyunsaturated fats.
5. Also, have client choose between high saturated fatty acid and high PUFA foods. If client chooses the high PUFA food, no further teaching is required in that area.

Continued

Client Education

- Butter contains more saturated fats than margarine; it contains cholesterol, whereas margarines do not (except margarine-butter blends).
- Reduce dietary cholesterol intake to less than 300 mg daily by limiting meats, cheeses, whole milk, and eggs.
- Because of lack of information regarding long-term consequences of high PUFA intake, the Committee on Diet and Health of the Food and Nutrition Board recommends that PUFA not exceed 10% of intake (NRC, 1989b).
- A few fruits and vegetables contain a small amount of fat. For example, bananas contain a trace of fat (0.55 gm, or 0.5% fat by weight and 6% of the kilocalories); avocados contain 31 gm fat (15% by weight and 86% of the kilocalories). Both are good sources of several vitamins and minerals.
- Teach clients to read labels and determine kilocalories for an accurate amount of fat rather than the weight. To determine fat content, multiply the gm of fat by 9 to determine the kilocalories provided by fat in that food. Then divide this number by the total kilocalories of the product and multiply by 100. If the food contains less than 30% fat, it is generally a wise choice. Fats and oils that are 100% fat are necessary to provide adequate PUFAs and fat-soluble vitamins; therefore, food items are averaged together to determine if an item that exceeds 30% fat would cause the day's or week's intake to exceed the overall 30% desired fat level.
- A "low cholesterol diet" is a misnomer. A cholesterol-free product can still be high in saturated fat, which will elevate the blood cholesterol. Dietary saturated fat has a greater effect on serum cholesterol than dietary cholesterol.
- Children under the age of 2 are growing rapidly; fat restriction is potentially unsafe for this age group because of uncertainties about amounts of energy, cholesterol, and EFAs required for growth. After 2 years of age, a "prudent" diet is desirable.

HYPER- AND HYPO- STATES

Some conditions related to fat will be observed in nursing practice. The following conditions suggest alteration of the amount and/or type of fat in the diet: obesity, gallbladder disease, diabetes mellitus, fatty infiltration of the liver, **hyperlipidemia,** and certain types of cancer. Fat content of the diet is modified in malabsorption syndromes, such as cystic fibrosis. Fats may be poorly tolerated in gallbladder and pancreatic diseases (see Chapter 26). Fat intake is increased for those who need to gain weight.

Hyperlipidemia is elevated concentrations of any or all of the serum lipids, especially triglycerides and/or cholesterol.

Obesity

Excessive fat stores are a common disorder in the US. Although the cause is overconsumption of all energy nutrients, kilocalories from fat are so concentrated that relatively small quantities may rapidly increase kilocaloric intake. Kendall et al (1991) found that weight loss can occur by reducing the dietary fat without any other food restrictions. In one study, it was found that men who normally consume a larger percentage of fat have more body fat stores and consume more kilocalories than men with a low fat intake (Tremblay et al, 1989).

Blood Lipid Levels

Elevated blood lipids are related to diet. Hyperlipidemia is associated with heart disease. Although many factors can affect blood lipid levels, the strongest dietary determinant of blood cholesterol level is the total fat content of the diet (NRC, 1989b). Reduction of the total dietary fat content to below 30% of the intake helps lower saturated fat content of the diet. Cholesterol and fatty acid content also affect serum lipid levels but to a lesser extent.

What affects blood lipid levels the most?

Cancer

Thirty to 40% of all cancers in men and 60% of all cancers in women have been attributed to diet; fat has been linked more frequently to cancer than any other dietary factor (AICR, 1992). Epidemiological studies of human populations indicate a correlation of total fat intake and cancer of the breast and colon and, to some extent, prostate. Evidence linking dietary fat and particular fatty acids with risk of cancer has elicited considerable interest and debate because of the diversity of findings. Inconsistencies in findings of studies may be the result of differences in fatty acid composition of fats, time of exposure, and tumor sites. Different mechanisms may be involved in tumor development at different sites.

Dietary fat may influence carcinogenesis by controlling immune function. At some stages of carcinogenesis, saturated fatty acids are more important, whereas tumor growth appears to be affected by total fat intake. Metastasis may depend on the tumor type and site and on the dietary regimen (Erickson & Hubbard, 1990). A high intake of linoleic acid promotes metastasis (Chapkin et al, 1989; Erickson & Hubbard, 1990).

The incidence of colon cancer is strongly correlated with per capita consumption of red meat and animal fat in various countries (Willett et al, 1990). Despite many uncertainties about the relationship between dietary fat and cancer risk, the consensus of opinion is to limit fat intake with increased consumption of fish and chicken and concurrent decrease of high-fat meats.

Nursing Applications

1. A client with inadequate fat intake will be thin in appearance, will have dry skin and dull hair, and be sensitive to cold temperatures. If these signs and symptoms are noted, suggest a dietary consultation and/or monitor fat intake.
2. To determine obesity from edema, palpate the skin: If obesity is the cause, it will have a flabby, not mushy consistency.

Client Education

- A high intake of fat can lead to obesity. Advise the client that 10% of the total kilocalories should come from saturated fats, with the remaining 20% from monounsaturated and polyunsaturated fatty acids.
- Diets high in fat may lead to obesity, coronary heart disease, and possibly breast and colon cancer and strokes.

NUTRITION UPDATE 5–1: OMEGA-3 FATTY ACIDS

One of the newest and most exciting nutrition topics is omega-3 fatty acids. Interest was sparked in the 1970s when several studies indicated the typical diet of the Greenland Eskimos was rich in seafood, high in protein, fat, and cholesterol. Yet heart disease was virtually nonexistent. These Eskimos had low levels of plasma triglycerides, long blood coagulation time, and low incidence of cancer. Although the Greenland Eskimos have less heart disease, their incidence of stroke is greater.

The presence of omega-3 fatty acids in the diet has been linked to reduction or amelioration of several chronic diseases: Atherosclerosis, rheumatoid arthritis, psoriasis, and inflammatory and immune disorders. Research on the effects of omega-3 fatty acids on blood lipid and lipoprotein levels is promising, but the mechanism by which these unsaturated fatty acids reduce the risk of heart disease is unknown. Flaten et al (1990) were able to lower triglycerides with fish oil supplementation. The effects of omega-3 fatty acids on HDL and LDL cholesterol levels have been variable (Harris et al, 1991; Childs et al, 1990; Green et al, 1990). Studies of the effect of fish oils on blood pressure have yielded inconsistent results. If these unsaturated fatty acids lower blood pressure, the effect is minimal. Fish consumption may have a favorable effect on blood platelets and other blood clotting mechanisms, reducing the risk of clot formation (Li & Steiner, 1991).

EPA has an antiinflammatory effect on prostaglandin function or synthesis. Findings indicating a beneficial role of omega-3 fatty acid intake in rheumatoid arthritis are promising, with reduction in the number of painful joints (Kremer et al, 1985). There is no consensus, however, to support prevention or treatment of this disease. Omega-3 fatty acids may result in a slowing of tumor growth and protection against some types of cancer. The amount to elicit a beneficial effect is unknown.

The health benefits of fish oil remain unproved, but fish oil preparations are being aggressively promoted as a cure-all for a variety of diseases (Ballard-Barbash & Callaway, 1987). OTC products provide the client with little information regarding the source of omega-3 fatty acids. Some fish oil preparations are made from fish livers, which can be high in pesticides, heavy metals, and other environmental contaminants. They may contain potentially toxic amounts of the fat-soluble vitamins A and D and appreciable quantities of cholesterol. Fish oil capsules are expensive, and there are no controls on their manufacture.

A recommended safe level of fish or fish oil has not been determined. A dosage of 10 gm/day of fish oil for clients with non–insulin dependent diabetes mellitus had a negative effect on blood glucose and low-density lipoprotein cholesterol values (Hendra et al, 1990). Therefore, a recommended level needs to be established to avoid deleterious effects. Because of these concerns regarding the effectiveness and safety of fish oil preparations, consumption of fish 2 to 3 times/week is recommended rather than fish oils.

There are other adverse consequences of fish oil supplements. Regular intake may cause excessive bleeding or wound healing problems, which could be especially dangerous for clients receiving anticoagulant or aspirin therapy.

Nursing Applications

1. Assess diet or supplemental intake of omega-3 fatty acids, especially diabetic clients who are at risk of complications as described in the text.
2. If client is taking anticoagulants or aspirin, evaluate use of omega-3 fatty acids. These clients may be prone to bleeding problems or poor wound healing.
3. Do not advocate the indiscriminate use of omega-3 fatty acids.

Client Education

- Omega-3 fatty acids should not be taken unless ordered by a physician.
- Read labels of omega-3 fatty acid supplements. If made from livers, do not

buy because high levels of pesticides or heavy metals may be present. Eat fish instead.
- There are currently no regulations or controls on manufacturing omega-3 supplements.
- High sources of omega-3 fatty acids (EPA and DHA) include mackerel, dogfish, Atlantic salmon, herring, lake trout, and tuna (presented in order of highest to lowest) (Nettleton, 1991).

SUMMARY

Lipids are important sources of energy in the diet and are the body's principal form of energy storage. They furnish more than twice as many kilocalories (9 kcal/gm) as proteins or carbohydrates. When more kilocalories are consumed than the body needs, the excess is stored as adipose tissue (3500 kcal = 1 lb of fat); this adipose tissue is oxidized for energy when the diet is deficient in kilocalories.

The EFA required in the diet is linoleic acid, supplied by safflower, corn, soybean, and cottonseed oils and nuts, such as almonds and walnuts. From this, the body can make other fatty acids it needs—linolenic and arachidonic acids. Omega-3 fatty acids from fish oils appear to have many health benefits, but supplements may have undesirable effects. Cholesterol is an essential constituent of all cells but is not a dietary necessity.

Fats are furnished in the diet mainly from meat, whole milk products, and added fats, such as margarine and salad dressings. Polyunsaturated fats are supplied from vegetable oils. Cholesterol is found only in animal products, especially organ meats, shellfish, and eggs.

NURSING PROCESS IN ACTION

A 50-year-old client is admitted to the hospital with complaints of chest pain. Laboratory values indicate elevated blood cholesterol levels. He states he eats whatever he wants. He realizes that some foods are high in fat and should be avoided, but he is unable to identify any he is willing to eliminate from his diet. When questioned about fat requirements and different types of fat, he says that he does not understand all of those big medical terms. He also indicates that his parents ate what they wanted without all these problems and concerns.

Nutritional Assessment

- Readiness/willingness to learn.
- Knowledge level concerning fat principles and how these relate to his diagnosis.
- Total amount of fat intake.
- Typical foods eaten.
- Type of dietary habits: who purchases and prepares the food, where he lives, where most meals are eaten.
- Weight and height, IBW, blood pressure.

Dietary Nursing Diagnosis

Altered health maintenance RT lack of knowledge of fat principles; diet and how it relates to condition.

Nutritional Goals

Client will follow/adhere to a low-fat, low-cholesterol diet, list foods high and low in fat, and state how disease may improve or deteriorate with diet.

Nutritional Implementation

Intervention: Explain how diet affects his condition—(1) saturated fat increases rate of fatty deposits in the arteries, (2) high cholesterol intake adversely affects this process, (3) roles of fat.
Rationale: Knowledge increases compliance.

Intervention: Teach the difference between PUFA and saturated fats—(1) use actual food labels, (2) provide a list of foods high and low in these 2 fats, (3) keep fat intake to less than 30% of total kcal, (4) 10% from saturated fats and 20% from PUFA.
Rationale: If client knows the difference between the 2 types of fat, he can make informed choices to help decrease progression of heart disease.

Intervention: Explain the difference between fat and cholesterol—(1) provide a list of foods high and low in cholesterol, (2) limit cholesterol intake to 300 mg or less a day, (3) explain that "cholesterol-free" does not necessarily mean "fat-free."
Rationale: Serum cholesterol lowering may help slow effects of heart disease.

Intervention: Monitor lipid levels (cholesterol less than 200 gm/dl, HDLs 30 to 80 mg/dl, LDLs 62 to 185 mg/dl). Use these as motivators to stay on healthy diet.
Rationale: These values can provide concrete evidence for motivation and compliance.

Intervention: Involve client in care by allowing him to select his menu.
Rationale: Participation increases compliance.

Intervention: Weigh client.
Rationale: Ideal body weight can help minimize adverse effects of heart disease.

Intervention: Teach client how to read nutrition labels (use an actual food label for teaching) and calculate grams and/or kilocalories of fat—use margarine that lists the first ingredient as either liquid oil or H_2O.
Rationale: Labels can be misleading to clients. Accurate information can promote healthy food choices and lower incidence of heart disease.

Intervention: Teach him how to decrease the amount of fat and saturated fats in the diet—(1) eat smaller servings of meat, (2) trim visible fat from meats, (3) use more poultry and fish, (4) avoid fried foods.
Rationale: These are all ways to decrease intake of fat, thereby decreasing progression of atherosclerosis. The use of more fish will increase intake of omega-3 fatty acids.

Intervention: Review labels to point out information provided in Table 1–2.
Rationale: Knowledge that is practical increases compliance.

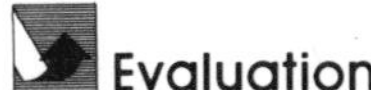

Evaluation

If client lists foods higher and lower in fat; can choose a low-fat, low-cholesterol diet from a restaurant menu; and consumes a low-fat, low-cholesterol diet, nursing care was effective. In addition, if client can choose the healthiest low-fat, low-cholesterol choices from 3 food labels; states how fat and cholesterol can lead to further deterioration of his disease; and verbalizes that fat speeds up the progression of fatty deposits, nursing care was successful. Other factors to evaluate include a decrease in blood lipid levels to within levels listed in care plan, and client can plan a diet that is low in fat and cholesterol.

STUDENT READINESS

1. Define lipid, hydrogenation, triglyceride, and lipoprotein to a client.
2. A client wants to know foods to consume to increase (1) polyunsaturated fats and (2) decrease saturated fats. Name 3 sources for each.
3. In observing physical properties of fats, how could you make an intelligent guess about the polyunsaturated and saturated fat content of a food?
4. What unsaturated fatty acid is essential in the diet? What are the functions of unsaturated fatty acids in the body?
5. Compare the labels of 3 brands of stick margarine, 3 brands of tub margarine, and 2 brands of diet margarine. How do they differ in their P/S ratio?
6. List the functions of fat in the diet.
7. What is ketosis? Why does it occur?
8. Describe the role of cholesterol in the body.
9. Calculate the kilocaloric value of the following items:

   2 slices bacon (8 gm fat, 4 gm protein)
   1 tbsp margarine (12 gm fat)
   1 tbsp whipped margarine (8 gm fat)
   1 tbsp mayonnaise (6 gm fat)
   1 tbsp lard (13 gm fat)

10. A client asks if it is possible to lose or gain 1 pound of body fat per day? What would you say?
11. Calculate the grams of fat a client could consume on a (1) 1500-kilocalorie diet and (2) 2000-kilocalorie diet to meet the Dietary Guidelines.
12. List 5 points you think a client should know about fats in general.

REFERENCES

American Academy of Pediatrics. Appendix K: Composition of human milk: Normative data. *In* Forbes GB, ed. *Pediatric Nutrition Handbook.* Elk Grove Village, IL, American Academy of Pediatrics, 1985, pp. 363–368.

American Dietetic Association (ADA). *Lowfat Living. A Guide to Enjoying a Healthy Diet.* Chicago, The American Dietetic Association, 1988.

American Institute for Cancer Research (AICR). *Diet and Cancer . . . What's the Link?* Washington, DC, American Institute for Cancer Research, 1992.

American Medical Association Council on Scientific Affairs (AMA). Saturated fatty acids in vegetable oils. *JAMA* 1990 Feb 2; 263(5):693–695.

Anonymous. Soy oil nutritionally related to fish oil. *Nutr Today* 1989 Mar/Apr; 24(2):4–5.

Ballard-Barbash R, Callaway CW. Marine fish oils: Role in prevention of coronary artery disease. *Mayo Clin Proc* 1987 Feb; 62(2):113–118.

Chapkin RS, et al. Linoleic acid metabolism in metastatic and nonmetastatic murine mammary tumor cells. *Cancer Res* 1989 Sept 1; 49(17):4724–4728.

Childs MT, et al. Divergent lipoprotein responses to fish oils with various ratios of eicosapentaenoic acid and docosahexaenoic acid. *Am J Clin Nutr* 1990 Oct; 52(4):632–639.

Erickson KL, Hubbard NE. Dietary fat and tumor metastasis. *Nutr Rev* 1990 Jan; 48(1):6–14.

Flaten H, et al. Fish oil concentrate: Effects on variables related to cardiovascular disease. *Am J Clin Nutr* 1990 Aug; 52(2):300–306.

Green P, et al. Effects of fish-oil ingestion on cardiovascular risk factors in hyperlipidemic subjects in Israel: Randomized, double-blind crossover study. *Am J Clin Nutr* 1990 Dec; 52(6):1118–1124.

Harris WS, et al. Effects of four doses of n-3 fatty acids given to hyperlipidemic patients for six months. *J Am Coll Nutr* 1991 Jun; 10(3):220–227.

Hendra TJ, et al. Effects of fish oil supplements in NIDDM subjects: Controlled study. *Diab Care* 1990 Aug; 13(8):821–829.

Kendall A, et al. Weight loss on a low-fat diet: Consequences of the imprecision of the control of food intake in humans. *Am J Clin Nutr* 1991 May; 53(5):1124–1129.

Kremer JM, et al. Effects of manipulation of dietary fatty acids on clinical manifestations of rheumatoid arthritis. *Lancet* 1985 Jan 26; 1(8422):184–187.

Leaf A, Weber, PC. Cardiovascular effects of n-3 fatty acids. *N Engl J Med* 1988 Feb 25; 318(9):549–557.

Li L, Steiner M. Dose response of dietary fish oil and supplementations on platelet adhesion. *Arterioscler Thromb* 1991 Jan/Feb; 11(1)39–46.

Mela DJ. Nutritional implications of fat substitutes. *J Am Diet Assoc* 1992 Apr; 92(4):472–476.

Morrison RM. The market for fat substitutes. *Nat Food Rev* 1990 Apr–June; 13(2):24–30.

National Research Council (NRC). *Recommended Dietary Allowances.* 10th ed. Washington, DC, National Academy Press, 1989a.

National Research Council (NRC). *Diet and Health: Implications for Reducing Chronic Disease Risk.* Report of the Committee on Diet and Health, Food and Nutrition Board. Washington, DC, National Academy Press, 1989b.

Nettleton JA. Omega-3 fatty acids: Comparison of plant and seafood sources in human nutrition. *J Am Diet Assoc* 1991 Mar; 91(3):331–337.

Putnam, JJ. Food consumption. *Nat Food Rev* 1990 July/Sept; 13(3):1–9.

Raper N. Nutrient content of the U.S. food supply. *Food Rev* 1991 July/Sept; 14(3):13–18.

Rolls BJ. Effect of covert fat replacement with Olestra on 24-hour food intake in lean adults. *FASEB J* 1991 March 15; 5(5):A1077.

Stephen AM, Wald NJ. Trends in individual consumption of dietary fat in the United States, 1920–1984. *Am J Clin Nutr* 1990 Sept; 52(3):457–469.

Thomson ABR. Intestinal aspects of lipid adsorption. *Nutr Today* 1989 Aug; 24(4):16–20.

Tremblay A, et al. Impact of dietary fat content and fat oxidation on energy intake in humans. *Am J Clin Nutr* 1989 May; 49(5):799–805.

Willet WC, et al. Relation of meat, fat and fiber intake to the risk of colon cancer in a prospective study among women. *N Engl J Med* 1990 Dec 13; 323(24):1664–1670.

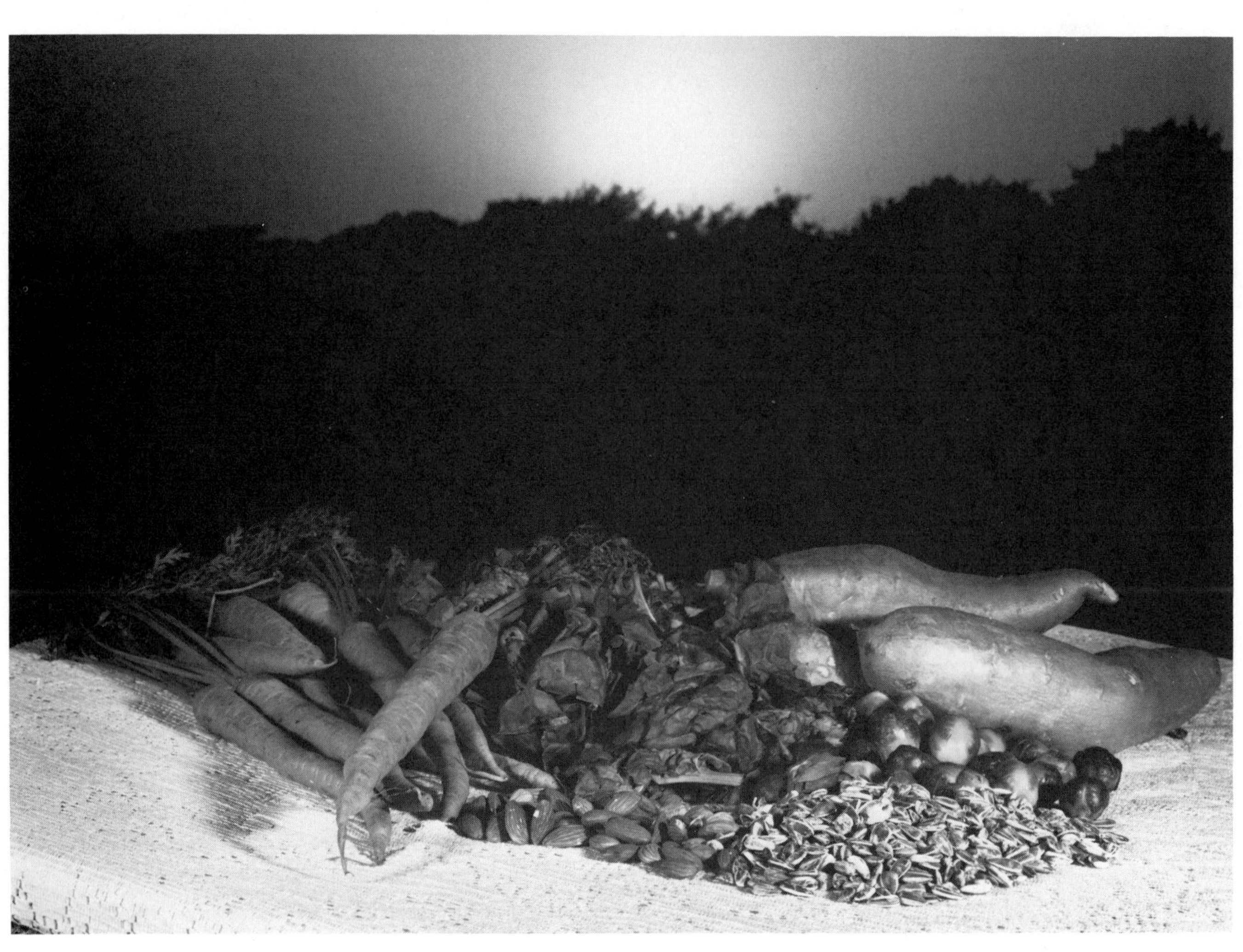

CHAPTER 6

Fat-Soluble Vitamins: The Miracle Workers

OUTLINE

OBJECTIVES

THE STUDENT WILL BE ABLE TO:

- Define and describe the fat-soluble vitamins.
- Identify functions, deficiencies, surpluses or toxicities, and symptoms of each fat-soluble vitamin.
- Select food sources for each fat-soluble vitamin.
- Identify nursing application principles for each of the fat-soluble vitamins.
- Discuss client teaching tips for fat-soluble vitamins.

TEST YOUR NQ (True/False) -- ELP guide

1. Fat-soluble vitamins are stored in the body.
2. A deficiency of vitamin K can lead to bleeding problems.
3. Vitamin E depresses response to iron therapy.
4. Fat-soluble vitamins include K, A, D, and E.
5. Animal foods are the principal dietary source of beta carotene.
6. Xerophthalmia occurs with a deficiency of vitamin A.
7. Vitamin D is called the sunshine vitamin.
8. An excess of vitamin D causes rickets.
9. Vitamin E is found in vegetable oils and green leafy vegetables.
10. Vitamin K is the antidote for heparin overdose.

Vitamin is a general term for a number of unrelated organic substances present in foods in small amounts. They are necessary for normal metabolic and physiological functions.

Vitamins are the catalysts for all reactions using proteins, fats, and carbohydrates for energy, growth, and cell maintenance. Because only small amounts of these chemicals obtained from food facilitate millions of processes, they may be regarded as "miracle workers." Vitamins do not provide energy or building materials for the body. Nutrients never work single-handedly but in partnership with each other.

Eating fats, carbohydrates, and proteins without enough vitamins means the energy cannot be used. The opposite is also true. These vitamins cannot be used without an adequate supply of fats, carbohydrates, proteins, and even minerals.

Do vitamins provide energy?

Most vitamins come in several forms with only one form performing a specific task, making them even more difficult to identify. These organic substances are easily destroyed by heat, oxidation, and chemical processes used in their extraction.

REQUIREMENTS

Although these chemical substances are vital to life, they are required in minute amounts. Vitamins are like hormones because of their potent effects, but they must come from an outside source because they cannot be produced by the body. Each vitamin is essential even though the amount may vary from 2 to 4 mcg for vitamin B_{12} to as much as 45 to 60 mg/day of vitamin C, or a 10,000-fold difference.

Even though the RDAs list the amounts of vitamins for different ages and sexes, many factors, such as tobacco, alcohol, caffeine, drugs, and stress, modify a client's requirements. Periods of unusually rapid growth; pregnancy or lactation; fever; and recovery from accidents, disease, surgery, or burns are all considered stressful. Therefore, requirements for most of the vitamins, especially the water-soluble ones, are increased. Dietary energy components affect some vitamin requirements, for example, a protein-rich diet or a high-carbohydrate or high-kilocalorie diet increases vitamin requirements.

What are some factors that may modify requirements?

DEFICIENCIES

Nutritional deficiencies may be a result of decreased intake, inadequate absorption or utilization, increased requirements, excretion, or destruction. Nutrients are codependent; a deficiency of one may cause deficiency symptoms of another because it relies on a metabolic product from the initial vitamin deficit.

If adequate amounts of the nutrient are not available to sustain biochemical functions, a nutritional deficiency occurs.

Although specific vitamin deficiency syndromes are relatively rare in the US, several groups are at risk: the elderly, those who consume minimal amounts of food, and clients with a chronic debilitating condition (for example, cancer, AIDS). Because vitamin levels in the blood are often nondiagnostic, nutritional deficiency is identified on the basis of clinical signs and symptoms and response to vitamin supplementation. Based on this information, nurses must be knowledgeable about vitamin requirements and deficiencies. For ease of reading, the fat-soluble and water-soluble vitamins are presented in 2 chapters.

What groups of clients are prone to vitamin deficiencies?

SIMILARITIES OF FAT-SOLUBLE VITAMINS

Although the 4 fat-soluble vitamins (A, D, E, and K) differ in function, utilization, and sources, they have several similar characteristics in common: (1) they are soluble in fat or fat solvents; (2) they are fairly stable to heat, as in cooking; (3) they do not contain nitrogen; (4) they are absorbed in the intestine along with fats and lipids in foods; and (5) they require bile for absorption.

Fat-soluble vitamins are different from water-soluble vitamins mainly because larger amounts can be stored in the body. Vitamins A and D are stored for long periods of time; hence minor shortages may not be identified until drastic depletion has occurred. For example, vitamin A can be stored in the liver to meet the basic needs for at least a year; **dietary deficiencies** may occur for some time before the shortage is obvious.

Dietary deficiencies occur when foods consumed do not provide recommended amounts for that nutrient.

Because several forms of each of the fat-soluble vitamins can be used by the body, in the past, vitamins A, D, and E were measured by their biological activity based on the growth of animals. International units (IUs) do not always represent the absorption rates of humans. Because various forms of vitamins A and E have varying activity levels, the RDAs for these vitamins were determined based on the biological effectiveness of each. Following measurement of all active forms of the vitamins, they are converted to micrograms or milligrams and totaled to indicate the amount of the vitamin in that food. Thus, retinol equivalents (RE) reflect the vitamin A activity in foods, and tocopherol equivalents (TE) reflect vitamin E ac-

Name 3 similarities of fat-soluble vitamins. Describe how they differ from water-soluble vitamins.

TABLE 6–1

SUMMARY OF FAT-SOLUBLE VITAMINS

Vitamin	Daily Allowances	Important Sources	Physiological Functions	Deficiency Symptoms	Toxicity Symptoms
Vitamin A Retinol; provitamin A (beta-carotene); anti-infective vitamin	Infants 0–1: 375 mg RE Children 1–3: 400 mg RE Children 4–6: 500 mg RE Children 7–10: 700 mg RE Males 11 and over: 1000 mg RE Females 11 and over: 800 mg RE Pregnancy: 800 mg RE Lactation: 1200–1300 mg RE	Liver and other organ meats; egg yolk; green, yellow, or orange vegetables and fruits; tomatoes; whole milk and cheese; cream; fortified margarine; fatty fish; fish oils	Production of rhodopsin (visual purple) Forms and maintains the integrity of mucosal epithelium to ensure healthy functioning of eyes, skin, hair, teeth, gums, various glands, and mucous membranes Synthesizes glycoprotein or mucus Important in immune function	Night blindness; dry skin; keratinization of epithelium; follicular hyperkeratosis; keratomalacia; faulty bone and tooth development; skin and mucous membrane infections; xerophthalmia; blindness and death	Bulging of the fontanelle; headaches; anorexia; hair loss; skin changes; pruritus; diplopia; dry mucous membrane; bone abnormalities; liver damage
Vitamin D Calciferol; vitamin D_2 (ergocalciferol); vitamin D_3 (cholecalciferol); calcitriol; antirachitic factor	Infants 0–0.5: 7.5 mcg Infants 0.5–1: 10 mcg Children 1–10: 10 mcg Males and females 11–24: 10 mcg Males and females over 25: 5 mcg Pregnancy and lactation: 10 mcg	Fortified milk; fortified margarine; fish oils; liver; butter; and egg yolk Synthesized in skin by ultraviolet light	Regulator of blood calcium and phosphorus levels; mineralization of bones and teeth	Children: rickets—soft and fragile bones; enlarged joints; bowed legs; and deformities of the chest, spine, and pelvis Infants: tetany Adults: osteomalacia (soft bones)	Early symptoms: anorexia; nausea; vomiting; diarrhea; bloody stools; polyuria; muscular weakness; lassitude; and headache More serious symptoms: renal failure and calcification
Vitamin E Tocopherol; alpha-, beta-, and gamma-tocopherol	Infants 0–0.5: 3 mg Infants 0.5–1: 4 mg Children 1–3: 6 mg Children 4–10: 7 mg Males 11 and over: 10 mg Females 11 and over: 8 mg Pregnancy: 10 mg Lactation: 11–12 mg	Vegetable oils and margarines; whole grains; wheat germ; green leafy vegetables; and nuts	Antioxidant; stability of cell membranes	RBC hemolysis and abnormal fat deposits Deficiency is unlikely In premature infants, anemia may occur requiring iron, folate, and tocopherol	Possibly may cause increased serum lipids and cholesterol
Vitamin K K—menadione; K_1—phylloquinone, from food sources; K_2—menaquinone, synthesized in GI tract and from animal tissues; K_3—synthetic menadinone: water-soluble and requires no bile salts for absorption (called the coagulation factor and antihemorrhagic vitamin)	Infants 0–0.5: 5 mcg Infants 0.5–1: 10 mcg Children 1–3: 15 mcg Children 4–6: 20 mcg Children 7–10: 30 mcg Males and females 11–14: 45 mcg Males 15–18: 65 mcg Males 19–24: 70 mcg Males over 25: 80 mcg Females 15–18: 55 mcg Females 19–24: 60 mcg Females over 25: 65 mcg Pregnancy and lactation: 65 mcg	Green leafy vegetables; kale; cauliflower; cabbage; egg yolk; soybean oil; and liver	Production of prothrombin, a compound required for normal blood clotting	Hypoprothrombinemia and prolonged blood clotting times; hemorrhagic disease of the newborn; and hemorrhages. Deficiency usually associated with disease states or from drug therapy	Kernicterus

tivity. Although many food tables still list IUs, conversions are being made to the more accurate weight measurements in micrograms or milligrams. A summary of the fat-soluble vitamins is provided in Table 6–1.

NURSING APPLICATIONS

1. Assessment is crucial to determine requirements for vitamins. Assess for the following: tobacco and alcohol use, excessive caffeine use, medications, stress, surgery, or burns. If present, vitamin requirements may be elevated.
2. Physical assessment is more diagnostic for vitamin deficiencies than laboratory values.
3. Evaluate nutrient intake of groups at high risk for developing nutritional deficiencies by questioning elderly clients, poverty/low income clients, and clients with chronic diseases. A dietary consultation may be necessary.

Client Education

- Although no vitamin contains kilocalories, some vitamins are essential to the production of energy.

VITAMIN A

Retinol is the dietary source of vitamin A from animal sources, and beta-carotene is the principal carotenoid present in plant pigments. Retinoic acid is the most biologically active form.

What is vitamin A called if it comes from animal versus plant sources?

Physiological Roles

Vitamin A has many hormonal-like roles in the body, but the main functions relate to the health and integrity of the body orifices and their linings. It is also required for normal bone growth and development and for facilitating the transcription of DNA into RNA.

Vision

Retinal combines with opsin, a protein in the eye, to form **rhodopsin. Night blindness** may be the result of inadequate vitamin A to permit rhodopsin production. This condition takes years to develop in an adult but occurs much sooner in children because they have fewer body stores.

Retinol is converted to retinal in the eye. Rhodopsin is a light-sensitive pigment that allows the eye to adjust to changes in light. Night blindness is an inability to adapt to bright lights when the eyes are adapted to darkness.

Growth

Vitamin A is necessary for growth of both soft tissues and bones. In soft tissues, vitamin A increases synthesis of cell proteins that stimulate growth and influence metabolism. Its function in cellular reproduction may be the reason a deficiency state results in sterility or inability to reproduce. In skeletal tissue, vitamin A is necessary for resorption of old bone and synthesis of bone.

Epithelial Tissue

One of the most important functions of vitamin A is to maintain the integrity of the epithelial cells. Deterioration of epithelial tissues incurs damage to mucous membranes and loss of cilia, which constantly help keep membrane surfaces clean.

Epithelial tissue includes the cellular covering of internal and external surfaces.

Mucus functions as a lubricant throughout the body, including the eye, where it attacks bacteria. One of the first organs affected by dietary deficiency is the cornea of the eye, resulting in night blindness. In addition to preventing entry of bacteria into the body, vitamin A is important in the formation of T lymphocytes or immune cells.

Cancer

Free radicals or peroxides are produced by cells and tissues using free oxygen. These free radicals have unpaired electrons seeking to combine with whatever is available. They attack cell membranes or DNA, producing a chain reaction with the formation of more free radicals. Unchecked by an antioxidant, free radicals can damage both the structure and function of cell membranes. PUFAs in the cell membrane are very sensitive to attack by free radicals.

Carotene has consistently been associated with cancer prevention because of its importance to the development and integrity of cells. Studies suggest that vitamin A and beta-carotene reduce the incidence of lung, breast, oral mucosa, esophageal, and bladder cancers by functioning as an **antioxidant** in preventing cell membrane damage from **free radicals** (Weisburger, 1991). Studies are complicated by a difference in the effects of preformed vitamin A and the precursor beta-carotene.

Currently it is uncertain whether beta-carotene or some other factor in fruits and vegetables is anticarcinogenic. Supplementation is not advisable other than increasing consumption of fruits and vegetables as indicated in the US Dietary Guidelines and basic food groups.

Requirements

Describe the functions of vitamin A.

What is the RDA for vitamin A in men and women?

The RDA for vitamin A is 1000 mcg RE for men and 800 mcg RE for women. The need for vitamin A is increased during periods of rapid growth and with GI problems affecting its absorption or conversion and hepatic diseases limiting vitamin A storage or conversion of beta-carotene to its active form.

Average intake in the US meets the RDA. Inadequate intake occurs in lower socioeconomic groups due to decreased vegetable and fruit intake.

Sources

Vitamin A, as preformed retinol, is found in milk fat and butter (sometimes retinol is added to skim milk and margarine), eggs, meat, cod liver oil, and liver. Beta-carotene or provitamin A is also present in yellow, orange, and green leafy vegetables (spinach, turnip greens, broccoli) (Table 6–2). Beta-carotene is deep red in pure form and derives its name from carrots, from which it was first isolated. Chlorophyll covers up the carotenoids in green vegetables. Most yellow, orange, and dark green fruits and vegetables are high in carotene or vitamin A content. The deeper the color, the more vitamin A activity.

Name sources for retinol and beta-carotene.

Absorption and Excretion

Absorption is optimal when body stores are depleted and when optimal amounts of other interrelated nutrients are present. The presence of vitamin E and the hormone thyroxine also enhance the use of vitamin A.

The liver stores approximately 90% of vitamin A. When vitamin A is released into the blood stream and enters the cell of a target tissue, it is bound to a special transport substance, retinol-binding protein. Retinol-binding protein requires zinc for its synthesis. Adequate serum proteins are necessary to mobilize vitamin A from the liver.

TABLE 6–2

FOOD SOURCES OF VITAMIN A

Food	Portion	Vitamin A (RE)	Kilocalories (per serving)
Beef liver	3 oz	9018	137
Baked sweet potato	1	2488	118
Raw carrots	1	2025	31
Mangos	1	806	135
Cooked spinach	½ cup	798	29
Butternut squash (baked)	½ cup	718	41
Cooked dandelion greens	½ cup	615	18
Cantaloupe	1 cup	516	56
Cooked collard greens	½ cup	509	31
Dried apricots	½ cup	471	155
Cooked turnip greens	½ cup	396	15
Raw spinach	1 cup	376	12
Baked winter squash	½ cup	365	40
Papaya	1 cup	282	55
Cooked mustard greens	½ cup	212	11
Cooked broccoli	½ cup	174	26
Skim milk	1 cup	150	86
Romaine lettuce	1 cup	146	9
Butter	1 tbsp	105	100
Raw apricot	1	92	17
Whole milk	1 cup	92	150
Whole egg	1	84	77
Half-and-half cream	¼ cup	79	79
Tomato	1	77	24
Canned oysters	3 oz	77	59

Nutrient data from Nutritionist III software, version 7.0. N-Squared Computing, Salem, Oregon.

Hyper- and Hypo- States

Toxicity

When present in high concentrations, unbound vitamin A causes damage to cell membranes, especially in erythrocytes and **lysosomes.** Large amounts of vitamin A supplements can exceed the storage capacity of the liver and binding capability of retinol-binding protein; free vitamin A enters the blood stream and exerts its toxic effects on cell membranes.

Lysosomes—intracellular bodies that contain hydrolytic enzymes that promote the breakdown of materials taken into the cells.

Maternal consumption of vitamin A supplements has been associated with fetal birth defects. Vitamin A readily accumulates in the body; excessive vitamin A intake before conception may contribute to teratogenic risk.

Toxicity from excessive intake of food sources is possible but does not occur too often. Overzealous mothers have unintentionally induced vitamin A toxicity in children by providing too much vitamin A supplement. Toxicity is evident in infants by bulging of the fontanelle as a result of increased cerebrospinal fluid pressure. One of the peculiarities of vitamins is that the symptoms of an overdose frequently resemble those caused by a deficiency. For vitamin A, these include headache, vomiting, diplopia, **alopecia,** dryness of the mucous membranes, desquamation, bone abnormalities, and liver damage. Toxicity symptoms usually appear only when excessive intakes, or more than 10 times the RDA, occur over a sustained period.

Alopecia—hair loss.

Although carotenoids are not known to be toxic, overconsumption may result in **hypercarotenemia** as a result of carotene storage in fatty tissue.

Hypercarotenemia is accompanied by yellow pigmentation of the skin occurring first on the palms of the hands and soles of the feet.

Deficiency

Inadequate vitamin A results in degeneration of epithelial cells in the eye and cessation of tear secretion. Lids are swollen and sticky with pus, and eyes are sensi-

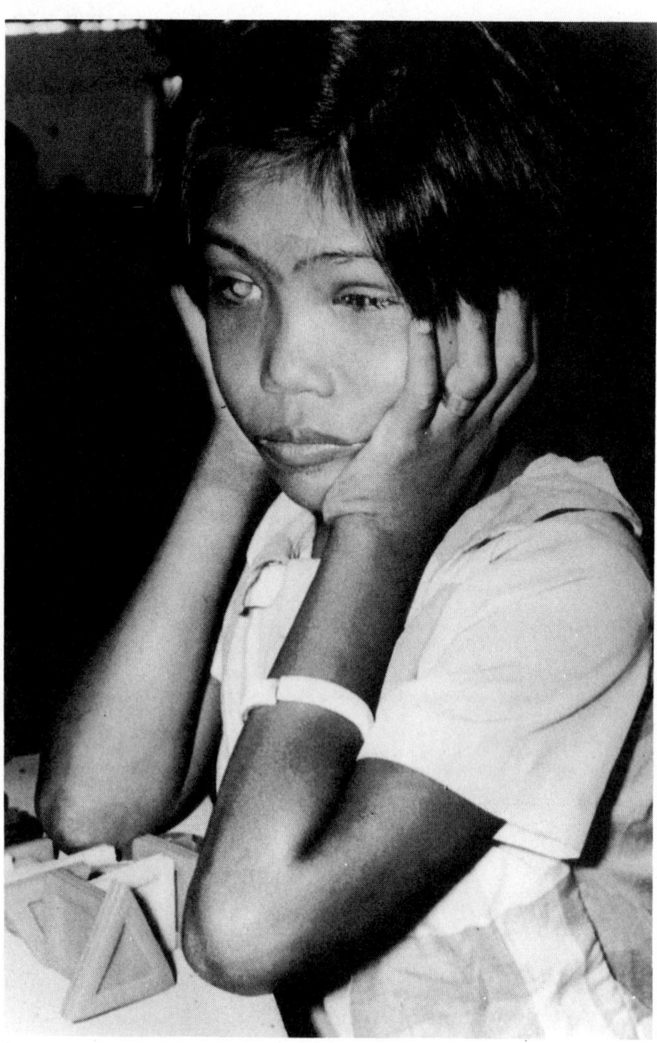

Figure 6–1 Blindness from xerophthalmia. If this girl had been given food containing vitamin A, she need not have lost her sight. (Courtesy of WHO/Helen Keller International.)

Xerophthalmia is abnormally dry and thickened surface of the conjunctiva and cornea as a result of a vitamin A deficiency.

Xeroderma is dry, rough, scaly skin.

Keratinization is production of hardened eruptions around the hair follicles by the epithelial tissues. In follicular hyperkeratosis caused by vitamin A deficiency, the skin is like goose flesh on the buttocks and arms.

Describe what happens to the body with excessive intake of vitamin A.

Describe what happens when vitamin A intake is deficient.

tive to light in **xerophthalmia,** sometimes resulting in blindness because of vitamin A deficiency. The first symptom of xerophthalmia is night blindness, followed by the occurrence of xerotic spots on the conjunctiva, called Bitot's spots. These ulcers of the eye may spread and result in blindness if left untreated (Fig. 6–1).

Degeneration of epithelial cells results in dry, scaly skin as a result of inability to produce mucus. This occurs not only in epithelial cells, but also in the intestines and lungs. **Xeroderma** can progress until the whole body is covered with flaky, scaly skin similar to dandruff. It is followed by **follicular hyperkeratosis.**

Keratinization may also affect the respiratory and GI tract. In both areas, degeneration of epithelial cells results in increased infections.

Inadequate dietary intake is the primary reason for vitamin A deficiency, found most commonly in children under 5 years of age. It may also result from chronic fat malabsorption. Vitamin A deficiency is rarely seen in the US but is a major nutritional problem in Third World countries. Even mild vitamin A deficiency is directly associated with at least 16% of all deaths in children 1 to 6 years of age in Asia. This may be related to depressed immune response. Deficiency in adults results in night blindness and follicular hyperkeratosis followed by elevated cerebrospinal fluid pressure, loss of sense of taste and smell, and abnormal vestibular function (balance).

NURSING APPLICATIONS

1. Assess for signs of vitamin A deficiencies (loss of night vision, keratomalacia, corneal ulceration, Bitot's spots), especially in the young and the elderly. When in doubt, consult the physician and/or dietitian.
2. Hypercarotenemia may be distinguished from jaundice by the fact that sclera retains its normal white color in hypercarotenemia.
3. Jaundice or celiac disease or any disorder that affects fat absorption also affects fat-soluble vitamin absorption, making these clients prone to vitamin A deficiency.
4. The alcoholic or alcoholic-cirrhotic client may be deficient in vitamin A because of the effects of ethanol and impaired liver function. Retinol-binding protein and vitamin A excretions are reduced when the liver is not healthy.
5. Vitamin A toxicity can be masked, especially when protein-energy malnutrition is present. Therefore, closely monitor these clients for signs and symptoms of vitamin A toxicity.
6. Chronic vitamin A deficiency leads to microcytic anemia.
7. Beta-carotene or other factors in fruits and vegetables may have an inhibitory role in early stages of carcinogenesis but not in later stages of skin and breast cancers (Greenberg et al, 1990; Hislop et al, 1990). Do not suggest vitamin A supplements to clients with late stage cancer.
8. Excessive intake of vitamin E or C may decrease absorption of vitamin A. Do not encourage use of vitamin E and C supplements or vitamin E- or C-rich foods if client is deficient in vitamin A.

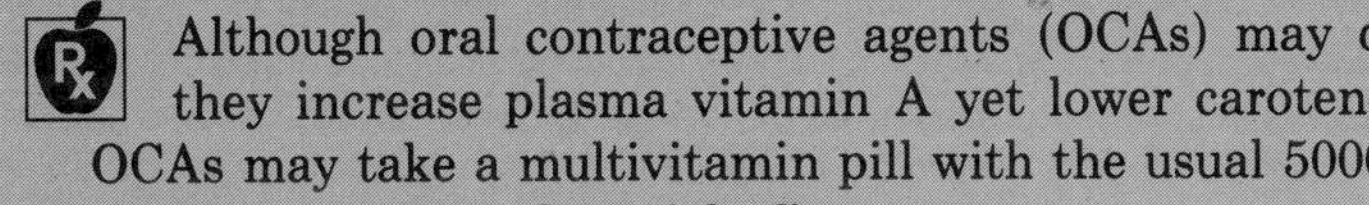

Although oral contraceptive agents (OCAs) may deplete some vitamins, they increase plasma vitamin A yet lower carotene levels. Women using OCAs may take a multivitamin pill with the usual 5000 mcg IU (1000 RE) of vitamin A without harmful effects.

Client Education

- Inform clients that vitamin A from animal sources is better used by the body.
- Explain to clients that vitamin prescriptions should be followed explicitly; severe life-threatening liver damage can result from increasing the amounts.
- Discourage clients from taking more than the RDA in OTC vitamin preparations unless specifically advised to do so by a physician or dietitian.
- Recommend storing vitamins in a cool, dark place to prevent deterioration.

VITAMIN D

Although vitamin D has been called a vitamin, it is more appropriately classified as a **hormone.** Skin cells are able to make vitamin D when exposed to ultraviolet light or sunshine. The precursor 7-dehydrocholesterol present in the skin is converted to vitamin D_3 or cholecalciferol by ultraviolet irradiation. Vitamin D from food, ergocalciferol (vitamin D_2) or cholecalciferol (vitamin D_3), is biologically inert. Further processing occurs in the liver with the conversion of vitamin D_2 or D_3 into 25-hydroxycholecalciferol (calcidiol) and a final change to the active form of 1,25-dihydroxycholecalciferol (calcitriol) by the kidney (Fig. 6–2).

Hormone is a substance produced by cells of the body and transported in the blood stream to another site, where it has a specific regulatory effect.

What are the steps to produce calcitriol, the active form of vitamin D?

Physiological Roles

Vitamin D is intricately related to calcium and phosphorus, each being required for optimal use of the other. The primary role of vitamin D is mineralization of

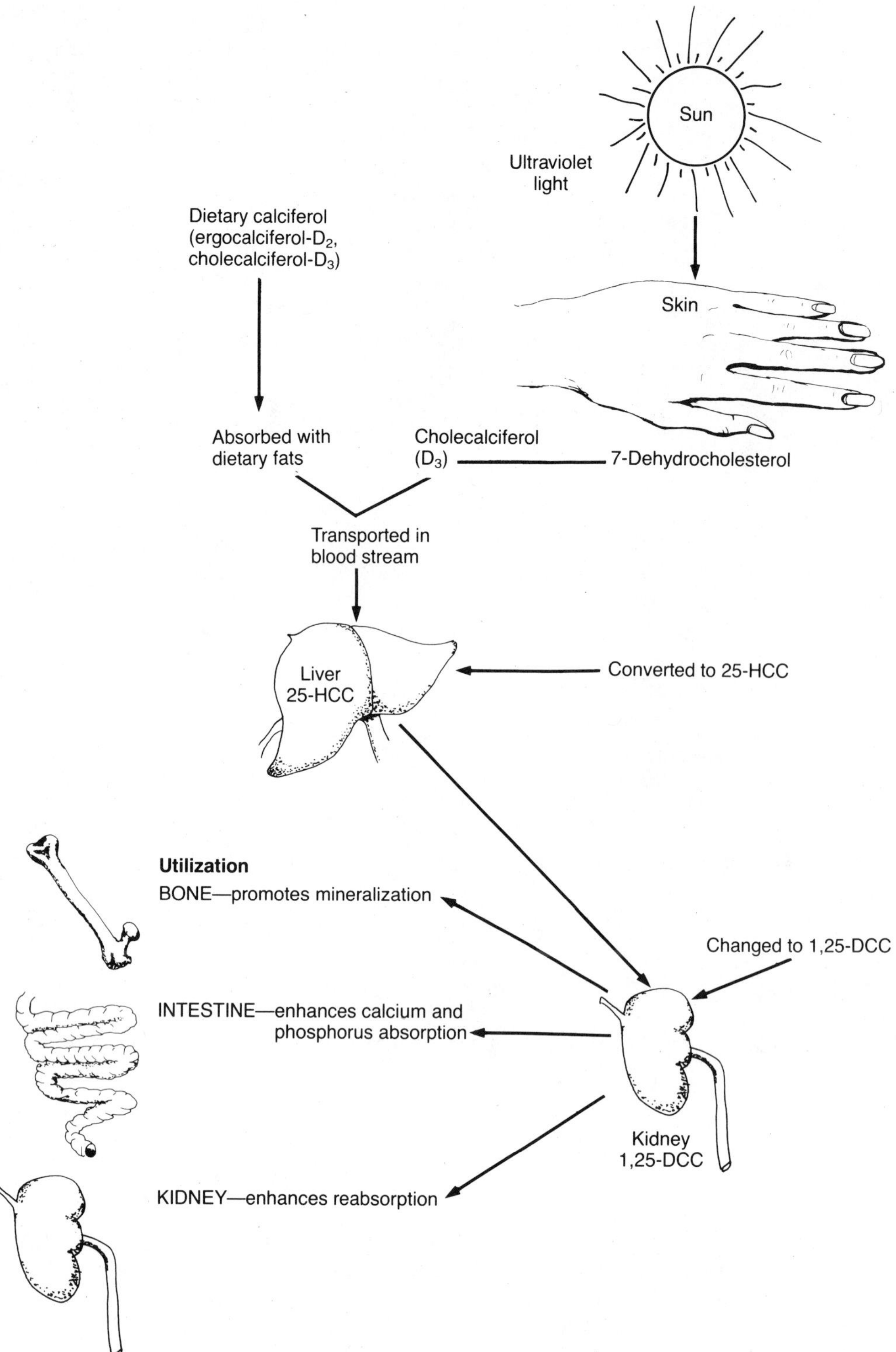

Figure 6–2 Vitamin D metabolism. 25-HCC, 25-hydroxycholecalciferol; 1,25-DCC, 1,25 dihydroxycholecalciferol.

bones and teeth and regulation of blood calcium and phosphorus levels. It functions with the parathyroid and thyroid (calcitonin) hormones to regulate intestinal absorption of calcium and phosphorus, enhance renal calcium and phosphorus reabsorption, and regulate skeletal calcium and phosphorus reserves.

Hematopoietic—formation of red blood cells (RBCs).

Vitamin D may also be involved in the functioning of **hematopoietic** cells, the skin, cardiovascular function, cancer cells of various origins, islet cells of the pancreas, and immune responses (Quesada et al, 1989; Reichel et al, 1989; Rigby, 1988; Sowers et al, 1988).

What are the roles of vitamin D?

Requirements

The current RDA for vitamin D is 5 mcg (200 IU) for adults. Vitamin D requirement is difficult to determine. When sufficient sunlight is available, the client does not require an exogenous source of vitamin D. Because many Americans have limited exposure to sunlight, however, and many factors can interfere with ultraviolet light–dependent synthesis of vitamin D in the skin, vitamin D is considered an essential dietary nutrient.

What is the RDA for vitamin D?

Sources

Sunshine

The body's ability to produce enough vitamin D (sometimes called the sunshine vitamin) from sunlight is the reason the sun has been known as a source of health. Most clients experience an increase in vitamin D during the summer months, with a lower amount during the winter because of less sun exposure.

In addition to geographical and seasonal factors, ultraviolet light from the sun may be blocked by air pollution, clothing, synthetic sunscreens, and indoor lifestyles. The use of sunscreens and moderation in sun exposure are important to protect against skin cancer.

Signs of deficiency are also commonly found in elderly clients consuming inadequate diets with little exposure to sunshine. By age 70, the skin generally produces vitamin D at only half the level that it did at age 20 (Kavookjian et al, 1990).

Food

Even though adequate quantities of this vitamin may be derived from exposure to sunlight, additional food sources are necessary in most cases. Natural content of vitamin D in foods is limited and variable; food tables do not normally list the vitamin D content. A diet composed of the best (unfortified) food sources of vitamin D would supply only slightly more than 2.5 mcg daily.

Foods are not legally required to be fortified, but about 98% of the milk in the US is fortified to obtain 10 mcg cholecalciferol (400 IU) per quart. Milk fortification is prevalent because of its popular consumption among children, and the calcium and phosphorus content of milk is beneficial for absorption and use of vitamin D. Because fortification is optional, it cannot be taken for granted.

Other foods such as margarine, infant cereals, prepared breakfast cereals, chocolate beverage mixes, and cocoa may also be fortified (Table 6–3). Nutrition labels

TABLE 6–3

FOOD SOURCES OF VITAMIN D

Food	Portion	Vitamin D (mcg)	Kilocalories (per serving)
Broiled herring	3 oz	15	134
Broiled salmon	3 oz	11	155
Fortified milk	1 cup	2.6	86–150
Margarine, diet	1 tbsp	1.5	50
Margarine, regular	1 tbsp	1.1	101
Egg yolk	1	0.6	59

Nutrient data from Nutritionist III software, version 7.0. N-Squared Computing, Salem, Oregon.

Name food sources of vitamin D.

can be used to assess daily intake of vitamin D; this information plus the amount of exposure to sunlight must be considered before giving vitamin D supplements.

Absorption

As with other nutrients, optimal absorption occurs when all closely interrelated nutrients (particularly calcium) are present in sufficient quantities. Conversely, diets high in fiber can result in less absorption of vitamin D.

Hyper- and Hypo- States

Toxicity

Vitamin D can be toxic if too much is ingested. Intakes of 5 times the RDA for vitamin D have been associated with signs of toxicity in young children and adults. Early symptoms of calciferol poisoning include hypercalcemia, hyperphosphatemia, and enhanced bone resorption, leading to deposition of calcium in soft tissues and irreversible kidney and cardiovascular damage. Detection of these symptoms with immediate dosage reduction is imperative.

What are signs and symptoms of vitamin D toxicity? Who is prone to this?

The most common reason for vitamin D toxicity is prolonged intake of pharmacological doses. Toxicity from excessive vitamin D may arise when a concentrated calciferol preparation that is 50 times more potent than cod liver oil is mis-

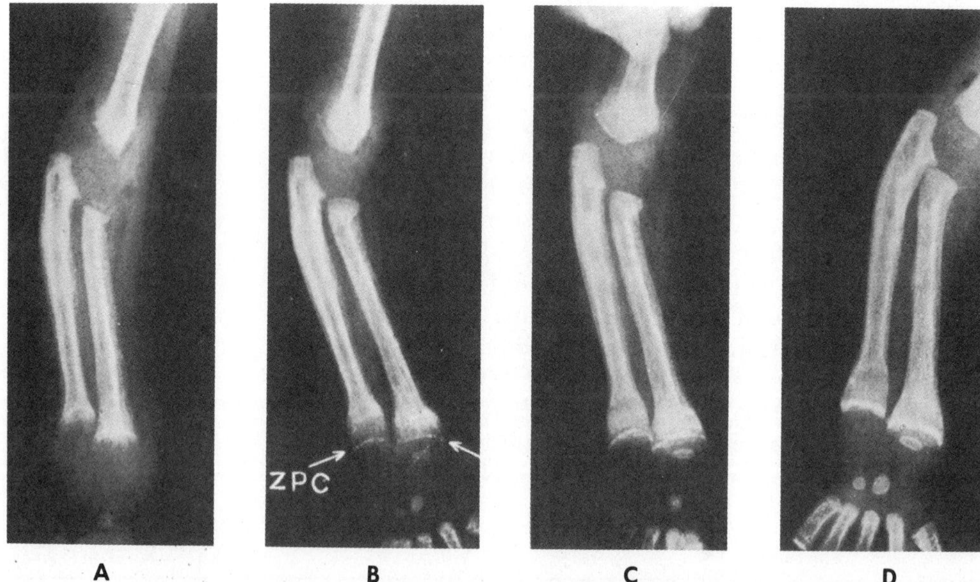

Figure 6–3 *A*, Active rickets; cupping and fraying of distal ends of radius and ulna; double contour along lateral outline of radius (periosteal osteoid). The two dense zones in the shaft of the ulna are calluses of greenstick fractures. *B*, Healing rickets after 12 days of treatment with vitamin D. Zones of preparatory calcification; above them in the rachitic metaphyses, there is beginning calcification. *C*, Healing rickets after 18 days of treatment. The zones of preparatory calcification are well defined, and the rachitic metaphyses appear well calcified. The epiphysis of the radius has become visible. *D*, Healing rickets after 29 days of treatment. Zones of preparatory calcification, rachitic metaphyses, and shafts have become united. (From Behrman RE, Vaughan VC. *Nelson Textbook of Pediatrics.* 14th ed. Philadelphia, WB Saunders, 1992.)

takenly given. An infant on a commercial formula and a vitamin supplement can easily ingest 2 to 4 times the RDA of vitamin D.

Deficiency

Vitamin D deficiency is most frequently seen in children and the elderly. Plasma vitamin D is significantly lower in older clients than in a younger population; it is consistently higher for men than women among the elderly. Supplements may be recommended along with calcium to prevent osteoporosis. When supplementation is recommended by a physician, care must be used to prevent toxic overdoses.

Vitamin D deficiency affects the skeletal structure in both children and adults. Laboratory values indicating serum calcium or phosphorus above or below normal values, the failure of bones to grow properly in length, and x-ray films showing abnormal epiphyses (growing points) of the bones indicate deficiencies (Fig. 6–3). Because vitamin D is intricately related to calcium and phosphorus functions, a change in any of these 3 nutrients affects the others.

Rickets

Rickets, caused by vitamin D deficiency, usually occurs in children between 1 and 3 years of age and is characterized by weak bones.

The name **rickets** came from the word "wrikken," meaning to bend or twist. Rachitic deformities such as bowlegs or knock-knees develop. The epiphyses of bones do not develop normally in children, so bones are twisted and warped. Other bone changes include a row of bead-like protuberances on each side of the narrow, distorted chest (pigeon breast) at the juncture of the ribs and costal cartilage (rachitic rosary), which predisposes the client to lung diseases (Fig. 6–4). A narrow pelvis is also observed, making future childbearing difficult in women.

Rickets develops during a time of extremely rapid growth when clients have had only a brief period to acquire vitamin D stores. Adequate intake during pregnancy and lactation is important because vitamin D can be passed from the mother to the infant before birth and in breast milk. Rickets is rare in the US but occa-

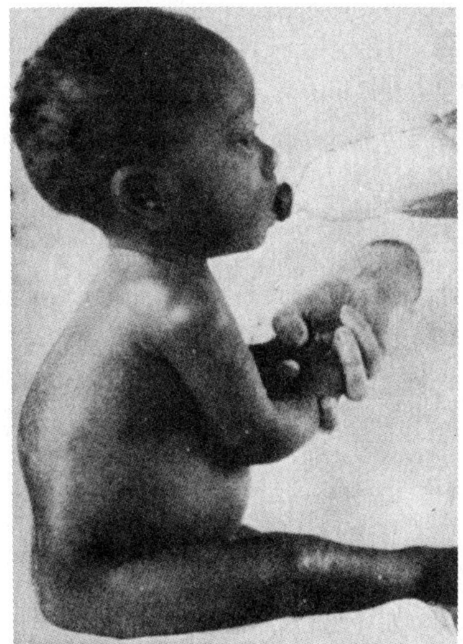

A

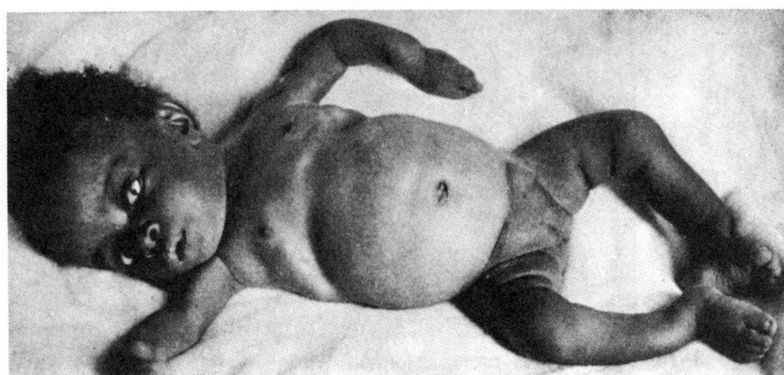

B

Figure 6–4 *A*, Rachitic spinal curvature, well marked when the child is sitting. (From Behrman RE, Vaughan VC. *Nelson Textbook of Pediatrics.* 13th ed. Philadelphia, WB Saunders, 1987.) *B*, Deformities in rickets, showing curvature of the limbs, potbelly, and Harrison groove.

Describe what happens in rickets.

sionally occurs among blacks, especially Muslims because of total dietary restrictions of animal-derived products.

Osteomalacia

Osteomalacia is a condition of decreased bone mineralization or softening of the bones, which may lead to deformities of the limbs, spine, thorax, and pelvis.

Vitamin D deficiency in adults is called **osteomalacia**; it is also intricately related to calcium intake. The main symptoms are skeletal pain and muscle weakness, resulting in kyphosis or uneven gait. The condition is more prevalent in women of child-bearing age with calcium depletion because of multiple pregnancies or inadequate intake or in women who have little exposure to the sun.

NURSING APPLICATIONS

1. Assess for vitamin D toxicity and deficit, especially in young children, women, and the elderly.
2. Vitamin D supplements should be given only in prescribed dosage because clients vary widely in their susceptibility to vitamin D toxicity. Do not recommend that clients buy vitamin D supplements.
3. When supplemental doses of vitamin D are used, cloudiness or a red color of the urine may indicate toxicity, so monitor color of urine.
4. An overdose of vitamin D is potentially lethal. In an acute overdose, induction of emesis or gastric lavage is beneficial if the overdose is discovered within a short time. Administration of mineral oil may increase fecal excretion.
5. Conditions that may lead to vitamin D deficiency include any abnormalities that (1) interfere with intestinal absorption (e.g., diarrhea, steatorrhea, celiac disease, and biliary obstruction) or (2) abnormalities in calcium balance and bone metabolism caused by disease states such as renal failure. Evaluate the client's physical status for risk of vitamin D deficiency.
6. Clients not exposed to sunlight should be monitored for adequate vitamin D intake and/or supplementation to maintain adequate stores of vitamin D. Evaluate client's living environment or hobbies to determine exposure to sunlight.
7. Determine the use of sunscreens. Consistent use of sunscreens may contribute to vitamin D deficiency in some clients (Matsuoka et al, 1988).

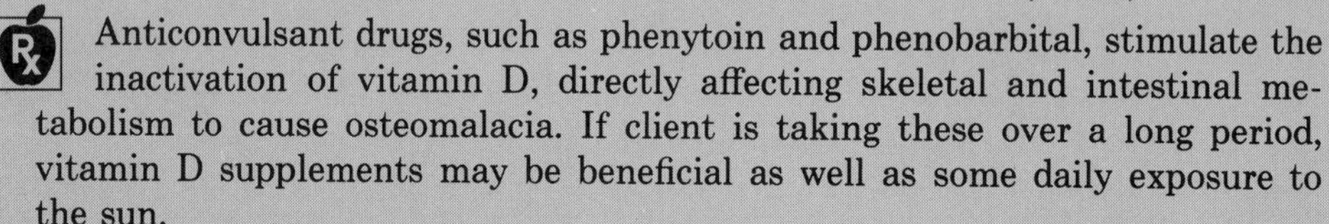

Anticonvulsant drugs, such as phenytoin and phenobarbital, stimulate the inactivation of vitamin D, directly affecting skeletal and intestinal metabolism to cause osteomalacia. If client is taking these over a long period, vitamin D supplements may be beneficial as well as some daily exposure to the sun.

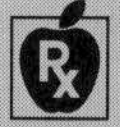

Hypercalcemia and hypoparathyroidism may result from vitamin D supplementation with thiazide medications.

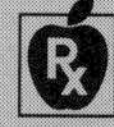

Cimetidine (a histamine-2 receptor antagonist) may disrupt vitamin D metabolism (Odes et al, 1990).

Client Education

- The bright sunlight between 11 AM and 2 PM offers maximum conversion. As little as 10 to 15 minutes exposure to the sun results in adequate conversion for light-skinned people.
- Toxicity may result from excessive intake of fortified foods.
- Contact the physician if urine becomes cloudy or red.
- Explain the importance of taking or giving the exact prescribed dose to avoid toxicity.

VITAMIN E

Four different tocopherols are collectively called vitamin E. Biological activity of the tocopherols varies; alpha-tocopherol is the most potent.

Physiological Roles

Vitamin E is the most important lipid-soluble antioxidant (Bjørneboe et al, 1990). Thus, vitamin E protects the integrity of normal cell membranes, effectively prevents hemolysis of RBCs, and protects vitamin A and unsaturated fatty acids from oxidation.

Vitamin E supplementation has been shown to improve immune response in healthy elderly clients; this effect may be mediated by increases in **interleukin-2** and a decrease in **prostaglandin E_2** (Meydani et al, 1990). There may be some association between serum tocopherol (vitamin E) levels and cancer risk, particularly GI cancers (Knekt et al, 1991).

Interleukin-2—promotes the growth of white blood cells.

Prostaglandin E_2—suppresses white blood cells.

Describe the roles of vitamin E.

Requirements

The RDA for vitamin E is 10 mg alpha-tocopherol for men and 8 mg for women. High intakes of linoleic acid or other PUFAs increase the requirement for vitamin E. Most polyunsaturated oils also contain vitamin E, but when stores are

TABLE 6–4

FOOD SOURCES OF VITAMIN E

Food	Portion	Vitamin E (mg)	Linoleic Acid (gm)	Kilocalories (per serving)
Sunflower seeds	¼ cup	19	11.8	205
Corn oil	1 tbsp	11	7.9	120
Mayonnaise, low kilocalorie	1 tbsp	8.1	NA	40
Commercial mayonnaise	1 tbsp	8	5.2	99
Almonds	¼ cup	8	3.4	192
Salad dressings (vinegar/oil, French, Russian, blue cheese, thousand island, sesame seed, Italian)	1 tbsp	7–8	2.6–4*	60–77*
Cooked sweet potato	½ cup	7.6	0.2	172
Cooked lima beans	½ cup	6.9	0.1	94
Margarine	1 tbsp	6.5	4.7	100
Walnuts	1 tbsp	6.1	10.5	190
Pecans	¼ cup	5.4	4.3	180
Safflower oil	1 tbsp	5.2	10.1	120
Iceberg lettuce	1 cup	4.3	0.2	70
Peanuts	¼ cup	4.2	5.6	209
Whipped margarine	1 tbsp	4.2	2.1	70
Mixed nuts	¼ cup	4.1	3.6	204
Bran cereal	½ cup	3.9	NA	106
Cashews	¼ cup	3.8	2.6	197
Peanut butter	1 tbsp	3.2	2.3	94
Cooked spinach	½ cup	3.1	0.01	29
Canned green peas	½ cup	2.2	0.1	80

* Lower kilocalories if reduced or low kilocalorie products are used.
NA, not available.
Nutrient data from Nutritionist III software, version 7.0. N-Squared Computing, Salem, Oregon.

List the RDA for vitamin E for men and women and the effect on requirements when clients consume increased amounts of PUFAs.

low or when chemical processes have destroyed vitamin E, the requirement increases more than for similar amounts of saturated fats in the diet.

Sources

Vitamin E is available from vegetable oils and margarine made from them; whole-grain or fortified cereals; wheat germ and nuts; green leafy vegetables; and some fruits such as apples, apricots, and peaches (Table 6–4). Meats, fish, and animal fats contain very little vitamin E.

Vitamin E is stable to heat but readily destroyed by oxidation and ultraviolet light. Normal cooking temperatures are not destructive, but some is lost in freezing and processing. (This is unusual; most nutrients are preserved by freezing.)

Fruits and vegetables provide about 20% of vitamin E in the diet, with oils also contributing about 20%. Mean intake of vitamin E is close to the RDA, but many clients consume lower amounts (Murphy et al, 1990). Vitamin E and linoleic acid are available in similar proportions in foods, as shown in Table 6–4.

Name food sources of vitamin E.

Absorption and Excretion

Absorption of vitamin E is relatively inefficient, ranging from 20 to 80% in healthy clients. Efficiency of absorption depends on the body's ability to absorb fat and appears to decline as the amount of dietary vitamin E increases.

Following its transport to the liver in chylomicrons, it is secreted into the blood with VLDLs and transferred to LDLs and HDLs following metabolism of VLDLs.

Hyper- and Hypo- States

Toxicity

Lack of research on excessive amounts of vitamin E prevents prediction of toxic levels; however, vitamin E is relatively nontoxic. Oral vitamin E supplementation results in few side effects even at doses as high as 3200 mg/day (Bendich & Machlin, 1988). Large doses exacerbate the coagulation defect produced by vitamin K deficiency but not in normal clients. Many claims have been made regarding the benefits of vitamin E in a variety of disorders; therefore, many clients take vitamin E supplements well in excess of the RDA.

Deficiency

Because vitamin E is widely distributed in foods, dietary deficiencies seldom occur if a well-balanced, varied diet is consumed. Deficiency occurs in premature infants and clients who are unable to absorb fats normally. Plasma vitamin E concentration in a newborn infant is about one-third of an adult's and that of a low birth weight infant is even lower. Premature infants born with inadequate reserves develop an anemia that requires treatment with iron, folic acid, and tocopherol. When plasma vitamin E is below normal, RBCs are susceptible to excessive hemolysis. The high oxygen concentration in incubators increases the stress on the erythrocytes causing hemolysis.

Which clients are prone to vitamin E deficiency?

NURSING APPLICATIONS

1. Assess for toxicities or deficiencies.
2. Vitamin E may help the immune system function better, so assess intake of vitamin E in hospitalized clients.
3. Vitamin E is useless in the treatment of sterility, or prevention of abortions or toxemia during pregnancy. It is a misnomer to call vitamin E the "reproduction vitamin" because all vitamins are necessary for reproduction. Clarify any misconceptions the client may have.
4. Vitamin E supplementation is not recommended for clients with vitamin K deficiency or with known coagulation defects or those receiving anticoagulation therapy.
5. Because chronic fat malabsorption reduces the absorption of fat-soluble vitamins, vitamin E supplementation should be administered early to provide the most benefit.

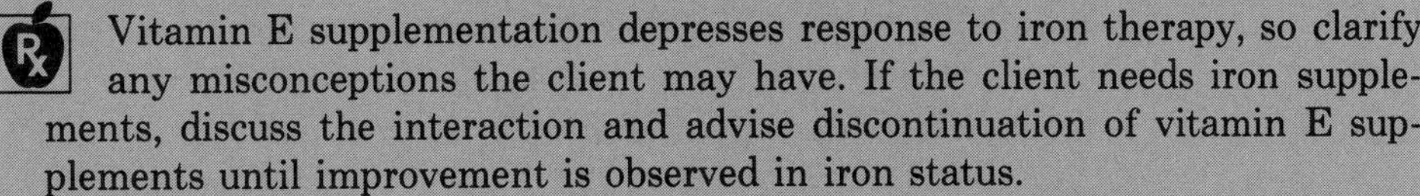

Vitamin E supplementation depresses response to iron therapy, so clarify any misconceptions the client may have. If the client needs iron supplements, discuss the interaction and advise discontinuation of vitamin E supplements until improvement is observed in iron status.

Client Education

- When oils are reused in frying, heavy losses of vitamin E occur.
- An increase in fruit and vegetable selections would provide low-fat sources of vitamin E.
- High levels of vitamin E supplementation should be taken only with proper medical supervision.

VITAMIN K

Three forms of vitamin K have been identified, all belonging to a group of chemical compounds known as quinones. The naturally occurring vitamins are K_1 (phylloquinone), which occurs in green plants, and K_2 (menaquinone), which is formed by *Escherichia coli* bacteria in the large intestine and is found in animal tissues. The fat-soluble synthetic compound menadione (K_3) is 2 to 3 times as potent as the natural vitamin.

Where does each of the 3 forms of vitamin K come from?

Physiological Roles

Vitamin K functions principally as a catalyst for synthesis of blood-clotting factors, including prothrombin. Vitamin K–dependent proteins have also been identified in bone, kidney, and other tissues. These proteins bind calcium and may be involved in bone crystal formation and possibly synthesis of some phospholipids.

What are the functions of vitamin K?

Requirements

The RDA for adult men is 80 mcg and 65 mcg for women. The US food supply provides an average of 300 to 500 mcg of vitamin K.

What are vitamin K requirements for men and women?

Sources

Even though limited amounts of vitamin K are stored in the body, a shortage of vitamin K is unlikely because it is derived from both food and microflora in the

TABLE 6–5

FOOD SOURCES OF VITAMIN K

Food	Portion	Vitamin K (mcg)	Kilocalories (per serving)
Cooked Brussels sprouts	½ cup	287	33
Cooked spinach	½ cup	142	29
Raw cabbage	1 cup	104	16
Milk	1 cup	10	86–150

Nutrient data from Nutritionist III software, version 7.0. N-Squared Computing, Salem, Oregon.

gut. Green leafy vegetables are high in vitamin K, but meats and dairy products provide significant amounts (Table 6–5).

What are sources of vitamin K?

Bacterial flora in the jejunum and ileum synthesize vitamin K and provide about half of the body's requirement. Synthesis of vitamin K by intestinal bacteria, however, does not provide adequate amounts of the vitamin. For example a restriction of dietary vitamin K can alter clotting factors (Suttie et al, 1988).

Absorption and Excretion

Vitamin K absorption decreases with high levels of vitamin E supplementation. Small amounts of vitamin K stores have a rapid turnover. Ordinarily 30 to 40% of the amount absorbed is excreted via bile into the feces as water-soluble metabolites, with approximately 15% excreted in the urine.

Hyper- and Hypo- States

Hemolytic anemia—anemia caused by toxic agents.

Hyperbilirubinemia—elevated serum concentrations of bilirubin.

Kernicterus—elevated levels of bilirubin accompanied by neural symptoms.

No toxicity symptoms have been documented from oral intake of vitamin K. The synthetic menadione, however, may cause **hemolytic anemia**, **hyperbilirubinemia**, and **kernicterus** in the newborn.

Primary vitamin K deficiency is uncommon, but disease or drug therapy may cause deficiencies. In vitamin K deficiency, blood clotting time is prolonged, making clients prone to bleeding problems.

Fat Malabsorption

Any condition of the biliary tract affecting the flow of bile prevents vitamin K absorption. Bleeding tendencies are increased with obstruction of the bile ducts, jaundice, or gallbladder disease. Severe bleeding may occur during or after an operation for bile duct obstruction. Clients receive an injection of vitamin K or a water-soluble analog.

Vitamin K deficiency is common in celiac disease and sprue (which affect absorption in the small intestine) and other diarrheal diseases (such as ulcerative colitis) as a result of malabsorption. Intravenous administration of vitamin K may be indicated.

Newborn Infants

Anoxia—total lack of oxygen.

Prothrombin concentrations and other clotting factors are low for approximately 1 week after birth, and newborn infants are usually given a single dose of vitamin K intramuscularly immediately after birth to prevent hemorrhage. Newborn infants may develop hemorrhagic disease secondary to vitamin K deficiency because the gut is sterile during the first few days after birth. Premature and **anoxic** infants and infants of mothers taking anticoagulants are most susceptible to development of hemorrhagic disease of the newborn because of poor placental transfer of vitamin K or trauma at birth. Commercial infant formulas normally contain vitamin K in sufficient quantity to prevent deficiency. Breast milk contains only 20% of the RDA requirement of 5 mcg/day; vitamin K prophylaxis at birth is important.

Why is vitamin K prophylaxis necessary for infants? What are some toxic symptoms of vitamin K? What are symptoms of deficiency?

NURSING APPLICATIONS

1. Dosage of vitamin K (menadione) for infants is critical because an overdose may cause irreversible brain damage. Double check dose with another nurse if any questions arise.
2. Suggest water-soluble forms of vitamins K_1 and K_2 for clients unable to absorb the fat-soluble form.
3. Excessive amounts of vitamin A and/or vitamin E have a detrimental effect on vitamin K. Assess vitamin supplements taken. Discourage the use of vitamins A and E if client is prone to vitamin K deficiencies.
4. Vitamin K should never be confused with the symbol "K" used to designate potassium. If information is confusing or unclear, double check with another nurse or a physician.

Rx Cholestyramine, prescribed for hyperlipidemia, binds with bile salts; clients being treated with this drug are at risk of vitamin K deficiency, so assess for any bleeding problems such as petechiae (pinpoint, flat red spots) or ecchymosis (bruising).

Rx Antibiotic therapy inhibits vitamin K–producing intestinal microflora and appears to be a factor in the origin of vitamin K deficiency, especially with impaired hepatic or renal function (Alperin, 1987). Cancer clients especially need to be assessed for this.

Rx Clients receiving Warfarin (Coumadin) drugs may develop serious hemorrhaging problems if high intakes of vitamin E are taken simultaneously. Vitamin K is the antidote for warfarin overdose.

Client Education

- A lack of vitamin K may lead to bleeding problems.
- Large amounts of vitamin K–rich foods are contraindicated for clients on dicumarol or warfarin therapy.
- Vitamin K is stable to heat, so cooking does not affect vitamin K content of foods.

SUMMARY

The fat-soluble vitamins, summarized in Table 6–1, are unique because they are stored in the body for long periods of time. However, this increases the chances of toxicity particularly from overdoses of vitamins A and D.

Deficiencies can occur with fat-soluble vitamins but may take months or years to develop. Because fat-soluble excesses and deficiencies can be determined more readily from a thorough physical assessment rather than from diagnostic tests, nurses need to be knowledgeable about the requirements, sources, and functions of fat-soluble vitamins.

NURSING PROCESS IN ACTION

A healthy client comes to the clinic seeking information about vitamin K. He is not sure what foods he should eat or what to look for if an excess or deficiency should develop.

Nutritional Assessment

- Income.
- Living arrangements, working, and storage facilities.
- Knowledge about vitamin K.
- Beliefs about fat-soluble vitamins.
- Physical status, especially bleeding problems.
- Use of OTC or prescribed supplements or medications.
- Emotional state.

Dietary Nursing Diagnosis

Health seeking behavior RT inadequate/insufficient knowledge about vitamin K.

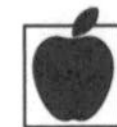

Nutritional Goals

Client will state beliefs/information about vitamin K and consume foods high in vitamin K.

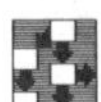

Nutritional Implementation

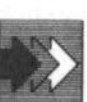

Intervention: Teach the following: (1) Forms—vitamin K_1 occurs in plants, vitamin K_2 is formed in the body, and vitamin K_3 is a synthetic compound. (2) Role—helps in blood clotting. (3) Sources—green leafy vegetables, meats, dairy products, and bacteria in the gut.

Rationale: This provides the client with a basic knowledge base about vitamin K.

Intervention: Instruct not to take high dosages of vitamin E or A.

Rationale: Vitamin K absorption decreases with high dosages of vitamin E or A.

Intervention: Explain hyper- and hypo- states: (1) Deficiency rarely occurs only because of diet but results from other disease processes, for example, fat malabsorption, gallbladder disease. (2) If deficiency is present, bleeding problems develop, such as petechiae, purpura, or ecchymosis.

Rationale: Because vitamin K is fat soluble, it is stored in the body, and toxicity may occur if too much is ingested. Knowledge increases likelihood that if deficiencies develop, treatment will be sought earlier.

Evaluation

If client consumes green leafy vegetables, kale, and cauliflower, goals were met. Additionally, if client states that supplements are not necessary and large doses may interfere with absorption of other nutrients and if he develops bleeding problems and seeks help, nursing care helped achieve desired outcomes. Lastly, he should also verbalize information concerning excesses and deficits of vitamin K.

STUDENT READINESS

1. Which fat-soluble vitamins are the most toxic? What are the symptoms of toxicity? What treatment is recommended for each?
2. A client asks why food is fortified with vitamin D. How would you respond?
3. Plan a 1-day menu that meets the RDA for vitamin A.
4. Janie is excited about vitamin E. She wants to be sure her intake is generous, so she bought a vitamin E supplement. When she discovers that you are studying nutrition, she starts to brag about her plan. How would you respond?
5. Keep a record of your food intake for 1 day. Use the table of nutrient values of foods in the Appendix for the amounts of vitamin A. Was your diet adequate? What are some food choices you could make for improvement?

REFERENCES

Alperin JB. Coagulopathy caused by Vitamin K deficiency in critically ill hospitalized patients. *JAMA* 1987 Oct 9; 258(14):1916–1919.

Bendich A, Machlin JJ. Safety of oral intake of vitamin E. *Am J Clin Nutr* 1988 Sept; 48(3):612–619.

Bjørneboe A, et al. Absorption, transport and distribution of vitamin E. *J Nutr* 1990 March; 120(3):233–242.

Greenberg ER, et al. A clinical trial of beta carotene to prevent basal-cell and squamous-cell cancers of the skin. The skin cancer prevention study group. *N Engl J Med* 1990 Sept 20; 323(12):789–795.

Hislop TG, et al. Diet and histologic types of benign breast disease defined by subsequent risk of breast cancer. *Am J Epidemiol* 1990 Feb; 131(2):263–270.

Kavookjian H, et al. Vitamin D deficiency contributes to hip fractures. *Am Fam Phys* 1990 Apr; 41(4):1231.

Knekt R, et al. Vitamin E and cancer prevention. *Am J Clin Nutr* 1991 Jan; 53(suppl):283S-286S.

Matsuoka LY, et al. Chronic sunscreen use decreases circulating concentrations of 25-hydroxy-vitamin D. *Arch Dermatol* 1988 Dec; 124(12):1802–1804.

Meydani SN, et al. Vitamin E supplementation enhances cell-mediated immunity in healthy elderly subjects. *Am J Clin Nutr* 1990 Sept; 52(3):557–563.

Murphy AP, et al. Vitamin E intakes and sources in the United States. *Am J Clin Nutr* 1990 Aug; 52(2):361–367.

Odes HS, et al. Effect of cimetidine on hepatic vitamin D metabolism in humans. *Digestion* 1990; 46(2):61–64.

Quesada JM, et al. Immunologic effects of vitamin D (Letter). *N Engl J Med* 1989 Sept 21; 321(12):833.

Reichel H, et al. The role of the vitamin D endocrine system in health and disease. *N Engl J Med* 1989 Apr 13; 320(15):980–991.

Rigby WFC. The immunobiology of vitamin D. *Immunol Today* 1988 Feb; 9(2):54–58.

Sowers MFR, et al. Relationship between dihydroxy vitamin D and blood pressure in a geographically defined population. *Am J Clin Nutr* 1988 Oct; 48(4):1053–1056.

Suttie JW, et al. Vitamin K deficiency from dietary vitamin K restriction in humans. *Am J Clin Nutr* 1988 March; 47(3):475–480.

Weisburger JH. Nutritional approach to cancer prevention with emphasis on vitamins, antioxidants, and carotenoids. *Am J Clin Nutr* 1991; 53 (Suppl):226S-237S.

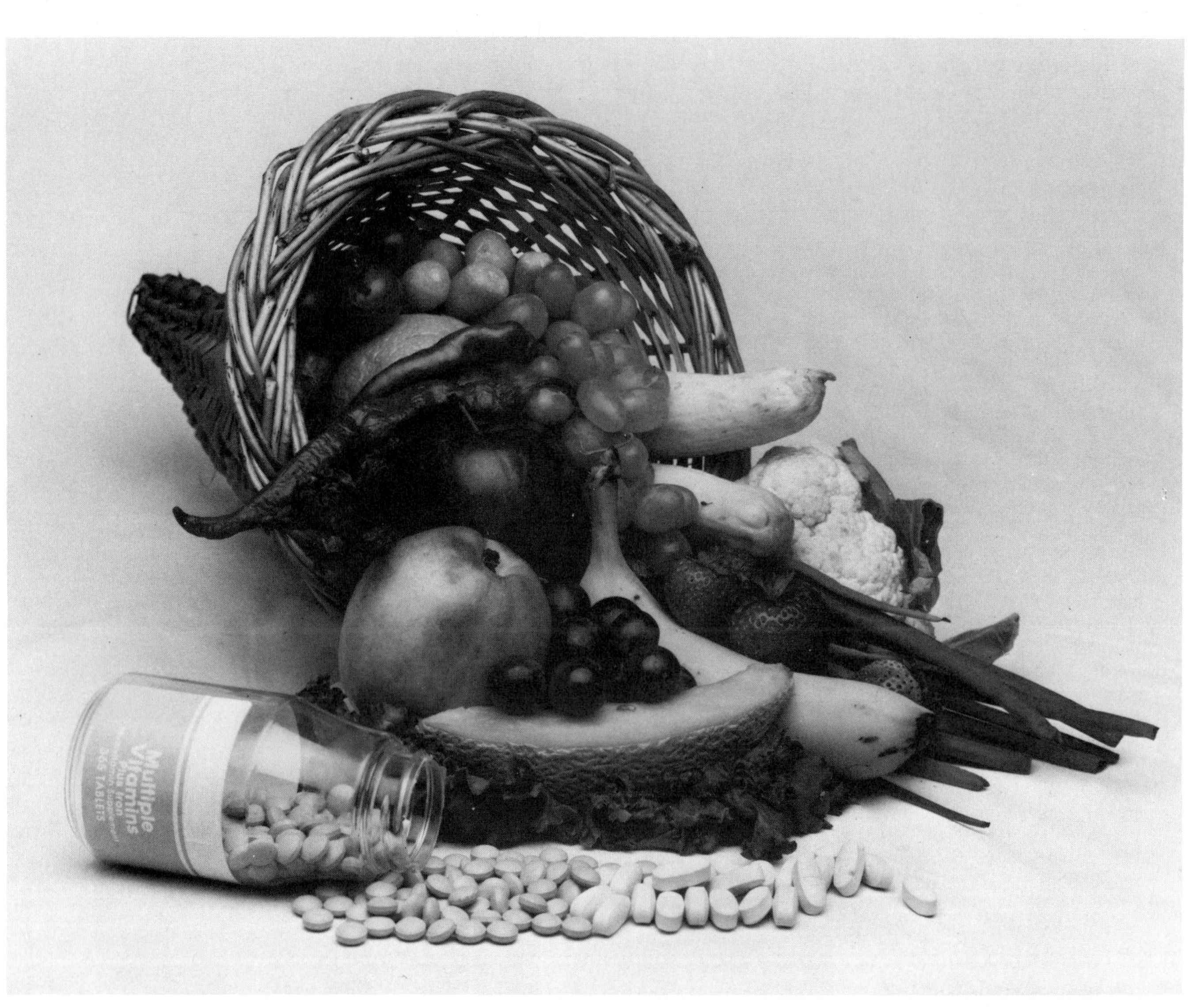
Multiple
Vitamins
Plus Iron
365 TABLETS

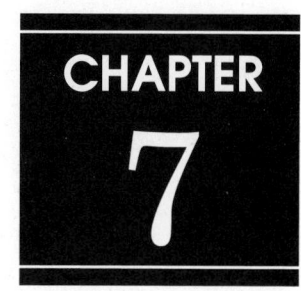

Water-Soluble Vitamins: More Miracle Workers

OUTLINE

I. CHARACTERISTICS OF WATER-SOLUBLE VITAMINS
II. VITAMIN C
  A. Physiological Roles
  B. Requirements
  C. Sources
  D. Hyper- and Hypo- States
  Nursing Applications
III. THIAMIN
  A. Physiological Roles
  B. Requirements
  C. Sources
  D. Hypo- States
  Nursing Applications
IV. RIBOFLAVIN
  A. Physiological Roles
  B. Requirements
  C. Sources
  D. Hypo- States
  Nursing Applications
V. NIACIN
  A. Physiological Roles
  B. Requirements
  C. Sources
  D. Hyper- and Hypo- States
  Nursing Applications
VI. VITAMIN B_6
  A. Physiological Roles
  B. Requirements
  C. Sources
  D. Absorption and Excretion
  E. Hyper- and Hypo- States
  Nursing Applications
VII. PANTOTHENIC ACID
  A. Physiological Roles
  B. Requirement

C. Sources
D. Hypo- States
Nursing Applications
VIII. BIOTIN
A. Physiological Roles
B. Requirement
C. Sources
D. Hypo- States
Nursing Applications
IX. FOLATE
A. Physiological Roles
B. Requirements
C. Sources
D. Absorption and Excretion
E. Hypo- States
Nursing Applications
X. VITAMIN B_{12}
A. Physiological Roles
B. Requirements
C. Sources
D. Absorption and Excretion
E. Hyper- and Hypo- States
Nursing Applications
XI. PSEUDOVITAMINS
Nursing Applications
XII. NUTRITION UPDATE 7–1: SUPPLEMENTS
A. Vitamin Megadoses
1. Megadoses of Niacin
Nursing Applications

OBJECTIVES

THE STUDENT WILL BE ABLE TO:

- Compare the characteristics of water-soluble vitamins with those of fat-soluble vitamins.
- Discuss the pros and cons of vitamin supplementation.
- Differentiate between scientific facts versus food fads concerning vitamins.
- Discuss the role and sources of vitamin B_{12} for vegetarians.
- Compare and contrast the function, sources, surpluses or toxicities, deficiencies, and symptoms of each water-soluble vitamin.
- Identify nursing application principles for each of the water-soluble vitamins.
- Discuss client teaching tips for water-soluble vitamins.

TEST YOUR NQ (True/False)

1. Vitamin pills containing 10 times the RDA are a better buy.
2. A daily intake of water-soluble vitamins is necessary.
3. Vitamin C is needed for wound healing.
4. Vitamin B_6 is the sunshine vitamin.
5. Beriberi is caused by niacin deficiency.
6. Strict vegetarians may be prone to vitamin B_{12} deficiency.
7. Clients with hypercholesterolemia should take niacin supplements.

8. Whole grains are high in thiamin.
9. Carrots are high in folate.
10. Riboflavin is furnished by foods in the grain group.

CHARACTERISTICS OF WATER-SOLUBLE VITAMINS

Vitamins B complex and C are all water soluble. In contrast to vitamin C and fat-soluble vitamins, the B vitamins all contain nitrogen. The water-soluble vitamins have vital roles as coenzymes necessary for almost every cellular reaction in the body (Fig. 7–1).

Unless otherwise indicated in the following discussion, water-soluble vitamins are readily absorbed in the jejunum. As a rule, absorption efficiency decreases with high concentrations. The body stores very small amounts of each of these vitamins, and therefore, few water-soluble vitamins produce toxic symptoms. Because of their limited storage, daily intake is important. A summary of water-soluble vitamins is provided in Table 7–1.

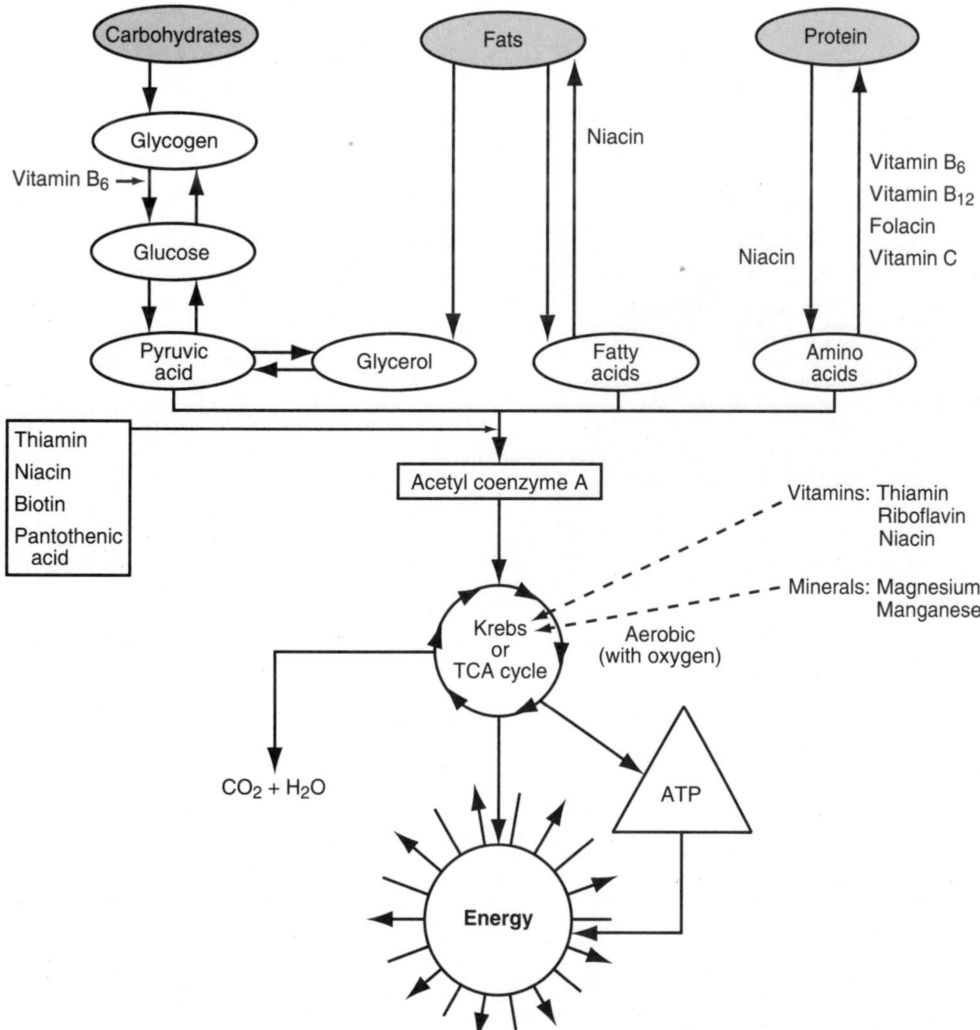

Figure 7–1 The role of vitamins in nutrient metabolism. TCA, tricarboxylic acid; ATP, adenosine triphosphate.

TABLE 7–1

SUMMARY OF WATER-SOLUBLE VITAMINS

Vitamin	Recommended Daily Allowances	Important Sources	Physiological Roles	Hypovitaminosis or Deficiency Symptoms
Vitamin C or ascorbic acid	Males and females (15–51+): 60 mcg Males and females (11–14): 50 mg Pregnancy: 70 mg Lactation: 90–95 mg Infants: 30–35 mg Children (1–10): 40–45 mg	Citrus fruits; strawberries; cantaloupe; tomatoes; sweet peppers; cabbage; potatoes; turnip greens; broccoli; mango; peaches; pineapple	Antioxidant; maintains integrity of capillaries; promotes healing of wounds and fractures; aids tooth and bone formation; increases iron absorption and protects folate; and helps form collagen for healthy connective tissue	Bruise and hemorrhage easily; incomplete or slow wound healing; gingivitis (loose teeth, gums that bleed easily, and sore mouth); anemia; scurvy
Thiamin (vitamin B_1)	0.5 mg/1000 kcal Males (11–14): 1.3 mg (15–50): 1.5 mg (51+): 1.2 mg Females (11–50): 1.1 mg (51+): 1 mg Pregnancy: 1.5 mg Lactation: 1.6 mg Infants: 0.3 mg Children (1–10): 0.7–1 mg	Pork; liver; chicken; beef; whole grains; enriched cereals; legumes	Coenzyme for metabolism of energy nutrients, especially important in carbohydrate metabolism	Poor appetite; fatigue; depression; apathy; polyneuritis; cardiac failure; Wernicke-Korsakoff syndrome; beriberi
Riboflavin (vitamin B_2)	0.6 mg/1000 kcal Males (11–14): 1.5 mg (15–18): 1.8 mg (19–50): 1.7 mg (51+): 1.4 mg Females (11–50): 1.3 mg	Milk; liver; meat; fish; enriched cereal products	Coenzyme for metabolism of energy nutrients, especially important in protein metabolism	Dermatitis; glossitis; cheilosis; hypersensitivity to light
Niacin (tryptophan is precursor; also called nicotinic acid and nicotinamide)	Men and women: 6.6 mg/1000 kcal or minimum 13 niacin equivalents Males (11–14): 17 mg (15–18): 20 mg (19–50): 19 mg (51+): 15 mg Females (11–50): 15 mg (51+): 13 mg Pregnancy: 17 mg Lactation: 20 mg Infants: 5–6 mg Children (1–10): 9–13 mg	Liver; poultry; beef; fish; eggs; whole grains; enriched cereals; legumes; seeds; nuts	Coenzyme in metabolism of energy nutrients; important in electron transport	Dermatitis; decreased energy; weakness; apathy; mental confusion; anorexia; and pellagra (dermatitis, diarrhea, depression or dementia, and death)
Pyridoxine (vitamin B_6), pyridoxal, and pyridoxamine	0.016 mg/gm protein Males (11–14): 1.7 mg (15–51+): 2 mg Females (11–14): 1.4 mg (15–18): 1.5 mg (19+): 1.6 mg Pregnancy: 2.2 mg Lactation: 2.1 mg Infants: 0.3–0.6 mg Children (1–10): 1–1.4 mg	Pork; organ meats; beef; poultry; fish; corn; legumes; seeds; grains; wheat; potatoes; bananas; green leafy vegetables and green beans	Coenzyme especially important in protein metabolism; converts tryptophan to niacin; hemoglobin synthesis; and integrity of CNS	Nervous irritability; seborrhea-like skin lesions; weakness; anemias (hypochromic, microcytic, and of pregnancy); impaired immune responses; and convulsions (in infants)
Pantothenic acid	ESADDI: Infants: 2–3 mg Children (1–3): 3 mg Children (4–6): 3–4 mg Children (7–10): 4–5 mg Children (11+) and adults: 4–7 mg	Present in all plant and animal foods; meats; legumes; whole grains	Coenzyme in metabolism of carbohydrate, protein, and fat Formation of some hormones and nerve regulating substances	Deficiency seen only with severe multiple B-complex deficits

TABLE 7–1

SUMMARY OF WATER-SOLUBLE VITAMINS *Continued*

Vitamin	Recommended Daily Allowances	Important Sources	Physiological Roles	Hypovitaminosis or Deficiency Symptoms
Biotin	ESADDI Infants: 10–15 mcg Children (1–3): 20 mcg Children (4–6): 25 mcg Children (7–10): 30 mcg Children (11+) and adults: 30–100 mcg	Liver; meat; egg yolk; cereals; milk Synthesized by microorganisms in GI tract	Coenzyme in metabolism of energy nutrients	Depression and anorexia; glossitis; dermatitis
Folate, folic acid, folacin, and tetrahydrofolic acid	3 mcg/kg Males and females (11–14): 150 mcg Males (15–51+): 200 mcg Females (15–51+): 180 mcg Pregnancy: 400 mcg Lactation: 280–260 mcg Infants: 25–35 mcg Children (1–10): 50–100 mcg	Green leafy vegetables; liver; beef; fish; legumes; whole grains	Coenzyme, especially important in purines, pyrimidines, nucleic acid, RBC maturation	Megaloblastic anemia; glossitis; diarrhea; poor growth; frequent infections; depression; mental confusion
Vitamin B_{12}, cyanocobalamin, and hydroxycobalamin	Males and females (11–51+): 2 mcg Pregnancy: 2.2 mcg Lactation: 2.6 mcg Infants: 0.3–0.5 mcg Children (1–10): 0.7–1.4 mcg	Only in animal foods: liver; meat; salt-water fish; oysters; milk; and eggs Synthesized by microorganisms in the GI tract	Coenzyme in nucleic acid synthesis, RBC maturation; myelin synthesis	Pernicious or megaloblastic anemia; peripheral neuropathy

ESADDI, estimated safe and adequate daily dietary intakes.

VITAMIN C

Physiological Roles

Vitamin C functions as an antioxidant in numerous reactions in the body. As a coenzyme, it has numerous metabolic roles. It is important in the production of **collagen,** which plays a vital role in wound healing. Vitamin C strengthens the tissues and promotes capillary integrity. Vitamin C facilitates development of RBC by enhancing iron absorption and utilization. It has a coenzymatic function in the metabolism of amino acids, and biosynthesis of thyroxine, epinephrine, bile acids, and steroid hormones. Vitamin C can also affect immune responses via functions of leukocytes and macrophages.

Collagen is the basic protein substance of connective tissue that helps support body structures such as skin, bones, and tendons.

Based on epidemiologic evidence, ascorbic acid intake may be associated with a lower risk of gastric and esophageal cancer. Functioning as an antioxidant, vitamin C may combine with nitrite, thus reducing the risk of stomach cancer. Such conclusions are based on consumption of vitamin C–rich foods (Weisburger, 1991).

What are the roles of vitamin C?

Requirements

The RDA for adults is established at 60 mg daily. The requirement for vitamin C is increased under many situations in which it is directly involved (e.g., healing and infections). It is detrimentally affected by many drugs (e.g., tobacco and aspirin) that increase requirements. Smokers may benefit from an intake of 200 mg vitamin C (Schectman et al, 1991).

What is the RDA for vitamin C?

TABLE 7–2

FOOD SOURCES OF VITAMIN C

Food	Portion	Vitamin C (mg)	Kilocalories (per serving)
Hot chili peppers	½ cup	182	30
Guava	1	165	46
Strawberries	1 cup	106	123
Currants	½ cup	102	36
Navel orange	1 cup	95	76
Grapefruit	1	91	74
Raw kohlrabi	1 cup	87	38
Papaya	1 cup	87	55
Kiwi	1	75	46
Cantaloupe	1 cup	68	56
Raw sweet pepper	1	66	20
Fresh orange juice	½ cup	62	56
Cooked broccoli	½ cup	58	22
Mango	1	57	135
Tomato paste	½ cup	56	110
Low-kilocalorie cranberry juice	½ cup	54	24
Cooked Brussels sprouts	½ cup	48	30
Canned hot chili peppers	½ cup	46	17
Cranberry juice	½ cup	45	72
Raw cabbage	1 cup	43	10
Raw cauliflower	½ cup	36	12
Green peas	½ cup	31	181
Baked sweet potatoes	1	28	118
Collard greens	½ cup	23	31
Tomato juice	½ cup	22	21
Cooked asparagus	½ cup	22	25
Raw cabbage	½ cup	21	22
Baked potato	1	20	145
Sauerkraut	½ cup	17	22
Baked butternut squash	½ cup	16	41
Watermelon	1 cup	15	51
Pineapple juice	½ cup	15	65
Cooked okra	½ cup	13	26
Fresh pineapple	½ cup	12	38

Nutrient data from Nutritionist III software, version 7.0. N-Squared Computing, Salem, Oregon.

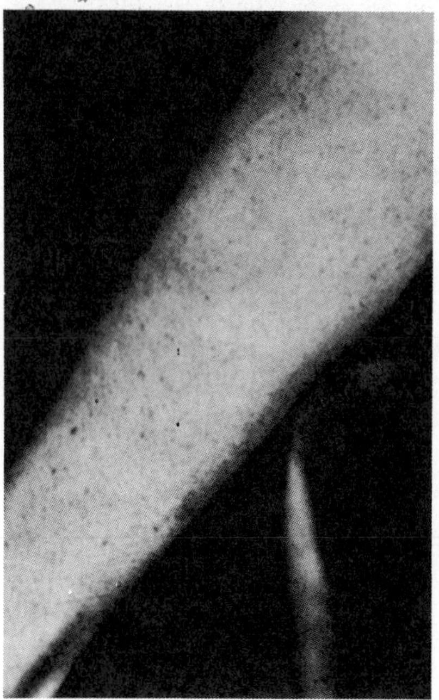

Figure 7–2 Perifollicular hemorrhages on the leg of a 16-year-old boy with scurvy. (From Merck Report, Rahway, NJ, May, 1956.)

Sources

The RDA can usually be met by choosing one serving of foods known as excellent sources (citrus fruits, cantaloupe, green pepper, broccoli, Brussels sprouts, strawberries, and mango). Good sources include peaches, pineapple, cabbage, potatoes, sweet potatoes, and tomatoes and may require at least 2 choices to meet the RDA (Table 7-2).

What are excellent and good sources of vitamin C?

Hyper- and Hypo- States

Megadoses of ascorbic acid have been promoted as increasing resistance to colds and other respiratory diseases. These claims have not been well substantiated or reproducible. Excessive intakes are well tolerated by most clients. Adverse effects reported, however, include diarrhea, hypoglycemia, **oxaluria,** and dependency or rebound effect. Although vitamin C increases iron absorption, large amounts interfere with absorption of vitamin B_{12}.

Scurvy, caused by vitamin C deficiency, is characterized by **petechiae,** bleeding gums, follicular hyperkeratosis, fatigue, and depression (Fig. 7-2). Scurvy can mimic several serious disorders, such as deep vein thrombosis, vasculitis, and systemic bleeding (Fig. 7-3). Initially, scorbutic clients may be extensively evaluated for other disorders. Symptoms may develop within 60 to 90 days with total elimination of vitamin C from the diet.

Vitamin megadose is defined as more than 10 times greater than the RDA.

Oxaluria—an excess of oxalate in the urine.

Petechiae—small pinpoint round red spot caused by submucous hemorrhage.

What are some adverse effects of excess/deficient amounts of vitamin C?

NURSING APPLICATIONS

1. Elderly clients, especially those who live alone or who avoid acidic foods to control esophageal reflux; clients undergoing peritoneal dialysis or hemodialysis; smokers; and drug abusers are at greatest risk to become scorbutic. Therefore, assess for deficiency: nose bleeds, melena (vomitus or stools containing blood), loose teeth, bleeding gums, petechiae (especially lower legs and back), and anemia.
2. Decreased collagen synthesis is evident in slow wound healing, defects in tooth formation, bleeding gums, bone fractures, and rupture of capillaries. Assess for vitamin C intake.
3. Because vitamin C enhances iron absorption, routine use of intravenous fluids containing the usual 3 gm of ascorbic acid should be avoided in iron-overloaded clients, such as alcoholics.
4. Clients who form kidney stones should avoid high doses of vitamin C.
5. In clients taking large doses of vitamin C, a sudden reduction in vitamin C may lead to scurvy. Intake should be gradually tapered.
6. Evaluate the amount of vitamin C supplements taken. If vitamin C intake is high, vitamin B_{12} deficiency could occur and the client should be monitored for this.

Client Education

- Storage is important for the vitamin's preservation. Fruit juices kept in an airtight container that is appropriate for the amount stored retain more vitamin C. The vitamin C content of 2 cups of juice in a pint container with an airtight lid is protected better than that of a pint of juice in a gallon container.
- Inform clients who smoke that they need 200 mg rather than 60 mg of vitamin C (Schectman et al, 1991).
- Ascorbic acid is another name for vitamin C.

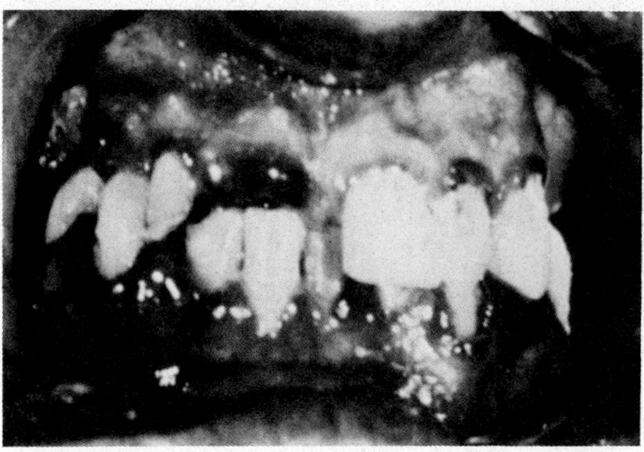

Figure 7–3 Gingival enlargement as a result of ascorbic acid deficiency. (From Nizel AE, Pappas AS. *Nutrition in Clinical Dentistry*. 3rd ed. Philadelphia, WB Saunders, 1989.)

THIAMIN

Physiological Roles

What is the role of thiamin?

Thiamin functions as a coenzyme in the metabolism of energy nutrients via the Krebs cycle to produce energy. This role makes it crucial for normal functioning of the brain, nerves, muscles, and heart. The main effects of thiamin deficiency, however, are disturbances of carbohydrate metabolism, which is impossible without thiamin.

Requirements

What is the requirement for thiamin, and what is it based on?

Because thiamin is a coenzyme in the Krebs cycle, the requirement is based on the total kilocalories needed. Those engaged in rigorous physical activity burn more energy, so more thiamin is required. The RDA for adults is 0.5 mg/1000 kcal or a minimum intake of 1 mg/day for clients consuming <2000 kcal/day. USDA surveys indicate that adult men consume adequate amounts of thiamin; the average intake of women is slightly below the RDA.

Sources

What are sources of thiamin?

Thiamin is widely distributed in foods, and intake of a variety of foods, including whole grains or enriched grains, can ensure adequate amounts (Table 7–3). Approximately 40% of thiamin intake is provided by grain products or unrefined and enriched cereals and grains. In the meat group, pork is an exceptionally good source. Other good sources include nuts and legumes.

Hypo- States

Thiaminase—an active enzyme that inactivates thiamin. Cooking deactivates thiaminases.

Because thiamin is required for the metabolism of carbohydrates, proteins, and fats, a wide range of symptoms develops with an insufficient intake. Primary dietary deficiency usually occurs in Third World countries, where polished rice is the staple diet. In developed countries, thiamin deficiency is secondary to alcoholism, ingestion of raw fish containing microbial **thiaminases,** chronic febrile states, and total parenteral nutrition (McCormick, 1988). Thiamin deficiency has been

TABLE 7–3

FOOD SOURCES OF THIAMIN

Food	Portion	Thiamin (mg)	Kilocalories (per serving)
Brewers yeast	1 tbsp	1.3	25
Lean broiled pork chop	3 oz	0.83	218
Sunflower seeds	¼ cup	0.82	205
Baked ham	3 oz	0.62	151
Wheat germ	¼ cup	0.54	103
Cooked oatmeal	1 cup	0.26	145
Cooked Eastern oysters	3 oz	0.25	117
Black beans	½ cup	0.21	114
Baked acorn squash	½ cup	0.17	58
Baked potato	1	0.16	145
Cooked split peas	½ cup	0.15	115
Kidney beans	½ cup	0.14	113
Watermelon	1 cup	0.13	51
White bread	1	0.12	67
Orange	1	0.11	62
Lean broiled sirloin steak	3 oz	0.11	176
Green peas	½ cup	0.10	59
Whole-wheat bread	1	0.10	69
Peanuts	¼ cup	0.09	209
Baked winter squash	½ cup	0.09	40
Blackeyed/cowpeas	½ cup	0.08	80
Cooked asparagus	½ cup	0.06	25
Cantaloupe	1 cup	0.06	56

Nutrient data from Nutritionist III software, version 7.0. N-Squared Computing, Salem, Oregon.

classified as an alcohol-related disease, but it can also occur in malnourished homeless people and Southeast Asian immigrants to the US (Skelton & Skelton, 1990).

Thiamin is called the morale vitamin because short-term deficiency causes clients to become depressed, irritable, anorexic, fatigued, and unable to concentrate. In addition to loss of stamina, clients with thiamin deficiency lose interest in their work. The brain and central nervous system (CNS), almost entirely dependent on glucose for energy, are seriously impaired when thiamin is not available.

Severe thiamin deficiency results in beriberi, which causes extensive damage to the nervous and cardiovascular systems.

Beriberi means "I cannot" because clients with this thiamin deficiency cannot move easily. There are 2 forms of beriberi: severe muscle wasting results in dry beriberi, whereas wet beriberi is accompanied by edema (Fig. 7–4). Additional symptoms of wet beriberi include **dyspnea, hepatomegaly,** and **oliguria** with resultant cardiac failure.

Dyspnea—difficulty breathing. Hepatomegaly—enlarged liver. Oliguria—decreased urine output.

The classic chronic form of dry beriberi presents with impairment of both sensory and motor function without involvement of the CNS. Other symptoms include muscular weakness, deep muscle pain in the calf, peripheral paralysis, tachycardia, and enlarged heart. Deficiency symptoms appear suddenly and are frequently devastating in infants.

Nystagmus—involuntary rapid movement of the eyeball. Ataxia—uncoordinated muscle movements.

Beriberi associated with alcoholism is characterized by mental confusion, **nystagmus,** and **ataxia.** These symptoms, similar to those seen in Wernicke-Korsakoff syndrome, occur most frequently in malnourished alcoholics. This syndrome usually occurs in alcoholics because alcohol intake increases thiamin requirement when total nutrient intake is poor. Thiamin deficiency has also been documented with long-term total **parenteral** feeding (Seligmann et al, 1991) and use of the diuretic furosemide (Zak et al, 1991). Early diagnosis is essential, so thiamin therapy is initiated early in the course of the disease. A quick response to thiamin therapy confirms the diagnosis.

Parenteral feeding—providing nutrients intravenously.

What groups of clients are prone to decreased thiamin? How is the brain affected with thiamin deficiency? Describe the differences between wet and dry beriberi.

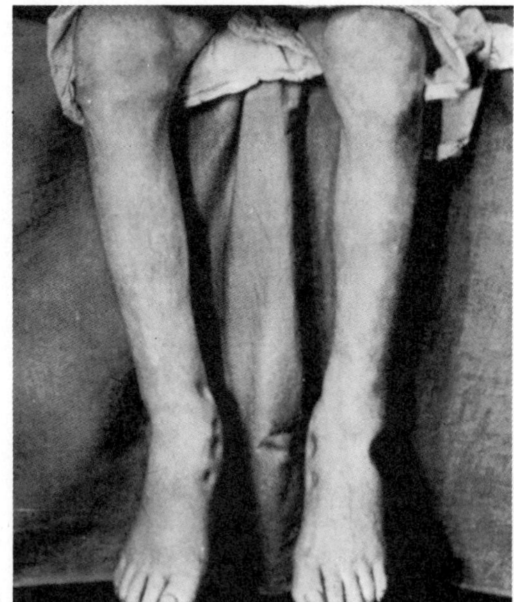

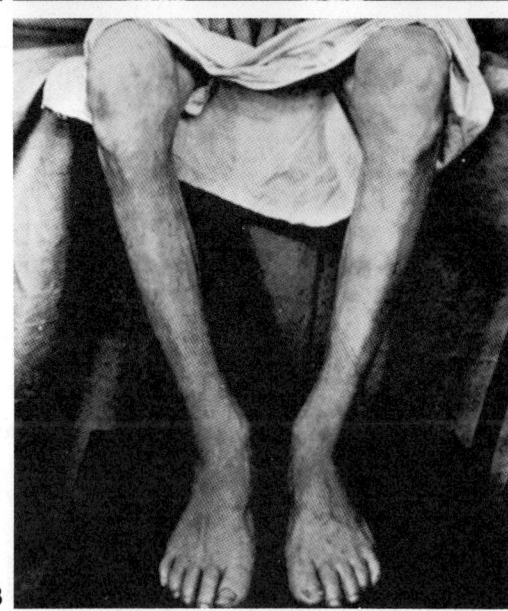

Figure 7–4 Client before and after treatment for vitamin B_1 deficiency (so-called wet beriberi). *A*, Swelling of the legs and marked pitting edema in the ankle region. *B*, Ten days after initiation of thiamin therapy, during which the client lost 40 pounds. Presumably this weight loss was due to the loss of fluid because the general nutritive state was greatly improved. (From Spies. *Rehabilitation Through Better Nutrition.* Philadelphia, WB Saunders, 1947.)

NURSING APPLICATIONS

1. A careful dietary history, including that of alcohol consumption, along with a detailed physical assessment of the cardiovascular and neurological systems, helps identify the early stages of thiamin deficiency: vasodilation (ruddy skin), salt retention (dependent edema), dyspnea, palpitations, and neuropathy (tingling and numbness in extremities, decreased feeling).
2. Vitamin deficiencies seldom occur in isolation. If a deficiency is suspected or diagnosed, observe for symptoms of other vitamin B deficiencies.
3. Carbohydrate loading or a very high carbohydrate diet and high physical activity slightly increase thiamin requirement. If intake and activity levels are high, assess diet for thiamin adequacy. (Generally, increased intake results in high levels of thiamin consumption.)
4. Beriberi heart failure occurs in clients who continue hard physical work, maintaining a high cardiac work load, so advise clients with beriberi to decrease physical activity and rest frequently.

5. Although immediate clinical response to thiamin therapy is often dramatic, ultimate recovery may be incomplete, and relapses may occur, especially if the precipitating factors persist. Recovery is usually extremely slow after prolonged paralysis. Based on this, offer emotional support to the client to prevent depression or hopelessness.
6. Thiamin deficiency is often an unsuspected cause of lactic acidosis. If client has lactic acidosis for no apparent reason, request that the physician evaluate for thiamin deficiency.

Client Education

- Raw fish contains an active enzyme, thiaminase, which destroys thiamin.
- Another name for thiamin is vitamin B_1.

RIBOFLAVIN

Physiological Roles

Riboflavin functions as a coenzyme in the metabolism of energy nutrients to release cellular energy. It is also involved in the **deamination** process. Closely related to the metabolism of protein, all conditions requiring increases in protein (e.g., burns or growth spurts) lead to additional riboflavin requirements. Riboflavin is also essential for healthy eyes, as a part of an enzyme in tissue reproduction, and in hydrogen transport.

Deamination—removal of the amino group from an amino acid.

What are the roles of riboflavin?

Requirements

The NRC has recommended a minimum intake of 1.2 mg/day for all adults (0.6 mg/1000 kcal), with an allowance of 1.7 for men and 1.3 for women. This level is influenced by the kilocaloric requirements of individuals. Additionally, when nitrogen balance is positive, more riboflavin is retained.

What are the requirements for riboflavin?

Sources

Although milk and milk products are excellent sources of riboflavin, approximately 30% of the dietary intake is furnished by foods in the grain group (Table 7–4). Meat, poultry, and fish also provide about one-fourth of the dietary requirement.

What are food sources of riboflavin?

Hypo- States

The body carefully guards its limited riboflavin stores. Even in severe deficiency, as much as one-third of the normal amount is present in the liver, kidney, and heart. Uncomplicated riboflavin deficiency is uncommon but is encountered in clients with multiple nutrient deficiencies related to poor nutrient absorption or utilization. Since riboflavin is essential to the functioning of vitamin B_6 and niacin, riboflavin deficiency also results in symptoms related to deficiency of these nutrients.

Ariboflavinosis is caused by riboflavin deficiency. Cheilosis is cracks and sores around the corners of the mouth; the skin is scaly with red lesions. Glossitis is inflammation of the tongue. Normochromic—color of erythrocytes is normal; normocytic—size and shape of erythrocytes are normal.

TABLE 7–4

FOOD SOURCES OF RIBOFLAVIN

Food	Portion	Riboflavin (mg)	Kilocalories (per serving)
Beef liver	3 oz	3.48	137
Braunschweiger sausage	3 oz	1.30	305
Cooked Eastern oysters	3 oz	1.30	117
Ricotta cheese	1 cup	0.45	340
Cheddar cheese	1 cup	0.42	455
Milk	1 cup	0.40	86–150
Buttermilk	1 cup	0.38	99
Low-fat cottage cheese	1 cup	0.37	164
Brewers yeast	1 tbsp	0.34	25
Raw mushrooms	1 cup	0.31	18
Almonds	¼ cup	0.25	192
Baked lean pork loin	3 oz	0.22	204
Cooked spinach	½ cup	0.21	21
Cooked beet greens	½ cup	0.21	20
Canned salmon	3 oz	0.16	118
Lean beef	3 oz	0.15	151
Turkey breast	3 oz	0.11	115
Cooked asparagus	½ cup	0.09	25
Cooked broccoli	½ cup	0.07	26

Nutrient data from Nutritionist III software, version 7.0. N-Squared Computing, Salem, Oregon.

What happens in the body with a riboflavin deficiency?

The symptoms associated with **ariboflavinosis** include **cheilosis** and angular stomatitis; **glossitis** and dermatitis; and **normochromic, normocytic** anemia. These symptoms, especially glossitis and dermatitis, may actually be secondary to vitamin B_6 deficiency.

NURSING APPLICATIONS

1. Hyperthyroidism, fevers, the added stress of injuries or surgery, and malabsorption syndromes increase riboflavin requirements. Assess clients with these conditions for deficiencies: cheilitis (inflammation of the lips), glossitis, and dermatitis.
2. Clients with increased nitrogen losses that are due to catabolism have increased riboflavin excretion. If intake does not appear to provide adequate amounts of riboflavin, increase the riboflavin provided either orally or intravenously.
3. The sensitivity of riboflavin to light may result in decomposition of the vitamin during phototherapy of hyperbilirubinemic infants. Observe for signs and symptoms of riboflavin deficiency in infants receiving phototherapy.

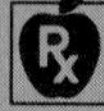

Phenothiazines and antibiotics increase excretion of riboflavin, so monitor for a deficiency in these clients.

Client Education

- Another name for riboflavin is vitamin B_2.
- Enriched products provide more riboflavin than their whole-grain counterparts.
- Lighted display cases have the potential for decomposition of riboflavin when milk is marketed in translucent plastic containers (Hoskin, 1988).
- A mixed diet that contains a pint of milk and 4 to 6 ounces of meat daily assures an adequate riboflavin supply.

NIACIN

Physiological Roles

The term niacin is loosely used to refer to 2 compounds, nicotinic acid and nicotinamide. Both compounds are used by the body. Niacin is crucial as a coenzyme in the production of energy (ATP). It functions with riboflavin in **gluconeogenesis** and **glycolysis.** Its role in tissue respiration via electron transport is very important.

Gluconeogenesis—synthesis of glucose from noncarbohydrate sources. Glycolysis—the conversion of glucose to lactate and then to energy storage in the form of ATP.

What are the roles of niacin?

Requirements

The body obtains niacin not only directly from the diet, but also indirectly from the conversion of an amino acid, tryptophan, and possibly also from that synthesized by intestinal microorganisms. RDAs are given in terms of niacin equivalents that include dietary sources of niacin plus its precursor, tryptophan. Approximately 1 mg of niacin may be formed from 60 mg of dietary tryptophan. The RDA niacin equivalent for adults is between 13 and 19 mg (6.6 mg/1000 kcal) daily. Niacin requirements are related to kilocaloric intake.

What is the requirement for niacin? How can the body obtain niacin?

Sources

Tryptophan is found mainly in milk, eggs, and meats. Niacin is widely distributed in plant and animal foods. Good sources include meats, cereals, legumes, seeds, and nuts (Table 7–5). With foods high in niacin plus those having tryptophan, it is easy to meet the RDA for niacin equivalents. Approximately 65% of the niacin in the US diet is provided by meat, milk, and eggs (NRC, 1989).

What are sources of niacin?

Hyper- and Hypo- States

Supplemental doses of nicotinic acid (3 to 6 gm/day) have been recommended to lower serum cholesterol and triglyceride levels. (Nicotinamide will not function in

TABLE 7–5

FOOD SOURCES OF NIACIN

Food	Portion	Niacin (mg)	Kilocalories (per serving)
Beef liver	3 oz	9.12	137
Baked chicken breast	3 oz	6.65	156
Broiled halibut	3 oz	6.06	119
Broiled lean lamb chop	3 oz	5.57	200
Canned salmon	3 oz	5.56	118
Turkey, white meat	3 oz	5.35	168
Peanuts	¼ cup	5.15	212
Canned tuna	3 oz	4.93	116
Sardines	3 oz	4.47	177
Broiled lean sirloin	3 oz	3.65	176
Brewers yeast	1 tbsp	3	25
Turkey, dark meat	3 oz	3	188
Raw mushrooms	1 cup	2.88	17
Cooked shrimp	3 oz	2.20	84
Baked potato	1	2.18	145
Peanut butter	1 tbsp	2.09	94
Wheat bran	¼ cup	2.04	32

Nutrient data from Nutritionist III software, version 7.0. N-Squared Computing, Salem, Oregon.

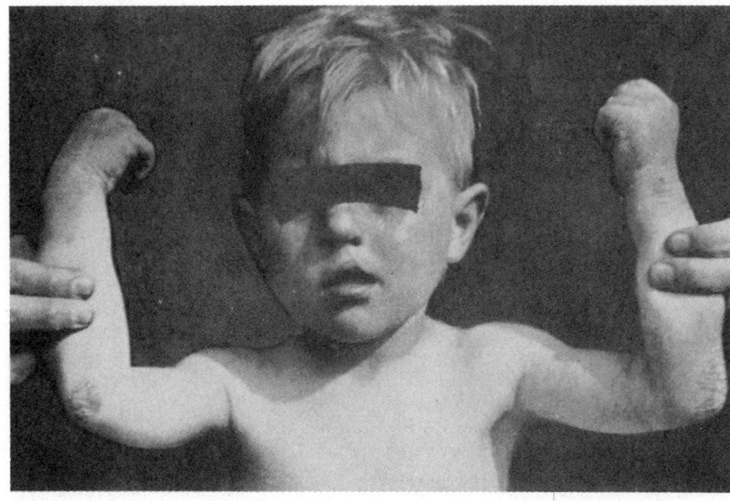

Figure 7–5 Pellagra in a 3-year-old boy, showing lesions on the hands and elbows and an early lesion over the nose and malar eminences. (From Behrman RE, Vaughan VC. *Textbook of Pediatrics.* 14th ed. Philadelphia, WB Saunders, 1992.)

this role.) The use of 250 mg of nicotinic acid daily results in the vitamin functioning as a vasodilator, producing flushing of the skin, nausea, itching, tachycardia, fainting, and blurred vision. Larger doses may lead to serious problems, including abnormal liver function and gout (see Nutrition Update 7–1).

Niacin deficiency results in pellagra, involving tissue degeneration of the skin, GI tract, and nervous system.

Pellagra is usually associated with a maize (corn) diet but may occur in alcoholics. Pellagra has been referred to as "the 3 D's—dermatitis, diarrhea, and depression or dementia." Pellagra means "rough skin," and the skin may look like goose flesh. The most striking and characteristic symptom of pellagra is a reddish skin rash, especially on the face, hands, or feet, that always appears on both sides of the body at the same time; i.e., it is bilaterally symmetrical (Fig. 7–5). It flares up when the skin is exposed to strong sunlight. Deficiency also affects mucous membranes; lesions in the GI tract result in diarrhea and less vitamin absorption. The tongue becomes scarlet and raw with fissures. Neurological symptoms include depression, apathy, headache, fatigue, and loss of memory.

NURSING APPLICATIONS

1. Assess clients, especially alcoholics and immigrants, for niacin deficiency: dementia (irritable and nervous), fatigue, depression, decreased memory, dermatitis (especially areas exposed to the sun), diarrhea, and raw scarlet tongue.
2. Because riboflavin deficiency often accompanies pellagra, supplemental riboflavin should accompany niacin treatment.
3. Niacin and thiamin may affect the appetite; however, weight-conscious clients should not avoid these vitamins. Evaluate client's beliefs concerning these 2 vitamins. If inaccurate information is given, provide correct information to prevent the development of a deficiency.

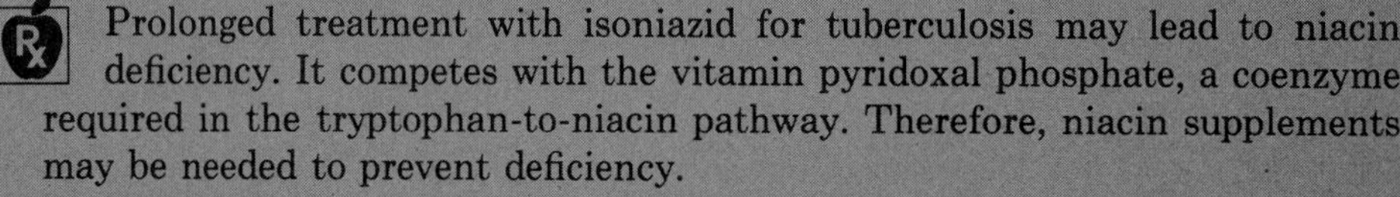

Prolonged treatment with isoniazid for tuberculosis may lead to niacin deficiency. It competes with the vitamin pyridoxal phosphate, a coenzyme required in the tryptophan-to-niacin pathway. Therefore, niacin supplements may be needed to prevent deficiency.

Client Education

- Clients should understand that a frequent side effect of a therapeutic dose of nicotinic acid is flushing. This should be discussed with the physician.
- Nicotinic acid and niacinamide are correct terminology for niacin and should not be confused with nicotine.
- Corn products are relatively deficient in tryptophan.

VITAMIN B_6

Vitamin B_6 is the term commonly used for a group of 3 compounds—pyridoxine, pyridoxal, and pyridoxamine. All 3 forms can be used by the body in its role as a coenzyme.

What are the 3 forms of vitamin B_6?

Physiological Roles

Several essential roles for vitamin B_6 have been identified: (1) coenzyme in protein metabolism, (2) conversion of tryptophan to niacin, (3) hemoglobin synthesis, (4) synthesis of unsaturated fatty acids from essential fatty acids, (5) energy production from glycogen, and (6) proper functioning of the nervous system including brain cells.

Name 4 functions of vitamin B_6.

Requirements

The current RDA for vitamin B_6 is 2 mg/day for men and 1.6 mg/day for women. The requirement for vitamin B_6 increases with protein intake because of its major role in amino acid metabolism. The average daily intake is slightly lower than the RDA for both men and women.

What is the RDA for vitamin B_6 in men and women?

Sources

Beef, poultry, fish, and pork are good sources of vitamin B_6. Other good sources include some fruits, nuts, whole-grain products, and vegetables (Table 7–6). Foods

TABLE 7–6

FOOD SOURCES OF PYRIDOXINE (VITAMIN B_6)

Food	Portion	Pyridoxine (mg)	Kilocalories (per serving)
Beef liver	3 oz	0.77	137
Banana	1	0.66	105
Navy peas	½ cup	0.53	113
Baked potato	1	0.47	145
Baked chicken breast	3 oz	0.47	167
Salmon	3 oz	0.39	157
Turkey	3 oz	0.39	145
Tuna fish	3 oz	0.37	116
Sunflower seeds	¼ cup	0.28	205
Watermelon	1 cup	0.23	51
Cooked spinach	½ cup	0.22	21
Baked flounder	3 oz	0.20	99
Brewers yeast	1 tbsp	0.20	25
Cantaloupe	1 cup	0.18	56
Pinto beans	½ cup	0.13	118
Cauliflower	½ cup	0.13	15
Cooked broccoli	½ cup	0.11	22
Raw spinach	1 cup	0.11	12
Cooked asparagus	½ cup	0.11	22
Wheat germ	1 tbsp	0.09	26
Peanuts	¼ cup	0.09	214

Nutrient data from Nutritionist III software, version 7.0. N-Squared Computing, Salem, Oregon.

What are good sources of vitamin B_6?

from animal and plant sources provide 48 and 52% of the total vitamin B_6 intake, respectively (Kant & Block, 1990).

Absorption and Excretion

Phosphorylation—the process of adding a phosphate group.

Absorption of vitamin B_6 differs from that of other B complex vitamins. It requires ATP for its absorption. All 3 forms of the vitamin are converted to an absorbable form by an intestinal enzyme. They are absorbed by the mucosal cells, which contain an enzyme that results in their **phosphorylation.** Body stores are small, and repletion is gradual.

Hyper- and Hypo- States

Ataxia—gait disorders.
Severe sensory neuropathy—impairment of sensations of touch, vibration, temperature, and pinprick.
Hypotonia—decreased strength.

Numerous studies have been presented regarding the benefits of providing supplemental amounts of vitamin B_6 in coronary heart disease, cancer, and premenstrual syndrome. Because of inconsistent findings, supplemental amounts are not currently recommended. Acute pyridoxine toxicity is low; however, studies of routine consumption of megadoses (more than 2 gm for 2 months or more) have documented such side effects as **ataxia** and **severe sensory neuropathy** and, in some instances, bone pain and muscle weakness (Dalton & Dalton, 1987). Pyridoxine given for neonatal seizures was reported to cause **hypotonia** requiring assisted ventilation (Kroll, 1985). In most cases, when megadose supplementation is discontinued, clients recover normal function.

What are the side effects of excessive amounts of vitamin B_6? List the symptoms of vitamin B_6 deficiency. How is vitamin B_6 affected by food processing of infant formulas and by OCAs?

Deficiency rarely occurs alone; vitamin B_6 deficiency is most commonly observed along with several other B vitamins. Clinical signs include CNS abnormalities or epileptiform convulsions, dermatitis with cheilosis and glossitis, impaired immune responses, and anemia.

Seizures have developed in infants fed a commercial infant formula in which vitamin B_6 was destroyed during processing. The mother's body stores of vitamin B_6 are critical to the well-being of the newborn infant. OCAs taken before conception may result in low vitamin B_6 plasma concentrations of the mother during pregnancy and in breast milk. A daily intake of 2 mg of vitamin B_6 may be recommended for women taking OCAs, especially if a pregnancy is planned in the near future.

NURSING APPLICATIONS

1. Assess clients for toxicity or deficiency.
2. Intake of this vitamin may decrease with increasing age and decreasing education and income status (Kant & Block, 1990). Therefore, offer foods high in vitamin B_6, and monitor for deficiency signs and symptoms.
3. Although serum levels are low in clients with chronic renal failure, supplementation may not be warranted (Pike et al, 1990), so do not panic if levels are low.
4. Any infant with intractable seizures should be diagnostically considered for vitamin B_6 deficiency. Even though it is rare, an increased requirement for this vitamin within the CNS can cause such seizures.

Rx Drugs that affect the metabolism of vitamin B_6 should be accompanied by a vitamin B_6 supplement. These drugs include isoniazid (for tuberculosis), cycloserine (antibiotic for tuberculosis), and penicillamine (for Wilson's disease, lead poisoning, kidney stone, arthritis). Secondary vitamin B_6 deficiency may occur if vitamin B_6 is not given with these drugs.

Excessive pyridoxine can reduce clinical benefits of levodopa therapy in Parkinson's disease. Assess vitamin supplementation of clients taking levodopa. If OTC supplements are being taken, discuss the interaction. Encourage client to limit intake of foods fortified with vitamin B_6. If the physician has ordered the supplement, monitor the client for desired effects of levodopa. If desired effects are not seen, consult with physician.

Client Education

- Do not take vitamin B_6 supplements unless ordered by a physician.
- Adequate daily intake of vitamin B_6 is important.

PANTOTHENIC ACID

Physiological Roles

Pantothenic acid is similar to the other B vitamins in its metabolic roles. Pantothenic acid is involved in the Krebs cycle with carbohydrates, fat, and protein metabolism in the form of coenzyme A. Additionally, it is important in gluconeogenesis, synthesis and degradation of fatty acids, and formation of certain hormones and nerve-regulating substances.

What are the roles of pantothenic acid?

Requirement

In 1989, the NRC subcommittee concluded that there is insufficient evidence to establish an RDA for pantothenic acid. They have established that an intake of 4 to 7 mg/day should be safe and adequate for adults.

What is the recommended intake of pantothenic acid?

Sources

Pantothenic acid is synthesized by most microorganisms and plants. It is particularly abundant in animal foods, legumes, and whole-grain cereals. Usual intake of pantothenic acid in the US is reported to be 5 to 10 mg/day (NRC, 1989).

What are sources of pantothenic acid?

Hypo- States

Semisynthetic—consumable items produced by chemical manipulation of naturally occurring substances.

Naturally occurring dietary deficiency of pantothenic acid has not been documented. Deficiency symptoms have been induced in clients using a metabolic antagonist or **semisynthetic** diets devoid of pantothenic acid. The resulting symptoms include postural hypotension, rapid heart rate on exertion, anorexia and constipation, and numbness and tingling of the extremities.

What signs and symptoms occur with pantothenic acid deficiency?

NURSING APPLICATIONS

1. Assess clients for deficiencies. Pantothenic acid deficiency rarely occurs alone, so assess for other vitamin deficiencies as well.
2. Pantothenic acid may help in wound healing, so be sure client is eating a well-balanced diet.

Client Education

- Distribution of this vitamin is widespread.
- Diets including whole-grain unprocessed foods contain more pantothenic acid.

BIOTIN

Physiological Roles

Describe how biotin is used by the body.

Biotin functions as a coenzyme in metabolism of the energy nutrients, assisting in the addition of carbon dioxide molecules to other compounds. As such, it is important for gluconeogenesis, synthesis of fatty acids, catabolism of some amino acids, and synthesis of purines.

Requirement

List the ESADDI for biotin.

Dietary requirement of biotin is uncertain because microflora synthesize it. ESADDI for biotin has been established at 30 to 100 mcg for adults.

Sources

What are 3 rich sources of biotin?

Although biotin is widely distributed in foods, its availability in foods is low compared with other water-soluble vitamins. Rich sources of biotin include egg yolk, liver, and cereals. GI microflora probably provide part of the body's needs (Table 7–7).

Hypo- States

Avidin is a biotin-binding glycoprotein substance present in raw egg white.

What can cause biotin deficiency? What happens in biotin deficiency?

Biotin deficiency can be produced by the ingestion of **avidin.** Avidin is denatured by heat; therefore, cooked egg white does not present a problem. Symptoms include anorexia, nausea, vomiting, glossitis, pallor, depression, and a dry scaly dermatitis. Seborrheic dermatitis of infants under 6 months of age has been documented as biotin deficiency. The condition is corrected with approximately 5 mg/day of biotin.

TABLE 7–7

FOOD SOURCES OF BIOTIN

Food	Portion	Biotin (mcg)	Kilocalories (per serving)
Cooked cauliflower	½ cup	10.7	15
Egg yolk	1	7.6	59
Brewers yeast	1 tbsp	6.4	25
Watermelon	1 cup	6.4	51
Peanut butter	1 tbsp	6.4	94
Cooked spinach	½ cup	5.7	21
Cantaloupe	1 cup	4.8	56
Banana	1	4.6	105

Data from Nutritionist III software, version 7.0. N-Squared Computing, Salem, Oregon.

NURSING APPLICATIONS

1. Assess clients for deficiencies: scaly dermatitis, depression.
2. Clients on prolonged intravenous therapy may be prone to this deficiency, so monitor closely.

Client Education

- Drinking or eating large amounts of raw egg whites over a long period of time may lead to biotin deficiency.
- Eggs should be cooked to decrease avidin's binding capacity and minimize danger of *Salmonella* poisoning.
- A balanced diet that includes a variety of foods contains adequate amounts of biotin, so supplements are unnecessary.

FOLATE

The generic term folate encompasses several compounds that have nutritional properties similar to those of folic acid. Several different metabolically active forms have been identified.

Physiological Roles

Folate functions as a coenzyme for approximately 20 enzymes. As such, it has an important role in synthesis of purine and pyrimidine bases in RNA and DNA. Its functions in the maintenance of normal levels of mature red cells (erythropoiesis) and choline synthesis are interrelated with vitamin B_{12}.

Describe important functions of folate.

Requirements

The RDA is 200 mcg for men and 180 mcg for women. Average intake is 305 mcg/day for men and 189 mcg/day for women (Bailey, 1990). Folate requirements are increased during growth and development, such as adolescence, pregnancy, and lactation, as a result of its role in DNA formulation.

What is the RDA for folate for men and women?

Sources

Rich sources of folate include liver, green leafy vegetables, legumes, and some fruits (grapefruit and oranges), as shown in Table 7–8.

Absorption and Excretion

Dietary folates must undergo some changes for their absorption. The intestinal enzyme that accomplishes this requires a slightly acidic pH and is activated by the presence of zinc. Alcohol consumption, oral contraceptives, and other drugs may interfere with absorption.

TABLE 7–8

FOOD SOURCES OF FOLATE

Food	Portion	Folate (mcg)	Kilocalories (per serving)
Brewers yeast	1 tbsp	313	25
Beef liver	3 oz	184	137
Pinto beans	½ cup	147	118
Cooked asparagus	½ cup	132	22
Cooked spinach	½ cup	131	21
Sunflower seeds	¼ cup	82	205
Romaine lettuce	1 cup	76	9
Orange juice	½ cup	55	56
Dry roasted peanuts	¼ cup	53	214
Sliced beets	½ cup	45	26
Cooked broccoli	½ cup	39	22
Navy peas	½ cup	33	113
Cooked turnip greens	½ cup	33	25
Cooked cauliflower	½ cup	32	15
Cantaloupe	1 cup	27	56
Egg yolk	1	24	59
Banana	1	22	105
Wheat germ	1 tbsp	20	26
Baked potato	1	14	145
Peanut butter	1 tbsp	13	94

Nutrient data from Nutritionist III software, version 7.0. N-Squared Computing, Salem, Oregon.

Folate is transported in the blood primarily bound to albumin. The liver is the primary storage site, with total body storage of 5 to 10 mg.

Hypo- States

Deficiency symptoms first appear in rapidly dividing cells, such as in the GI tract, RBCs, and white blood cells. Protein synthesis is also altered. Anemia from folate deficiency develops because cells cannot divide as a result of their inability to produce DNA. Hence RBCs do not develop normally; they become extremely large (megaloblastic) yet cannot transport oxygen to the cells. Further discussion of megaloblastic anemia is in Chapter 18. Other clinical symptoms of folate deficiency in addition to lethargy include glossitis, diarrhea, and poor growth.

Numerous medications interfere with folate absorption or metabolism (Table 7–9). Methotrexate, used in cancer chemotherapy, resembles folate and interferes with folate metabolism. This results in decreased DNA synthesis—not only the rapidly growing cancer cells, but also intestinal and epithelial cells. Diarrhea, vomiting, and hair loss are commonly seen.

TABLE 7–9

DRUGS THAT MAY NEGATIVELY AFFECT FOLATE STATUS

Anticonvulsants
Oral contraceptives
Analgesics
Cancer chemotherapeutic agents
Anti-inflammatory agents
H_2 receptor blockers
Antacids

NURSING APPLICATIONS

1. Assess clients, especially those with cancer, for deficiency (megaloblastic anemia).
2. Factors that increase metabolic rate, such as infection and hyperthyroidism, or increased cell turnover, such as hemolytic anemia, rapid tissue growth in a fetus, or malignant tumor, increase the requirement. Assess for folate intake by questioning client and monitoring intake. Additionally, evaluate client's physical status for folate deficiency.
3. Folate supplementation in pernicious anemia results in a remission of hematological abnormalities but not the neurological deficits. Therefore, a correct diagnosis must be made before the correct treatment can be ordered.

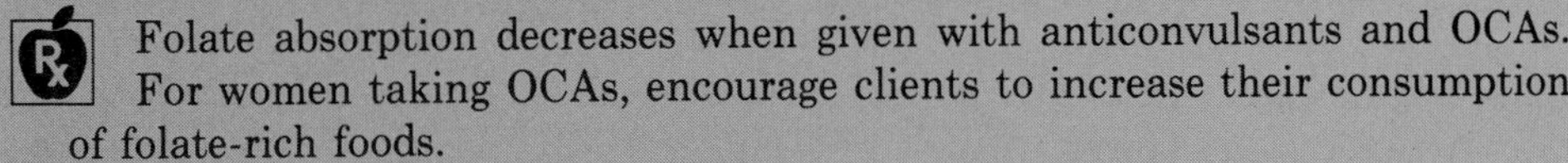

Folate absorption decreases when given with anticonvulsants and OCAs. For women taking OCAs, encourage clients to increase their consumption of folate-rich foods.

Folate supplementation should be closely monitored in clients being treated for convulsions with phenytoin (Dilantin). Clients taking anticonvulsants should be carefully monitored if folate supplements are taken; high intakes can decrease effectiveness of the medication.

Client Education

- Folate may be called folic acid or folacin.
- Prolonged cooking destroys folate.
- Folate is easily destroyed by food processing, so raw vegetables provide more folate than cooked ones.

VITAMIN B_{12}

Vitamin B_{12} or cobalamin represents a complex group of compounds that contain cobalt. The metabolism of vitamin B_{12} is closely correlated with folate metabolism.

Physiological Roles

Vitamin B_{12} functions as a coenzyme in conjunction with folate metabolism in nucleic acid synthesis. It also functions in the catabolism of certain amino acids and odd-chain fatty acids. Vitamin B_{12} is essential for hematopoiesis and **myelin** synthesis.

Myelin is a lipid substance that insulates nerve fibers.

Requirements

The RDA for adults is small, 2 mcg daily. Dietary intake frequently exceeds the RDA. A high vitamin B_{12} intake results in accumulation in the liver with increasing age, but this may be desirable because vitamin B_{12} intake declines in the elderly because of lower absorption rates (NRC, 1989).

Describe vitamin B_{12} roles and requirements.

Sources

Microorganisms (bacteria, fungi, and algae) can synthesize vitamin B_{12}. Vitamin B_{12} is not found in plants unless they are contaminated by microorganisms

TABLE 7–10

FOOD SOURCES OF VITAMIN B_{12}

Food	Portion	Vitamin B_{12} (mcg)	Kilocalories (per serving)
Beef liver	3 oz	60.5	137
Cooked Eastern oysters	3 oz	32.5	117
Cooked lean beef	3 oz	2.2	175
Cooked shrimp	3 oz	1.3	84
Protein fortified low-fat milk	1 cup	1.1	137
Broiled lean pork chop	3 oz	0.8	295
Whole egg	1	0.5	75
Baked chicken breast	3 oz	0.3	167
Cheddar cheese	1 oz	0.2	114

Nutrient data from Nutritionist III software, version 7.0. N-Squared Computing, Salem, Oregon.

What are sources of vitamin B_{12}?

(legumes and root vegetables). More than 80% of the dietary vitamin B_{12} is provided by meat and animal products (Table 7–10). GI flora produce small amounts of absorbable vitamin B_{12}.

Absorption and Excretion

R-binder is a protein produced by the salivary glands.

Intrinsic factor is secreted by the parietal cells in the stomach.

How is vitamin B_{12} absorbed in the body? What 2 elements are necessary?

In the stomach, free vitamin B_{12} combines with salivary **R-binder.** In the small intestine, trypsin (pancreatic enzyme) removes the R-binder, and vitamin B_{12} combines with **intrinsic factor** (Herbert & Colman, 1988). Absorption of vitamin B_{12} occurs at specific receptor sites in the ileum and is possible only if it is bound to intrinsic factor. Without R-binder and/or intrinsic factor, absorption of vitamin B_{12} is drastically reduced. The percentage absorbed decreases with increased dietary intake. The vitamin is recycled from bile and other intestinal secretions.

Hyper- and Hypo- States

Double-blind crossover study is a test in which neither the client nor the observer is aware of the substance being administered.

No benefits are seen from large quantities of vitamin B_{12}, but no harmful effects have been observed either. Injections of vitamin B_{12} are popular treatments for fatigue and weakness, with few clients meeting accepted medical criteria for its use. In a **double-blind crossover study** using vitamin B_{12} or placebo injections, clients reported that both treatments seemed to increase their energy but that neither therapy improved their functional status or decreased their symptoms (fever, generalized weakness, fatigue, or impaired memory) (Kaslow et al, 1989).

Achlorhydria—decreased production of HCl in the stomach.

A deficiency of vitamin B_{12} is rarely caused by insufficient dietary sources (unless strict vegan diets are followed). Lack of intrinsic factor is the primary cause of deficiency. As with folate-induced anemia, many macrocytes are present in the blood stream. The condition is also referred to as macrocytic, megaloblastic anemia. Pernicious anemia occurs more frequently in the elderly related to **achlorhydria** and decreased synthesis of intrinsic factor by the parietal cells.

What are some reasons vitamin B_{12} deficiency develops?

Neurological symptoms occur as a result of demyelination of the spinal cord and brain and optic and peripheral nerves. Orthostatic hypotension may occur (Lossos & Argov, 1991). Deficiency symptoms are rapidly corrected with vitamin B_{12} injections.

In a totally vegan community, children assessed to be deficient in vitamin B_{12} had stunted growth (Miller et al, 1991).

NURSING APPLICATIONS

1. Assess for deficiency: megaloblastic anemia, neurological deficits (abnormal sensations such as burning and prickling), weakness, and personality changes.
2. Concomitant ingestion of megadoses of ascorbic acid via foods or tablets can destroy substantial amounts of vitamin B_{12} and produce vitamin B_{12} deficiency. If client is prone to or has vitamin B_{12} deficiency, assess intake of vitamin C. If high, advise client to decrease vitamin C intake to approximate RDA levels.
3. Clients who have had permanent gastric surgery or ileal damage require monthly injections of vitamin B_{12} for life. Be sure client is aware of this.

Client Education

- Because vitamin B_{12} is found only in meat products, vegans (i.e., strict vegetarians) require a daily supplement of 1 mcg or vitamin B_{12}-fortified foods.
- Vitamin B_{12} shots are not a panacea against "tired blood."

PSEUDOVITAMINS

Other substances that resemble the B vitamins are sometimes touted as important. No deficiencies of these substances have been observed in clients, and no recommendations for intakes have been advised because they exist abundantly in foods and/or are formed within the body. They have been identified, however, as specific agents in various reactions within the body.

Choline is sometimes called a B vitamin. It has been identified as a coenzyme in metabolism, but no deficiencies have been observed. Infants may be vulnerable to choline deficiency, so some manufacturers add choline to their milk-based formulas.

Vitamin B_{12} and folate are involved in the biosynthesis of choline from methionine. Therefore, adequate intakes of these vitamins must be considered in relationship to an assessment for possible choline deficiency. Although choline is **lipotropic,** high doses of choline are ineffective in the treatment of fatty liver. High doses cause "fishy" body odor, gastric distress, and vomiting.

Lipotropic agents decrease fatty deposits in the liver.

Carnitine is essential in the oxidation of long-chain fatty acids. Because of endogenous synthesis from the amino acids, lysine and methionine, by the liver and kidney, healthy adults do not require a dietary source of carnitine. However, premature or newborn infants and clients who are critically ill or have renal or liver conditions may not be able to synthesize adequate quantities. Dietary sources of carnitine are meat and dairy products. Most infant formulas are supplemented with carnitine to levels similar to that of human milk. Carnitine supplements in clients with a secondary carnitine deficiency have shown improvement in symptoms such as progressive muscle disease, cardiomyopathy, hypoglycemia, and hyperammonemia (Borum, 1990). Many tube feeding formulas contain carnitine.

Also called pangamic acid, vitamin B_{15} is a substance that has been isolated but does not fit the prerequisites of a vitamin.

p-Aminobenzoic acid (PABA) is not a specific vitamin but rather a part of folate. Clients are unable to synthesize PABA and to attach it to the other part of the folate molecule if PABA is provided in its free state. PABA functions well as a sunscreen to prevent skin damage.

Bioflavonoids have been shown to act as antioxidants by protecting ascorbic acid and other components from oxidation. Most flavonoids are located in the skin or peel of many fruits and vegetables. They are not considered vitamins, and average intake is about 1000 mg daily (Herbert, 1988).

Bioflavonoids—flavonoids that have biological activity.

Describe choline's roles, clients prone to deficiency, vitamins necessary for choline synthesis, and possible effects of high doses. What are good sources of carnitine? What clients may need exogenous sources of carnitine? What do bioflavonoids do?

NURSING APPLICATIONS

1. Neonates and chronically ill clients with progressive muscle weakness seem to benefit from carnitine supplementation to enhance their tolerance to metabolic stress. Suggest formulas that contain added carnitine.
2. Choline as part of acetylcholine affects nerve transmission and motor functions. Provide safety measures to prevent client injury.

Client Education

- An excellent source of choline is egg yolks.
- Pills sold at health food stores containing bioflavonoids may contain a mutagen (agent that can cause a change in genetic material).

NUTRITION UPDATE 7–1: SUPPLEMENTS

Approximately one-half of all Americans consume vitamin-mineral supplements (Subar & Block, 1990), with an expenditure of $2.92 billion in 1986 (Anonymous, 1987). No single class of drugs is the target of as much quackery, misunderstanding, misrepresentation, and misuse as vitamins. Many clients consider vitamins safe to take in any amount, but each year, thousands of cases of vitamin poisoning occur, especially in children. Some supplements used far exceed the RDA. Usually physicians are not consulted. Clients become their own diagnosticians by self-prescribing vitamin supplements for various health problems and may delay seeking competent medical attention. Vitamins A, B_6, and C and several minerals (zinc and selenium) have the highest potential for toxicity.

The American Medical Association (AMA) Council (1987) recommends that doses of supplemental vitamins should range from 50 to no more than 150% of the US RDA. Vitamin preparations containing more than 2 times the US RDA for any vitamin should be limited to the treatment of specific circumstances under medical supervision.

According to the AMA (1987) and the American Dietetic Association (1987), certain conditions justify consideration of therapeutic use of vitamins: (1) Women with excessive menstrual bleeding may need iron supplements; (2) pregnant or lactating women require more iron, folic acid, and calcium; (3) weight reduction or low kilocalorie diets (below 1500 kilocals) may not provide adequate nutrients; (4) vegetarians may not receive adequate calcium, iron, zinc, and vitamin B_{12}, (5) newborns should receive a single dose of vitamin K to prevent abnormal bleeding; and (6) certain disorders or diseases (such as specific vitamin deficiency diseases, malabsorption, prolonged illness, enteral and parenteral nutrition, alcoholism, burns, renal failure and dialysis, and certain genetic diseases) and some medications may interfere with nutrient intake, digestion, absorption, metabolism, or excretion and thus alter requirements and warrant consideration of therapeutic use of vitamin-mineral preparations. Public health nutrition will be served best by the insistence on a scientifically sound basis for vitamin supplementation and therapy. The use of a variety of foods as a basis for good nutrition should be emphasized by all health care practitioners.

Vitamin Megadoses

Large doses of vitamins are sometimes advocated with intakes of 20 to 600 times the RDAs. A megavitamin is actually a misnomer because the amounts are so high that the particular vitamin functions as a drug rather than as a nutrient. A well-established principle of pharmacologic therapy is that all substances are potentially toxic if the dose is large enough.

The Council on Scientific Affairs of the AMA (1987) states that megadose vitamin therapy is based only on anecdotal or nonscientific evidence. This can contribute to false hopes and needless financial expenditure and may result in direct toxic effects or hinder metabolic interactions among vital nutrients.

Megadoses of Niacin

In a best-selling book, *The 8-Week Cholesterol Cure,* Kowalski (1990) indicated that nicotinic acid intake produces a significant lowering of total cholesterol levels. The book fails to carry adequate warning about the potential health problems that can result from taking large doses of this form of niacin. As a result of this promotion, many clients have self-prescribed niacin (either form) rather than follow a stringent low-cholesterol, low-fat diet. Niacin can be purchased without a prescription, so clients may self-prescribe larger amounts than recommended without medical supervision.

In addition to the side effects already mentioned with the use of large doses of nicotinic acid, long-term use may lead to jaundice or activation of peptic ulcer. As little as 750 mg daily may precipitate **hepatotoxicity** and **cholestatic jaundice** (DiPalma & Thayer, 1991). Regular crystalline or short-acting nicotinic acid is absorbed rapidly, causing unpleasant flushing, itching, and short-lived blurred vision. On the other hand, sustained-release nicotinic acid is absorbed gradually but is much more toxic to the liver. This form is not recommended for long-term therapy. Numerous incidences of toxic symptoms have been treated, with resolution of the problems when supplemental use of the vitamin was discontinued.

Hepatotoxicity—causing destruction of liver cells.
Cholestatic jaundice—abnormality of bile flow in the liver.

NURSING APPLICATIONS

1. Assess daily food intake and use of vitamin supplements. Healthy clients do not need vitamin supplements if they eat a well-balanced diet from the basic food groups.
2. If the client insists on supplements, encourage using a single supplement that provides both vitamins and minerals in quantities that do not exceed the US RDA/RDIs.
3. Megadoses of vitamin C can lead to a false-positive glucose tolerance test.
4. Nicotinic acid is an inexpensive effective way to treat hypercholesterolemia, but when taken in therapeutic doses, it should be used only with a prescription under a physician's supervision. Do not advocate indiscriminate OTC use of niacin.
5. Diabetic clients frequently have an elevated serum cholesterol level. The effects of supplementation with nicotinic acid in this group of clients may result in a rise in blood glucose. Garg and Grundy (1990) concluded that niacin should be used with caution for non–insulin-dependent diabetes mellitus. Closely evaluate client's blood glucose level. If elevated, notify the physician. The niacin dose may have to be changed or even discontinued.
6. Researchers have tested the effect of niacin in dilating blood vessels to prevent a second incidence of myocardial infarction in clients with coronary heart disease. Although the incidence of a second nonfatal infarction was reduced, various arrhythmias outweighed potential benefits. Question physician's or client's use of niacin to prevent a second heart attack.

Continued

Client Education

- The desirable way to obtain recommended levels of nutrients is by eating a variety of foods.
- Before opting for supplementation, attempts should be made to correct dietary practice by improving food selections.
- Nutrients obtained from dietary sources rather than by supplementation reduce the potential risk for both nutrient deficiencies and nutrient excesses.
- Many vitamins can become toxic if large amounts are taken.
- Treat these supplements like other medications; keep them in a safe place inaccessible to children.
- If it is suspected that a child has swallowed an excess of vitamins or minerals, telephone the poison control center, even if the child appears to be all right.

SUMMARY

Vitamins function primarily in enzyme systems that facilitate the metabolism of proteins, fats, and carbohydrates. All of the nutrients—fats, carbohydrates, proteins, minerals, and vitamins—are interdependent, which means all must be present at the same time for metabolic functions to proceed. With their intricate codependence, overdosing of any nutrient is just as harmful as a deficiency.

Water-soluble vitamins are fragile, cannot be stored in the body for long periods of time, and are absolutely crucial for optimum health (see Table 7–1). Not only do all of the food groups need to be included in the daily intake, but also variety from each food group is equally important. Nurses need to be knowledgeable about water-soluble vitamins because excesses and deficiencies can be more readily diagnosed from a thorough physical assessment of signs and symptoms rather than from diagnostic tests.

NURSING PROCESS IN ACTION

A healthy client comes to the clinic seeking information about vitamin C. She is not sure what foods she should eat or what to look for if an excess or deficiency develops.

 Nutritional Assessment

- Income.
- Living arrangements, cooking and storage facilities.
- Knowledge level about vitamin C.
- Beliefs about water-soluble vitamins.
- Physical status, especially any bleeding problems.
- Use of any OTC or physician-prescribed supplements/medications.
- Emotional state.

 Dietary Nursing Diagnosis

Health seeking behavior RT inadequate/insufficient knowledge about vitamin C.

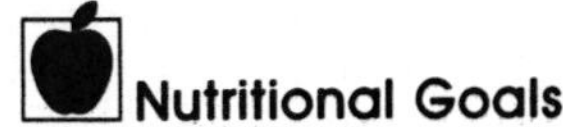

Client will consume foods high in vitamin C and state beliefs/information about vitamin C.

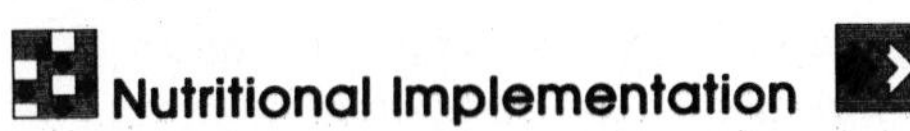

Intervention: Teach the following about vitamin C: (1) roles, (2) requirements, (3) sources.
Rationale: This provides client with a sound knowledge base about vitamin C.

Intervention: Explain hyper- and hypo- vitamin C states.
Rationale: Diarrhea, hypoglycemia, oxaluria, and rebound effect may occur with megadoses. Large amounts of vitamin C decrease absorption of vitamin B_{12}. Because vitamin C helps maintain capillary integrity, a reduction of vitamin C causes bleeding problems. Following large doses, scurvy may develop unless the amount is gradually decreased.

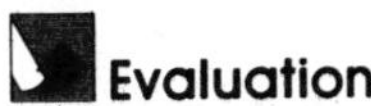

Client should consume citrus fruits, strawberries, cantaloupe, and mangos. Additionally, client should state that supplements are not necessary for vitamin C and large doses may interfere with absorption of other nutrients, or if she does develop any bleeding problems, she will seek help. Lastly, client should verbalize information concerning excesses and deficiencies of vitamin C.

STUDENT READINESS

1. Name 2 water-soluble vitamins most involved in the metabolism of fats, proteins, and carbohydrates to form energy (ATP) through the Krebs cycle.
2. Match the conditions associated with the appropriate vitamin deficiency:

Thiamin	Ascorbic acid	Megaloblastic anemia
Riboflavin	Cheilosis	Beriberi
Niacin	Scurvy	Pellagra
Vitamin B^{12}		

3. How do water-soluble vitamins differ from fat-soluble vitamins? What do these differences mean as you teach clients about nutrition?
4. What are the disadvantages of taking vitamin megadoses?
5. Name 3 foods that are good sources for each of these vitamins: thiamin, riboflavin, and B_{12}. Name 3 excellent sources of vitamin C.
6. What would you teach a vegetarian about vitamin B_{12}?

CASE STUDY

Mr. A. K. has been diagnosed to have pernicious anemia. His RBCs are macrocytic and normochromic, and he shows evidence of nervous system damage, with impaired judgment, hallucinations, and decreased reflexes. He has started on vitamin B_{12} injections and has been informed that these will have to be continued indefinitely. After discharge, Mr. A. K. discontinues the injections for which he has to travel to the clinic, and he uses high-dose supplements of multivitamins.

1. Why were the vitamin B_{12} injections originally prescribed?
2. What is the possible outcome of Mr. A. K.'s self-medication attempts?
3. Develop a tentative nursing diagnosis from this history and at least 1 goal.
4. Why are clients who have had a gastrectomy at risk to develop pernicious anemia?

REFERENCES

American Dietetic Association (ADA) Task Force. Recommendations concerning supplement usage. *J Am Diet Assoc* 1987 Oct; 87(10):1342–1343.

American Medical Association (AMA) Council on Scientific Affairs. Vitamin preparations as dietary supplements and as therapeutic agents. *JAMA* 1987 Apr 10; 257(14):1929–1936.

Anonymous. $2.9 billion for vitamins. *FDA Consumer* 1987 Apr; 21(3):4.

Bailey LB. The role of folate in human nutrition. *Nutr Today* 1990 Sept/Oct; 25(5):12–19.

Borum PR. Carnitine and lipid metabolism. *Contemp Nutr* 1990; 15(8):1–2.

Dalton K, Dalton MJT. Characteristics of pyridoxine overdose neuropathy syndrome. *Acta Neurol Scand* 1987 July; 76(1):8–11.

DiPalma JR, Thayer WS. Use of niacin as a drug. *Annu Rev Nutr* 1991; 11:169–187.

Garg A, Grundy SM. Nicotinic acid as therapy for dyslipemia in non–insulin-dependent diabetes mellitus. *JAMA* 1990 Aug 8; 264(6):723–726.

Herbert VD. Pseudovitamins. *In* Shils ME, Young VR (eds): *Modern Nutrition in Health and Disease.* Philadelphia, Lea & Febiger, 1988, pp 471–477.

Herbert VD, Colman N. Folic acid and vitamin B_{12}. *In* Shils ME, Young VR (eds): *Modern Nutrition in Health and Disease.* Philadelphia, Lea & Febiger, 1988, pp 388–416.

Hoskin JC. Effect of fluorescent light on flavor and riboflavin content of milk held in modified half-gallon containers. *J Food Protection* 1988 Jan; 51(1):19.

Kant AK, Block G. Dietary vitamin B_6 intake and food sources in the US population: NHANES II, 1976–1980. *Am J Clin Nutr* 1990 Oct; 52(4):707–716.

Kaslow JE, et al. Liver extract–folic acid–cyanacobalamin vs placebo for chronic fatigue syndrome. *Arch Intern Med* 1989 Nov; 149(11):2501–2503.

Kowalski R. *The 8-Week Cholesterol Cure.* New York, HarperCollins, 1990.

Kroll JS. Pyridoxine for neonatal seizures: An unexpected danger. *Dev Med Child Neurol* 1985 June; 27(3):377–379.

Lossos A, Argov Z. Orthostatic hypotension induced by vitamin B_{12} deficiency. *J Am Geriatr Soc* 1991 June; 39(6):601–602.

McCormick DB. Thiamin. *In* Shils ME, Young VR (eds): *Modern Nutrition in Health and Disease.* Philadelphia, Lea & Febiger, 1988, pp 355–361.

Miller DR, et al. Vitamin B_{12} status in a macrobiotic community. *Am J Clin Nutr* 1991 Feb; 53(2):524–529.

National Research Council (NRC). *Recommended Dietary Allowances.* Washington, DC, National Academy Press, 1989.

Pike S, et al. Lack of effect of vitamin B_6 supplementation of the lipoprotein profile of postmenopausal chronic hemodialysis patients. *J Am Diet Assoc* 1990 July; 90(7):968–972.

Schectman G, et al. Ascorbic acid requirements for smokers: Analysis of a population survey. *Am J Clin Nutr* 1991 May; 53(6):1466–1470.

Seligmann H, et al. Thiamine deficiency in patients with congestive heart failure receiving long-term furosemide therapy: A pilot study. *Am J Med* 1991 Aug; 91(2):151–155.

Skelton WP, Skelton NK. Deficiency of vitamins

A, B, and C. *Postgrad Med J* 1990 March; 87(4):293–310.

Subar AF, Block G. Use of vitamin and mineral supplements: Demographics and amounts of nutrients consumer. The 1987 Health Interview Survey. *Am J Epidemiol* 1990 Dec; 132(12): 1091–1101.

Weisburger JH. Nutritional approach to cancer prevention with emphasis on vitamins, antioxidants, and carotenoids. *Am J Clin Nutr* 1991; 53(suppl): 226S–237S.

Zak J, et al. Dry beriberi: Unusual complications of prolonged parenteral nutrition. *JPEN* 1991 March/Apr; 15(2):200–201.

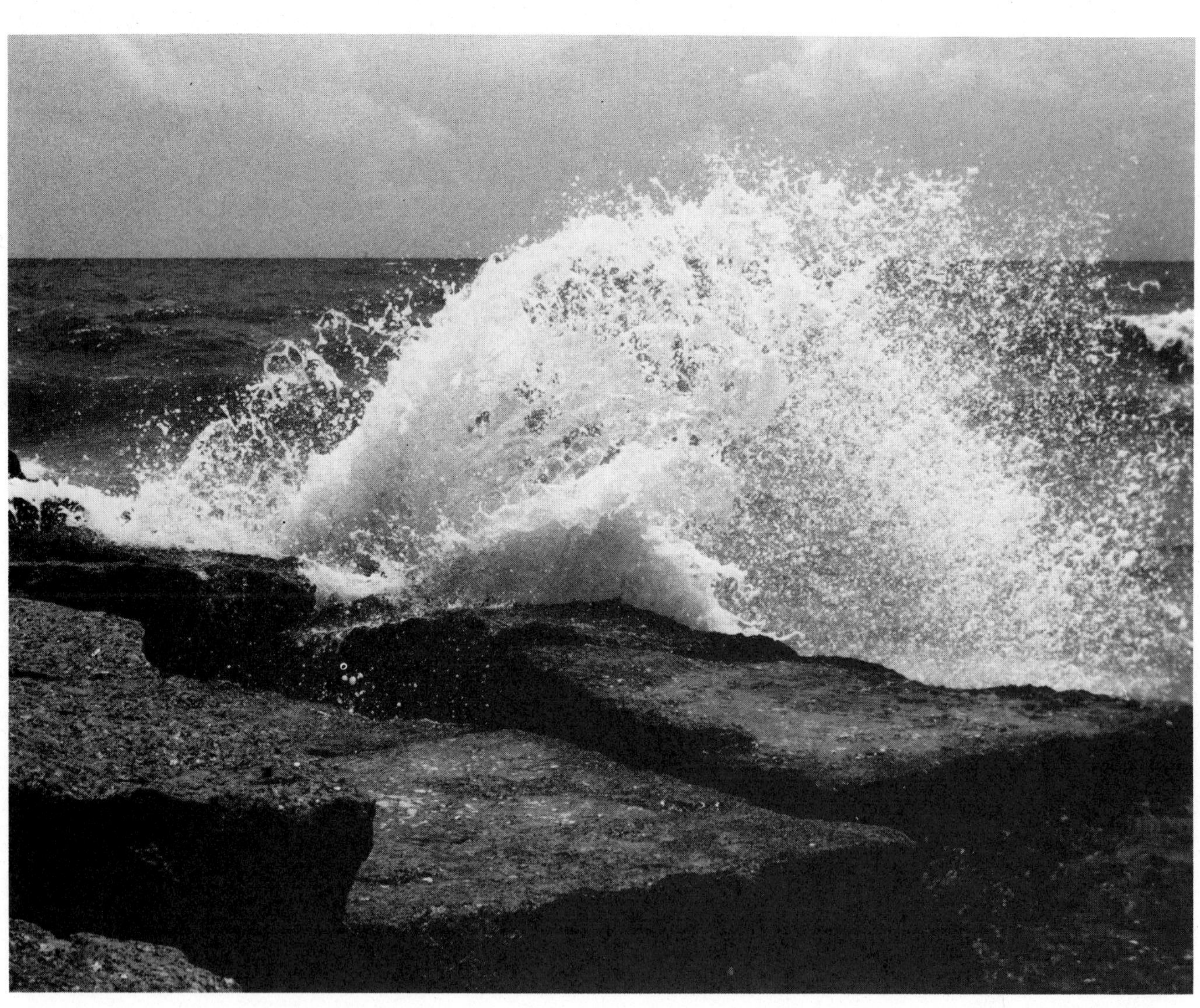

CHAPTER 8

Fluid and Electrolytes: The Balancers

OUTLINE

- I. FLUIDS
  - A. Physiological Roles
  - B. Requirements and Regulation
  - C. Absorption
  - D. Sources
  - E. Hyper- and Hypo- States
    - 1. Fluid Volume Excess
    - 2. Fluid Volume Deficit
  - *Nursing Applications*
- II. ELECTROLYTES
- III. SODIUM
  - A. Physiological Roles
  - B. Requirements and Regulation
  - C. Sources
  - D. Hyper- and Hypo- States
    - 1. Hypernatremia
    - 2. Hyponatremia
  - *Nursing Applications*
- IV. POTASSIUM
  - A. Physiological Roles
  - B. Requirements and Regulation
  - C. Sources
  - D. Hyper- and Hypo- States
    - 1. Hyperkalemia
    - 2. Hypokalemia
  - *Nursing Applications*
- V. ACID–BASE BALANCE
  - A. pH of Foods
  - *Nursing Applications*

OBJECTIVES

THE STUDENT WILL BE ABLE TO:

- Identify the importance of the nursing tasks in maintaining a client's fluid balance.
- Explain fluid and electrolyte balance.
- Explain why and which foods are acid-forming or base-forming.

- Discuss the roles, imbalances, and sources of water, sodium, and potassium.
- Discuss nursing application principles for fluid and electrolyte imbalances.
- Identify nutritional information for clients with fluid and electrolyte imbalances.

TEST YOUR NQ (True/False)

1. Thirst is the primary regulator of fluid intake.
2. Orange juice is a base-forming food.
3. Water is the most abundant component in the body.
4. Solid foods do not provide water.
5. Normal serum sodium levels are 3.5 to 5 mEq/L.
6. Sodium helps regulate acid–base balance.
7. Potassium is principally found in extracellular fluid.
8. Broccoli is a good source of potassium.
9. The most common cause of potassium deficiency in healthy clients is inadequate intake.
10. Sodium is lost in sweat.

FLUIDS

ICF includes all the fluid in the cell, chiefly present in muscle tissue. ECF consists of water outside the cells. Interstitial fluid, located between cells and in body cavities, includes joints, pleura, and the GI tract. Intravascular fluid is within the blood vessels.

Solutes—dissolved substances in fluid.

Osmosis is movement of water from an area of lower solute concentration to a higher solute concentration. When solute concentrations in the body are different, water moves across the membrane.

Osmolarity—number of solutes per liter of solution. Osmolality—number of solutes per kilogram of solution.

Solutions that have a greater osmolality than plasma are hypertonic, those with less are hypotonic, and those with a similar osmolality are isotonic.

What are the 2 main fluid compartments? What is the difference between osmolarity and osmolality?

Water is the most abundant component in the body. It represents 50 to 60% of the total body weight in an adult. At birth, water constitutes approximately 75 to 80% of body weight (Guyton, 1991). Because such a large percentage of the infant's body is water, fluid loss is more significant. Total body water decreases with age. Adipose tissue contains less water than does muscle; therefore, the presence of increased fat results in lower amounts of total body water. Thus, women, with inherent larger fat stores, contain less water as compared with men, who have a higher percentage of lean muscle tissue.

Body fluids are distributed within 2 major compartments: **Intracellular fluid (ICF)** constitutes 60% of the body's fluid weight, and **extracellular fluid (ECF)** can be subdivided into **interstitial** and **intravascular fluid** (Fig. 8–1). Fluid compartments are separated from one another by the presence of membranes. These membranes serve as barriers in that they prevent movement of certain substances; however, they do not completely isolate the compartments. Water is essentially unrestricted in its movement from compartment to compartment. Certain **solutes,** such as glucose, amino acids, and oxygen, also cross membranes freely. These membranes, which are referred to as semipermeable, allow maintenance of solute concentration by their selectivity.

When 2 compartments are separated by semipermeable membranes and movement of some solutes is restricted, **osmosis** occurs. **Osmolarity** and **osmolality** describe the total solute concentration, which determines osmotic pressure. Osmolality is the measurement most often used in clinical practice. The osmolality of plasma is approximately 290 to 300 mOsm/kg of water; solutions are referred to as **hypertonic, hypotonic,** or **isotonic** with respect to serum osmolality.

Physiological Roles

Water has important physiological roles, as follows: (1) acts as a solvent enabling chemical reactions to occur by actually entering into some reactions, such as

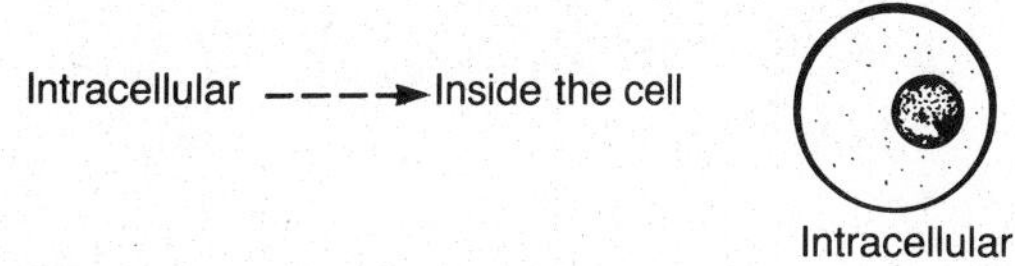

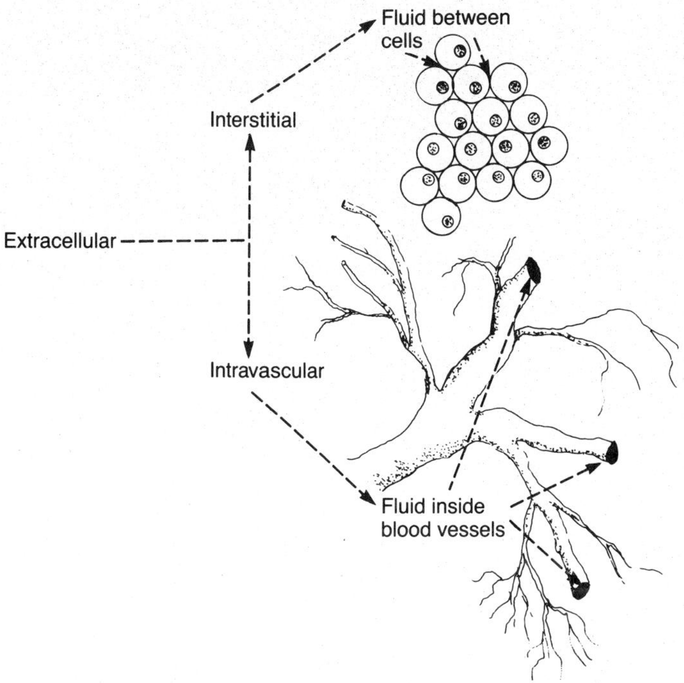

Figure 8–1 Fluid compartments.

hydrolysis; (2) maintains the stability of all body fluids, as the principal component and medium for fluids, secretions, and excretions (such as blood, lymph, gastric secretions, urine, and perspiration); (3) enables nutrients to be transported to the cells and provides a medium for excretion of waste products; (4) acts as a lubricant between cells to permit movement without friction; and (5) regulates body temperature by evaporating perspiration from the skin. A few days without water can be fatal; negative fluid balance has serious detrimental effects on many physiological functions.

Name 3 roles of water.

Requirements and Regulation

An intake of approximately 2500 to 3000 ml of fluid is required daily. Therefore, water must be supplied regularly for metabolic use and to compensate for daily losses. Water is lost through a variety of routes: (1) urine, (2) perspiration, (3) water vapor in expired air, and (4) feces. Urine production depends on the amount of fluid intake and the type of diet eaten; however, waste products must be kept in solution, and obligatory urine output is 400 to 600 ml/day. Approximately 1 ml/kg body weight/hour of urine output is normal.

Water losses in the form of sweat can vary greatly. A rise in body temperature is accompanied by increased sweating and insensible water loss through increased respiration. Strenuous exercise can greatly affect the amount of water lost through the skin. Vapor in expired air varies with the rate of respiration. The presence of inflammation in the tracheobronchial tree also elevates the respiration rate. Ap-

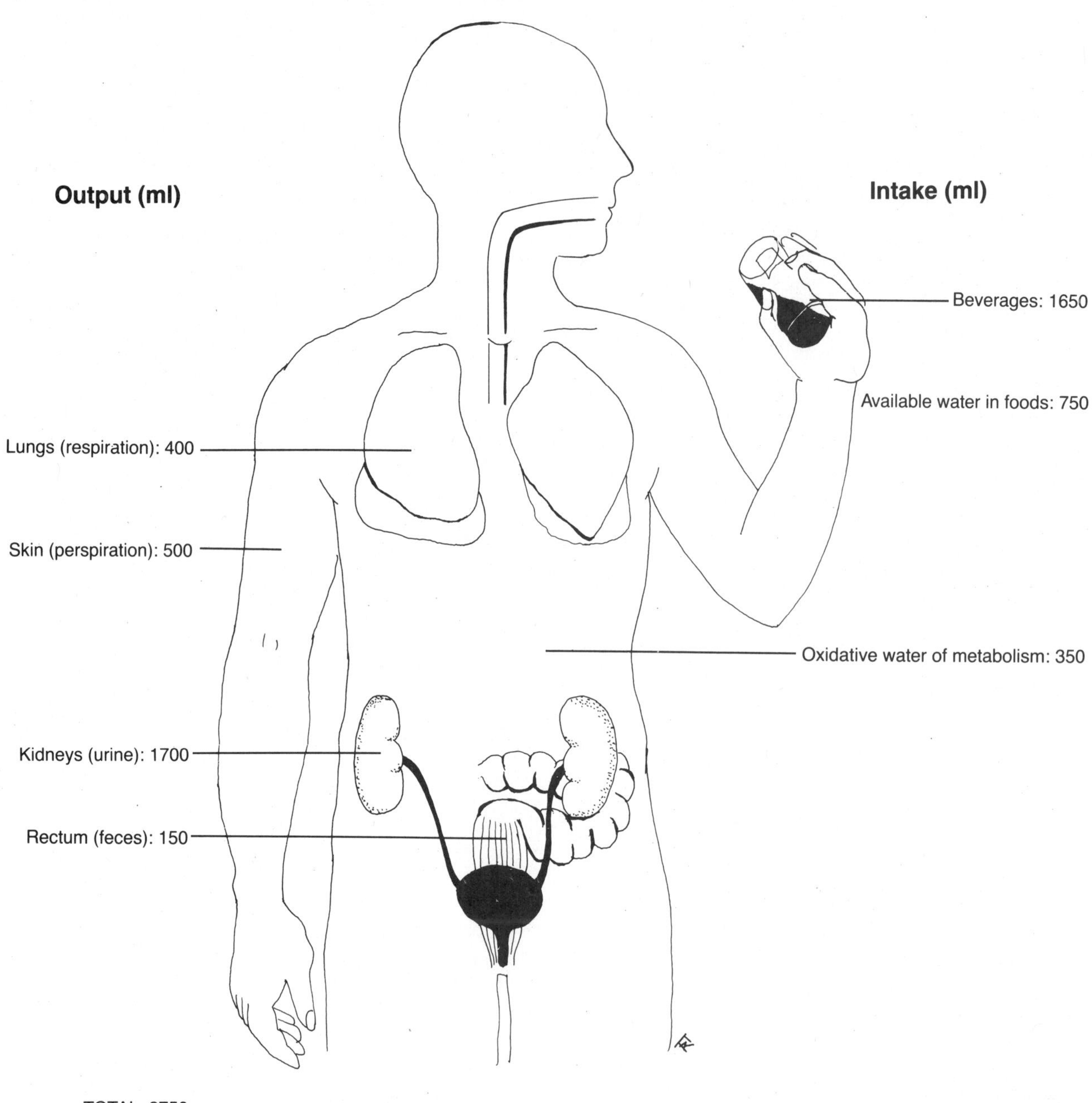

Figure 8–2 Fluid intake and output.

proximately 100 to 200 ml of water are lost each day in feces; this is dramatically increased in clients with diarrhea. Water losses result in stimulation of water intake via thirst and decreased kidney output to maintain fluid balance.

Normal fluid requirements, shown in Figure 8–2, can be drastically changed in different climatic environments, with various exercise levels, or with illnesses such as diarrhea or vomiting. The body cannot store water, so the amount lost must be replaced.

Osmoreceptors, located in the hypothalamus, are sensitive to changes in serum osmolality levels.

Thirst is the primary regulator of water intake. When as little as 2% of body water is lost, **osmoreceptors** are stimulated, creating a physiological desire to ingest liquids.

Stimulation of the osmoreceptors not only causes thirst, but also increases the production of vasopressin or **antidiuretic hormone (ADH)** from the pituitary gland. This hormone causes the retention of water only (Metheny, 1992). Conversely, if there is too much water in the body, ADH secretion is inhibited, and excess water is eliminated.

ADH causes the body to retain fluid and decrease urinary output.

Decreased blood volume also stimulates the release of renin, which leads ultimately to the increased release of aldosterone by the adrenal cortex. This results in retention of sodium and water by the kidneys.

Name 3 ways water is lost. How do ADH and aldosterone affect body water?

Absorption

No digestion is necessary for water absorption; it is transported fully in both directions across the intestinal mucosa by osmosis. As much as 1 L can be absorbed from the small intestine in 1 hour. Normally almost all the fluid is reabsorbed, with only about 100 ml excreted in the feces daily.

How is water absorbed?

Sources

Both liquids and solid foods provide water. Surprisingly, some fruits and vegetables have a higher percentage of water than milk, and meats are more than half water (Table 8–1). Water is also liberated in the process of metabolism and is available to the body. The metabolism of fats produces approximately twice as much water as the metabolism of protein and carbohydrate; about 300 to 350 ml/day are supplied from this process.

Name sources of water available for physiological needs.

Hyper- and Hypo- States

Regulation of fluid intake and fluid excretion by the kidneys usually maintains fluid balance in the body. However, imbalances, namely **fluid volume excess (FVE)** and **fluid volume deficit (FVD),** may occur.

Fluid Volume Excess

FVE mainly occurs in the ECF compartments secondary to an increase in the total body sodium content (Fig. 8–3). Because water follows sodium, this excess sodium leads to an increase in total body water. Excess fluid moves into the interstitial compartment causing edema.

FVE is the relatively equal gain of water and sodium in relation to their losses. FVD results from relatively equal loss of sodium and water.

Obviously overloading a client with fluids will cause this problem. Typically, overloading involves overinfusion with 0.9% normal saline (NS) intravenous (IV)

TABLE 8–1

PERCENTAGE OF WATER IN FOODS

Food	Percent Water
Fruits and vegetables	70–99
Milk	88
Eggs	75
Cooked meats	50–70
Hard cheese	37–40
Bread	35
Margarine and butter	16
Nuts	5
Dry cereals and crackers	4
Shortening, oils, and sugar	0

Data from *Nutritive Value of Foods,* U.S. Department of Agriculture, Home Garden Bull. No. 72, Washington, DC, 1964.

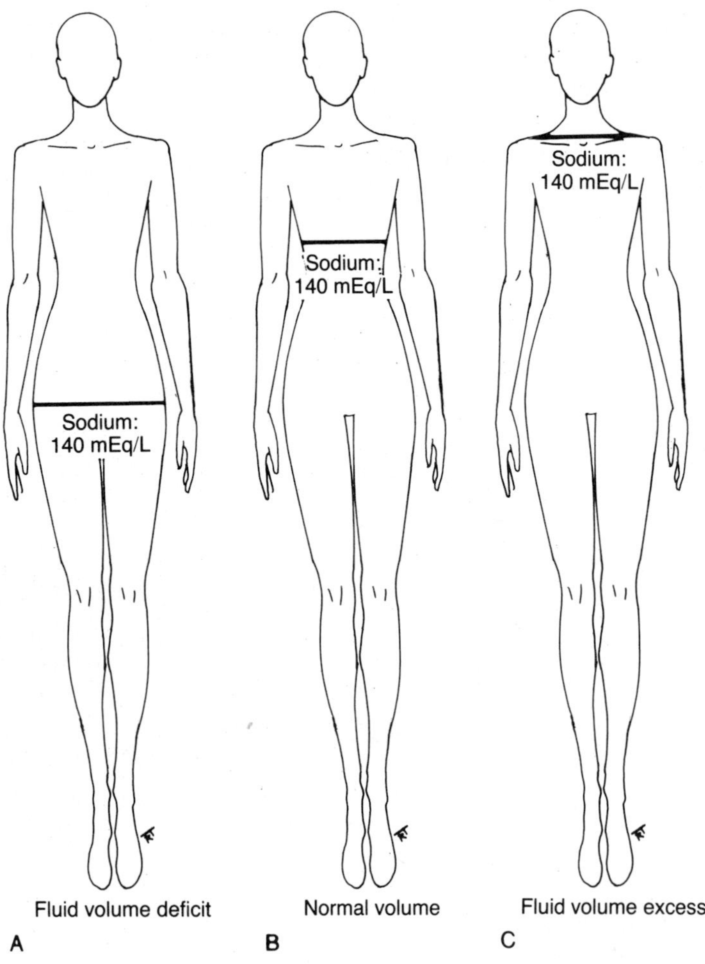

Figure 8–3 Fluid-volume disturbances. As compared with *(B)* normal body fluids, in *(A)*, fluid volume deficit (FVD), equal percentages of water and sodium losses occur, producing an isotonic depletion. In *(C)*, fluid volume excess, both water and sodium are retained, producing an isotonic expansion.

solutions, or administering 3 and 5% NS. Excessive ingestion of sodium may also lead to FVE.

Congestive heart failure, chronic renal failure, chronic liver disease, and high levels of steroids may also predispose clients to FVE because retention of sodium causes water retention. Diseases that cause a loss of protein and lower albumin levels (malnutrition and renal diseases) may also contribute to FVE because the osmotic forces ordinarily exhibited by proteins and albumin are lacking.

TABLE 8–2

HELPFUL HINTS FOR FLUID RESTRICTION

1. Carefully limit fluids at mealtime.
2. Within dietary limitations, encourage fatty foods to help decrease the desire for fluid with the meal. (For instance, margarine may help a person to swallow a roll without having to "wash it down" with liquids.)
3. Encourage the intake of moist foods. This would include raw vegetables and fruits. In contrast, mashed potatoes can be very dry. Gravies and sauces added to foods can help, if allowed on the diet.
4. Give small amounts of fluid at a time.
5. Eliminate salty foods and concentrated sweets such as candy, which produce thirst.
6. Give medications at one time, so small amounts of total fluids are used in taking medications.
7. Give medications at mealtime, when appropriate.
8. Offer ice chips because ice is sometimes more satisfying than water. Ice chips should be approved by the physician because they could be a hazard by adding solute free fluid.
9. Encourage gum chewing because salivary flow is stimulated.
10. Keep the mouth clean by brushing the teeth frequently and rinsing the mouth.

Common manifestations of FVE include rapid weight gain, puffy eyelids, distended neck veins, elevated blood pressure, and crackles auscultated in lungs. Peripheral edema, especially of the ankles and legs, is also observed.

Treatment involves correction of the underlying problems or therapy for the specific disease. Treatment may involve fluid and/or sodium restriction (Table 8–2) or the use of diuretics. Skin care is important because edematous skin is more prone to breakdown. Therefore, turning every 2 hours is recommended.

Fluid Volume Deficit

In FVD, serum osmolality is not affected (sodium and water ratio remain relatively equal); thus, ADH and aldosterone secretions are not activated (see Fig. 8–3). Inadequate fluid intake, if prolonged, can result in FVD. FVD, however, is usually associated with excessive loss of fluids from the GI tract (vomiting, diarrhea, GI suction, drainage tubes), urinary tract (diuretics, **polyuria**), or skin (sweating). Fever increases utilization of electrolytes and increases fluid losses in expired air and **diaphoresis.**

Polyuria—excessive urination.

Diaphoresis—excessive sweating.

Decreased intake can result from obvious reasons such as anorexia, nausea, and fatigue. Other less obvious reasons include an inability to (1) obtain water, such as with impaired movements; (2) activate the thirst mechanism, as in **hypodipsia;** or (3) swallow, as in neuromuscular problems or unconsciousness.

Hypodipsia—diminished thirst.

Common characteristics of FVD include weight loss, hypotension, and orthostatic hypotension. Classic signs are decreased skin turgor, dry tongue with longitudinal wrinkles, dry skin and mucous membranes, and decreased urinary output.

Treatment involves replacing lost fluid. If FVD is mild, the client is more likely able to tolerate oral fluids. IV therapy is indicated in moderate and severe FVD, using either isotonic (0.9% NS) or hypotonic (0.45% NS) IV solutions.

What are some causes, symptoms, and treatments for FVE and FVD?

NURSING APPLICATIONS

1. Direct measurement of the total amount of body water is not possible. Laboratory findings are of little value. Therefore, the nurse must assess physical signs for fluid deficit or excess.
2. The decrease of fluid reserves in the geriatric client and the greater surface area to body mass in the infant place these groups at greater risk for FVD. Assess infants and geriatric clients frequently.
3. The larger percentage of extracellular fluid in the newborn as compared with that of the adult leaves the newborn more vulnerable to FVD than an adult (Metheny, 1992). Monitor intake and output (I&O) closely in infants and assess fontanels (depressed).
4. In infants, glucose-electrolyte replacement fluids are given orally unless FVD is severe. In this case, IV solutions are given.
5. Insensible water loss equals approximately 1000 ml/m^3 of body surface area daily for bedridden clients. This amount is higher if respiration is increased or when fever is present. Offer fluids frequently to these clients.
6. Monitor I&O. If heavy perspiration losses necessitate clothing and bed linen changes, this important information should be recorded in I&O charting.
7. When vomiting is persistent, water is withheld because the gastric juices are rich in electrolytes. Just replacing water increases the risk of water excess, so do not give plain water. Without a physician's approval, water or ice chips are withheld from a client receiving GI suction to prevent water excess.
8. If fluid restriction is necessary, follow guidelines in Table 8–2.

Continued

9. To encourage fluid intake, offer preferred liquids, place within reach, and praise efforts.
10. Monitor weight changes. Rapid weight changes generally indicate loss/gain of water rather than fatty tissue because 480 ml (2 cups) of fluid result in a weight loss/gain of 1 lb.
11. Many antipsychotic drugs increase ADH secretion, increasing the risk of ECF in psychiatric clients. Regularly assess clinical signs and symptoms of clients taking these medications.

Client Education

- Beverages containing caffeine increase urine production.
- Inadequate water intake may result in constipation.
- Lying down enhances elimination of edematous fluid (Schrier, 1992).
- The water supply and use of water softeners are "hidden" sources of sodium that may make edema worse.
- High-protein diets require larger amounts of water to eliminate the higher levels of waste products.

ELECTROLYTES

Ions having positive charges are cations, and negatively charged ions are anions. Cations are sodium, potassium, calcium, and magnesium; anions include chloride, bicarbonate, and phosphate.

Where is the majority of potassium and sodium found in the body?

Compounds or ions that dissociate in solution are known as **cations** or **anions.** Because electrolyte concentration in plasma is so small, it is expressed as milliequivalents per liter (mEq/L). Electrolytes are important in both water balance and acid–base balance.

Electrolyte distribution is different in ICF and ECF compartments. The principal cation in plasma and interstitial fluid is sodium; the principal anion is chloride. The principal cation in ICF is potassium; the principal anion is phosphate. The major difference between intravascular and interstitial fluid is the large amount of proteins in the former. Because sodium and potassium are the major cations, these will be discussed further.

SODIUM

Physiological Roles

What are the roles of sodium?

Sodium's important physiological roles include (Innerarity & Stark, 1990) (1) maintaining normal ECF osmolality by affecting the concentration, excretion, and absorption of potassium and chloride and water distribution; (2) regulating acid–base balance; and (3) facilitating impulse transmission in nerve and muscle fibers.

Requirements and Regulation

Because sodium is so readily available in foods, no RDA has been established. The NRC (1989) estimates a safe minimum intake might be set at 22 mEq (500 mg) per day. This amount is increased in the face of abnormal losses. Sodium regulation involves several mechanisms. To keep the ECF concentration normal, the sodium–potassium pump is constantly moving sodium from the cell to the ECF. Through the release of aldosterone from the adrenal cortex, sodium is reabsorbed or excreted

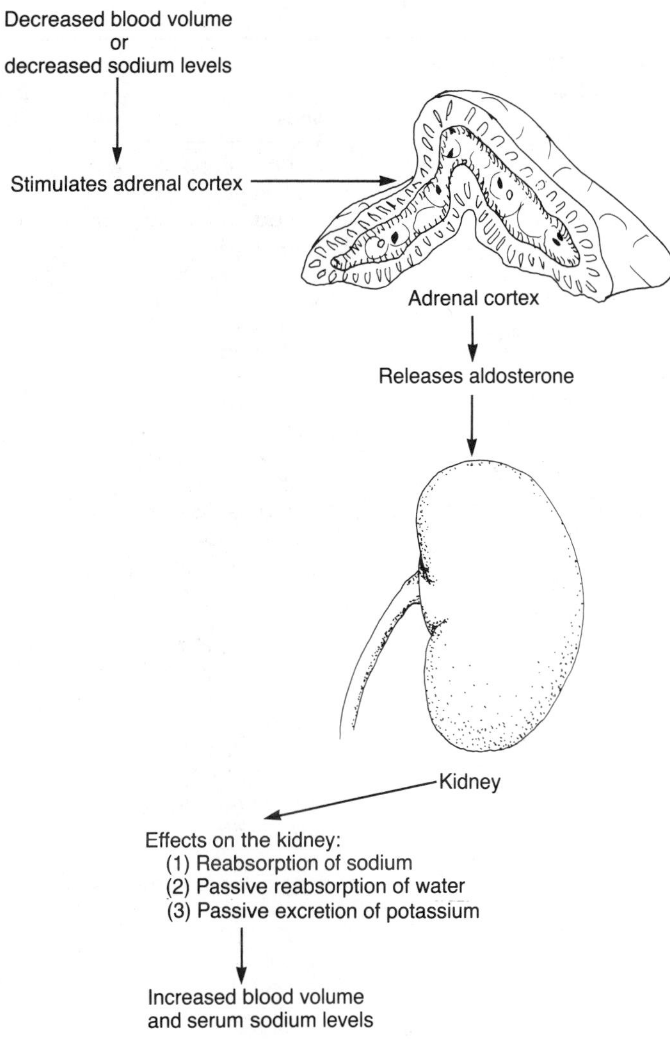

Figure 8–4 **Effects of aldosterone on sodium levels.**

in the kidneys depending on the body's need (Fig. 8–4). The kidneys can adjust sodium excretion to match sodium intake despite great variations in intake (Innerarity & Stark, 1990). Thus, if serum sodium is high, aldosterone is inhibited, and sodium is excreted; the opposite is true for depressed serum sodium levels.

What are the requirements for sodium, and how is it regulated?

Sources

Sodium is naturally available from foods and fluids regularly ingested (Table 8–3). Other sources include IV fluids. An IV solution of 0.9% NS provides 154 mEq/L of sodium; lactated Ringers (LR) solution provides 130 mEq/L. "Hidden" sources include drinking water, baking powder, antibiotics, and OTC medications (antacids, cough medicines, laxatives).

What are some sources of sodium?

Hyper- and Hypo- States

Serum sodium levels in the body range from 135 to 145 mEq/L. Serum sodium concentration is an index of water deficit or excess, not an index of sodium levels of

TABLE 8–3

SODIUM CONTENT OF YOUR FOOD*

Foods	Approximate Sodium Content (in milligrams)	Some Major Points About the Table
Breads, cereals, and grain products		Unprocessed grains are naturally low in sodium. Ready-to-eat cereals vary widely in sodium content. Some have no salt added at all. Others are higher in sodium than most breads
Cooked cereal, pasta, rice (unsalted)	Less than 5 per ½ cup	
Ready-to-eat cereal	100–360 per oz	
Bread, whole-grain or enriched	110–175 per slice	
Biscuits and muffins	170–390 each	
Vegetables		Most canned vegetables, vegetable juices, and frozen vegetables with sauce are higher in sodium than fresh or frozen ones cooked without added salt
Fresh or frozen vegetables (cooked without added salt)	Less than 70 per ½ cup	
Vegetables, canned or frozen with sauce	140–460 per ½ cup	
Fruit		Fresh, frozen, and canned fruits and fruit juices are low in sodium.
Fruits (fresh, frozen, or canned)	Less than 10 per ½ cup	
Milk, cheese, and yogurt		A serving of milk or yogurt is lower in sodium than most natural cheeses, which vary widely in their sodium content. Processed cheeses, cheese foods, and cheese spreads contain more sodium than natural cheeses. Cottage cheese falls somewhere between natural and processed cheeses
Milk and yogurt	120–160 per cup	
Buttermilk (salt added)	260 per cup	
Natural cheeses	110–450 per 1½-oz serving	
Cottage cheese (regular and low-fat)	450 per ½ cup	
Process cheese and cheese spreads	700–900 per 2-oz serving	
Meat, poultry, and fish		Most fresh meats, poultry, and fish are low in sodium. Canned poultry and fish are higher. Most cured and processed meats such as hotdogs, sausage, and luncheon meats are even higher in sodium because sodium is used during processing to preserve them
Fresh meat, poultry, finfish	Less than 90 per 3-oz serving	
Cured ham, sausages, luncheon meat, frankfurters, canned meats	750–1350 per 3-oz serving	
Fats and dressings		
Oil	None	
Vinegar	Less than 6 per tbsp	
Prepared salad dressings	80–250 per tbsp	
Unsalted butter or margarine	1 per tsp	
Salted butter or margarine	45 per tsp	
Salt pork, cooked	360 per oz	
Condiments		
Catsup, mustard, chili sauce, tartar sauce, steak sauce	125–275 per tbsp	Condiments such as soy sauce, catsup, mustard, tartar sauce, chili sauce, pickles, and olives are high in sodium
Soy sauce	1000 per tbsp	
Salt	2000 per tsp	

TABLE 8–3

SODIUM CONTENT OF YOUR FOOD*
Continued

Foods	Approximate Sodium Content (in milligrams)	Some Major Points About the Table
Snack and convenience foods		Most "convenience" foods are quite high in sodium. Frozen dinners and combination dishes, canned soups, and dehydrated mixes for soups, sauces, and salad dressings contain a lot of sodium.
Canned and dehydrated soups	630–1300 per cup	
Canned and frozen main dishes	800–1400 per 8-oz serving	
Unsalted nuts and popcorn	Less than 5 per oz	
Salted nuts, potato chips, corn chips	150–300 per oz	Many low-sodium or reduced-sodium foods are available as alternatives to those processed with salt and other sodium-containing ingredients. Check the label for the sodium content of these foods
Deep-fried pork rind	750 per oz	

* This table shows the sodium content of some types of foods. The ranges are rough guides; individual food items may be higher or lower in sodium.

From US Department of Agriculture, Human Nutrition Information Service. *Nutrition and Your Health. Dietary Guidelines for Americans: Avoid Too Much Sodium.* Home and Garden Bull. No. 232-6. Washington, DC, 1986.

the body. Sodium blood levels are significantly higher than potassium because sodium is the major cation in intravascular fluid. **Hypernatremia** or **hyponatremia** usually is a result of hormonal imbalances or increased fluid losses or retention. "True" hypernatremia or hyponatremia, or imbalances caused by too much or too little sodium intake, rarely occurs in adults.

A serum sodium level above 145 is hypernatremia, and a level below 135 is hyponatremia.

Hypernatremia

A gain of sodium in excess of water or loss of water in excess of sodium can predispose to hypernatremia. Because water and sodium are so closely related, a change in one causes a change in the other. Thus, hypernatremia can be associated with FVD or FVE.

Loss of hypotonic fluid without adequate water replacement is the major cause of hypernatremia. Excessive solute loading, i.e., high protein tube feedings or supplements, or IV infusion of too much sodium, may lead to hypernatremia. Water deprivation (unconscious, debilitated clients or infants), insensible water loss (exposure to dry heat, sweating, hyperventilation), and watery diarrhea lead to loss of water in excess of sodium. Infants are more prone to watery diarrhea, whereas elderly clients are susceptible to water deprivation. If **polyuria** is not balanced with increased water intake, hypernatremia may occur.

Polyuria—increase in urination.

Symptoms of hypernatremia are a result of fluid moving from the ICF to the ECF to try to equalize sodium and water balance. This movement of fluid causes the tissue cells to shrink. Cells in the CNS shrink, producing hallucinations, disorientation, lethargy, and possible coma. Other signs are extreme thirst; dry, sticky tongue and oral mucous membranes; convulsions; and fever.

Gradually lowering sodium concentrations over 48 hours or longer is the preferred treatment. Typically, hypotonic fluids (D_5W or 0.45% NS) are administered. If shock is present, however, isotonic fluid (0.9% NS) is given.

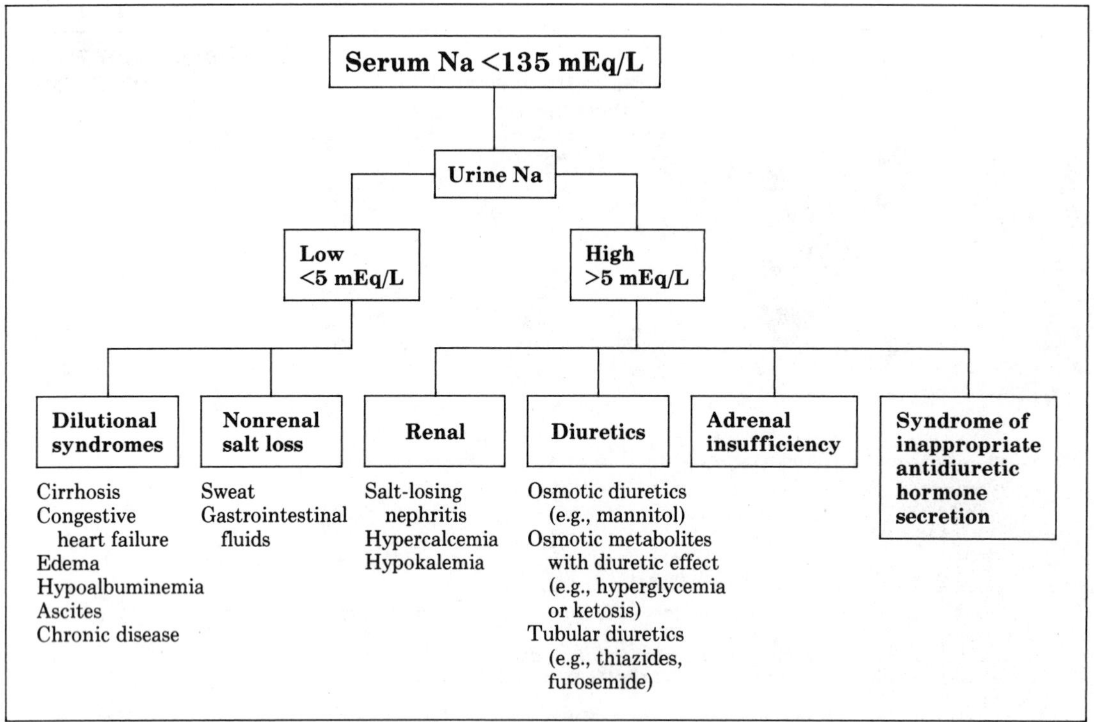

Figure 8–5 Diagnostic tree for hyponatremia. (Adapted with permission of Ross Laboratories, Columbus, OH 43216. Nutrients in Enteral Feeding. © 1989, Ross Laboratories.)

Hyponatremia

Hyponatremia may develop when sodium losses exceed water losses or when fluids are retained, leading to a greater concentration of water than sodium. Because of the change in ECF osmolality, sodium moves from the ECF to the ICF and water enters the ICF, causing cellular edema. This can cause problems especially in the cranium, where there is no room for expansion.

Heat exhaustion in unacclimatized clients may result from sodium deficit. Hyponatremia may also occur in clients who drink excessive quantities of water for psychiatric reasons or when excessive amounts of diuretics are given. Hyperglycemia may precipitate hyponatremia because the elevated blood glucose level draws water into the vascular space (edema), causing a dilutional effect. This is not a reflection of true body sodium. On the other hand, excessive loss of electrolytes in adrenal insufficiency causes a true sodium deficit. Syndrome of inappropriate release of ADH (SIADH) may also lead to hyponatremia because of the retention of water only. AIDS clients are also prone to hyponatremia because of SIADH (Agarwal, 1989). As shown in Figure 8–5, urinary sodium concentration is essential in determining the cause of hyponatremia.

Early symptoms of hyponatremia are nausea and abdominal cramps. Other symptoms are the result of cellular swelling: headache, confusion, lethargy, and coma. Even though there is cellular edema, peripheral edema is not present. This is because the water is primarily retained within cells rather than in the interstitial compartment.

Acute hyponatremia usually causes few problems unless the serum sodium concentration falls below 120 mEq/L. Chronic hyponatremia is usually well tolerated, especially in clients with chronic diseases such as tuberculosis and cancer. Thus, hyponatremia may or may not be treated, depending on the precipitating cause and severity.

Because dilutional hyponatremia (see Fig. 8–5) is characterized by normal or increased total body sodium and even greater retention of total body water, increasing sodium would only worsen the condition. These conditions may be treated with diuretics and/or restriction of fluid and sodium intake.

Hyponatremia associated with nonrenal salt loss often requires treatment with dietary or IV sodium. When renal losses of sodium are excessive (>5 mEq/L), additional sodium may be provided except when this is precipitated by medications. Replacing sodium orally, nasogastrically, or parenterally can be complicated by the plasma and/or water volume. If plasma volume is below normal, isotonic fluids are administered IV (LR or NS). However, 3 to 5% NS is prescribed if plasma volume is normal or excessive.

If treatment of hyponatremia is confusing, use Figure 8–5 as a reference tool, and remember the general rule of thumb: In hyponatremia, either sodium is decreased or water is increased (Metheny, 1992).

What is the normal blood level for sodium, for hyponatremia, for hypernatremia? What are the causes, symptoms, and treatment for hypernatremia? What are the causes, symptoms, and treatment for hyponatremia?

NURSING APPLICATIONS

1. Assess clients for the signs and symptoms of hypernatremia and hyponatremia.
2. An often neglected client that needs assessing for hypernatremia is the client undergoing abortion by instillation of hypertonic saline infusion.
3. To determine hyponatremia, assess the laboratory value (low sodium) and check for finger printing. (For finger printing, roll a finger over the sternum; the finger print will be visible on the client's skin.)
4. A serum sodium level above 170 mEq/L may produce permanent brain damage, so notify the physician for orders.
5. Weigh daily and monitor I&O.
6. Monitor and record vital signs.
7. To evaluate care for hypernatremic and hyponatremic clients, evaluate laboratory results. Sodium levels should normalize.

Client Education

- Stress the importance of either decreasing or increasing sodium intake.
- Dietary sodium restriction is rarely the cause of hyponatremia. (In most conditions, as little as 22 mEq dietary sodium maintains normal serum sodium concentrations.)
- Salt tablets are usually unnecessary to replace lost sodium. If needed, the recommendation is 2 gm table salt for each 2 lb of weight loss.
- To convert milligrams of sodium to milliequivalents, divide the number by 23 (the atomic weight of sodium). Example:

$$1000 \text{ mg sodium} \div 23 = 43 \text{ mEq sodium}$$

- Table salt is not the same thing as sodium.
- Explain the "hidden" sources of sodium if indicated.

POTASSIUM

Physiological Roles

Potassium has the following important physiological roles (Innerarity & Spark, 1990): (1) Maintains cell (ICF) osmolality, (2) Directly affects muscle contraction

TABLE 8–4

POTASSIUM CONTENT OF SELECTED FOODS

Food	Portion	Potassium (mg)	Kilocalories (per serving)
Dried apricots	½ cup	896	155
Baked potato	1	610	145
Dried prunes	½ cup	600	193
Cantaloupe	1 cup	494	56
Dried pears	½ cup	480	236
Banana	1	451	105
Baked winter squash	½ cup	448	40
Cooked spinach	½ cup	420	21
Dried peaches	½ cup	413	100
Pinto beans	½ cup	400	118
Milk	1 cup	377	86–150
Split peas	½ cup	355	116
Lima beans	½ cup	347	85
Broiled sirloin steak	3 oz	343	176
Kidney beans	½ cup	337	115
Blackeyed/cowpeas	½ cup	319	112
Baked butternut squash	½ cup	291	41
Cooked beets	½ cup	266	26
Orange juice	½ cup	236	56
Cooked broccoli	½ cup	228	22
Cooked zucchini	½ cup	228	14
Cooked cauliflower	½ cup	200	15
Cooked asparagus	½ cup	196	25
Watermelon	1 cup	186	51
Stewed tomatoes	½ cup	125	40

Nutrient data from Nutritionist III software, version 7.0. N-Squared Computing, Salem, Oregon.

What are the physiological roles of potassium?

(especially cardiac) and electrical conductivity of the heart, (3) facilitates transmission of nerve impulses, and (4) regulates acid–base balance.

Requirements and Regulation

What are the requirements for potassium? How are potassium levels regulated?

Similar to sodium, there is no RDA for potassium. Minimum requirement to maintain normal body stores and normal plasma concentration is 40 to 50 mEq/day. Potassium deficiency rarely occurs from a normal American diet because potassium is present in practically all foods.

The sodium–potassium pump regulates potassium levels. Depending on cellular needs, potassium is constantly moving either into or out of cells.

Aldosterone indirectly affects potassium serum levels. If aldosterone is released, sodium is reabsorbed, but potassium is excreted. Subsequently, if aldosterone is inhibited, potassium is retained in the body (see Fig. 8–4). Approximately 80% of ingested potassium is excreted in the urine. The rest is lost through feces or sweat.

Sources

Name 3 sources of potassium.

Sources of potassium are naturally available from foods and fluids regularly ingested (Table 8–4). Processed foods usually contain lower levels of potassium than fresh products. Potassium supplements (orally and parenterally) are another source.

Hyper- and Hypo- States

A normal range for serum potassium is 3.5 to 5 mEq/L. Because this is such a narrow range, minor deviations can be life-threatening. Abnormal levels are referred to as **hyperkalemia** or **hypokalemia.**

An increase in potassium (>5) is called hyperkalemia; a deficit (<3.5) is hypokalemia.

Hyperkalemia

Hyperkalemia results from 3 causes: (1) impaired renal excretion, (2) increased shift of potassium out of the cells, or (3) increased potassium intake. Acute or chronic renal failure impairs potassium excretion, resulting in potassium being retained in the body. This is logical because 80% is excreted through the kidneys. Increased serum potassium levels can result from an increased dietary intake, excessive administration of potassium supplements orally or parenterally, or excessive use of potassium-containing salt substitutes. Burns, trauma, crushing injuries, increased catabolism, and acidosis cause potassium to leave the cell and enter the blood stream.

Hyperkalemia is life-threatening because cardiac arrest can occur. Symptoms include muscle weakness (the first sign), tingling and numbness in extremities, diarrhea, bradycardia, abdominal cramps, confusion, and electrocardiogram changes (tented T-waves). To help remember these symptoms, think of elevated potassium levels as irritating to the body.

Treatment for hyperkalemia involves restricting or removing potassium. Restricting potassium can be initiated through dietary means as well as discontinuing parenteral IV sources. Removal of potassium can be accomplished by administering (1) sodium polystyrene sulfonate (Kayexalate) either orally or rectally (potassium is removed from the body by exchanging sodium for potassium in the GI tract), (2) glucose and insulin (insulin lowers potassium levels by moving it into the cell, and glucose helps prevent hypoglycemia from the insulin), or (3) sodium bicarbonate (moves potassium into the cell by reducing the acidosis). Calcium gluconate can also be prescribed. This drug does not move potassium into the cell but protects the heart while the previously mentioned therapies are being initiated (Metheny, 1992).

Hypokalemia

Excessive losses or inadequate intake of potassium can result in hypokalemia. Excessive losses include GI, renal, and skin losses. Because potassium is contained in intestinal fluid, it is evident why diarrhea causes hypokalemia. Potassium is also contained in gastric fluid. However, hypokalemia usually occurs in vomiting and gastric suctioning because potassium is lost in the urine as the kidneys try to conserve hydrogen ions to stabilize acid–base balance. Drugs are the main culprit of excessive renal losses. Potassium-losing diuretics (furosemide [Lasix] and hydrochlorothiazide [Esidrix, HydroDIURIL]) and antibiotics (carbenicillin and amphotericin B) are the major offenders. Some potassium is lost through sweat; excessive perspiration can lead to hypokalemia.

Because potassium is the major ICF cation, deficits can affect every body system. Death from cardiac or respiratory arrest can occur. Clinical manifestations are anorexia, absence of bowel sounds, muscle weakness in the legs, leg cramps, and electrocardiogram changes (flattened T-waves or U-waves present).

Prevention is the best treatment. Information concerning dietary measures to increase potassium content should be provided to clients at risk. If hypokalemia develops, supplementation of potassium is advised; usually dietary means alone are not sufficient. Oral supplementation is preferred, but IV replacement may be necessary.

Name the normal blood range for potassium, for hypokalemia, and for hyperkalemia. Explain the causes, symptoms, and treatment for hyperkalemia and hypokalemia.

NURSING APPLICATIONS

1. Be aware of factors that can cause potassium to elevate but should not be treated: blood sample was allowed to hemolyze or client was allowed to clench fist while the sample was being drawn.
2. Do not give IV potassium until renal function is evaluated because renal excretion is how the body eliminates potassium.
3. Administer oral sodium polystyrene sulfonate (Kayexalate) with sorbitol to enhance potassium removal; if ordered rectally, use an indwelling urinary catheter with the balloon inflated to promote administration and retention.
4. Give calcium carbonate slow IV push and place client on cardiac monitor.
5. A serum potassium level above 5.5 mEq/L is a medical emergency, so notify the physician for orders.
6. Never give potassium IV push or bolus because this could prove fatal.
7. To evaluate care of hyperkalemic or hypokalemic clients, monitor serum potassium levels, which should return to normal.

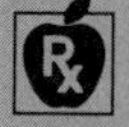
Indomethacin (Indocin) and piroxicam (Feldene) may produce hyperkalemia in some clients. Assess clients with arthritis closely.

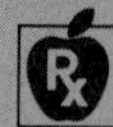
Administer potassium supplements with 4 oz of fluid or with food to prevent gastric irritation.

Client Education

- Involve client and family in food choices.
- Stress the importance of either increasing or decreasing potassium.
- Read labels; salt substitutes may be high in potassium. Consult your physician or dietitian before using potassium-containing salt substitutes.

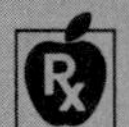
Encourage clients taking potassium-wasting diuretics to consume high-potassium foods if they are not taking a potassium supplement.

ACID–BASE BALANCE

An acidic solution would have a pH of less than 7, and a basic (alkaline) solution would have a pH over 7.

The **acidity** or **alkalinity** of a solution is measured by pH, or the concentration of hydrogen ions. Acids donate hydrogen ions; bases accept hydrogen ions. Because the concentration of hydrogen ions is so small, a scale of 1 to 14 is used that has an inverse relation to the actual concentration. As the hydrogen ion concentration goes up, the numbers on the pH scale go down.

The primary by-products of metabolism are acids; therefore, the body must have some means to prevent dramatic pH changes. Chemicals present within the body can both accept and donate the hydrogen ion as necessary to maintain the blood pH within a narrow range (7.35 to 7.45); these include bicarbonate, **carbonic acid,** phosphate, and protein. The blood is slightly alkaline because there is more base (bicarbonate) than acid (carbonic acid) in the blood. When the pH is higher (7.46 to 7.8), the body is in a state of alkalosis; below normal (6.8 to 7.34) is a sign of acidosis. Life can exist between 6.8 to 7.8 pH.

Carbonic acid—carbon dioxide in a liquid solution.

What is the normal blood pH? What is a blood pH of 7.2 called? Of 7.5?

pH of Foods

Because acidity is a chemical measurement of the number of hydrogen ions, it has nothing to do with taste sensations. If the metabolism of food results in more cations (calcium, magnesium, potassium, sodium) than anions (chloride, sulfur, phosphates), the food is said to be alkaline. Conversely, if the metabolism of a food results in more anions than cations, the food is acidic.

When some foods are eaten, such as lemons, they taste acidic because they contain some free organic acids. When oranges or lemons with their acids are oxidized in the body, however, the result is carbon dioxide, water, and a residue of potassium. Because potassium is a cation, orange juice is a **base-forming food.**

Protein foods, such as meat and eggs, leave residues of sulfur and phosphorus or **acid ash.** Fats, sugar, and starches contain no residue and do not form excess cations or anions to affect the acid–base balance of the body. When a variety of foods is consumed from the food groups, the residue produced is reasonably balanced.

Plums, cranberries, and prunes contain an organic acid that the body cannot metabolize. Intake of these substances should slightly acidify the urine and are sometimes used to change the pH of the urine.

Vegetables, fruits, and some nuts result in an alkaline residue or ash and are considered base-forming foods.

Acid-forming or acid ash foods include meats, eggs, fish, and seafood.

List foods that produce (1) alkaline ash and (2) acid ash.

NURSING APPLICATIONS

1. The body's normal pH is 7.35 to 7.45. Nurses can monitor these values through a blood test called arterial blood gases (ABGs).
2. In healthy clients, acid ash or alkaline foods do not alter the body's serum pH but can be used to alter the body's urine pH. Therefore, monitor pH of urine on the urinalysis report.
3. Remember not to confuse blood pH and urine pH. These measure different systems and have different values.

Client Education

- Cranberry juice is beneficial for clients with urinary tract infections.
- Avoid excessive intake of antacids and bicarbonate because this can result in alkalosis (too much base).

SUMMARY

All processes of life are dependent on an intricate balance of the chemicals dissolved in body fluids. Accurate assessment of intake and output must include all sources of water gains and losses. Therefore, the nurse plays an important role in helping to maintain fluid-electrolyte balance when any of the body's mechanisms fail. Adequate water intake is more important than sufficient kilocalories.

The 2 main cations (sodium and potassium) are usually regulated within their normal ranges. However, changes can occur (hyper- or hypo- states), and nurses must be alert to assess and treat these alterations.

NURSING PROCESS IN ACTION

A client has severe diarrhea and poor intake for 4 days. On admission, she weighed 136 lb; normal weight was around 145 lbs. Poor skin turgor and low urine output were observed.

Nutritional Assessment

- Vital signs, especially BP (orthostatic hypotension), pulse, and temperature.
- Mucous membranes, tongue characteristics.
- IBW, % of weight loss.
- Elevated urine specific gravity, BUN, and hematocrit.
- Fluid likes and dislikes.
- Mental changes.

Dietary Nursing Diagnosis

Fluid volume deficit RT diarrhea and poor fluid intake.

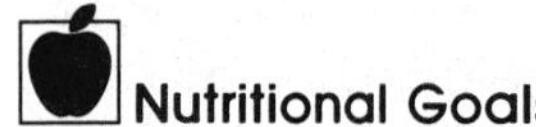

Nutritional Goals

Client will have good skin turgor and moist mucous membranes, with return of laboratory values to normal.

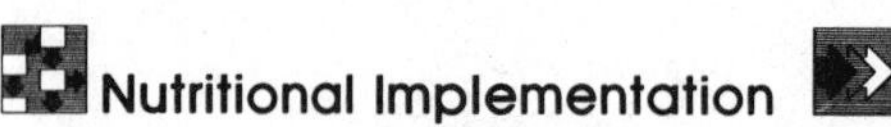

Nutritional Implementation

Intervention: Monitor I&O.
Rationale: Output is exceeding intake and needs to return to normal ratio of I&O (equal). Monitoring I&O will determine whether dehydration is resolving or becoming worse.

Intervention: Weigh client daily.
Rationale: Daily weights are an indicator of fluid loss or gain because 480 ml results in a positive or negative change of 1 lb.

Intervention: Administer antidiarrheal medication as ordered.
Rationale: Antidiarrheal medications prevent loss of fluid by decreasing diarrhea.

Intervention: Administer 0.9% NS IV fluids as prescribed.
Rationale: IV fluids replace lost fluid, and client has a poor intake.

Intervention: Offer favorite fluids.
Rationale: Client is more apt to drink her favorite fluid and replace fluid loss.

Intervention: Explain the need for fluid intake.
Rationale: Knowledge and involvement in care increase compliance.

Intervention: Offer mouth care frequently.
Rationale: In FVD, mucous membranes become sticky and dry, thereby leading to decreased intake because of taste and pain and possible infection because of cracks in the integrity of oral mucous membranes.

Intervention: Explain that coffee, tea, and colas need to be avoided.
Rationale: Beverages containing caffeine increase urine production, thus contributing to more fluid loss.

Intervention: Monitor skin turgor.
Rationale: Skin turgor is an indication of fluid status.

Intervention: Monitor BUN, specific gravity, and Hct.

Rationale: Decreased fluid decreases the glomerular filtration rate, thereby interfering with clearance of nitrogenous waste, so BUN increases; therefore, the goal is for the BUN to decrease. Because the kidneys conserve fluid during FVD, specific gravity is increased; the goal is for the specific gravity to decrease. Hematocrit is the percentage of fluid in relation to formed cells in the blood. Therefore, because fluid is decreased, the hematocrit is elevated; the goal is for the hematocrit to decrease.

Evaluation

Desired outcomes include urinary volume increases to 40 to 60 ml/hr; vital signs return to within normal parameters; skin turgor improves; mucous membranes are moist; and specific gravity, hematocrit, and BUN return to normal levels.

STUDENT READINESS

1. Define intracellular and extracellular fluid. What are the principal electrolytes found in each?
2. Write down your daily intake of fluid. How does this compare with the required intake?
3. What determines whether food produces acid or alkaline ash?
4. What can cause hypernatremia and hyponatremia? How are these disorders treated?
5. What can cause FVD or FVE? How are these conditions treated?

CASE STUDY:

A 45-year-old female client who was taking Lasix came into the emergency room with complaints of muscle weakness and inability to carry out activities of daily living. The physician ordered electrolytes drawn. Results were potassium, 2.5 mEq/L; sodium, 130 mEq/L. She was admitted to your unit.

1. What are the normal serum ranges for sodium and potassium?
2. Why do you think the physician admitted her?
3. What signs and symptoms would you expect to assess?
4. What foods would you tell her to increase?
5. Why were both her sodium and potassium levels decreased?
6. What nursing interventions are appropriate for this client? Give rationales.
7. How would you evaluate your care of this client?

REFERENCES

Agarwal A, et al. Hyponatremia in patients with acquired immune deficiency syndrome. *Nephron* 1989 Dec; 53(4):317–321.

Guyton AC: *Textbook of Medical Physiology.* 8th ed. Philadelphia, WB Saunders, 1991.

Innerarity S, Stark J. *Fluids and Electrolytes: A Study and Learning Tool.* Springhouse PA, Springhouse, 1990.

Metheny, N. *Fluid and Electrolyte Balance: Nursing Considerations.* 2nd ed. Philadelphia, JB Lippincott, 1992.

National Research Council (NRC). *Recommended Dietary Allowances.* Washington, DC, National Academy Press, 1989.

Schrier R. *Renal and Electrolyte Disorders.* 4th ed. Boston, Little, Brown, 1992.

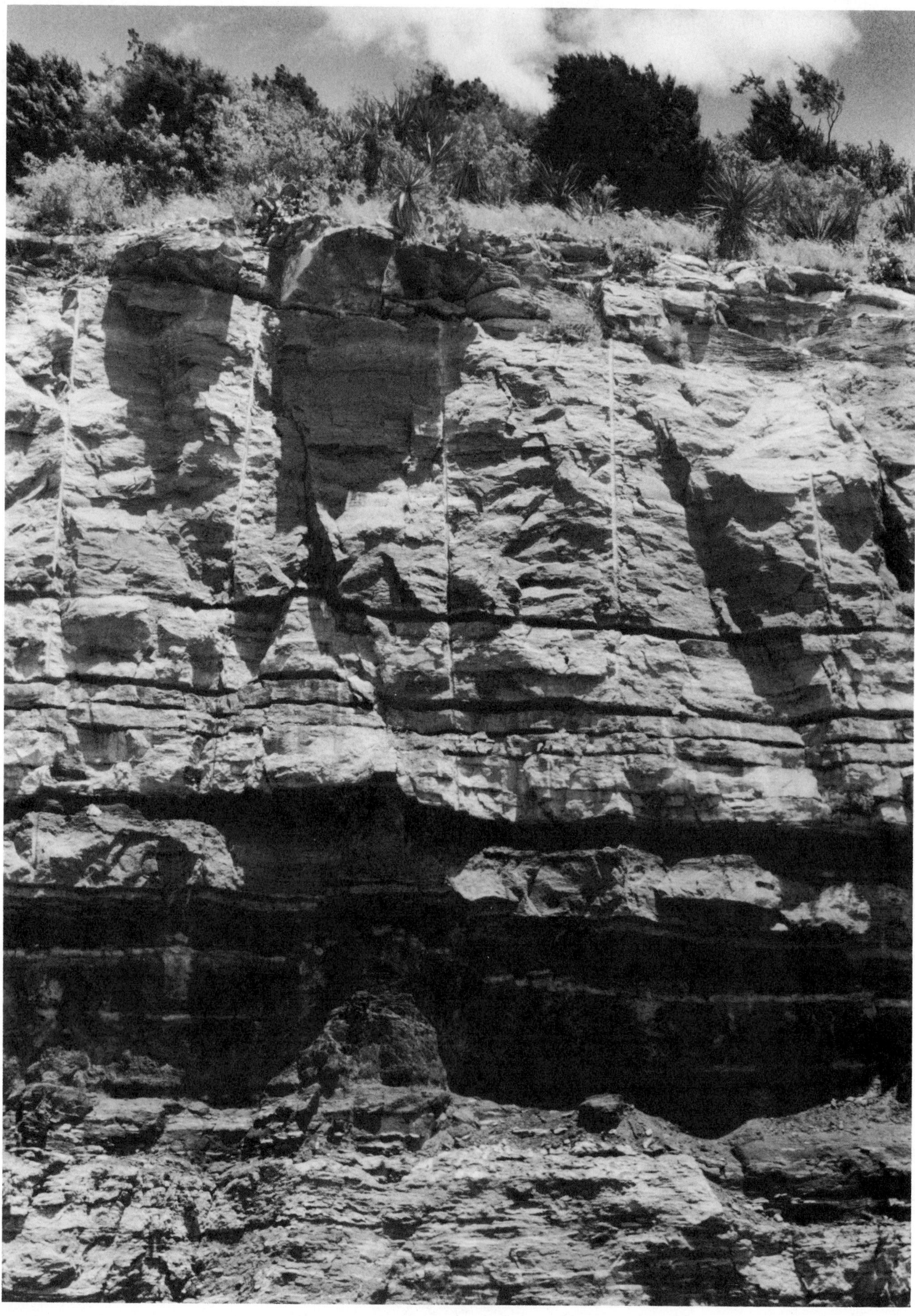

CHAPTER 9

Minerals: The Unique Workers/Substances

OUTLINE

- I. CALCIUM
  - A. Physiological Roles
  - B. Requirements and Regulation
    - 1. Calcium Balance
    - 2. Calcium-to-Phosphorus Ratio
  - C. Absorption and Excretion
  - D. Sources
  - E. Hyper- and Hypo- States
    - 1. Hypercalcemia and Hypocalcemia
    - 2. Excessive Calcium Intake
    - 3. Inadequate Calcium Intake
  - *Nursing Applications*
- II. PHOSPHORUS
  - A. Physiological Roles
  - B. Requirements
  - C. Absorption and Excretion
  - D. Sources
  - E. Hyper- and Hypo- States
  - *Nursing Applications*
- III. MAGNESIUM
  - A. Physiological Roles
  - B. Requirements
  - C. Sources
  - D. Hyper- and Hypo- States
  - *Nursing Applications*
- IV. SULFUR
  - A. Physiological Roles
  - B. Requirements and Sources
  - C. Hyper- and Hypo- States
  - *Nursing Applications*
- V. IRON
  - A. Physiological Roles
  - B. Requirements
  - C. Absorption and Excretion
  - D. Sources
  - E. Hyper- and Hypo- States
  - *Nursing Applications*

VI. COPPER
  A. Physiological Roles
  B. Requirements
  C. Absorption and Excretion
  D. Sources
  E. Hyper- and Hypo- States
  Nursing Applications
VII. ZINC
  A. Physiological Roles
  B. Requirements
  C. Absorption and Excretion
  D. Sources
  E. Hyper- and Hypo- States
  Nursing Applications
VIII. MANGANESE
  A. Physiological Roles
  B. Requirements
  C. Sources
  D. Hyper- and Hypo- States
  Nursing Applications
IX. IODINE
  A. Physiological Role
  B. Requirements
  C. Sources
  D. Hyper- and Hypo- States
  Nursing Applications
X. MOLYBDENUM
  Nursing Applications
XI. FLUORIDE
  A. Physiological Roles
  B. Requirements
  C. Sources
  D. Hyper- and Hypo- States
  Nursing Applications
XII. SELENIUM
  A. Physiological Roles
  B. Requirements
  C. Sources
  D. Hyper- and Hypo- States
  Nursing Applications
XIII. CHROMIUM
  A. Physiological Roles
  B. Requirements
  C. Sources
  D. Hyper- and Hypo- States
  Nursing Applications
XIV. COBALT
  Nursing Applications
XV. OTHER TRACE MINERALS
  Nursing Applications

OBJECTIVES

THE STUDENT WILL BE ABLE TO:

- List the minerals found in the body with their main physiological roles and sources.
- Describe causes and symptoms of mineral excess or deficits.
- List 3 trace elements found in the body that are probably better considered as contaminants than physiological necessities.
- Discuss the pros and cons of fluoridation of the water supply.

- Describe advantages and disadvantages of mineral supplementation.
- Describe client education tips for minerals.
- Discuss nursing applications for minerals.

TEST YOUR NQ (True/False)

1. Meats are good sources of phosphorus.
2. Women and the elderly should always take iron supplements.
3. Bone meal or dolomite is a good calcium supplement.
4. Large doses of zinc increase virility and improve the sex drive.
5. There is no RDA for sulfur.
6. Heme iron is provided by meat sources and is readily absorbed.
7. All women should take calcium supplements to prevent osteoporosis.
8. Calcium absorption is increased when a sugar is present.
9. Nuts, beans, and green leafy vegetables are good sources of magnesium.
10. Goiter is the result of iodine deficiency.

Minerals have many functions. The numerous mineral elements in the body account for only about 4% of total body weight, or 6 lbs for a 150-lb person. Minerals are subdivided into those required in larger amounts, i.e., major minerals, and those required in smaller amounts, i.e., micronutrients or trace elements (Table 9–1). Despite the small amounts required, trace elements are just as important as the major minerals.

Minerals are inorganic elements required to perform varied roles.

Even in the US where food is abundant, many clients consume a diet inadequate in minerals. Intake of 11 essential minerals is assessed annually by the FDA. Reports have revealed low levels of calcium, magnesium, iron, zinc, copper, and manganese (i.e., less than 80% of the RDAs or below the ESADDI) for more than 3 out of the 18 RDA age-sex groups. Young children, teenage girls, and adult and older women are at risk of low intakes. Copper intake was low for all groups (Pennington & Young, 1991).

On the other hand, sodium intake continues to exceed the estimated minimum requirements. This is of concern because of its relationship to hypertension. Potas-

TABLE 9–1

MINERAL ELEMENTS IN THE BODY

Major Minerals (> 100 mg or more/day)	Trace Elements (< 100 mg daily)	Possible Essential Trace Elements (No RDA)	Trace Elements (Unknown Function or Contaminants)
Calcium (Ca)	Iron (Fe)	Nickel (Ni)	Aluminum (Al)
Phosphorus (P)	Copper (Cu)	Tin (Sn)	Barium (Ba)
Sodium (Na)	Zinc (Zn)	Silicon (Si)	Strontium (St)
Potassium (K)	Manganese (Mn)	Vanadium (V)	Mercury (Hg)
Magnesium (Mg)	Iodine (I)	Boron (Bo)	Silver (Ag)
Chlorine (Cl)	Molybdenum (Mo)	Cadmium (Cd)	Gold (Au)
Sulfur (S)	Fluorine (Fl)	Arsenic (As)	Antimony (Sb)
	Selenium (Se)	Lead (Pb)	Others
	Chromium (Cr)		
	Cobalt (Co)		

sium, phosphorus, selenium, and iodine intake was adequate for all groups (Pennington & Young, 1991).

CALCIUM

Physiological Roles

Osteoblasts produce bone minerals to strengthen bone and fill the cavities; osteoclasts resorb bone in microscopic cavities.

Name the roles of calcium.

At least 99% of the body's calcium is found in the skeleton and teeth. The calcium deposited in teeth remains permanently. However, calcium (as well as phosphorus) in the bone functions as a "savings account" for maintaining serum calcium levels. Bone is constantly changing as the **osteoblasts** deposit fresh calcium salts where new stresses have developed and where **osteoclasts** are removing calcium deposits.

Only 1% of the calcium is found in blood, but as such, it controls body functions such as blood clotting, transmission of nerve impulses, muscle contraction and relaxation, membrane permeability, and activation of enzymes.

Requirements and Regulation

What is the adult RDA for calcium?

The RDA for calcium has been established at 800 mg/day for adults. During growth periods, from 11 to 24 years of age, and during pregnancy and lactation, the estimated requirement is higher (1200 mg/day) because peak bone mass appears to be related to calcium intake during periods of bone mineralization. By age 40, bone resorption begins to exceed formation, resulting in gradual loss of bone mass. In 1984, as a result of a conference on osteoporosis sponsored by the National Institutes of Health, the group recommended 1000 mg of calcium per day for nonpregnant adults and suggested that individuals at risk of osteoporosis consume 1500 mg per day (Consensus Conference, 1984).

Calcium Balance

Calcitriol is the active form of vitamin D.

Calcitonin is a hormone secreted by the thyroid gland; its action is antagonistic to parathyroid hormone.

What are the functions of calcitriol and calcitonin?

Despite wide variations in calcium intake, serum calcium is relatively constant because each cell has a vital need for calcium. Bones are used as calcium reserves if the serum calcium level drops. If calcium withdrawal from the bones exceeds the deposits, calcium imbalance occurs. Decreased bone density caused by insufficient calcium is a slow process.

A decrease in serum calcium activates release of parathyroid hormone by the parathyroid gland. In response, **calcitriol** synthesis results in (1) increased calcium absorption, (2) decreased urinary excretion of calcium, (3) increased excretion of phosphorus, and (4) calcium withdrawal from bones. **Calcitonin** is released when serum calcium levels increase, causing decreased bone loss and decreasing synthesis of calcitriol.

Calcium-to-Phosphorus Ratio

Serum levels of calcium and phosphorus have an inverse relationship, called the serum calcium-to-phosphorus (Ca:P) ratio. If the calcium level goes up, the phosphorus goes down, and vice versa. This acts as a protective mechanism to prevent high combined concentrations with subsequent calcification of soft tissue and stone formation. Normal serum calcium level is about 10 mg/dl, and normal phosphorus level is 4 mg/dl.

A normal serum calcium and phosphorus value multiplied together is 40. Calcification and stone formation may result when the calcium and phosphorus level is greater than 75. Sufficient phosphorus intake is necessary to decrease the loss of calcium with all intake levels. The ideal dietary calcium-to-phosphorus ratio for adults is 1:1; during periods of growth, a ratio of 1:1.5 is advisable. This ratio does not warrant as close attention under normal conditions as in conditions such as renal disease.

Why is there an inverse relationship between calcium and phosphorus? What are the normal serum levels for calcium and phosphorus?

Absorption and Excretion

Calcium balance, i.e., an intake that equals excretion, is not solely dependent on adequate amounts of calcium intake. Under normal conditions, less than one-third of the calcium consumed is absorbed.

Absorption occurs in the upper part of the intestine and is affected by many factors (Fig. 9–1). Calcium absorption from various dairy products is similar (Recker et al, 1988), whereas calcium present in dark green leafy vegetables is not readily absorbed. During periods of increased needs, especially during growth and pregnancy and lactation, calcium absorption may increase to 50% of intake. Calcium absorption decreases with age, probably because of decreased gastric acidity. The rate of absorption is lowest in postmenopausal women because of diminished estrogen levels. The presence of calcitriol, parathyroid hormone, and sugars (such as glucose and lactose) has a positive effect on calcium absorption (Knowles, 1988; Wood et al, 1987).

Although several plant foods contain large amounts of calcium, absorption is poor. Oxalates in vegetables and phytates from wheat bran bind the calcium to reduce absorption, but they do not interfere with calcium absorption from other foods. Excessive dietary fiber also interferes with calcium absorption.

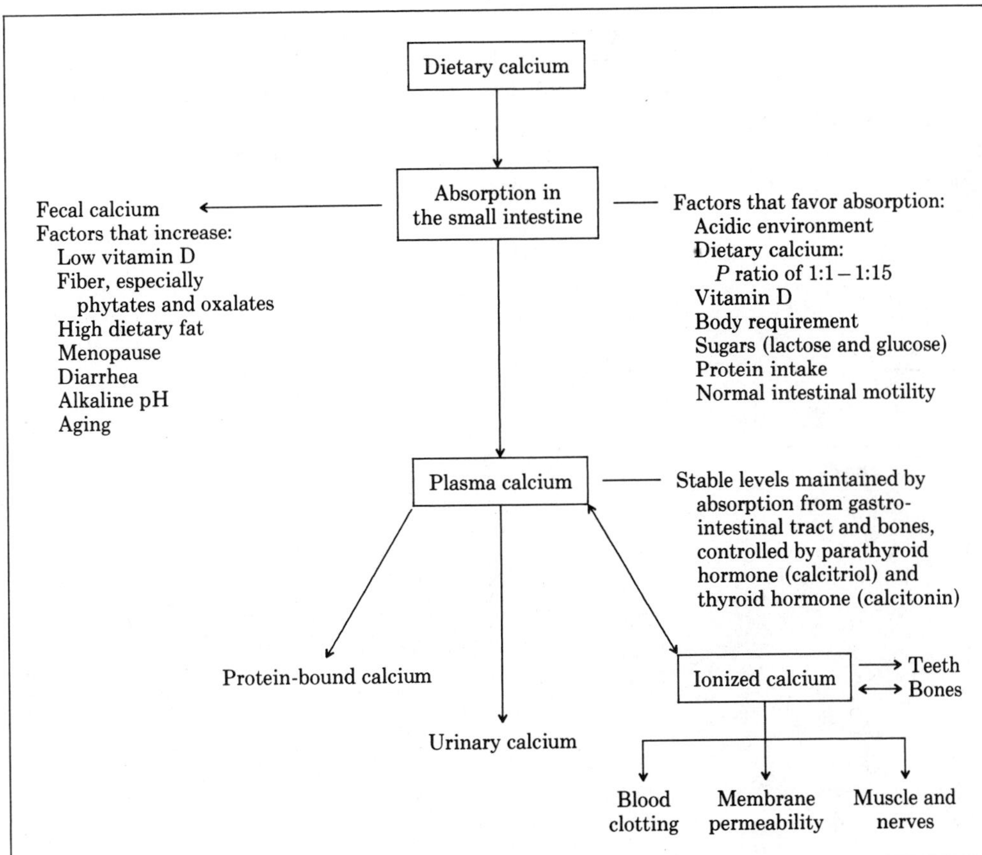

Figure 9–1 Calcium absorption and utilization.

Bioavailability is the amount of the nutrient available to the body based on its absorption.

Explain what can enhance or decrease calcium absorption.

Previously many professionals in the scientific community thought that protein and phosphorus adversely affected calcium **bioavailability.** High-protein foods typically eaten in the US have a high phosphorus content. The usual intake does not cause calcium loss, whereas a diet low in protein and phosphorus may have adverse effects on calcium balance in the elderly (Spencer et al, 1988).

Sources

Milk and other dairy products supply most of the available calcium (Table 9–2). Not only are they excellent sources because of their high calcium content, but inherent lactose content enhances calcium absorption. Table 9–3 lists portion sizes for various foods to provide approximately 300 mg of calcium. Table 9–2 contains a more extensive list of foods with their calcium content.

Consumers in the US spent over $177 million on calcium supplements in 1987 (Hegarty & Stewart, 1988). In addition to all the pharmaceutical products available, food manufacturers fortify products such as fruit juice, soft drinks, and breakfast cereal. This strong trend toward the use of calcium supplements is especially prevalent in the older population. Benefits may be less than expected, partly because of limited bioavailability of supplemental calcium. Calcium carbonate, lactate, citrate, gluconate, phosphate, and citrate malate are all absorbed reasonably well. Calcium citrate malate (available only in orange drink) may be the most effective supplement available (Dawson-Hughes et al, 1990).

Name sources of calcium.

Hyper- and Hypo- States

Clinical conditions are associated with excesses and deficiencies of calcium. Hypercalcemic and hypocalcemic conditions (too much or too little calcium) are critical metabolic conditions and can lead to loss of consciousness, fatal respiratory failure, or cardiac arrest. These problems are seldom caused directly by calcium intake; however, bone density can be adversely related to intake.

TABLE 9–2

CALCIUM AND PHOSPHORUS CONTENT OF SELECTED FOODS

Food	Portion	Calcium (mg)	Phosphorus (mg)	Kilocalories (per serving)
Romano cheese	3 oz	904	644	329
Swiss cheese	3 oz	815	512	320
Cheddar cheese	3 oz	611	434	341
American cheese	3 oz	521	632	317
Nonfat plain yogurt	1 cup	452	355	127
Canned sardines	3 oz	325	417	177
Milk	1 cup	300	232	121
Buttermilk	1 cup	285	219	99
Canned salmon	3 oz	181	280	118
Low-fat cottage cheese	1 cup	138	302	164
Turnip greens	½ cup	125	28	25
Cooked spinach	½ cup	123	51	21
Cooked oysters	3 oz	76	236	117
Cooked broccoli	½ cup	36	46	22
Cooked shrimp	3 oz	33	116	84

Nutrient data from Nutritionist III software, version 7.0. N-Squared Computing, Salem, Oregon.

TABLE 9–3

CALCIUM EQUIVALENTS

The following foods contain approximately 300 mg calcium:*
1 cup milk
1 ½ oz cheddar cheese
2 cups cottage cheese
1 cup yogurt
1 ½ slices processed cheese
1 ½ cups ice cream
1 ½ cups dark green leafy vegetables†
4 oz salmon
2 ½ oz sardines

* The RDA for calcium is 800 mg for persons 24 years and older.
† Calcium from vegetable sources is not as easily absorbed by the intestine and is not as effective in fulfilling calcium requirements.

Hypercalcemia and Hypocalcemia

Because calcium exists in the blood ionized and bound to protein, determination of serum proteins is needed so the calcium value can be properly interpreted. A depressed concentration of total calcium can be due to hypoproteinemia, but nurses are concerned with the concentration of ionized calcium. A general rule of thumb for reassessing "pseudohypocalcemia" is that for every 1 gm albumin below 4 gm, calcium is lowered by 0.8 mg.

Tetany is a neuromuscular disorder of uncontrollable muscular cramps and tremors.

Hypocalcemia results in **tetany,** involving the muscles of the face, hands, feet, and eventually the heart. Depressed serum calcium levels may be caused by hypoparathyroidism, some bone diseases, certain kidney diseases, and low serum protein levels.

Why should the nurse assess protein levels when monitoring serum calcium? What causes hypocalcemia, and what does this result in? Who is most prone to hypercalcemia and why? What can cause adult hypercalcemia?

Hypercalcemia is observed in infants most frequently between 5 and 8 months of age. It is caused by overdoses of cholecalciferol or excessive amounts of vitamin D preparations. Treatment involves providing a low-calcium diet with no vitamin D. Hyperparathyroidism, certain types of bone disease, vitamin D poisoning, sarcoidosis, cancer, or prolonged excessive intake of milk may cause adult hypercalcemia.

Excessive Calcium Intake

Excessively high calcium intake may cause constipation, increase the risk of urinary stone formation in hypercalciuric men, and inhibit iron and zinc absorption (NRC, 1989).

Inadequate Calcium Intake

Dietary deficiency of calcium is frequently observed. This could be due to (1) uninformed choices or just not selecting adequate amounts, (2) the mistaken belief that adults do not need milk, or (3) economic hardships plus a lack of knowledge regarding inexpensive sources of calcium-rich foods.

Rickets is the result of inadequate amounts of calcium deposits in the bone during childhood.

Rickets, discussed in Chapter 7 in connection with vitamin D deficiency, results in porous, soft bones. Calcium intake may be adequate, but absorption is poor because of inadequate vitamin D.

Osteoporosis is an age-related disorder characterized by decreased bone mass, causing bones to be more susceptible to fracture.

Osteoporosis is caused by numerous factors, including decreased estrogen, inadequate calcium intake, and lack of weight-bearing activity. The relationship of calcium intake to bone density indicates a protective effect solely in women reporting high "lifetime" calcium intake, not by just increasing intake following menopause (Cauley et al, 1988). Building bone during the formative years is the best insurance against osteoporosis. Initial signs may be loss of calcium in the jawbone, resulting in loose teeth and gum disease. The condition, however, usually goes undetected until pain or spontaneous fracture occurs. Osteoporosis is discussed further in Chapter 18.

Numerous scientists have investigated the role of dietary calcium in blood pressure regulation. Despite the fact that high blood pressure is more prevalent in clients with a low calcium intake, not all clients have the same response to calcium supplementation. Although some are responsive to calcium supplementation, others experience a rise in blood pressure. Because there is no way to predict blood pressure response, recommendation of calcium supplements to treat hypertension is inappropriate at this time (Clark, 1989).

What results from increased calcium intake; what results from decreased intake?

NURSING APPLICATIONS

1. Fatty acids form insoluble soaps with calcium, so clients unable to absorb fats have low calcium absorption and are prone to brittle bones. Move these clients carefully.
2. When serum calcium is low, calcium supplementation is usually not needed. Low serum calcium may be a result of low protein (especially albumin) or inadequate parathyroid hormone secretion. Correction of the primary problem is necessary rather than calcium supplementation. Therefore, check the serum protein and albumin and parathyroid hormone levels before becoming concerned over the calcium level.
3. Immobilization from a fracture immediately starts bone depletion. In the young client, recovery of calcium deposits is usually rapid, but the geriatric client may never regain bone density. Get these clients up and around as soon as possible.
4. No benefits have been observed for fracture healing when increased calcium or hormones are taken. In fact, urinary stones may occur. Thus, do not give calcium supplements unless ordered. If supplements are ordered, monitor for flank pain. If it occurs, strain urine for possible stone excretion. Consumption of calcium in the amounts recommended in the RDA is appropriate. (Calcium-rich foods are not eliminated but limited to 2 to 3 cups daily.)
5. Clients with a family history of kidney stones should consult a physician before increasing calcium intake.
6. Assess a client with hypercalcemia (as determined by laboratory values greater than 5.8 mg) for deep bone pain or flank pain and increased urine output. Interventions include monitoring I&O, straining urine for stones, limiting high-calcium foods, and encouraging fluid intake.
7. Assess clients with hypocalcemia (serum calcium less than 4.5 mg) for pathological fractures, tingling in extremities, and tetany. Nursing care consists of administering calcium supplements and initiating safety precautions for seizures.
8. Interventions for osteoporosis include offering calcium-rich foods. Encourage exercise, and administer estrogen replacement as ordered.
9. Clients who do not smoke use calcium more efficiently. If a client smokes, recognize that more calcium may be needed.

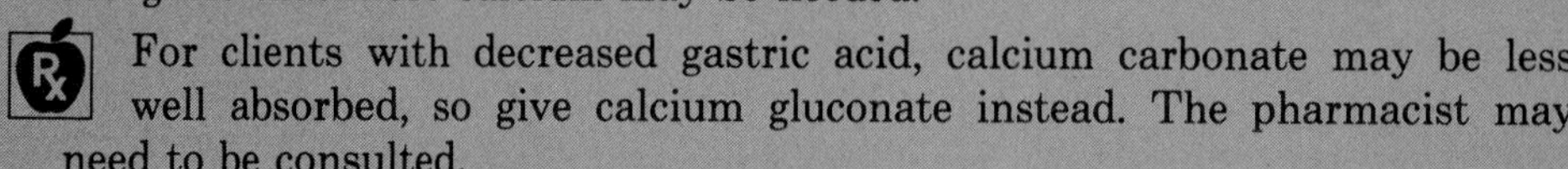

For clients with decreased gastric acid, calcium carbonate may be less well absorbed, so give calcium gluconate instead. The pharmacist may need to be consulted.

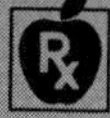

For older clients with decreased gastric acid, give calcium with meals or a snack to enhance calcium absorption.

Client Education

- Calcium supplement absorption can be enhanced if taken with some form of sugar: Lactose, dextrose, or sucrose enhances its absorption (Knowles, 1988; Wood et al, 1987). Vitamin D also enhances absorption.
- Consider each supplement for the amount of elemental calcium provided (actual amount of calcium in the supplement), cost per tablet, and expected compliance. Poor compliance may be expected if several tablets are necessary, the supplement is too expensive, or it causes GI problems. More than 500 mg per tablet may cause constipation.
- Encourage exercise because weight-bearing exercise has a positive effect on normal calcium deposits in bone.
- If a client's usual calcium intake is low, encourage increased consumption of dairy products first if tolerated. If the client dislikes milk, powdered milk can be added to many items, or other high-calcium foods can be used.
- The use of dolomite as a calcium supplement is questionable. Dolomite, produced from the animal bones that have accumulated lead, can result in lead poisoning. A client must always question whether such supplements have appropriate sanitation and quality control.
- If a calcium tablet does not readily dissolve in a 25% vinegar in water solution, it probably will not dissolve in the body.
- After menopause, calcium supplements have been shown to diminish bone loss when coupled with estrogen replacement therapy.

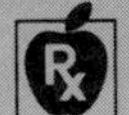

Calcium intake decreases the effectiveness of tetracycline if taken concurrently.

PHOSPHORUS

Physiological Roles

Phosphorus is the second most abundant mineral in the body, with about 85% in the skeleton and teeth. Its presence in all body cells is necessary for almost every aspect of metabolism, including (1) the transfer and release of energy stored as ATP; (2) a component of DNA and RNA; (3) cell permeability as phospholipids; and (4) metabolism of fats, carbohydrates, and proteins.

Name the roles of phosphorus.

Requirements

The RDA for phosphorus is 800 mg for adults over 25 years of age, the same as for calcium. The ideal intake of Ca:P ratio is 1:1. Because phosphorus is more readily available, intake is generally 1.5 times higher than calcium.

List the requirement for phosphorus.

Absorption and Excretion

Approximately 60 to 70% of the dietary phosphorus is absorbed in the jejunum. Its absorption can be inhibited by the same dietary factors that affect calcium absorption, i.e., phytate, excessive amounts of fats, iron, aluminum, and calcium. The kidneys excrete excessive amounts of phosphorus to maintain optimum body levels.

What can inhibit phosphorus absorption?

Sources

List sources of phosphorus.

Phosphorus is so abundant in foods that deficiencies have not been observed. A diet adequate in calcium and protein contains enough phosphorus because it is present in the same foods (see Table 9–2). In addition to its presence in milk products, meats are also a good source of phosphorus. Because of its wide use as a food additive in baked goods, cheese, processed meats, and soft drinks, dietary restriction of phosphorus is extremely difficult.

Hyper- and Hypo- States

What are some causes of hypophosphatemia and hyperphosphatemia? What are the clinical symptoms of each?

Hypophosphatemia (serum level below 1.8 mg/dl) may occur with long-term ingestion of aluminum hydroxide antacids, which interfere with phosphorus absorption, or in certain stress conditions in which the calcium-to-phosphorus balance is disturbed. Even relatively small phosphorus depletions can cause increased calcium excretion, resulting in negative calcium balance and bone loss. Intestinal conditions, such as sprue and celiac disease, can result in phosphorus malabsorption deficiencies. The principal clinical symptom of hypophosphatemia is muscle weakness.

Hyperphosphatemia (serum level above 2.6 mg/dl) may occur in cases of hypoparathyroidism or renal insufficiency (see Chapters 28 and 29). Excessive amounts of phosphorus bind with calcium, resulting in tetany and convulsions.

NURSING APPLICATIONS

1. Low phosphate levels may occur in clients with use of diuretics, total parenteral nutrition, or alcohol withdrawal. Assess these types of clients closely.
2. Normal serum levels are 1.8 to 2.6 mEq/L, so monitor laboratory values for increases or decreases.
3. If the client has hyperphosphatemia, sodium phosphate enemas and vitamin D supplements are not appropriate, so question order if written.
4. Avoid the use of sodium phosphate/biphosphate enemas in children because hyperphosphatemia has been reported.

Client Education

- Phosphorus is so widespread in foods that educating clients about phosphorus is limited to disease states such as renal disease when a dietary restriction is necessary (see Chapters 28 and 29).

MAGNESIUM

Physiological Roles

Describe the roles of magnesium.

Magnesium is vitally important in structural integrity of heart muscle as well as other muscles and nerves. Bones contain almost two-thirds of the body's magnesium. Magnesium also has an important function in enzyme action fundamental to the production of energy (ATP).

Requirements

The RDA for magnesium is 280 mg/day for women and 350 mg/day for men. Between 1982 and 1989, average intake of magnesium was 195 mg for women and

TABLE 9–4
MAGNESIUM CONTENT OF SELECTED FOODS

Food	Portion	Magnesium (mg)	Kilocalories (per serving)
Sunflower seeds	¼ cup	128	205
Sesame seeds	¼ cup	126	206
Cashews	¼ cup	89	197
Cooked spinach	½ cup	79	21
Wheat germ	¼ cup	69	103
Navy beans	½ cup	54	130
Beet greens	½ cup	49	20
Blackeyed/cowpeas	½ cup	43	112
Baked potato	1	39	145
Sliced beets	½ cup	31	26
Lima beans	½ cup	29	85
Cooked shrimp	3 oz	29	84
Cooked broccoli	½ cup	19	22

Nutrient data from Nutritionist III software, version 7.0. N-Squared Computing, Salem, Oregon.

301 mg for men 25 to 30 years of age (Pennington & Young, 1991). Dietary surveys consistently indicate magnesium intake is lower than the RDA, but magnesium deficiency has not been observed in healthy Americans (NRC, 1989).

What is the RDA for magnesium in men and women?

Sources

Whole-grain products, nuts, beans, and green leafy vegetables are some of the best sources of magnesium (Table 9–4). Magnesium is part of the chlorophyll molecule; therefore, green leafy vegetables are good sources. Bananas, a popular fruit, are a good source of magnesium. Enrichment does not replace the magnesium removed from refined grains.

Name food sources of magnesium.

Hyper- and Hypo- States

A significant number of clients with serum magnesium abnormalities are clinically unrecognized (Whang & Ryder, 1990). Because kidneys regulate plasma magnesium levels, toxicity has only been associated with kidney failure.

In certain diseases or under stressful conditions, deficiencies may occur. Magnesium in bone is not available to replace serum magnesium deficits. A deficiency may result from numerous disease states: GI abnormalities with diarrhea, renal disease, general malnutrition, and alcoholism or medications that interfere with magnesium conservation. Symptoms of a magnesium deficiency are neuromuscular dysfunction, personality changes, muscle spasm, convulsions (especially in infants), hyperexcitability, tremors, anorexia, nausea, apathy, and cardiac arrhythmias.

What causes hypermagnesemia and hypomagnesemia problems? What are the symptoms of low magnesium?

NURSING APPLICATIONS

1. Normal serum magnesium level is 1.5 to 2.5 mEq/L, so monitor laboratory values for increases or decreases.
2. Hypomagnesemia has been found in about one-third of infants of diabetic mothers. This was related to the severity of maternal diabetes and premature birth (Shils, 1988). Assess infants for signs and symptoms of hypomagnesemia, especially in cases of prematurity and uncontrolled maternal diabetes.
3. Chronic alcoholics may require magnesium therapy after an acute attack of delirium tremens because of high urinary losses of magnesium.

Continued

4. Nursing care for hypomagnesemia involves administering intravenous magnesium sulfate and providing foods high in magnesium.
5. Hypermagnesemia results in drowsiness, vasodilation, and loss of deep tendon reflexes. Treatment consists of alleviating renal failure by use of dialysis or giving calcium gluconate as ordered (calcium counteracts magnesium) or administering diuretics with fluid.

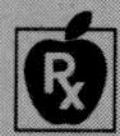
Obstetrical clients who receive magnesium sulfate must be monitored for excess magnesium.

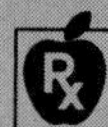
Decreased food intake and/or impaired absorption and use of certain diuretics may be contributing factors to hypomagnesemia. Encourage a well-balanced diet with liberal use of foods high in magnesium. Administration of magnesium may be useful for some clients (Shils, 1988).

Client Education

- Diets high in unrefined grains and vegetables provide more magnesium than diets including a lot of refined foods, meats, and milk products.
- If gravida is given magnesium sulfate, the infant may be lethargic.
- If renal dialysis clients need antacids, emphasize the use of aluminum-based or calcium-based antacids rather than magnesium hydroxide.

SULFUR

Physiological Roles

Name the roles of sulfur.

Sulfur is a constituent in the cytoplasm of all body cells. It is principally found combined with protein compounds and structural proteins in cartilage, tendons, and bone matrix and keratin in hair and nails. It also has an important role in acid–base balance. One of the most important functions of sulfur is its ability to neutralize toxins by combining with them to form harmless compounds that can be excreted.

Requirements and Sources

No RDA has been established for sulfur because it is readily available in protein foods that are essential for an adequate diet.

Hyper- and Hypo- States

No problems have been observed because sulfur is so readily available.

NURSING APPLICATIONS

1. Sulfur may be associated with cysteine renal stones; strain the urine if stones are suspected.
2. Sulfur deficiency is rarely seen as long as protein intake is adequate.

Client Education

- Sulfur should not be confused with sulfa drugs or sulfites (used as a food additive).

IRON

Physiological Roles

Every body cell contains iron; approximately 4 gm (less than 1 tsp) are present in the entire body. Iron is a major component of hemoglobin, which transports oxygen from the lungs to the tissues. It also catalyzes many oxidative reactions within cells and participates in the final steps of energy metabolism. Other roles include (1) conversion of beta-carotene to vitamin A, (2) synthesis of collagen, (3) formation of purines as part of nucleic acid, (4) removal of lipids from the blood, (5) detoxification of drugs in the liver, and (6) production of antibodies.

Virtually all functional iron is bound to protein, present in the blood as **hemoglobin,** transferrin, and ferritin; in every cell as cytochrome; and in muscle cells as **myoglobin** (Fig. 9–2). Hemoglobin in the blood and myoglobin in cells transport

Hemoglobin and myoglobin are iron-containing proteins combined with iron; they bind oxygen.

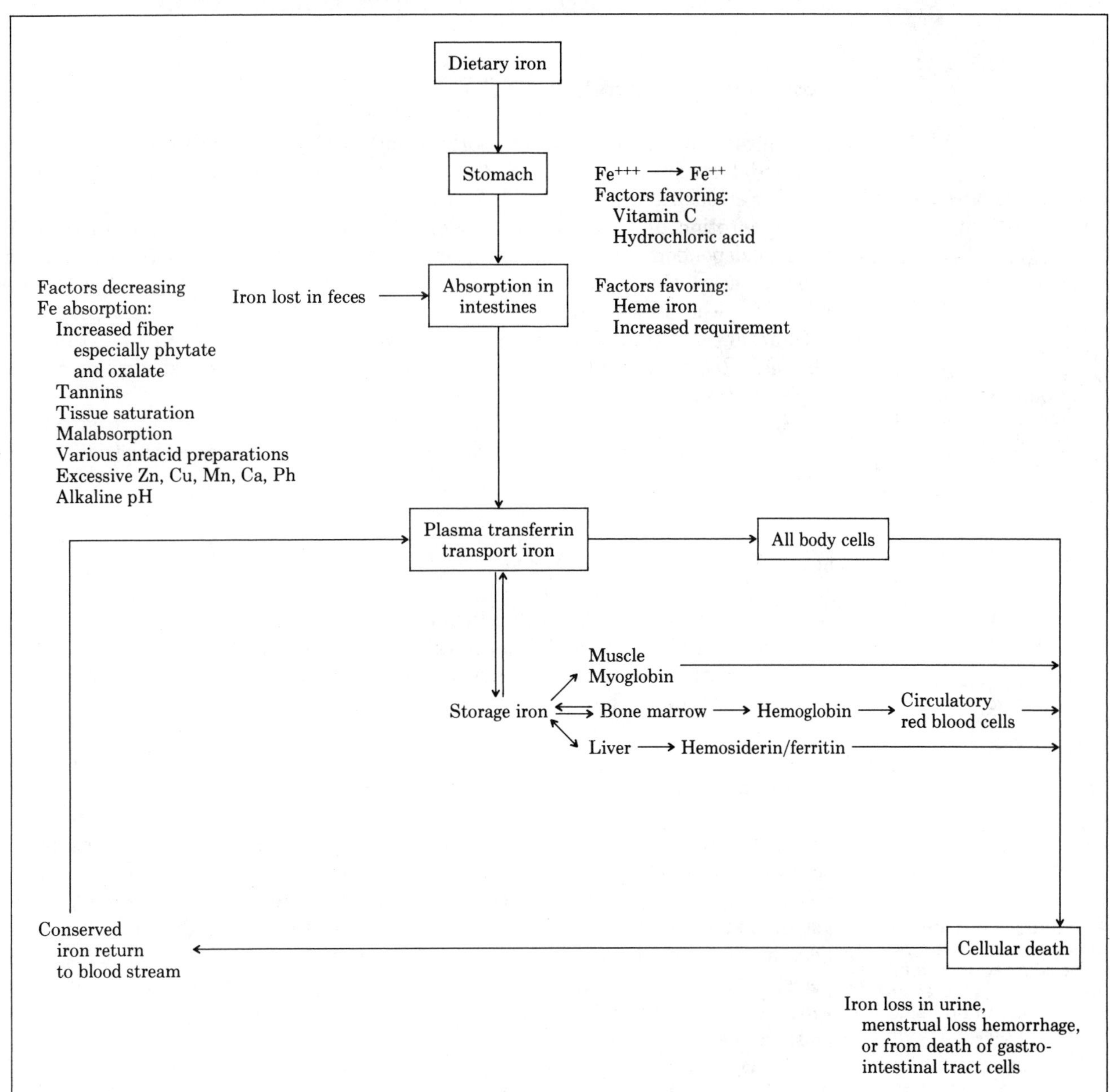

Figure 9–2 Iron absorption and utilization.

Name the roles of iron. What are the functions of hemoglobin, transferrin, ferritin, and myoglobin, and how do these relate to iron?

oxygen and carbon dioxide to and from the tissues. Transferrin transports iron to the bone marrow and various storage sites.

Storage iron represents about one-third of the body's iron. Iron is stored within the ferritin molecule. Approximately 60% of all ferritin is stored in the liver, with the remainder in the spleen and bone marrow.

Requirements

RBCs are also referred to as erythrocytes.

What are the iron requirements for men and women?

The recommendations are 15 mg/day for women and 10 mg/day for men. The RDA is higher for women than for men due to blood loss related to menstruation. During the reproduction phase of a woman's life, iron loss is at least double that of a man or of a postmenopausal woman. The RDA is based on the approximation that 10% of dietary iron is absorbed. The demand for iron replenishment is constant because the life of an **RBC** is 120 days. When the cell dies, iron is released and transported in the blood by transferrin to various storage sites.

Absorption and Excretion

Heme iron is provided by meat sources that contain hemoglobin and myoglobin molecules. Non-heme iron is the type of iron present in eggs, milk, and plants.

Which iron is better absorbed? Explain the difference between heme and non-heme iron. How can acidic conditions and calcium affect iron absorption?

Similar to calcium, iron is poorly absorbed. Most of the iron in food is in the oxidized form of ferric iron (Fe^{+++}), although some ferrous iron (Fe^{++}) has been found. Ferrous iron is absorbed better than ferric iron.

Absorption of **heme iron** parallels the body's need; absorption of **non-heme iron** is dependent on intraluminal and meal composition as well as physiological need. In a healthy client, as little as 10% may be absorbed, compared with an anemic client who uses as much as 50%. Acidic conditions enhance iron absorption, but calcium and manganese interfere with its absorption (Cook et al, 1991; Hallberg et al, 1991; Rossander-Hulten et al, 1991). Factors affecting iron absorption are listed in Figure 9–2.

Combinations of food can enhance iron absorption. A meal of roast beef (rich in iron) with potatoes (rich in vitamin C) and a tossed green salad (rich in folate) increases iron absorption.

Sources

List sources of heme and non-heme iron.

Iron is probably the most difficult mineral to obtain in adequate amounts in the American diet. Although liver is the best source of iron, meats (especially beef), egg yolk, dark green vegetable, and enriched breads and cereals all contribute significant amounts (Table 9–5).

Hyper- and Hypo- States

Hemosiderin is a form of storage iron that is more concentrated than ferritin. Hemosiderin is increased in the body when hemosiderosis occurs.

The body cannot easily eliminate excess iron; possibly this explains poor absorption rates. It is unusual for the body to overcome its regulation of intestinal absorption. Iron overload can occur, however, if ingestion of iron is extremely elevated. **Hemosiderosis,** a hereditary disorder, occurs when excessive iron accumulates in the body. This may occur with (1) excessive iron intake, (2) multiple blood transfusions, and (3) a failure to regulate absorption. Inexpensive red wines contain wide variations in iron content (10 to 350 mg/L) and have been associated with hemosiderosis.

Elevated iron stores have been associated with increased risk of coronary heart disease (Salonen et al, 1992). More studies are needed to confirm this finding, but iron and vitamin C supplements should not be taken indiscriminately and without depressed laboratory findings.

TABLE 9–5

IRON CONTENT OF SELECTED FOODS

Food	Portion	Iron (mg)	Kilocalories (per serving)
Cooked oysters	3 oz	11.4	117
Beef liver	3 oz	5.8	137
Spinach	½ cup	3.2	21
Blackstrap molasses	1 tbsp	3.2	45
Dried apricots	½ cup	3.1	155
Lean beef sirloin	3 oz	2.9	176
Cooked shrimp	3 oz	2.6	84
Navy beans	½ cup	2.6	113
Lean round steak	3 oz	2.5	163
Kidney beans	½ cup	2.3	115
Lean rib lamb chop	3 oz	1.8	200
Ground hamburger	3 oz	1.8	231
Sauerkraut	½ cup	1.7	22
Cooked oatmeal	½ cup	1.6	145
Seedless raisins	½ cup	1.5	218
Prune juice	½ cup	1.5	91
Veal, rib cut	3 oz	1.2	185
Chicken leg	3 oz	1.2	157
Whole-wheat bread	1 slice	0.94	67
Green peas	½ cup	0.81	59
Lean ham	3 oz	0.80	134
Lean pork loin chop	3 oz	0.80	218
Bologna, pork	3 oz	0.7	210
Broccoli	½ cup	0.6	26
White tuna	3 oz	0.5	116
Chicken breast	3 oz	0.4	67
Cod fish	3 oz	0.4	89
Peanut butter	1 tbsp	0.3	94

Nutrient data from Nutritionist III software, version 7.0. N-Squared Computing, Salem, Oregon.

Iron deficiency anemia continues to be a worldwide problem. A deficiency can lead to various symptoms, such as microcytic anemia, fatigue, faulty digestion, blue sclerae, pale conjunctiva, and tachycardia. Iron deficiency anemia may be caused by inadequate dietary intake of iron; accelerated iron demand; increased iron losses; or inadequate absorption secondary to diarrhea, decreased acid secretions, or antacid therapy. Iron deficiency is frequently the result of postnatal feeding practices and has a serious impact on growth and on mental and psychomotor development in infants and children. Iron deficiency anemia is further discussed in Chapter 18.

What can predispose to hemosiderosis? What can cause iron deficiency anemia?

NURSING APPLICATIONS

1. Despite the prevalence of iron deficiency anemia, supplements are not recommended without laboratory testing to indicate a deficiency. Monitor laboratory results before initiating supplements.
2. Hemosiderosis is common among chronic alcoholics who may drink more than 1 L of inexpensive wine daily. Therefore, assess an alcoholic's amount and type of alcohol intake.
3. Clients who receive numerous blood transfusions can develop iron toxicity; monitor for hemosiderosis.
4. Give moderate amounts of iron-rich and iron-fortified foods to men who absorb excess iron.
5. Few clients realize the potential danger from ferrous sulfate supplements. In 1988, the American Association of Poison Control Centers National Data Collection System reported 19,676 ingestions of iron-containing products, of which 83.9% were children under 6 years of age (Litovitz & Schmitz, 1989).

Continued

Evaluate client's knowledge by questioning client's use of supplements and where supplements are stored.

Client Education

- A vitamin C–rich food with supplements or with meals increases absorption of iron, especially non-heme iron (Hallberg et al, 1989; Hunt et al, 1990). Take iron with orange juice or tomato juice or vitamin C–enriched juices such as apple juice.
- If iron-containing grains or vegetables are consumed with small amounts of heme iron, absorption of the non-heme iron doubles (Monsen, 1988).
- Coffee and tea decrease the absorption of iron. No decrease in iron absorption occurs when coffee is drunk 1 hour before a meal.
- Keep iron supplements out of reach of children.
- Iron supplements cause stools to turn black.

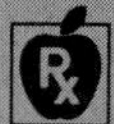 Avoid taking iron supplements with milk because the calcium in milk interferes with iron absorption.

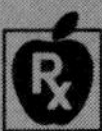 When a calcium supplement is taken with an iron supplement between meals, only calcium carbonate does not affect the absorption of iron (Cook et al, 1991).

COPPER

Physiological Roles

Neurotransmitters transmit messages through the CNS.

What are the roles of copper?

Copper is essential for the formation of RBCs and connective tissue. Copper is a cofactor of many enzymes that function in oxidative reactions and production of **neurotransmitters** (including norepinephrine and dopamine).

Requirements

What is the ESADDI for copper?

The National Research Council has established ESADDI of copper to be 1.5 to 3 mg/day for adults. Most adults consume about 1 mg/day (Pennington & Young, 1991).

Absorption and Excretion

What enhances and decreases copper absorption?

Approximately one-third of dietary copper is absorbed, with absorption occurring in the stomach and duodenum. Absorption is enhanced by a low pH and decreased with large amounts of calcium and zinc. Copper is principally excreted through bile in feces.

Sources

Name sources of copper.

Copper is widely distributed in foods. The richest sources include shellfish, oysters, crabs, liver, nuts, sesame and sunflower seeds, legumes, and cocoa (Table 9–6).

Hyper- and Hypo- States

Copper toxicosis is seldom encountered. Oral copper is an emetic, and as little as 10 mg of oral copper can produce nausea (Solomons, 1988). Serum copper levels are elevated in clients with rheumatoid arthritis, myocardial infarction, conditions requiring administration of estrogen, and pregnancy.

TABLE 9–6

ZINC AND COPPER CONTENT OF SELECTED FOODS

Food	Portion	Zinc (mg)	Copper (mg)	Kilocalories (per serving)
Eastern oysters	3 oz	155	7.58	117
Pacific oysters	3 oz	14.1	1.34	69
All bran cereal	1 cup	11.2	0.98	212
Broiled lean sirloin	3 oz	5.6	0.13	176
Beef liver	3 oz	5.2	3.84	137
Lean veal chop	3 oz	5.1	0.12	185
Lean hamburger patty	3 oz	4.6	0.06	231
Lean lamb chop	3 oz	4.5	0.12	200
Wheat germ	¼ cup	3.5	0.23	103
Cheddar cheese	1 oz	2.6	0.09	341
Lean pork chop	3 oz	2.5	0.08	218
Chicken leg	3 oz	2.4	0.07	157
Lean ham	3 oz	2.2	0.07	134
Pork bologna	3 oz	1.7	0.06	210
Canned clams	3 oz	1.0	N/A	38
Milk	1 cup	0.95	0.02	121
Whole egg	1	0.6	0.01	75
Cod fish	3 oz	0.5	0.03	89
Whole-wheat bread	1 slice	0.5	0.09	67
Baked potato	1	0.5	0.34	145
Chicken breast	3 oz	0.4	0.02	67

N/A, Not available.
Nutrient data from Nutritionist III software, version 7.0. N-Squared Computing, Salem, Oregon.

Wilson's disease represents a special case of copper toxicosis in which an inborn error of metabolism permits large amounts of copper to accumulate in the liver, kidney, brain, and cornea. Copper concentration in the cornea leads to a characteristic brown or green ring called the Kayser-Fleischer ring.

Prolonged copper deficiency has resulted in a form of anemia not corrected by iron supplements. Most copper deficiencies have been detected under unusual conditions, such as total parenteral nutrition or with zinc supplementation. Deficiency results in hematologic abnormalities, low white blood cell count, glucose intolerance, decreased skin and hair pigmentation, and mental retardation.

Some signs of copper deficiencies have been noted in cases of children recovering from protein-energy malnutrition on a diet mainly composed of milk. Failure to grow, anemia, and disturbances in bone development are the assessed manifestations; copper supplementation reverses the symptoms.

What is Wilson's disease? What are the causes and symptoms of copper deficiency?

NURSING APPLICATIONS

1. Assess clients who consume zinc supplements for copper deficiency.
2. Anemia not corrected with iron supplements may be due to copper deficiency. Monitor RBC laboratory reports. If clients do not improve when taking iron, copper may need to be added.

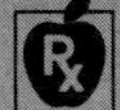

Zinc supplements exceeding 1500 mg/day decrease copper absorption, possibly leading to anemia-related fatigue (Greger, 1987). Evaluate client's dose and energy level.

Client Education

- High dietary fiber intakes increase the dietary requirement for copper.
- Large amounts of vitamin C supplements (1000 mg) decrease serum bioavailability of copper (Eisenberg, 1989).

ZINC

Physiological Roles

What are the functions of zinc?

Zinc is a cofactor in over 120 enzymes that perform a variety of functions affecting cell growth and replication; sexual maturation, fertility, and reproduction; night vision; immune defenses; and taste and appetite.

Requirements

What is the requirement for zinc in men and women?

The NRC has recommended an intake of 15 mg daily for men and 12 mg for women. The US food supply currently provides approximately 12.3 mg zinc daily (Moser-Veillon, 1990). Although some concerns have been expressed about marginal intakes, zinc deficiencies in Americans consuming a variety of foods have not been reported.

Absorption and Excretion

Approximately 40% of dietary zinc is absorbed. Absorption is highly dependent on several factors, including body size; total dietary zinc; and the presence of other potentially interfering substances, such as calcium, fiber, and phosphate salts. The main protein source of zinc in meals is a primary determinant in the amount of zinc absorbed because many substances in plant products (fiber, phytate) interfere with zinc absorption (Sandstrom et al, 1989). The higher quality of protein, the more zinc is absorbed.

Zinc is lost in the feces. Abnormal losses from diarrhea or ileostomies increase zinc requirements.

Sources

List sources of zinc.

Protein-rich foods are good sources of zinc. Lamb, beef, crustaceans (especially oysters), eggs, and leafy and root vegetables contain significant amounts of zinc. Foods with a high zinc content are also high in copper (see Table 9–6).

Hyper- and Hypo- States

Consumption of high levels of zinc normally causes vomiting and diarrhea, epigastric pain, lethargy, and fatigue but can result in renal damage, pancreatitis, and even death. Supplementation is recommended only under medical supervision.

Zinc deficiencies may be caused by a number of problems other than dietary intake, as shown in Table 9–7. Those at particular risk of zinc deficiency include clients whose zinc requirements are relatively high (such as during periods of rapid growth), elderly clients, total vegetarians whose diets consist primarily of cereal protein and/or poor overall nutrient intake, and clients with severe malabsorption (diarrhea) or other chronic health problems.

What are symptoms of high zinc levels? What are causes and symptoms of zinc deficiency? What clients are prone to zinc deficiency?

In developing countries, severe zinc deficiency has been related to large consumption of inhibitors, which adversely affects zinc absorption, rather than inadequate zinc intake. Growth failure and hypogonadism in adolescent boys and increased incidence of pregnancy complications are principal manifestations of zinc deficiency (Sandstead, 1991). Other clinical manifestations of zinc deficiency are listed in Table 9–8. When zinc deficiency is diagnosed, zinc supplementation is vital.

TABLE 9–7

CAUSES OF ZINC DEFICIENCY

Zinc deficiency may be related to:

Dietary deficiency
- Poor food selection
- Poor appetite
- Total parenteral nutrition

Decreased absorption
- High fiber
- High phytate
- High dietary iron-to-zinc ratio
- Pica or geophagia
- Malabsorption syndromes
- Alcoholic cirrhosis
- Pancreatic insufficiency
- Chronic renal disease

Increased loss
- Thiazide diuretics
- Alcoholism
- Oral penicillamine therapy

Genetic disorders
- Sickle cell disease
- Thalassemia

NURSING APPLICATIONS

1. Adverse effects, i.e., vomiting, diarrhea, lethargy, anemia, renal damage, and death, have been reported with chronic consumption of 15 mg zinc supplements; these doses are approximately 100% of the RDA (Fosmire, 1989). If client confirms ingestion of zinc supplements, assess dosage level. If 15 mg or above, monitor for listed adverse effects.
2. Clients with abnormalities of taste because of zinc deficiency may respond to supplementation, but additional zinc is not effective in restoring normal taste acuity associated with other conditions.
3. Zinc supplementation to improve immune function is controversial because of its beneficial effect on one measure of cellular immune function while simultaneously having an adverse effect on another measure of cellular immunity (Bogden et al, 1990).
4. Supplementation in zinc-depleted clients is beneficial for wound healing but unnecessary for normal subjects. Zinc supplementation may be helpful in sickle cell anemia. Give zinc only to clients who will benefit from supplementation.
5. Zinc supplementation interferes with use of iron and copper and adversely affects HDLs (Broun et al, 1990; Fosmire, 1990; Yadrick et al, 1989). Do not advocate indiscriminate use of zinc.

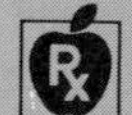 When zinc supplements are taken as a simple salt without food, about 65% is absorbed compared with the usual 40% absorbed in the presence of food. If ordered, give between meals.

Client Education

- Relatively small amounts of animal protein can significantly improve the bioavailability of zinc from a legume-based meal (Sandstrom et al, 1989).
- Fruits and vegetables are low in zinc, whereas peanuts and peanut butter are high.
- Meats are the preferred source of zinc because of its bioavailability.
- No evidence exists that zinc supplementation increases virility and improved sex drive.
- If a well-balanced diet is consumed, zinc supplements are rarely needed and may be harmful.

TABLE 9–8

CLINICAL MANIFESTATIONS OF ZINC DEFICIENCY

Mild	Moderate	Severe
Decreased sperm count	Growth retardation	Dermatitis with pus-containing blisters
Increased serum ammonia	Delayed sexual maturation	Baldness
Weight loss	Skin lesions	Diarrhea
	Impaired wound healing	Behavioral disturbances
	Impaired taste	Infections
	Poor appetite	Death
	Night blindness	

MANGANESE

Physiological Roles

What are the roles of manganese?

Manganese is essential in several enzyme systems and important for bone development, prevention of osteoporosis, insulin production, and other metabolic functions.

Requirements

What is the requirement for manganese?

The ESADDI is 2 to 5 mg/day. Average intake for adults is 2 to 3 mg/day (Pennington & Young, 1991). The absorption of iron and manganese is inversely proportional, so a large amount of one causes a reduction in the other.

Sources

What are sources of manganese?

Foods high in manganese are whole-grain cereals, legumes, leafy vegetables, and tea. The bioavailability of manganese from meats, milk, and eggs makes these important sources despite their smaller quantities.

Hyper- and Hypo- States

Manganese madness—severe psychotic symptoms and neuromuscular symptoms that resemble those of parkinsonism.

Manganese deficiencies have never been reported in clients consuming a normal diet. Manganese dust can be an environmental hazard. Miners have developed **"manganese madness"** (Levander, 1988).

NURSING APPLICATIONS

1. Inhaling manganese dust can be toxic. Assess if client's job increases possibility of inhalation (i.e., factory or coal miners).
2. Before deciding a client is psychotic or has Parkinson's disease, determine client's vocation. If the client is a miner, manganese may be the culprit.

Client Education

- Phytate and fiber in bran, tannins in tea, and oxalic acid in spinach inhibit the absorption of manganese.
- Manganese should not be confused with magnesium.

IODINE

Physiological Role

Iodine is a part of thyroxine, the hormone secreted by the thyroid gland. Thyroxine regulates the basal metabolic rate.

What is the role of iodine?

Requirements

The adult RDA for iodine is 150 mcg daily. Because iodine is related to metabolic rate, needs are increased during periods of accelerated growth, especially during pregnancy and lactation.

What are the requirements for iodine, and when are requirements increased?

Sources

The only natural source of iodine is seafood and plants grown near the ocean. The best safeguard for an adequate intake is the use of iodized salt.

What are sources of iodine?

Hyper- and Hypo- States

Very high levels of iodine may cause adverse effects in some clients. Excessive amounts of iodine can result in enlargement of the thyroid gland similar to the condition produced by deficiency. Thyroiditis, hypothyroidism, hyperthyroidism, **goiter,** and sensitivity reactions have occurred related to excessive iodine through foods, dietary supplements, topical medications, and iodinated contrast media (Pennington, 1990).

Goiter is the result of iodine deficiency whereby the thyroid gland enlarges to compensate for the deficiency.

Iodine deficiency has virtually been eliminated in the US because of iodine fortification of salt. A deficiency may cause profound metabolic and emotional influences ranging from a mild deceleration of catabolic functions, with sensitivity to cold, dry skin, mildly elevated blood lipids, to mild depression of mental functions. Endemic goiter occurs where the soil and/or water is low in iodine content (Fig. 9–3).

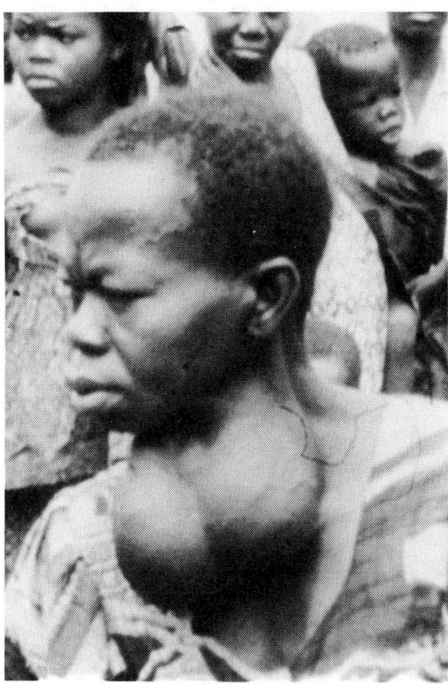

Figure 9–3 Goiter resulting from iodine deficiency. (Courtesy of Food and Agricultural Organization of the United Nations. Photo by Marcel Ganzin.)

With insufficient iodine intake, the thyroid cannot produce adequate amounts of thyroxine. The pituitary gland continues to secrete thyroid stimulating hormone, resulting in further hypertrophy and engorgement of the thyroid gland. Goiter is usually associated with iodine deficiency but may be caused by excessively large intake of **goitrogens.** Raw turnips and rutabagas contain goitrogens.

Goitrogens are substances that interfere with the synthesis of thyroid hormone production by the thyroid.

Goiter is the main disorder from low-iodine intake. Other iodine deficiency disorders include stillbirths, abortions, and congenital anomalies; endemic **cretinism** usually characterized by mental retardation and deaf mutism related to fetal iodine deficiency; and impaired mental function.

An iodine deficiency during pregnancy may result in a disorder in the infant called cretinism.

NURSING APPLICATIONS

1. Assess client's allergies. Clients allergic to shellfish should not be given iodine-based diagnostic tests.
2. Severe hypothyroidism is termed myxedema, and hyperthyroidism is called Graves' disease.

Client Education

- Sea salt has been advocated by health food promoters, but much of the iodine is lost in processing.
- Confirm from package labeling that iodized salt is being purchased.

MOLYBDENUM

What are sources and requirements for molybdenum?

Molybdenum functions as an enzyme cofactor. Legumes, whole-grain cereals, and organ meats are good sources. ESADDI for molybdenum is 75 to 250 mcg. Except for deficiency reported during administration of total parenteral nutrition, molybdenum deficiency has not been documented in the US.

NURSING APPLICATIONS

1. Assess clients on long-term total parenteral nutrition for molybdenum deficiency.
2. Consumption of large quantities of molybdenum may result in copper deficiency, making the client prone to anemia. Evaluate intake by questioning the client.

Client Education

- Meats and whole grains are good sources of molybdenum.

FLUORIDE

Physiological Roles

What is the function of fluoride?

Notoriety for fluoride has come through its protection of teeth. Fluoride has been called a "bone seeker" because of its presence in bone and dental enamel.

Requirement

Because of its toxicity, fluorine has a very narrow ESADDI of 1.5 to 4 mg.

Sources

All foods contain some fluoride, but the amounts are insignificant (less than 1 ppm) except for seafood, which may have 5 to 10 ppm. Food is not a major source of fluoride for adults, but infant foods are often fortified with fluoride.

Fluoridation of community water contributes to fluoride intake and is a practical, cost-effective means of achieving significant decreases in the prevalence of dental caries. Current fluoridation of drinking water at the level of 1 mg/L is safe.

What are sources of fluoride?

Hyper- and Hypo- States

Mottling of tooth enamel results from slight overexposure during tooth formation (approximately 3 to 4 times the amount necessary to prevent caries) (Fig. 9–4). Further increases may result in toxicity (fluorosis) and bone deformities.

The ingestion of large amounts of fluoride in adults can result in adverse effects on skeletal tissue. These changes may gradually increase in severity, eventually resulting in a general increase in bone density and considerable calcification of ligaments in the neck and vertebral column.

A lack of fluoride results in increased dental caries. The protective effect against caries is greatest during tooth formation. The American Dental Association recommends use of a fluoride supplement until calcification of all teeth is completed (about age 13). The American Academy of Pediatrics recommends continued use until eruption of the third molars (about age 16). Continued supplementation into adulthood may even be beneficial in maintaining the integrity of teeth (Jong, 1991).

What are symptoms of too much fluoride?

NURSING APPLICATIONS

1. An increase in fluoride intake is beneficial during development of skeletal tissue and teeth. Encourage fluoride-fortified foods, water, or supplements for infants and fluoridated water for children and adolescents.
2. Growth of cariogenic bacteria is reduced by the presence of fluoride. Suggest use of toothpastes or mouthwashes with fluoride for oral care.
3. Sodium fluoride has been used to treat osteoporosis. Although some studies suggest satisfactory skeletal strength in clients treated with fluoride, its efficacy and long-term safety are unproved. Do not advocate its use to postmenopausal women.

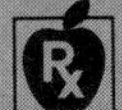
If fluoride and calcium supplements are given concurrently, absorption of both is decreased.

Client Education

- Excess fluoride can cause brittle bones that break easily.
- Studies have found no association between fluoride supplementation and cancer in humans (Mahoney et al, 1991; Mason, 1991).

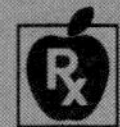
Aluminum antacids decrease fluoride absorption.

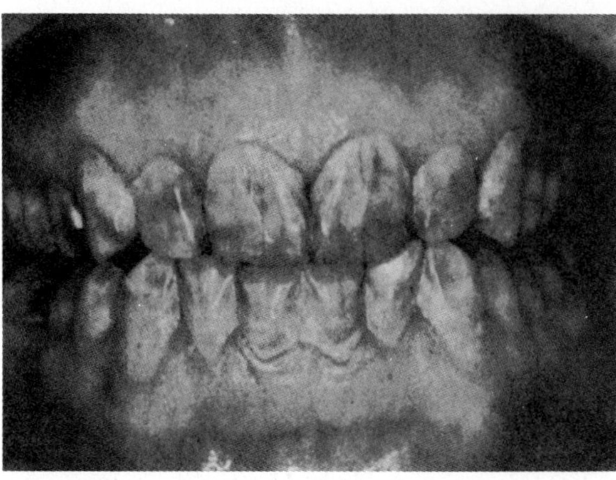

Figure 9–4 Mottled tooth enamel caused by fluorosis. (From Nizel AE. *Nutrition in Preventive Dentistry Science and Practice.* 2nd ed. Philadelphia, WB Saunders, 1981.)

SELENIUM

Physiological Roles

What are the roles of selenium?

Selenium functions mainly as a cofactor for an antioxidant enzyme, which protects membrane lipids, proteins, and nucleic acids from oxidative damage. Selenium works hand in hand with vitamin E; a deficiency of either increases the requirement for the other. Although selenium has been suspected as a carcinogen, it may actually be an anticarcinogen (Clydesdale, 1989).

Requirements

What is the selenium requirement for men and women?

The RDA establishes the adult requirement at 70 mcg for men and 55 mcg for women. Selenium intake is believed to be adequate (Pennington & Young, 1991).

Sources

What are sources of selenium?

Seafood, kidney, and liver are rich in selenium. Other meats are also good sources. Selenium intake correlates closely with kilocaloric and protein intake. Selenium in dairy products and eggs is more readily absorbed than from other foods.

Hyper- and Hypo- States

Both toxicity and deficiency have been seen in animals from irregular distribution of selenium in soil, but these are rarely seen in humans. Routine ingestion of 2 to 3 mg selenium can cause toxic symptoms of nausea and vomiting, weakness, dermatitis, hair loss, and garlic breath. Cirrhosis of the liver may also develop.

What are symptoms of selenium toxicity? What is Keshan disease?

In the People's Republic of China, an endemic cardiomyopathy is associated with severe selenium deficiency called Keshan disease. Fatality rate is as high as 80% in infants and children and women of child-bearing age. Oral selenium prophylaxis is extremely effective in reducing but not completely eliminating Keshan disease.

NURSING APPLICATIONS

1. Assess where client lives: Northeastern, Pacific Northwest, and extreme Southeastern US regions are prone to selenium deficiency, as are clients visiting from eastern Finland, parts of New Zealand, and the People's Republic of China.
2. Decreased selenium levels may cause heart damage, resulting in a heart attack.

Client Education

- Selenium supplements should not be taken by cancer clients unless specified by a physician because of possible toxicity.

CHROMIUM

Physiological Roles

Chromium is involved in carbohydrate and lipid metabolism, especially in the utilization of glucose. Chromium is a cofactor for insulin, so a deficiency causes insulin resistance.

What are the roles of chromium?

Requirements

The ESADDI requirement of a healthy adult has been estimated between 50 and 200 mcg/day. Chromium is poorly absorbed; whether or not intestinal absorption compensates for increased demand is unclear.

What is the ESADDI for chromium?

Sources

Chromium is found in meats, whole-grain cereals, and brewer's yeast. Refined cereals are depleted of chromium.

What are sources of chromium?

Hyper- and Hypo- States

Deficiency states are rare and slow to develop. Chromium toxicity has been caused by industrial exposure, resulting in liver damage and lung cancer.

NURSING APPLICATIONS

1. Assess clients employed in industry for chromium toxicity.
2. Adequate amounts of chromium may improve glucose tolerance in some people with elevated blood glucose levels if their body still secretes insulin (McBride, 1991). However, it does not replace the need for medicine in most people, so give medicine as ordered.
3. Infection causes depressed serum chromium levels, so do not be alarmed if laboratory values of chromium are decreased in clients being treated for infection.
4. Serum chromium levels decline with age, possibly contributing to glucose problems seen in noninsulin-dependent diabetes mellitus (NIDDM).

Continued

Client Education

- Because sucrose consumption results in increased insulin levels, body chromium can be conserved by using table sugar in moderation (USDA, 1989).
- Do not take chromium supplements unless ordered by a physician.

COBALT

What are the functions of cobalt? What deficiency is unknown in humans?

The only known function of cobalt is as an essential component of vitamin B_{12}. As such, it is also necessary for the formation of RBCs. Cobalt deficiency is unknown in humans because it is derived from bacterial synthesis. No RDA is necessary (NRC, 1989).

NURSING APPLICATIONS

Refer to Chapter 7 for Nursing Applications of vitamin B_{12}, which contains cobalt.

Client Education

- Cobalt therapy, a form of radiation therapy, is beneficial in treatment of certain cancers but is not related to the nutrient cobalt.

OTHER TRACE MINERALS

Other trace minerals found in the body include arsenic, nickel, silicon, boron, cadmium, lead, lithium, tin, vanadium, aluminum, and mercury. Requirements, however, have not been quantified. No deficiency has been observed in humans for these elements except for boron. Boron is present in water, fruits, vegetables, nuts, and legumes.

Cadmium, lead, lithium, tin, and vanadium deficiency in animals result in impaired reproduction and depressed growth. If they are required, they are easily met by amounts naturally occurring in foods, water, and air.

Other trace elements listed in Table 9–1 are found in the body. It is unknown whether they are necessary or if they are contaminants. More attention has been given to them as contaminants in the environment and foods. Some are considered to have no harmful effects and are used therapeutically, such as aluminum in antacids.

NURSING APPLICATIONS

1. Boron is necessary for the development and maintenance of strong healthy bones, so be sure children and adolescents are consuming a well-balanced diet.
2. Boron deficiency affects development of osteoporosis (Nielson, 1988), so correct this deficiency quickly, especially in postmenopausal women.

Client Education

- Supplements of these trace elements are not encouraged until further research is performed.
- Consumption of a variety of foods and fluids helps obtain these trace minerals.
- Unrefined foods generally provide more trace minerals than do highly refined foods.

SUMMARY

Mineral elements differ from other nutrients because they are available from sources other than food intake. Air pollution, direct contact of the skin, or sources such as drinking water complicate assessment.

Supplements in excess of the RDAs or ESADDIs are dangerous. Large intakes of some minerals may be toxic and interfere with the absorption and/or metabolism or other minerals. A synopsis of the minerals is provided in Table 9–9.

TABLE 9–9

SYNOPSIS OF MINERAL ELEMENTS

Mineral	Physiological Roles	Hyper- and Hypo- States	Food Sources	Recommended Amounts
Calcium	Structural part of bones and teeth Blood clotting Transmission of nerve impulses Muscle activity Membrane permeability Cofactor for enzyme function	*Hyper:* Renal calculi Calcification of soft tissues Inhibits absorption of iron and zinc *Hypo:* Rickets Osteoporosis Tetany	Milk and other dairy products Dark green leafy vegetables Salmon; sardines Fortified orange juice	Infants 0–0.5: 400 mg 0.5–1: 600 mg Children 1–10: 800 mg Males and females: 11–24 1200 mg over 25: 800 mg Pregnancy and lactation: 1200 mg
Phosphorus	Structural part of bones and teeth Energy storage Component of DNA and RNA Metabolism of fats, carbohydrates, and proteins	*Hyper:* Tetany Convulsions Renal insufficiency *Hypo:* Increased calcium excretion, bone loss Muscle weakness	Milk and dairy products Meats Whole grains Legumes Nuts	Infants 0–0.5: 300 mg 0.5–1: 500 mg Children 1–10: 800 mg Males and females 11–25: 1200 mg over 25: 800 mg Pregnancy and lactation: 1200 mg
Magnesium	Cardiovascular function Structural part of bones and teeth Enzyme function Muscle and nerve function	*Hyper:* Weakness *Hypo:* Neuromuscular dysfunction Personality changes Muscle spasm Convulsions Hyperexcitability, tremors, anorexia, apathy Decreased tendon reflexes Cardiac arrhythmias	Whole-grain products Nuts Beans Green leafy vegetables Bananas	Infants 0–0.5: 40 mg 0.5–1: 60 mg Children 1–3: 80 mg 4–6: 120 mg 7–10: 170 mg Males 11–14: 270 mg 15–18: 400 mg 19 and over: 350 mg Females 11–14: 280 mg 15–18: 300 mg 19 and over: 280 mg Pregnancy: 320 mg Lactation: 340–355 mg

Table continued on following page

TABLE 9–9

SYNOPSIS OF MINERAL ELEMENTS *Continued*

Mineral	Physiological Roles	Hyper- and Hypo- States	Food Sources	Recommended Amounts
Sulfur	Structural proteins in cartilage, tendons, and bone matrix; keratin in hair and nails Part of amino acids and vitamins Acid–base balance Neutralizes toxins	*Hyper:* None *Hypo:* None	Protein foods	None
Iron	Transports oxygen Catalyzes oxidative reactions Energy metabolism Synthesis of collagen Conversion of beta-carotene to vitamin A Formation of purines Removal of lipids Detoxification of drugs Production of antibodies	*Hyper:* Hemochromatosis Hemosiderosis *Hypo:* Microcytic, hypochromic anemia	Liver Meats, egg yolk Dark green vegetables Enriched breads and cereals	Infants 0–0.5: 6 mg 0.5–1: 10 mg Children 1–10: 10 mg Males 11–18: 12 mg 19 and over: 10 mg Females 11–50: 15 mg over 51: 10 mg Pregnancy: 30 mg Lactation: 15 mg
Copper	RBC formation Connective tissue Cofactor in enzyme functions for protein metabolism and oxidative reactions	*Hyper:* Nausea *Hypo:* Anemia Decreased skin and hair pigmentation Failure to grow Disturbances in bone development	Shellfish Liver Nuts Sesame and sunflower seeds Legumes Cocoa	ESADDI: Infants 0–0.5: 0.4–0.6 mg 0.5–1: 0.6–0.7 mg Children 1–3: 0.7–1 mg 4–6: 1–1.5 mg 7–10: 1–2 mg 11: 1.5–2.5 mg Adults: 1.5–3 mg
Zinc	Cofactor for over 120 enzymes affecting growth and replication, sexual maturation, fertility and reproduction, night vision, immune responses, and taste and appetite	*Hyper:* Vomiting, diarrhea Epigastric pain Lethargy and fatigue Renal damage Pancreatitis *Hypo:* Growth failure Hypogonadism Wound healing Impaired taste Poor appetite Infections	Meats Eggs Crustaceans Leafy and root vegetables	Infants 0–1: 5 mg Children 1–10: 10 mg Males over 11: 15 mg Females over 11: 12 mg Pregnancy: 15 mg Lactation: 16–19 mg
Manganese	Part of enzymes Bone development Insulin production	*Hyper:* Unknown from food intake *Hypo:* Unknown	Whole-grain products Legumes Leafy vegetables Tea Meats Milk Eggs	ESADDI: Infants 0–0.5: 0.3–0.6 mg 0.5–: 0.6–1 mg Children 1–3: 1–1.5 mg 4–6: 1.5–2 mg 7–10: 2–3 mg 11+: 2–5 mg Adults: 2–5 mg
Iodine	Part of thyroid hormone Regulates basal metabolic rate	*Hyper:* Enlargement of thyroid gland Thyroiditis, hypothyroidism Goiter and hyperthyroidism *Hypo:* Goiter Poor growth Cretinism Congenital anomalies, stillbirths	Iodized salt Saltwater fish	Infants 0–0.5: 40 mcg 0.5–1: 60 mcg Children 1–3: 70 mcg 4–6: 90 mcg 7–10: 120 mcg Males and females over 10: 150 mcg Pregnancy: 175 mcg Lactation: 200 mcg

TABLE 9–9

SYNOPSIS OF MINERAL ELEMENTS *Continued*

Mineral	Physiological Roles	Hyper- and Hypo- States	Food Sources	Recommended Amounts
Molybdenum	Enzyme cofactor	*Hyper:* Unknown *Hypo:* Unknown	Legumes Whole grains Organ meats Milk	ESADDI: Infants 0–0.5: 15–30 mcg 0.5–1: 20–40 mcg Children 1–3: 25–50 mcg 4–6: 30–75 mcg 7–10: 50–150 mcg over 11 and adults: 75–250 mcg
Fluoride	Structural component of bones and teeth, increasing hardness	*Hyper:* Mottling of tooth enamel Fluorosis Bone deformities *Hypo:* Increased risk of dental caries	Seafood Fluoridated water	ESADDI: Infants 0–0.5: 0.1–0.5 mg 0.5–1: 0.2–1 mg Children 1–3: 0.5–1.5 mg 4–6: 1–2.5 mg over 7: 1.5–2.5 mg Adults: 1.5–4 mg
Selenium	Cofactor of antioxidant enzymes	*Hyper:* Nausea and vomiting Hair loss Liver disease *Hypo:* Muscle pain and weakness Heart disease	Seafood Liver Meats Dairy products Vegetables–varies with soil	Infants 0–0.5: 10 mcg 0.5–1: 15 mcg Children 1–6: 20 mcg 7–10: 30 mcg Males 11–14: 40 mcg 15–18: 50 mcg over 19: 70 mcg Females 11–14: 45 mcg 15–18: 50 mcg over 19: 55 mcg Pregnancy: 65 mcg Lactation: 75 mcg
Chromium	Cofactor for insulin Involved in carbohydrate and lipid metabolism	*Hyper:* Unknown *Hypo:* Possibly decreased glucose tolerance	Meats Whole-grain products Brewer's yeast	ESADDI: Infants 0–0.5: 10–40 mcg 0.5–1: 20–60 mcg Children 1–3: 20–80 mcg 4–6: 30–120 mcg 7–10: 50–200 mcg 11+ and adults: 50–200 mcg
Cobalt	Component of vitamin B_{12}	*Hyper:* Unknown *Hypo:* Associated vitamin B_{12} deficiency	Vitamin B_{12} sources	None

NURSING PROCESS IN ACTION

A 69-year-old woman is admitted with osteoporosis. She admits to taking calcium supplements occasionally when she can afford them. She does not like to walk or drink milk.

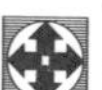 Nutritional Assessment

- Calcium, vitamin D intake.
- Protein and caffeine intake (increases calcium excretion).

- Smoking and drinking habits.
- Exercise habits.
- Fractures, especially sites in thoracic and lumbar vertebral bodies and neck and intertrochanteric regions of femur and distal radius.
- Use of diuretics and glucocorticoids (increases chance of osteoporosis).
- Level of income and cultural or religious influences.
- Dietary beliefs and habits.
- Knowledge base about osteoporosis, calcium, and exercise.
- Support groups or significant others.
- Weight, race, body frame (small-framed whites are at most risk).
- Serum levels of calcium, protein, albumin.

Dietary Nursing Diagnosis

Altered health maintenance RT inadequate knowledge about nutritional therapy for osteoporosis.

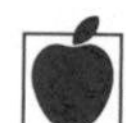

Nutritional Goals

Client will describe alterations/modifications needed in diet to help prevent adverse effects of osteoporosis.

Nutritional Implementation

Intervention: Check serum levels of calcium and compare with protein/albumin levels.
Rationale: Pseudohypocalcemia may be occurring if protein/albumin is low. For every 1 gm albumin below 4 gm, calcium will be lowered 0.8 mg.

Intervention: Give calcium with meals or snack. Take with sugar, estrogen, and vitamin D.
Rationale: This enhances calcium absorption.

Intervention: Offer foods high in calcium, i.e., powdered milk, cheese, yogurt.
Rationale: Because client dislikes milk, alternate sources of calcium need to be provided.

Intervention: Offer calcium fortified orange drink.
Rationale: Calcium citrate maleate, used in fortification of orange drink, is well absorbed and is a good source of calcium for this client who dislikes milk.

Intervention: Encourage diet high in calcium (1000 to 1500 mg) and vitamin D (100 to 500 mg per day).
Rationale: Calcium slows the rate of bone loss; vitamin D is needed for calcium absorption.

Intervention: If the client is unable or unwilling to consume adequate dietary calcium, administer calcium supplements as ordered, preferably calcium carbonate.
Rationale: Adequate calcium is essential to arrest bone loss, and calcium carbonate is the most readily absorbed calcium supplement.

Intervention: Discourage use of dolomite.
Rationale: Dolomite may cause lead poisoning because of the high level of lead in animal bone.

Intervention: Give estrogen if ordered.
Rationale: Estrogen prevents the estrogen-dependent component of bone loss.

Intervention: Monitor for excessive use of fiber/fiber supplements.
Rationale: High fiber intake may increase fecal calcium.

Intervention: Inquire about factors in the home environment that could predispose to falls, e.g., throw rugs, slippery bathtubs, electrical cords.
Rationale: Prevention may safeguard the client against falling and resulting in a fracture.

Intervention: Give calcitonin, fluoride, and etidronate diphosphonate if ordered.
Rationale: These drugs may augment bone, reverse osteoporosis, and reduce incidence of vertebral compression fractures (Miller, 1990). However, calcium-rich foods or enteral feeding formulas should be withheld for 2 hours after giving etidronate disodium.

Intervention: Refer to National Osteoporosis Foundation.
Rationale: The National Osteoporosis Foundation is a valuable resource for clients.

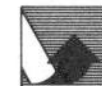

Evaluation

Desired outcomes include: client verbalizes methods to increase calcium and vitamin D in the diet.

STUDENT READINESS

1. A client claims that she dislikes milk. How would you advise her to obtain the needed calcium?
2. What are the main physiological roles of iron, fluoride, selenium, and zinc?
3. How do trace elements differ from vitamins?
4. How would you respond to a remark that milk is only for babies?
5. Name other minerals or vitamins that either are required for metabolism of the mineral or function in such similar ways that they are called "sparers" for each other.

   A. Calcium: ______ and ______
   B. Selenium: ______
   C. Sodium: ______
   D. Zinc:______ and ______
6. How can iron absorption be increased?
7. Name some trace elements that may be useful as well as toxic to clients.
8. A client who is slightly overweight and anemic is advised that red meats contain more kilocalories than chicken and fish. Therefore, she decided to delete red meats from her diet. What advice would you offer her?

Case Study:

Mrs. J. M. has been admitted to the unit for chronic alcoholism. On admission, she is noted to have hyperactive deep tendon reflexes and tremors. Laboratory data on admission reveal decreased serum magnesium.

1. What signs would you expect to see during a physical assessment?
2. What is the effect of increased calcium intake on serum magnesium?
3. What other conditions may lead to decreased serum magnesium levels?
4. What effect would increased vitamin D have on serum magnesium?

Case Study:

Mr. A. C. comes to the local health clinic complaining of headaches, nausea, and constipation for the past 6 weeks. As the nurse gathers assessment data, she learns that Mr. A. C. sustained a tibial fracture 12 months before this visit. Following the fracture, the client attempted to enhance the healing process by increasing his intake of vitamin D and calcium. Laboratory data reveal a serum calcium of 12.8 mg/dl.

1. What is the normal range for serum calcium?
2. What is the RDA for calcium?
3. What foods are good sources of calcium?
4. What are the sequelae of an elevated serum calcium?
5. What nursing diagnoses might be derived from the assessment data?
6. What would you teach Mr. A. C. about calcium, vitamin D, and phosphorus?

REFERENCES

Bogden JD, et al. Effects of one year of supplementation of zinc and other micronutrients on cellular immunity in the elderly. *J Am Coll Nutr* 1990 June; 9(3):214–225.

Broun ER, et al. Excessive zinc ingestion: A reversible cause of sideroblastic anemia and bone marrow depression. *JAMA* 1990 Sept 19; 264(11):1441–1443.

Cauley JA, et al. Endogenous estrogen levels and calcium intakes in postmenopausal women. Relationships with cortical bone measures. *JAMA* 1988 Dec 2; 260(21):3150–3155.

Clark K. Calcium and hypertension: Does a relationship exist? *Nutr Today* 1989 July/Aug; 24(4):21–26.

Clydesdale FM. The relevance of mineral chemistry to bioavailability. *Nutr Today* 1989 March/Apr; 24(2):23–30.

Consensus Conference. Osteoporosis. *JAMA* 1984 Aug 10; 252(6):799–806.

Cook JD, et al. Calcium supplementation: Effect on iron absorption. *Am J Clin Nutr* 1991 Jan; 53(1):106–111.

Dawson-Hughes B, et al. A controlled trial of the effect of calcium supplementation on bone density in post-menopausal women. *N Engl J Med* 1990 Sept 27; 323(13):878–1883.

Eisenberg S. Diet supplements: Wisdom or folly. *Food Tech* 1989 Aug; 43(8):46,50.

Fosmire GJ. Possible hazards associated with zinc supplementation. *Nutr Today* 1989 May/June; 24(3):15–18.

Fosmire GJ. Zinc toxicity. *Am J Clin Nutr* 1990 Feb; 51(2):225–227.

Greger JL. Mineral bioavailability/new concepts. *Nutr Today* 1987 July/Aug;22(4):4–9.

Hallberg L, et al. Iron absorption in man: Ascorbic acid and dose-dependent inhibition by phytate. *Am J Clin Nutr* 1989 Jan; 49(1):140–144.

Hallberg L, et al. Calcium: Effect of different amounts on non heme- and heme-iron absorption in humans. *Am J Clin Nutr* 1991 Jan; 53(1):112–119.

Heaney RP, et al. Meal effects on calcium absorption. *Am J Clin Nutr* 1989 Feb; 49(2):372–376.

Hegarty V, Stewart B. The cost of calcium supplements. *N Engl J Med* 1988 Aug 18; 319(7):449.

Hunt JR, et al. Ascorbic acid: Effect on ongoing iron absorption and status in iron-depleted young women. *Am J Clin Nutr* 1990 Apr; 51(4):649–655.

Jong AW. Duration of fluoride supplementation (questions and answers). *JAMA* 1991 Aug 14; 266(6):850.

Knowles JB. Response of fractional calcium absorption in women to various coadministered oral glucose doses. *Am J Clin Nutr* 1988 Dec; 48(6):1471–1474.

Levander OA. Selenium, chromium and manganese. (C) Manganese. *In* Shils ME, Young VK (eds). *Modern Nutrition in Health and Disease.* 7th ed. Philadelphia, Lea & Febiger, 1988, pp 274–277.

Litovitz TL, Schmitz BF. 1988 Annual Report of the American Association of Poison Control Centers National Data Collection System. *Am J Emerg Med* 1989 Sept; 7(5):495–545.

Mahoney MC, et al. Bone cancer incidence rates in New York State: Time trends and fluoridated drinking water. *Am J Public Health* 1991 Apr; 81(4):475–479.

Mason JO. From the Assistant Secretary for Health, U.S. Public Health Service. A message to health professionals about fluorosis. *JAMA* 1991 June 12; 265(22):2939.

McBride J. Chromium supplementation helps keep blood glucose levels in check. *J Am Diet Assoc* 1991 Feb; 91(2):178.

Miller P. Osteoporosis: New developments in prevention and treatment. *Phys Assist* 1990 June; 14(6):17–28.

Monsen ER. Iron nutrition and absorption: Dietary factors which impact iron bioavailability. *J Am Diet Assoc* 1988 July; 88(7):786–790.

Moser-Veillon RB. Zinc: Consumption patterns and dietary recommendations. *J Am Diet Assoc* 1990 Aug; 90(8):1039–1093.

National Research Council (NRC). *Recommended Dietary Allowances.* 10th ed. Washington, DC, National Academy Press, 1989.

Nielson FH. Possible future implications of ultratrace elements in human health and disease. *In* Prasad AS (ed). *Essential and Toxic Trace Elements in Human Health and Disease. Current Topics in Nutrition and Disease.* Vol 18. New York, Alan R. Liss, 1988.

Pennington JAT. A review of iodine toxicity reports. *J Am Diet Assoc* 1990 Nov; 90(11):1571–1579.

Pennington JAT, Young BE. Total diet study nutritional elements, 1982–1989. *J Am Diet Assoc* 1991 Feb; 91(2):179–183.

Recker RR, et al. Calcium absorbability from milk products, an imitation milk, and calcium carbonate. *Am J Clin Nutr* 1988 Jan; 47(1):93–95.

Rossander-Hulten L, et al. Competitive inhibition of iron absorption by manganese and zinc in humans. *Am J Clin Nutr* 1991 July; 54(1):152–156.

Salonen JT, et al. High stored iron levels are associated with excess risk of myocardial infarction in Eastern Finnish men. *Circulation* 1992 Sept; 86(9):803–811.

Sandstead HH. Zinc deficiency. A public health problem? *Am J Dis Child* 1991 Aug; 145(8):853–859.

Sandstrom B, et al. Effect of protein level and protein source on zinc absorption in humans. *J Nutr* 1989 Jan; 119(1):48–53.

Shils ME. Magnesium. *In* Shils ME, Young, VK (eds). *Modern Nutrition in Health and Disease.* 7th ed. Philadelphia, Lea & Febiger, 1988, pp 159–192.

Solomons NW. Zinc and copper. *In* Shils ME, Young VK (eds). *Modern Nutrition in Health and Disease.* 7th ed. Philadelphia, Lea & Febiger, 1988, pp 238–262.

Spencer H, et al. Do protein and phosphorus cause calcium loss? *J Nutr* 1988 June; 118(6):657–660.

Tilkian SM, et al. *Clinical Implications of Laboratory Tests.* 4th ed. St. Louis, CV Mosby, 1987.

US Department of Agriculture (USDA). Too many sweets can drain your body of chromium. *J Am Diet Assoc* 1989 Sept; 89(9):1289.

Whang R, Ryder KW. Frequency of hypomagnesemia and hypermagnesemia. *JAMA* 1990 June 13; 263(22):3063–3064.

Wood RJ, et al. Effects of glucose and glucose polymers in calcium absorption in healthy subjects. *Am J Clin Nutr* 1987 Oct; 46(10):699–701.

Yadrick MK, et al. Iron, copper, and zinc status: Response to supplementation with zinc or zinc and iron in adult females. *Am J Clin Nutr* 1989 Jan; 49(1):145–150.

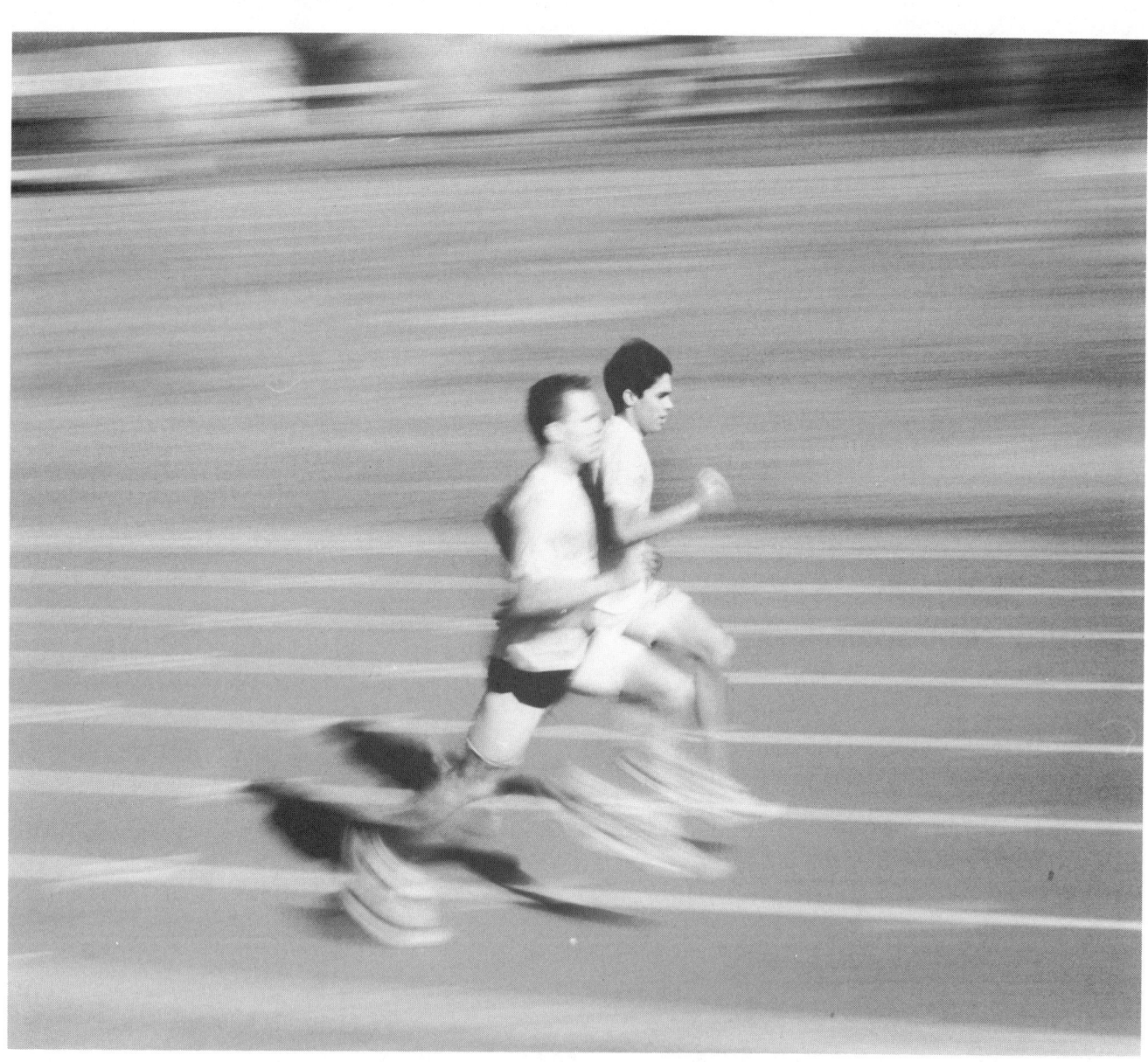

Energy Requirements: Normal, Physically Challenged, and Athletic

CHAPTER 10

OUTLINE

I. METABOLIC INTERRELATIONSHIPS
II. ALCOHOL METABOLISM
III. ENERGY PRODUCTION
IV. ENERGY MEASUREMENT
   A. Storage of Energy Sources
V. METABOLIC ENERGY
   A. Kilocalorie Intake
   B. Role of Carbohydrates
   C. Glycogen
   D. Lactate
   E. Role of Fats
   F. Adenosine Triphosphate
   Nursing Applications
VI. BASAL METABOLISM
   A. Factors Affecting Basal Metabolic Rate
      1. Sleep: The Ebb of Life
      2. Age
      3. Pregnancy and Lactation
      4. Surface Area
      5. State of Health
      6. Body Composition
      7. Sex
      8. Endocrine Glands: Chemical Messengers
      9. Temperature
      10. Fasting and Starvation
   Nursing Applications
VII. MEASUREMENT OF POTENTIAL ENERGY
VIII. ENERGY REQUIREMENTS
   A. Basal Metabolic Rate
   B. Voluntary Work and Play
   C. Thermogenic Effect
   D. Basal Energy Expenditure or Resting Energy Expenditure
IX. HYPER- AND HYPO- STATES
   A. Maintaining Energy Balance
      1. Physiological Factors
      2. Psychological Factors
      3. Energy Expenditure
   B. Inadequate Energy Intake
   Nursing Applications

X. ENERGY NEEDS OF THE PHYSICALLY CHALLENGED
   Nursing Applications
XI. NUTRITIONAL NEEDS OF THE ATHLETE
   A. Energy Balance
   B. Protein
   Nursing Applications
   C. Other Nutrients
   Nursing Applications
   D. Beverages
      1. Fluid and Electrolyte Replacement
      2. Sugar Content
      3. Alcohol
   E. Pregame Meals
      1. Liquid Meals
   Nursing Applications

OBJECTIVES

THE STUDENT WILL BE ABLE TO:

- Calculate energy needs according to the client's weight and activities.
- Explain the sources of energy.
- Identify factors affecting basal metabolic rate.
- Explain how nutrient needs of sports activities differ from normal activities.
- Assess factors affecting energy balance.
- Identify client teaching interventions for energy balance.
- Describe nursing principles for regulating energy balance.

TEST YOUR NQ (True/False)

1. A kilocalorie is 1000 times larger than a calorie.
2. Even during sleep, the body requires energy.
3. BMR stands for blood malnutrition reaction.
4. A malnourished client will have a low BMR.
5. The hypothalamus controls hunger and satiety.
6. Hunger is the same as appetite.
7. Salt tablets should be taken when heavy sweating occurs.
8. Clients who exercise moderately should drink commercially prepared beverages to replace electrolytes.
9. The best food before an athletic event to enhance muscle replacement is a steak.
10. Vitamins are a source of energy.

METABOLIC INTERRELATIONSHIPS

As you may have observed in your study of earlier chapters, a discussion of any of the nutrients cannot be isolated from the others because of their concurrent distribution in foods and many points of interaction in digestion, absorption, and metabolism (Fig. 10–1). Lipids do not contribute significantly to the synthesis of amino acids, but glycerol from triglycerides can be used for synthesis of carbohy-

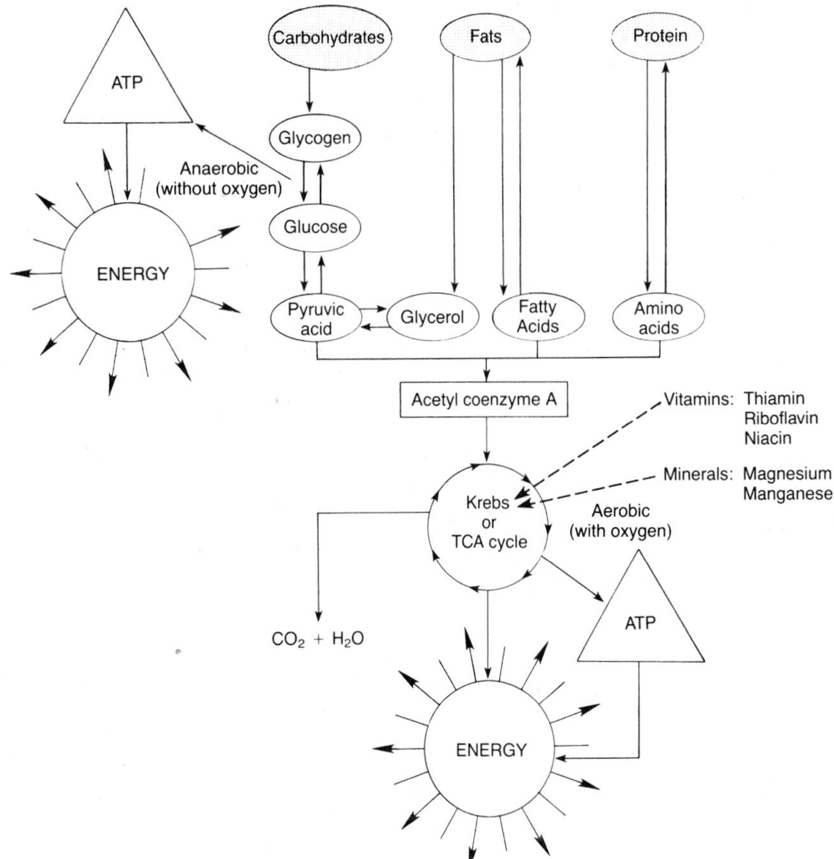

Figure 10–1 Simplified version of energy production in the body. Potential energy from the storage of glycogen is dependent on the increased intake of carbohydrates. Because this pathway is anaerobic (without oxygen), it can be used without delay. The major pathway of energy production is through the Krebs cycle, which is dependent on adequate coenzymes of certain vitamins and minerals plus oxygen (aerobic). ATP, Adenosine triphosphate; TCA, tricarboxylic acid.

drates. Even though fat is a good source of energy, carbohydrate is the preferred fuel. However, the body cannot metabolize excessive quantities of fat without some side effects, including ketosis, hyperlipemia, and fatty liver.

Carbohydrates also assist lipids to enter the Krebs cycle and can be used in forming NEAA. Fatty acids and some of the amino acids can be converted to glucose. Proteins contribute to the synthesis of some lipids, for example, lipoproteins. Not only are these 3 energy nutrients necessary, but also without the essential vitamins and minerals involved in the digestion, absorption, and metabolism of carbohydrate, protein, and fat, all processes are hindered.

Catabolism from all classes of foodstuffs involves oxidation through the Krebs cycle to produce energy. A sufficient quantity of kilocalories in the diet from carbohydrate or lipids influences protein metabolism. In some situations, one nutrient can be substituted for another because of the interrelationships. For example, a decrease in carbohydrate increases lipolysis; a protein excess can be used for energy.

A detailed discussion of metabolic interrelationships is beyond the scope of this text. These interrelationships are important, and for optimal utilization of nutrients, food sources of all the nutrients should be incorporated into every diet. The easiest way to accomplish this is to include a variety of foods from all the food groups.

ALCOHOL METABOLISM

Although alcohol is also considered a drug, the kilocalories it provides can be used by the body for energy, providing approximately 7 kcal/gm. Kilocaloric content of alcoholic beverages can be calculated by using Table 10–1. The metabolism of

TABLE 10-1

KILOCALORIC VALUE OF ALCOHOLIC BEVERAGES

For gin, rum, vodka, and whiskey
To estimate the kilocalories, multiply the number of ounces by the proof and then again by the factor 0.8
Example: 2 oz × 86 proof × 0.8 kcal/proof/oz = 137.6 kcal
For beer and wines
To estimate the kilocalories, multiply the ounces by the percentage of alcohol and then by the factor 1.6
Example: 6 oz × 9% (0.09) × 1.6 kcal/%/oz = 86 kcal

ethanol is an energy-wasteful process, but the reason is not fully understood. Alcohol consumed in excess of 50 gm/day provides less than 7 kcal/gm, but in moderate social drinking (less than 2 drinks/day for men and 1 for women), the energy from alcohol is efficiently used (Lieber, 1991).

Alcohol provides an alternate fuel that is oxidized instead of fat. This substitution of alcohol results in accumulation of lipids, leading to fatty liver. There is little information on how much alcohol can be consumed without risk of liver damage. Habitual consumption of ethanol in excess of energy needs probably favors lipid storage and weight gain (Suter et al, 1992). In the average-sized woman (nonpregnant), 20 gm/day is probably safe, but 60 gm/day is not. In the average-sized man, 40 gm/day is probably safe, but 80 gm/day is not. Problems associated with alcohol intake are discussed in Chapters 20 and 26.

ENERGY PRODUCTION

Energy is the ability, or power, to do work.

Without energy from chemical reactions, people could not bat an eye, wiggle a toe, or think a thought. **Energy** from food is converted into forms of energy the body can use: electrical for the brain and nerves, mechanical for muscles, thermal for body heat, and chemical for synthesis of new compounds.

Physiological sources of energy are carbohydrates, protein, fat, and alcohol.

After foods are chewed and digested, the **body's sources of energy** are converted to glucose, fatty acids, and amino acids. These basic nutrient units are delivered to cells, where, at the direction of specific enzymes and various cofactors, they can be used. As discussed in Chapter 4, glycolysis is the metabolism of glucose to produce ATP, or the form of energy used to drive energy-requiring cellular processes. However, this is an inefficient method of energy production.

Aerobic—requiring oxygen.

The more efficient way to produce energy requires oxygen from the atmosphere. **Aerobic** oxidation occurs through the Krebs cycle within the mitochondria (known as the powerhouse of the cell). These chemical reactions constitute the energy cycle causing organic nutrients to be catabolized into the carbon dioxide and water from which they were originally formed. This process releases the energy that held these constituents together (see Fig. 10-1). These reactions may be simply seen as:

$$\text{carbon dioxide} + \text{water} + \text{sunlight (energy)} \longrightarrow \text{glucose} + \text{oxygen}$$

followed by the reverse:

$$\text{glucose} + \text{oxygen} \longrightarrow \text{carbon dioxide} + \text{water} + \text{energy}$$

The coenzyme forms of thiamin, niacin, and riboflavin are indispensable throughout the energy-releasing pathway. Since thiamin and niacin are particularly essential in many reactions to release energy, the RDAs for these B vitamins are based on the number of kilocalories consumed. Other cofactors essential for energy release include magnesium and potassium.

What are the body's sources of energy? Where does aerobic oxidation occur? List the coenzymes needed for the energy-releasing pathway.

ENERGY MEASUREMENT

The potential energy value of foods and the energy exchanges within the body are expressed in terms of the **kilocalorie (kcal).** Although kilocalorie is the proper terminology and is being used more frequently, it has formerly been used interchangeably with Calorie or large calorie (abbreviated Cal). One kilocalorie is 1000 times larger than the small calorie (abbreviated cal).

A kilocalorie is the amount of heat required to raise the temperature of 1 kg of water 1° C.

The **joule (J)** is more popularly used in countries using the metric system. During this transition time of converting to the metric system in the US, both the kilocalorie and kilojoule (kJ) are used. The equivalents are shown in the margin.

The joule is also used for expressing energy values in nutrition.

Carbohydrate, fat, protein, and even alcohol are chemical sources of energy for humans. (Vitamins and minerals are not energy sources but are necessary for energy-producing reactions.) The physiological energy values commonly used are 4 kcal/gm (17 kJ) carbohydrate, 9 kcal/gm (38 kJ) fat, 4 kcal/gm (17 kJ) protein, and 7 kcal/gm (29 kJ) alcohol.

1 kcal = 4.18 kJ.

How many kilocalories equal a kilojoule? What are the energy values for carbohydrate, fat, and protein? When excessive food intake occurs, how is this stored in the body?

Storage of Energy Sources

Whether excessive food intake is in the form of protein, carbohydrate, alcohol, and/or fat, most of the excessive energy intake is stored as adipose tissue. Glycogen stores are another storage form of energy. However, normal glycogen stores provide only 1200 to 1800 kcal. A limited amount of protein is available in the metabolic pool of amino acids. Protein stored in lean muscle mass is generally not considered a good source of kilocalories.

METABOLIC ENERGY

Kilocalorie Intake

Even during sleep, the body requires energy for the obvious minimum tasks of respiration and circulation as well as many intricate activities within each cell. Increasing kilocalorie intake from carbohydrates and fats will not produce optimum energy without adequate protein intake. Energy use is remarkably sensitive to both the quantity and the quality of dietary protein.

What nutrient is necessary for efficient energy use?

Role of Carbohydrates

Dietary carbohydrates assure optimal glycogen stores and are digested faster than other energy nutrients. Carbohydrates require less oxygen for their metabolism. Cells in the brain, RBC, and renal medulla require glucose as their energy source. Liver glycogen stores maintain a source of glucose for physiological requirements if the dietary carbohydrate is adequate. One safety mechanism is the synthesis of glycogen from some amino acids to provide the necessary glucose if insufficient carbohydrate is consumed.

What cells require glucose?

Glycogen

Glycogen stores in the liver are a ready source of energy via glycogenolysis. The amount of glycogen stores varies greatly and is dependent on the amount of dietary carbohydrate.

Lactate

Muscle glycogen does not form blood glucose but instead forms lactate. Because lactate is a fairly strong acid, the presence of large quantities in the blood stream tends to reduce the alkaline reserves and cause acidosis (which the buffer systems try to prevent). This in itself is an automatic stimulus to increase the respiration rate so more oxygen facilitates oxidation of lactate. As work intensity increases, a client exhales faster to remove excess carbon dioxide formed from lactate oxidation. Logically the body is limited in its ability to inhale enough oxygen to oxidize the lactate as quickly as it is formed.

An oxygen debt is incurred when oxygen demand exceeds oxygen supply, which must be replaced during the recovery period.

What happens to the body when lactate is elevated?

With prolonged strenuous exercise, lactate momentarily accumulates faster than the body can supply oxygen to oxidize it, resulting in **oxygen debt.** Muscle cell glycogen is lowered, whereas lactic acid concentration is elevated. The client may become fatigued since there is insufficient energy to activate the muscle. During the recovery period, oxidative processes operate at high levels for up to 1 hour to replenish glycogen stores and other forms of cellular energy.

Role of Fats

Although carbohydrate plays a dominant role in heavy exercise when the muscle's oxygen supply is limited, fat provides about half the energy during steady-state work. Fats can be stored in body depots in virtually inexhaustible amounts; however, their slower rate of metabolism makes them a less efficient source of quick energy.

Adenosine Triphosphate

ATP is an instant source of cellular energy for mechanical work, transport of nutrients and waste products, and synthesis of chemical compounds.

Metabolism of the basic nutrients can result in the release of energy, which is stored as **adenosine triphosphate (ATP).** ATP units, also called high-energy phosphate compounds, are the currency or "money" the body uses for energy. Since ATP can be metabolized without oxygen, the reaction is classified as anaerobic. The body must always have a supply of ATP, and several systems within the body ensure a constant supply.

NURSING APPLICATIONS

1. Assess intake of thiamin, riboflavin, niacin, magnesium, and potassium that are required to help produce energy. If intake is deficient, problems such as fatigue may develop.
2. Low-carbohydrate diets are not as effective in supporting exertion as a high intake of complex carbohydrates. Thus, in athletic clients, advise the use of complex carbohydrates.
3. Glycogen stores are depleted with a carbohydrate-poor diet even when high levels of fat and protein are eaten. A client who ingests a carbohydrate-poor diet will have decreased energy reserves and be prone to prolonged healing periods and fatigue.

4. Because thiamin is essential for carbohydrate metabolism, a thiamin deficiency is closely linked to aberrations of brain function. Monitor for confusion or altered thought processes.
5. The trained athlete is capable of longer periods of sustained work before becoming fatigued and accumulating an oxygen debt. At rest, the athlete's heartbeat may be below 60. This is not abnormal since the cardiovascular system has been conditioned.

Client Education

- Intake of foods containing thiamin, riboflavin, niacin, magnesium, and potassium are essential to help the body function properly.
- Prolonged strenuous exercise produces fatigue because of the buildup of lactic acid.
- For maximum work output, it is best to alternate periods of intense work with short rest periods, such as 10 minutes of intense work with short rest periods.
- Teach clients how to figure kilocalorie content of foods. For example, if a food contains 10 gm of fat (fat supplies 9 kcal/gm), 10 gms × 9 kcal/gm = 90 kcal. The same principle applies to calculating the amount of kilocalories from carbohydrate or protein, using 4 kcal/gm. The kilocalories from carbohydrate, protein, and fat are added to determine total kilocalories in the food.

BASAL METABOLISM

A client's **basal metabolic rate (BMR)** is lowest while lying down, awake, rested, and relaxed in a comfortable environment, not having eaten for 12 to 15 hours. Since digestion and absorption require energy, the basal metabolic rate is the amount of energy required when the body is in a **post-absorptive state.**

BMR is the energy required for the involuntary physiological functions to maintain life, including respiration, circulation, and maintenance of muscle tone and body temperature.

Postabsorptive state—when digestive and absorptive processes are minimal.

Factors Affecting Basal Metabolic Rate

Various factors can increase or decrease the BMR, which determines the kilocaloric needs.

Sleep: The Ebb of Life

After a few hours of sleep, the metabolic rate is lowest because muscles are more relaxed. About 10% less energy is needed for the BMR during this relaxed state.

Age

From birth through age 2, growth results in the highest BMR, which decreases until the puberty growth spurt, and is followed by a gradual decline for the rest of the life cycle (Fig. 10–2).

Pregnancy and Lactation

During the last trimester of pregnancy, BMR increases about 15 to 30%. The amount of energy necessary to produce milk for lactation increases the BMR as much as 40%.

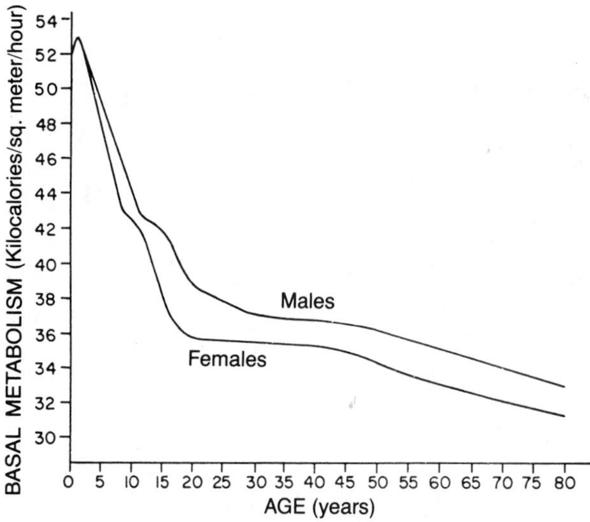

Figure 10–2 Normal basal metabolic rates at different ages for each sex. (From Guyton AC. *Textbook of Medical Physiology.* 8th ed. Philadelphia, WB Saunders, 1991.)

Surface Area

The more surface exposed, the greater the BMR. Because of greater surface area, a tall, thin person would require more energy than a short, heavy one of similar weight.

State of Health

Certain illnesses and diseases may increase or decrease the BMR. Clients recovering from a wasting illness require extra energy to build new tissue. Additionally, the activity level may be influenced by such conditions as lack of sleep or exhaustion, tenseness, fatigue, or depression.

Body Composition

In adulthood, lean body mass is the best single predictor of the BMR. Because cells in muscles and glands are more active than those in bone and fat, body composition influences the BMR (Broeder et al, 1992).

Although muscle tone is an important factor in metabolism, the state of tension or relaxation also has an effect. Athletes, who have better muscle tone than sedentary people, require more kilocalories than the nonathletic person of similar size and shape. Therefore, more food may be eaten by athletes without weight gain.

Sex

Sex hormones indirectly influence BMR. Girls generally use less energy than boys. As adults, the amount of lean body tissue versus fat tissue is a distinguishing factor; normally women have more fat tissue and use fewer kilocalories. Therefore, differences in BMR may be primarily related to typical variations in body composition rather than directly related to gender.

Endocrine Glands: Chemical Messengers

Thyroid problems as the cause of obesity are rare. Thyroxine, the iodine-containing hormone from the thyroid gland, has a greater influence on the rate of internal processes than secretions from any other gland.

Adrenal glands affect metabolism to a lesser degree. Stimulations by fright, excitement, or even joy can cause a temporary rise in the BMR by releasing catecholamines, particularly epinephrine. The pituitary gland accounts for about a 15 to 20% increase in the BMR during growth of children and adolescents.

Temperature

BMR can be affected by body temperature or climate. The BMR is slightly higher in cooler climates to maintain normal body temperature. When a fever is present, the BMR increases 7% for each 1° F rise above normal body temperature.

Fasting and Starvation

Clients who are undernourished or fasting for long periods of time have a lower than normal BMR. This is a result of decreased muscle mass as well as an adaptive body process to conserve energy.

Name 4 factors that affect BMR and state how they affect BMR.

NURSING APPLICATIONS

1. For healthy men, the BMR usually ranges from about 1500 to 1800 kcal daily, whereas approximately 1200 to 1350 kcal is needed for women. Supply at least this amount of energy to prevent further deterioration of physical status. A dietary consultation or supplemental feedings may be needed to maintain this level.
2. Because of accelerated BMR, a fever increases energy requirements as much as 100 to 125 kcal/day for each 1° F above normal body temperature for an average-sized person. Therefore, if temperature is 101° F, offer an additional 300 to 375 kcal/day.
3. Shivering is the body's way of asking for more energy or heat. Offer extra clothing, a warmer room environment, or a warm snack.
4. The BMR almost doubles in hyperthyroidism, in which too much thyroxine is secreted. The BMR may also be 30 to 50% below normal when too little thyroxine is secreted, as in hypothyroidism (see Chapter 28). If any of these conditions is diagnosed, adjust kilocalories accordingly.
5. Increased thyroxine activity can cause vitamin deficiencies because the quantity of many of the different enzymes is increased: Vitamins are essential parts of some of these coenzymes. Without supplementation, thiamin and vitamins B_{12} and C may become deficient. Porous bones may result from greater losses of calcium and phosphorus caused by increased thyroxine activity.
6. A naturally higher BMR is a reason why children do not feel as cold as adults under the same weather conditions. Do not overdress or underdress a child based on an adult's perception.
7. Unless physical activity is above average, the BMR represents the largest proportion of a client's energy requirement. Determination of BMR can be used to evaluate adequacy of kilocaloric intake.

Client Education

- BMR may be elevated or depressed. A high BMR requires more kilocalories, with fewer kilocalories necessary for a low BMR.
- The BMR decreases about 2% every 10 years after age 25, and many clients gain weight because previous eating habits are maintained without increasing activity.

MEASUREMENT OF POTENTIAL ENERGY

The amount of energy, or kilocalories, available in a food may be precisely calculated by placing a weighed amount of food inside a bomb **calorimeter.** As it is burned, the increase in water temperature indicates the heat given off or the potential (free) energy of that food.

Calorimeter is used to measure kilocalories.

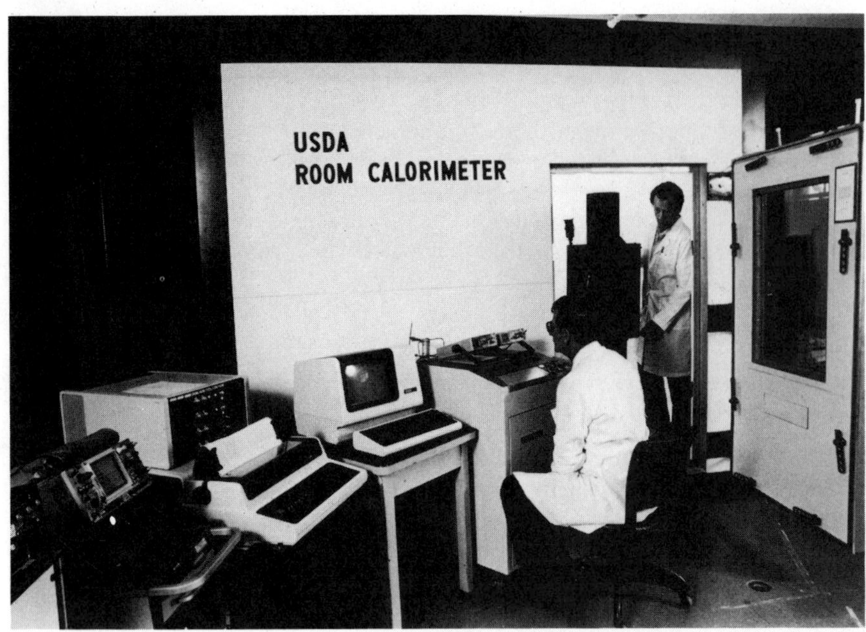

Figure 10–3 One of six in the world, the U.S. Department of Agriculture's room calorimeter, when complete, will measure heat given off (kilocalories used) by human subjects. In testing the calorimeter, one researcher steps inside while another reviews the computer output. (Courtesy of U.S.D.A.'s *Food News for Consumers* 1986 (summer); 3(2):5.)

Coefficient of digestibility is the amount of energy used in digestion.

Measurement of heat produced by a body or food is called direct calorimetry.

Describe the difference between bomb calorimetry and direct calorimetry.

Not all the free energy is available to the body. The **coefficient of digestibility** reduces the actual amount of energy that is physiologically available.

Room calorimeters have been built to learn about energy consumption and expenditure (Fig. 10–3). Computers record the amount of energy supplied by foods and how a person makes use of the energy by **direct calorimeter.** Heat sensors in the walls measure how many kilocalories are expended by the body while living in the chamber.

ENERGY REQUIREMENTS

Basal Metabolic Rate

There are several methods of determining the BMR. For most clients, the BMR accounts for 65 to 70% of the body's energy requirement. Determining the exact BMR is still inexact, but many general guidelines have been formulated. One quick guideline for adults is:

10–11 × ideal weight (lbs) = kcal needed for BMR daily

Voluntary Work and Play

The most variable factor affecting total energy needs is muscle activity, which is influenced by the physical activity level. This is normally 20 to 30% of the daily energy requirement.

The tired feeling after a period of mental work usually is due to tension rather than use of stored energy. Mental activity uses almost no extra energy (about 3 to 4 kcal/hr). Half of a glass of skim milk or an apple furnishes the total amount of energy required for 1 hour, including BMR and mental activity. The best criterion to evaluate energy expenditures is based on body weight, the amount of time involved, and the degree of intensity of the activity (Table 10–2). Exercise of adequate intensity and duration may also enhance BMR (Molé, 1990).

TABLE 10–2

KILOCALORIC EXPENDITURE FOR VARIOUS ACTIVITIES

Kcal/Hr for 150-lb Body Weight	Kcal/Hr for 150-lb Body Weight
100–200 kcal/hr	*400–450 kcal/hr*
Billiards	Disco dancing
Golf	Square dancing
Music Playing	Hunting (carry load)
200–250 kcal/hr	Lawn mowing (hand)
Jazzercise, light	Bicycling (11 mph)
Walking (20–26 min/mile)	Wood chopping, sawing
Aerobics, light	Jogging (14 min/mile)
Shuffleboard	*450–500 kcal/hr*
Gardening	Tennis, singles
Canoeing (2.5 mph)	Jogging (13 min/mile)
Archery	Water skiing
Sailing	*500–550 kcal/hr*
Fishing	Hiking, mountain
Bicycling (6 mph)	Fencing
Golf (pull cart)	Bicycling (12 mph)
Lawn mowing (power)	Football, touch
250–300 kcal/hr	Canoeing (5 mph)
Bowling	Swimming, slow
Jogging (17 min/mile)	Aerobics, heavy
Housework	Calisthenics, heavy
Calisthenics, light	Jazzercise, heavy
Weight lifting, light	Skiing, downhill
Badminton, doubles	*550–600 kcal/hr*
Row boating (2.5 mph)	Boxing, sparring
300–350 kcal/hr	Bicycling (13 mph)
Jazzercise, medium	Jogging (12 min/mile)
Aerobics, medium	Racquetball, social
Carpentry	Tennis, vigorous
Golf (carry clubs)	*600–650 kcal/hr*
Tennis, doubles	Weight lifting, heavy
Jogging (15 min/mile)	Backpacking
Volleyball	Swimming, fast
Badminton, singles	Basketball, nonvigorous
Horseback trotting	*650–700 kcal/hr*
Roller skating	Ice hockey, vigorous
350–400 kcal/hr	Climbing, mountain
Table tennis	Racquetball, vigorous
Fishing (wading)	Jogging (10 min/mile)
Hiking (cross-country)	Handball, vigorous
Bicycling (10 mph)	Skiing, cross-country
Ditch digging (hand)	*700–800 kcal/hr*
Ice skating (10 mph)	Jogging (9 min/mile)
	Basketball, vigorous
	Over 800 kcal/hr
	Running (5–8 min/mile)
	Rowing (11 mph)
	Boxing, competition
	Swimming, competition

Data from FIT III software, N-Squared Computing, Salem, OR.

Thermogenic Effect

The thermogenic effect (formerly called specific dynamic action) of food refers to the increased heat production resulting from the metabolism of food.

Food digestion requires energy. The thermogenic effect of a mixed diet is estimated to be about 10% of the energy required for BMR.

TABLE 10–3

BASAL ENERGY EXPENDITURE USING THE HARRIS-BENEDICT EQUATION

Men: 66 + (13.7 × kg) + (5 × cm) − (6.8 × yr) = kcal
Women: 655 + (9.6 × kg) + (1.7 × cm) − (4.7 × yr) = kcal

Example: Man, weight 180 lbs (82 kg), 6′ (183 cm), 36 years old
66 + (13.7 × 82 kg) + (5 × 183 cm) − (6.8 × 36 yrs) =
66 + 1123 + 915 − 245 = 1859 kcal

Additional factors are added for activity and injury:

Activity Factor		*Injury Factor*	
Bed rest	1.2	Minor surgery	1.2
Sedentary	1.25	Skeletal trauma	1.35
Ambulatory	1.3	Major sepsis	1.6
Aerobic activity (3 times/wk)	1.3	Severe burns	2.1
Aerobic activity (5 times/wk)	1.5		
True athlete	1.7		

Example: activity level, ambulatory; injury factor, broken femur (skeletal trauma)
1859 (BEE) × 1.25 (activity) × 1.35 (injury) = 3137 kcal/day

Basal Energy Expenditure or Resting Energy Expenditure

BEE and REE are the estimated kilocaloric requirement for BMR plus additional kilocalories needed for thermogenic effect, voluntary activities, and any increased needs from catabolic (disease states, fever) or anabolic (growth, pregnancy) processes.

Basal energy expenditure (BEE) and **resting energy expenditure (REE)** are often used interchangeably. However, there are subtle differences in their usage. As a general rule, BEE is obtained using the Harris-Benedict formula. The Harris-Benedict equation has been the standard used for many years and is fairly accurate in predicting the energy requirements of healthy, nourished clients. Its reliability in the malnourished client has been questioned but for lack of a better guideline is still used. The formula takes into consideration sex, weight, height, and age, as shown in Table 10–3. Also, factors can be added for specific dynamic action (food digestion), activity level, and disease state.

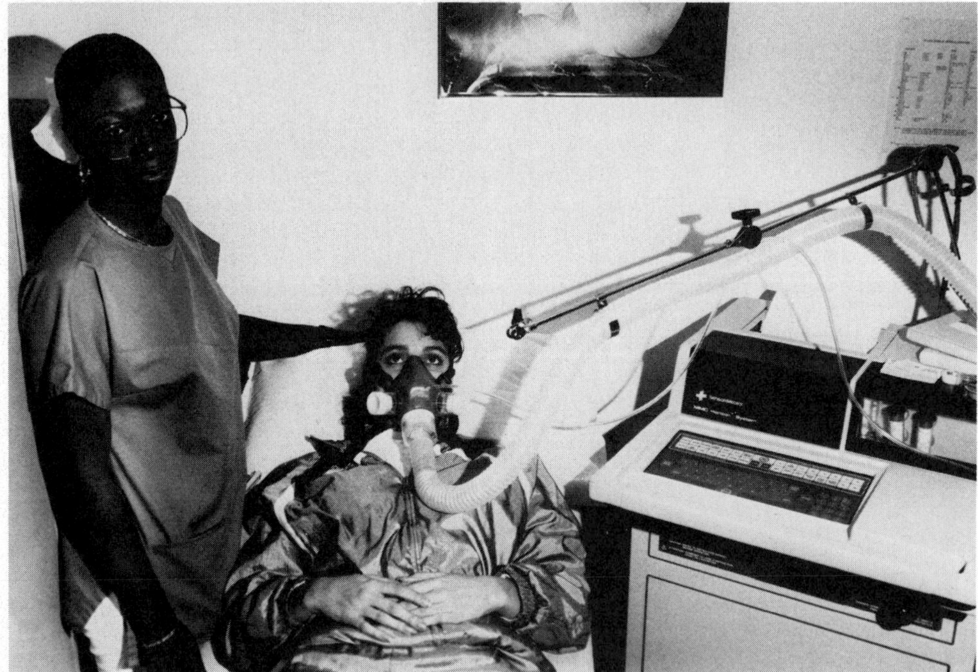

Figure 10–4 The metabolic cart is used to measure resting energy expenditure of clients to provide adequate amounts of kilocalories.

TABLE 10–4

CALCULATION OF TOTAL ENERGY NEEDS

1. Determine IBW (see Appendix C-1)
2. Basal metabolic needs 10–11 kcal × IBW = kcal for BMR
   Example: IBW, 180 lbs
   10 kcal/lb × 180 = 1800 kcal for BMR
3. Add a factor for kilocalories needed for voluntary activities
   Sedentary—30%
   Light—50%
   Moderate—75%
   Very active—100%

Example: Client's activity level, light (sedentary job with routine workouts 3 times a week)
1800 kcal for BMR × 0.50 kcal for light activity = 900 kcal for light activity
1800 kcal for BMR + 900 kcal for light activity = 2700 total kcal daily requirement

IBW, Ideal body weight; BMR, basal metabolic weight.

Estimating the energy needs of a hospitalized client is a time-consuming and inexact process. BEE is more accurately predicted by **indirect calorimetry.** Portable metabolic carts are available specifically for this function. The metabolic cart (Fig. 10–4) is an indirect calorimeter using a computer programmed to calculate exact kilocaloric requirements. The client inhales air from the room through one valve and exhales into the computer through the second valve. By measuring the amount of oxygen consumed and the amount of carbon dioxide exhaled, the kilocalories used daily are determined. The term REE is generally associated with use of a metabolic cart to determine kilocaloric requirement. This form of indirect calorimetry precisely determines the metabolic state and permits the physician or dietitian to design the most effective nutritional regimen (Makk et al, 1990), which is especially effective for clients with severe burns or trauma that causes **hypermetabolism.**

Measurements of oxygen consumption and carbon dioxide production are used to determine kilocaloric requirement in indirect calorimetry.

Hypermetabolism—elevated metabolic rate.

In the 1989 RDAs, the National Research Council has recommended energy allowances for reference adults with light to moderate activity levels, as shown in the Table on the inside front cover. These recommended allowances can be adjusted for increased physical activity and body size.

To figure the total energy expenditure, (1) calculate the basal metabolism based on ideal body weight and (2) add the energy costs of voluntary activities, as shown in Table 10–4.

List methods used to determine BEE/REE.

HYPER- AND HYPO- STATES

The proper energy balance for stable weight is maintained when the kilocaloric intake equals the amount of energy needed for body processes and physical activities (Fig. 10–5). One pound of body fat is equivalent to 3500 kcal. When more kilocalories are consumed than the body needs, the excess is stored as fat, resulting in weight gain. A negative energy balance results in weight loss.

Many healthy clients are able to control energy intake to balance energy output with little effort; their **appetite** controls food intake to balance energy expenditure.

Appetite or the desire to eat is related to the pleasurable sensations of eating.

On the other hand, overweight clients have a difficult time losing extra pounds and maintaining their energy balance to keep off unwanted pounds. Weight control can be approached by either decreasing the number of kilocalories consumed or increasing physical activities. Generally, a combination of both is most effective (see Chapter 19).

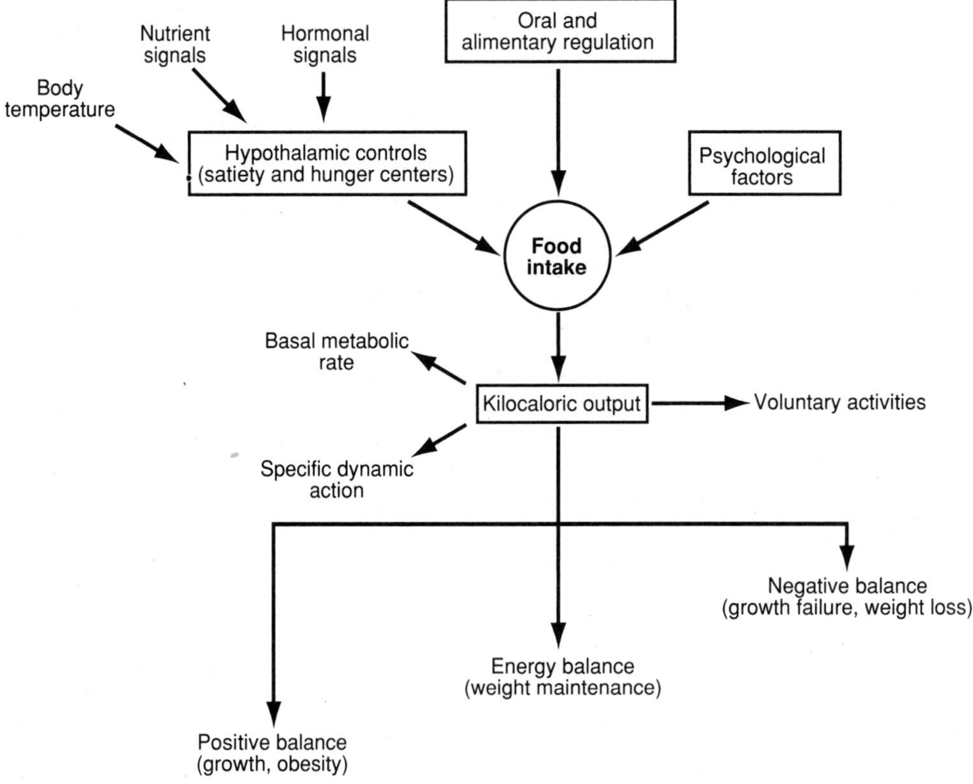

Figure 10–5 Factors affecting energy balance.

Maintaining Energy Balance

Energy balance is maintained when the kilocalorie intake equals the amount of energy needed for body processes and physical activities. This statement sounds innocent and simple. However, very few Americans are able to maintain energy balance at an appropriate body weight.

Hunger is the physiological drive to eat.

Many factors enter into this unbalanced equation; because it is a complex system, there are no easy answers. **Hunger** is regulated by a complex network of factors (see Fig. 10–5). The opposite of hunger is satiety. Appetite is frequently used in the same sense as hunger, but it usually implies desire for specific types of food. Hunger and appetite greatly affect weight balance.

Intake has generally been regarded as the key to weight regulation. Most clients' weights tend to remain stable for long periods. Even small daily deviations from balance could result in gradual significant fluctuations in fat stores. (One hundred additional kilocalories daily would result in a 10-lb weight gain over a year's time and a 100-lb increase over 10 years.) Most clients are unaware of changing their intake or physical activity level to maintain stable weight. Klesgas et al (1992) determined in a longitudinal study that high fat intake and increases in total energy intake were related to higher weight gain in women; in men, however, dietary fat intake was related to weight gain. Thus, nurses need to be aware of the complexities of maintaining energy balance to prevent undesirable weight gain or loss.

Physiological Factors

The hypothalamus, located in the middle of the brain, is especially important in controlling hunger. Within the hypothalamus, there is a satiety and a hunger center.

Stimulation of the hunger center causes insatiable hunger (hyperphagia), but damage to this area results in no desire for food. Stimulation of the satiety center results in complete satiety. If the satiety center of the hypothalamus is destroyed, the appetite becomes voracious, resulting in obesity. The feeding center stimulates the drive to eat, whereas the satiety center inhibits the feeding center.

Metabolic factors control the feeding center. Hypoglycemia causes hunger, which has led to the glucostatic theory of hunger and feeding regulation. An increase in the blood glucose level activates the satiety center and deactivates neurons in the hunger center.

Several mechanisms affect the amount eaten at a particular meal. Distention of the stomach results in inhibitory signals to suppress the feeding center, reducing the desire to eat. The release of cholecystokinin in response to fat in the duodenum has a strong direct effect on the feeding center to cease eating. Food in the stomach and duodenum causes the secretion of glucagon and insulin, both of which suppress the feeding center.

Additionally, the hypothalamus is responsive to body temperature. Cold temperatures result in increased food intake, resulting in increased metabolic rate and increased fat for insulation.

The relationship between exercise and food intake is unclear. Exercise has been reported to increase, decrease, or have no effect on appetite. As a general rule, acute exercise decreases food intake following the exercise, but regular exercise promotes increased kilocaloric intake.

Nutrient and hormonal signals affect the brain and liver to stimulate satiety and feeding centers in the brain (Table 10–5). Numerous studies have shown that physiological control of energy intake is unreliable. Therefore, energy balance must be adjusted through some other mechanism.

How do metabolic factors affect the feeding center? What mechanisms affect the amount eaten at a particular meal? What effect does exercise have on eating?

Psychological Factors

Appetite is affected by the fact that eating is rewarding or pleasurable and makes us feel good. The eating behavior of obese clients is believed to be influenced more by external cues, including time, taste, smell, and sight of food than the behavior of clients of normal weight. Greater weight usually means the client is responding to feelings and emotions rather than actual hunger. Boredom is a frequent reason for the eating habits of the obese.

Energy Expenditure

Contrary to popular opinion, obese women have a similar or higher metabolic rate than less obese women (Owen et al, 1987; Garrow, 1986). The effect of this is less weight gain for a given increase in kilocaloric intake. However, obese clients who have lost weight often have a lower BMR at their reduced weight than clients who have never been obese; this factor may partially explain the frequent weight

TABLE 10–5

STIMULI AFFECTING FOOD INTAKE

	Food Intake	
Signal	***Increased***	***Decreased***
Food odors	Pleasant	Repulsive
Taste	Desirable	Offensive
Climate (temperature)	Cold	Hot
Gastrointestinal	Hunger pains	Distention
		Cholecystokinin
		Glucagon
Glucose level	Low	High
Lipoprotein	High	Low
Nutrient stores	Decreased	Increased

gain that is prevalent following weight loss (Leibel & Hirsch, 1984). Genetics may also play a role in BMR. Some families have low metabolic rates, but not all family members are obese (Ravussin et al, 1988). Infants of overweight mothers had a lower BMR by 3 months of age; these infants later became obese (Roberts et al, 1988).

Exercise tolerance of obese clients is less than normal, but any activity uses more kilocalories because of the amount of additional mass that has to be moved. Not all inactive clients are obese, so activity level does not appear to be an important factor in the development of obesity. BMR as a result of body composition affects energy expenditure for activities.

In summation, weight loss resulting from a specific kilocaloric deficit is invariably smaller than expected. Conversely, overconsumption fails to produce weight gains anticipated. Adjustments in energy expenditure appear to be adaptive.

Inadequate Energy Intake

Inadequate amounts of energy may result in a depressed rate of growth in children and weight loss in adults. Intentional weight loss may be helpful or harmful, depending on the methods used for losing weight (discussed in Chapter 19). Decreased fat stores are normally the goal, but loss of muscle may be an undesirable side effect.

Inadequate energy intake may result in malnutrition and become a serious problem in the face of a physiologically stressful situation (see Chapter 21). Inadequate intake may be intentional, as in the case of anorexia nervosa which is a psychological disorder in which the client does not perceive that he or she is undernourished. Inadequate intake causes a vicious downhill situation due to metabolic imbalances that decrease hunger and may become life-threatening without proper treatment (see Chapter 20).

NURSING APPLICATIONS

1. Assess emotional factors. Depression and other emotional factors result in overeating and decreased activity in some clients.
2. A positive energy balance is desirable during periods of growth; therefore, a proportionately larger amount of energy is needed for pregnant women and children.
3. When nutrient stores decrease, the feeding center of the hypothalamus becomes active, and the client becomes hungry; when nutrient stores are abundant, the client feels satiated and loses the desire to eat. If the hypothalamus is injured in any way (as in a head injury or stroke), hunger and satiety may be altered.
4. If kilocalories are underestimated, the body must use stored energy (fat and protein), making the client at risk for malnutrition. If excessive kilocalories are given, the body converts excess kilocalories to fat. Evaluation of energy requirement is needed to prevent malnutrition or obesity.

Client Education

- Exercise may enhance the BMR by increasing the amount of lean body mass, which uses more kilocalories.
- To gain 1 lb of fat, a client must consume 3500 kcal more than he or she uses.
- To lose 1 lb of weight, energy intake must be 3500 kcal less than the number of kilocalories used.
- Boredom may trigger the desire to eat for some clients.
- A decrease from prior activity level or additional kilocaloric intake may result in weight gain.

ENERGY NEEDS OF THE PHYSICALLY CHALLENGED

Extra energy costs result from various deformities of the joints of the trunk and lower extremities. Since more energy is required, a hemiplegic or amputee's movements at 1 to 2 miles/hr require almost the same amount of energy as normal clients walking at 3 miles/hr.

Energy costs vary with the efficiency of the prosthetic design and weight as well as with the age of the amputee. Wheelchair ambulation by amputees requires no more energy than normal walking at the same speed. For the paraplegic using crutches, the expenditure is 2 to 4 times greater than that of a normal client walking at the same speed.

NURSING APPLICATIONS

1. Assess physical activity of the physically challenged and determine kilocalories needed.
2. Evaluate effectiveness of care by monitoring client's weight and choices of food.

Client Education

- One of the major problems for the physically challenged is excessive body weight. Three ways to combat this problem include:
  1. Encourage mobility by increasing favorite activities and offering suggestions to initiate appropriate new activities.
  2. Explain the various kilocalorie levels of different foods and kilocalories used so the client understands precisely how weight is controlled.
  3. Plan meals and snacks together for optimum nutrients within the kilocalorie limit for weight maintenance.

NUTRITIONAL NEEDS OF THE ATHLETE

Athletic competition places unusual and unique demands on the body for energy. Nutrient composition is similar to the Dietary Guidelines for Americans, with 15 to 20% of energy as protein, 30% as fat, and 50 to 55% as carbohydrate (ADA, 1987).

Energy Balance

Gymnasts and figure skaters have a fairly low energy requirement, with participants in marathon and cross-country running sports requiring over 4000 kilocalories. It is not unusual for vigorous exercise training programs to require from 3000 to 6000 kilocalories daily. When more than 4000 kilocalories are required, larger amounts of energy-dense foods, such as sugar and fat, are used to obtain sufficient energy.

Most male and female athletes compete best if their body fat is between 8 to 10% and 12 to 14%, respectively. For most clients, recommended body fat levels are 15 to 18% for men and 20 to 25% for women; average percentages are 23% for American men and 32% for women (Bailey, 1991).

Ordinarily exercise is conducive to maintaining bone density, but **amenorrhea** occurs in 10 to 20% of women who exercise regularly and in up to 50% of competitive athletes (Nieman, 1990). This menstrual dysfunction appears to be a complex interplay of factors, including a direct effect of exercise on sex hormones, a decrease

Amenorrhea—without menstruation.

What can cause amenorrhea, and what are secondary effects of amenorrhea?

in body fat, or a response to malnutrition or over-restrictive dietary modification (Henderson, 1991; Shangold et al, 1990). Treatment with hormonal replacement and nutritional strategies is recommended because of lower bone density, increased stress fractures, and long-term risk for osteoporosis (Drinkwater et al, 1990).

Protein

The recommendation of 1 gm protein/kg body weight is slightly higher than the RDA, but this is usually automatically met with increased kilocalorie intake. Despite the fact that excessive protein consumption has not been demonstrated to enhance athletic performance, many athletes take protein supplements.

NURSING APPLICATIONS

1. Although athletes may be heavier than their "ideal" body weight, they are not considered obese. Do not reduce kilocalories for the overweight athlete, as this may cause the athlete to lose muscle mass.
2. Excessive protein intake exceeding 2 gm/kg/day has several disadvantages, such as displacing carbohydrate intake and causing hypercalciuria and dehydration; therefore, nurses must inquire about protein consumption and determine amount ingested. If high, assess carbohydrate intake and urine for calcium.
3. In athletes, assess for dehydration. Excess nitrogen from protein supplements is excreted along with water, with resulting possibility of dehydration.
4. Amenorrhea should be a sign for nurses to encourage increased energy intake to avoid detrimental life-long effects on bone integrity.

Client Education

- If weight loss is desired, fat should be reduced instead of carbohydrate or protein.
- Extreme fluctuations in weight should be avoided.
- When adequate amounts of carbohydrates are not consumed everyday, glycogen stores become depleted, detrimentally affecting endurance and performance. To help prevent glycogen depletion during endurance events, an athlete must consume at least 60% of total daily kilocalories from carbohydrates (Wheeler, 1989).
- Carbohydrate feedings during exercise are associated with improved exercise performance (Murray et al, 1991).
- Discuss the risks associated with amenorrhea with clients and encourage them (1) to consume adequate amounts of calcium daily (1500 mg/day), (2) to consume adequate intake of kilocalories and dietary fat (30%), and (3) to consider gaining weight (Shangold et al, 1990).

Other Nutrients

Any nutrient deficiency can impair athletic performance, but advantages of nutrient supplementation over the RDA have not been established. Increased nutrient intake is not necessary during athletic events as long as additional kilocalories are provided for the extra demands, and the proportions of nutrients maintain the desired balance. An exception, however, is that along with increased energy requirements, there are increased requirements for thiamin (a minimum of 1 mg for intake between 1000 and 2000 kcal), riboflavin (0.6 mg/1000 kcal), and niacin (not less than 13 niacin equivalents for intakes of less than 2000 kcal). This is consistent

What nutrients need to be increased in the athlete's diet?

with the RDAs, since the requirements for these B vitamins are based on kilocaloric requirement. Without sufficient quantities of these vitamins, energy nutrients cannot be completely metabolized for their available energy.

NURSING APPLICATIONS

1. Assess intake of fruits and vegetables to help protect against potassium depletion that is frequently observed.
2. If the client is not gaining strength as expected, assessment of total food intake must be part of the overall evaluation, e.g., adequate rest and mental and physical condition.
3. Serum testosterone levels are significantly lower with low body fat, loss of body fat, and weight loss. As a result, decreased strength and endurance as well as decreased sex drive during rigid dietary restriction for weight loss have been reported. Perform a holistic assessment including sexuality issues.
4. Be aware of the signs of eating compulsion and obsession in athletes. If emphasis on leanness and strict weight control is indicated, refer client for nutritional and/or psychological counseling.
5. Iron needs are slightly higher in athletes due to increased iron losses. Iron-deficiency anemia frequently occurs in athletes because of increased RBC destruction, GI blood loss, iron loss in sweat, and decreased iron absorption (Kris-Etherton, 1990). Monitor RBC and hemoglobin levels and iron intake.

Client Education

- Female athletes need to make an exerted effort to consume adequate amounts of calcium and iron.
- Iron-rich foods are important to maintain the oxygen-carrying capacity of the blood. Laboratory values should be monitored regularly detect to anemia.

Beverages

Nutrition during athletic events has 2 goals: (1) maintain an adequate level of hydration and (2) provide energy to delay the onset of fatigue.

Fluid and Electrolyte Replacement

Beverages should minimize physiological imbalances that occur during exercise and prevent injury and/or enhance performance. Since the typical American diet supplies ample sodium, chloride, potassium, and magnesium to replace sweat lost, plain cool water is recommended.

Sufficient water replacement is the most critical factor during athletic events since as little as 2 to 3% of body weight loss through sweating can cause measurable impairments in circulatory and thermal regulatory function (Table 10–6). Further loss can cause cramps and heat exhaustion and even heat stroke.

Thirst cannot be regarded as an indicator for water replacement. Sweat loss of 1 lb (2.2 kg) of body weight is equal to 2 cups (480 ml) of water. Weighing nude before and after events to determine fluid needs is the most accurate method of adequate water replacement.

Electrolytes rarely require replacement unless the event is of long duration. Sodium and potassium are lost in very small quantities; they can be maintained or replaced easily by foods or beverages high in these electrolytes before and after events. Many of the commercially available beverages marketed for athletic events contain electrolytes and some carbohydrate. Marathon runners particularly must protect themselves from too much as well as too little fluid. Water intoxication and

What is the most needed nutrient during athletic events?

TABLE 10–6

GUIDELINES FOR FOOD AND BEVERAGE INTAKE FOR ENDURANCE ACTIVITIES

High carbohydrate (60–65% of kcal)	Maximizes glycogen stores to maintain blood glucose levels during competition	
Low fat	Gastric emptying is delayed with high fat	
Low protein	High levels of protein may cause dehydration	
Moderate salt	High salt levels may cause intracellular dehydration and increase water losses	
Low bulk	High-fiber foods increase GI bulk, which can precipitate discomfort or diarrhea	
Adequate fluid	Adequate fluids are imperative to maintain hydration, both before and during the event. Proposed schedule for fluids:	
	2 hr before event:	16 oz water
	20 minutes before:	16 oz water
	Every 10–15 min during the event:	4–6 oz water
	Within 15–30 min after the event:	Carbohydrate-containing beverage providing 2 gm carbohydrate/kg body weight

dilutional hyponatremia are possible in duration events with intakes of large quantities of free water.

Sugar Content

Carbohydrate ingestion during endurance athletic events (lasting 90 minutes or longer) may help maintain blood glucose and enhance performance (Davis et al, 1990; Davis et al, 1988). On the other hand, a moderate amount of sugar intake before exercise may cause an insulin response with subsequent accelerated glycogen depletion and hypoglycemia. Carbohydrate content of these beverages should not exceed 10% (Kris-Etherton, 1990).

Sports drinks containing glucose polymers are available, such as Bodyfuel 450 (Vitex Foods), Exceed (Ross), and MAX (Coca-Cola). These glucose polymer solutions have a lower osmolality than solutions of glucose, fructose, or sucrose. Therefore, when equivalent amounts of carbohydrate are given, glucose polymer solutions do not cause the fluid imbalance that results in GI distress. The use of these fluids with added carbohydrate and electrolytes during prolonged exercise appears to decrease free fatty acids in the serum, which may increase the availability of glucose to the liver and adipose tissue (Deuster et al, 1992).

Alcohol

What are the recommendations for carbohydrate and alcohol content for athletes?

No beneficial effect of alcohol ingestion has been shown on athletic performance. Negative effects include diuresis, impairment of psychomotor coordination, and impairment of thermoregulation in cold temperatures. Endurance, muscle strength, and power may be adversely affected by alcohol intake; therefore, its use is not recommended for athletes.

Pregame Meals

The composition of the meal before a competitive event affects performance. The stomach and upper bowel should be empty to prevent gastric distress; liver and muscle glycogen reserves should be as high as possible. Table 10–6 indicates some important features of the pregame meal for high-intensity activities lasting more than 1 hour. Glycogen loading, begun about a week before the event, as described in Chapter 4, may allow longer periods of maximum workload.

The most hallowed of the time-honored fads, the precompetition steak, is undesirable because of the slow digestive process required. A light meal taken 3½ to 4 hours before the event ensures gastric emptying to avoid cramping. The ideal meal contains 300 to 1000 kcal with primarily complex carbohydrates, minimal fats, and 3 to 4 cups of fluid, as shown in Table 10–6. A sample breakfast and lunch menu pattern is shown in Figure 10–6.

Liquid Meals

Lowered performance caused by pregame nausea, muscle and leg cramps, and depleted glycogen stores have resulted in the use of liquid meals to relieve these problems. Liquid meals may be taken up to 1 hour before an event without harmful effects. They are satisfying, can provide adequate kilocalories, and are absorbed rather quickly. These do not replace the fluid benefits of plain water. If any extra supplements are taken with these liquid meals to give extra protein or carbohydrate, the higher concentrations can backfire, causing cramping and diarrhea.

SAMPLE MEALS FOR PRE-EVENT ENDURANCE ACTIVITIES

Breakfast Menu	Carbohydrate	kcal	Lunch/Dinner Menu	Carbohydrate	kcal
3/4 cup orange juice	20	84	Chicken and pasta salad	23	230
1 cup raisin bran cereal	37	154	8 Saltine crackers	16	100
1/2 English muffin	15	77	1/2 cup dried apricots	40	155
1 tsp Margarine	0	34	2 sugar cookies	18	140
2 tbsp apple butter	18	74	1/2 cup 1% milk	6	51
1 cup 1% milk	12	102	16 oz water	0	0
8 oz water	0	0			
TOTALS	102	525		103	676

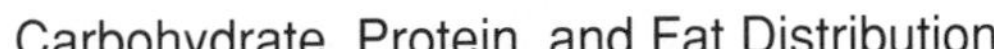

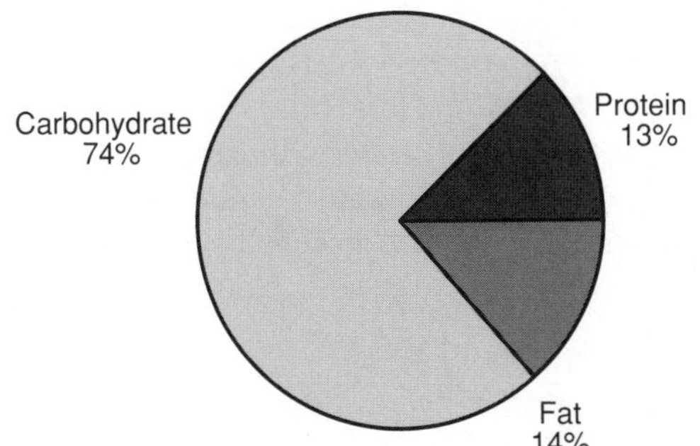

Carbohydrate, 102 gm; protein, 17, gm; fat, 9 gm

Carbohydrate, Protein, and Fat Distribution

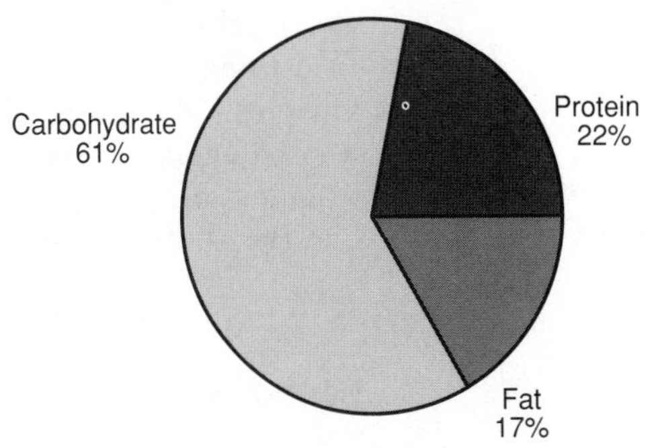

Carbohydrate, 103 gm; protein, 37, gm; fat, 13 gm

Figure 10–6 Sample meals for pre-event endurance activities.

NURSING APPLICATIONS

1. When the body cannot be cooled through sweat, heat stroke and death are likely possibilities. During high humidity weather, assess client's skin. If skin is dry and temperature is elevated, heat stroke is suspected; remove to cool location. Nursing care is essential to prevent death.
2. Water intake before exercise of moderate intensity is essential in terms of temperature regulation and cardiovascular homeostasis (Lamb & Brodowicz, 1986). If a client does not drink enough water during exercise or competition, monitor temperature, heart rate, and blood pressure. If the body does not have enough water, these parameters will be abnormal and stabilization will be needed.

Client Education

- Emphasize the importance of adequate fluids (see Table 10–6).
- Some commercially prepared beverages and fruit juices usually have a high osmolarity and should be diluted to enhance gastric emptying. Their use is warranted only for heavy exercise or high temperature-humidity index (ADA, 1987).
- Water is the preferred source of fluids. If water is disliked, the above-mentioned diluted beverages can be used.
- Whether a light meal (high in complex carbohydrates) or a liquid meal is chosen before an athletic event is up the athlete. There is no evidence that one is significantly better for all athletes.
- The normal diet can replace the salt lost in sweat more satisfactorily than salt tablets.
- Depending on the length and the level of the activity, athletic performance diminishes/depletes glycogen stores. Without carbohydrates, glycogen levels can remain exhausted as long as 5 days. With adequate carbohydrate intake, muscle glycogen is resynthesized to normal levels within 24 hours. Within 15 to 30 minutes following exercise, a source of carbohydrate, such as orange juice, is recommended to replenish glycogen stores.
- Liquid meals do not replace fluid requirements.
- Other factors that play an important role in athletic performance include genetics, training, and motivation. Good nutrition is important but cannot replace any of these other factors.

SUMMARY

Clients use fats, carbohydrates, protein, and even alcohol as fuel for the chemical, mechanical, electrical, and thermal energy necessary to maintain life. When food intake is increased for higher energy production, thiamin, niacin, and riboflavin must also be consumed in larger amounts. The final assessment of achieving desired energy levels may be determined by the maintenance of normal body weight or adjustments in body weight as desired by the client (excluding anorexic clients) and the ability to perform in sports and/or work activities.

NURSING PROCESS IN ACTION

A 17-year-old girl is a competitive swimmer and is training for a long-distance competition. She has questions about what she should be eating to allow her to compete at her maximum level.

Nutritional Assessment

- BMR, kilocalories needed, activity level, body fat.
- Height, weight, weight changes, stress fractures, curvature of the spine.
- Sexual history: onset of menses, estimation of flow, sexual activity.
- Iron, RBC, and hemoglobin levels.
- Mental and physical condition.
- Intake of carbohydrate, fats, protein, vitamins, (thiamin, riboflavin, and niacin), and minerals (iron and calcium).
- Willingness/motivation to learn.
- Knowledge base for nutritional needs of an athlete.
- Beliefs about weight control, especially compulsions or obsessions with eating and losing weight.

Dietary Nursing Diagnosis

High risk for altered health maintenance RT inadequate/insufficient knowledge of nutritional needs for athletes.

Nutritional Goals

Client will discuss the importance of nutrition and explain/consume the types of foods she should eat.

Nutritional Implementation 

Intervention: Determine nutrient composition of food eaten.
Rationale: Athletes need 15 to 20% of energy as protein, 30% as fat, and 50 to 55% as carbohydrate.

Intervention: Increase kilocalorie consumption.
Rationale: Lack of kilocalories can result in amenorrhea and loss of bone integrity among competitive women athletes. Inadequate intake associated with weight loss lowers estrogen levels.

Intervention: Discuss why protein supplements may be harmful.
Rationale: Excessive protein consumption has not been demonstrated to enhance athletic performance, is frequently used as a substitute for carbohydrates, and causes hypercalciuria and dehydration.

Intervention: Suggest foods high in thiamin, riboflavin, and niacin (grains and cereals) and calcium (milk and dairy products).
Rationale: Without sufficient quantities of these vitamins, energy nutrients cannot be completely metabolized for their available energy. Calcium is needed to prevent bone loss and osteoporosis.

Intervention: Eat fruit and vegetables with each meal.
Rationale: This protects against potassium depletion that is frequently observed.

Intervention: Offer foods high in iron (meats) with vitamin C.
Rationale: The vitamin C will enhance iron absorption, and foods will replace needed iron to produce hemoglobin. Iron deficiency anemia frequently occurs in athletes because of increased RBC destruction, GI blood loss, and decreased iron absorption.

Intervention: (1) Stress the importance of fluid intake using Table 10–6. (2) Weigh nude before and after an event.
Rationale: (1) As little as 2 to 3% of body weight loss through sweating can cause measurable impairments in circulatory and thermal regulatory function.

Sweat loss of 1 lb of body weight is equal to 2 cups of water. (2) This is the best technique to determine adequate water replacement.

Intervention: Discuss the undesirable effects of alcohol intake.
Rationale: Diuresis, impairment of psychomotor coordination, and impairment of thermoregulation in cold temperatures can occur. Endurance and muscle strength may also be adversely affected.

Intervention: Discuss amounts and types of appropriate foods and appropriate time for precompetition meal.
Rationale: The stomach and upper bowel should be empty to prevent gastric distress; liver and muscle glycogen reserves should be as high as possible.

Intervention: After the event, consume high-carbohydrate foods.
Rationale: Athletic performance depletes glycogen stores, demanding carbohydrate intake to replace those depleted amounts.

Evaluation

If she can state the importance of nutrient, kilocalorie, and fluid consumption for athletic events; eats grains and cereals, dairy products, fruit and vegetables, and iron-rich foods; and abstains from alcohol, desired outcomes were met. Additionally, she could plan/consume a high-carbohydrate precompetition and postcompetition meal from a list of foods given her. Also, anemia would not be experienced.

STUDENT READINESS

1. Define the following: calorimetry, energy, thermogenic effect, basal metabolism, BEE.
2. Figure your total kilocaloric needs for 1 day (BMR plus estimated voluntary energy expenditures plus thermogenic effect).
3. What activities could you do to lose 1 lb per week? How long will you need to do each of these activities?
4. Assuming height and weight are the same, is the BMR higher or lower in:
   a. Men or women?
   b. An athlete or a sedentary person?
   c. A person 40 years old or one who is 20 years old?
   d. A woman who is not pregnant or one who is pregnant?
5. How many kilocalories of protein, fat, and carbohydrate are in 1 cup of homogenized milk that contains 8.5 gm protein, 8.5 gm fat, and 12 gm carbohydrate?
6. A boxer achieved a dramatic weight loss of about 18 kg (39.6 lb) in about 60 days. A strict diet, heavy exercise, thyroid supplements, and a diuretic drug produced his large weight loss. His defeat in a boxing match shocked some of his fans. What happened to his physical condition?

CASE STUDY

Jay G. is a 16-year-old high school athlete. He is on the football and baseball teams. He has been told by his classmates that he needs to eat a high-protein, low-carbohydrate diet. His mother is concerned about this approach to diet and contacts her best friend who is a nurse.

1. What do you think the nurse told this mother?
2. How many additional grams of protein does an athlete need each day above the recommended allowances?

3. For increased energy expenditures, what should be the primary source of nutrients?
4. What is the effect of a high-protein intake?
5. What is the desirable percentage of body fat for a male athlete? A female athlete?
6. Which vitamins are important in the production of energy?

REFERENCES

American Dietetic Association (ADA). Position of the American Dietetic Association: Nutrition for physical fitness and athletic performance for adults. *J Am Diet Assoc* 1987 July; 87(7):933–934.

Bailey C. *The New Fit or Fat.* Boston, Houghton-Mifflin, 1991.

Broeder CE, et al. The effects of aerobic fitness on resting metabolic rate. *Am J Clin Nutr* 1992 Apr; 55(4):795–801.

Davis JM, et al. Fluid availability of sports drinks differing in carbohydrate type and concentration. *Am J Clin Nutr* 1990 June; 51(6):1054–1057.

Davis JM, et al. Carbohydrate-electrolyte drink: Effects on endurance cycling in the heat. *Am J Clin Nutr* 1988 Oct; 48(4):1623–1630.

Deuster PA. Hormonal responses to ingesting water or a carbohydrate beverage during a 2 hr run. *Med Sci Sports Exerc* 1992 Jan; 24(1):72–79.

Drinkwater BL, et al. Menstrual history as a determinant of current bone density in young athletes. *JAMA* 1990 Jan 26; 263(4):545–548.

Garrow JS. Physiological aspects of obesity. *In* Brownell KD, Foreyt JP, eds.: *Handbook of Eating Disorders.* New York, Basic Books, 1986:45–62.

Henderson RC. Bone health in adolescence: Anorexia and athlete amenorrhea. *Nutr Today* 1991 March/Apr; 26(2):25–29.

Klesgas RC, et al. A longitudinal analysis of the impact of dietary intake and physical activity on weight change in adults. *Am J Clin Nutr* 1992 Apr; 55(4):818–822.

Kris-Etherton PM. Nutrition and athletic performance. *Nutr Today* 1990 Sept/Oct; 25(5):35–37.

Lamb DR, Brodowicz FR. Optimal use of fluids of varying formulations to minimize exercise-induced disturbances in homeostasis. *Sports Med* 1986 July-Aug; 3(4):247–274.

Leibel RL, Hirsch J. Diminished energy requirements in reduced-obese patients. *Metabolism* 1984 Feb; 33(2):164–170.

Lieber CS. Perspectives: Do alcohol calories count? *Am J Clin Nutr* 1991 Dec; 54(6):976–982.

Makk LJ, et al. Clinical application of the metabolic cart to the delivery of total parenteral nutrition. *Crit Care Med* 1990 Dec; 18(12):1320–1327.

Molé PA. Impact of energy intake and exercise on resting metabolic rate. *Sports Med* 1990 Aug; 10(2):72–87.

Murray R, et al. Responses to varying rates of carbohydrate ingestion during exercise. *Med Sci Sports Exerc* 1991 June; 23(6):713–718.

Nieman DC. *Fitness and Sports Medicine: An Introduction.* Rev. ed. Menlo Park, CA, Bull Publishing, 1990.

Owen OE, et al. A reappraisal of the caloric requirements of men. *Am J Clin Nutr* 1987 Dec; 46(6):875.

Ravussin E, et al. Reduced rate of energy expenditure as a risk factor for body weight gain. *N Engl J Med* 1988 Feb 25; 318(8):467–472.

Roberts SM, et al. Energy expenditure and intake in infants born to lean and overweight mothers. *N Engl J Med* 1988 Feb 25; 318(8):461–466.

Shangold M, et al. Evaluation and management of menstrual dysfunction in athletes. *JAMA* 1990 Mar 23–30; 263(12):1665–1669.

Suter PM, et al. The effect of ethanol on fat storage on healthy subjects. *N Engl J Med* 1992 Apr 9; 326(15):983–987.

Wheeler KB. Sports nutrition for the primary care physician. The importance of carbohydrate. *Physician Sportsmed* 1989 May; 17(5):106–117.

SECTION

II

Orientation to Clinical Nutrition

Once you know which nutrients are essential and where to find them, you will need nutritional skills to work with clients in the community and in the hospital. You are probably familiar with the nursing process; this can be used to provide optimal nutritional care in various settings in which you may work. Frequently clients in acute care settings and in their own homes are unable to receive their nourishment in a traditional manner; thus, they may be fed via a tube into their stomach or through their veins. This information will provide you with the practical knowledge of clinical nutrition skills to perform either method safely.

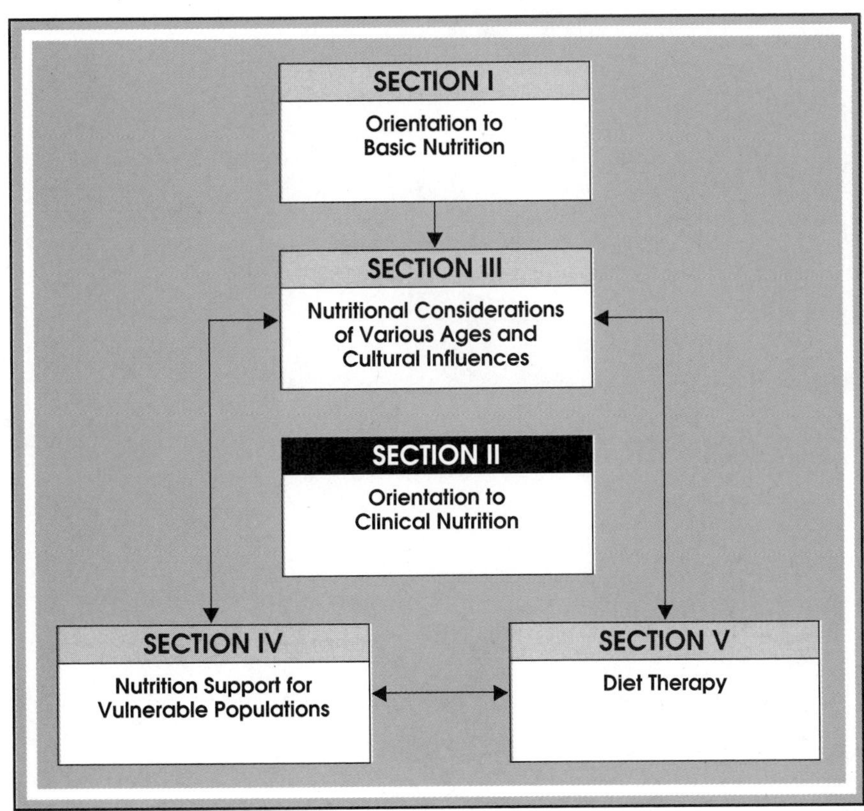

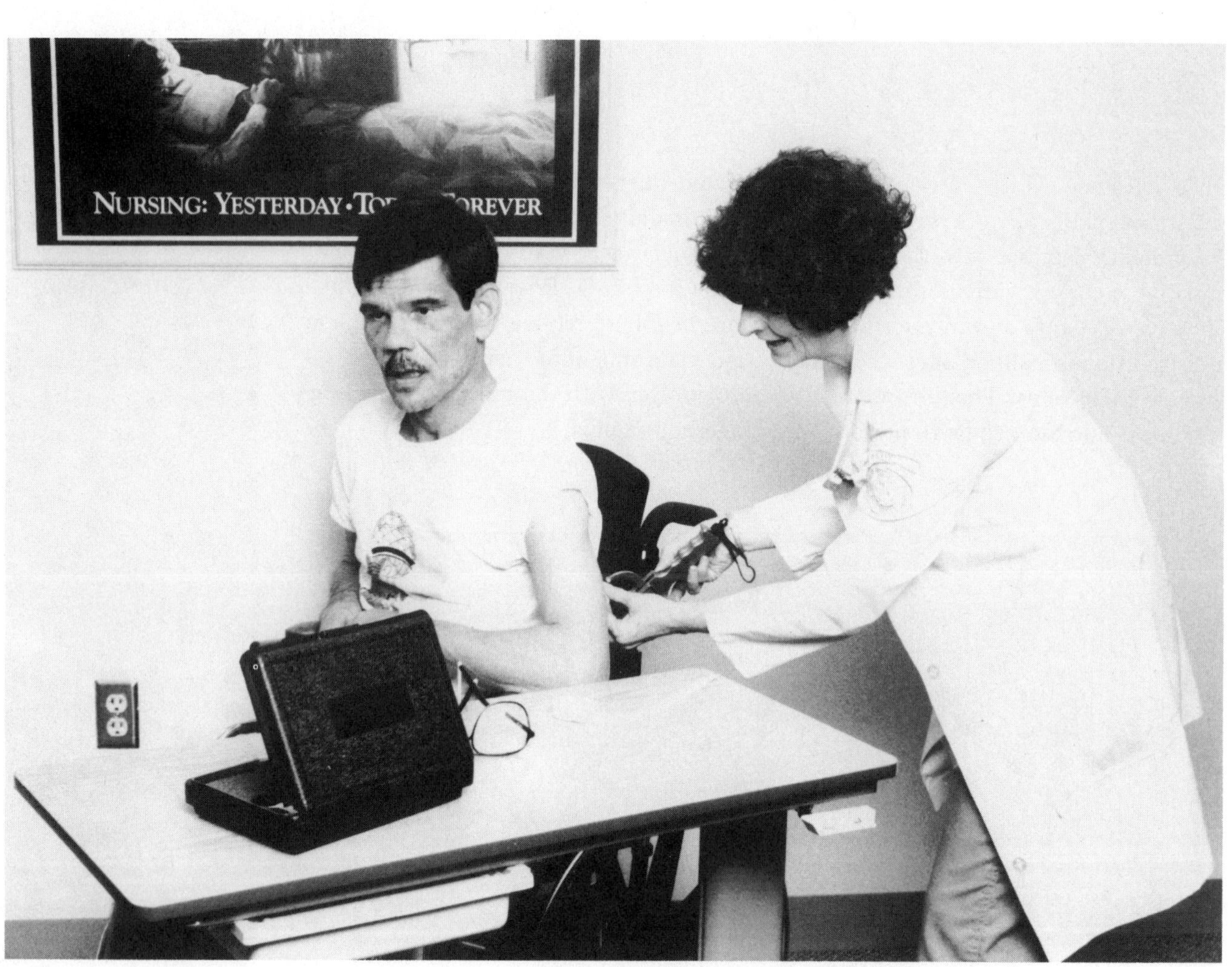
NURSING: YESTERDAY · TO
OREVER

Nutritional Applications of the Nursing Process

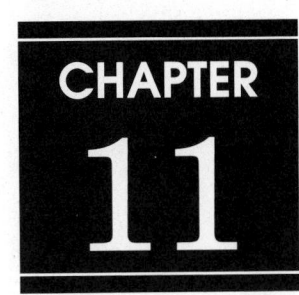

OUTLINE

I. ASSESSMENT
   A. Diet History
      1. Dietary Intake
   B. Anthropometric Measurements
      1. Height
      2. Weight
      3. Frame
      4. Height and Weight Tables
      5. Calculation of Desirable Body Weight
      6. Body Mass Index
      7. Weight Loss
      8. Skinfold Measurements
      9. Mid-Arm Circumference
   C. Physical Assessment
   D. Laboratory Information
      1. Vitamin Levels
      2. Protein Levels
   E. Immunological Testing
      1. Total Lymphocyte Count
      2. Skin Antigen Testing
   F. Nutrition Screening
II. DIAGNOSIS
III. PLANNING
IV. IMPLEMENTATION
   A. Client Education
   B. Referrals
V. EVALUATION
VI. NUTRITION UPDATE 11–1: DUBIOUS NUTRITIONAL ASSESSMENT TECHNIQUES

OBJECTIVES

THE STUDENT WILL BE ABLE TO:

- Describe each component of the nursing process and how it relates to nutrition.
- Perform a nutritional assessment.
- Describe important facets of a nutritional assessment.
- Identify physiological and psychological factors that have nutritional implications.

- State the nurse's role in a nutritional assessment.
- Write appropriate nutritional nursing diagnoses.
- Identify steps in the planning phase.
- Describe possible nursing interventions that relate to nutritional implementation.
- Evaluate nutritional goals.
- Apply the nursing process to clients with alterations in nutritional status.
- Identify 3 referrals for nutrition support.

TEST YOUR NQ (True/False)

1. Assessment and interventions are the same thing.
2. Nutritional deficits can affect all systems of the body.
3. Teaching and referrals are examples of nutritional interventions.
4. The first step of the nursing process is diagnosis.
5. Clients need to participate in setting their nutritional goals.
6. Giving a client his or her meal tray is an example of planning.
7. Laboratory tests can be helpful in assessing nutritional status.
8. Evaluation of nutritional goals indicates whether interventions were successful or not.
9. A diet history involves eating with a client.
10. Nutritional referrals can be community or in-hospital.

The nursing process provides an orderly, systematic, and scientifically based approach to client care and is analogous to the scientific or problem-solving method. Thus, nursing care is based on a logical thought process rather than intuition or generalizations about clients.

The nursing process is composed of 5 components: assessment, diagnosis, planning, implementation, and evaluation. Even though the nurse always starts with assessment and works through to evaluation, the parts are interrelated. Therefore, the process is not linear; during assessment, evaluation can also be occurring (Fig. 11–1).

All the components are client-centered: the nurse assesses the client, diagnoses, plans, implements the collaborated plan, and evaluates the results with the client. Since the client is dynamic, the process has to be flexible in consideration of individual differences and changing health status. Any client may have an altered nutritional status; the nursing process can be adapted to assist the nurse in addressing both dietary and nutritional problems of clients.

The nurse, who has more "hands-on" time with clients than anyone else involved in their care, observes their physical and mental condition, listens to their problems, and fills most of their needs. Nurses are in a unique position to observe food intake, assess nutritional status, evaluate the response and attitudes of the client to diet therapy, and support the dietary teaching and regimen ordered. When facilities/clinics do not have a dietitian, a nurse shares the responsibility with a physician for meeting the client's nutritional needs and dietary counseling. A basic knowledge of nutrition enables the nurse to make sound assessments, to know when to make appropriate referrals, and to work effectively as a team member with dietitians.

What are the 5 steps of the nursing process? What are specific tasks nurses can do, because of their unique position, to assist in nutritional care of clients?

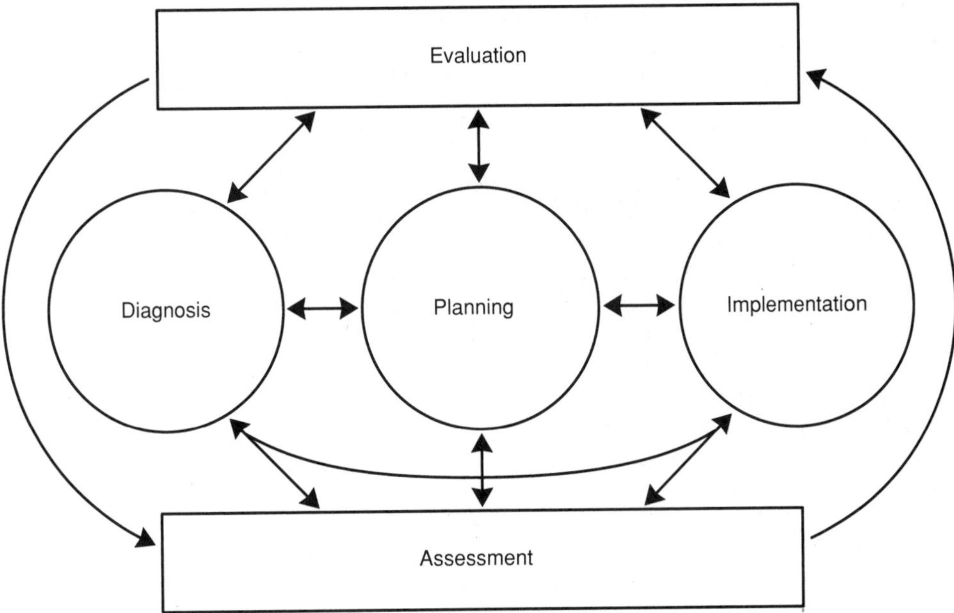

Figure 11–1 The nursing process: Each step is interrelated.

ASSESSMENT

Although **assessment** is the first step of the process, it is continuous. During assessment, the nurse gathers **subjective** and **objective** data from the client and other sources (charts, other health care members, significant others). The key to successful assessment is the acquisition of information in a manner that allows each succeeding step to be built on a solid foundation.

A nutritional assessment is used to determine **nutritional status.** Since many physical and laboratory findings can be secondary to another disease or condition, it is important that all aspects are considered to rule out other precipitating factors. For instance, hypoalbuminemia can be caused by an underlying illness, surgery, or a nutritional problem. Nutritional assessments on admission or soon thereafter are important in identifying clients who are at high risk of developing nutritional disruptions or who have actual nutritional problems (Kamath et al, 1986). Early implementation of nutrition support lowers costs associated with secondary complications that result in needless client suffering and sometimes fatal consequences. Therefore, both the hospital and clients experience benefit from optimal nutritional care.

Depending on the facility and its policies, the nutritional assessment may be completed by a nurse, **registered dietitian (RD),** or **dietetic technician (DTR).** Typical data gathered, which will help to determine adequacy of intake, absorption, or utilization and altered requirements, are shown in Figure 11–2. In most instances, nurses gather much of the data necessary for a nutritional assessment; this information must be coordinated with other team members for effective implementation of nutritional care.

Assessment—systematic, organized gathering of information about the client. Subjective data—cannot be verified by others; obtained through hearing what client or significant others say about their feelings and perceptions. Objective data—verified by others and confirmed via the senses, i.e., visual, tactile, or smell; involve findings from physical assessment and laboratory results. Nutritional status—condition of health as determined by evaluation of diet history, anthropometric measurements, physical examination, and laboratory data. An RD has been specifically trained in foods and nutrition with a BS degree and supervised work experience to interpret nutrition information. A DTR has an associate degree in nutrition care and food service management that combines academic instruction with clinical experience. What is the purpose of a nutritional assessment? Why are these assessments important? Who performs them?

Diet History

Subjective information gathered in a diet history can be used to determine nutritional adequacy of the client's usual intake (Table 11–1). In addition to actual foods eaten, factors influencing intake, such as other family members, economic

NUTRITION ASSESSMENT DATA

Nutritional History Information

Client's Name ____________________ Room Number ________

Age ________ Sex ________ Admission Date ____________

___ Yes ___ No 1. Have you lost more than 10 lbs. in the last 6 months without trying to lose weight? (Pediatrics, any weight loss)

___ Yes ___ No 2. Have you had a recent appetite loss causing you to miss meals for 5 days or more?

___ Yes ___ No 3. Is your appetite good? If not, please explain: ____________

___ Yes ___ No 4. Do you have daily problems with vomiting or diarrhea?

___ Yes ___ No 5. Do you have frequent problems with constipation? What have you used for this? ____________

___ Yes ___ No 6. Do you have problems with dry mouth?

___ Yes ___ No 7. (If wearing dentures): Do your dentures fit properly?

___ Yes ___ No 8. Have you experienced problems chewing or swallowing your food?

___ Yes ___ No 9. Do any foods disagree with you? Specify: ____________

10. Do you have any of the following medical conditions?

___ Yes ___ No a. Crohn's disease or ulcerative colitis?

___ Yes ___ No b. Chronic renal failure?

___ Yes ___ No c. Chronic liver disease?

___ Yes ___ No d. Cancer?

___ Yes ___ No e. Diabetes?

___ Yes ___ No f. Pressure sores?

___ Yes ___ No 11. Have you had surgery in the last month or a chronic illness lasting more than 3 weeks?

___ Yes ___ No 12. Have you had a temperature higher than 100.4° F for more than 3 days?

13. Are you presently restricting any of the following items in your diet?

___ Yes ___ No a. Salt?

___ Yes ___ No b. Sugar?

___ Yes ___ No c. Fat?

___ Yes ___ No d. Protein?

___ Yes ___ No e. Special (for example, food allergies)? Specify: ____________

14. Are you presently taking any of the following medications:

___ Yes ___ No a. Steroids? (Prednisone or cortisone)

___ Yes ___ No b. Antibiotics?

___ Yes ___ No c. Vitamins?

___ Yes ___ No d. Insulin?

Completed by: ____________

Relation to Client: ____________

Anthropometric Information

1. Height ________ inches (________ cm)
2. Weight ________ lbs. (________ kg)
3. Head circumference ________ cm

Completed by: ____________

Figure 11–2 Sample form for nutrition assessment data.

Laboratory Information

Serum albumin ____________ gm/dl
Serum transferrin ____________ mg/dl
Serum cholesterol ____________ mg/dl
Serum triglycerides ____________ mg/dl

Hemoglobin ____________ gm/dl
Hematocrit ____________%
White blood cell ____________ μl
Lymphocytes ____________%
Total Lymphocyte Count ____________

Summary:

____

____

Recommendations: ______________________________

Completed by: ____________

TABLE 11–1

DIET HISTORY

- I. Fluids
  - A. Usual fluid intake amount
  - B. Recent changes in amount (increased, decreased, or unchanged)
  - C. Beverage preferences
  - D. Frequency of intake
  - E. Beverages not tolerated
- II. Nutrition
  - A. Teeth/mouth
    1. Condition of teeth
    2. Dentures
    3. Chewing difficulties
    4. Soreness in mouth
    5. Difficulty in swallowing
    6. Problems with choking
    7. Recent changes in taste
  - B. Recent weight changes
  - C. Appetite/food preferences
    1. Recent appetite changes (increased, decreased, or unchanged)
    2. Favorite foods
    3. Foods disliked
    4. Foods not tolerated and why
    5. Food allergies
    6. Where meals are taken
    7. Who purchases and prepares the food
    8. Snacking habits
    9. Number of feedings daily
    10. Vitamin or mineral supplements
    11. Budgeting problems
    12. Alcohol intake (type and amount)
    13. Personal or religious restrictions (e.g., kosher or vegetarian)
  - D. Diet
    1. Type of special diet
    2. Problems or concerns with diet
- III. Gastrointestinal problems
  - A. Excessive belching or heartburn
  - B. Indigestion
  - C. Nausea
  - D. Vomiting
- IV. Elimination
  - A. Bowels
    1. Constipation or diarrhea
    2. Recent changes in bowel movements
    3. Frequency of bowel movements
    4. Use of laxatives or enemas or other practices
  - B. Difficulty of urination
    1. Recent changes (increased, decreased, or unchanged)
- V. Current medications

status, religion, culture, education, and social and recreational activities, are important in understanding overall dietary intake. Mobility, independence, and transportation indicate the client's ability to obtain and prepare foods. A knowledge of the client's occupation and daily activities can indicate general kilocaloric needs. Financial problems frequently have significant nutritional impact. The nurse attempts to determine what the client is eating and why specific foods are eaten. Other possible data must be assessed: concurrent disease, drugs, diagnostic tests, or genetic effects modifying a client's absorption, utilization, requirement, destruction, or excretion of nutrients. Most of these facts are generated from the diet history.

Ample time is allowed during the assessment for the client to ask questions and to present problems and frustrations. Mutual respect and understanding are necessary. Open-ended questions are asked in an indirect manner. (Rather than "What did you eat for breakfast yesterday?" ask, "Tell me when you first ate yesterday and what you ate.") Listening can be the most effective method to encourage the client to provide adequate information. However, questions may need to be inserted to keep the conversation on track and to obtain relevant or needed information. After obtaining a dietary pattern, identify some good things about the pattern and praise those things; negative and critical judgments about current practices are not helpful.

Emotional factors should not be ignored. Thorough questioning may reveal psychological handicaps to eating or food preparation; a depressed client may have no energy to eat.

In addition to revealing food preferences and quality and quantity of nutrients, a good diet history should disclose information regarding inadequate food and fluid intake, abnormal fluid losses, recent weight changes, and increased nutrient losses and requirements.

The diet history is important because the intake of foods and the interrelationships of diet, medications, lifestyle, and physiological/psychological conditions identified help to recognize actual or high-risk nutritional problems. If the nurse is skilled in collecting information and the client is reliable, the history can be extremely beneficial in assessing nutritional status. Additionally, information is obtained to help make recommendations and dietary changes that are workable and realistic for the client. Table 11–2 identifies risk factors that may be assessed in the client's diet history.

What is the purpose of a diet history? What types of data need to be assessed?

Dietary Intake

There are several techniques for determining actual and habitual dietary intake. This information can be collected by interview (recall) or by a record the client maintains. A nutrient intake record is used to provide a rough estimate of actual nutrient intake that can be compared with standards (RDA, food guide pyramid, Dietary Guidelines for Americans). Frequently, only key nutrients—kilocalories, protein, fat, dietary fiber, calcium, and vitamins A and C—may be used as indices to assess overall nutrient intake. Based on information from the second National Health and Nutrition Examination Survey, screening intake for food group consumption can provide meaningful information about nutrient quality of food intake (Kant et al, 1991). This minimizes time and expense involved in such studies.

In the 24-hour dietary recall, a record of all foods and amounts eaten for the previous day may be obtained by interview or by self-administered questionnaire.

The **dietary recall** or **food diary** is more precise than a diet history for determining intake for a short period. The 24-hour dietary recall is easier and quicker than other methods but less accurate than a food diary. It minimizes the risk of client's modifying intake to look good but is subject to accuracy of recall. Clients may need cues such as food models and measuring utensils to report actual amounts eaten accurately. For more valid information, a weekend day should be included in a food diary. Maintaining a food diary may be subject to changes from ordinary patterns but is useful in involving clients in behavioral strategies for changing eat-

TABLE 11–2

RISK FACTORS FOR NUTRITIONAL PROBLEMS

Diet history	
Chewing or swallowing difficulties (including ill-fitting dentures, dental caries, and missing teeth)	Inadequate food budget
Inadequate food intake	Inadequate food preparation facilities
Restricted or fad diets	Inadequate food storage facilities
No oral intake for 5 or more days	Physical disabilities
Intravenous fluids (glucose/saline solutions) for 7 or more days	Elderly living and eating alone
Medical history	
Overweight	Kidney disease
Underweight	GI problems (hiatal hernia, ulcers, lactose intolerance)
Recent weight loss or gain	Diabetes
Recent major illness	Thyroid or parathyroid disease
Recent major surgery	Adrenal disease
Surgery of the GI tract	Pancreatic insufficiency
Anorexia	Radiation therapy
Nausea/vomiting	Mental disability
Diarrhea/constipation	Teenage pregnancy
Alcoholism	Multiple pregnancies
Cancer	
Liver disease	
Medication history	
Aspirin	Antineoplastic agents
Antibiotics	Steroids
Antacid	Digitalis
Antidepressants	Laxatives
Antihypertensives	Diuretics (thiazides)
Anti-inflammatory agents	Potassium chloride
Warfarin sodium	Vitamin or other nutrient preparations
Anticonvulsants	

ing behaviors. The shorter period a diary is maintained, the less information will be revealed, but longer periods become too tedious, leading to noncompliance or poorly maintained records. Using either the dietary recall or food diary, totals of nutrients eaten are compared with a standard guide to determine the adequacy of the diet.

A food diary is maintained for 3 to 7 days and consists of a record of foods eaten, the amounts, method of preparation, where the food is eaten, and time of intake.

The **food frequency form** is also a quick method to assess adequacy of intake compared with the food groups. Approximately 40 to 80 types of foods may be listed. It is more of a descriptive assessment tool, as portion sizes are not indicated. This information can be easily analyzed and translated to estimate nutritional adequacy of the diet.

The food frequency form is a food checklist to ascertain the number of times per day, week, or month that specific foods or categories of foods are eaten.

Diet intake records or kilocalorie counts are frequently indicated for hospitalized clients for monitoring kilocalorie, protein, and other nutrient intake or for nitrogen balance tests. Accuracy is important for valid conclusions. In most facilities, nursing staff is responsible for documenting the amounts/percentage of each food eaten for evaluation by the dietitian/dietetic technician. All foods eaten within the designated time period should be documented, including foods provided by family and friends and snacks. These data may be used to justify more aggressive nutritional support or its withdrawal. This intake record is not appropriate for determining adequacy of intake outside the facility.

What is the difference between dietary recall and a food diary? What is the nurse's responsibility for kilocalorie counts?

Anthropometric Measurements

Anthropometric measurements are human body measurements that provide an objective assessment that can be compared with established standards.

Appropriateness of weight is normally determined by **anthropometric measurements.** These measurements are used to compare a client's value with a nor-

Malnutrition is due to faulty nourishment from a deficiency, imbalance, or excess of nutrients. Nutritional deficiencies can be a deficit of energy and/or nutrients. Overnutrition is an excess of 1 or more nutrients; kilocalories are most frequently consumed in excessive amounts.

What body components should nurses assess? What should be measured directly for all clients?

mal value to identify adequate nutritional status or **malnutrition** and to detect loss or gain of body components relative to previous measurements.

Body components of interest include height, weight, lean body mass, and fat stores. Height and weight are important parameters that should be measured directly and accurately for all clients. Many methods can be used to determine appropriate body weight. In children, physical growth (height and weight) is one of the best indicators of nutritional adequacy. Growth charts for infants and children are discussed in Chapter 15.

Height

Height and weight can be obtained from the client or family if direct measurements are impossible, but these are usually inaccurate (Rowland, 1990). A fixed measuring guide attached to a vertical flat surface, such as a wall, is a more accurate measurement of height than the measuring rod on platform scales. A movable right-angle headboard is lowered onto the crown of the head. The client is measured standing as straight as possible, with bare or stocking feet close together, legs straight, shoulders relaxed, looking straight ahead. As the client takes a deep breath, the height is recorded to the nearest 0.1 cm or ⅛ inch. Two measurements made in immediate succession should be within 1 cm or ½ inch.

Any significant spinal curvature present should be noted. The curvature of the spine should not be measured but rather a straight line through the trunk area, which is accomplished by the client standing as straight and tall as possible.

If the client is unable to stand upright without assistance, other methods are used to determine height. Knee height changes little with increasing age and is commonly used. While lying supine, the length between the left knee and ankle is measured (both joints are at a 90-degree angle) with a sliding broad-blade caliper. Using the client's knee height, sex, and age, body height can be calculated:

How should height be measured? If the client is unable to stand, how should height be measured?

$$\text{Male} = 64.19 - [0.04 \times \text{age (yr)}] + [2.02 \times \text{knee ht (cm)}]$$

$$\text{Female} = 84.88 - [0.24 \times \text{age (yr)}] + [1.83 \times \text{knee ht (cm)}]$$

Weight

Body weight is one of the most expedient and helpful indicators of nutritional status. Although weight is considered the cornerstone of a good nutritional assessment, accurate weights are frequently the most difficult parameter to obtain. It is a nonspecific measure of all body components, including fat, protein, and water. An accurate weight can be compared with standards to determine whether the client is overweight, normal, or underweight.

Because of its significance in assessing nutritional status, care must be taken to obtain accurate weights. All scales should be professionally calibrated at least semiannually in addition to adjustment of the 0 balance on the horizontal beam of the scale before each use. Use of calibrated lever-balance or beam balance scales that are appropriate for the client's mobility status is important. In a clinic setting, clothing should be minimal without shoes. Clients in the hospital should be weighed at the same time of day, preferably before breakfast and after voiding. Wheelchair scales are used if the client is able to sit (Fig. 11–3); bed scales are necessary for bedridden clients. By checking current weight against the previous weight, weighing technique errors can be spotted and corrected immediately. For clients who are weighed daily, consistency of the following practices results in more accurate weight: same time of day, clothing, and scales.

What is one of the most helpful indicators of nutritional status? What 3 factors should stay consistent to obtain accurate weights?

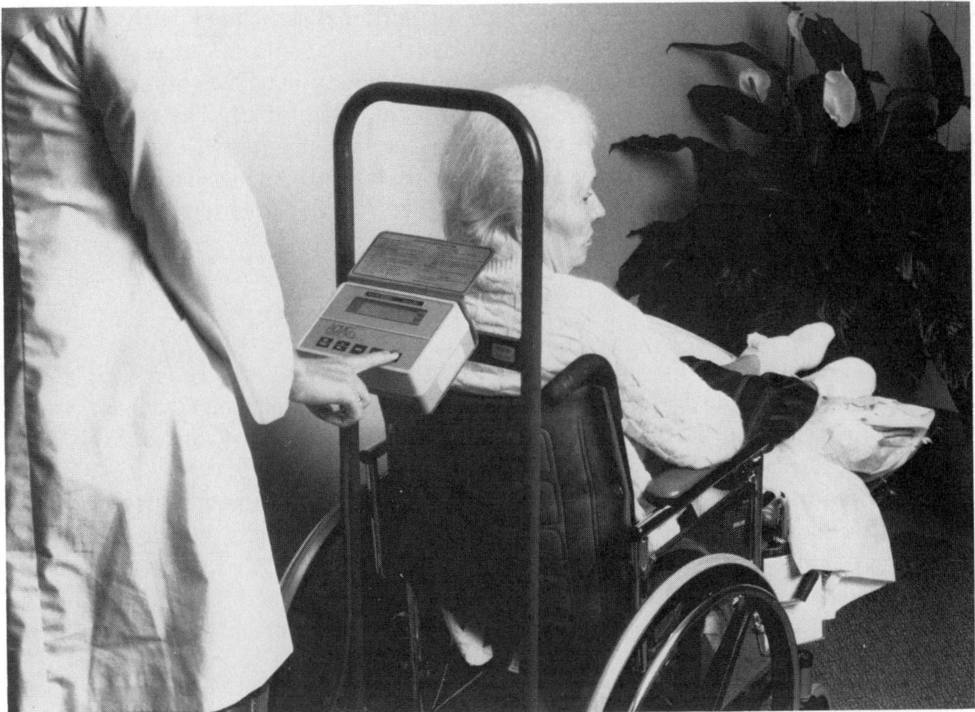

Figure 11–3 Wheelchair scale. Use an appropriate scale for client's mobility status.

Frame

Since weight is directly related to bone structure, frame size is another aspect that must be considered when determining appropriate weight. In the development of the Metropolitan Life Insurance Tables, frame size was not measured. These weights were derived from estimates of the population proportions having varying frame sizes.

The simplest technique for determining frame size is determined by wrist measurement. The wrist is measured at its smallest circumference distal to the styloid process of the radius and ulna (Fig. 11–4) and then classified as shown in Appendix C–4.

Height and Weight Tables

Height-weight tables developed by the life insurance companies, such as the Metropolitan Height and Weight Table, are widely used (see Appendix C–1). Life insurance height-weight charts were developed to predict mortality on the basis of

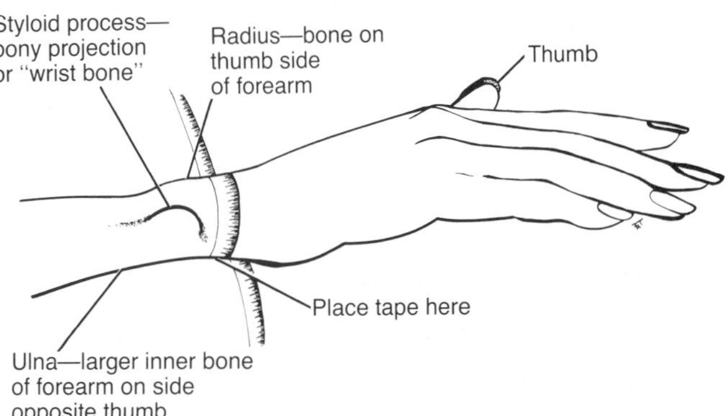

Figure 11–4 Measurement of wrist circumference to determine frame size.

weight and are not predictive of medical conditions associated with increased weight. They can best be used as a screening tool in a nutritional assessment since such information as body fat and edema are not identified. Weights in the 1985 standards are heavier for a given height than in the 1959 tables. The relatively low 1959 Metropolitan weights may be more appropriate for clients with other risk factors such as hypertension or diabetes mellitus (Schulz, 1986). Deviations from the ideal body weight (IBW) indicate the degree of depletion or overweight.

$$\frac{\text{actual weight}}{\text{IBW}} \times 100 = \%\ \text{IBW}$$

Table 11–3 indicates the classification of these deviations. To re-emphasize, weights or classification of weight based solely on weight and height do not reflect body fat or hydration status and are limited in their reliability for making judgments about health status.

What can deviations from the normal IBW indicate? What are drawbacks of using standard weight-height tables for nutritional assessments?

Another drawback of the standard weight-height tables is the lack of age-specific information. In the US, weights of both sexes gradually increase from age 20 until after age 50 to 60, when they begin to decline. With increasing age, fat stores increase with loss of lean body mass. Energy requirements established by the NRC are based on weights that are age-related. Whether normal weight should remain the same as age advances is unclear.

Calculation of Desirable Body Weight

In the health field, an easy popular tool is used to estimate desirable weight:

Women — 100 lbs for the first 60 in. (5 ft). Add 5 lbs for each additional inch over 60 in.

Men — 106 lbs for the first 60 in. (5 ft). Add 6 lbs for each additional inch over 60 in.

What is a quick method to determine desirable weight for women and men?

An additional 10% is added or subtracted for large or small frame, respectively. For paraplegics, 5 to 10% is subtracted, and for quadriplegics, 10 to 15% is subtracted. Again, these are unscientific measures and can provide only an estimate of appropriate weight.

Body Mass Index

BMI is calculated by dividing weight in kilograms by the square of height in meters.

Body mass index (BMI) estimates total body mass but shows the highest correlation with actual body fat (Revicki & Israel, 1986). BMI minimizes the effect of height and is useful for descriptive and comparison purposes. Classification of BMI is shown in Appendix C–2. As shown in Figure 11–5, a BMI between 20 and 25 is an acceptable weight for height. A BMI of 25 to 30 kg/m^2 is approximately 20% above desirable. Although this is classified as obesity, clients are at low risk for health problems. Clients with BMIs between 35 and 40 are at high risk, and those with a BMI greater than 40 kg/m^2 have a very high risk (Bray, 1992). These numbers correlate well with normal mortality ratios derived from life insurance tables.

TABLE 11–3

CLASSIFICATION OF WEIGHT BASED ON DEVIATIONS FROM IDEAL BODY WEIGHT

% Ideal Body Weight	Indication
> 120	Obesity
110–120	Moderately overweight
80–90	Moderate depletion
< 70	Severe depletion

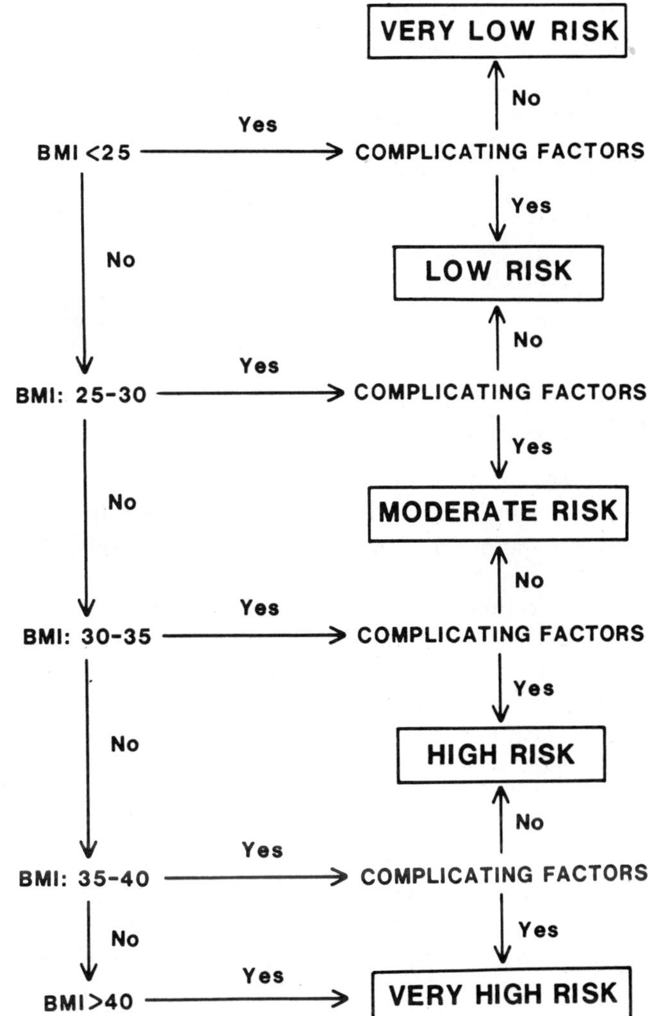

Figure 11–5 Risk classification algorithm. The client is first placed into a category based on body mass index. The presence or absence of complicating factors determines the degree of health risk. Complicating factors include elevated abdominal to gluteal ratio (male = 0.95, female = 0.85), diabetes mellitus, hypertension, hyperlipidemia, male sex, and age less than 40 years. (From Bray GA. Classification and evaluation of the obesities. *Med Clin North Am* 1989; 73(1): 161–183. Copyright George A. Bray, 1987.)

BMIs less than 20 for men or 19 for women, classified as underweight (Bray, 1990), are associated with risk factors such as respiratory disease, tuberculosis, digestive disease, and some cancers. Again, the major weakness of the use of BMIs is the lack of distinction between heaviness resulting from adiposity and muscularity and edema.

Weight Loss

Weight loss can be an ominous sign, indicating use of lean body mass (muscle and organ tissue) for energy. If fluid loss is not significant, weight loss is a better indicator of current nutritional status; it reflects loss of vital body protein stores (muscle and organ tissue) for energy. This occurs rapidly when kilocaloric intake is grossly inadequate. During a high-stress condition, and especially if IV dextrose solutions are being administered, protein stores are catabolized. Weight status may be maintained, falsely indicating adequate nutrition, because water and collagen replace fat and muscle tissue being catabolized. This common finding in PEM occurs particularly in obese clients.

What does weight loss indicate? Why may weight status be maintained even though protein is being catabolized? What do daily weights reflect? What is a significant weight loss?

The rate of weight loss is important (Table 11–4). Very rapid weight loss indicates more severe nutritional consequences. For nutritional assessment, a 10% involuntary weight loss over a 6- to 12-month period or 5% in 1 month is significant. Daily weight fluctuations reflect body fluid changes. Trends over a period of time are more helpful for indicating nutritional status.

TABLE 11–4

EVALUATION OF WEIGHT CHANGE

Time	Significant Weight Loss (%)	Severe Weight Loss (%)
1 wk	1 to 2	>2
1 mo	5	>5
3 mo	7.5	>7.5
6 mo	10	>10

$$\text{Percent weight change} = \frac{(\text{Usual weight} - \text{Actual weight})}{\text{Usual weight}} \times 100$$

From Blackburn GL, Thornton PA. Nutritional and metabolic assessment of the hospitalized patient. *JPEN* 1977 Jan–Feb; 1(1):11–22.

Skinfold Measurements

Why can skinfold thickness indicate energy reserves?

Assessment techniques can help confirm or discredit visual appraisals. The amount of body fat, indirectly measured by skinfold measurements, is also an indirect indicator of previous kilocaloric balance (intake versus requirement). Since 50% of fat stores are subcutaneous, the skinfold thickness indicates energy reserves. Special skinfold calipers are required for this technique. Triceps and subscapular skinfold measurements are most commonly used. Three consecutive measurements at each site are averaged. The nondominant arm is normally measured (Fig. 11–6). Percentiles for triceps skinfold (TSF) are shown in Appendix C–6. Body fat increases with age, but the sum of skinfold measurements remains constant, indicating that fat accumulates at other than subcutaneous sites.

Mid-Arm Circumference

Somatic proteins include all skeletal muscles. MAC is an index of the arm's total area and reflects kilocaloric adequacy.

MAMC is a measurement of protein stores or the amount of muscle.

Body fat and **somatic proteins** are assessed by **mid-arm circumference (MAC)** (see Fig. 11–6). Using a mathematical equation, the amount of subcutaneous fat (measured by skinfold thickness) can be subtracted from the MAC to estimate the lean tissue in the arm, called the **mid-arm muscle circumference (MAMC).** This can also be determined by using the nomogram in Appendix C–5. MAMC correlates well with other estimates of body protein status, such as serum albumin.

What is the difference between MAC and MAMC?

Disuse atrophy, common in clients confined to bed, produces changes similar to those seen when muscles are catabolized for energy and must be considered. Visual observation of muscle in the scapular, pelvic, and calf areas may indicate muscle wastage. Percentiles of MAC and MAMC are in Appendix C–7.

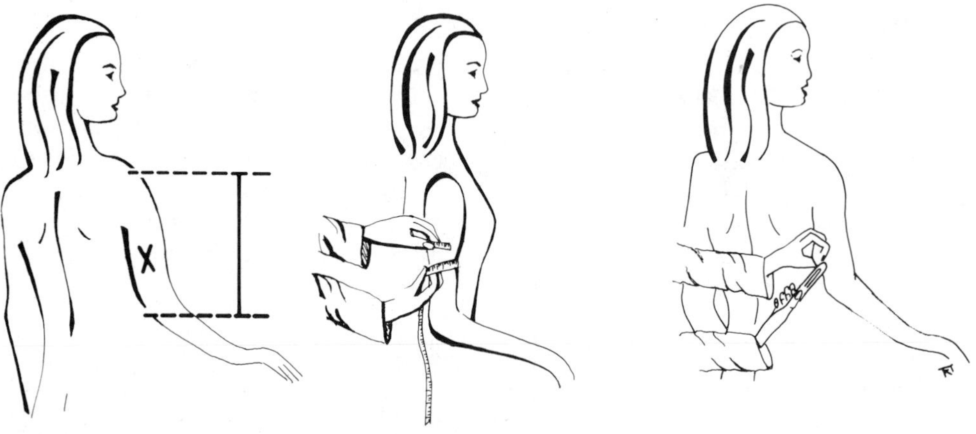

(1) Measure and mark mid-point (2) Measure circumference of mid-upper arm (3) Measure skin-fold thickness of triceps

Figure 11–6 Measuring mid-arm circumference and triceps skin-fold thickness.

Physical Assessment

A physical assessment can reveal existing nutritional deficiencies (Table 11–5). However, signs of malnutrition are often nonspecific; different problems may produce the same specific clinical finding. For this reason, clinical findings must correlate with other assessment parameters, laboratory data, and diet history. Losses of protein and fat stores are usually accompanied by vitamin and mineral depletion.

Signs of malnutrition are most frequently evident in the skin, eyes, mouth, skeleton, and nervous system (see Table 11–5). A close look at these areas is important for a thorough assessment. Even well-nourished clients can develop nutritional problems in a short time: PEM may evolve within 2 weeks; water-soluble vitamin deficiencies may be seen in 1 to 2 months. Mineral deficiencies (iron, calcium, magnesium, and zinc) accompany stress situations and anorexia. Even though this occurs rapidly, it is not the result of a client's not eating properly for 1 day; it is a reflection of improper long-term nutritional habits or a stressful condition. Clinical assessment and judgments are as important as any test but should be used concurrently with dietary and biochemical assessments.

How long does it take for PEM or water-soluble vitamin deficiencies to develop?

TABLE 11–5

CLINICAL NUTRITION EXAMINATION

Clinical Findings	Consider Deficiency of*	Consider Excess of	Frequency†
Hair, nails			
Flag sign (transverse depigmentation of hair)	Protein		Rare
Easily pluckable hair	Protein		Common
Sparse hair	Protein, biotin, zinc	Vitamin A	Occasional
Corkscrew hairs and unemerged coiled hairs	Vitamin C		Common
Transverse ridging of nails	Protein		Occasional
Skin			
Scaling	Vitamin A, zinc, essential fatty acids	Vitamin A	Occasional
Cellophane appearance	Protein		Occasional
Cracking (flaky paint or crazy pavement dermatosis)	Protein		Rare
Follicular hyperkeratosis	Vitamins A, C		Occasional
Petechiae (especially perifollicular)	Vitamin C		Occasional
Purpura	Vitamins C, K		Common
Pigmentation, desquamation of sun-exposed areas	Niacin		Rare
Yellow pigmentation sparing sclerae (benign)		Carotene	Common
Eyes			
Papilledema		Vitamin A	Rare
Night blindness	Vitamin A		Rare
Perioral			
Angular stomatitis	Riboflavin, pyridoxine, niacin		Occasional
Cheilosis (dry, cracking, ulcerated lips)	Riboflavin, pyridoxine, niacin		Rare
Oral			
Atrophic lingual papillae (slick tongue)	Riboflavin, niacin, folate, vitamin B_{12}, protein, iron		Common
Glossitis (scarlet, raw tongue)	Riboflavin, niacin, pyridoxine, folate, vitamin B_{12}		Occasional
Hypogeusesthesia, hyposmia	Zinc		Occasional
Swollen, retracted, bleeding gums (if teeth are present)	Vitamin C		Occasional

Table continued on following page

TABLE 11–5

CLINICAL NUTRITION EXAMINATION
Continued

Clinical Findings	Consider Deficiency of*	Consider Excess of	Frequency†
Bones, joints			
Beading of ribs, epiphyseal swelling, bowlegs	Vitamin D		Rare
Tenderness (subperiosteal hemorrhage in child)	Vitamin C		Rare
Neurological			
Headache		Vitamin A	Rare
Drowsiness, lethargy, vomiting		Vitamins A, D	Rare
Dementia	Niacin, vitamin B_{12}		Rare
Confabulation, disorientation	Thiamin (Korsakoff's psychosis)		Occasional
Ophthalmoplegia	Thiamin, phosphorus		Occasional
Peripheral neuropathy (e.g., weakness, paresthesias, ataxia, and decreased tendon reflexes, fine tactile sense, vibratory sense, and position sense)	Thiamin, pyridoxine, vitamin B_{12}	Pyridoxine	Occasional
Tetany	Calcium, magnesium		Occasional
Other			
Parotid enlargement	Protein (consider also bulimia)		Occasional
Heart failure	Thiamin ("wet" beriberi), phosphorus		Occasional
Sudden heart failure, death	Vitamin C		Rare
Hepatomegaly	Protein	Vitamin A	Rare
Edema	Protein, thiamin		Common
Poor wound healing, decubitus ulcers	Protein, vitamin C, zinc		Common

* In this table, "protein deficiency" is used to signify kwashiorkor.
† These frequencies are an attempt to reflect the authors' experience in the setting of a US medical practice. Findings common in other countries but virtually unseen in usual medical practice settings in the US (e.g., xerophthalmia and endemic goiter) are not listed.
From Weinsier AL, et al. *Handbook of Clinical Nutrition.* 2nd ed. St. Louis, CV Mosby, 1989.

Laboratory Information

Laboratory data provide objective information for nutritional status and are warranted especially if the diet history is questionable or unavailable. Laboratory findings are remarkably accurate, indicating existing and potential problems. However, use of laboratory assessments requires knowledge of the purpose of each test, awareness of normal values, and knowledge of other factors that may cause abnormalities. Marginal nutritional deficiencies can be detected before overt clinical signs appear. A thorough inspection of laboratory values sometimes reveals a direct relationship between a client's diet and his or her physical condition. In general, clinical and dietary assessments can be substantiated from laboratory data by confirming suspicions or indicating possible causes (Fig. 11–7).

Biochemical indicators of nutritional status use blood and urine analyses. Urine is routinely checked for specific gravity, protein, glucose, pH, and acetone. As a general rule, urinary excretion levels fluctuate more than serum levels, reflecting recent rather than usual intake.

What do urinary excretion levels indicate? What can be assessed to determine electrolyte balance, carbohydrate metabolism, and lipid metabolism?

Laboratory tests for hemoglobin, hematocrit, total protein, serum albumin or prealbumin, and total lymphocyte count (TLC) collectively reflect protein nutriture. Determinations of sodium and potassium, glucose, and cholesterol and triglyceride levels are indicative of electrolyte balance, carbohydrate metabolism, and lipid metabolism, respectively. These tests are discussed in therapeutic chapters with the

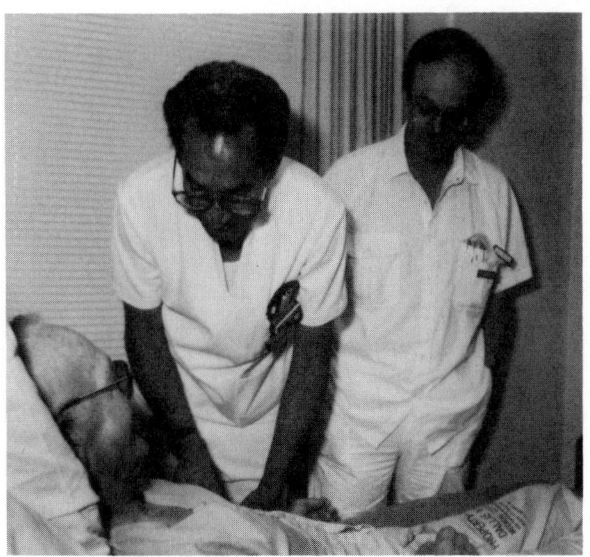

Figure 11–7 Nurses taking a blood sample as part of a nutrition investigation at the Dallas Veterans Administration Medical Association. (Courtesy of Eugene R. Davies.)

disease or condition in which abnormalities are normally observed. Routine laboratory tests used for determining nutritional status are shown in Table 11–6.

Vitamin Levels

Although some mineral (calcium, chloride, phosphorus, magnesium) levels are easy to determine, elaborate testing techniques are required for determining most vitamin and other mineral levels. These tests are expensive, and many hospitals are

TABLE 11–6

ROUTINE LABORATORY TESTS USED IN NUTRITIONAL ASSESSMENT

Test Normal Values	Nutritional Use	Causes of Normal Value Despite Malnutrition	Other Causes of Abnormal Value
Serum albumin 3.5 to 5.5 gm/dl	2.8 to 3.5—Compromised protein status < 2.8—Possible kwashiorkor Increasing value reflects positive nitrogen balance	Dehydration Infusion of albumin, fresh frozen plasma, or whole blood	*Low* Common— Infection and other stress, especially with poor protein intake Burns, trauma Congestive heart failure Fluid overload Severe hepatic insufficiency Uncommon—Nephrotic syndrome Zinc deficiency Bacterial overgrowth of small bowel
Total iron binding capacity 270 to 400 mcg/dl	< 200—Compromised protein status, possible kwashiorkor Increasing value reflects positive nitrogen balance More labile than albumin	Iron deficiency	*Low* Similar to albumin *High* Iron deficiency
Prothrombin time < 2 sec beyond "Control," or 70 to 100% of "Control" activity	Prolongation—Vitamin K deficiency		*Prolonged* Anticoagulant therapy—Warfarin (Coumadin) Severe liver disease

Table continued on following page

TABLE 11–6

ROUTINE LABORATORY TESTS USED IN NUTRITIONAL ASSESSMENT *Continued*

Test Normal Values	Nutritional Use	Causes of Normal Value Despite Malnutrition	Other Causes of Abnormal Value
Serum creatinine 0.6 to 1.6 mg/dl	< 0.6—Muscle wasting due to kilocalorie deficiency Reflects muscle mass		*High* Despite muscle wasting: Renal failure Severe dehydration
24-hr urinary creatinine 500–1200 mg/day (standardized for height and sex)	Low value—Muscle wasting due to kilocalorie deficiency	> 24-hr collection Decreasing serum creatinine	*Low* Incomplete urine collection Increasing serum creatinine Muscle wasting resulting from paralytic atrophy
24-hr UUN < 5 g/day—depends on level of protein intake	Determine level of catabolism (as long as protein intake is ≥ 10 mg below calculated protein loss) 5 to 10 gm/day = mild catabolism (e.g., after elective surgery) 10 to 15 gm/day = moderate catabolism (e.g., in infection, major surgery) > 15 gm/day = severe catabolism (e.g., in severe sepsis, major burns) Estimate protein balance Protein balance = Protein intake − Protein loss where Protein loss = (24-hr UUN (gm) + 4) × 6.25 Exception—Adjustment required in burn clients and others with large nonurinary nitrogen losses		*Low* Active fluid retention Increasing BUN Incomplete urine collection *High* High protein intake Corticosteroid therapy Active diuresis Decreasing BUN > 24-hr urine collection GI bleeding
BUN 8 to 23 mg/dl	< 8—Possibly inadequate protein intake > 12—Possibly adequate, even excessive, protein intake If serum creatinine is normal, use BUN If serum creatinine is elevated, use BUN/creatinine ratio		*Low* Severe liver disease Anabolic state *High* Despite poor protein intake: Renal failure (use BUN/creatinine ratio) Congestive heart failure GI hemorrhage Corticosteroid therapy Dehydration Shock
TLC* > 1500/mm³	< 1500—Possible immunocompromise associated with protein-energy malnutrition, especially kwashiorkor Significant limitation—marked day to day fluctuation		*Low* Severe stress, e.g., infections, with "left shift" Corticosteroid therapy Renal failure Cancer, e.g., colon *High* Despite malnutrion: Infections Leukemia, myeloma Cancer, e.g., stomach, breast Adrenal insufficiency

* TLC = white blood cell count × % lymphocytes.
From Weinsier RL, et al. *Handbook of Clinical Nutrition.* 2nd ed. St. Louis, CV Mosby, 1989.

TABLE 11–7

ASSESSMENT OF VISCERAL PROTEINS

Protein	Function	Half-Life	Normal	Degree of Malnutrition		
				Mild	*Moderate*	*Severe*
Albumin (gm/dl)	Carrier protein; maintains colloid osmotic pressure	21 days	> 3.5	3–3.5	2.5–3	< 2.5
Transferrin (mg/dl)	Transports iron	8–10 days	> 200	180–200	160–180	< 160
Prealbumin (mg/dl)	Transports thyroxin and retinol-binding protein	2–3 days	> 15	10–15	5–10	< 5
Total lymphocyte count (mm³)	Reflects immune status		> 1500	1200–1500	800–1200	< 800

not equipped to evaluate them on a routine basis. Some tests include those for urinary thiamin, riboflavin, vitamin B_{12} and N′-methylnicotinamide (niacin), and serum levels for carotene and vitamins A and C. Dietary deficiency of a vitamin results in decreased excretion (or conservation) before laboratory changes or physical signs of deficiency are evident. By early detection of vitamin deficiency from laboratory tests, more serious complications can be prevented.

Protein Levels

Laboratory evaluation of protein status can be determined by several tests: serum proteins and 24-hour urine urea nitrogen excretion. **Visceral protein** stores are reflected in serum albumin, transferrin, and prealbumin levels (Table 11–7). Plasma proteins are affected by stress and renal and hepatic disease. Albumin, synthesized in the liver, transports small molecules (including many medications, hormones, and vitamins) and provides 70% of **colloid osmotic pressure** of plasma. When colloid osmotic pressure decreases, peripheral edema may develop. A low colloid osmotic pressure in the intestinal villa leads to decreased absorption of nutrients. Albumin levels are more stable and correlate better with changes in MAMC. Low serum levels indicate rate of synthesis, catabolism, loss into interstitial fluids, and abnormal external loss in some cases (Table 11–8). Clients with depressed serum albumin levels (< 3.4 gm/dl) on hospital admission have longer stays and are more likely to die (Herrmann et al, 1992).

Visceral protein stores are all body proteins, i.e., those in internal organs and blood, other than muscle tissue.

Colloid osmotic pressure is affected by nondiffusable particles, especially protein, that influence the force that pulls water through a semipermeable membrane toward the more concentrated solution.

TABLE 11–8

FACTORS THAT AFFECT RELIABILITY OF SERUM ALBUMIN LEVELS AS A NUTRITIONAL MARKER

Hydration status (dehydration falsely elevates level; FVE may depress levels)
Abnormal capillary loss of albumin (caused by surgery or other trauma)
Protein depletion caused by albumin loss (burns, some types of renal disease)
Liver dysfunction (depressed synthesis)
Pregnancy (related to FVE)
Bed rest (FVE causes a concurrent decreased level)
Long half-life (21 days)
Chronic malnutrition (remains relatively high)

FVE = fluid volume excess.

Anergy is a decreased reaction to specific antigens.

Serum transferrin and albumin levels are closely correlated. Serum albumin is a good indicator of long-term nutritional status if there is no current illness or condition. However, transferrin, an iron-carrying protein, has a shorter half-life, and its measurement is more sensitive of current status. Low levels indicate protein deficiency, which is accompanied by increased risks of **anergy,** sepsis, and mortality. Although low levels of albumin do place the client at increased risk, physiological stress such as infection or surgery may also cause low albumin and transferrin levels. Malnutrition is not indicated, but clients need adequate nutrition support to prevent further decreases. Significant physiological stress causes protein levels to remain low.

Prealbumin is more sensitive for recent nutritional problems and correlates better with nitrogen balance than albumin or transferrin (Rammohan & Juan, 1989; Winkler et al, 1989). Thus a prealbumin level is a better indicator of visceral protein anabolism.

A 24-hour urine urea nitrogen (UUN) clearance test can be used to determine the extent of protein catabolism and adequacy of protein intake. Urea is the major waste product of protein catabolism. (Ammonia, a toxic substance, is changed to urea in the liver and excreted in the urine.) In catabolic clients (negative nitrogen balance), protein breakdown is much higher than rates of synthesis; approximately three-fourths of the ingested nitrogen is excreted. The following formula is used to calculate estimated nitrogen balance (ENB):

$$\text{ENB} = \frac{\text{protein input (gm)}}{6.25} - [\text{24-hr UUN (gm)} + 4]$$

What do low levels of albumin indicate? Which is more sensitive of current nutritional status: albumin or transferrin? What is a better indicator of visceral protein anabolism?

To determine protein and kilocaloric adequacy, an estimate of protein intake (preferably over the previous 2 or 3 days) is necessary. A 3-day average, using the preceding formula, should be positive by more than 0.04 gm of nitrogen/kg/day to assure positive nitrogen balance. If the value obtained is a negative number, more protein is needed.

Immunological Testing

Assessment may also include measuring immune response. Two different types of laboratory tests are used: TLC and skin antigen testing.

Total Lymphocyte Count

The immune status is reflected in the TLC. A depressed TLC predisposes clients to infection. TLC can be calculated from the complete white blood count (WBC) and the percentage of lymphocytes by using the following formula:

$$\text{TLC} = \text{percent of lymphocytes (use decimal)} \times \text{WBC}$$

What range indicates moderate nutritional problems; what range indicates severe nutritional problems?

Moderate nutritional problems are characterized by a TLC between 800 and 1200 mm^3 (see Table 11–7). Below 800 mm^3, clients are considered to be severely malnourished and anergic. TLC is affected by many medical conditions and fluctuates significantly.

Skin Antigen Testing

Intradermal skin tests of recall antigen-mumps, *Candida albicans,* and streptokinase-streptodornase (SK-SD) are administered to determine cellular immune response. The tuberculin skin test may be used as a control. A healthy client will have a response within 24 hours; the malnourished client may have a delayed or no response. Numerous factors commonly observed in critically ill clients can alter cutaneous hypersensitivity; therefore, this testing has fallen in disfavor as a critical assessment tool.

Nutrition Screening

Because of the emphasis on cost containment, unnecessary tests and measurements or elaborate dietary histories are discouraged. However, all clients should be interviewed within 24 hours after admission with a simple, brief but effective screening procedure to identify those who need more intensive nutritional work-up (Roubenoff et al, 1987). The goal of **nutrition screening** is to identify clients who may benefit from nutritional intervention and thereby decrease length of hospitalization. Table 11–9 lists commonly available information and routines that provide minimal nutrition screening. Each institution organizes the screening process to use

Both nutrition screening and nutrition assessment evaluate indicators related to client outcomes, such as length of stay, complication rate, and death. However, screening indicators must meet stringent cost and time criteria.

TABLE 11–9

MINIMAL SCREENING OF NUTRITIONAL STATUS

	Medical and Socioeconomic	Dietary	Anthropometric Measurements	Clinical Evaluation	Laboratory Evaluation
Infants	Birth weight Length of gestation	Bottle- or breast-fed Supplemental feedings (fluids, solids, method of preparation, weaning, self-feeding) Source of iron Vitamin supplements	Weight Length Overall rate of growth Head circumference	Skin color, turgor Malformations	Hematocrit Hemoglobin
Children	Birth weight Chronic/recent illness Physical activity	Food intake* Appetite Feeding jags, pica Snacking habits Vitamin/mineral supplements Arrangements for eating away from home	Weight Height Arm circumference Overall rate of growth	Skin color, turgor Muscle tone Subcutaneous fat Dental caries	Hematocrit Hemoglobin BUN
Adolescents	Medical history/allergies Socioeconomic data Physical activity Family history Medications	Food intake* (assess for excessive salt or sugar) Where and when foods are eaten Snacking habits Fad diets (especially girls) Vitamin/mineral supplements Alcohol intake	Weight Height Recent weight changes	General appearance of hair, skin, eyes Muscle tone Subcutaneous fat Dental caries	Hemoglobin Urine protein Blood glucose
Adults	Medical history Age Number in family Socioeconomic data Physical activity Family history Medications	Food intake* (assess for saturated fat, cholesterol, sugar, salt; iron and calcium in women) Snacking habits Vitamin/mineral supplements Alcohol intake	Weight Height Recent weight changes	General appearance and maintenance of hair, skin, eyes, muscles Dental caries Blood pressure	Hemoglobin Albumin Transferrin Blood glucose Urinary pH Cholesterol
Elderly persons	Chronic illness or disability Use of tobacco, alcohol, drugs Source of income; amount for food Any physical changes (bleeding, bowel/urinary patterns, fainting, headaches)	Food intake* and patterns Supplements (protein, vitamins, minerals) Who purchases and prepares food Changes in food habits Taste changes Dietary restrictions	Weight Height Recent weight changes	Skin color, pallor Blood pressure Dentition	Hemoglobin Blood glucose Urinalysis Feces

* Question about the frequency of use of foods in the Food Guide Pyramid.

the expertise of personnel as appropriate. The ultimate goal is to make use of the limited time of all personnel and provide adequate nutritional care to clients. In most instances, nurses gather much of the data necessary for a nutrition screening.

A client should be referred to the dietitian or metabolic specialist for further assessment of any of the following conditions:

1. A recent weight loss of more than 5%.
2. A low serum albumin and transferrin level.
3. Low TLC or immune function.

DIAGNOSIS

Diagnosis is the step in which client problems and strengths are identified.

The nurse analyzes and interprets gathered data to form a nursing **diagnosis.** Since nurses make inferences from the data, it is imperative that they (1) be able to differentiate normal from abnormal, (2) not draw conclusions based on inadequate data, and (3) not approach data gathering or the analysis of the data with preconceived notions about the client's status.

A nursing diagnosis is a statement of an actual or high-risk health problem within the scope (legally and educationally) of nursing practice (Gordon, 1987). Thus, in nutrition, a nursing diagnosis is a description of an actual or high-risk nutritional problem in which the nurse is licensed to initiate treatments. Nursing diagnoses are composed of 3 parts: problem; its etiology, or cause; and signs and symptoms. This is referred to as the PES format (Alfaro, 1990; Gordon, 1987). The components, problem and etiology, are joined together by the words "related to" (RT). The signs and symptoms are validating data for the problem. The signs and symptoms are connected to the nursing diagnosis with the words "as evidenced by" (AEB). One example of nutrition/dietary nursing diagnosis is altered nutrition: more than body requirements RT imbalance of intake versus activity expenditure AEB, weight 110% above IBW, and client statements, "I hate exercising" and "Food is my only enjoyment in life." Other nursing diagnoses are listed in Table 11–10. Since signs and symptoms are specific to each client's situation, only the 2-part nursing diagnosis (problem and etiology) is used in this text.

In many instances, the problem is collaborative; the nurse must collaborate with someone of another discipline. Collaborative problems focus on physiological complications the client may experience. The nurse's role is to monitor, detect, and manage these complications (Carpenito, 1991). In the acute care setting, collaboration with many disciplines, especially food service and dietitians, or a multidisciplinary team is essential for optimal client care (Table 11–11). Team members support one another not only to ask for help from others, but also to offer their advice and expertise. Mutual respect and an understanding of each other's roles, capabilities, and responsibilities are essential for optimal client care.

PLANNING

Client goals/outcomes are the healthy alternatives to the diagnoses/problem state. The expected goals are the guideposts that identify whether the problem is resolved or reduced.

The planning stage involves 3 steps: (1) setting priorities, (2) determining **client goals,** and (3) writing a care plan. Setting priorities means addressing life-threatening diagnoses first. If none are life-threatening, some factors to consider in deciding which diagnosis to approach first include (1) the diagnosis causing the most concern or hardship for the client; (2) which diagnosis, if resolved, would improve the client's health status and other occurring problems; and (3) which diagnosis is potentially life-threatening. Of course, actual problems would be addressed

TABLE 11–10

NUTRITIONAL NURSING CARE PLAN

Possible Nutrition Nursing Diagnoses

Activity intolerance	Fatigue	Oral mucous membrane, altered
Anxiety	Fear	Poisoning, high risk for
Aspiration, high risk for	Fluid volume deficit	Self-esteem, situational low
Body image disturbance	Fluid volume excess	Sensory-perceptual alterations: gustatory, olfactory
Breast-feeding, effective	Health maintenance, altered	Skin integrity, impaired
Breast-feeding, ineffective	Health seeking behaviors (specify)	Swallowing, impaired
Constipation	Knowledge deficit (specify)	
Diarrhea	Noncompliance	
Family coping, compromised		

Written Care Plan

Diagnosis	*Goals*	*Interventions*	*Evaluations*
Altered nutrition: less than body requirements RT anorexia AEB eating only 15% of ordered meals, stating "I don't feel hungry" and weighing 90% of IBW	Client will gain 1 lb/wk until desired body weight is attained	1. Offer favorite food 2. Weigh weekly 3. Suggest supplement to physician/dietitian 4. Offer kilocalorie-dense foods, i.e., milkshakes, custards	Goal met; client gained 1 lb this week
Altered nutrition: more than body requirements RT imbalance of intake versus activity expenditure AEB weight 110% of IBW, "I hate to exercise" and "Food is my only enjoyment in life"	Client will lose 1 lb/week until desired body weight is attained	1. Discuss low-kilocalorie, low-fat foods 2. Encourage exercise 3. Weigh weekly 4. Teach relationships of intake, exercise, and weight gain	Goal not met; client did not lose 1 lb this week because client didn't exercise. Discuss with client motivation to lose weight. Do not be harsh or judgmental. Offer support. Problem solve other ways to exercise such as walking, playing golf, or joining an exercise group

RT = related to; AEB = as evidenced by.

before potential or high-risk ones. Since the client is dynamic and changing, these priorities may change. As for nutrition, these same techniques are used to prioritize dietary nursing diagnoses. For instance, a brittle diabetic client with frequent episodes of hypoglycemia, retinopathy, nephropathy, and hyperlipidemia would need many changes in food choices. However, the most imminent problem is stabilizing the blood glucose.

Client goals are then derived from the nursing diagnosis to direct nursing care (see Table 11–10). Client goals are often used interchangeably with the terms "client outcomes" and "objectives." These goals determine nutritional nursing care. Nutritional goals must be client centered and realistic; thus, collaboration with the client is essential, as everyone does not want to achieve the same degree of wellness. A nutritional goal for the previously mentioned dietary nursing diagnoses would be "client will lose 1 lb per week (until the desired weight is reached)." Even this will

TABLE 11–11

TEAMWORK AND NUTRITION

Professional or Specialist	Nutritional Input
Physician	Makes the diagnosis Reviews laboratory results for decisions about medications, diets, and other treatments Discusses disease changes and implications of lifestyle on food intake
Nurse	Assists client with tray and/or eating Documents food and fluid intake Reports new diets or diet changes promptly Assesses status and monitors client progress in physical condition and eating behavior Projects a positive attitude to the client/family about food and the dietary department Teaches and reinforces diet therapy instructions from other team members
Dietitian	Reviews chart for relevant information Assesses nutritional status Plans nutritional care Counsels client, family, and staff
Pharmacist	Offers information regarding drug-food interactions Checks contraindications of drug content with client's condition, i.e., sodium content
Speech/language therapist	Assesses swallowing problems Recommends appropriate diet texture/NPO status as appropriate Recommends appropriate feeding techniques for swallowing problems Treats client to strengthen oral-motor muscles to improve swallowing difficulties
Occupational therapist	Helps client with eating handicaps Assesses and assists client with activities of daily living, such as meal preparation and cooking May teach kilocalorie expenditures and activity costs for energy conservation
Physical therapist	Teaches appropriate exercises to strengthen problem areas and to improve total health
Social worker	Finds assistance for nutrition problems, such as food stamps and Meals on Wheels
Psychologist	Helps client in adjusting to frustrations affecting needed changes in lifestyle Leads discussion with staff about their own problems related to case work

be affected by client's personal goals; although IBW for a client weighing 250 lbs may be 180 lbs, the client may think that 200 lbs is a more realistic long-term goal.

What are the 3 steps within the planning stage? How are goals developed?

Lastly, the nurse develops a care plan. This written care plan involves developing strategies or nursing interventions to achieve goals and eliminate the cause of the nursing diagnosis. In the nutritional care plan, the nurse develops nutritional interventions to meet the specified goal (increase or decrease weight) and eliminate the cause, i.e., anorexia or imbalance of intake and physical activity (see Table 11–10). This written care plan is vital for continuity of care.

IMPLEMENTATION

Implementation is the action step.

Implementation is the actual followthrough of specified interventions to accomplish the set goals, i.e., implementing nutritional nursing interventions. This includes not only direct care of the client, but also collaboration and coordination with the client and other health care workers. Typical nutritional interventions include monitoring intake and weight, serving diet ordered or recommending change if needed, supplementing diet as ordered and providing physical (opening cartons) and emotional (communicating empathy) support of diet regimen. Two other important nutritional interventions are client education and referrals.

Client Education

Teaching can be defined as "activities by which the teacher helps the student to learn." The ultimate goal of teaching is **learning.** The actual changes of behavior that result from teaching may not be immediately visible, so teaching may be described as activities intended to produce learning. The 3 domains of learning include (1) the cognitive domain, which is concerned with the intellectual aspect or the acquisition of facts (the effects of insulin, the signs and symptoms of hypoglycemia or hyperglycemia); (2) the psychomotor domain, which is concerned with the acquisition of new skills (self-administration of insulin); and (3) the affective (emotional) domain, which reflects the client purposefully choosing the desired behavior over other alternatives. Each domain must be addressed to guide a client to change a behavior. A planned learning experience uses a variety of methods, such as teaching, **counseling,** and behavior modification techniques that influence knowledge and health behaviors. Table 11–12 summarizes tips for helping clients change eating patterns for a healthier lifestyle. Nutritional counseling is generally more effective than teaching in eliciting dietary changes as a result of collaborative efforts of counselor and client to establish realistic workable goals achievable by the client.

Learning is defined as a change of behavior.

Nutritional counseling is helping people with present or high-risk nutritional problems, whether they exist because of inadequate knowledge or motivation or both.

In many situations, a dietitian is available to offer nutritional counseling; however, in many outpatient and community clinics and home health care organizations, the nurse is given the responsibility of counseling clients regarding dietary habits. Thorough knowledge of basic nutrition principles are prerequisites to effective counseling. Interpretation of the principles of nutrition into practical terms that the client can understand is a vital skill. (Instructing the client to decrease salt intake is not sufficient; instead, specific foods that are low in salt, liked by the client, affordable, and readily available, must be discussed.)

An understanding of factors that influence food behaviors and use of counseling techniques to help clients make appropriate changes are important (Fig. 11–8). A good counselor establishes a rapport to make the client feel comfortable and does not use threats or commands. The counselor recognizes that changing dietary habits is a process, but it is unrealistic to expect immediate and lasting changes from a few

TABLE 11–12

COUNSELING SKILLS TO PROMOTE DIETARY COMPLIANCE

Relate: Develop a positive relationship with clients—they need to know that you care
Communicate: Be certain that clients understand what you are saying—ask them to repeat the message that you gave
Motivate: Set realistic short-term goals for making dietary changes
Educate: Develop/seek educational aids to help clients keep track of daily eating patterns and medication regimens
Collaborate: Enlist the support of the client's family or refer clients to self-help and support groups
Facilitate: Change the client's diet gradually, and keep medication regimens as simple as possible
Innovate: Give a token reward for goals achieved; have clients contribute favorite recipes appropriate for the diet; provide a small lending library of consumer-appropriate books
Calculate: Chart the number of clients who are successfully reaching their goals for blood pressure control, lower cholesterol levels, and weight loss

Data from National Heart, Lung, and Blood Institute. Patient Education: Eight Moves to Help Your Patients Improve Adherence. *Infomemo* 1991 Spring: 9.

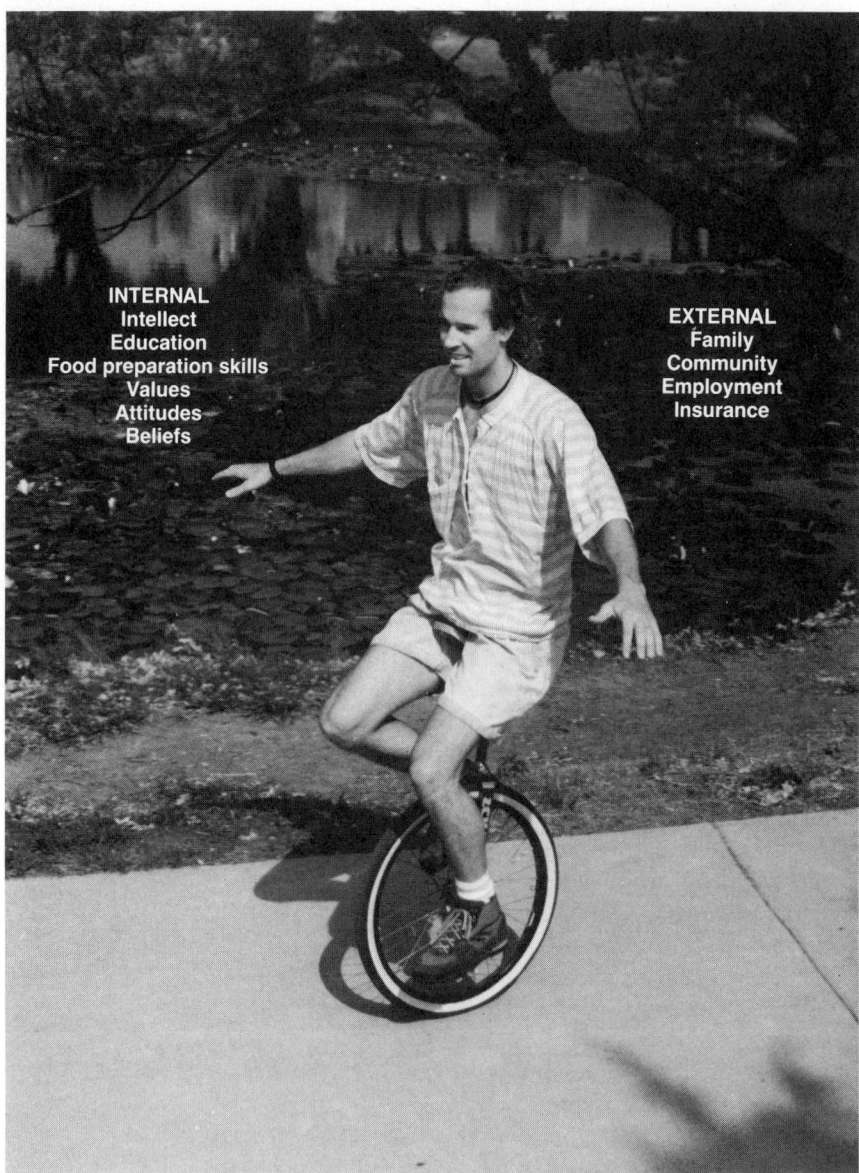

Figure 11–8 Factors that influence health-promoting eating behaviors. All these factors influence the individual's ability to solve problems and change behaviors for a proper balance between habits and practices to achieve optimal nutritional status. (Courtesy of Doug Davis.)

counseling sessions. The client must recognize that there is a health risk, see its link to eating patterns, and be provided enough information to identify required changes.

Dietary counseling requires frequent interaction with the client. The goal is to produce a desirable change in food choices. Counseling is client centered by eliciting the client's opinions and feelings about specific recommendations. Goals are agreed on by both nurse and client at the outset. Cues that indicate confusion, disinterest, or denial of the need to learn should be observed. Tactful inquiries are made to determine the client's understanding and learning, for example, "What have you learned," rather than "what is the correct way of dieting?" The counselor must be able to organize the client's ideas into a meaningful pattern and take into consideration the client's lifestyle and knowledge level.

Counseling techniques that involve more than one of the senses and seek the active participation of the client have more impact. Thus, when the nurse uses a variety of modalities to present material (including those commercially produced), learning can be enhanced. Determining the accuracy, appropriateness, visibility, and length of materials are part of the preparation necessary by the nurse actually performing the counseling. Some topics addressed by nurses are how nutrition is affected by or may affect health and the importance of maintaining healthy eating habits; foods to avoid or increase; cooking principles, procedures, and techniques to maintain optimal nutrient content; and client's nutritional status.

What are some techniques a nurse can use to teach or counsel clients? What are topics nurses will address?

Referrals

Frequently special assistance is needed by clients. A variety of nutrition resources are available to help financially, to assist with food budgeting, or to teach basic nutrition and meal planning (Table 11–13). It is important for nurses to identify clients or families with nutritional needs and to help them participate in available programs (Table 11–14). One of the best sources is the city or county health department. State and local health departments usually have various programs to provide nutrition services, such as Well Baby Clinics and Family Health Centers. The health department and county hospitals are excellent resources for information about the various programs available.

The federal government administers several nutrition programs through the Department of Agriculture (USDA) and the Department of Health and Human Services (DHHS). The food stamp program provides coupons to low-income households that meet certain requirements. Food stamp coupons are free to clients who qualify. The program is designed to assist low-income households purchase a nutritious diet and is adjusted annually based on income and household size. Local welfare offices administer the program and are widely distributed throughout the US. Average participation was about 22.5 million persons in 1991 (Matsumoto, 1991).

Special Supplemental Food Program for Women, Infants, and Children (WIC) is designed to prevent nutritional problems. WIC is available to pregnant and lactating women, infants, and children up to 5 years of age who are considered to be at nutritional risk. Criteria for nutritional risk are evidence of iron deficiency, inadequate weight gain during pregnancy, teenage pregnancy, failure to thrive, poor growth patterns, and inadequate dietary patterns based on a scoring system of a 24-hour dietary recall. The WIC program is usually available through county and city health departments. Total participation in this program was 4.76 million in 1991 (Matsumoto, 1991). In addition to the supplemental foods, health care and nutrition education are provided.

The school breakfast and lunch programs provide nutritious meals for children at school. Nutritional standards for the school lunch require that lunch must fur-

TABLE 11–13

RELIABLE NUTRITION RESOURCE GUIDE

Type of Information	Title	Resource
General food or nutrition question	Registered dietitian, nutritionist, home economist	Hospital; local or state health department; extension service of a land-grant university
More technical questions	Professor, registered dietitian	Nutrition or home economics department of a university or college
Questions on food preparation and preservation	Home economist	USDA–County Cooperative Extension Service; gas or electric company
Special diets	Registered dietitian	Hospital; local or state public health departments; volunteer health organization (e.g., a diabetes association)

TABLE 11–14

REFERRAL CHART FOR COMMUNITY NUTRITION RESOURCE

Population Group	Risk Factor	Referral Source	Contact
Pregnant and lactating women	Low income	Food stamps	Welfare office
	Anemia, inadequate weight gain, age-related risk factor, inadequate diet, adolescent pregnancy, inadequate health care, or lack of food and nutrition information	WIC Program	City, county, or state health department
		Maternity and Infant Care Project	State health department
		EFNEP	Land-grant universities
		Prenatal education	Prenatal clinic or private health care team
Infants	Low birth weight, failure to thrive, or poor growth patterns	WIC Program	City, county, or state health department
	Inadequate health care	Children and Youth Project	State health department
Children	Poor growth patterns, inadequate diet, or anemia	WIC Program (up to 5 years of age)	City, county, or state health department
	Low income	Children and Youth Project (up to 18 years of age)	State health department
		Headstart (preschool)	Local community action project
		School Lunch	Board of education
		School Breakfast	Local community action project
General adult	Obesity	Weight Watchers International, Thin Within, Dieters workshop, TOPS, and other weight reduction groups	Local chapters
	Hyperlipidemia, cardiovascular disease, or hypertension	American Heart Association	Local chapter
	Diabetes	American Diabetes Association	Local chapter
	Low income	Food stamps	Welfare office
	Lack of food and nutrition information	EFNEP	Land-grant universities
	General consumer information for all populations*	Community nutrition groups and community cooperatives	Local groups
		American Dietetic Association	1 800 366-1655
		Center for Science in the Public Interest	1755 S St. NW Washington, DC 20009
		Nutrition Foundation	888 Seventeenth Street NW Washington, DC 20006
		Society for Nutrition Education	2001 Killebrew Dr. Ste. 340 Minneapolis, MN 55425
		US Government Printing Office	Superintendent of Documents Washington, DC 20402
Elderly	Low income	Food stamps	Welfare office
		Congregate meal sites	Social service agency
	Homebound	Meals on Wheels	Social service agency
	Diabetes	American Diabetes Association	Local chapter
	Obesity	Weight reduction groups	Local chapters
	Cardiovascular disease	American Heart Association	Local chapter

* This is only a partial listing. Programs may vary in different parts of the US.
From Finkelhor S. Nutrition resources. *Med Clin North Am* 1979; 63(5):1117.

nish at least one-third of the RDAs for children. Free and reduced-price meals are provided based on household income and size. Additionally, attempts to adhere to Dietary Guidelines for Americans (low in fats, salt, and sugars) are being implemented.

The Nutrition Program for the Elderly provides both group meals and home-delivered ones. Besides providing a hot meal to the elderly (containing one-third of the RDAs), a variety of social services are also available.

The Expanded Food and Nutrition Education Program (EFNEP) is designed to help lower socioeconomic groups with all aspects of nutrition. EFNEP is available through county extension services of land-grant universities and assists with meal planning, budgeting, cooking, and other food and nutrition-related problems. Nutrition aides, who are low-income homemakers, are trained to visit with other low-income clients/families in their homes to assist in providing well-balanced meals.

Headstart is a preschool educational program for low-income families. Meals are furnished for the children, and nutrition education is available for the parents.

Local chapters of many health-related organizations furnish free or inexpensive literature, audiovisual material, and health-oriented programs on various topics. They can be located in the telephone directory. Frequently local churches provide free meals or other help. Referrals can also be in-hospital such as the social worker, dietitian, metabolic specialist, or nutrition support team. Other referrals are listed in Appendix E-1.

Name 5 nutrition referrals available and the type of clients they serve.

EVALUATION

In this final step, a nurse determines the extent to which the nutritional goals have been achieved. For example, a nurse would weigh the client weekly to determine if a weight loss or gain of 1 lb occurred. If so, nutritional interventions were effective. If not, the nurse would reinitiate the process, reassess, and make the necessary changes (see Table 11-10). This is called modifying or revising the care plan. A change in the environment, equipment, or procedure may be needed. Difficult as it is to set aside personal biases, this is important to evaluate problems with the goals or process effectively. Any step of the nursing process may be deficient: (1) insufficient and inappropriate data were initially gathered, (2) nursing diagnosis was inaccurate, (3) outcomes were not realistic for the client, (4) nursing interventions were not suitable for the diagnosis, or (5) interventions were not implemented as planned. The evaluation component helps determine effectiveness of care. Its purpose is not to blame or find fault but to provide high-quality client care, in this case, high-quality nutritional care.

NUTRITION UPDATE 11-1: DUBIOUS NUTRITIONAL ASSESSMENT TECHNIQUES

Clients with chronic illnesses such as cancer, arthritis, AIDS, and multiple sclerosis are especially vulnerable to quackery. Nutritional quacks frequently use invalid diagnostic tests and questionable therapies that may cause the client to defer treatment by a reputable health care professional.

Leukocytotoxic (cytotoxic) tests are supposedly used to determine food allergies. Food extracts are added to a blood sample; an adverse reaction of white cells indicates allergy to the particular food. These tests are essentially useless and are potentially harmful since they produce both false-positive and false-negative results and may lead to unnecessary extensive dietary restrictions (see Chapter 23).

An amalgameter is reportedly used to diagnose "amalgam toxicity" from mercury-containing tooth fillings, which allegedly cause cancer and multiple sclerosis. None of the devices used are valid (Jarvis, 1989), nor does removal of the fillings eliminate the diseases. Special nutrition supplements marketed to be anti-amalgam are not approved by the FDA (Vitamin Pushers, 1986).

Live cell analysis is a drop of blood examined under a darkfield microscope that client and practitioner view together via a video camera. Interpretations are totally erroneous. For instance, separation of red cells is due to "impaired oxygen delivery and carbon dioxide removal caused by excess dietary fat"; red cells that are not round are said to be caused by "toxins" entering the body; lack of white cell movement is interpreted as decreased immunity; and spicules (small needle-like bodies caused by drying or contamination of specimens) may signify liver or bowel toxicity. The use of darkfield microscopy for live cell analysis and interpretations is unreliable.

The examination of lines, colors, and irregularities of a client's iris results in a diagnosis and prescription by an iridologist. Diagnoses are based on 19 different charts that are very inconsistent. If the client confirms that a problem exists in the named organ, the practitioner claims credit for diagnosis, but if the client denies a problem in that organ, the practitioner indicates a weakness or propensity to disease there.

Hair analysis has been a popular tool for determining nutritional status. New analytical techniques have resulted in laboratories diagnosing medical problems and prescribing therapies, but more frequently vitamin and mineral supplements are advised. Hair analysis has a number of potential pitfalls, including contamination by sweat, environmental pollutants, cosmetics (e.g., shampoos, bleaches, or dyes), and other factors. Several other factors alter the mineral content of hair — age, sex, hormonal levels, and disease. Concentrations of copper and zinc are variable with increasing distance from the scalp (the farther from the scalp, the higher the values). Hair analysis appears to be of no value in assessing vitamin status. On the other hand, hair analysis for certain heavy metals, such as methyl mercury, arsenic, cadmium, and lead, can be very sensitive. Results of hair analysis are of little value and should not be relied on as the sole criterion of nutritional status for therapeutic recommendations.

SUMMARY

The nursing process, consisting of 5 interrelated steps (assessment, diagnosis, planning, implementation, and evaluation), can be adapted to provide effective nutritional care. Since each step involves the client, flexibility is necessary, and some steps may occur simultaneously. The first step in the process, assessment, determines how well the rest of the process flows. Therefore, nutritional assessment is the cornerstone for nutritional care. Nutritional counseling and referrals are important interventions based on screening performed by the nurse. Adapting the nursing process to provide nutritional care is easy for a nurse and beneficial for a client. Nutrition can affect every system in the body, therefore, a nurse's ability to use this process may shorten a hospital stay, improve quality of life, or lengthen a client's life.

NURSING PROCESS IN ACTION

You may be wondering how you can remember all this information, much less apply it in your nursing care process. Although situations have been presented for applying the Nursing Process in Action for other chapters, Figure 11–9 will assist

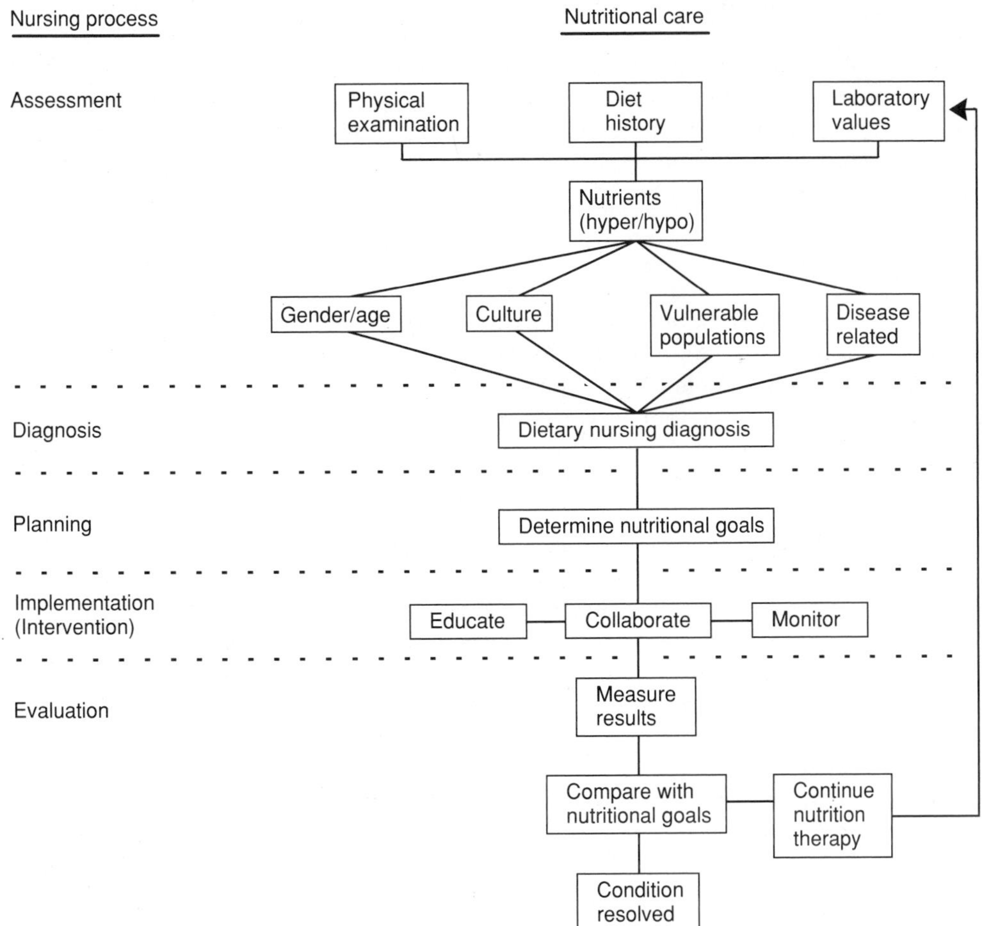

Figure 11–9 Sample nursing process for nutritional care.

you in integrating nutritional care into the nursing process with minimal difficulties. The flow chart shows the relationship between nutrition and the nursing process so optimal nutritional care will become a normal aspect of your routine nursing care.

Assessment

As you have learned from this chapter, there are 3 major assessment areas to determine a client's nutritional status: physical, dietary, and laboratory. Remember, physical involves not only a head to toe assessment, but also anthropometric measurements. Findings from all 3 of these areas will determine whether nutrient(s) are hyper-/hypo- states. To assist you in relating these 3 assessment areas to clients in the clinical area, the following chapters have italicized headings termed *physical, dietary,* and *laboratory* to organize your care.

In referring to Figure 11–9, the 4 boxes below hyper-/hypo- states are client specific and will vary depending on the type of client for whom you are caring. As you have previously learned, age, gender, and culture affect basic nutrition and food choices. Additionally, the RDAs are age and gender specific. Vulnerable populations and disease-related issues that affect nutrient(s) in hyper-/hypo- states are discussed in future chapters. As you will learn, these 2 factors can directly or indirectly affect nutrient hyper-/hypo- status. Generally, most clients in vulnerable populations are more prone to specific nutrient deficiencies or excesses, whereas in disease-related factors, the disease process may actually cause acute or chronic nutrient problem(s).

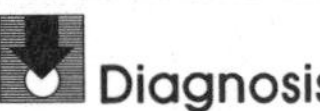

Diagnosis

From all of the assessment data, a nutritional nursing diagnosis is determined for your client. To ease you into this transition from assessment data to nursing diagnosis, each chapter concludes with a Nursing Process in Action, and the diagnosis state is labeled "dietary nursing diagnosis." This heading will be familiar to you because it has been in prior chapters.

Planning

Determining nutritional goals is derived from the nutritional nursing diagnosis. Of course, goal setting is a mutual effort between you and your client. Just as with diagnosis, a heading labeled "nutritional goals" in the Nursing Process in Action will help you set realistic, individualized goals.

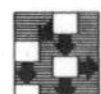

Implementation

Nutritional implementation for any nutritional problem in the clinical area involves 3 major interventions: educate, collaborate, and monitor. In nutrition, education is paramount. For you to educate clients, a separate section labeled "client education," another familiar heading, will provide information you can use to teach clients/families. Collaboration is necessary, not only with clients/families, but also with other health care workers, i.e., physicians, dietitians, pharmacists, social workers, speech-pathologists, and physical therapists. Monitoring clients' physical condition, dietary intake, and laboratory test results is needed in the clinical area because this determines if clients are improving or deteriorating and allows modifications in the plan of care to be made if necessary.

Evaluation

Evaluating your care of clients with nutritional problems is essential. Therefore, you need to measure a client's responses and then compare those results with the nutritional goals. If goals are met, the condition is resolved, and nutritional care is completed. However, if goals are not met, or only partially met, nutritional therapy is continued as you start the whole nursing process over, beginning with assessment. To facilitate this crucial function, in subsequent chapters an "evaluation" heading will appear in the text and continue as a section in the Nursing Process in Action. Desired client results/outcomes will be presented, thereby allowing evaluation of nutritional care to be performed in the clinical area.

If you follow this diagram in the clinical area, nutritional care will become a part of your everyday nursing care.

STUDENT READINESS

1. List the steps of the nursing process as they may relate to nutrition.
2. Name 2 examples of objective and 2 examples of subjective data for nutrition.
3. List the 3 components of a nursing diagnosis.
4. What is the purpose of nutritional goals?
5. Why should the nurse know what diet a client is receiving?
6. Why should nurses be informed about the types of food allowed or avoided on certain diets?
7. List observations for a nurse to chart about food intake.
8. What does evaluation accomplish, especially in nutrition?

9. A client asks you what anthropometric measures are. How would you respond?
10. A client has low blood count for the following: albumin, TLC, and transferrin. What would you suspect?
11. What are some referrals nurses could use for nutritional problems?

REFERENCES

Alfaro R. *Applying Nursing Diagnosis and Nursing Process: A Step by Step Approach.* 2nd ed. Philadelphia, JB Lippincott, 1990.

Bray GA. Pathophysiology of obesity. *Am J Clin Nutr* 1992 Jan; 55(1 Suppl):488S–494S.

Bray GA. Obesity. *In* Brown ML, ed. *Present Knowledge in Nutrition.* Washington, DC, Nutrition Foundation, 1990:23–38.

Carpenito LJ. *Handbook of Nursing Diagnosis.* 4th ed. Philadelphia, JB Lippincott, 1991.

Gordon M. *Nursing Diagnosis: Process and Application.* 2nd ed. New York, McGraw-Hill, 1987.

Herrmann FR, et al. Serum albumin level on admission as a predictor of death, length of stay, and readmission. *Arch Intern Med* 1992 Jan; 152(1):125–130.

Jarvis W. Dubious health assessments. *Nutr and the MD* 1989 Feb; 15(2):1–3.

Kamath SK, et al. Hospital malnutrition: A 33-hospital screening study. *J Am Diet Assoc* 1986 Feb; 86(2):203–206.

Kant AK, et al. Food group intake patterns and associated nutrient profiles of the U.S. population. *J Am Diet Assoc* 1991 Dec; 91(12):1532–1537.

Matsumoto M. Domestic food assistance costs are rising. *Nat Food Review* 1991 Oct/Dec; 14(4):40–42.

Rammohan M, Juan D. Effects of a low calorie, low protein diet on nutritional parameters, and routine laboratory values in non-obese young and elderly subjects. *J Am College Nutr* 1989 Dec; 8(6):545–553.

Revicki DA, Israel RG. Relationship between body mass indices and measure of body adiposity. *Am J Pub Health* 1986 Aug; 76(8):992–994.

Roubenoff R, et al. Malnutrition among hospitalized patients. *Arch Intern Med* 1987 Aug; 147(8):1462–1465.

Rowland ML. Self-reported weight and height. *Am J Clin Nutr* 1990 Dec; 52(6):1125–1133.

Schulz LO. Obese, overweight, desirable, ideal: When to draw the line in 1986. *J Am Diet Assoc* 1986 Aug; 88(8):939–942.

Vitamin Pushers. *Consumers Report* 1986 March; 51(3):170–175.

Winkler MF, et al. Use of retinol-binding protein and prealbumin as indicators of the response to nutrition therapy. *J Am Diet Assoc* 1989 May; 89(5):684–687.

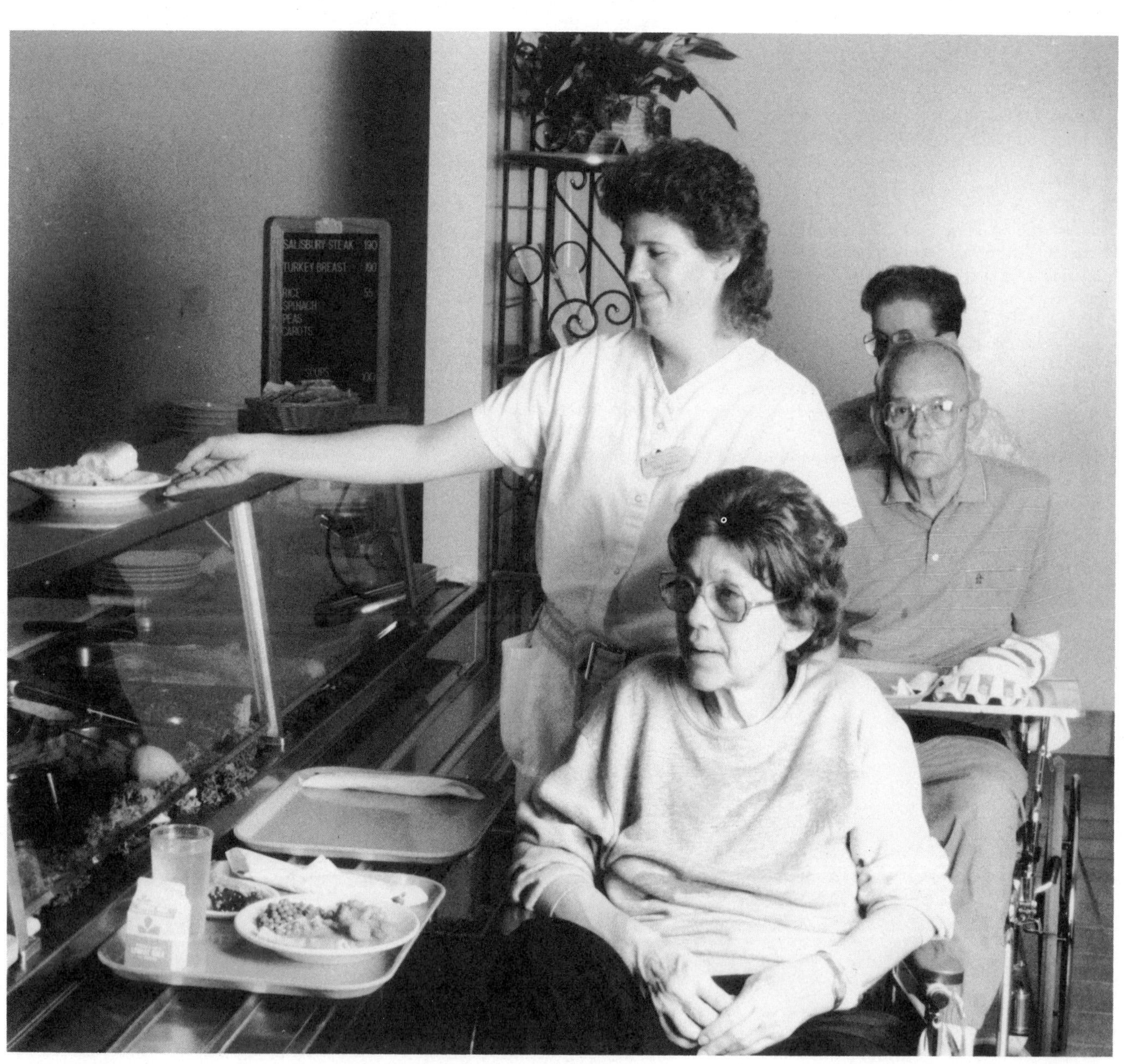
SALISBURY STEAK 190
TURKEY BREAST 190
RICE 55
SPINACH
PEAS
CAROTS

Basic Dietary Management Of Hospitalized Clients

CHAPTER 12

OUTLINE

I. DIET THERAPY
- A. Purposes

II. DIET MANUAL
- A. Diet Prescription
- *Nursing Applications*

III. FACTORS AFFECTING NUTRITIONAL STATUS
- A. Illness and Psychosocial Needs
- B. Illness and Appetite
- C. Illness and Nutrition

IV. NUTRITION TEAMWORK
- *Nursing Applications*

V. BASIC DIET MODIFICATIONS
- A. Clear Liquid Diet
  1. Indications
  2. Characteristics
  3. Supplementation
  4. Contraindications
- *Nursing Applications*
- B. Full Liquid Diet
  1. Indications
  2. Characteristics
  3. Supplementation
  4. Contraindications
- *Nursing Applications*
- C. Soft Diet
  1. Indications
  2. Characteristics
- *Nursing Applications*
- D. Mechanical Soft (Dental Soft) Diet
  1. Indications
  2. Characteristics
- *Nursing Applications*
- E. Pureed Diet
  1. Indications
  2. Characteristics

Nursing Applications
F. Dysphagia Diets
Nursing Applications
G. Regular or General Diet
1. Indications
2. Characteristics
Nursing Applications
H. Diet as Tolerated
Nursing Applications
VI. PROMOTING FOOD INTAKE
A. Increasing Frequency of Feedings
B. Assisting with Menu Selections
C. Providing a Pleasant Environment
D. Preparing the Client
E. Serving the Trays
F. Feeding the Client
G. Monitoring Fluid Intake
Nursing Applications

OBJECTIVES

THE STUDENT WILL BE ABLE TO:

- Identify the purposes of diet modifications.
- Explain the effect of illness on appetite and nutritional status.
- Define the basic diet modifications.
- List nutritional information that should be recorded on the client's chart.
- Properly prepare the client for feeding.
- Discuss the role of nursing in implementing and evaluating the nutritional care plan.
- Demonstrate proper procedures for serving trays.
- Determine when clients' dietary orders should be changed.
- Recognize that effective nutritional intervention is dependent on nursing care as well as collaboration with dietitians and the dietary department.
- Apply nursing principles to the various types of diets and dietary management.
- Describe client teaching points for the above.

TEST YOUR NQ (True/False)

1. A clear liquid diet provides adequate nutrients.
2. The nurse plays a vital role in explaining to clients the expectations of the dietary regimen in their overall care.
3. All fruit juices are allowed on a clear liquid diet.
4. A soft diet is appropriate for a client with dysphagia problems.
5. The soft diet can contain adequate amounts of nutrients except for fiber.
6. A diet prescription is as vital to the client's physical recovery as a drug prescription.
7. The purpose of diet therapy is to decrease nutritional deficiencies.
8. Communication among the nutritional care team is vital.
9. On a full liquid diet, raw eggs or egg whites are added to increase protein intake.
10. A fat-restricted diet may be used for clients with liver disease.

With current knowledge about the importance of nutrition and its effects on health, nurses cannot afford to ignore a client's nutritional status. A knowledge of dietary factors that must be modified because of the prescribed diet order assists nurses in guiding and motivating clients. Information learned in Section I helps the nurse understand basic dietary principles and how personal food choices may affect health.

Subsequently the diet prescription is as vital to the client's physical recovery as a drug prescription. Nutrition is an integral component of total client care, affecting the recovery process as much as other therapies. Following a diet prescription requires considerable self-discipline and is never an easy task. During illness, acceptance of the diet prescription is complicated because appetite is generally decreased, whereas requirements are increased.

DIET THERAPY

A therapeutic or modified diet may be regarded as an alteration in the normal diet to treat the disease or illness. Recommended nutrient allowances for healthy clients are a primary consideration, then necessary adaptations for specific disease conditions are made. Usually the diet is an adjunct to medical or surgical care; in instances such as phenylketonuria, it may be the principal treatment. Hospitals serve 10 to 20 different diets per meal to meet the various therapeutic requirements of clients. Examples of normal and modified diets are shown in Table 12–1.

Physical problems may require different routes for nutrition support, such as tube feedings because of an inability to swallow or total parenteral nutrition (TPN) via the veins because of severe GI dysfunction. If the GI tract is functional, the oral method of feeding is preferred to other feeding modalities.

Purposes

The purposes for diet therapy can be any one or a combination of the following:

1. To prevent genetically predisposed conditions such as heart disease.
2. To maintain/achieve normal or optimal nutritional status when requirements are increased (diarrhea, fever, surgery, or trauma).
3. To correct nutritional deficiencies that may occur, e.g., anemia.
4. To correct body weight in overweight or underweight clients.
5. To provide rest for the body or for certain organs, e.g., a low-protein diet for kidney disease.
6. To adjust nutrient intake to a level the body can properly metabolize, e.g., the diabetic diet.

What are the purposes for a therapeutic diet?

DIET MANUAL

Under Medicare's Conditions of Participation for Hospitals and the Joint Commission Accreditation for Healthcare Organizations, hospitals are required to have an up-to-date diet manual that has been jointly approved by the medical and dietary staffs. A copy of the adopted manual is usually available in the main office,

TABLE 12–1

COMMON NORMAL AND THERAPEUTIC DIETS

Diet	Purpose	Conditions When Used
Normal nutrition		
Regular	To provide nutritionally adequate diet for clients with no restrictions	Unrestricted
High-protein, high-kilocalorie	To provide increased nutrient requirements	Unrestricted
High-protein, high-kilocalorie for pregnancy	To meet increased nutrition requirements of mother and fetus	Pregnancy
High-protein, high-kilocalorie for lactation	To meet increased nutritional needs of the lactating woman	Lactation
Geriatric	To provide dietary adjustments related to the aging process	Older clients
Vegetarian	To provide adequate nutrients for clients who exclude meat, milk, and/or egg products*	Client preferences
Modification in consistency		
Clear liquid	To provide fluids and minimize residue	Presurgical or postsurgical; various laboratory tests
Full liquid	To provide nourishment in liquid form	Presurgical or postsurgical, transitional diet
Pureed	To provide adequate nutrients in a form tolerated by client	Oral problems or dental surgery, swallowing problems
Soft	To provide easily digested foods	Transitional diet
Dysphagia	To provide food in a form tolerated to decrease the risk of aspiration	Swallowing disorders
Mechanical soft	To provide food modified in texture and consistency for chewing problems	Edentulous clients and those with loose-fitting dentures; oral surgery
Kilocalorie-controlled diets		
Diabetic	To meet nutritional needs for diabetes (maintain stable serum glucose and prevent complications); based on exchange lists	Diabetes mellitus
Weight reduction	To provide adequate nutrition with kilocalorie level below energy requirement	Overweight
Reactive hypoglycemia	To decrease rate of absorption and use of carbohydrates and decrease insulin secretion	Reactive and functional hypoglycemia
Gastrointestinal Diets		
Bland†	To eliminate foods that cause pain and those that stimulate increased gastric secretion and motility	Gastric or duodenal ulcers, gastritis, irritable bowel (acute stage), or irritation of the GI tract
Low fiber and residue	To lower fiber intake to decrease fecal material in the lower GI tract	Pre– and post–GI surgery, colon obstruction, diverticulitis, radiation therapy
High-fiber	To provide high fiber and bulk to promote regular elimination and increase stool volume	Diverticular disease, irritable bowel syndrome (stable condition), and atonic gastrectomy
Postgastrectomy	To decrease symptoms of dumping syndrome	Recent partial or total gastrectomy
Lactose-controlled	To reduce lactose intake	Lactose intolerance or lactase deficiency
Gluten-restricted	To restrict foods that contain gluten	Celiac disease, nontropical sprue, idiopathic steatorrhea

TABLE 12–1
COMMON NORMAL AND THERAPEUTIC DIETS *Continued*

Diet	Purpose	Conditions When Used
Fat-modified diets		
Fat-controlled for hyperlipoproteinemia	To decrease cholesterol and fat intake	Clients at high risk for cardiovascular disease or elevated cholesterol or triglyceride level
Fat-restricted (25–50 gm)	To reduce total fat intake	Liver disease, gallbladder and pancreatic disorders
Mineral-modified diets		
Sodium-controlled (1, 2, 3–4 gm)	To decrease sodium intake	Prevention and control of edema and for hypertension; chronic renal disease and congestive heart failure
Potassium restricted	To provide lower levels of potassium	Clients unable to excrete potassium adequately, as in chronic renal failure
High potassium	To increase amount of potassium	Use of some diuretics and some cortical steroids, hypokalemia
Calcium restricted	To restrict calcium intake	Hypercalcemia and hypercalciuria (hyperparathyroidism, sarcoidosis)
Oxalate restricted	To restrict foods that contribute to increasing oxalate levels	Calcium oxalate renal stones and enteric hyperoxaluria; iliac disease or intestinal resection or bypass
High iron	To increase or maintain iron storage	Microcytic anemia
Protein-modified diets		
Protein restricted (21, 40, or 60 gm)	To decrease toxic nitrogenous breakdown products	Compromised liver or kidney function

* Elimination of meat, dairy, or egg products is determined by client preference, as discussed in Chapter 3.
† This is an obsolete diet, but is occasionally ordered by physicians.

at the head nurse's desk for the convenience of physicians and nurses, at all nursing stations, and, of course, in the dietary department.

The American Dietetic Association (ADA) has prepared the *Handbook of Clinical Dietetics* (1992), which documents the scientific basis for dietary modification in treatment of specific disorders and includes food lists and sample menus for various modified diets. A more comprehensive diet manual is the *Manual of Clinical Dietetics* (ADA, 1992).

Each facility selects its own manual, which may be developed locally to reflect regional food patterns. A good diet manual states the exact regimen to be followed with clearly defined restrictions. This avoids decisions being made by those who are not sufficiently trained. Slight variations in diet manuals occur, but overall principles will be consistent. Diet manuals are developed to provide:

1. Guidance for food preparation.
2. Information about available dietary regimens for particular conditions and their nutritional adequacy. (Inadequate diets are usually labeled as such, so missing nutrients can be supplemented or the diet can be changed as soon as possible.)
3. Samples of foods allowed and avoided.
4. Standards for monitoring the client by allied professional staff members.

Why are facilities required to have a diet manual? What information is provided in the diet manual?

Diet Prescription

In most instances, physicians order an appropriate diet for every client admitted, whether it is a regular (normal) or modified diet. In some facilities, registered dietitians are permitted to write a diet order. The diet should be based on the client's symptoms, laboratory tests, and nutritional needs.

Just as medications are not dispensed without a physician's order, clients should not be fed without a verbal or written order from the physician or registered dietitian. The diet prescription, like one for drugs, should specify the type of nutrients, amount (kilocalories or dosage), frequency or time of administration (if different from normal mealtimes), any nutrient supplementation indicated, and any texture modification (chopped, ground, pureed).

Depending on the client's condition, the order may vary from **NPO** to any of the specific therapeutic diets, or combinations thereof, or a regular diet. Records of this order are sent by the nurse's station to the dietary department. As the client's condition changes, the diet order may change.

NPO—nothing per os, or nothing by mouth.

NURSING APPLICATIONS

Assessment

Physical—for symptoms of specified disease.
Dietary—for nutritional needs and diet order.
Laboratory—for pertinent ordered laboratory tests for admitting diagnosis.

Interventions

1. Consult with the physician or dietitian as needed. For example, laboratory values indicate a low protein level in a client who has recently undergone surgery and has lost 5 lbs. He has been on a clear liquid diet for 3 days. Supplements or diet changes may be indicated to provide more protein.
2. Inform the physician and dietitian of client's condition and oral intake.
3. Encourage clients to eat; this is necessary to promote anabolism.
4. Know where the diet manual is located, and use it to be knowledgeable of what foods are or are not permitted on various diets in your facility.
5. Monitor and document client's food intake.
6. Present a positive acceptance of the prescribed diet. Since nutrition is a vital component of client care and can affect the recovery process, nurses need to encourage clients to eat without personal biases. Preconceived feelings about foods or the diet can be detected by clients and may influence their acceptance.

Client Education

- Use the diet manual to teach the client about foods allowed or to be avoided.
- Explain the importance and rationale of the diet to client for better compliance.

FACTORS AFFECTING NUTRITIONAL STATUS

Illness and Psychosocial Needs

Not only are the nutritional needs of the client important in the healing process, but also physiological, cultural, economic, emotional, and spiritual needs need to be considered. Hospitalization itself may elicit psychological stress in addition to the stress that accompanies most illnesses or health problems. The client entering a hospital or any other type of institution is in a formidable environment. He or she is unfamiliar with the surroundings and routines; apprehensive or frightened about what is going to happen; and dependent on others for his or her care, meals, and all other needs. These factors can contribute to poor dietary intake.

Since each client is coping with this stress in his or her own unique way, any of the following behaviors may be exhibited: defensiveness, self-centeredness, anger, depression, withdrawal, or irritability. Acceptance of hospital routine is more difficult for some clients. In general, illness does not bring out the best in anyone. Many become finicky and frequently make special demands. They may prefer their cultural patterns from childhood. Stress seems to strengthen a fear of trying new or disliked foods and may result in the rejection of anything but familiar ones. It is beyond the scope of this book to cover the different problems and their interpretation; the classic article by Luckmann and Sorensen (1975) is highly recommended for an understanding of the subject.

Frequently, food comes under attack because this is something the client knows about—how to feed himself or herself. Institutional mealtimes are not a social experience as they ordinarily are in the home. The food pattern, preparation, and times are different from most clients' regular food habits (Fig. 12–1). Eating in bed from a tray can be an awkward task.

Opinions about food are very strong; a certain food that is intensely disliked may provoke a client to refuse everything. A brief dietary history on admission can help avoid some of these conflicts. Criticisms of the food may be a way to draw attention. They should be acknowledged and appropriate changes made if possible. Generally clients have different opinions and food preferences; they are better satisfied if allowed to choose from a selective menu. Consider distinctive qualities of a client's background, such as religious, cultural, ethnic, and financial factors, that may influence acceptance or rejection of foods.

List psychosocial factors that may affect intake during hospitalization.

Illness and Appetite

Decreased appetite is prevalent during illnesses because of apathy, anorexia, drugs, inactivity, or many other reasons. A modified diet is for the comfort and treatment of clients, but it may cause distress rather than provide immediate comfort if clients are not given some explanation for the diet. Therefore, an understanding of the underlying disease conditions that require a dietary change and the desired physiological results is needed by the nurse and client.

Illness and Nutrition

Since stress can be both the cause and the consequence of poor intake, stress should be assessed. Intense stress or anxiety can reduce the absorption of a variety of nutrients, particularly protein and vitamin C. Although increased intake of nutrients is not a remedy for stress, nutrient losses can be replaced. Deficiency of any of the essential nutrients diminishes the body's resistance, which can initiate or aggravate other diseases. Supplying excessive amounts of nutrients is rarely of value unless a deficiency exists.

Different physiological conditions increase losses of various electrolytes and nitrogen; others increase metabolic rate, thereby increasing nutrient requirements; still others affect the body's ability to handle some nutrients. In general, disease states usually increase nutrient requirements of many nutrients; on the other hand, lack of appetite, vomiting, and pain often interfere with intake of sufficient quantities of nutrients. (Metabolic processes that affect utilization of specific nutrients may result in dietary restriction of these nutrients with further deleterious effects on intake). Drug therapy profoundly affects intake, absorption, and use of nutrients.

What are some factors that may affect food acceptance during illness? Is a client's nutrient requirement reflected in the client's appetite?

TYPICAL HOSPITAL REGULAR DIET

Sample Menu

Breakfast

6 oz pineapple juice
1 banana
1 cup bran flakes
8 oz fruit flavored yogurt
1 slice whole wheat toast
with 1 tsp margarine and jelly
1 cup low fat 2% milk
coffee, 1 tsp nondairy creamer and sugar

Lunch

3.5 oz lean broiled pork chop
1/2 cup scalloped potatoes
1/2 cup boiled carrots
1/2 cup coleslaw with 2 tbsp mayonnaise
1 whole wheat roll
1 tsp margarine
1 baked apple
coffee/tea

Dinner

6 oz beef stroganoff on 1/2 cup noodles
1/2 cup broccoli with 1/4 cup cheese sauce
relishes: cherry tomato, radishes, cucumber slices, celery sticks
1 slice cream pie with blueberries
1 slice whole wheat bread
1 tsp margarine
1 cup 2% low-fat milk
tea

Bedtime Snack

1 cup 10% fat ice cream

Nutrient	RDA: male 25 to 50 years	Actual	% RDA
kcal	===================*	2972 kcal	102
Protein	===================*==================	119 gm	188
Carbohydrate	===================**	394 gm	109
Fat	===================****	115 gm	119
Cholesterol	==================	268 mg	89
Fiber-dietary	===================***	33 gm	114
Vitamin A	===================*====================	3415 RE	342
Thiamin	===================*=================	2.8 mg	186
Riboflavin	===================*====================	4.0 mg	234
Niacin	===================*=======	25 mg	133
Vitamin B_6	===================*=============	3.4 mg	170
Folate	===================*====================	430 mcg	215
Vitamin B_{12}	===================*====================	7.0 mcg	351
Pantothenic acid	===================*=======	7.6 mg	138
Vitamin C	===================*====================	125 mg	209
Vitamin D	===================*===================	9.6 mcg	192
Vitamin K	===================*====================	362 mcg	452
Sodium	===================*============	3940 mg	164
Potassium	===================*====================	5354 mg	268
Calcium	===================*====================	1743 mg	218
Phosphorus	===================*====================	2051 mg	256
Magnesium	===================*=======	478 mg	137
Iron	===================* ===============	37 mg	368
Zinc	===================**	16 mg	107
Copper	===============	1.8 mg	81
Manganese	===================*====================	6.6 mg	188
Selenium	===================*=========	0.1 mg	147
	^0 ^50 ^100 ^150 ^200		

Carbohydrate, Protein, and Fat Distribution

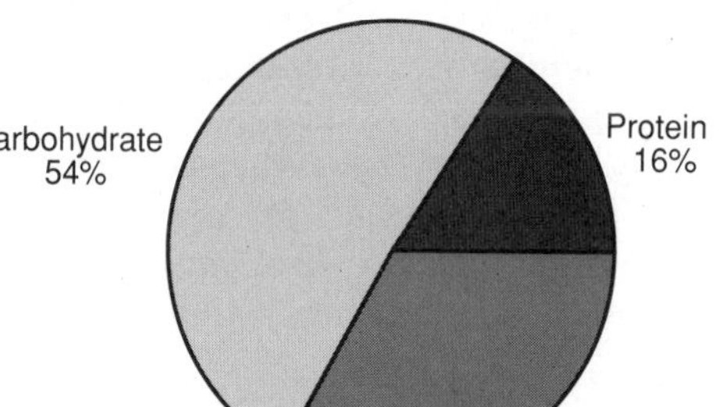

Figure 12–1 Typical hospital regular diet. (RDA, Recommended dietary allowance; RE, retinol requirements) (Nutrient data from Nutritionist III, version 7.0 software, Salem, Oregon.)

NUTRITION TEAMWORK

Before nursing nutritional care can be implemented, it is important that all team members are working together. Communication among the team (departments, client, family) is vital. For instance, if an Asian family brings in soy sauce for a client to use on the food when the physician has ordered a 3- to 4-gm sodium diet, it is likely the sodium intake will exceed the level ordered.

Successful nutrition management requires complementary teamwork between the client and family, physician, nurse, dietary department, and dietitian or dietetic technician. Sometimes the cooperative efforts of this team are less obvious than

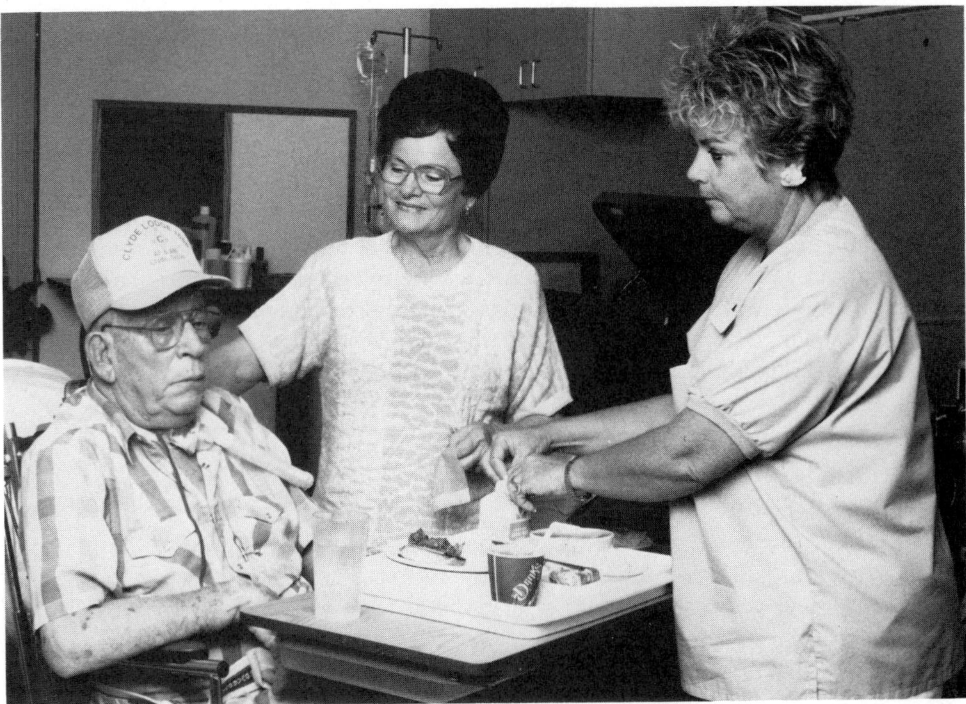

Figure 12–2 The nurse has an important role in the client's intake.

others; the shared responsibility for the client varies only in degree, not in overall support. Observation, documentation, and communication are critical operating factors among these members for a successful outcome.

Providing nutritious, appetizing food is usually a function of the dietary department. The dietitian plans the diet and may assess the nutritional status of the client. Nursing service has an important role in seeing that the client eats the food, progresses toward improved health, and is satisfied with his or her dietary plan (Fig. 12–2).

The client should be involved in the decision-making process to determine the expected outcome or goals. Input from the client and family can provide additional information about food habits or problems that may affect client cooperation. Foods brought in by family and friends must comply with the diet prescription. When all factors are considered, the diet will be more acceptable and is more likely to be followed on discharge.

Although the client needs to know what foods to avoid, emphasis should be placed on foods that are allowed as well as enjoyed. A positive emphasis can help to motivate the client. Motivation is best ensured by the client's understanding and knowledge. An awareness of the role of the diet in his or her health and recovery process or in minimizing the discomforts of the disease will more likely elicit cooperation from the client.

Because of close contact with the client and family, the nurse can frequently motivate the client to eat or to follow a diet at home. Through informal but "planned" conversations during meals, the client can learn more about the diet and nutritional needs. Patience, tact, kindness, ingenuity, and firmness bolster client morale. Continual education throughout the hospital stay by input from both nursing and dietary staffs is much more effective than one formal diet instruction just before discharge. Usually, formal diet instruction may be provided by dietary staff, but nursing service can have a great impact on client cooperation by reinforcing the expectations of the dietary regimen.

Uneaten food on the tray does not provide nourishment. Monitoring intake may be necessary when problems with intake are observed. Nurses are usually with the client at mealtimes; therefore, their attitude and understanding of nutritional concepts can influence whether the client eats. Observing, listening, and reporting are vital nursing responsibilities that provide essential information for the dietitian. Observations can be made regarding how well the client eats, what kinds and amounts of food are refused, and the client's attitude toward the food. Mealtime observations are essential to any care plan. When a client states he or she will eat something, yet it lies untouched on the tray, more adjustments must be made. By listening, the nurse can learn which foods are preferred and why. Without communication between the nursing staff and the dietary department about the client's needs and preferences, success in providing nutrition support is minimal.

Who is included in the nutrition team? What is a nurse's role on the nutrition team?

NURSING APPLICATIONS

Assessment

Physical—for emotional status, type of illness, drugs taken, stress level.

Dietary—for dietary history, especially regarding likes and dislikes and cultural or religious preferences; adequacy of food intake.

Interventions

1. Individualize nutritional care. Treatment varies depending on whether a client overeats when stressed as compared with one who has no appetite when stressed.
2. If intake appears to be low in protein and vitamin C foods, encourage client to choose foods that furnish these nutrients.
3. Raise the head of the bed or position in chair for meals.
4. Chart how well the client eats, kinds and amounts of food refused, and client's attitude toward food.
5. Focus on the positive, not the negative, i.e., "Look, you can still have..." rather than "Well, you can't have this, this, or that."
6. Allow client to choose from menu selections; do not choose for the client unless necessary.
7. Accept criticism of food casually.
8. Remind physicians of how many meals have been missed because of testing or how long the client has been on IV feedings or nutritionally inadequate diets (either the diet or the intake may be inadequate).

Client Education

- Eat foods high in protein and vitamin C to offset the effects of stress and immobilization associated with hospitalization unless contraindicated, such as in renal disease.
- A client's input is vital to the nutritional care team.
- Teach client about diet during "peak" learning times—i.e., while making menu selections, watching food commercials, reading food advertisements, and serving the tray.

BASIC DIET MODIFICATIONS

Despite numerous diet modifications available for various abnormal conditions, most hospital diets are based on a regular diet with variations in texture and consistency. As shown in Tables 12–2 and 12–3, hospital diets are designed to follow a sequence. Normally the client is NPO for a few hours before surgery. After surgery, clear liquid diets help the client return to normal absorption and digestion patterns. The full-liquid diet is then instituted, followed by the soft and then the regular diet.

TABLE 12–2

FOODS ALLOWED IN PROGRESSIVE HOSPITAL DIETS

Food Group	Regular	Mechanical Soft	Soft or Light	Full Liquid	Clear Liquid
Milk and milk products	All	All	All types of milk products; mild cheese	Milk and milk beverages, eggnog, milkshakes, yogurt, ice cream, pudding, custard	None
Meat and protein foods	All	Eggs, tender meats or meats processed by grinding or chopping, peanut butter, creamed meats, casseroles	Tender or ground chicken, fish, beef, lamb, liver, veal, eggs, simple casseroles, smooth peanut butter	Pureed meats added to cream soups	None
Fruits and vegetables	All	All juices, all pureed fruits and vegetables, applesauce, banana, cooked or canned tender fruits and vegetables; potatoes	Cooked vegetables and vegetable juices, potatoes, fruit juices, cooked and canned fruits (without seeds, coarse skins, or fiber), bananas, orange and grapefruit sections without membrane	Strained fruit juices, whipped potatoes, vegetable juices, vegetable puree in soup	Clear fruit juices, such as apple, cranberry, grape, other strained fruit juices, vegetable water
Grain	All	Cooked cereals, dry cereals served with milk, cooked noodles, rice, enriched and whole-wheat bread, refined crackers, simple cakes, plain cookies served with a beverage	Whole-grain or enriched breads and cereals without seeds or nuts or coarse cereals such as bran, noodles, rice, spaghetti, macaroni, crackers, melba toast, zwieback, graham crackers, plain cookies, cake	Cooked refined cereals, strained or blended gruels	None
Other beverages	All	All	All	All	Carbonated beverages, tea, coffee, clear fruit-flavored drinks, lemonade
Soups	All	All	Broth, strained cream soups	Cream soup, broth	Clear broths, bouillon, consomme
Fat	All	Butter, margarine	Butter, margarine, bacon, mild salad dressings	Margarine, butter, cream	None
Sweets	All	Pudding, pie, sherbet, gelatin desserts	Gelatin, sherbet	Clear candies, honey, sugar, popsicles, plain sugar-sweetened gelatin, syrup, sherbet	Syrup, clear candies, honey, sugar, popsicles, sugar sweetened gelatin, ices
Miscellaneous	All	Seasonings, cream sauce, gravy	Mild seasonings, gravy, plain sauces	Salt, spices in moderation, flavorings	Salt

The main concern is to provide continuous nutrition support to the fullest degree possible for the prevailing circumstances. However, if dietary modification is not required, nutritional care is supplied by a regular diet that provides clients' optimal nutritional requirements and meets their psychological and aesthetic needs for appetite appeal. Since the regular diet has no restrictions or nutrient inadequacies, it is presented last.

What is the normal diet progression following surgery and why?

TABLE 12–3

MENUS FOR PROGRESSIVE DIETS

Regular	Mechanical Soft	Soft	Full Liquid	Clear Liquid
Breakfast				
Pineapple juice	Pineapple juice	Pineapple juice	Strained pineapple juice	Apple juice
Banana	Banana	Banana		
Bran flakes	Bran flakes or oatmeal	Corn flakes	Cream of wheat with margarine and sugar	Chicken broth
Fruit-flavored yogurt	Fruit-flavored yogurt	Fruit-flavored yogurt		High-kilocalorie fruit-flavored gelatin
Whole wheat toast with margarine and jelly	Whole wheat toast with margarine and jelly	Whole wheat toast with margarine and jelly		
Low-fat (2%) milk	Low-fat (2%) milk	Low-fat (2%) milk	Homogenized or low-fat (2%) milk	
Coffee with nondairy creamer and sugar	Coffee with nondairy creamer and sugar	Coffee with nondairy creamer and sugar	Coffee with nondairy creamer and sugar	Coffee or tea with sugar
Mid-morning nourishment				
			Milkshake	Carbonated beverage
Lunch				
Broiled lean pork chop	Ground/chopped pork chop	Broiled lean pork chop	Strained cream soup	Beef broth
Scalloped potatoes	Scalloped potatoes	Scalloped potatoes		
Boiled carrots	Boiled carrots	Boiled carrots		
Coleslaw	Cranberry juice	Cranberry juice	Tomato juice	Cranberry juice
Whole wheat roll	Whole wheat roll	Whole wheat roll		
Margarine	Margarine	Margarine	Margarine	
Baked apple	Peeled baked apple	Peeled baked apple	Vanilla pudding	High-kilocalorie, fruit-flavored gelatin
Coffee or tea with sugar/nondairy creamer	Coffee or tea with sugar/nondairy creamer	Coffee or tea with sugar/nondairy creamer	Coffee or tea with sugar, lemon, and cream	Coffee or tea with sugar, lemon
			Homogenized or low-fat milk	
Mid-afternoon nourishment				
			Vanilla pudding	Tea with sugar and lemon
			Grape juice	Popsicle
Dinner				
Beef stroganoff on noodles	Tender/chopped beef stroganoff on noodles	Beef cubes in bouillon on noodles	Beef broth with strained pureed beef	High-protein broth
Steamed broccoli with cheese sauce	Steamed chopped broccoli with cheese sauce	Yellow squash		
Relishes (cherry tomatoes, radishes, cucumbers, celery sticks)	Sliced tomatoes	Tomato juice	Fruit-flavored gelatin	Grape juice
Cream pie with blueberries	Cream pie with blueberries	Cream pie with blueberry sauce	Ice cream	Popsicle

TABLE 12–3

MENUS FOR PROGRESSIVE DIETS
Continued

Regular	Mechanical Soft	Soft	Full Liquid	Clear Liquid
Whole wheat bread	Whole wheat bread	Whole wheat bread		
Margarine	Margarine	Margarine		
Low-fat (2%) milk	Low-fat (2%) milk	Low-fat (2%) milk	Homogenized or low-fat (2%) milk	
Tea or coffee with sugar, lemon, non-dairy creamer	Tea or coffee with sugar, lemon, non-dairy creamer	Tea or coffee with sugar, lemon, non-dairy creamer	Tea or coffee with sugar, lemon, non-dairy creamer	Tea or coffee with sugar, lemon
Evening nourishment				
Ice cream	Ice cream	Low-fat (2%) milk Graham crackers	Eggnog	High-kilocalorie gelatin

Clear Liquid Diet

Indications

The **clear liquid diet** provides clear fluids requiring minimal digestion to relieve thirst, prevent dehydration, maintain electrolyte balance, yield minimal bowel residue, and test the ability to tolerate oral feedings. The clear liquid diet is inadequate in all nutrients and should be used for only a brief period of time (24 to 48 hours) following periods of acute vomiting or diarrhea or surgery.

Only clear liquids or substances that liquefy at room temperature (e.g., gelatin) are allowed.

Broth provides some sodium, carbonated beverages provide sugar, and fruit juices provide a small amount of carbohydrate and potassium. Commercial gelatin products and sweetened beverages are good sources of fluid and provide some kilocalories; at the same time, their electrolyte content is insufficient to be of practical value in replacing electrolytes lost from vomitus and diarrheal fluid.

What are the indications for a clear liquid diet?

Characteristics

The amount of fluid in a given feeding on the clear liquid diet is usually restricted to 30 to 60 ml/hr at first, gradually increasing the amount as tolerance improves. These should be provided frequently (approximately every 2 hours).

Some facilities allow only apple juice on the very strict clear liquid diet; others may allow all juices except prune and tomato. (Some juices, e.g., orange, may not be well tolerated, causing stomach distention.) The most preferred items on this diet are tea, ginger ale, and apple juice.

Some facilities allow only decaffeinated coffee, whereas others serve regular coffee. Such policies should be verified in the diet manual.

Give some examples of clear liquid foods.

Supplementation

A growing trend is to increase the nutrient intake during this period. A few institutions have even phased out the clear liquid diet because of its nutritional inadequacies in favor of specific items that promote optimum nutrition and decrease the length of stay in the hospital. Several supplements of high-nutrient content are appropriate. High-protein broth mixes (Delmark, Ross) provide high-quality protein and more kilocalories yet contain half as much sodium as a standard broth. Citro-

Osmolality—number of osmotically active particles per kilogram of a solvent; the osmolality of body fluids is approximately 300 mOsm/kg. Carbohydrates, electrolytes, and free amino acids increase the osmolality of a product.

source (Sandoz), Surgical Liquid Diet (Ross), or Forta (Ross) beverages are nutritionally balanced and are suggested for use until the client can tolerate normal foods of higher nutrient content. These beverages have a specified **osmolality,** an important concern when clients have been NPO for extended periods (possibly receiving parenteral feedings) or when diets are advanced postoperatively.

Contraindications

Ingestion of large amounts of fluids with a high osmolality can cause body fluids to enter the intestine to dilute hyperosmotic fluids; this fluid imbalance may result in nausea, diarrhea, and other GI distress. Fluids having a high osmolality (>500 mOsm/kg) may need to be diluted with water before ingestion to avoid this (Table 12–4). These problems are more prevalent in clients following gastric surgery, in debilitated clients, and in those who have not had any oral intake for several days. Special attention must be given to clients with diabetes mellitus or functional hypoglycemia to maintain blood glucose control (see Chapters 27 and 28). Following gastric surgery or myocardial infarction, caffeine-containing beverages (coffee, tea, and colas) may be undesirable since caffeine stimulates hydrochloric acid secretion and increases the heart rate.

What clients are more prone to problems with clear liquid diets?

NURSING APPLICATIONS

Assessment

Physical—for thirst, dehydration, vomiting, diarrhea, type of surgery, nausea.

Dietary—for beverage preferences.

Interventions

1. For clients with congestive heart failure, use the high-protein or low-sodium broth mixes.
2. Notify physician or dietitian if this diet is used for more than 48 hours.

Client Education

- Some fruit juices, e.g., orange, may not be well tolerated, causing stomach distention.

TABLE 12–4

APPROXIMATE OSMOLALITY OF SOME COMMON LIQUID FOODS

Food Item	mOsm/kg
Tea	8
Diet cola	43
Tea with 1 tsp sugar	106
Milk	277
Chicken broth	389
Ginger ale	565
Orange juice (strained)	601
Lemon-lime soda	640
Apple juice	705
Cola	714
Gelatin dessert	735
Cranberry juice	836
Grape juice	1170
Sherbet	1230

Data from Bell SJ. Osmolality of beverages commonly provided on clear and full liquid menu. *Nutr Clin Pract* 1987 Dec; 2(6):241–244.

Full Liquid Diet

Indications

The **full liquid diet** is frequently used for clients (1) postoperatively as a transition between clear liquid and solid foods, (2) unable to chew or swallow solid foods following dental surgery or surgery of the face-neck area, and (3) unable to tolerate solid foods due to stricture or anatomical irregularity. The full liquid diet has traditionally been used as a step in the progression from clear liquids to solid foods, but often this is unnecessary (see Table 12–2).

Foods that are liquid or liquefy at room temperature, including all items on the clear liquid diet plus milk and some milk-containing products, make up the full liquid diet.

Following tonsillectomy or throat surgery, a cold semiliquid diet may be used because it is chemically, mechanically, and thermally nonirritating to the throat (see Chapter 25).

What are some indications for a full liquid diet?

Characteristics

The main criterion for foods on the full liquid diet is that they "pour." The diet should be smooth, easy to swallow, require no chewing, and become liquid at room or body temperature. Protein and energy levels are easily increased if desired. The goal is for maximum nutrients per serving, so each serving can be fortified with other foods as much as possible. The diet can be supplemented with commercial products such as Ensure (Ross) or Instant Breakfast (Carnation) to provide adequate nutrients. Four to 6 feedings or more per day may be provided to increase client intake.

A variety of foods may be used, including milk, plain frozen desserts, pasteurized eggs, fruit juices, vegetable juices, cereal gruels, broth, milk, and egg substitutes. The use of whole raw eggs or egg whites is not advisable because of the danger of *Salmonella* infection. Frequently, a pasteurized, commercial eggnog preparation or other high-protein supplement is recommended. Many clients who are ill may refuse milk products for various personal beliefs. Pinnock et al (1990) found no overall association between milk or dairy products and nasal secretions for adults with a cold. The client's temperature has no bearing on the ability to tolerate milk. Milk is easily digested and provides little residue. Milk in moderation is not constipating, but if the diet is lacking bulk and fiber, constipation can result.

A dental liquid diet may be necessary for long periods of time for those who have wired jaws. The goal is to provide nutritional requirements through nutrient-dense liquids and blenderized foods. Blended foods are not always appealing and may become monotonous to some clients. Freeze-dehydration in combination with blenderizing has produced commercially available items with identifiable taste and improved acceptability, i.e., beef burgundy, beef stroganoff, beef with gravy, beef with spaghetti, chili, and chicken and pork concoctions.

Give some examples of full liquid foods.

Supplementation

A vitamin-mineral supplement plus high-kilocalorie, high-protein supplements are recommended if the full liquid diet is to be used for more than a few days. The protein level of the full liquid diet may be augmented by including nonfat dry milk in allowable foods or using commercial nutrition supplements (see Chapter 13). Pureed meats can be added to bouillon or tomato juice to increase protein content.

For additional kilocalories, butter or fortified margarine may be added to hot liquids, and **glucose polymers** may be dissolved in fruit juices. Glucose polymers (Polycose, Ross; Sumacal, Sherwood), which are not as sweet as sucrose, can provide more kilocalories without significantly affecting the taste of the food.

Glucose polymers, commercially available carbohydrate supplements composed of glucose, maltose, and dextrins, can be mixed with most foods and beverages to increase the kilocaloric content.

How can additional kilocalories be added to a full liquid diet?

Contraindications

If a low-sodium diet is indicated, low-sodium soups, eggnogs, and custard can be offered. The full liquid diet may be contraindicated for clients who are **lactose-**

Clients who have a deficiency of the enzyme lactase to hydrolyze lactose are lactose-intolerant and develop GI cramping, flatus, and diarrhea when lactose is consumed.

What clients need special attention if on a full liquid diet?

intolerant or have had GI surgery causing a temporary lactose intolerance (see Chapter 23). Lactose-hydrolyzed milk or lactose-free supplements may be substituted. Because of its high concentration of simple carbohydrates and hyperosmolality, the full liquid diet may be contraindicated following gastric surgery.

Special attention should be given to planning full liquid diets for clients with diabetes mellitus or functional hypoglycemia to provide proper amounts of carbohydrate. Since this diet tends to be high in cholesterol, modifications can be implemented if it is to be used on a long-term basis for clients with hyperlipidemia. Skim milk can be substituted for whole milk, and polyunsaturated fats and oils can be used.

NURSING APPLICATIONS

Assessment

Physical—for chewing problems, type of infection, fever, type of surgery or disease process.
Dietary—for anorexia, kilocaloric intake.
Laboratory—for high cholesterol and triglyceride levels and high glucose levels.

Interventions

1. If a client likes milk and has a cold or cough, offer milk.
2. Monitor for diarrhea, bloating, and flatus in clients on full-liquid diets. If observed, consult the dietitian or physician since the client may be lactose intolerant.
3. If lipid level is elevated, offer skim milk.

Client Education

- Milk and dairy products do not increase mucus production.
- Cool liquids may be used to help lower a high temperature.

Soft Diet

Indications

A soft diet, consisting of liquid and solid foods that contain a limited amount of indigestible carbohydrate and no tough connective tissue, is designed for clients unable to tolerate a regular diet.

Stenosis—contracted or narrowed opening.

What types of clients need a soft diet?

A **soft diet** is used in the diet progression between a liquid and general diet, for debilitated clients unable to consume a general diet, and for clients with mild GI disturbances. Distention caused by bulky food and bowel movements may elicit pain. This is typical in acute GI disturbances or following surgery. The diet is indicated whenever inflammatory changes have progressed to **stenosis** of the intestinal or esophageal lumen or, in some instances, of esophageal varices.

Characteristics

Foods are cooked simply. Tender meats or those tenderized in the cooking process are used to decrease the amount of connective tissue. These are low in residue and readily digested. Fried foods and rich pastries are omitted. Other high-fat, highly seasoned foods, such as corned beef and frankfurters, salad dressing, nuts, and coconut, as well as strong seasonings (garlic, barbecue sauce) are avoided.

Vegetables must be cooked, not raw. Dried beans and peas and corn are excluded. Strongly flavored vegetables, such as onions, leeks, and radishes, and vegetables of the cabbage family (Brussels sprouts, cauliflower, broccoli, and turnips) have commonly been omitted. These "gas-forming" vegetables are more likely to cause discomfort when cooked improperly. To minimize these effects, such vegetables should be cooked quickly; the cooking utensil is kept uncovered; vegetables are drained and served promptly. Rather than prohibit all strongly flavored vegetables, options by the staff and clients should be exercised. Some fresh fruits such as bananas, grapefruit, or orange sections without membrane and most canned or cooked fruits are permitted. All others are avoided as well as brans, coarse grains, and alcoholic beverages.

The diet is likely to be deficient in fiber, which compounds the problems of abnormal bowel movements associated with bed rest, medications, anesthesia, and inadequate food and fluid intake. Small frequent feedings may be helpful if gas and distention are a problem.

Some facilities define a light or convalescent diet separately from a soft diet. Others use these terms interchangeably. The diet manual can be consulted to distinguish hospital policy.

List examples of foods allowed on a soft diet. What is this diet usually lacking?

NURSING APPLICATIONS

Assessment

Physical—for inability to consume a general diet, GI disturbances, constipation, type of surgery.

Dietary—for food preferences allowed on soft diet, cooking techniques.

Intervention

1. Monitor bowel movements. Clients may become constipated on a soft diet because of a lack of fiber.

Client Education

- Broiled and baked foods are allowed on a soft diet.
- Fried foods, rich pastries, highly spiced foods, and raw vegetables are eliminated to prevent GI discomfort.

Mechanical Soft (Dental Soft) Diet

Indications

A **mechanical soft** diet is used for the client who has no teeth or who has difficulty in chewing or swallowing that may be due to the absence of several teeth, loose dentures, sore gums, cancer of the head or neck region, esophageal repair, or certain neurological disorders.

A mechanical soft diet provides foods that are easy to chew and swallow.

What type of clients would benefit from a mechanical soft diet?

Characteristics

This diet may be used indefinitely since it is adequate in all nutrients. Any regular foods the client is able to masticate are allowed; others are chopped, ground, or pureed as needed. Since pureed foods are not as well received as chopped or ground foods, individualization according to the client's tolerance and acceptance and other restrictions is the key to client acceptance.

Foods that may need to be avoided or modified include tough meats; fruits or vegetables with membranes, tough skins, or tough fibers; hard rolls; nuts; and caramels.

NURSING APPLICATIONS

Assessment

Physical—for location of cancer, condition of teeth or dentures, and mucous membranes.
Dietary—for food intake and acceptance of diet.

Intervention

1. Check food tray to determine client's acceptance of diet.

Client Education

- This diet can be used as long as needed with no ill effects.

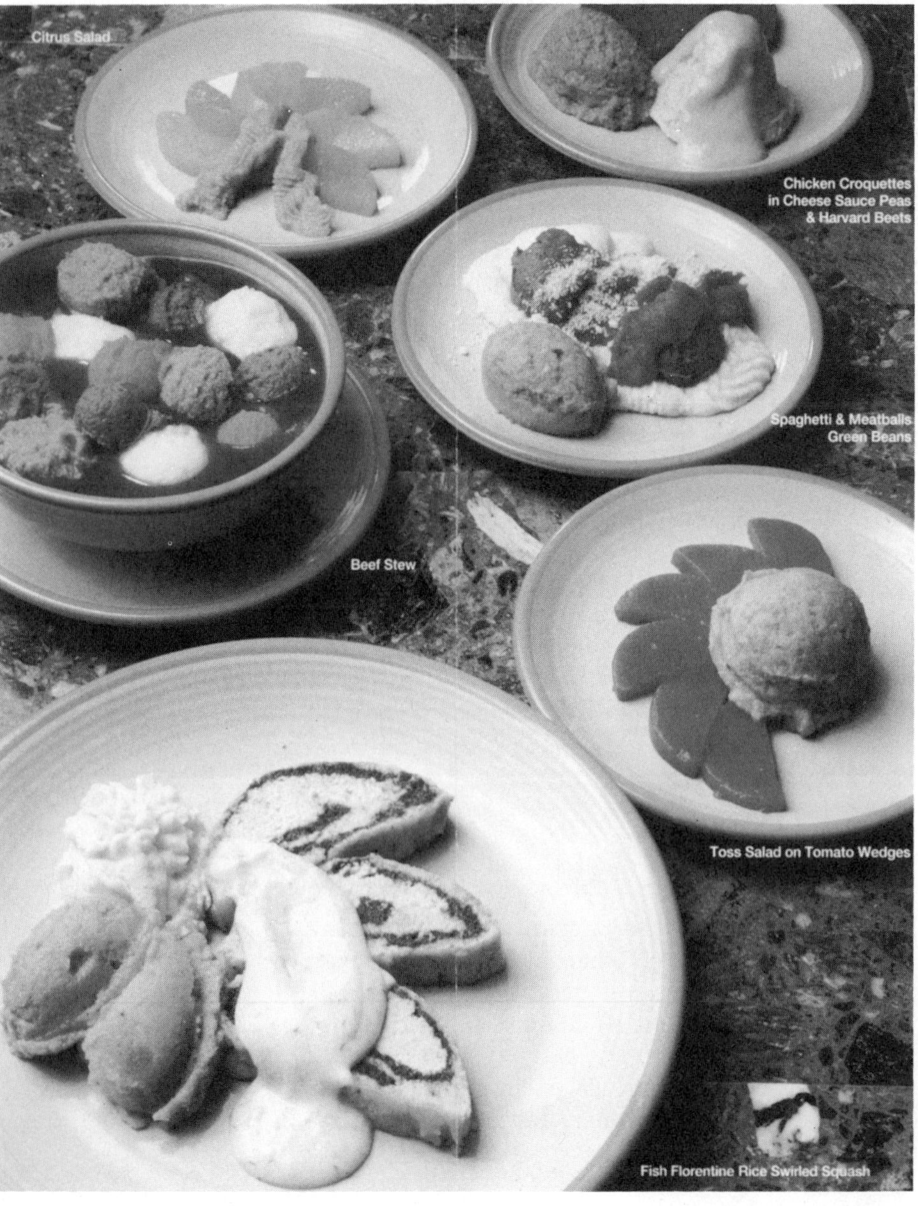

Figure 12–3 Pureed foods can be presented attractively. (Courtesy of Anderson Benner Associates, 3915 Spring Bloom Ct., Sugar Land, TX 77479.)

Pureed Diet

The **pureed diet** is similar to the full liquid diet except foods are semi-liquid instead of more free-flowing. Consistency may be varied according to the client's preference and ability. (More liquid consistency may be called dental liquid.) The nurse and dietitian should evaluate this with the client.

Easily swallowed foods that are soft, smooth, and require no mastication are classified as pureed.

Indications

Clients with neurological disorders who may need retraining in swallowing without aspiration may require this diet; those with wired or fractured jaws would also be candidates. Cancer clients with head and neck abnormalities and stroke clients may also require pureed foods.

What types of clients need pureed foods?

Characteristics

Normally a soft diet is the basis for the pureed diet, and adjustments can be made for any therapeutic regimen (for example, diabetes, low salt, low fat). Special attention may be required for optimal food intake. These clients particularly may be under more stressful conditions than others, which may compromise ability to take foods and result in less absorption of available nutrients. Liquids such as milk, gravies, or sauces may be added when the foods are blended to increase palatability and nutritional value. Various fats and sweeteners can be used to provide additional kilocalories.

Component pureeing is advocated to present foods more attractively. Pureed foods can be made to resemble their natural form using an instant food thickener to thicken to the appropriate consistency and using cake decorating techniques (Fig. 12–3).

Component pureeing—each menu item is pureed separately then reassembled in a casserole dish topped with a sauce.

NURSING APPLICATIONS

Assessment

Physical—for neurological disorders, wired or fractured jaw, head and neck cancer, cerebrovascular accident.
Dietary—for food intake and preferences.

Interventions

1. Serve pureed foods attractively to make the meal as enjoyable as possible. This will pay off with improved acceptance.
2. When client is on pureed diet, keep your comments upbeat, i.e., "Your carrots are ready; this looks appetizing; would you rather have your vegetable before eating your meat?" Negative comments such as "This looks like baby food" or "How can you eat this stuff?" may affect the client's acceptance of the food.

Client Education

- The texture of the food is modified to eliminate the need for chewing and/or to ease the swallowing process.

Dysphagia Diets

Dysphagia diets probably vary more from institution to institution than any other diets. Facilities vary as to the number of levels of dysphagia diets. When a dysphagia diet is ordered, usually the speech-language pathologist will be providing

Dysphagia diets are ordered for life-threatening problems in the normal passage of food from the mouth to the stomach.

TABLE 12–5

SAMPLE MENUS FOR DYSPHAGIA DIETS*

Meal	Pureed	Pureed with Texture	Finely Chopped Foods	Chopped Foods
Breakfast	Pureed banana	Mashed banana	Sliced ripe banana	Ripe banana
	Pureed oatmeal with margarine, sugar, and cinnamon	Cooked oatmeal with margarine, sugar, and cinnamon	Rice Krispies	Rice Krispies
	Smooth fruit-flavored yogurt/pureed scrambled egg	Chunky fruit-flavored yogurt/soft scrambled egg	Chunky fruit-flavored yogurt/soft scrambled egg	Chunky fruit-flavored yogurt/soft scrambled egg
			Bread with margarine and jelly	Toast with margarine and jelly
Lunch	Pureed cream of chicken soup with finely crushed crackers	Pureed cream of chicken soup with crushed crackers	Cream of chicken soup with crumbled crackers	Cream of chicken soup with crackers
	Pureed baked pork chop with gravy	Finely ground baked pork chop with gravy	Finely chopped baked pork chop with gravy	Chopped pork chop with gravy
	Mashed potatoes	Finely chopped well-cooked scalloped potatoes	Tender chopped scalloped potatoes	Scalloped potatoes
	Pureed carrots with margarine	Finely chopped cooked carrots with margarine	Tender cooked diced carrots with margarine	Tender cooked carrots
	Applesauce	Chunky applesauce	Peeled baked apple	Peeled baked apple
Dinner	Pureed beef stroganoff with gravy	Finely ground beef stroganoff with gravy	Finely chopped beef stroganoff with gravy	Chopped beef stroganoff with gravy
	Pureed buttered noodles with gravy	Mashed buttered noodles with gravy	Chopped buttered noodles	Buttered noodles
	Pureed broccoli with cheese sauce	Chunky pureed broccoli with cheese sauce	Tender cooked finely chopped broccoli with cheese	Cooked broccoli with cheese sauce
	Pureed peaches with whipped topping	Finely chopped peaches with whipped topping	Diced peaches with whipped cream	Sliced peaches with whipped cream
	Pureed cream pie with strained blueberry glaze	Cream pie with graham cracker crust and blueberry glaze	Cream pie with graham cracker crust and blueberry sauce	Cream pie with blueberries
Evening snack	Chocolate pudding	Chocolate pudding	Chocolate pudding	Chocolate pudding

* Fluids are omitted from the menu because thickness is dependent on the order (e.g., thin, nectar-like, honey-like, or pudding-like consistency).

swallowing training and will recommend specific techniques to facilitate a safe swallow. The nurse should follow these guidelines for anything provided orally (medications, fluids). There is an increased risk of aspiration if the diet is not followed; nurses should be especially aware of the texture level ordered and what types of food are or are not appropriate. Further discussion of conditions causing dysphagia and interventions are found in Chapter 25.

Dysphagia diets normally require an order for texture of foods and thickness of liquids (Table 12–5). Liquids are the most difficult texture to control, especially in the oral stage of the swallow. Liquids can be thin (water, apple juice, milk, tea, coffee, sherbet), medium thick (vegetable juice, nectars, eggnog, cream soups, ice cream), or spoon thick (yogurt, pudding).

When aspiration is a high risk, the client may be NPO or receive only pureed foods. Clients displaying moderate disruption may be allowed some increased texture, but foods must be cohesive to avoid loss of control, pocketing, and/or choking.

For clients exhibiting mild disruption in the oral and/or pharyngeal transit of food, minced (or ground) and soft foods that require little chewing and are easy to control in the mouth are allowed. This level includes finely chopped meats with gravy or sauce, soft meat salads, cottage cheese, chopped legumes, finely chopped canned and cooked fruits, hot cereals, moistened dry cereal, soft bread without crust or seeds, and cream pies (without coconut or nuts).

A further upgrade in texture is for clients displaying minimal difficulty with swallowing. It is essentially a regular diet with slight alterations to increase safety. Soft textured foods are allowed, with meats coarsely chopped. Foods that do not soften easily are avoided, such as raw carrots, celery, raisins, raw apples, peas, corn, nuts, popcorn, and melba toast.

NURSING APPLICATIONS

Assessment

Physical—for neurological disorders such as a cerebral vascular accident, ability to swallow.

Dietary—for attitude and acceptance of dietary restrictions.

Interventions

1. Consult and follow speech pathologist's and RD's orders.
2. Check for pocketing by observing the inside of the client's mouth. Pocketing usually occurs on the affected/weaker side.
3. Monitor color of secretions. Green secretions or secretions that resemble the same color as the food may indicate aspiration is occurring. A blue, dusky skin color, increased respiration rate, and crackles on lung auscultation are also indicators of aspiration.

Client Education

- As the swallowing process improves, the diet will be changed.

Regular or General Diet

Self-selected diets offered by the facility allow the client some options. The regular diet normally meets the basic nutrient requirements to maintain healthy body tissues plus additional demands necessary for new growth and repair (see Fig. 12–1).

Indications

This diet is ordered for the client without restrictions or modifications.

Characteristics

Individual preferences, tolerances, and aversions vary considerably among clients. Some clients associate (sometimes correctly or mistakenly) problems with an intolerance to a particular food or group of foods and refuse to eat it. There is no reason to push such food when substitutes can be found.

Diet As Tolerated

On admission or postoperatively, the order may read "diet as tolerated." Postoperatively the clear liquid to regular diet progression is the standard routine. However, the diet-as-tolerated order permits a client's preferences to be considered at the discretion of the nurse and dietitian. For instance, a client who refuses to eat congealed gelatin and apple juice but who feels "in the mood" for chicken soup and crackers should be allowed to select them. On the other hand, if the request postoperatively is pizza, judicious nurses would advise against such foods, which are slower to digest and could cause problems.

On admission, the diet-as-tolerated order also requires consultation with the client. Digestive problems or strong preferences can influence the ingestion of many foods; this warrants consideration of the foods given for nourishment. This order is an excellent opportunity for interaction between the nurse, dietitian, and client to plan a diet that is eaten, well tolerated, and therefore nourishing.

NURSING APPLICATIONS

Assessment

Physical—for type of illness.
Dietary—for food preferences.

Interventions

1. Allow the client to choose entrees.
2. If allowed by the facility, involve family members in bringing client's favorite foods.

Client Education

- Adequate intake of all nutrients is essential to promote faster recovery.

PROMOTING FOOD INTAKE

Adequate nutrition may mean the difference between a speedy recovery and a prolonged hospital stay. Although all diets need a variety of foods for promoting optimal health, restrictive therapeutic diets may make this harder to achieve. Without a wide variety, the needed nutrients may not be provided. Consequently, inadequate amounts of nutrients to meet the requirements may cause therapeutic measures to be unsuccessful and affect the outcome. Promoting adequate intake includes providing a pleasant eating environment; helping the client obtain nutritious, palatable food by assisting with the meal service; and helping the client eat.

Increasing Frequency of Feedings

During illness, small frequent meals served 4 to 6 times a day may be better accepted in the following situations:

1. Food intolerance caused by acute illness or surgery (anorexia, vomiting, diarrhea, or stress).
2. Reduced capacity as a result of partial or total gastrectomy, hiatal hernia, poor intake for an extended period of time, or continuous enteral feedings.
3. Increased need for kilocalories and nutrients.

4. Specific disease conditions (one should increase fluids for urinary tract infections but restrict fluids in cases of renal failure, congestive heart failure, or increased intracranial pressure).
5. Satiety and comfort (i.e., full or clear liquid diets have limitations to the amount that can be consumed at one time but have a low-satiety value).

Including the basic food groups in each meal (or even in snacks as far as possible) helps the body to obtain optimal nutritive value from each food eaten. To assure frequent feedings, noting proper time intervals for scheduled feedings (approximately every 2 hours) in the nursing care plan may help.

Federal regulations require a time lapse between the last meal of one day and the first meal of the next to be not more than 14 hours. Meals should be 1½ to 3 hours apart, or not more than 5 hours apart between 7:00 AM and 10:00 PM. The kilocalories should be divided among these meals. Items such as juice or ice cream may be counted as snacks but do not constitute a meal.

Describe how to promote food intake. What are some reasons to increase frequency of feedings?

Assisting with Menu Selections

In some institutions, clients can select from a menu, whether on a therapeutic or regular diet. Although it is thought that this provides an opportunity to order preferred foods, some problems arise. Assistance is needed for clients who have visual problems or difficulty in reading or writing. Some are apathetic; these selections become a chore. Institutional food terminology is fairly standardized but may be unfamiliar to clients; some are hesitant to select unfamiliar items.

When menus are filled out, clients may not be hungry and do not know how they will feel the next day. Thus, they may fail to select enough food. Occasionally, every item on the menu is checked; this would result in too many kilocalories. Finicky eaters may not find anything on the menu that whets their appetite. Many clients need guidance in selecting their foods to assure that they receive an appropriate amount.

An excellent learning opportunity occurs when clients on modified diets are allowed to select from a menu. Explanations can be given why certain foods are not on the diet or why only limited amounts are allowed.

What types of clients may need help with menu selections?

Providing a Pleasant Environment

Nursing service is generally responsible for helping the client obtain and enjoy the foods by creating a pleasant environment for eating. If possible, ambulatory clients should be taken to a dining room, where the social experience during mealtime is more conducive to eating. Some facilities have cafeterias or dining rooms for clients. These areas should be bright, cheerful, and seasonally decorated.

Some clients who are clumsy or have difficulty chewing or swallowing may be embarrassed and prefer to eat alone. The perceptive nurse is aware of and respects these feelings.

Preparing the Client

In many circumstances, tray service is necessary. If proper preparations are completed before tray service, food can be delivered faster, reaching the client at its proper temperature. Clients in pleasant surroundings, ready to eat when the tray arrives, are more likely to eat. The nurse should avoid scheduling unpleasant proce-

TABLE 12–6

TIPS FOR PROMOTING FOOD AND FLUID INTAKE

Preparing the client for the meal

Make the client as comfortable as possible—raise the bed if permitted. Sitting in an armchair is the preferred position for eating
Offer bedpans and urinals ahead of time, and remove them before mealtime
Try to ensure that the room is clean and free of odors
Wash the client's face and hands, provide necessary oral hygiene, insert dentures
Clear the bed tray and place it in front of the client
Determine if visitors hinder or help nutritional intake. Some visitors are a hindrance to the client's eating and should be asked to leave; others encourage the client to eat or even feed him or her

Tray service

Check the client's name with the name on the tray
Always check the food on the tray to be sure the correct diet is being served
Check the tray to be certain everything needed is on the tray. (In some instances, if the client has not circled sugar, salt, pepper, or margarine, these items will be omitted)
Serve trays promptly so the food is at an appropriate temperature
Serve trays first to the clients who require less assistance
Remove tray cover before setting the tray in front of the client, especially if client is experiencing nausea. The combined odors of the foods can be offensive
Position everything on the tray so it is within easy reach
Remove covers from foods. Open food containers, butter bread, pour beverages, cut meat, and otherwise assist, as needed. This is especially necessary when one arm cannot be used
Encourage the client to eat, but do not rush him or her
Place a hand towel over the chest to protect the gown or pajamas for those with coordination problems or who are slightly reclining on the bed
Remove the tray promptly when the client has finished eating
After the client has finished eating, provide an opportunity for proper mouth care and washing his or her hands
If the tray cannot be eaten immediately because of tests or treatment, make arrangements to keep the food at the proper temperature or to receive the tray at a later time

Feeding the client

Sit down while feeding the client and appear at ease and unhurried
For blind clients, attractively describe the food. Caution them about foods that seem to be very hot, and identify each food before placing it in their mouth. Many blind clients can feed themselves if they know where the food is located on the tray. The items can be described in relation to the numbers on a clock
Offer small amounts of food at a time, encouraging the client to chew the food well
Find out how the client prefers to eat the items: Some eat all of one food; others alternate one food with another. However, studies indicate switching from one food to another during a meal generally increases intake
Use flexible straws for those who cannot use a cup
Allow ample time for the client to chew and swallow or rest between mouthfuls
Try to be neat and not spill foods; wipe the client's mouth with a napkin as needed during the meal
Converse in a pleasant and supportive manner to make the client feel more at ease

Promoting fluid intake

Be familiar with a client's beverage preferences and offer them frequently, if they are permitted on the diet
Offer fluids frequently throughout the day
Serve fluids in small glasses
Offer fluid alternatives such as ice cream or gelatin
Use a straw for beverage intake with bedfast clients

dures, such as painful dressing changes and postural drainage, around mealtime. Remember, the objective with hospitalized clients is usually to entice them to eat despite a poor appetite. Suggestions for making sure the client is ready to eat when the tray arrives are listed in Table 12–6.

Serving the Trays

Preparation of the trays is usually the responsibility of the dietary department, but interdepartmental cooperation assures better care of the client. An attractive tray served in a warm, cheerful manner helps ensure its being eaten. This gives the nurse an opportunity to learn more about the client, discuss the diet, and see how well the food is tolerated. Certain procedures ensure that the proper tray is served in the right manner so it can be eaten by the client, as shown in Table 12–6.

Foods brought in by family and friends should be judged for their suitability for the client's diet and condition. If these items interfere with the intake of nutritious foods or are contradictory to the prescribed diet, they should be discouraged.

Feeding the Client

Most clients prefer to feed themselves, but acutely ill or handicapped clients warrant being fed. To encourage their self-esteem, clients should be allowed to do as much as they are capable of doing (see Table 12–6). Providing unnecessary assistance can be offensive to clients or nudge them into a dependent role. Occasionally, clients will not eat rather than request assistance. In determining how much assistance is necessary, consider both the client's nutritional needs and the physical ability.

The types of food served may affect one's ability to self-feed. Gelatin, baked custard, and peas are difficult to spoon if only one hand can be used. Sometimes finger foods are easier for clients to handle and permit more independence.

Monitoring Fluid Intake

Tissue hydration is essential for normal physiological functions. Included in fluid intake are substances taken into the body that are liquids at body temperature, such as gelatin, ice cream, and other frozen liquids.

Normal fluid intake should be 1500 to 2000 ml, or approximately 2 qts daily. Fever, infection, and increased losses from sweating or diarrhea increase fluid requirements. Although thirst normally regulates a client's fluid intake to maintain proper fluid and electrolyte balance, clients are sometimes too weak to get themselves a drink. Bedridden clients may purposely curtail fluid intake to avoid bothering the nurse for a bedpan.

When oral fluid is not sufficient, parenteral infusions are necessary; these should not routinely replace oral intake. Measures to promote fluid intake are presented in Table 12–6.

Before an operation and for various testing procedures, fluid may be withheld for 8 to 10 hours. However, sufficient amounts of fluid should be offered before and after these periods.

During certain disease conditions, fluids may be limited. The total allotment should be divided proportionately over the 24-hour period. It is usually advisable to serve fluids between meals rather than at mealtimes. Denying a client's request for fluids is hard to do; tips to alleviate problems associated with limited fluid intake are given in Chapter 8, Table 8–1.

What may increase fluid requirements? When are parenteral fluids necessary?

NURSING APPLICATIONS

Assessment

Physical—for ability to fill out the menu; type of illness or surgery; sensory problems, especially visual; I&O.

Dietary—for adequacy in nutrients and kilocalories; any restrictions, family's/client's acceptance of ordered diet.

Interventions

1. Assist client in filling out menu as needed.
2. Monitor verbal and nonverbal cues to determine eating place for client. If client turns away or tightens muscles/hands, this client does not want to eat in public. Accept this decision.
3. Follow suggestions in Table 12–6.
4. Large quantities of food can be upsetting to some—they become discouraged just looking at it or become concerned about food waste. If this occurs, alert the dietitian to the problem.
5. Discuss any unresolved dietary problems with a dietitian.

Evaluation

* Anytime the client does not eat well, whether he or she is self-feeding or being fed, try to determine the cause and a remedy. Recording is the best way to communicate this information with other team members.
* Make judgments about the quantity of food served by determining whether the client is satisfied afterward. If it is not adequate, offer substitutions, snacks, or nutritional supplements as appropriate.
* Evaluate the client's lifestyle to determine if any nutritional care is needed after discharge, such as Meals on Wheels or food stamps.
* Evaluate a client's health for maintenance or improvement (overweight client loses weight; client with kidney disease eats low-protein diet; or client verbalizes high-fiber foods to help decrease constipation).

Client Education

- Explain the institution's policies about feedings: tray service versus cafeteria style, time of meals, selective menus, whether or not the client will be allowed to sit up for meals, and so forth.
- Explain nutrition terms as the need arises.

SUMMARY

The client's food should be appetizing and enjoyable as well as suitable for his or her physical condition and served in an atmosphere conducive to eating. A conscientious nurse with a fundamental knowledge of dietary principles can help elicit client cooperation and diet adherence. When this is questionable for any reason, the physician and the dietitian should be consulted.

For optimal nutrition planning, implementation, and evaluation, the nurse's input is invaluable. Information about the client is obtained during discussions with the client and family and during physical observations. A record of food intake and the client's attitude to the food or diet is important as well as information regarding cultural, religious, and social background. Physical observations include a record of weight changes, poorly fitting dentures, arthritic problems, and other problems that may interfere with food intake. The nurse's role involves providing informal, correct dietary information about the implementation and reason for a diet, ensuring a pleasant environment for eating, assisting clients to obtain their food, and encouraging food intake.

NURSING PROCESS IN ACTION

An elderly edentulous man is admitted to the hospital. On assessment, the nurse finds that he has eliminated many foods because they are hard to chew. He also does not enjoy cooking and hates eating alone. His physical condition is stable. Diet as tolerated is ordered.

Nutritional Assessment

- Visual acuity.
- Ability to cut food.
- Motivation for dentures.
- Food preferences, nutrients and food intake, diet ordered.
- Signs and symptoms of malnutrition.
- Beliefs about eating and aging.
- Anthropometric measurements, including body weight and height.
- Psychological factors: anxiety, depression, grief, anger, and others.
- Economic and educational status.
- Oral assessment.

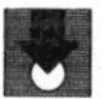

Dietary Nursing Diagnosis

Altered nutrition: high risk for less than body requirements RT possible decreased intake secondary to no teeth and psychological factors.

Nutritional Goals

Client will maintain his body weight and not experience nutritional complications.

Nutritional Implementation 

Intervention: Refer to the dietitian.

Rationale: The dietitian can reinforce the importance of eating well for improved health and well-being and offer suggestions for easy to prepare healthy foods.

Intervention: Discuss preferences for and feelings about tough meats, fruits or vegetables with membranes, nuts, and hard rolls. If the client enjoys some of these items, suggest ways of modifying them. For example, suggest he soften hard rolls or cookies in gravy or beverage.

Rationale: These are the types of food that may be avoided because of chewing problems. Including these items in any form will improve intake.

Intervention: Serve mechanical soft diet.

Rationale: This diet may be used indefinitely since it is adequate in all nutrients and may be preferred by edentulous clients (but this should always be confirmed with the client).

Intervention: Stay with the client while he eats or have him eat in dining room or with another client if allowed.

Rationale: One reason he gave for not eating was he disliked eating alone. This may be a viable option for him to increase intake.

Intervention: Monitor bowel movements.

Rationale: Since he is elderly and on a mechanical soft diet, he is prone to constipation because of loss of muscle tone and lack of fiber, respectively.

Intervention: Allow client to feed himself.

Rationale: He is physically stable, and this will allow him to maintain his independence and self-esteem.

Intervention: Encourage fluid intake, especially water.

Rationale: Fluid is a nutrient, and some elderly are less sensitive to the thirst regulation by the hypothalamus.

Intervention: Refer to social worker, Meals on Wheels, and Senior Citizen agency before discharge.

Rationale: The social worker may be able to assist with nutritional needs by informing him of food stamps, supplemental security income program, and federal and state nutrition programs for the elderly. Senior Citizen agencies can provide not only nutrition support via congregate meals, but also emotional and social support. Meals on Wheels could bring food to his home if needed.

Intervention: Determine willingness for dentures.

Rationale: If client is receptive, this would provide mechanical means for adequate chewing.

Evaluation

If client's weight remains stable and no nutritional complications occurred such as malnutrition, nausea, vomiting, or PEM, the desired goals were met. Additionally, eating 80 to 100% of meals, enjoying eating, developing no oral lesions, and wearing dentures would also indicate goals were achieved. Naturally, weighing and monitoring client's physical and emotional status for the conditions discussed are warranted for effective evaluation.

STUDENT READINESS

1. Discuss how illness affects dietary intake and body requirements.
2. What is diet therapy? What are the purposes of diet therapy?
3. (a) Write a day's menu plans for each of these diets with modifications based on the general diet: general, mechanical soft, soft, full liquid, and clear liquid. (b) Explain the rationale for each of the dietary modifications and describe foods allowed and avoided.
4. Review 2 other diet manuals besides your facility's manual. (Ask the dietitian where to get these.) How are they different? Why do these changes occur? Rank them in order of your preferences, and state reasons for these decisions.
5. What are some available options for clients who constantly complain about the food?
6. How can the nursing and dietetic staffs work together for the utmost benefit to the client?
7. How can a nurse be influential in the client's food intake?
8. What should the nurse do to ensure adequate nutrition for a client?

REFERENCES

American Dietetic Association (ADA). *Handbook of Clinical Dietetics.* 2nd ed. Chicago, American Dietetics Association, 1992.

American Dietetic Association (ADA). *Manual of Clinical Dietetics.* 4th ed. Chicago, American Dietetic Association, 1992.

Luckmann J, Sorensen KC. What patients' actions tell you about their feelings, fears, and needs. *Nursing* 1975 Feb; 5(2):54–61.

Pinnock CB, et al. Relationship between milk intake and mucus production in adult volunteers challenged with rhinovirus-2. *Am Rev Respir Dis* 1990 Feb; 141(2):352–356.

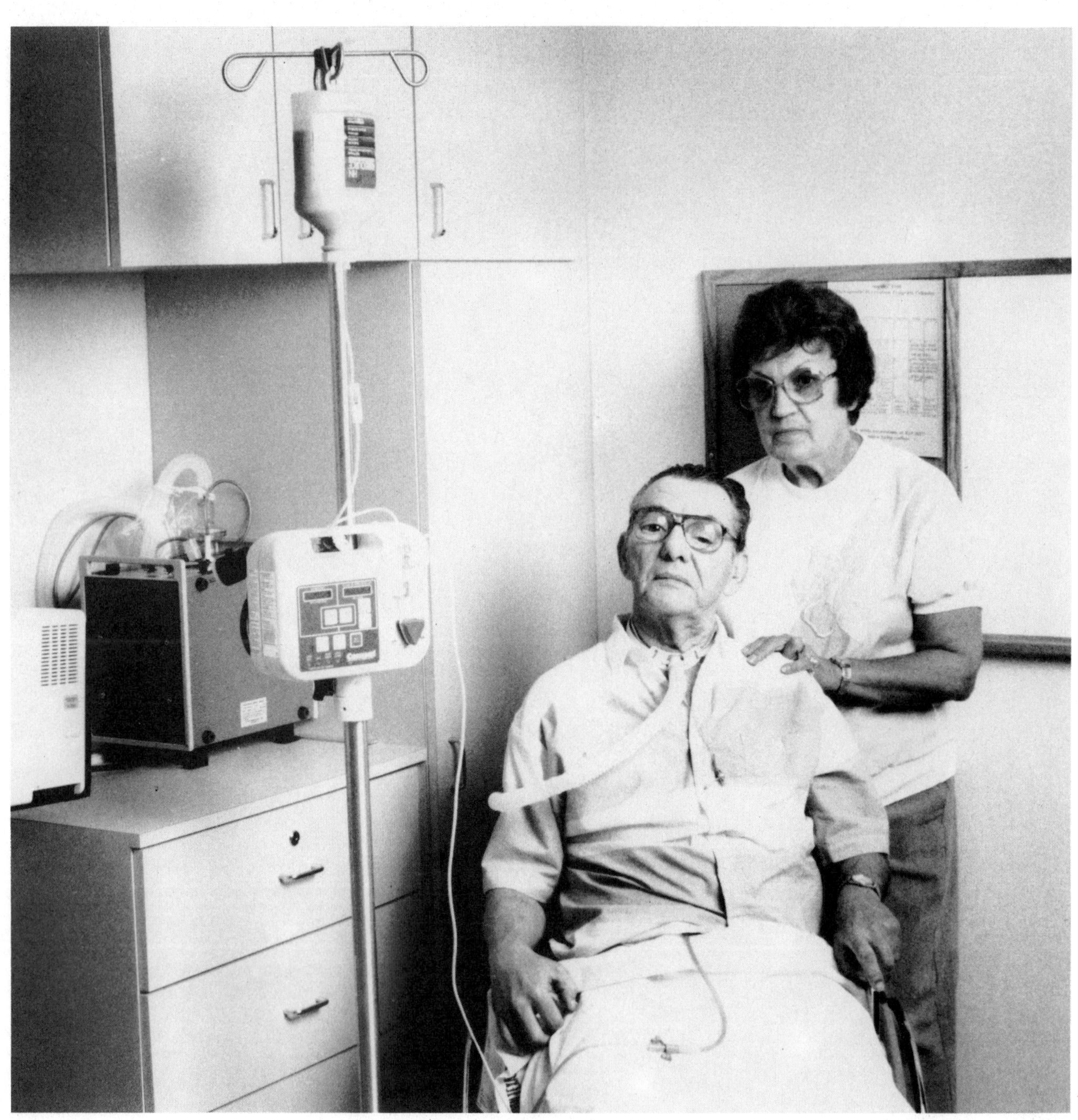

Methods of Nutrition Support: Enteral and Parenteral Nutrition

CHAPTER 13

OUTLINE

- V. **HOME ENTERAL NUTRITION**
  - A. **Determining Appropriate Clients**
  - B. **Psychosocial Adjustments**
  - C. **Determining Appropriate Regimen**
  - D. **Training for Home Therapy**
  - E. **Follow-up**
  - *Nursing Applications*
- VI. **PARENTERAL NUTRITION**
  - A. **Indications for Use**
  - B. **Routes for Total Parenteral Nutrition**
  - *Nursing Applications*
  - C. **Composition of Parenteral Solutions**
    - 1. **Kilocalories**
    - 2. **Carbohydrate**
    - 3. **Fat Emulsions**
    - 4. **Protein**
    - 5. **Vitamins**
    - 6. **Electrolytes and Trace Minerals**
  - *Nursing Applications*
  - D. **Methods of Delivery**
  - E. **Nutrition Support Team**
  - F. **Parenteral Feeding Order**
  - G. **Principles and Procedures for Total Parenteral Nutrition**
  - *Nursing Applications*
  - H. **Complications**
    - 1. **Sepsis**
    - *Nursing Applications*
    - 2. **Hyperglycemia and Hypoglycemia**
    - *Nursing Applications*
    - 3. **Lipid Overload**
    - *Nursing Applications*
    - 4. **Other Problems**
    - *Nursing Applications*
- VII. **HOME PARENTERAL NUTRITION**
  - A. **Determining Clients Appropriate for Home Feedings**
  - B. **Psychosocial Adjustments**
  - C. **Training for Home Parenteral Nutrition**
  - D. **Follow-up**
  - *Nursing Applications*
- VIII. **TRANSITIONAL FEEDINGS**
  - A. **Parenteral to Oral Feeding**
  - B. **Parenteral to Tube Feeding**
  - C. **Tube to Oral Feeding**
  - *Nursing Applications*
- IX. **NUTRITION UPDATE 13–1: CUSTOMIZING FORMULAS TO BOOST IMMUNITY**

OBJECTIVES

THE STUDENT WILL BE ABLE TO:

- Describe when supplemental, tube, parenteral, and/or transitional feedings are required.
- State the advantages of enteral feedings over parenteral feedings.
- Identify the various routes and methods of delivery for tube feedings.
- Explain the cause, prevention, and treatment of hyperglycemic hyperosmolar nonketotic dehydration.
- Describe nursing techniques for administering tube, parenteral, or transitional feedings that affect a client's comfort and adaptation.
- Describe complications and treatments commonly associated with total parenteral nutrition (TPN) and enteral feedings.

- Apply nursing applications for enteral, parenteral, and transitional feedings.
- Describe client education information concerning enteral, parenteral, and transitional feedings.

TEST YOUR NQ (True/False)

1. CPN is a form of TPN.
2. Standard IV solutions are considered a method of nutrition support.
3. Elemental formulas should be given when the GI tract is not wholly functional.
4. Intake of liquid nutrition supplements is enhanced if formulas are at room temperature.
5. A formulary records a client's food intake.
6. TPN feedings are administered into the subclavian vein.
7. Sepsis is a complication of TPN.
8. When changing from tube to oral feeding, tube feedings can be discontinued when the client consumes 1000 kcal/day.
9. Clients currently on TPN can go home.
10. The head of the bed should be elevated 15 degrees when administering tube feedings.

NUTRITION SUPPORT

The catabolic stresses of illness, surgery, trauma, and some therapeutic measures demand aggressive nutrition support: Anywhere from 2000 to 4000 kcal/day are required for recovery; few clients can afford to remain NPO for extended periods without developing malnutrition. Standard dextrose IV solutions are not considered a form of nutrition support; a liter of D_5W (5% dextrose in water) provides only 170 kcal. These dextrose solutions are necessary to prevent or correct more imminent problems of fluid and electrolyte balance; they provide little in terms of required nutrients.

When adequate amounts of nutrients and/or kilocalories are not ingested, somatic and visceral proteins are used for energy. Visceral protein losses lead to poor wound healing, **immunosuppression,** and increased risk of sepsis and other problems.

Immunosuppression—diminished ability to fight infection.

How long a client can withstand inadequate nutritional intake is influenced by many factors: age, previous state of health and nutrition, degree of trauma, and presence of sepsis. A well-nourished adult in a moderately catabolic state usually can tolerate up to 14 days of starvation without encountering significant problems. However, if the client is between 60 to 70 years old, tolerance of starvation is no more than 10 days; for a client over 70, tolerance drops to no more than 7 days (Sax & Fischer, 1988).

When previous food intake and/or accelerated catabolism have resulted in weight loss and less than normal body stores, nutrition support should be implemented as early as possible. Nutrition support should be initiated in the critically ill following 7 to 10 days of partial starvation if not earlier. Prolonged nutrient deprivation prolongs the effects of critical illness.

A general timetable for implementation of nutrition support has been proposed by Rombeau et al (1989a): (1) The client has been without nutrition for 5 to 7 days;

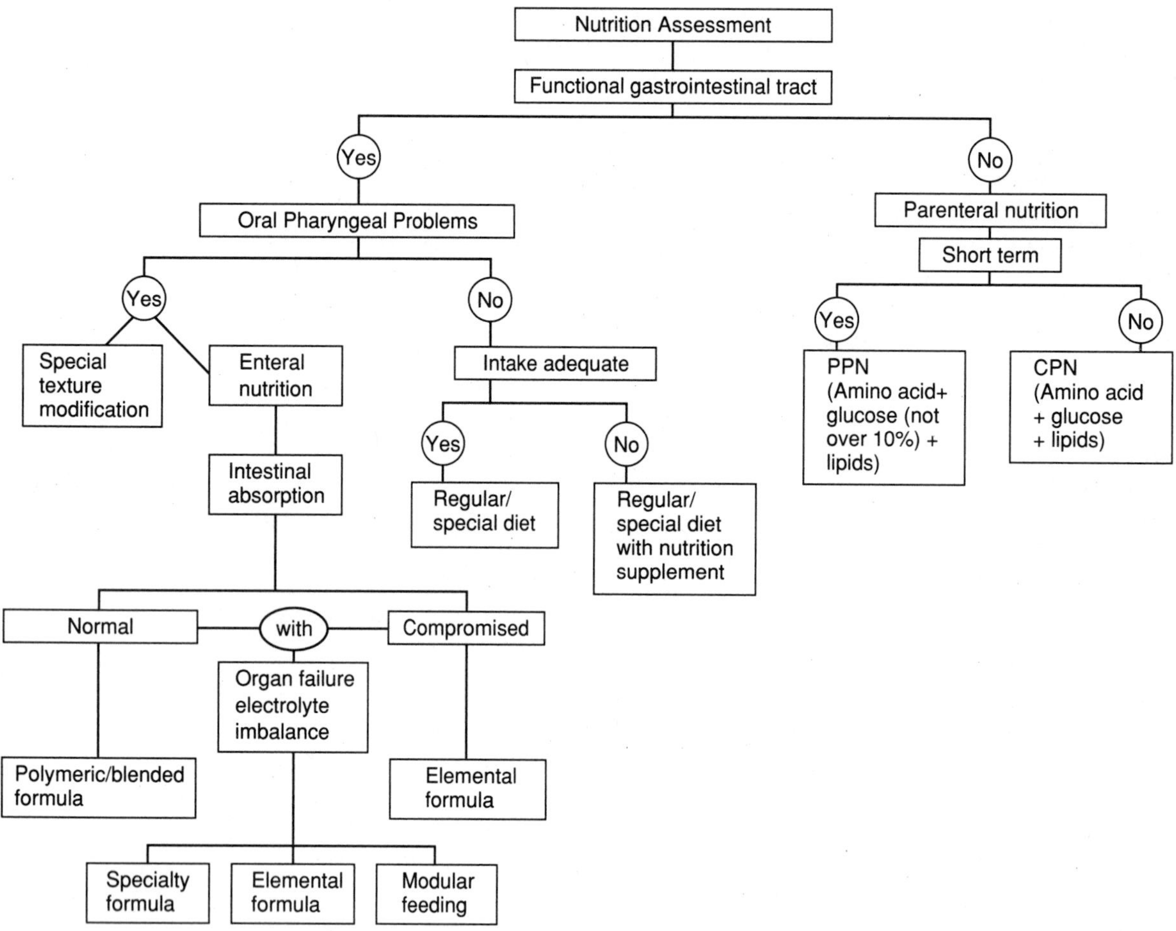

Figure 13–1 **Decision tree for nutrition support. PPN, Peripheral parenteral nutrition; CPN, central parenteral nutrition.**

Enteral nutrition is technically defined as the provision of liquid formulas into the GI tract by tube or orally, but the term usually denotes feedings by tube.

Parenteral (intravenous) nutrition is provided when nutrient needs cannot be met solely by enteral intake as a result of GI dysfunction.

How many days of starvation can a well-nourished adult withstand; if 60 to 70 years old; if over 70? What is the general timetable for nutrition support?

(2) the duration of illness is anticipated to be more than 10 days; and (3) the client is malnourished (unintended loss of >10% of usual body weight).

Assessment of clients whose intake is inadequate (either because they cannot or do not ingest sufficient nutrients) aids in precisely tailoring a plan to provide adequate nutrition support using a variety of feeding modalities. The most appropriate method of providing nutrition support is with oral feedings, using regular foods, frequent feedings, or foods modified in texture and/or flavor. If adequate intake is not achieved, oral supplements of nutritionally complete formulas can be an adjunct to the normal diet (Fig. 13–1).

When nutritional status cannot be maintained on oral feedings, nutrition support in the form of **enteral** and **parenteral nutrition** should be considered. Enteral feedings can provide adequate nutrients when the client is unable to take food orally, but adequate bowel function is retained. When the GI tract is incapacitated or should be rested, parenteral feedings are in order (see Fig. 13–1).

OBJECTIVES OF NUTRITION SUPPORT

The main goal of nutrition support is to provide an optimum amount of nutrients and kilocalories to prevent malnutrition from becoming a comorbidity or comortality factor in the disease process. Other goals include (Talbot, 1991):

1. Do no harm physically or psychologically.

TABLE 13–1

CLASSIFICATION OF ENTERAL FORMULAS

Type	Commercial Preparations	Comments
Blenderized	Compleat B (Sandoz) Formula 2 (Cutter) Vitaneed (Sherwood)	Blended natural foods; ready-to-use
Polymeric milk-based	Meritene (Sandoz) Instant Breakfast (Carnation) Sustacal Powder (Mead Johnson)	Pleasant-tasting oral supplements; provide intact nutrients
Polymeric lactose-free	Ensure, Jevity, Osmolite (Ross) Sustacal liquid, Isocal, Ultracal (Mead Johnson) Fibersource, Resource (Sandoz) Entrition, Nutren (Clintec) Attain, Comply (Sherwood)	May be used as tube feeding, meal replacement, or oral supplement; made with intact protein isolates, oligosaccharides and starches, and fats; provide 1 kcal/ml (others available providing up to 2 kcal); in adequate quantities meet RDIs for vitamins and minerals; ready-to-use; isotonic (except Ensure and Sustacal)
Elemental or monomeric formulas	Vital HN (Ross) Vivonex T.E.N. (Sandoz) Criticare HN (Mead Johnson) Travasorb (Clintec) Peptamen (Clintec) Reabilan (O'Brien)	Partially digested nutrients for feeding; hypertonic (except for Reabilan and Peptamen); require reconstitution (except for Peptamen, Reabilan, and Criticare)

2. Improve nutritional assessment indices, especially albumin, transferrin, prealbumin, and TLC.
3. Prevent single and multiple nutrient deficiencies.
4. Promote organ integrity and function.
5. Ameliorate clinical manifestations of the disease.
6. Favorably affect the disease process.
7. Positively influence client outcome.

List 3 objectives for nutrition support.

TYPES OF ENTERAL FORMULAS

Several types of formulas* are available to meet nutritional needs for different disease states, feeding modes, and digestive and absorptive functions (Table 13–1). With more than 50 medical food products available, the formulations differ in **osmolality;** digestibility; kilocaloric density; protein, fat, lactose, and carbohydrate content; viscosity; and other nutrients (see Appendix A–2). Changes are constantly made (new formulas and composition of old formulas) as a result of new knowledge.

Osmolality—concentration of electrically charged particles per kilogram of solution.

* The FDA has defined formulas as foods that are "formulated to be consumed or administered enterally under the supervision of a physician that is intended for the specific dietary management of a disease or condition for which distinctive nutritional requirements, based on recognized scientific principles, are established by medical evaluation." As such, medical foods are excluded from food labeling regulations.

Blended Formulas

Normal foods are blended to a liquid consistency for use as a tube feeding. Baby foods may be used with the addition of some liquid. Since the proportions of carbohydrate, protein, and fat are similar to a regular diet, the feeding is well tolerated by clients with a normally functioning GI tract. Some clients prefer blended foods because of better palatability, variety, and reduced cost.

If the particle size is too large or the mixture too thick, the feeding tube may become clogged. Other problems include bacterial contamination and inconsistency of nutrient composition.

Blended products are commercially available (see Table 13–1). These contain natural foodstuffs plus additional vitamins and minerals and moderate amounts of fiber.

Polymeric Formulas

Polymeric formulas provide intact nutrients (whole proteins and long-chain triglycerides), which require a normally functioning GI tract.

Commercially prepared **polymeric formulas** can be used to increase nutrient intake orally or to provide complete nutrition via tube feeding. Polymeric formulas are either milk-based or lactose-free. Some polymeric formulas are flavored, increasing their acceptance as oral supplements; they may be generically referred to as nutrition supplements. Oral supplemental feedings may be used anytime nutrient requirements exceed the amount of nutrients the client is able to ingest.

Formulas are available as a powder to be mixed with milk or water and in ready-to-use liquid form. These have extended shelf life and are relatively palatable.

Because of the prevalence of lactose intolerance, most commercially prepared formulas are lactose-free. A limited number contain lactose (see Table 13–1).

The sources or components of carbohydrate, protein, and fats vary, as shown in Table 13–2. Most polymeric formulas contain 1 kcal/ml but may contain up to 2 kcal/ml. When the client is given 1000 to 2000 ml of formula, the RDIs for vitamins and minerals are met. (Although the RDIs are used as a standard, these amounts may not be adequate for many hospitalized clients.) Many provide fiber, which is believed to help maintain gut integrity and bowel function, especially when formulas are the sole source of nutrition support (Frankenfield & Beyer, 1991; Shankardass et al, 1990). Besides their convenience, commercially prepared formulas are microbiologically safe and are consistent in their nutrient content and osmolality.

Elemental formulas, also called monomeric diets, require minimal digestion because basic nutrients are ready-to-absorb and do not overly stimulate pancreatic, biliary, and intestinal secretions.

Elemental Formulas

When the GI tract is not wholly functional (as in short gut syndrome) or when fecal residue should be minimal (as before an operation), **elemental formulas** may be needed. Older products are powders that are mixed with water to form hyper-

TABLE 13–2

COMPONENT SOURCES OF ENTERAL FORMULAS

Carbohydrates	Protein	Fats
Hydrolyzed corn starch	Casein	Corn oil
Corn syrup	Soy protein	MCT
Maltodextrin	Beef	Canola oil
Sucrose	Nonfat milk	Safflower oil
Glucose oligosaccharides	Lactalbumin	Soy oil
Glucose polymers	Egg white	Sunflower oil
	Free amino acids	
	Whey	

tonic solutions; some newer products are ready-to-use liquids. The protein source is a balanced mixture of short-chain peptides or pure amino acids. Newer products have a lower osmolality than those containing solely amino acids. The carbohydrate is glucose or dextrins. Older formulas contain very little fat, but several newer products use a large percentage of MCT oils. Electrolytes, minerals, and trace elements are also present.

Nutrients from elemental formulas are rapidly absorbed in the proximal small intestine and are adequately absorbed even in some cases of short bowel syndrome. For clients with a normally functioning GI tract, there is no evidence that elemental formulas are superior to polymeric formulas. Elemental formulas are 2 to 4 times more expensive than most 1 kcal/ml formulas. They are sometimes given indiscriminately, even though the less expensive polymeric formulas would be beneficial for clients.

The high osmolality of elemental formulas can cause an osmotic effect, drawing fluid into the GI tract to dilute the concentration of the formula. The result is gastric distention, nausea, diarrhea, and dehydration. Adequate fluid intake is essential.

Because of their amino acid and peptide content, elemental formulas are not very palatable and are usually administered by tube. Incorporating even meager quantities of these formulas into clear liquids can significantly increase nutrient density of clear liquid diets.

Modular Feeding Components

Individual nutrients (protein, carbohydrate, and fat components) can be used to supplement nutrient content of foods or commercial formulas or can be combined to tailor nutrition support for the specific requirements of disease states. Most of these contain a single energy nutrient, as shown in Table 13–3, without any vitamins or minerals.

Specialty Formulas

Special formulations are designed for clients with normally functioning GI tracts but with metabolic problems. Many have been formulated for oral consumption. Increasing numbers of these special formulations are appearing on the market in response to growing knowledge of nutritional requirements in certain disease states, i.e., renal and liver disorders, respiratory failure, immune incompetence, diabetes, and conditions causing hypermetabolism. Some of these formulas are listed along with their intended use in Appendix A–2 and are discussed with the condition for which they are formulated.

List the types of enteral formulas and the purposes for each.

TABLE 13–3

MODULAR FEEDING COMPONENTS*

Formula	Kilocaloric Density	Protein (% kcal)	Fat (% kcal)	Carbohydrate (% kcal)
Carbohydrate				
Polycose (Ross)	2 kcal/ml			100
Moducal (Mead Johnson)	3.8 kcal/gm			100
Fat				
M.C.T. oil (Mead Johnson)	8.3 kcal/ml		100	
Microlipid (Sherwood)	4.5 kcal/ml		100	
Protein				
Casec (Mead Johnson)	3.7 kcal/gm	95	5	0
ProMod (Ross)	4.2 kcal/gm	71	19	10
Propac (Sherwood)	4 kcal/gm	76	18	6

* Not nutritionally complete.

NURSING APPLICATIONS

Assessment

Physical—for lactose intolerance; if so, offer lactose-free formulas; abdominal distention, nausea, diarrhea, or dehydration, weight (twice weekly).
Dietary—for formula ordered.

Interventions

1. If weight fluctuates significantly, consult the physician or dietitian for adding nutrition supplement or modular components or changing formula.
2. Monitor I&O (oral and formula intake).
3. If formula is to be taken orally, (a) serve very cold to enhance acceptability of the formula; (b) leave at the bedside in a chilled container for easy access; (c) offer a variety of flavors to prevent flavor fatigue; (d) encourage supplements to replace coffee or tea if given at mealtime; (e) if an elemental formula is needed, cover and offer with a straw to minimize smell and taste bud contact.

Evaluation

* Determine effectiveness of care by evaluating weight, fluid and formula intake, and client's acceptability of diet. Additionally, no distention, nausea, vomiting, or dehydration should occur.

Client Education

- Formulas help tissues heal and prevent weight loss by providing needed nutrients in combinations the body can use.
- These formulas are nutritionally well balanced and provide more nourishment than most individual foods.
- Clients should not consume nutrition supplements for about 1 to 2 hours before mealtime to promote appetite for regular foods.
- Small amounts of elemental formulas taken slowly over a period of time can improve nutrient intake significantly.

ENTERAL NUTRITION (TUBE FEEDINGS)

If the GI tract is functional, it should be used, even if oral intake is not feasible. Enteral nutrition is a convenient, economical method of nutrition support when clients are unable to ingest adequate nutriment orally to meet their metabolic needs (Fig. 13–2). It can be used as the only feeding method, as a supplement to oral intake, or in conjunction with parenteral nutrition.

Advantages

The advantages of feedings that use the gut are obvious. They are physiologically more natural, less expensive, and nutritionally more complete than routine IV solutions. Nutrients administered via the gut are used efficiently; metabolic upsets are less likely to occur.

Bowel rest for any reason (for example, starvation, GI tract dysfunction, and so forth) leads to atrophy in the small and large bowel (including absorptive cells, mucus-secreting cells, and enzyme secretions). It is not certain whether the provision of enteral feedings helps maintain GI integrity by promoting anatomic (villous structure) or immune functions, but **bacterial translocation** is decreased. The endotoxins from translocation of bacteria can trigger a hypermetabolic response and

Bacterial translocation is the passage of viable resident bacteria from the GI tract into lymph nodes and other internal organs.

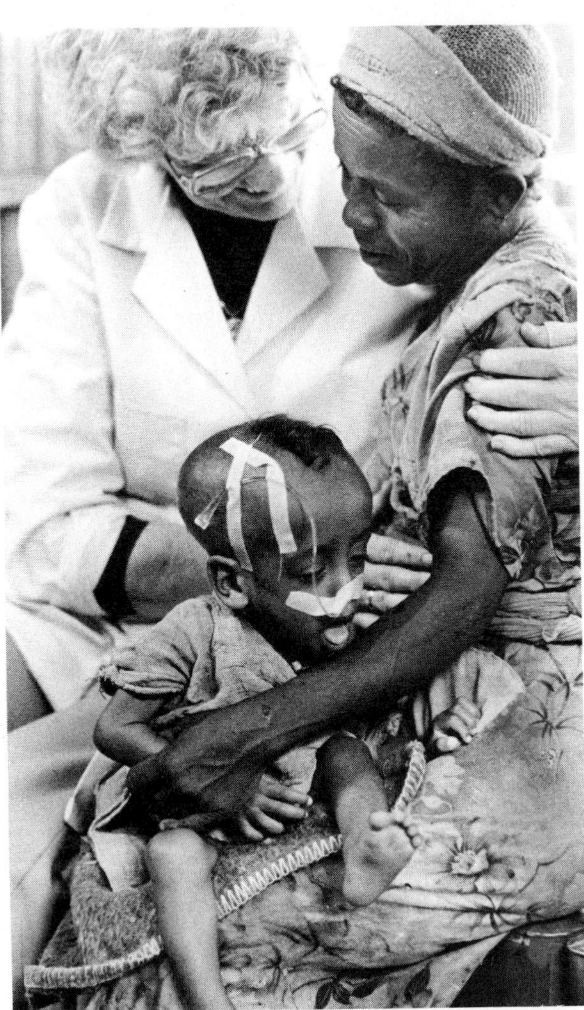

Figure 13–2 A missionary volunteer nurse comforts a mother whose 12-pound, 22-month-old child came to the feeding–health care center in Rabel, Ethiopia, on the verge of death. The baby was fed with a nasogastric tube because his blood vessels were too small for normal intravenous feeding. (From Foreign Mission Board, Southern Baptist Convention, Richmond, VA. Photo by Don Rutledge.)

induce a septic state, ultimately resulting in multiple system organ failure (Alexander, 1990). Early initiation of enteral feeding is associated with maintenance or more rapid establishment of positive nitrogen balance, lessened hypermetabolic response, prevention of paralytic ileus, and reduced costs (Bowers, 1992).

List 2 advantages of enteral feedings.

Indications for Use

The uses for tube feedings have expanded in recent years, benefiting many clients with conditions that prevent adequate intake but who have a functional GI tract. Enteral nutrition is usually helpful following major trauma or burns, radiation therapy, limited chemotherapy, liver failure, and severe renal dysfunction. It may be warranted in clients with physical and neurological impairments or for mental disturbances. Used both pre-operatively and postoperatively, it provides nutrition support to promote anabolism and prevent **cachexia** and malnutrition.

Cachexia—state of malnutrition and ill health characterized by marked anorexia, early satiety, weight loss, tissue wasting, anemia, organ dysfunction, and ultimately death.

When are enteral feedings indicated?

Routes for Administration

Enteral nutrition can be administered through a number of routes (Fig. 13–3). The route chosen depends on anticipated duration of feeding, condition of the GI

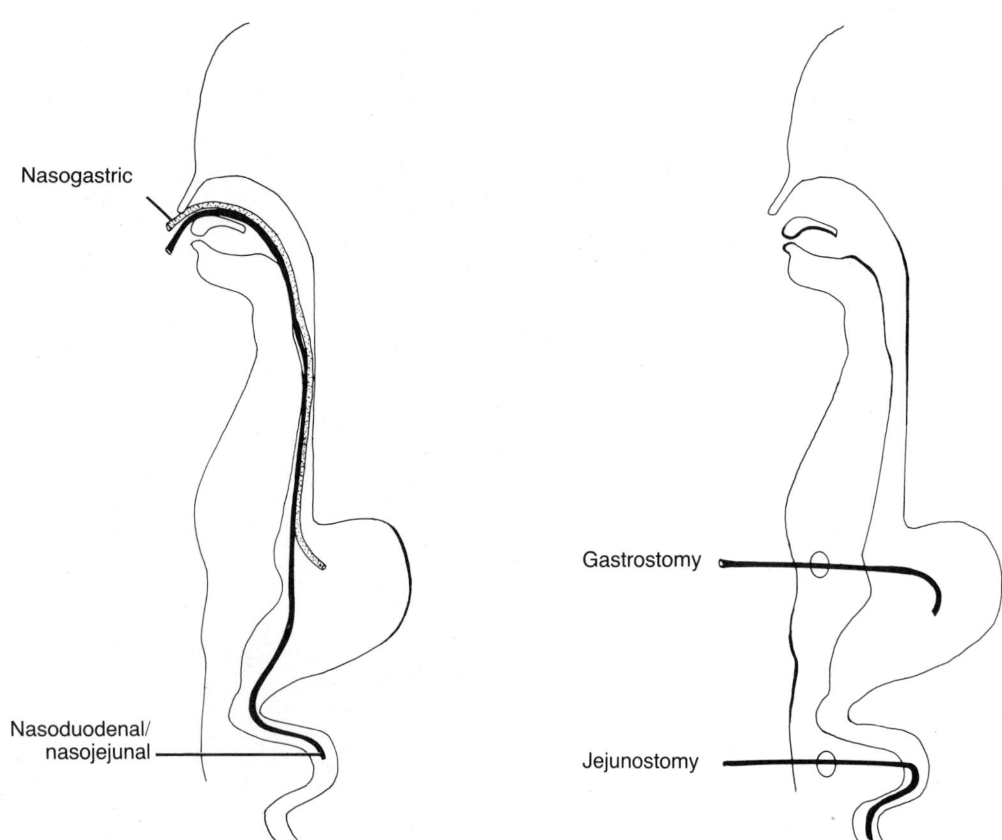

Figure 13-3 Types of enteral feedings. *Nasogastric tube.* A tube is passed through the nose into the stomach. *Nasoduodenal/nasojejunal.* Weighted tube is passed through the nose into the duodenum/jejunum. *Gastrostomy.* Temporary or permanent opening (stoma) into the stomach for a feeding tube. *Jejunostomy.* Stoma directly into the jejunum for feeding.

tract, and potential for aspiration. Smaller, soft-bore tubes made of polyurethane or silicone elastomers are available in several sizes and come with stylets to facilitate their placement.

The most common route is a nasogastric (NG) tube inserted into the stomach (intragastric route). This is satisfactory for short-term feeding, but the presence of the tube interferes with normal functioning of the LES. Reflux esophagitis is a problem; regurgitation and aspiration are risks, especially in comatose and mechanically ventilated clients. Although oral intake with a NG tube is feasible, intake is generally adversely affected due to esophageal irritation and discomfort. On the other hand, intragastric feeding permits full use of digestive and absorptive functions and lessens the chances of a hyperosmolar solution causing gastric distention, nausea, and vomiting.

Longer, more flexible weighted tubes can also be passed to the duodenum (nasoduodenal) and the jejunum (nasojejunal). Intact nutrients can still be digested. However, mercury-weighted or tungsten-weighted tubes normally used must be radiographed for placement; this is a real disadvantage due to frequent inadvertent **extubations.** (Feedings may be omitted while waiting for x-ray confirmation). Rates of self-extubation have been reported anywhere from 4.6 to 67% (Mobarhan & Trumbore, 1991; Abernathy et al, 1989; Ciocon et al, 1988). In the past, it was believed that regurgitation and aspiration were lessened with postpylorus feedings, but a more recent study indicated that these complications are not decreased (Strong et al, 1992).

Extubation is removal of the tube.

Placement of permanent feeding access is indicated for long-term enteral feeding. For a gastrostomy, esophagostomy, or jejunostomy, the tube is surgically inserted at the appropriate location and sutured in place. An esophagostomy may be indicated in connection with head and neck surgery; gastrostomies are frequently used for oropharyngeal or esophageal obstruction or dysfunction; jejunostomies are commonly used for gastric stasis or severe problems with reflux. The percutaneous endoscopic placement of a gastrostomy (PEG) can be performed at the bedside with minimal sedation. If necessary, a gastrostomy can be used as access to insert a tube into the jejunum (PEJ) to minimize reflux and aspiration. A jejunostomy is sometimes placed during a laparotomy, especially for preoperative malnutrition, major upper abdominal operations, and the anticipated need postoperatively for chemotherapy or radiation therapy. PEG and PEJ tubes are rarely pulled out inadvertently by clients or medical personnel.

What are some routes for enteral feedings?

NURSING APPLICATIONS

Assessment

Physical—for type of tube.
Dietary—for diet order.

Interventions

1. Secure tubes properly because gastric tubes can migrate into the esophagus; gastrostomy tubes can move into the duodenum or jejunum; duodenal/jejunal tubes can displace into the stomach (Young & White, 1992).
2. Remember the following about tubes: Small-diameter tubes are easier for clients to swallow and are more comfortable for clients, but clogging is more likely. For ease of medications and formula delivery, large-bore tubes are better, but they reduce the competency of the LES. No. 8 or 9 French tubes are associated with less irritation and better tolerance.
3. If a PEJ or newly inserted PEG becomes inadvertently extubated notify the physician, as he must reinsert the tube. After the PEG tube is established, nurses may reinsert. NG tubes can be reinserted by nurses (Young & White, 1992).

Client Education

- Enteral feedings are a cost savings in that they are less expensive than parenteral feedings and help prevent malnutrition.
- Explain the type of tube, where the tip is located, and why it is needed.

Methods of Delivery

Formulas can be administered intermittently using **bolus feedings,** or continuous, or cyclic infusion. The best method of feeding depends on many factors, including the client's medical condition and tolerance and client preference. Facility policies and staffing are also important factors in determining method of delivery.

Bolus feedings, delivered only to the stomach, are normally given in 4 to 6 feedings daily and resemble normal meal-feeding patterns.

Bolus

Bolus-type feedings are more appropriate when tube feedings are used to supplement oral intake or for ambulatory clients. There are 2 methods of bolus feedings. About 300 to 400 ml of formula are rapidly administered over a short period of time (10 minutes) with a syringe. This type of bolus feeding is generally not recommended. Tolerance is dependent on the functional ability of the GI tract. These bolus feedings are associated with a high risk of gastric retention, pulmonary aspiration, nausea, vomiting, diarrhea, distention, and cramps.

In the recommended type of bolus feeding, intermittent feedings provide approximately 300 to 400 ml every 3 to 6 hours but are administered over a 30 to 60-minute period. An enteral feeding bag is normally used. An intermittent feeding

Accurate amounts of formula need to be delivered at a steady rate. Gravity systems use gravity, with a control mechanism to control the flow rate. The mechanical pump is an electrical device that accurately delivers the amount of formula at an even rate. Pumps are equipped with an alarm to indicate malfunction.

schedule requires minimal equipment, but **gravity systems** must be more closely monitored than a **mechanical pump.** In general, the feeding is better tolerated if the rate is 6 to 12 ml/min (Fleming & Nelson, 1988). For larger volumes that must be delivered over a 45 to 60-minute period, a pump may be advantageous. Intermittent feedings are a practical and inexpensive method of feeding for clients at home.

Since rapid bolus-type feedings are not recommended, the term "bolus feeding" in this text refers to intermittent bolus feeding. Bolus enteral feedings mimic normal meal patterns. These are frequently used for diabetic clients because of improved metabolic control.

Continuous

Continuous feedings are usually recommended if all of the client's nutrition is provided via enteral feeding and for critically ill clients or clients with feedings into the small bowel. These feedings are infused over the 24 hour period.

Continuous infusions are administered by a mechanical pump. The rate of administration is more dependable using a pump than the gravity drip method, which is subject to an uneven flow rate. Precise flow rates are important and are checked every 1 to 2 hours for accuracy. A small tube with a lumen smaller than a No. 8 French requires a pump for continuous infusion.

Mechanical pump infusions are necessary for feedings into the distal duodenum or proximal jejunum, elemental formulas, and clients who have limited absorptive area or who have a high risk for aspiration. Continuous infusions decrease the risk of abdominal distention. On the other hand, the client's mobility is restricted since the feeding is administered continuously. To overcome this restricted mobility, a portable, ambulatory pump can be used (Young & White, 1992).

It is currently believed that in an acute-care setting, continuous feedings are advantageous because they are used more efficiently and permit quicker achievement of kilocaloric goal (Skipper, 1989; Heymsfield et al, 1987).

Cyclic

Another type of continuous feeding is cyclic feedings infused over 8 to 16 hours either during the day or night. If clients are able to eat, nighttime cyclic feedings are preferred. Nighttime feedings allow for more freedom during the day. Conversely, daytime feedings are recommended for clients who have a greater chance of aspiration or tube dislodgment (McCrae & Hall, 1989).

Describe the different methods of delivery.

NURSING APPLICATIONS

Assessment

Physical—for type of tube.
Dietary—for diet order, method of delivery.

Interventions

1. If client has gastrostomy or PEG tube, monitor for "dumping syndrome" (nausea, vomiting, sweating, low blood glucose) if receiving bolus feedings. If this occurs, notify the physician.
2. If client has jejunostomy or PEJ tube, give only continuous feedings. If not ordered, consult the physician.
3. When possible, use a pump for more accurate flow rates, especially with viscous (thick) formulas (with fiber or 1.5 to 2 kcal/ml).

Client Education

- Explain the method of delivery.
- This feeding will supplement current intake (if applicable) or provide adequate amounts of required nutrients.

Enteral Feeding Order

The choice of formula and method and rate of delivery are crucial in the client's recovery. Assessment of many factors ultimately determines the best formula: diagnosis and preexisting medical conditions, nutritional requirements, tolerances, tube size and location, integrity of the GI tract.

An enteral feeding order should include (1) the type of formula (e.g., blended, polymeric, or elemental) or name of formula, (2) type of tube, (3) total volume and/or rate of feeding to be administered, (4) type of feeding (intermittent, continuous), (5) number of feedings per day, and (6) any other pertinent information such as the amount of protein or other nutrients desired. An example of an enteral feeding order is shown in Figure 13–4.

To avoid electrolyte imbalances or fluid overload, laboratory values and weight are monitored. The amount of sodium in the formula is of special consideration for clients with fluid retention, especially if sodium-containing antibiotics are necessary.

As a result of the numbers of formulas currently available, most facilities have instituted a **formulary** to limit the numbers of products stocked. Familiarity with the enteral feeding formulary for the facility prevents errors in administering substitutes.

An enteral feeding formulary is a list of interchangeable products or nutritionally equivalent products that can be substituted when the specified formula is not available.

What is included in the enteral feeding order?

Check items to be completed:

_____ 1a. Insert standard feeding tube
_____ b. Insert _______________ (specify tube).
_____ 2a. Obtain chest radiograph following tube insertion to confirm position.
_____ b. Confirm placement of tube by aspiration of gastric contents before feeding.
_____ 3. Head of bed elevated approximately 30 degrees during infusion and for 1 hour following feeding.
4. Type of formula to be used:
( ) 1 kcal/ml ( ) Elemental
( ) 1.5 kcal/ml ( ) Liver dysfunction
( ) 2 kcal/ml ( ) Renal dysfunction
( ) With fiber ( ) Pulmonary dysfunction
( ) No fiber
5. Type of feeding
a. Bolus: Give _______ ml over 30 minutes every _______ hours at _______ strength.
b. Continuous drip using enteral pump: Give _______ ml per hour for _______ hours at _______ strength. (Specific hours for infusion): _____
_____ 6. Flush tube with 20 ml water before and after formula infusion and medications and when tube is disconnected or feeding is stopped for any reason.
_____ 7. Minimum additional fluid needed daily _______ ml.
Add for fever, diarrhea, excess perspiration.
_______ a. Administer during nonfeeding times.
_______ b. Distribute over 24-hour period.
_____ 8a. Check gastric placement and residual every _______ hours. Replace residual in stomach.
b. If more than _______ ml, hold feedings for 1 hour and recheck. Notify physician if this occurs on 2 consecutive measurements of residual.
_____ 9. Change tubing and feeding bag every 24 hours.
_____ 10. Weigh every other day and record on chart.
_____ 11. I&O daily. Record number, volume, and consistency of bowel movements.
_____ 12. Obtain CBC, complete serum chemistry profile, TIBC, prealbumin, magnesium, UA.
_____ 13. Begin 24-hour urine for creatinine and BUN at 0700 on _______.
_____ 14. Contact physician for nausea, vomiting, abdominal distention, cramping, severe diarrhea or shortness of breath.

Figure 13–4 Sample form for enteral feeding standard orders. CBC, Complete blood count; TIBC, total iron-binding capacity; UA, urinalysis; BUN, blood urea nitrogen.

TABLE 13–4

CALCULATION OF FLUID REQUIREMENTS

Example: 55-year-old man who weighs 56 kg; fever of 100° F; moderately perspiring	
For the first 10 kg—100 ml for each kg	
	First 10 kg (100 ml × 10 kg) = 1000 ml
For the next 10 Kg—50 ml for each kg	
	Next 10 kg (50 ml × 10 kg) = 500 ml
Add 20 ml/kg for all weight above 20 kg if < 50 years	
Add 15 ml/kg for all weight above 20 kg if > 50 years	
	> 50 years 15 ml × (56 kg − 20 kg) = 540 ml
For fever—add 500 to 1500 ml/day	
Fever	*1000 ml*
For moderate perspiration—add 500 ml/day	
For profuse perspiration—add 1000 ml/day	
Moderate perspiration	*500 ml*
Total	*3540 ml*

Principles and Procedures for Tube Feedings

Tonicity refers to the relationship of the solution to the osmotic pressure of body fluids; isotonic solutions have the same osmolality as body fluids and do not cause rapid fluid shifts into or from the GI tract.

Feedings administered directly into the intestinal tract should be easily digestible, almost **isotonic** (about 300 mOsm/L), and dispensed slowly. The previous belief that formula should be diluted resulted in provision of very little nourishment and has been determined unnecessary.

The higher the osmolality, the greater the possibility exists that the formula will be poorly tolerated without implementing a reduced rate starter regimen. Thus, the solute load can be controlled by rate of infusion rather than formula dilution. If the client has had food in the GI tract in the previous 24 hours, a full-strength isotonic or slightly hypertonic formula (300 to 500 mOsm) at a rate of 50 to 75 ml/hr is appropriate. When nourishment has been withheld for longer than 7 days and the formula is hyperosmolar, the starter regimen may be initiated at a slower rate (30 to 50 ml/hr). The rate may be advanced by 15 to 25 ml/hr every 8 to 12 hours until optimal kilocaloric goal is reached.

The volume (rate) is increased as tolerated to achieve adequate nutrient, fluid, and electrolyte requirements as soon as possible. Three to 5 days may be required for the client's adaptation to the formula. Too rapid increases may have negative results (such as abdominal cramping, nausea, and diarrhea) and require starting the adaptive process over again. Even if feeding falls behind schedule, "catch-up" (increasing the rate) is not advisable.

Adequate fluid intake is imperative to prevent dehydration, especially in infants, children, and elderly clients. Elderly clients receiving hyperosmolar formula are especially prone to development of hypernatremia and FVD, as the formula may promote loss of water into the bowel (Bowman et al, 1988). Additional water is usually necessary to maintain a satisfactory urinary output. Fluid requirements can be determined using the guidelines provided in Table 13–4.

Although the physician may order a specific amount of fluid to be provided, nurses are more familiar with the client's changing status and must use judgment to adjust fluids when warranted by the client's status. Depending on the institution, this may be done by the nurse or dietitian independently or in consultation with the physician. Clients able to take fluids by mouth are encouraged to do so. Additional water is especially necessary with a larger protein and electrolyte load, additional fiber, hyperthermia, decreased renal concentrating ability, or extensive tissue breakdown. The amount of fluid necessary can be determined by fluid I&O, clinical signs, and laboratory data, such as BUN and sodium levels.

When clients are on intermittent tube feedings, check gastric residuals before each feeding to prevent overfilling, which can lead to vomiting and aspiration. If >100 to 150 ml are aspirated, or more than half of volume previously infused, the usual rule is to withhold the feeding and remeasure in an hour. Because of the useful gastric secretions and electrolytes, residuals are reinstilled immediately. After an hour, if residual is <100 ml, or less than half of previous volume, feeding is initiated. If excessive (>300 ml) residual persists, contact the physician and dietitian so the reason for slowed gastric emptying can be determined and the problem resolved. In continuous feedings, residuals are checked every 2 to 4 hours depending on facility policies. If residual is 2 to 3 times the hourly rate, notify the physician for appropriate changes. With many narrow-bore, pliable feeding tubes, residuals may be unreliable; question clients regarding fullness and examine for abdominal distention.

Describe formulas and rates for the following: client who has food in GI tract in the previous 24 hours, when nourishment has been withheld for longer than 7 days. How long may adaptation take? What can happen if too rapid increases occur? Is "catch-up" advisable? What clients are prone to dehydration with tube feedings? When is additional water warranted? Describe when residuals are measured for intermittent and continuous feedings. What should be done if a residual of 200 ml is obtained on an intermittent feeding; if 50 ml is obtained? When should the physician be notified of residuals in continuous feedings?

Nursing Applications

Assessment

Physical—for gastric residual, abdominal cramping, nausea, diarrhea, fever, abdominal distention, enteral feeding order, weight/weight changes.

Dietary—for type of feeding, osmolality of formula, fluid intake, length of time since oral intake (assess GI tolerance), adequacy of kilocalorie, protein in formula for client's needs.

Laboratory—for sodium, potassium, BUN, specific gravity of urine.

Interventions

1. If client has jejunostomy or PEJ tube, do not check for residual, as this is impractical.
2. Following tube insertion, allow 30 minutes before initiating the first feeding (water or formula).
3. Raise head of bed to 30 to 45 degrees during feedings and for 30 minutes to 1 hour after feeding to decrease risk of aspiration.
4. If feeding is placed distal to the pylorus, verify placement by radiograph before initiating feeding.
5. To prevent bacterial contamination of formula, follow guidelines provided in Table 13–5.
6. Chart volume of formula administered separately from other liquids given (Petrosino et al, 1989).
7. Do not increase rate even if feeding falls behind.
8. Never increase volume (rate) and formula concentration simultaneously. By initiating full-strength formula at a decreased rate and gradually increasing the rate, complications such as abdominal cramping, diarrhea, or electrolyte imbalances are lessened.
9. Do not dilute formula. If ordered, consult with physician or dietitian.
10. Shake formulas to make sure particles are in suspension.
11. Provide routine oral hygiene, i.e., brush the teeth and gums, use glycerin swabs to moisten lips and mucous membranes in the mouth.
12. Provide discharge planning for clients to be transferred to a nursing home or rehabilitation center to make any necessary transitions before discharge.

Evaluation

* Client should receive right formula, correct amount, using the method ordered. Client's weight should be maintained or increased, depending on condition.

Client Education

- Stress the importance of additional fluid intake. Outline exactly how much additional fluid is needed and how to administer.
- Explain purpose for checking residuals.

TABLE 13–5

SANITARY GUIDELINES FOR HANDLING ENTERAL FEEDING FORMULAS

1. Provide formulas in a closed system container, if available, to prevent bacterial contamination
2. Date, refrigerate, and discard open containers of formula if not used within 24 to 48 hr since bacterial growth may occur
3. Do not mix more than a 24-hr supply
4. Do not hang more than will be given in an 8-hr period
5. Change the infusion bag or bottle every 24 hr to avoid bacterial overgrowth
6. Use aseptic technique and basic principles of good hand washing to prevent bacterial contamination. Handle the bag and tubing as little as possible because bacteria are easily introduced where the delivery tubing connects with the client's feeding tube and whenever the system is open
7. Check expiration date on the formula. Do not use formula that has expired
8. Do not add new formula to formula already hanging

Complications

Serious complications from enteral feedings may occur; however, most can be averted or lessened if all team members are knowledgeable about their roles and signs and symptoms of complications. Specific tasks performed by team members vary between institutions; general guidelines are shown in Table 13–6. Nurses should be knowledgeable about nutritional requirements and physiological symptoms and monitor the client's responses. A form documenting all pertinent information on a single page should be used to document problems and signs and symptoms of complications (Fig. 13–5). This is an invaluable tool for problem solving. It is unnecessary for nurses to perform tasks normally assumed by dietitians, but some knowledge of the dietitian's role and why these functions are important enables nurses to assist the dietitian by providing appropriate documentation and knowing when to consult the dietitian.

TABLE 13–6

TEAM MEMBER ROLES FOR ENTERALLY FED CLIENTS

Responsibilities	Nurse	Physician	Dietitian
Monitor gastric residuals	X		
Irrigate enteral tube with water	X		
Refill feeding container at regular intervals	X		
Check feeding tube position/placement each shift	X		
Perform abdominal assessment each shift	X		
Document tolerance (constipation, distention, diarrhea)	X		
Change feeding container and tubing daily	X		
Elevate head of bed	X		
Record daily weight; maintain I&O	X		
Order tube placement radiographically		X	
Select access route, formula, and administration technique		X	X
Perform daily client examination		X	
Monitor appropriate laboratory values	X	X	X
Order administration of medications		X	
Determine appropriateness of crushing medications or obtain liquid form	X		
Anticipate potential complications	X	X	X
Monitor client's tolerance (constipation, distention, diarrhea)	X	X	X
Assess/recommend nutrient requirements			X
Teach about alternative method of feeding	X		X
Monitor psychosocial status	X		
Maintain tube care	X		
Assist with transitional phases of nutrition support (kilocalorie counts)	X		X

Client's Name ______________________

Room Number ______________ Date ______________

Time	Formula infused (ml)	H_2O (ml)	Residual (ml)	Distention	Flatulence	Emesis	Feces*	Elimination Aid†	Irrigation or medications (ml)	Weight
0000										
0100										
0200										
0300										
0400										
0500										
0600										
0700										
0800										
0900										
1000										
1100										
1200										
1300										
1400										
1500										
1600										
1700										
1800										
1900										
2000										
2100										
2200										
2300										
2400										

* Feces: S—Small, M—Medium, L—Large.
1. Watery. 2. Loose. 3. Soft, unformed. 4. Soft, formed. 5. Hard, formed. 6. Hard, dry.
† Elimination Aid: Supp—Suppository, E—Enema, L—Laxative.

Figure 13–5 **Nursing flow sheet for tube feeding.**

Most complications can be prevented by correct formula selection and proper administration techniques (Table 13–7). Some complications are diarrhea, aspiration, and obstructed tube.

TABLE 13–7

TROUBLE SHOOTING GUIDE FOR TUBE FEEDING

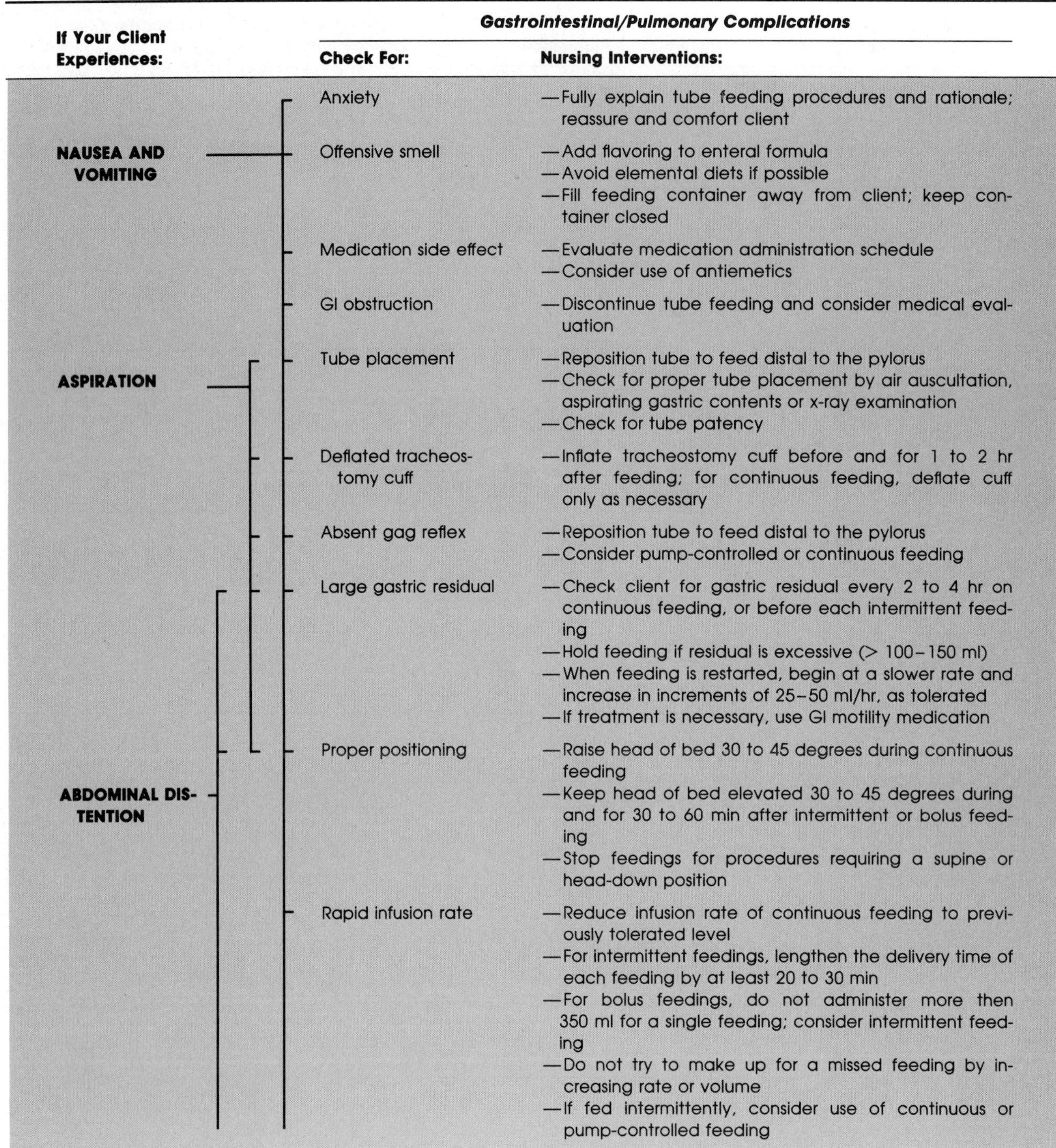

If Your Client Experiences:	*Gastrointestinal/Pulmonary Complications*	
	Check For:	**Nursing Interventions:**
	Anxiety	—Fully explain tube feeding procedures and rationale; reassure and comfort client
NAUSEA AND VOMITING	Offensive smell	—Add flavoring to enteral formula —Avoid elemental diets if possible —Fill feeding container away from client; keep container closed
	Medication side effect	—Evaluate medication administration schedule —Consider use of antiemetics
	GI obstruction	—Discontinue tube feeding and consider medical evaluation
ASPIRATION	Tube placement	—Reposition tube to feed distal to the pylorus —Check for proper tube placement by air auscultation, aspirating gastric contents or x-ray examination —Check for tube patency
	Deflated tracheostomy cuff	—Inflate tracheostomy cuff before and for 1 to 2 hr after feeding; for continuous feeding, deflate cuff only as necessary
	Absent gag reflex	—Reposition tube to feed distal to the pylorus —Consider pump-controlled or continuous feeding
	Large gastric residual	—Check client for gastric residual every 2 to 4 hr on continuous feeding, or before each intermittent feeding —Hold feeding if residual is excessive (> 100–150 ml) —When feeding is restarted, begin at a slower rate and increase in increments of 25–50 ml/hr, as tolerated —If treatment is necessary, use GI motility medication
ABDOMINAL DISTENTION	Proper positioning	—Raise head of bed 30 to 45 degrees during continuous feeding —Keep head of bed elevated 30 to 45 degrees during and for 30 to 60 min after intermittent or bolus feeding —Stop feedings for procedures requiring a supine or head-down position
	Rapid infusion rate	—Reduce infusion rate of continuous feeding to previously tolerated level —For intermittent feedings, lengthen the delivery time of each feeding by at least 20 to 30 min —For bolus feedings, do not administer more then 350 ml for a single feeding; consider intermittent feeding —Do not try to make up for a missed feeding by increasing rate or volume —If fed intermittently, consider use of continuous or pump-controlled feeding

TABLE 13–7

TROUBLE SHOOTING GUIDE FOR TUBE FEEDING *Continued*

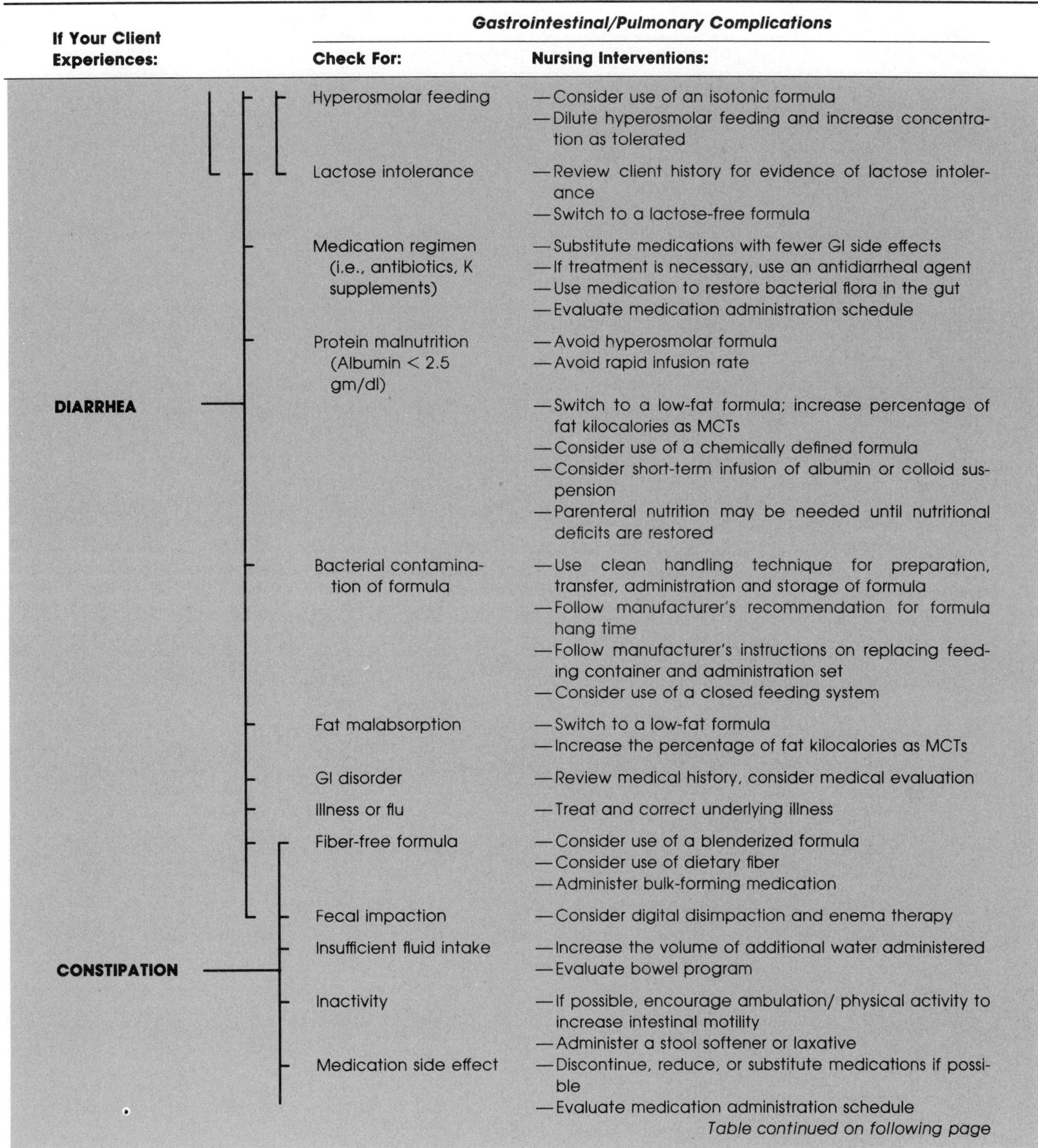

Gastrointestinal/Pulmonary Complications

If Your Client Experiences:	Check For:	Nursing Interventions:
DIARRHEA	Hyperosmolar feeding	—Consider use of an isotonic formula —Dilute hyperosmolar feeding and increase concentration as tolerated
DIARRHEA	Lactose intolerance	—Review client history for evidence of lactose intolerance —Switch to a lactose-free formula
DIARRHEA	Medication regimen (i.e., antibiotics, K supplements)	—Substitute medications with fewer GI side effects —If treatment is necessary, use an antidiarrheal agent —Use medication to restore bacterial flora in the gut —Evaluate medication administration schedule
DIARRHEA	Protein malnutrition (Albumin < 2.5 gm/dl)	—Avoid hyperosmolar formula —Avoid rapid infusion rate —Switch to a low-fat formula; increase percentage of fat kilocalories as MCTs —Consider use of a chemically defined formula —Consider short-term infusion of albumin or colloid suspension —Parenteral nutrition may be needed until nutritional deficits are restored
DIARRHEA	Bacterial contamination of formula	—Use clean handling technique for preparation, transfer, administration and storage of formula —Follow manufacturer's recommendation for formula hang time —Follow manufacturer's instructions on replacing feeding container and administration set —Consider use of a closed feeding system
DIARRHEA	Fat malabsorption	—Switch to a low-fat formula —Increase the percentage of fat kilocalories as MCTs
DIARRHEA	GI disorder	—Review medical history, consider medical evaluation
DIARRHEA	Illness or flu	—Treat and correct underlying illness
DIARRHEA, CONSTIPATION	Fiber-free formula	—Consider use of a blenderized formula —Consider use of dietary fiber —Administer bulk-forming medication
DIARRHEA, CONSTIPATION	Fecal impaction	—Consider digital disimpaction and enema therapy
CONSTIPATION	Insufficient fluid intake	—Increase the volume of additional water administered —Evaluate bowel program
CONSTIPATION	Inactivity	—If possible, encourage ambulation/ physical activity to increase intestinal motility —Administer a stool softener or laxative
CONSTIPATION	Medication side effect	—Discontinue, reduce, or substitute medications if possible —Evaluate medication administration schedule

Table continued on following page

TABLE 13–7

TROUBLE SHOOTING GUIDE FOR TUBE FEEDING *Continued*

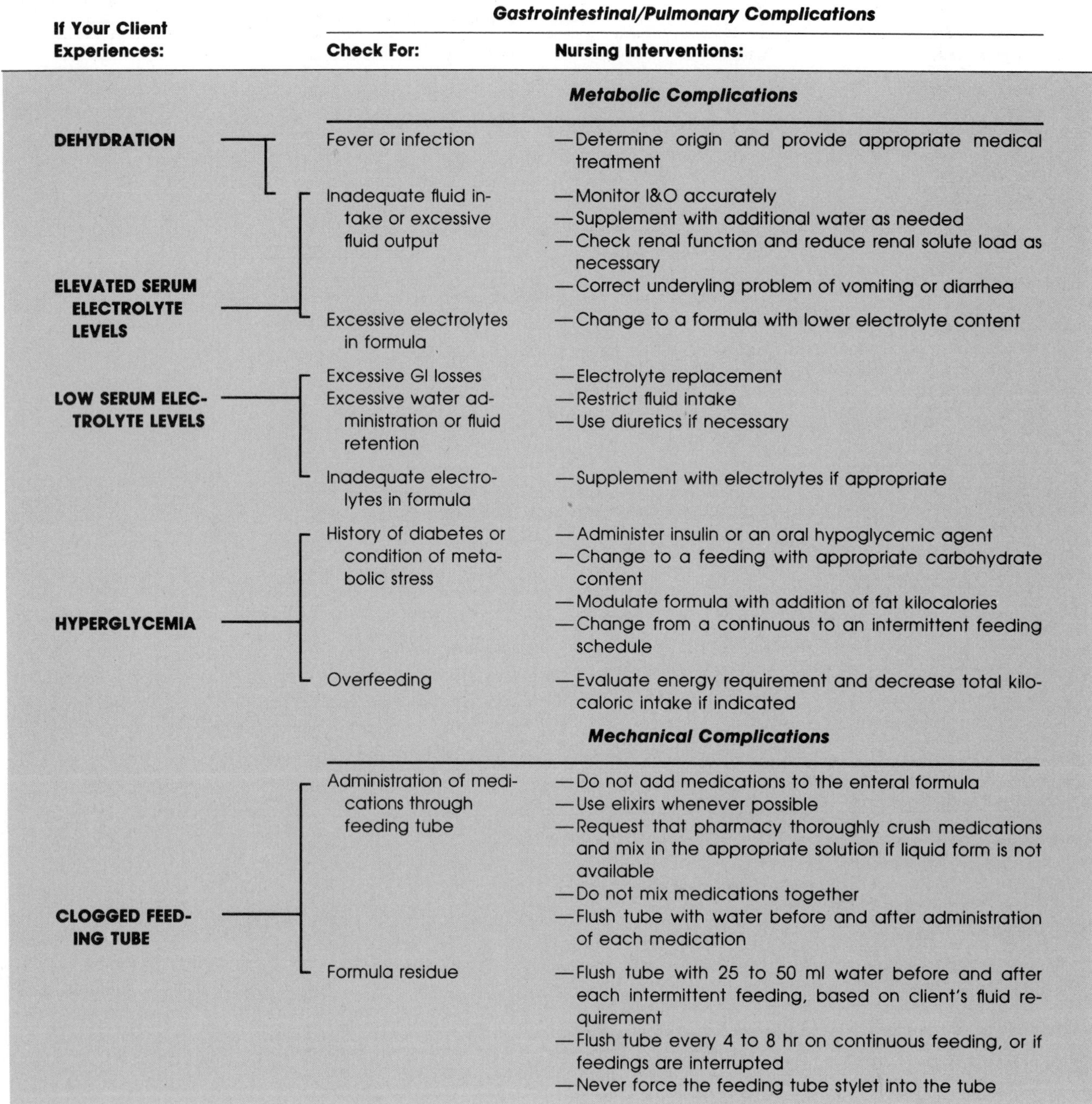

If Your Client Experiences:	Check For:	Nursing Interventions:
		Gastrointestinal/Pulmonary Complications
		Metabolic Complications
DEHYDRATION	Fever or infection	—Determine origin and provide appropriate medical treatment
DEHYDRATION; **ELEVATED SERUM ELECTROLYTE LEVELS**	Inadequate fluid intake or excessive fluid output	—Monitor I&O accurately —Supplement with additional water as needed —Check renal function and reduce renal solute load as necessary —Correct underlying problem of vomiting or diarrhea
ELEVATED SERUM ELECTROLYTE LEVELS	Excessive electrolytes in formula	—Change to a formula with lower electrolyte content
LOW SERUM ELECTROLYTE LEVELS	Excessive GI losses	—Electrolyte replacement
	Excessive water administration or fluid retention	—Restrict fluid intake —Use diuretics if necessary
	Inadequate electrolytes in formula	—Supplement with electrolytes if appropriate
HYPERGLYCEMIA	History of diabetes or condition of metabolic stress	—Administer insulin or an oral hypoglycemic agent —Change to a feeding with appropriate carbohydrate content —Modulate formula with addition of fat kilocalories —Change from a continuous to an intermittent feeding schedule
	Overfeeding	—Evaluate energy requirement and decrease total kilocaloric intake if indicated
		Mechanical Complications
CLOGGED FEEDING TUBE	Administration of medications through feeding tube	—Do not add medications to the enteral formula —Use elixirs whenever possible —Request that pharmacy thoroughly crush medications and mix in the appropriate solution if liquid form is not available —Do not mix medications together —Flush tube with water before and after administration of each medication
	Formula residue	—Flush tube with 25 to 50 ml water before and after each intermittent feeding, based on client's fluid requirement —Flush tube every 4 to 8 hr on continuous feeding, or if feedings are interrupted —Never force the feeding tube stylet into the tube

TABLE 13–7

TROUBLE SHOOTING GUIDE FOR TUBE FEEDING *Continued*

If Your Client Experiences:	Check For:	Nursing Interventions:
		Metabolic Complications
COUGHING OR VOMITING	Tube displacement	—Confirm tube placement by air auscultation, aspiration of gastric contents, or x-ray examination
NASAL IRRITATION	Tube exerting pressure on nostrils	—Use a smaller bore tube —Tape tube to assure no pressure is exerted on nostrils

Bernard M, Forlaw L. Complications and their prevention. *In* Rombeau JL, Caldwell MD eds. *Enteral and Tube Feeding.* Vol 1, Philadelphia, WB Saunders, 1984.
Blackburn GL, Bell SJ eds. *Nutritional Medicine: A Case Management Approach.* Philadelphia, WB Saunders 1989.
Breach CL. Tube feeding complications, part II: mechanical. *Nutritional Support Services* 1988, 8(5):28.
Davis PD, Dolin BJ, Flinn PJ. A tube feeding monitoring flow sheet. *Nutritional Support Services* 1988, 8(7):21.
Haynes-Johnson V. Tube feeding complications: causes, prevention and therapy. *Nutritional Support Services* 1986, 6(3):17.
Krey SH, Murray RL eds. Dynamics of Nutrition Support. Norwalk, CT, Appleton-Century-Crofts, 1986.
Metheny NM. Twenty ways to prevent tube feeding complications. *Nursing '85* 1985, 15(1):47.
From Sandoz Nutrition, Clinical Products Division, Minneapolis.

Diarrhea

Diarrhea has been reported in 5 to 30.6% of enterally fed clients (Silk & Payne-James, 1990); its incidence may be as high as 68% in intensive care clients (Benya & Mobarhan, 1991; Smith et al, 1990). Wide differences exist for a definition of diarrhea. Daily stool output quantified with a fecal output of greater than 250 gm/day is classified as diarrhea (Hart & Dabb, 1988). Diarrhea may originate from (1) hyperosmolar load that is due to the formula composition or medications, (2) bacterial overgrowth or contamination of formula, and/or (3) malnutrition. Contrary to popular opinion, in most cases, diarrhea is not caused by the formula. In 60% of cases, medications are responsible for diarrhea; in 30%, formula; and in 17%, *Clostridium difficile* (Edes et al, 1990).

Most oral medication solutions have an osmolality greater than 1000 mOsm/kg (Dickerson & Melnik, 1988). If these are not diluted, this hyperosmolar solution results in diarrhea. Medications in liquid form frequently contain sorbitol as sweetener, which increases risk of osmotic diarrhea. Potassium chloride (if not sufficiently diluted) or other diarrhea-inducing medications (especially magnesium-containing antacids) may also be culprits.

Malnutrition may affect formula tolerance in several ways. Anatomic changes in the GI tract (blunted villi height) may result in less intestinal disaccharidases and thus formula intolerance accompanied by diarrhea. Serum albumin levels less than 3 gm/dl are significantly correlated with development of diarrhea when tube feedings are initiated (Rolandelli et al, 1990). Hypoalbuminemia may promote development of intestinal mucosal edema due to reduced colloid osmotic pressure. However, not all clients with hypoalbuminemia experience diarrhea (Patterson et al, 1990).

The risk of diarrhea from bacterial contamination of formulas is affected by such variables as initial contamination, composition of solution (affecting the rate of bacterial growth), presence of preservatives, number of manipulations involved in the preparation process, and mode and duration of administration (hang time of the formula) (Levy et al, 1989). Life-threatening septic complications can result from contaminated enteral solutions; therefore, care must be taken in their preparation and administration to prevent contamination and inhibit excessive bacterial growth (see Table 13–5). Most formulas can be safely hung for 8 hours. Prefilled ready-to-use containers offer a decreased risk of contamination during handling, preparation, and transfer. To prevent unacceptable contamination levels, delivery sets need to be changed every 24 hr (Kohn, 1991).

TABLE 13–8

ANTIDIARRHEAL MEDICATIONS FOR DIARRHEA OF NONSPECIFIC CAUSE

Medication	Dosage
Opiates	
Natural	
Tincture of opium (10 mg/ml)	0.5–1.5 ml 1–3 × /day
Paregoric acid (0.4 mg/ml)	4–8 ml 1–2 × /day
Codeine	16–64 mg 1–2 × /day
Synthetic	
Diphenoxylate HCl (0.5 mg/ml) + atropine sulphate (0.005 mg/ml)(Lomotil)	Initial: 5 mg 1–2 × /day Maintenance: 2.5 mg 2 × /day
Loperamide HCl (Imodium)	Initial: 4 mg/BM Maintenance: 2 mg/BM
Anticholinergics	
Atropine sulfate	0.6–1 mg 3 × /day
Tincture of belladonna	12–15 drops/day
Propantheline bromide (Pro-Banthine)	15 mg 3 × /day
Adsorbents	
Kaolin (4.5 g/ml) + pectin (6 mg/ml) (Kaopectate)	45–180 ml/day
Cholestyramine (Questran)	4 gm 3 × /day
Bismuth subsalicylate (Pepto-Bismol)	60 mg (2 tab)/day
Lactobacillus acidophilus	4–8 cap (1 g)/day

BM, Bowel movement.
From Rombeau JL, et al. Diarrhea. *In* Blackburn GL, et al. *Nutritional Medicine: A Case Management Approach.* Philadelphia, WB Saunders, 1989: 65–72.

Antibiotics or infections frequently lead to *Clostridium difficile*–induced colitis (Mobarhan & Trumbore, 1991). Diarrhea related to pathogenic microorganisms due to antibiotics can be alleviated by oral vancomycin and IV or oral Metronidazole (Flagyl), which are specific for the organism, or *Lactobacillus acidophilus* (Lactinex granules) to restore the normal GI flora. Narcotic antidiarrheals (diphenoxylate, loperamide, camphorated opium, and codeine) should not be used for pathogen-induced diarrhea because they reduce GI motility and may increase the risk of sepsis by prolonging exposure to invading microbes (Silk & Payne-James, 1990). Decreased GI tract motility or use of H_2 blockers (decrease HCl secretion and increase gastric pH) can lead to bacterial overgrowth causing diarrhea.

What are some causes and treatments for diarrhea?

Treatment with kaolin pectate antidiarrheals has been effective in retarding diarrhea without organic cause (Rombeau et al, 1989b). Cholestyramine has been used to treat diarrhea associated with small bowel resection or diabetes mellitus (Skipper, 1989). Various pharmaceutical treatments for diarrhea are given in Table 13–8. A fiber-containing formula may be helpful; the fiber serves as a substrate for bacteria that normally absorb water and electrolytes (Silk & Payne-James, 1990).

NURSING APPLICATIONS

Assessment

Physical—for diarrhea, type of medicine taken, infections.
Dietary—for composition, contamination of formula.
Laboratory—for protein, albumin, prealbumin; electrolytes, BUN; stool cultures.

Interventions

1. Notify physician to lower feeding rate, then raise it more slowly. Stopping the feeding for 12 to 24 hours may be used as a last resort if diarrhea persists (Young & White, 1992).
2. If client is on intermittent feedings, suggest a trial of continuous feedings or more frequent feedings using less volume per feeding (Young & White, 1992).

3. If client is malnourished or septic, be sure the formula is isotonic. A glutamine-based formula may be indicated.
4. Dilute oral medications before giving.
5. Before adding new formula to delivery set, rinse delivery set with water (Kohn & Keithley, 1989).

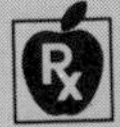 Give diphenoxylate (Lomotil) or loperamide HCl (Immodium) as ordered to stop diarrhea.

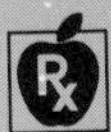 When possible, suggest using fiber-enriched formulas or adding psyllium hydrophilic mucilloid (Metamucil) to drug regimen.

Evaluation

* Diarrhea is prevented or minimized.

Client Education

- Taking yogurt, buttermilk, or Lactinex may help decrease diarrhea.
- Check antacids for ingredients; magnesium-containing antacids may cause diarrhea. If magnesium antacids are used, alternate with calcium-containing or aluminum-containing antacids (Kohn & Keithley, 1989).

Aspiration

Aspiration can occur because of an incorrectly placed tube. This can be avoided by confirming tip position with radiography, aspirating gastric residual with a syringe, or listening with a stethoscope while blowing air into the stomach. If gastric contents are aspirated through the tube, this is an adequate confirmation for tube placement. However, aspiration of gastric contents is frequently not possible through a small-bore feeding tube (Metheny et al, 1988a). In this case, x-ray confirmation is mandatory. Auscultation to determine tube location was ineffective in identifying feeding tube location in a study conducted by Metheny et al (1990). X-ray confirmation is always necessary for a nasal tube placed into the duodenum or jejunum.

Tubes may become displaced after x-ray confirmation, placing clients at risk for aspiration. Coughing and decreased level of consciousness, absent or diminished gag reflex, tracheal or nasotracheal suctioning, and upper airway intubation predispose clients to tube displacement (Metheny et al, 1987). Other risk factors are retching and vomiting. Softer, small-bore feeding tubes dislocate more easily than large-bore or firmer tubes. On the other hand, small-diameter feeding tubes are less likely to cause reflux than large-bore tubes.

What factors predispose tube displacement and thus aspiration?

NURSING APPLICATIONS

Assessment

Physical—for aspiration (acute onset of respiratory distress or crackles, fever, increased respiratory rate, increased heart rate), physical conditions that increase risk of aspiration, bowel sounds.
Dietary—for type of feeding.
Laboratory—for ABGs, sputum culture.

Interventions

1. For high-risk clients, suggest postpyloric continuous feedings with small-diameter, pliable tubes.
2. Mark tube at exit site, then monitor marking to be sure tube has not moved.

Continued

3. Check gastric residuals; if this is impractical (as with PEJ tubes), measure abdominal girth or check for abdominal distention.
4. Although results may not be reliable, check tube for placement.
5. Food coloring can be added to formula if client is at high risk for aspiration. This helps determine if aspiration occurs because food coloring is in secretions suctioned.
6. If aspiration occurs, suction immediately.

Evaluation

* Aspiration and aspiration pneumonia do not occur.

Client Education

- If severe coughing occurs during feeding, notify nurse or physician.
- If the tube becomes displaced, the marking on the tube will not be at the exit site. It will either be above or below this site.
- Teach about signs of aspiration.

Clogging

How can clogged tubes affect clients?

Obstructed tubes cause havoc for clients. Their feeding regimen is disrupted until the tube is cleared or replaced. If the tube has to be replaced, clients may not be as willing participants as during the first insertion. Considerable discomfort occurs as the tube is reinserted, not to mention increased costs. Clients are charged for another tube (if not reusable) and x-ray confirmation if needed (Kohn & Keithley, 1989). Some factors that promote clogged tubes are tube size (small diameter), viscous or high-osmolality formulas, and medications.

NURSING APPLICATIONS

Assessment

Physical—for type of tube, medication ordered.
Dietary—for type of formula.

Interventions

1. Use polyurethane tubes when possible rather than silicone since polyurethane clogs less (Metheny et al, 1988b).
2. Flush the tube with 20 to 50 ml water before and after each bolus feeding, every 4 hr with continuous feedings, after checking residuals, before and after administering drugs, and anytime the formula is stopped (Bockus, 1991).
3. Use liquid forms of medicine ordered. If liquid is not available, crush medicine and dissolve in 10 ml warm water. Consult the pharmacist as needed.
4. If tube becomes obstructed, irrigate with 60 ml water or crush a pancreatic enzyme and sodium bicarbonate and dissolve in 5 ml water (close to optimal pH of 6.9) (Marcuard et al, 1990).
5. Use a pump for viscous formulas or if a slow rate is ordered.

Evaluation

* Tube does not become clogged.

Client Education

- Prevention rather than treatment is the best method to avoid clogged tubes.
- Water is the best irrigant for clogged tubes, not colas, cranberry juice, or meat tenderizer.
- Do not crush time-released or enteric-coated medications.

Underfeeding and Overfeeding

If tube feeding is the only feeding modality used, the total energy level provided must be adequate to prevent PEM but not excessive to avoid complications of overfeeding (excessive carbon dioxide production, **cholestasis, hyperglycemia,** pulmonary edema, **lipogenesis,** hepatic complications, and others). Failure to administer adequate amounts has been attributed to interruptions for diagnostic tests and physical and respiratory therapy and clogged tubes (Petrosino et al, 1989). Since as many of 30 to 50% of hospitalized clients are malnourished, this significant problem may retard recovery.

Cholestasis—suppression of bile flow. Hyperglycemia—elevated serum glucose levels. Lipogenesis—production of body fat.

What can happen if underfeeding or overfeeding occurs?

NURSING APPLICATIONS

Assessment

Physical—for PEM, crackles, gurgling breath sounds (pulmonary edema), weight.
Dietary—for underfeeding or overfeeding, number of kilocalories needed.
Laboratory—for glucose, LFTs.

Interventions

1. Make sure flow rate is correct and maintained.
2. Consult with the dietitian if the amount provided is not maintaining client's weight or there are signs of overfeeding.
3. Coordinate schedule so feedings are not interrupted by various therapies (physical therapy, recreational therapy, and others).

Evaluation

* Underfeeding and/or overfeeding do not occur.

Client Education

• Underfeeding can cause problems as well as overfeeding.

Hyperglycemia

Hyperglycemia is one of the first detectable signs (other than nausea and abdominal cramps) related to diuresis caused by a hyperosmotic or high-kilocalorie (1.5 to 2 kcal/ml) formula. Hyperglycemia occurs in 10 to 30% of tube-fed adult clients. Elderly clients are prone to hyperglycemia because of glucose intolerance that occurs with aging. Clients on steroid therapy and diabetics are more intolerant of large carbohydrate loads and must be monitored more closely.

Formula rate or concentration may be decreased or insulin administered until blood glucose is approximately 200 mg/dl. If left unchecked, hyperglycemic hyperosmolar nonketotic (HHNK) dehydration and coma may result. The syndrome of HHNK develops when insulin reserves are adequate to prevent **ketosis** but inadequate to control serum glucose. The elevated blood glucose rises to cause osmotic diuresis and eventually dehydration. Because of careful monitoring of tube-fed clients, this complication is not frequently observed. In addition to insulin, adequate fluids are given to correct this situation.

Ketosis—the accumulation of ketones (acidic byproducts of lipid metabolism in the blood) that occurs when inadequate amounts of glucose are available for energy.

The onset of hyperglycemia in a client who has been adapted to the regimen with no complications can be a sign that an inadvertent amount of nutrient solution has been given. Flow rate should be checked, but if flow has fallen behind, rate should not be increased in an attempt to catch up. Hyperglycemia in a client whose glucose level was previously normal may also be an indication of sepsis.

What is the treatment for hyperglycemia?

NURSING APPLICATIONS

Assessment

Physical—for extreme thirst, lethargy, increased urine output, sepsis (high fever, subnormal temperature, chills), confusion, weight, skin turgor, mucous membranes, age.
Dietary—for hunger, kilocalories of formula.
Laboratory—for serum glucose, BUN, electrolytes; urine specific gravity.

Interventions

1. Monitor I&O and flow rate of feeding.
2. If a kilocalorie-dense formula (1.5 to 2 kcal/ml) is being used, suggest a lower kilocalorie formula.

Evaluation

* Blood glucose returns to within normal limits (WNL), and HHNK does not develop.

Client Education

- Hyperglycemia is high blood glucose.
- Explain signs of hyperglycemia and why it is commonly associated with illness and tube feedings. This does not mean the client is diabetic.

Refeeding Syndrome

Refeeding syndrome is characterized by fluid imbalance, hypophosphatemia, hypokalemia, hypomagnesemia, and hyperglycemia.

How can refeeding syndrome be prevented?

Malnourished clients or those who have been NPO for a prolonged period are at risk for **refeeding syndrome.** Electrolyte imbalances should be corrected before starting nutrition support. Refeeding syndrome can be prevented by initially providing basal energy requirements, with gradual increases over a 5- to 7-day period to kilocaloric goal. For clients at risk for refeeding syndrome, monitor serum and urinary electrolytes daily during the first week of nutrition support (Solomon & Kirby, 1990).

NURSING APPLICATIONS

Assessment

Physical—for signs of FVD, FVE, malnourishment, hypokalemia (muscle weakness, decreased bowel sounds).
Dietary—for time of last food intake, kilocaloric requirement.
Laboratory—for phosphate, potassium, magnesium, glucose, BUN, hematocrit.

Evaluation

* Refeeding syndrome is prevented because feedings were gradually increased.

Client Education

- The feedings will start out slow but will increase over time. This allows the body to adapt to refeeding without complications.

Formula–Drug Incompatibilities

The stomach responds to oral medications as it does to food, but tube placement beyond the stomach alters drug delivery method. Because of numerous incompatibilities, routine mixture of enteral formulas and medication is not advisable. Medications such as potassium chloride or pseudoephedrine hydrochloride are strongly acidic and cause clumping in an enteral formula. Bulk-forming agents congeal and occlude the tube. Since most drugs are best absorbed in the fasted state, optimal absorption is obtained when administered 2 hours before or after a feeding.

Liquid medications usually recommended are hyperosmolar. Intragastric administration may delay gastric emptying or result in dumping into the small bowel. Diluting the medication with 10 to 30 ml of tap water and flushing the tube before and after each medication can decrease the viscosity of the medication to facilitate its passage through the tube and prevent osmotic diarrhea (Melnik, 1990).

Warfarin (Coumadin) resistance has been reported in clients receiving enteral feedings (Brown, 1992). Initially this was attributed to the amount of vitamin K in the formula. Since the problem still exists despite decreases in the vitamin K content of formulas, it may be an interaction of vitamin K with the formula that decreases the effectiveness of warfarin (Kuhn et al, 1989).

Because of decreased serum concentrations of phenytoin (Dilantin), theophylline, and methyldopa in clients receiving concurrent enteral formulas, it is recommended that enteral feedings be stopped 1 hour before and 2 hours after administration of these medications (Fleisher et al, 1990; Splinter et al, 1990; Holtz et al, 1987).

NURSING APPLICATIONS

Assessment

Physical—for type of medicine ordered.
Dietary—for type of formula ordered.
Laboratory—for prothrombin time, theophylline and dilantin levels.

Interventions

1. Flush tube with 30 ml before and after administration of liquid or crushed medicines.
2. If on warfarin and enteral nutrition, monitor for clots since warfarin may be less effective.
3. Monitor clients with asthma and seizures for effectiveness of medicines if on enteral feedings.

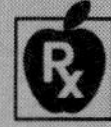
Provide theophylline, phenytoin, or methyldopa at times when formula is not being given.

Evaluation

* Clots do not occur in clients taking warfarin, and prothrombin time is prolonged; asthma clients do not have asthmatic attacks, and theophylline level is WNL; and seizure clients have no seizures, and dilantin level is WNL.

Client Education

- Do not mix medicines with formula.

HOME ENTERAL NUTRITION

In 1986, approximately 52,000 clients received home enteral nutrition (Hoffman, 1989). However, some clients may be overwhelmed with the demands imposed by the home enteral tube feedings (Fleming & Nelson, 1988).

Determining Appropriate Clients

Not all clients are appropriate for home feedings. A number of factors need to be assessed: (1) must be medically stable; (2) must successfully complete a feeding

Name 3 factors to assess for discharge to home on enteral feedings.

trial (tolerates 70% of feedings) without (a) weight loss, (b) elevated temperature, (c) urinary output less than 30 ml/hr, (d) diarrhea, (e) abdominal distention, (f) nausea, (g) vomiting, and (h) large (>100 ml) gastric residuals; (3) must have ability to administer the feeding or support person who will (Young & White, 1992); (4) must have economic resources available; and (5) must have follow-up available.

Psychosocial Adjustments

List possible psychosocial adjustments.

Enteral home feedings increase levels of stress and cause depression, grieving, and changes in body image. Enteral feedings are less stressful and produce fewer psychosocial problems than parenteral nutrition. Financial costs are a major determinant of stress levels.

Determining Appropriate Regimen

Definite changes in lifestyle are necessary for successful home enteral feedings. Flexibility and client involvement are key components in developing a successful plan.

When deciding on a home enteral regimen, the client's nutritional needs, access route, tolerance to different methods, and lifestyle and environment must be considered to foster compliance. The method of delivery should be a decision of the client and the family. The client and family are informed of advantages and disadvantages of all feasible options before making a decision. Formula cost and availability must be considered. Additionally, the client and family should have an active role in deciding the optimal home schedule. Bolus or cyclic feedings are used more frequently in home care clients, facilitating normal activities of daily living. Elderly clients prefer bolus feedings because of their simplicity (Nelson & Weckworth, 1989) and the ability to infuse them during the daytime and thus prevent being awakened or disturbed at night for feedings. Cyclic feedings that necessitate a mechanical pump may be given nocturnally to provide daily requirements, while allowing normal activities during the day. The expense and inconvenience of using a pump and all its related equipment must also be considered. Third-party payers require a letter of medical necessity justifying the need for a pump. Although enteral systems are more expensive than regular foods, home care costs are substantially less than hospital care, and individuals can return to a near-normal life.

Training for Home Therapy

Home feedings require that clients and families are taught specialized skills in the acute-care setting using an intensive training program with careful follow-up in the home setting by a home health agency. An interdisciplinary effort involving a physician, nurse, dietitian, psychiatrist, social worker, pharmacist, and discharge planner should all be knowledgeable about the problems clients are likely to face. Instructing qualifying clients and their caretakers in formula preparation, tube care, feeding administration, and related techniques is essential. Full attention and regard for client and family needs, including emotional, psychological, social, and financial needs, as well as medical and nutritional condition contribute toward a successful home enteral program.

The client and preferably at least another individual should be taught and assume full responsibility for feedings before dismissal. Clear, concise materials and written instructions before discharge contribute to the client's confidence and ease the transition. Information that clients must learn and demonstrate include (1) feeding formulation preparation and administrations, including clean technique for

Purpose and Instructions

This checklist will assist in identifying instructional responsibilities and aid in training clients in the skills needed for performing HEN.

- The nurse and dietitian will jointly instruct the client on tube feeding administration and care.
- Date and initial section when instruction/demonstration is completed.
- RNs: Document training in Nursing Notes.
- RDs: Document training in Progress Notes.
- Save checklist when client is discharged.

Initiation of HEN Program (Date and initial when completed)

__________ Anticipated dismissal date: ____________________

__________ Assign teaching roles

__________ Home enteral coordinator notified

Client Education

Introduction to HEN Program

__________ Discuss rationale for HEN

__________ Introduce manual: *Instructions for Tube Feeding at Home*

Equipment

Discuss purpose, assembly, use, care, and cleaning of equipment.

	DISCUSS	DEMONSTRATE	CLIENT DEMONSTRATE
■ Feeding tube	__________	__________	__________
■ Feeding bag	__________	__________	__________
■ Syringe	__________	__________	__________
■ Pump (if needed)	__________	__________	__________

Formulas—Fluids.

__________ Show formula.

__________ Discuss purpose, type, amount, concentration.

__________ Discuss preparation, hang time, storage.

__________ Select packaging.

__________ Discuss extra fluid needs.

Administration

	DISCUSS	DEMONSTRATE	CLIENT DEMONSTRATE
■ Method	__________	__________	__________
■ Position of client during feeding	__________	__________	__________
■ Tube placement check	__________	__________	__________
■ Residual check	__________	__________	__________
■ Tube irrigation	__________	__________	__________
■ Problem solving	__________	__________	__________
■ Home monitoring	__________	__________	__________
■ Medications	__________	__________	__________
■ Oral diet	__________	__________	__________

Transition to Home

Arrange for the following:

__________ Equipment

__________ Formula

__________ Home vendor

__________ Home health agency

__________ Physician, nurse, dietitian summaries

Figure 13–6 Home enteral feeding checklist. HEN, Home enteral nutrition. (Modified from Nelson JK, Fleming CR. Home enteral nutrition for the adult. *In* Rombeau JL, Caldwell MD, eds. *Clinical Nutrition Enteral and Tube Feeding*. 2nd ed. Philadelphia, WB Saunders, 1988.)

preparation, storage, infusion, and manipulation; (2) clean technique for tube and site care; and (3) recognition and appropriate response to complications, equipment maintenance, and malfunctions (Fig. 13–6). They must know how they are to obtain supplies necessary for the feeding and resources available for financial management.

Although sanitary techniques are important and should be discussed, procedures do not have to be as closely followed as in the hospital. Home enteral tube feeding costs can be decreased by reusing enteral feeding bags. When bags are used for intermittent or cyclic feedings (up to 15 hours), the tubing set-up can be carefully rinsed daily with either soapy water or diluted vinegar and a final tap water rinse and reused for up to 7 days without significant bacterial contamination (Grunow et al, 1989).

NG tube feedings are not recommended for home use, but they are occasionally necessary. These clients should be taught how to check proper placement of the tubing by withdrawing stomach contents. If they belch when pushing air into the tube, formula should not be infused. Changes in the length of tube outside the nose may mean that the tube has moved out of position and should not be used until proper position has been verified.

What should a client/family be taught to prepare them for home feedings?

Follow-up

Frequent in-home visits, telephone calls, and return appointments are routine methods of follow-up. Follow-up contacts are necessary since earlier discharges shorten teaching/learning time. Continuity of care is improved with home care because adaptation of clients and families can be assessed in the actual environment where feedings are occurring. Home care reinforces previously presented information and initiates new information.

Ever-changing health status and nutritional needs require routine monitoring indefinitely or until enteral feedings are discontinued. The client can maintain weight and intake records for the nurse to review. Other parameters to be monitored are similar to those monitored in the acute setting (see Fig. 13–5). Occasionally problems are encountered in maintaining access or with tolerance of the feedings, but many of these problems can be resolved at home with the help of the home health nurse.

NURSING APPLICATIONS

Assessment

Physical—for home environment, support of significant others, physical abilities, motivation, tolerance to feedings, psychological status.
Dietary—for type of feeding schedule.

Interventions

1. Provide assistance with problem solving and adjustments to the nutritional care plan.
2. Explore the fears and concerns of client/family.
3. Monitor for tube complications, poor therapy response, weight loss despite appropriate kilocalorie and protein levels provided, and inappropriate inventory (Gulledge et al, 1987). These are signs of noncompliance.

Evaluation

* Client/family should be able to describe/demonstrate preparation, feeding and cleaning technique, checking for residuals, and proper tube care. Complications and treatments should also be verbalized by client/family.

Client Education

- Inform about social worker for financial resources.
- Inform about psychological support groups.

PARENTERAL NUTRITION

If the GI tract is dysfunctional, **parenteral nutrition** (PN) is required. PN may be through **peripheral veins** or **central veins.** The terms, PN, **total parenteral nutrition (TPN),** and CPN are used interchangeably, but TPN is most widely accepted. TPN, especially when CPN is used, is frequently called **hyperalimentation.** However, this connection is erroneous because normally CPN provides only the nutriment needed to promote cell growth and repletion, not an excess. Under severe stress or trauma, clients may have increased kilocalorie needs as a result of hypermetabolism. These needs can be met via TPN.

PN indicates that veins are being used to provide nourishment in contrast to standard IV therapy that provides only glucose, electrolytes, and fluid.

Peripheral parenteral nutrition (PPN) uses smaller peripheral veins to infuse isotonic or hypotonic or slightly hypertonic (10%) solutions to preserve lean body mass. Central parenteral nutrition (CPN) uses a central vein to infuse hypertonic solutions.

TPN means that all necessary nutrients are being provided via veins.

Hyperalimentation means that nutrients are provided in excess of maintenance needs.

Indications for Use

Early recognition of problems that necessitate TPN and initiation of therapy are important. If the client is unable to tolerate enteral feedings within 7 to 10 days, an alternative form of nutrition support should be instituted to prevent subcutaneous fat and muscle protein from being used for energy.

TPN is appropriate for clients with a nonfunctioning GI tract or trauma requiring multiple surgeries that make it impossible to obtain sufficient amounts of nutrients enterally. Some specific conditions frequently (but not always) warrant TPN. Bowel resection or other GI surgery, intestinal ileus or obstruction, abdominal trauma, severe malabsorption, significant intolerance of enteral feeding, and long-term chemotherapy and radiation therapy may cause prolonged unavailability or unreliability of the GI tract (Fig. 13–7). Prolonged bowel rest is needed to permit healing of specific conditions: enteric fistulas, inflammatory bowel disease, intractable diarrhea, and acute pancreatitis.

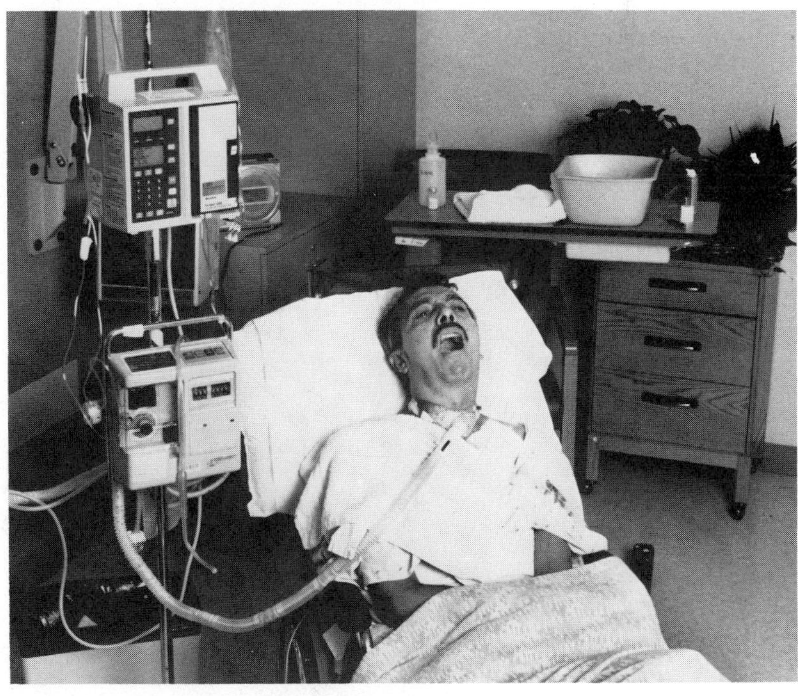

Figure 13–7 When a client is in a hypermetabolic state, malnutrition can develop rapidly. This young man was healthy and well-nourished when he left to serve in Desert Storm.

A thorough investigation of other alternatives is warranted before a final decision for TPN is made. A big problem with TPN therapy is its expense. The cost of TPN in the US varies between hospitals and areas of the country. Estimated cost of TPN in hospitals ranges from $75 to $500, with a median of approximately $200 daily (Katz & Oye, 1990; Perry et al, 1990). Outpatient costs are over $50,000 per year (Lin, 1991; Weiland, 1991). On the other hand, implementation of TPN is cost-effective when compared with the cost of malnutrition. For instance, the cost to heal one pressure sore, which is only one complication of malnutrition, ranges from $5000 to $40,000 (Mead Johnson, 1989).

What are some indications for TPN? What are the costs of TPN?

Routes for Total Parenteral Nutrition

In general, the objective of PPN is to prevent deterioration (achieve balance). Prevention of malnutrition rather than correction of nutritional deficits is the main goal of PPN (Worthington & Wagner, 1989). PPN is normally the route chosen when PN is anticipated for a short period of time (5 to 7 days). When enteral feeding is not possible, peripheral infusion is the safest route if peripheral veins are accessible. Because of limitations in fluid volumes tolerated (2000 to 3500 ml/day) and problems associated with infusion of hypertonic fluids, IV lipid emulsions must be used to provide adequate kilocalories. Moderately hypertonic dextrose solutions (10%) can be administered peripherally. PPN solutions containing amino acids, dextrose, and fat emulsions can provide up to 2000 kcal and 120 gm protein in 3500 ml (Fleming & Nelson, 1988). PPN is applicable when clients require only supplementary or low-kilocalorie support and when low concentrations of glucose and amino acids and/or lipids are sufficient.

If TPN is anticipated for longer than 7 days, CPN is recommended. When hypertonic solutions are given, fluid is drawn into the blood stream and can damage small peripheral veins. Peripheral infusions of highly hypertonic solutions (more than 10%) can cause sclerosis, phlebitis, clotting, and swelling. Therefore, when hypertonic solutions are necessary, CPN is advocated. High rates of blood flow through larger veins dilute solutions rapidly. The catheter is inserted into the superior vena cava or right atrium via the subclavian or internal jugular vein. Dextrose concentration can be the main energy source, with lipids provided 2 to 3 times weekly, but use of daily lipid infusions as a source of kilocalories has become a common practice.

What does PPN stand for, and when is it used? What are the advantages of CPN over PPN? What is the problem with administering hypertonic fluids into peripheral veins? What form of PN is necessary to use hypertonic solutions?

When nutrients are provided intravenously in sufficient quality and quantity for hypermetabolic clients who cannot be fed enterally, CPN is normally used since 2500 to 3000 ml of hypertonic glucose solutions can be given. The purpose of CPN is to provide nutrients to maintain or increase lean body mass over an extended period. CPN can provide needed energy; restore positive nitrogen balance; and replace essential vitamins, electrolytes, minerals, and trace elements.

NURSING APPLICATIONS

Assessment

Physical—for types of clients that are considered good candidates for PPN and CPN, muscle weakness and wasting, weight loss.
Dietary—for energy and nutrient requirement.
Laboratory—for glucose, protein, albumin.

Interventions

1. Consult with physician or dietitian if PPN or CPN is needed (clients who require increased amounts of nutrients because of multiple trauma, burns, and so forth).

2. For clients receiving PPN, monitor for phlebitis (redness, heat, and tenderness around insertion site or following vein). Discontinue if phlebitis occurs.

Client Education

- Explain the rationale for TPN.
- PPN prevents further deterioration, whereas CPN promotes cell growth and anabolism.

Composition of Parenteral Solutions

All the basic nutrients required by the body can be given intravenously: carbohydrates, proteins, fat emulsions, vitamins, water, electrolytes, and trace minerals.

Kilocalories

Energy needs can be met by various combinations of dextrose and/or fat emulsions. Kilocalories provided by energy nutrients can be determined using the equations shown in Table 13–9. Excessive energy intake has been shown to produce undesirable metabolic complications, such as hepatomegaly, liver dysfunction, and respiratory insufficiency. The metabolic cart, discussed in Chapter 10, is the best method of precisely determining kilocaloric requirements. The current trend is to match the kilocalories in the TPN solution closely with the client's kilocaloric requirements. Therefore, individualization is critical.

How are energy needs met with TPN? Why is it important to avoid excess kilocalories? What is the most precise method of determining kilocalories in the TPN solution?

Carbohydrate

The main source of carbohydrate in TPN solutions is dextrose. Since parenteral dextrose provides 3.4 kcal/ml, concentrated solutions are necessary, ranging from 10 to 70%. Table 13–10 shows the number of kilocalories provided by various

What is the main source of carbohydrate, and how many kilocalories per milliliter does it supply?

TABLE 13–9

ESTIMATING KILOCALORIES IN PARENTERAL SOLUTIONS

Glucose of amino acid solutions:*

$$\text{ml of solution} \times \text{concentration of nutrient in solution} = \text{gm glucose/amino acid infused} \times \text{physiologic fuel factor} = \text{kcal}$$

Example:

To determine the number of kcal/gm in 3000 ml of D_5W:

$$3000\ ml \times \frac{5\ mg\ glucose}{100\ ml} = 150\ gm\ glucose \times \frac{3.4\ kcal}{gm} = 510\ kcal$$

To determine the amount of protein in 2000 ml of 3.5% amino acid solution:*

$$2000\ ml \times \frac{3.5\ gm\ amino\ acid}{100\ ml} = 70\ gm\ amino\ acids/protein$$

Fat emulsions:

1 ml of 10% fat emulsion = 1.1 kcal/ml; number of ml × 1.1 = kcal

1 ml of 20% fat emulsion = 2.0 kcal/ml; number of ml × 2 = kcal

Example:

500 ml of a 20% fat emulsion = 500 ml × 2 kcal/ml = 1000 kcal

*Although the amount of protein supplied is important to determine adequacy, the number of kilocalories from protein is normally not counted because the protein is used for protein synthesis and anabolism.

TABLE 13–10

PARENTERAL DEXTROSE SOLUTIONS

Dextrose Solutions	Kilocalories/ Liter	Tonicity
5%	170	Isotonic
10%	340	Hypertonic
20%	680	Hypertonic
30%	1020	Hypertonic
50%	1700	Hypertonic
70%	2380	Hypertonic

dextrose solutions. When hypertonic dextrose solutions are given, insulin may be needed to prevent hyperglycemia.

Fat Emulsions

Lipid emulsions can be used in conjunction with carbohydrates and amino acids. Fat emulsions provide more than twice as much energy as protein or carbohydrate emulsions and have a low tonicity. Fat emulsions may be added "piggyback" into the amino acid/dextrose solution, or all 3 can be mixed in the same bag. These 3-in-1 mixtures are commonly called total nutrient admixture (TNA).

Fat emulsions are necessary when TPN continues more than 2 to 3 weeks to prevent EFA deficiency. However, this artificial method of feeding is more similar to a mixed meal profile and is physiologically more natural if lipids are provided daily. The use of both substrates avoids overloading metabolic pathways. Additionally, protein repletion is enhanced, glucose tolerance is improved, and fluid retention is reduced (Weinsier et al, 1989; Fleming & Nelson, 1988). Fat emulsions are especially recommended for clients with diabetes mellitus (for better glucose control and lower insulin requirements) and respiratory failure (less carbon dioxide produced from lipid oxidation).

Several fat emulsions are currently available in the US. They are derived from soybean and safflower oil. Lipid emulsions are isotonic and can be used to offset the high osmolality of the dextrose solution. A 10% solution provides 1.1 kcal/ml; a 20% solution provides 2 kcal/ml.

Coalescence is destabilization of the emulsion and is irreversible.

How many kilocalories per milliliter does each of the following provide: 10%, 20%? Why are fat emulsions required if TPN is needed for more than 3 weeks?

Lipid emulsions are complex pharmaceuticals to keep the fat particles emulsified in an aqueous solution. The stabilizer is egg yolk phospholipid. If fat particles aggregate, the particle size increases, with larger particles rising to the surface. This process is known as creaming and is reversible on gentle agitation. If the process proceeds, the large aggregates **coalesce.** A coalesced lipid solution administered to clients may result in capillary fat embolism.

Protein

When IV fluids are required for more than 3 to 4 days, protein solutions are recommended. These synthetic crystalline compounds contain both EAA and NEAA. They are well tolerated, enhance protein synthesis, and improve nitrogen balance when adequate amounts of both kilocalories and protein are provided.

Protein infusions can contribute to the kilocalories, but their objective is mainly for protein repletion. Thus, they are not usually relied on for kilocalories or administered in high concentrations because of increased urea production when metabolized for energy.

Amino acid concentrates are expensive, so minimal amounts are used to provide nitrogen requirements. Amino acids are commercially available in various concentrations, from 3 to 15%. The use of the new higher concentration (15%) allows higher protein levels when severe fluid restrictions are necessary. Although various specialized amino acid formulas are available for renal, hepatic, and trauma condi-

Why are minimal amounts of amino acid concentrates used?

tions, they have not proved to be more effective than general amino acid formulas (Heyman, 1990; Scholten et al, 1990).

Vitamins

Multivitamin preparations are essential for use in long-term TPN, but it is difficult to determine their optimal levels. Since the GI tract is bypassed, the RDAs are not appropriate. Maintenance levels for 12 vitamins have been recommended by the AMA (Table 13–11). Water-soluble vitamins (B complex and C) and water-miscible forms of fat-soluble vitamins (A, D, and E) are available as IV multivitamin preparations. These maintenance doses may not be sufficient to correct preexisting deficiencies or for increased requirements related to stress or disease.

Close monitoring of clinical signs and laboratory values is advisable to prevent deficiencies. IV multiple vitamin preparations do not contain vitamin K. Vitamin K is generally provided as phytonadione, 10 mg IM once a week.

What vitamin should be added?

Electrolytes and Trace Minerals

Sodium, potassium, chloride, phosphorus, magnesium, and calcium are essential and included in TPN therapy as indicated in Table 13–12. Serious complications have been reported when clients receiving TPN for extended periods did not receive trace elements (copper, chromium, molybdenum, iodine, selenium, and especially zinc). Particular attention should be given to the provision of zinc for clients who are stressed, have draining wounds, or excessive GI losses (Fig. 13–8). Trace mineral products are available as a single entity or combination to allow administration on an individualized basis.

Minerals such as boron, nickel, molybdenum, vanadium, aluminum, cadmium, and chromium have been documented as **contaminants** in TPN solutions and may contribute to the prevention of deficiencies (Ito et al, 1990; Berner et al, 1989).

Contaminants—unintentionally added from the environment or during processing.

Requirements vary with the client's condition; depleted catabolic states and anabolism increase the amount of trace elements needed. Laboratory values and clinical symptoms should be closely monitored. Usual ranges of daily needs for trace elements are shown in Table 13–13.

TABLE 13–11

AMERICAN MEDICAL ASSOCIATION'S VITAMIN RECOMMENDATIONS FOR PARENTERAL FEEDINGS

Vitamin	Up to Age 11	Age 11 and Older
A	2300 IU	3300 IU
D	400 IU	200 IU
E	7 IU	10 IU
Ascorbic acid	80 mg	100 mg
Folacin	140 mcg	400 mcg
Niacin	17 mg	40 mg
Riboflavin	1.4 mg	3.6 mg
Thiamin	1.2 mg	3 mg
B_6 (pyridoxine)	1 mg	4 mg
B_{12} (cyanocobalamin)	1 mcg	5 mcg
Pantothenic acid	5 mg	15 mg
Biotin	20 mcg	60 mcg

From AMA Department of Foods and Nutrition: *Guidelines for Multivitamin Preparations for Parenteral Use.* Chicago, Copyright 1975. American Medical Association.

TABLE 13–12

SUGGESTED APPROXIMATE DAILY INTRAVENOUS REQUIREMENTS* FOR MACROMINERALS

Ion	Units	Infants and Young Children (per kg/day)	Adults (per day)
Sodium*	mEq	3–5	60 and up
Potassium*	mEq	3–5	60 and up
Magnesium*	mEq	0.3–0.5	12–20 or higher
Calcium	mEq	1–2	10–25†
Phosphorus‡	mg	15–30	450 and up
Sulfur		§	§

* For clients with normal cardiovascular, renal, and intestinal function. The higher ranges are suggested for children with rapid growth rate and for adults with large GI losses and adequate renal functions. In such clients, periodic evaluation of serum, stool, and urine levels are indicated.

† The higher calcium intakes are indicated for children with rapid growth and adults with conditions predisposing to prior bone demineralization and chronic acidosis.

‡ As inorganic phosphate. Increased amounts are indicated when initiating TPN with large amounts of glucose to counteract resulting hypophosphatemia with serial serum monitoring. Phosphorus as phosphatide is present in IV fat. Increased amounts of phosphate have been recommended to decrease calciuria.

§ Supplied as methionine.

From Shils ME. Enteral (tube) and parenteral nutrition support. *In* Shils ME, Young VR, eds. *Modern Nutrition in Health and Disease.* 7th ed. Philadelphia, Lea & Febiger, 1988: 1023–1066.

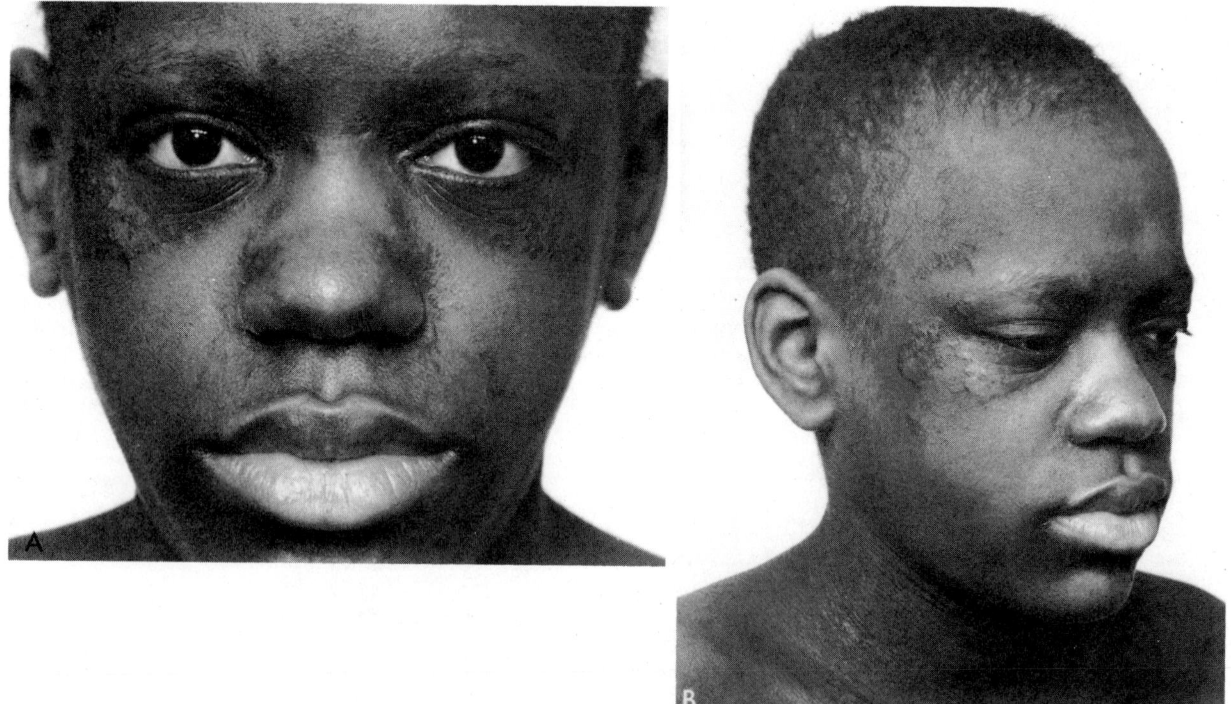

Figure 13–8 *A* and *B*, Skin manifestations of acute zinc deficiency during parenteral nutrition. Nonpruritic dermatitis about mouth and eyes and over nose and chin is evident. (From Grant JP. *Handbook of Total Parenteral Nutrition.* Philadelphia, WB Saunders, 1980.)

TABLE 13–13

SUGGESTED DAILY INTRAVENOUS INTAKE OF ESSENTIAL TRACE ELEMENTS

	Pediatric (mcg/kg)*	Stable Adult	Adult in Acute Catabolic State†	Stable Adult with Intestinal Losses‡
Zinc	300§ 100‖	2.5 to 4 mg	Additional 2 mg	Add 12.2 mg/L small-bowel fluid lost; 17.1 mg/kg of stool or ileostomy output.¶
Copper	20	0.5 to 1.5 mg		
Chromium	0.14 to 0.2	10 to 15 mcg		
Manganese	2 to 10	0.15 to 0.8 mg		20 mcg

* Limited data are available for infants weighing less than 1500 gm. Their requirements may be more than the recommendations because of their low body reserves and increased requirements for growth.
† Frequent monitoring of blood levels in these clients is essential to provide proper dosage.
‡ Premature infants (weight less than 1500 gm) up to 3 kg of body weight. Thereafter, the recommendations for full-term infants apply.
§ Full-term infants and children up to 5 years old. Thereafter, the recommendations for adults apply, up to a maximum dosage of 4 mg/day.
‖ Values derived by mathematical fitting of balance data from a 71-client-week study in 24 clients.
¶ Mean from balance study.
From AMA Department of Foods and Nutrition: Guidelines for essential trace element preparations for parenteral use. JAMA 241(May 11):2051, 1979. Copyright 1979, by American Medical Association.

NURSING APPLICATIONS

Assessment

Physical—for EFA deficiency (dry flaky skin, rash with small reddish papules and alopecia); zinc deficiency (lesions around the eyes, nose, mouth, buttocks); bleeding tendencies, sparse hair growth, and decreased wound healing ability.

Dietary—for composition of TPN solution, number of kilocalories needed; allergy to eggs.

Laboratory—for LFTs; serum glucose; protein, albumin, transferrin, prealbumin, TLC, BUN, creatine; electrolytes, especially calcium, magnesium, phosphorus levels; prothrombin time.

Interventions

1. Monitor I&O.
2. Refrigerate fat emulsions; remove from refrigerator at least 30 min before use. Liposyn can be stored at room temperature.
3. For 3-in-1 mixtures, do not use if appearance of oil globules or a "ring" is present (Worthington & Wagner, 1989).

Client Education

- Stress the importance of fat to prevent a deficiency and to provide more energy than dextrose or protein.
- Protein is provided to help tissues heal and grow.
- Dextrose or carbohydrate provides the body's main source of energy and allows protein to do its job (i.e., growth and repair).
- Hunger pains and food cravings may be experienced because signals to the CNS activated by the passage of food to the stomach are by-passed (Rodriguez, 1992). However, the body's physiological requirements are being met with these solutions.
- Lack of appetite may occur during TPN. This resolves in time.

24-HOUR DAILY PARENTERAL NUTRIENT ADMIXTURE ORDER FORM AND INTAKE RECORD

SEE INSTRUCTIONS ON BACK OF FORM

Date Due__________ Time Due__________ Bag#__________

Kilocalories per 24 hours (to nearest even numbered 200 kcal) __________

Check One	Formulas	% kcal Provided as: Dextrose	Amino Acids	Fat	Approximate Volume Per 1000 kcal
	Central Vein Nutrition				
	Standard	60	15	25	760 ml
	Intermediate Nitrogen	60	17	23	800 ml
	High Nitrogen	60	20	20	850 ml
	Restricted Carbohydrate	50	15	35	770 ml
	Restricted Carbohydrate - Intermediate Nitrogen	50	17	33	810 ml
	Restricted Carbohydrate - High Nitrogen	50	20	30	860 ml
	Low Carbohydrate - High Fat	42	16	42	790 ml
	Restricted Carbohydrate - Low Nitrogen	50	10	40	660 ml
	Standard - No Fat	85	15	0	740 ml
	High Nitrogen - No Fat	80	20	0	840 ml
	Peripheral Vein Nutrition	32	16	52	1420 ml

Additives	Suggested Adult Guidelines	Quantity Ordered
Sodium as Chloride	(60 + mEq/day)	mEq
Potassium as Chloride	(60 + mEq/day)	mEq
Phosphate as Potassium Buffer[1,2]	(20 – 40 mmol/day)	mmol
Sodium as Acetate		mEq
Potassium as Acetate		mEq
Phosphate as Sodium Buffer[1,2]		mmol
Calcium as Gluceptate[2]	(10 - 15 mEq/day)	mEq
Magnesium as Sulfate[2]	(8 - 20 mEq/day)	mEq
MVI-12	(10 ml/day)	ml
Ascorbic Acid	(1000 mg/day)	mg
Trace Elements[3]	(2 ml/day)	ml
Phytonadione	(10 mg/week)	mg
Insulin, Regular Human		units

Date __________

Time__________ Signature__________

For Nursing Use: (Please record information and initials)

Date & Time This Bag Started__________ Total Volume This Bag __________ Nurse Initials __________

Date & Time This Bag Stopped __________ Residual Volume This Bag When Stopped __________ Nurse Initials __________

N-128 (25483)

Figure 13–9 Example of a 24-hour daily parenteral nutrient admixture order form and intake record. (From Weinsier RL, et al. *Handbook of Clinical Nutrition.* 2nd ed. St. Louis, CV Mosby, 1989. Courtesy of University of Alabama at Birmingham.)

Methods of Delivery

Methods of TPN delivery are similar to enteral feedings: continuous or cyclic. Continuous infusion is the preferred method. However, cyclic (daytime or nighttime) infusions may be used, especially for home use.

Nutrition Support Team

Because of the complexity of a successful TPN program, some hospitals maintain a nutrition support team, consisting of a physician, nurse, pharmacist, and dietitian, with other medical personnel incorporated as needed. Team members may be responsible for technical aspects of care, initiate feeding, and closely monitor the client's condition, weight change, and daily fluid I&O. The nurse's role may encompass maintaining client care, educating the nursing staff, assisting with CPN catheter placement and care, and educating the client and family regarding this method of nutrition support. Institutions that have this teamwork report fewer complications of TPN therapy.

Name the members of the nutrition support team.

INSTRUCTIONS

1. Please use one of the specified formulas, if possible.
2. These complex mixtures may require up to four hours of preparation time. Please allow for this.
3. Orders received between 0600 and 1600 will be filled the same day. For TPN at other times, please order 1 liter units of Dextrose and Amino Acids utilizing the appropriate TPN order form.
4. Central Vein Formulas are prepared utilizing D70%W, Amino Acids 10%, and Fat Emulsion 20%. The Peripheral Vein Formula is prepared using D20%W, Amino Acids 8.5%, and Fat Emulsion 10%. The final total volume is determined by the formula selected, kilocalories required, and additives ordered. Approximate final volume and hourly infusion rate will be labeled on each bag. The infusion rate may require adjustment by the nurse so that the entire volume will be infused over a 24-hour period.

FOOTNOTES

1. Each 3 mmol of Phosphate buffer contains approximately 4 mEq of cation (Potassium or Sodium).
2. Upper limits of compatible electrolyte concentrations per 1000 ml final volume:

Calcium	10	mEq
Magnesium	20	mEq
Phosphate	15	mmol

3. Each 1 ml of Trace Elements Contains:

Zinc	2	mg
Copper	0.4	mg
Manganese	0.2	mg
Iodine	0.056	mg
Chromium	6.25	mcg
Sodium Chloride	9	mg

Figure 13–9 *Continued*

Unit nurses are responsible for constant delivery of nutrient solution and supplemental additives. They must also identify problems and initiate corrective action when needed. Emotional support is important for the client in adjusting to this drastically different method of feeding.

Parenteral Feeding Order

In general, TPN solutions are individualized to meet the specific requirements of each client. Figure 13–9 is an example of an order form for a typical central-vein solution. Infusion of nutrients is administered slowly at first to allow the body to adjust. The initial regimen depends on the client's condition and expected tolerance. If clients have been receiving dextrose infusions, TPN may be started at about 50 ml/hr and advanced at a rate of 25 ml/hr every 8 hours to reach full kilocaloric requirements within 2 to 3 days. Malnourished clients should be advanced to their kilocaloric goal over a 5- to 7-day period (Weinsier et al, 1989).

Blood glucose, electrolyte, and phosphorus levels are checked daily until they are stable, followed by monitoring 2 to 3 times a week. Lipid clearance is monitored by measuring serum triglyceride levels. If triglyceride level is above 300 to 350 mg/dl 6 hours after termination of first lipid infusion, fat emulsions should probably be limited to provision of EFA.

How long should it take for clients previously receiving routine IV solutions to reach kilocaloric requirements; for a malnourished client?

Principles and Procedures for Total Parenteral Nutrition

The infusion flow rate must be constant and uninterrupted. A pump is used for TPN administration to protect clients from air embolisms and erratic drip rates. If the rate is too slow, hypoglycemia may result with an insufficient amount of nutrients provided. Too rapid a flow rate could lead to hyperglycemia and osmotic diuresis. Trying to "catch up" to the proper rate is not permitted unless specified by the physician (usually 10 to 20% of the original rate). Careful monitoring of clinical and laboratory data is important (Table 13–14).

Is it acceptable to "catch up"?

TABLE 13–14

LABORATORY TESTS TO MONITOR IN PARENTERAL NUTRITION

Measure daily until stable, then 2 to 3 times weekly
- Electrolytes (sodium, potassium, chloride, carbon dioxide)
- Glucose
- Phosphorus
- Blood urea nitrogen, creatinine
- Triglycerides (if fat emulsions provided)

Measure 1 to 2 times weekly
- Complete blood count (CBC)
- Calcium, magnesium
- Liver function tests (LFT)
- Albumin/prealbumin/transferrin
- Prothrombin time (PT)

NURSING APPLICATIONS

Assessment

Physical—for weight daily, temperature.
Dietary—for parenteral feeding order, use of nutrition support team.
Laboratory—for glucose, electrolytes, phosphorus, triglycerides.

Interventions

1. Monitor I&O.
2. Check flow rate every hour.
3. Do not abruptly stop TPN unless the client is being fed enterally or orally.

Client Education

- Explain the purpose of nutrition support team.
- Discuss purpose of TPN, where catheter tip is located, and type of device used.

Complications

Sepsis

What may be an initial sign of sepsis?

Sepsis is one of the most frequent complications of TPN therapy. Strict aseptic techniques in preparation and storage of the infusion are essential to prevent bacterial contamination. One of the first signs of sepsis is glucose intolerance (provided that it was not a preexisting condition).

NURSING APPLICATIONS

Assessment

Physical—for temperature, chills, IV site for tenderness, redness, and drainage, enlarged lymph nodes.
Laboratory—for blood culture, tip of catheter culture, WBC with differential, glucose (usually an increase).

Interventions

1. Use aseptic technique when hanging solution and preparing tubing.
2. If infection occurs, notify physician. The tube may have to be removed and the tip cultured.

3. Give antibiotics as prescribed.

Evaluation

* Client does not experience sepsis, and IV site is clean and dry.

Client Education

- Explain the reason for aseptic technique.
- Notify the nurse if dressing becomes soiled.

Hyperglycemia and Hypoglycemia

Metabolic abnormalities related to the infusion of large amounts of glucose are common, including hyperglycemia and hypoglycemia. Excessive amounts of dextrose may result in **steatosis** and, unless appropriate action is taken, may prove fatal. If LFTs are elevated, notify physician for appropriate adjustments.

Abrupt termination of hypertonic dextrose infusion (which stimulates insulin secretion) results in hypoglycemia. The usual procedure is to reduce the infusion rate by 50% for ½ to 1 hour before discontinuation of TPN unless clients are receiving enteral (tube or oral) feedings. (PPN infusions do not need to be tapered).

Steatosis—fatty liver.

What may excess dextrose result in? How is hypoglycemia prevented in TPN client?

NURSING APPLICATIONS

Assessment

Physical—for hyperglycemia (deep, rapid breathing; increased urine output; lethargy), hypoglycemia (sweating, pallor, shaky feeling); I&O, skin turgor.
Dietary—for composition of formula and flow rate.
Laboratory—for blood glucose levels, LFTs, serum and urine osmolality.

Interventions

1. Monitor flow rate hourly.
2. Identify and closely monitor client at risk of developing hyperglycemia or hypoglycemia (early phase of injury, diabetes mellitus, pancreatic disease, hormonal abnormalities, liver disease, sepsis, surgery, the use of beta blockers, phenytoin, steroids, epinephrine, thiazide diuretics) (Orr, 1992).
3. If hyperglycemia develops, notify physician and give insulin as prescribed.
4. If hypoglycemic, if possible, give glass of milk. If severe, give dextrose as ordered.

Evaluation

* Client's blood glucose stays WNL.

Client Education

- Hyperglycemia does not mean the client is diabetic.
- Explain the reason for monitoring glucose.

Lipid Overload

Adverse reactions to lipid emulsions are usually observed with excessive doses. Acute reactions include fever, chills, vomiting, and pain in the chest or back. This usually occurs during the initial transfusion. A milder reaction is **pruritic urticaria.** Fat overload syndrome is characterized by hyperlipidemia, fever, focal seizures, **leukocytosis, hepatosplenomegaly,** shock, and spontaneous bleeding.

Pruritic urticaria—itchy skin rash. Leukocytosis—elevated levels of leukocytes (WBC). Hepatosplenomegaly—enlargement of the liver and spleen.

What are the symptoms of acute reactions; for fat overload?

TABLE 13–15

MAJOR METABOLIC COMPLICATIONS IN CLIENTS RECEIVING TOTAL PARENTERAL NUTRITION

	Presentations
Nutrient excess	
Glucose	Hyperglycemia, polyuria, polydipsia
Amino acids	Hyperammonemia in clients with liver disease Azotemia in renal failure
Calcium	Hypercalcemia, pancreatitis, renal stones
Vitamin D	Hypercalcemia, osteopenia, long bone pain
Nutrient deficiencies	
Copper	Neutropenia, anemia, scorbutic bone lesions, ↓ ceruloplasmin
Zinc	Nasolabial and perineal acrodermatitis, alopecia, ↓ T cell function, ↓ alkaline phosphatase
Chromium	Glucose intolerance
Selenium	Myalgias, cardiomyopathy, ↓ glutathione peroxidase
Molybdenum	Amino acid intolerance, tachycardia, tachypnea, central scotomas, irritability, ↓ uric acid
Essential fatty acids	Eczymoid dermatitis, ↑ linoleic acid and arachidonic acid
Vitamin A	Night blindness, ↓ dark field adaptation
Vitamin E	In vitro platelet hyperaggregation and H_2O_2-induced RBC hemolysis
Biotin	Dermatitis, alopecia, hypotonia
Thiamin	Wernicke's encephalopathy

From Fleming CR, Nelson J. Nutritional options. *In* Kinney JM, et al, eds. *Nutrition and Metabolism in Patient Care.* Philadelphia, WB Saunders, 1988:752–772.

NURSING APPLICATIONS

Assessment

Physical—acute reaction, itchy rash, enlarged liver, hypotension.
Dietary—for percentage of fat given in solution.
Laboratory—for triglycerides, cholesterol, WBC with differential, PT, and PTT.

Interventions

1. Give initial fat solution slowly. Follow facility guidelines.
2. If acute reactions or fat overload occurs, stop fat infusion and notify the physician.

Evaluation

* Lipid overload does not occur.

Client Education

- Explain the reason for administering initial fat solution slowly.

Other Problems

Other problems have been associated with excessive or deficient amounts of electrolytes and many of the vitamins and minerals (Table 13–15). Deficiency symptoms from many of the nutrients—copper, chromium, and biotin—were seldom or never observed before TPN therapy was developed.

NURSING APPLICATIONS

Assessment

Physical—for signs and symptoms listed in Table 13–15.
Dietary—for composition of solution.
Laboratory—for electrolytes and laboratory tests listed in Table 13–14.

Interventions

1. Use Table 13–15 to monitor for deficiencies or excesses. Notify physician/ nutrition support team if these are present.

Evaluation

* Complications with electrolytes, vitamins, and minerals were prevented.

Client Education

- Close monitoring of blood studies detects nutrient excess or deficit.
- Some nutrient deficiencies and excesses produce only physical symptoms, so a head-to-toe check every shift is necessary.

HOME PARENTERAL NUTRITION

For those who require TPN but not acute or extended medical care, home feedings can be managed effectively, safely, and economically for many clients. Increasing numbers of clients are being discharged using PN support at home. In 1986, approximately 14,300 clients received parenteral therapy at home (Hoffman, 1989). Most clients think that the ability to administer feedings at home improves daily living and helps to maintain quality of life by returning to a more normal lifestyle and allowing them to spend more time with their family. On the other hand, some clients are unable to adjust to the demands imposed by home TPN (Fleming & Nelson, 1988). With home parenteral nutrition, many clients are able to resume a somewhat normal lifestyle, but problems with chronic fluid, electrolyte, and micronutrient deficiencies, catheter sepsis, and insurance coverage often restrict optimal rehabilitation (Burnes et al, 1992).

How do clients feel about home parenteral feedings?

Determining Clients Appropriate for Home Feedings

Only some clients are appropriate for home feedings. A number of factors need to be assessed: (1) fairly stable medical condition, (2) ability to tolerate the full volume needed to meet nutrient requirements via parenteral feeding before discharge from the hospital, (3) psychosocial factors, such as willingness and motivation to administer the feeding, and support of family or significant others, (4) ability to understand and perform the therapy, (5) economic resources (feeding solutions and delivery devices must be affordable), and (6) availability of home follow-up and monitoring.

Name 3 factors to consider before client can go home with TPN.

Psychosocial Adjustments

In 1987, the Oley Foundation for Home Parenteral and Enteral Nutrition surveyed clients about psychosocial problems. More than half of 172 respondents indicated that depression, control, and independence are significant unresolved issues; other concerns included restricted food intake, relationships with spouse or significant others, body image, and sexual concerns (Rodriquez, 1992; Hoffman, 1989). Financial concerns have a major impact on the emotional well-being and lifestyle of

What are some psychosocial concerns of clients receiving PN?

clients, especially long-term home clients receiving PN (Heaphey, 1988). Nurses need to empathize with clients to reduce stress and discomfort.

Training for Home Parenteral Nutrition

Intensive training for the client and family for home parenteral feedings is similar to that provided for home enteral feedings. Training may take from 2 to 3 weeks in the hospital setting to teach (1) principles of asepsis, (2) catheter care, (3) care of parenteral nutrient solutions and pump, (4) parameters to monitor, and (5) problem solving. With adequate training, motivated persons not educated in the medical field are more than capable of performing the task of parenteral feedings successfully at home (Bisset et al, 1992).

Follow-up

Monitoring the client's hematologic status is dependent on the duration and stability of the clinical course. Initially the physician should obtain laboratory values every 2 weeks for at least the first 6 weeks. If the client's status improves and results normalize, frequency of testing may be decreased to every 6 months for long-term clients (Fleming, 1988). Catheter sepsis is the most common cause of rehospitalization; this may be related to noncompliance, but other factors such as bowel disease or age may also be involved (Burnes et al, 1992; Annual Report 1985 Data, 1987). Nutritional repletion of adult clients receiving PN at home has been favorable, with repletion of both fat and lean body mass; children receiving home parenteral support have shown either normal or an accelerated rate of growth (Bisset et al, 1992).

When is hematological testing performed?

NURSING APPLICATIONS

Assessment

Physical—for manual dexterity and willingness to learn feeding/caring techniques, home environment, support of significant others, psychosocial status.
Dietary—for type and amount of feeding.

Interventions

1. Involve the family/client in planning care.
2. Use the team approach for training the client and family.
3. Explore fears and concerns of client/family.

Evaluation

* Evaluate if the client/family is able to or wants to perform these techniques at home by monitoring body language, verbal responses, stress levels, and motivation levels.
* Return demonstration of the client/family's skills in preparing, administering solutions, caring for IV site and equipment; problem solving complications that may arise.

Client Education

- Inform client/family of home health care facilities, social workers, Medicare, support groups, and supplier of equipment and parenteral infusion.

TRANSITIONAL FEEDINGS

A change from one feeding mode to another is considered a transitional feeding or weaning period. This requires careful attention to maintain nutritional status while returning clients to their most normal intake possible. Despite the client's desire to return to oral feedings or complaints of hunger, oral intake to support nutritional requirements requires an adjustment period; early satiety is attributed to gastric atrophy. TPN infusions result in a decrease of voluntary food intake; for some clients, appetite may be suppressed for 1 to 2 weeks after infusions are stopped. Maintaining accurate intake records of oral intake is an important nursing function.

Parenteral to Oral Feeding

The client can be encouraged to take easily digested liquids. Small amounts of clear liquids with a low osmolality are usually well-tolerated. Initially the client is instructed to sip 1 to 2 oz (30 to 60 ml) at 20- to 30-min intervals, increasing to 3 to 6 oz as more volume is tolerated. After 24 hours, full liquids may be initiated in small amounts. Polymeric formulas or lactose-free liquids are recommended. If full liquids are tolerated, solid foods are introduced the next day. At this point, TPN can be decreased by 50%. When kilocaloric counts indicate client is consistently consuming two-thirds of total requirements, TPN can be discontinued. Between-meal supplements are usually needed to increase intake to this level. Only with complete documentation of oral intake (kilocalorie counts) can the infusion be decreased appropriately.

Describe the method for transition from parenteral to oral feeding.

Parenteral to Tube Feeding

Enteral formulas may be initiated at a reduced rate (25 to 50 ml/hr) to prevent hyperosmotic diarrhea and bloating. These can be advanced by 25 ml/hr every 8 hours until goal is reached. Isotonic formulas are usually recommended; they are essential to prevent GI intolerance in hypoalbuminemic clients. Occasionally elemental formulas may be needed. When at least one-third of the requirements are being provided by tube feedings, TPN may be decreased by one-half. IV feedings are discontinued after the client is stabilized on tube feeding at the desired rate to meet requirements.

Describe the procedure for changing from parenteral to tube feeding.

Tube to Oral Feeding

This transition may be surprisingly difficult for many clients. Be sure that the swallowing function is consistent and regular. Full liquids are initiated, followed by soft or pureed foods. Lactose intolerance and fat malabsorption are prevalent; initially lactose is excluded, and fat intake should be relatively low. When oral intake reaches 500 kcal or more, tube feedings can be proportionately and gradually decreased. (Tube feedings are provided at night, or feeding is stopped for at least 1 hour before and after meals to promote appetite.) When oral intake consistently exceeds two-thirds of the client's kilocalorie requirements, discontinue tube feedings.

Clients who have been on parenteral or continuous tube feedings for a long time may not feel hungry and experience early satiety. Clients may be encouraged to eat by providing favorite foods. Nutrient adequacy may be achieved earlier if oral nutrition supplements are provided.

Describe the procedure for transition from tube to oral feedings.

NURSING APPLICATIONS

Assessment

Physical—for swallowing ability before starting oral feedings.
Dietary—for kilocalorie intake.

Interventions

1. When starting with food, avoid foods that contain lactose or are high in fat and hyperosmolar clear liquids (see Chapter 12, Table 12–4).
2. Assist with kilocalorie counts.

Evaluation

* Desired results include client consuming his or her favorite foods with no complications.

Client Education

- Explain why transitional feeding is necessary.
- It is normal not to feel hungry right after parenteral or tube feedings. However, this should resolve. If it does not, the dietitian should be consulted.

NUTRITION UPDATE 13–1: CUSTOMIZING FORMULAS TO BOOST IMMUNITY

PEM has long been known to result in abnormalities in immune response. Aggressive nutrition therapy, or the use of enteral and parenteral feedings, has reduced the incidence of morbidity and mortality associated with uncomplicated malnutrition. However, other complications, including infections and sepsis, continue to be a problem. Whether the immune response is deficient because of the increased nutrient requirements or lack of specific nutrients in the defined formulas provided has been of concern. During the 1980s, nutrition research has focused on the role of individual nutrients on different aspects of immunocompetence.

The body's first line of defense against infection—the skin, GI tract, and mucous membranes—is usually effective in preventing entry of microorganisms into the body. Indeed, TPN has been associated with bacterial translocation of bacteria from the intestine to the lymph nodes (Alverdy et al, 1988). Nonuse of the GI tract is the suspected cause. By contrast, enteral feedings increase blood flow and preserve GI function, while decreasing mucosal atrophy, thereby supposedly preventing bacterial translocation.

IV protein solutions traditionally omit the amino acid glutamine because it is unstable. Glutamine plays an important role in GI metabolism, structure, and function. Glutamine catabolism markedly increases during physiological stress, such as trauma, sepsis, or burns. Enteral feedings containing glutamine preserve bowel integrity and thus prevent translocation of bowel organisms (Haw et al, 1991). The addition of glutamine to TPN mixtures enhances intestinal mucosal cell proliferation and improves intestinal immune function (Ziegler, 1992).

Other proteins have also been implicated in immune function. Arginine, another NEAA, is important in protein synthesis. Larger amounts of arginine are needed during physiological stress and rapid growth and development. A deficiency leads to compromised cellular immune function, particularly T cell function. Supplemental amounts result in increased thymic size and number of T lymphocytes. Incidence of infection is decreased. Small amounts have always been present in enteral formulas. Arginine supplementation in enteral formulas has resulted in an enhanced T lymphocyte response in surgical clients (Daly et al, 1988), accelerated wound healing, improved resistance to infection, and decreased body weight loss after injury (Gottschlich et al, 1986).

Nucleotides participate in nearly all biochemical processes and are precursors of DNA and RNA. ATP, a nucleotide, is a major substance used to transfer chemical energy. Nucleotides are available from protein-containing foods (meat, poultry, fish, milk, and eggs) and can be produced by the liver. Lymphocytes and intestinal epithelial cells are unable to synthesize nucleotides. During critical illness, decreased liver function may increase exogenous nucleotide requirements. A deficiency results in decreased delayed hypersensitivity responses and decreased resistance to infections (Fanslow et al, 1988). Nucleotide-free diets have been used in transplant clients because they impair the onset of macrophage phagocytic function and suppress immune responses, thus decreasing allograft rejection. Currently, most enteral and parenteral formulas contain casein-based proteins, which are nucleotide free.

The type and quantity of lipids provided affect immune function. Long-chain triglycerides have been used extensively in enteral and parenteral formulas. Excess amounts of linoleic acid (omega-6 fatty acid) are immunosuppressive, stimulating suppressor T cell activity. Omega-3 fatty acids, or eicosapentaenoic acid (EPA), are present in fish oil and can be made by the body from linolenic acid. EPAs are biochemical mediators that compete with or inhibit the immunosuppressive effects of linoleic acid. Because of a rate-limiting enzyme in EPA production from omega-6 fatty acids, a dietary source of EPA, such as fish oils, can favorably affect prostaglandin production, which is involved in inflammation, infection, tissue injury, and immune system modulation. Thus, a formula that provides a balance of omega-6 and omega-3 fatty acids may be beneficial, especially for clients with atherosclerosis, cancer, organ transplants, and arthritis.

Nutrition support can stimulate or suppress immunocompetence. Most importantly, enteral feedings initiated as soon as possible preserve the integrity of the GI tract. Providing higher than normal amounts of nutrients such as glutamine, arginine, dietary nucleotides, and omega-3 fatty acids can improve immune function. Excessive amounts of iron, zinc, fat, and linoleic acid have adverse effects. Since microorganisms need iron to survive, iron is not recommended. Some formulas have already been developed to maintain immune function in severely stressed clients. Others are certain to be produced and marketed. Whether these changes will significantly affect client mortality and morbidity remains to be seen.

SUMMARY

When clients have physical problems that interfere with the normal ability to ingest food orally, a plan for nutrition support is essential. Enteral and parenteral feedings are alternatives for clients who are unable or unwilling to receive adequate nourishment from a normal diet. Once a plan of nutrition support has been initiated, careful clinical and biochemical monitoring is essential to determine progress.

Enteral feedings use a functioning GI tract and are a physiologically natural method of feeding because they permit more efficient use of nutrients. Most tube feedings are commercial preparations made from intact nutrients. With sufficient energy intake, these provide 100% of the RDIs for vitamins and minerals.

PN is IV delivery of essential nutrients to maintain a client in nutritional equilibrium. It is indicated when enteral intake is impossible or potentially hazardous. Peripheral infusions of dextrose, amino acids, and fat emulsions can provide about 1800 kcal, a sufficient amount to maintain a client's ordinary needs. If larger amounts of kilocalories (2000 to 4000 kcal) are needed, TPN should be implemented.

NURSING PROCESS IN ACTION

An adult client is admitted with orders to initiate tube feedings. The client has not been eating well, and the physician thinks this is necessary to promote nutritional repletion for a needed surgical procedure. After tube insertion and initiation of feedings, the client becomes withdrawn. After much coaxing, the client states that the one thing she still enjoys in life is food and now she cannot even have that anymore.

Nutritional Assessment

- Feelings regarding tube feeding.
- Concerns related to tube feeding.
- Knowledge of tube feeding.
- Beliefs about food intake and mealtimes.
- Availability of support person/group.
- Allergies, especially lactose.
- Type of formula/feeding and amount of kilocalories needed.
- Anthropometric: weight and height.
- Physical: dehydration, diarrhea, bowel sounds, hyperglycemia and hypoglycemia.

Dietary Nursing Diagnosis

Self-concept disturbance RT inability to ingest and taste food.

Nutritional Goals

Client talks to nurse about her feelings about tube feedings and states the importance of these feedings.

Nutritional Implementation 

Intervention: Encourage client to vent feelings and concerns about feedings. Be nonjudgmental.

Rationale: Verbalization helps the client begin to problem solve by allowing expression of pent-up feelings in a conducive atmosphere of trust and acceptance.

Intervention: (1) Offer to watch TV with client or talk about hobby during mealtime; (2) place client at the nurses' station during mealtime; or (3) if client has a support person, encourage that person to visit during mealtimes.

Rationale: Diversional activities may help distract client's thoughts and feelings about loss of mealtime. Mealtimes are a social event for most clients.

Intervention: Monitor weight and praise weight gain or stress advantages in her physical status because of compliance with feedings.

Rationale: Positive feedback enhances the self-concept and self-image because praised behavior is repeated and the "good me" is reinforced.

Intervention: Allow her to chew some foods but not swallow, if possible, or chew sugar-free gum.

Rationale: Client's one desire in life is eating. This may be an acceptable compromise for her.

Intervention: If permitted, allow other clients with enteral feedings to visit her.

Rationale: This provides support to the client by emphasizing she is not alone; she can gain support from people who are experiencing the same thing.

Intervention: Teach the client about advantages and importance of tube feedings (why indicated) and remind her that the tube feedings are temporary.

Rationale: Knowledge increases compliance and decreases fear of the unknown.

Intervention: Monitor for psychological complications, i.e., depression, suicide, grieving. Refer to psychologist/psychiatrist as needed.

Rationale: Since she stated her main joy was eating, she experienced a loss.

Intervention: (1) Monitor for physical complications (see Table 13–7). (2) Check and record residual. (3) Use pump to infuse feeding.

Rationale: (1) Early recognition of complications may result in earlier treatment, thereby decreasing hospital stay and cost. (2) Checking residuals helps determine if amount provided is appropriate and is being emptied from the stomach. This prevents complications such as aspiration and gastric distention. (3) Pumps are more reliable than gravity drip.

Intervention: Refer to dietitian as needed to discuss nutrient requirements and ways to improve intake at home.

Rationale: Nutritional teamwork is a must to provide quality care and to assure this does not occur again.

Evaluation

If client expressed her positive and/or negative feelings and concerns to the nurse about the tube feedings, desired outcomes were achieved. At first, the client may have to be directly asked—"How do you feel?"—to describe feelings and concerns, but as the relationship develops, it is hoped that she will volunteer these feelings and concerns. In addition, these feelings and concerns may initially be negative, but later in her stay, feelings and concerns should become future oriented or positive—"this is going to help me get better quicker," or "this isn't as bad as I thought it would be." Her comments and behavior (i.e., accepting or refusing) also help determine how important she views feedings. Directly asking her, "What is the importance of these feedings?" or "Tell me the reason you are receiving these feedings?" helps nurses determine achievement of this goal.

STUDENT READINESS

1. List the different methods of feeding, and list 2 conditions that warrant using them.
2. What is an elemental formula, and for what conditions is it used?
3. What measures are taken to correct hyperglycemia in TPN? Why is it important?
4. You notice that a client in a nursing home is receiving 1800 kcal via intermittent tube feedings and has diarrhea. What are the possible causes and solutions for the problem?
5. The physician orders 1 kcal/ml formula via tube feeding for a bedridden client who has been on IV feedings for 3 days. What should you do in initiating the formula to prevent complications?
6. A TPN formula contains the following components: 500 ml of a 20% fat emulsion, 500 ml of an 8.5% amino acid solution, and 500 ml 30% dextrose. Calculate the amount of protein and energy provided.

CASE STUDY

Ms. B. D., a 23-year-old musician, has been admitted to the hospital for exacerbation of Crohn's disease (regional enteritis). Since her nutritional status is poor, the physician decides to use parenteral feedings during the acute phase of bowel inflammation. A subclavian venous catheter is inserted, and TPN is begun.

1. Describe a regimen that might be used as the TPN therapy is begun.
2. What laboratory values must be monitored and why?
3. What are the complications of TPN therapy? List nursing care for each.
4. Why is an infusion pump necessary for the administration of TPN?
5. What measures should the nurse take if the client does not receive the prescribed amount of TPN fluid?
6. List parameters to evaluate for determining if nursing care was effective.

REFERENCES

Abernathy GB, et al. Efficacy of tube feeding in supplying energy requirements of hospitalized patients. *JPEN* 1989 July/Aug; 13(4):387–391.

Alexander JW. Nutrition and translocation. *JPEN* 1990 Sept/Oct; 14(5):170S–174S.

Alverdy JC, et al. Total parenteral nutrition promotes bacterial translocation from the gut. *Surgery* 1988 Aug; 104(2):185–190.

Annual Report 1985 Data. Home Nutritional Support Patient Registry. The Oley Foundation. Albany, NY, 1987.

Benya R, Mobarhan S. Enteral alimentation: Administration and complications. *J Am Coll Nutr* 1991 June; 10(3):209–219.

Berner YN, et al. Selected ultratrace elements in total parenteral nutrition solutions. *Am J Clin Nutr* 1989 Nov; 50(5):1079–1083.

Bisset WM, et al. Home parenteral nutrition in chronic intestinal failure. *Arch Dis Child* 1992 Jan; 67(1):109–114.

Bockus S. Troubleshooting your tube feedings. *Am J Nurs* 1991 May; 19(5):24–30.

Bowers DF. The logistics of enteral nutrition support: Current practice for the initiation and progression of tube feeding. *In* Kudsk KA, Zaloga GP (Chairpersons). *Enteral Nutrition Support of the 1990s: Innovations in Nutrition, Technology, and Techniques.* Report of the Twelfth Ross Roundtable on Medication Issues. Columbus, OH, Ross Laboratory, Inc, 1992:30–34.

Bowman M, et al. Effect of tube-feeding osmolality on serum sodium levels. *Crit Care Nurs* 1988 Jan; 9(1):22–28.

Brown RO. Pharmacology in the ICU: Drugs and Enteral Nutrition. *In* Kudsk KA, Zaloga GP (Chairpersons). *Enteral Nutrition Support of the 1990s: Innovations in Nutrition, Technology, and Techniques.* Report of the Twelfth Ross Roundtable on Medication Issues. Columbus, OH, Ross Laboratory, Inc, 1992: 35–39.

Burnes JU, et al. Home parenteral nutrition—A 3-year analysis of clinical laboratory monitoring. *JPEN* 1992 July–Aug; 16(4):327–332.

Ciocon JO, et al. Tube feedings in elderly patients. *Arch Intern Med* 1988 Feb; 148(2):429–433.

Crocker KS, et al. Microbial growth in clinically used enteral delivery systems. *Am J Infec Control* 1986 Dec; 14(6):250–256.

Daly JM, et al. Immune and metabolic effects of arginine in the surgical patient. *Ann Surg* 1988 Oct; 208(10):512–521.

Dickerson R, Melnik G. Osmolality of oral drug solutions. *Am J Hosp Pharm* 1988 Apr; 45(4):832–834.

Edes TE, et al. Diarrhea in tube-fed patients: Feeding formula not necessarily the cause. *Am J Med* 1990 Feb; 88(2):91–93.

Fanslow WC, et al. Effect of nucleotide restriction and supplementation on resistance to experimental nurine Candidiasis. *JPEN* 1988 Jan/Feb; 12(1):49–52.

Fleisher D, et al. Phenytoin interactions with enteral feedings administered through nasogastric tubes. *JPEN* 1990 Aug/Sept; 14(5):513–516.

Fleming C. Home parenteral nutrition. *In* Jeejeebhoy K, ed. *Current Therapy in Nutrition.* Philadelphia, BC Decker, 1988:72–80.

Fleming CR, Nelson J. Nutritional options. *In* Kinney JM, et al, eds. *Nutrition and Metabolism in Patient Care.* Philadelphia, WB Saunders, 1988: 752–772.

Frankenfield DC, Beyer PL. Dietary fiber and bowel function in tube-fed patients. *J Am Diet Assoc* 1991 May; 91(5):591–596, 599.

Furst P, et al. Glutamine-containing dipeptides in parenteral nutrition. *JPEN* 1990;14(suppl) (4):118S–124S.

Gottschlich MM, et al. Therapeutic effects of a modular tube feeding recipe in pediatric burn patients. *Proc Am Burn Assoc* 1986; 18:84.

Grunow J, et al. Contamination of enteral nutrition systems during prolonged intermittent use. *JPEN* 1989 Jan/Feb; 13(1):23–25.

Gulledge A, et al. Psychosocial issues of home parenteral and enteral nutrition. *Nutr Clin Pract* 1987 Oct; 2(5):183–194.

Hart GK, Dabb GJ. Effect of a fecal bulking agent on diarrhea during enteral feeding in the critically ill. *JPEN* 1988 Sept/Oct; 12(5):465–468.

Haw MP, et al. Potential of parenteral and enteral nutrition in inflammation and immune dysfunction. *J Am Diet Assoc* 1991 June; 91(6):701–706, 709.

Heaphey R. Home nutritional support—current consumer concerns. *Nutr Support Services* 1988; 8(4):24.

Heyman MB. General and specialized parenteral amino acid formulations for nutrition support. *J Am Diet Assoc* 1990 March; 90(3):401–411.

Heymsfield SB, et al. Bioenergetic and metabolic response to continuous versus intermittent feeding. *Metabolism* 1987 June; 36(6):570–575.

Hoffman KC. Psychosocial concerns of home nutrition therapy consumers. *Nutr Clin Pract* 1989 Apr; 4(2):51–56.

Holtz L, et al. Compatibility of medications with enteral feedings. *JPEN* 1987 March/Apr; 11(2):183–186.

Ito Y, et al. Chromium content of total parenteral nutrition solutions. *JPEN* 1990 Nov/Dec; 14(6):610–614.

Katz SJ, Oye RK. Parenteral nutrition use at a university hospital. Factors associated with inappropriate use. *West J Med* 1990 June; 152(6):683–686.

Kohn CL. The relationship between enteral formula contamination and length of enteral delivery. *JPEN* 1991 Sept/Oct; 15(2):567–571.

Kohn CL, Keithley JK. Enteral nutrition: Potential complications and patient monitoring. *Nurs Clin North Am* 1989 June; 24(2);339–352.

Kuhn TA, et al. Recovery of warfarin from an enteral nutrient formula. *Am J Hosp Pharm* 1989 July; 46(7):1395–1399.

Levy J, et al. Contaminated enteral nutrition solutions as a cause of nosocomial bloodstream infection: A study using plasmid fingerprinting. *JPEN* 1989 May/June; 13(3):228–234.

Lin EM. Nutrition support: Making the difficult decision. *Cancer Nurs* 1991 Oct; 14(5); 261–269.

Marcuard SP, et al. Unclogging feeding tubes with pancreatic enzyme. *JPEN* 1990 March/Apr; 14(2):198–200.

McCrae JA, Hall NH. Current practices for home enteral nutrition. *J Am Diet Assoc* 1989 Feb; 89(2):233–240.

Mead Johnson Enteral Nutritionals and Consultant Dietitians in Health Care Facilities. *Preventing Pressure Sores.* Evansville, IN, Bristol-Myers Co, 1989.

Melnik G. Pharmacologic aspects of enteral nutrition. *In* Rombeau JL, Caldwell MD, eds. *Clinical Nutrition Enteral and Tube Feeding.* 2nd ed. Philadelphia, WB Saunders, 1990: 472–509.

Metheny N, et al. Effectiveness of the auscultatory method in predicting feeding tube location. *Nurs Res* 1990 Sept/Oct; 39(5):263–267.

Metheny N, et al. Measures to test placement of nasoenteral feeding tubes. *Western J Nurs Res* 1988a; 10(4):367–383.

Metheny N, et al. Effects of feeding tube properties and their irrigants on clogging rates. *Nurs Res* 1988b May/Jun; 37:165–169.

Metheny N, et al. Frequency of nasoenteral tube displacement and associated risk factors. *Res Nurs Health* 1987; 9:241–247.

Mobarhan S, Trumbore LS. Enteral tube feeding: A clinical perspective on recent advances. *Nutr Review* 1991 May; 49(5):129–140.

Nelson JK, Weckwerth JA. Home enteral nutrition. *In* Skipper A, ed. *Dietitian's Handbook of Enteral and Parenteral Nutrition.* Rockville, MD, Aspen, 1989: 311–326.

Orr ME. Hyperglycemia during nutrition support. *Crit Care Nurse* 1992 Jan; 12(1):64–70.

Patterson ML, et al. Enteral feeding in the hypoalbuminemic patient. *JPEN* 1990 July/Aug; 14(4):362–365.

Perry S, et al. The appropriate use of high-cost, high-risk technologies: The case of total parenteral nutrition. *QRB* 1990 June; 16(6): 214–217.

Petrosino BM, et al. Implications of selected problems with nasoenteral tube feedings. *Crit Care Nurs Quart* 1989 Dec; 12(3):1–18.

Rodriquez M. Effect of TPN on appetite. *Support Line* 1992 June; 14(3):11–12.

Rolandelli RH, et al. Critical illness and sepsis. *In* Rombeau JL, Caldwell MD, eds. *Clinical Nutrition Enteral and Tube Feeding.* 2nd ed. Philadelphia, WB Saunders, 1990: 288–305.

Rombeau JL, et al. Nutritional support. *In* Wilmore DW, et al, eds. *Care of the Surgical Patient. Vol 1, Critical Care.* New York, Scientific American, Inc., 1989a: Chapter 10, 1–40.

Rombeau JL, et al. Diarrhea. In Blackburn GL, et al. *Nutritional Medicine: A Case Management Approach.* Philadelphia, WB Saunders, 1989b: 65–72.

Sax HC, Fischer JE. Malnutrition. *In* Dent PL, et al, eds. *Surgical Tips.* New York, McGraw-Hill, 1988:137–161.

Scholten DJ, et al. Failure of BCAA supplementation to promote nitrogen retention in injured patients. *J Am Coll Nutr* 1990 Apr; 9(2):101–106.

Shankardass K, et al. Bowel function of long-term tube-fed patients consuming formulae with and without dietary fiber. *JPEN* 1990 Sept/Oct; 14(5):508–512.

Silk DBA, Payne-James, JJ. Complications of enteral nutrition. *In* Rombeau JL, Caldwell MD, eds. *Clinical Nutrition: Enteral and Tube Feeding.* 2nd ed. Philadelphia, WB Saunders, 1990: 510–531.

Skipper A. Monitoring and complication of enteral feeding. *In* Skipper A, ed. *Dietitian's Handbook of Enteral and Parenteral Nutrition.* Rockville, MD, Aspen, 1989: 293–309.

Smith CE, et al. Diarrhea associated with tube feeding in mechanically ventilated critically ill patients. *Nurs Res* 1990 May/June; 39(3):148–152.

Solomon SM, Kirby DF. The refeeding syndrome: A review. *JPEN* 1990 Jan/Feb; 14(1):90–97.

Splinter MY, et al. Effect of pH on the equilibrium dialysis of phenytoin suspension with and without enteral feeding formula. *JPEN* 1990 May/June; 14(3):275–278.

Strong RM, et al. Equal aspiration rates from postpylorus and intragastric-placed small-bore nasoenteric feeding tubes. A randomized prospective study. *JPEN* 1992 Jan/Feb; 16(1):59–63.

Talbot JM. Guidelines for the scientific review of enteral food products for special medical purposes. *JPEN* 1991 May/June; 15(3):99S–173S.

Weiland DE. Comparative uses and cost for TPN in the United States, Canada, and the United Kingdom (Letter). *JPEN* 1991 July/Aug; 15(4):498.

Weinsier RL, et al. *Handbook of Clinical Nutrition.* 2nd ed. St Louis, MO, CV Mosby, 1989.

Worthington PA, Wagner BA. Total parenteral nutrition. *Nurs Clin North Am* 1989 June; 24(2):355–370.

Young CK, White S. Preparing patients for tube feedings at home. *Am J Nurs* 1992 June; 24(2):46–53.

Ziegler TR. Current status of glutamine. Presentation at 16th Clinical Congress, American Society for Parenteral and Enteral Nutrition, Jan 1992.

Nutritional Considerations of Various Ages and Cultural Influences

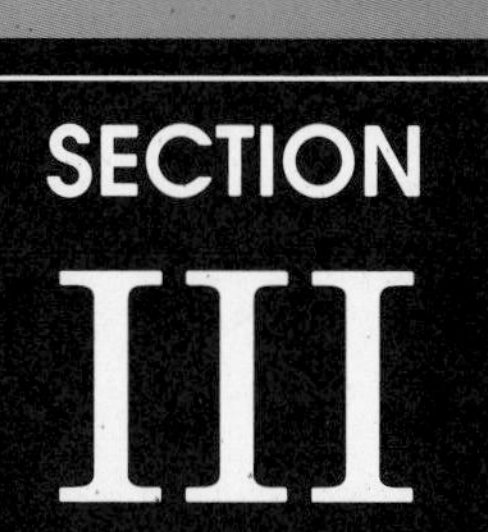

The amount of basic nutrients needed by clients, whether they are healthy or sick, is influenced by their age, sex, and body size. These factors, plus ethnic origin and socioeconomic factors, all affect food choices. Thus information presented in this section will help you to individualize client nutrient requirements based on their age and gender. You will also learn why clients choose the foods they prefer and how to guide clients in their food selections, whether they are on a regular diet or need a special diet.

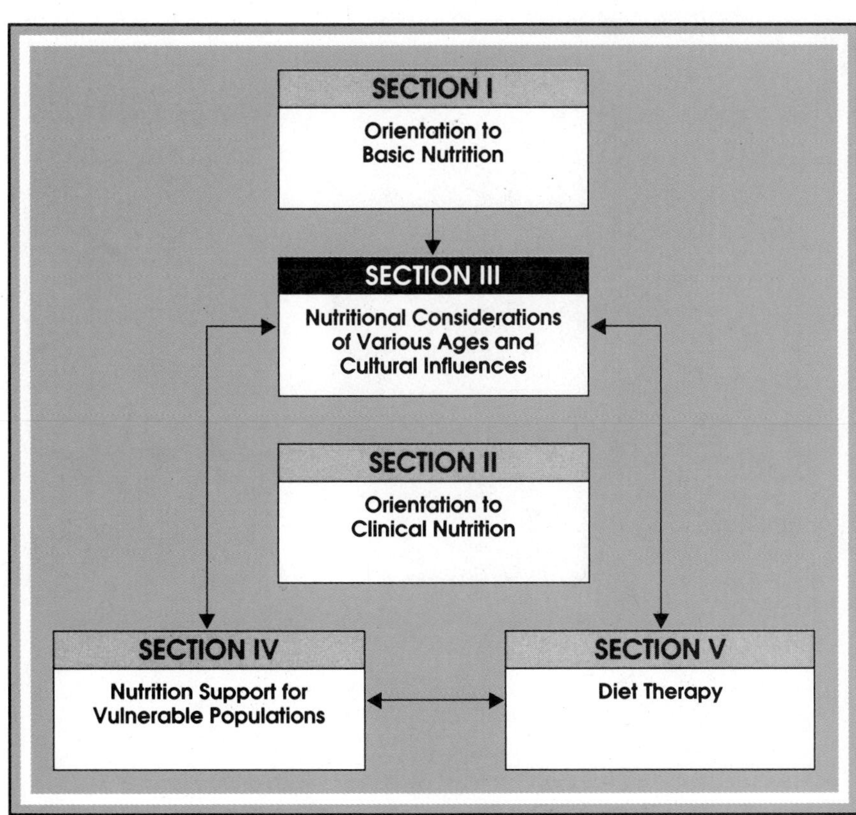

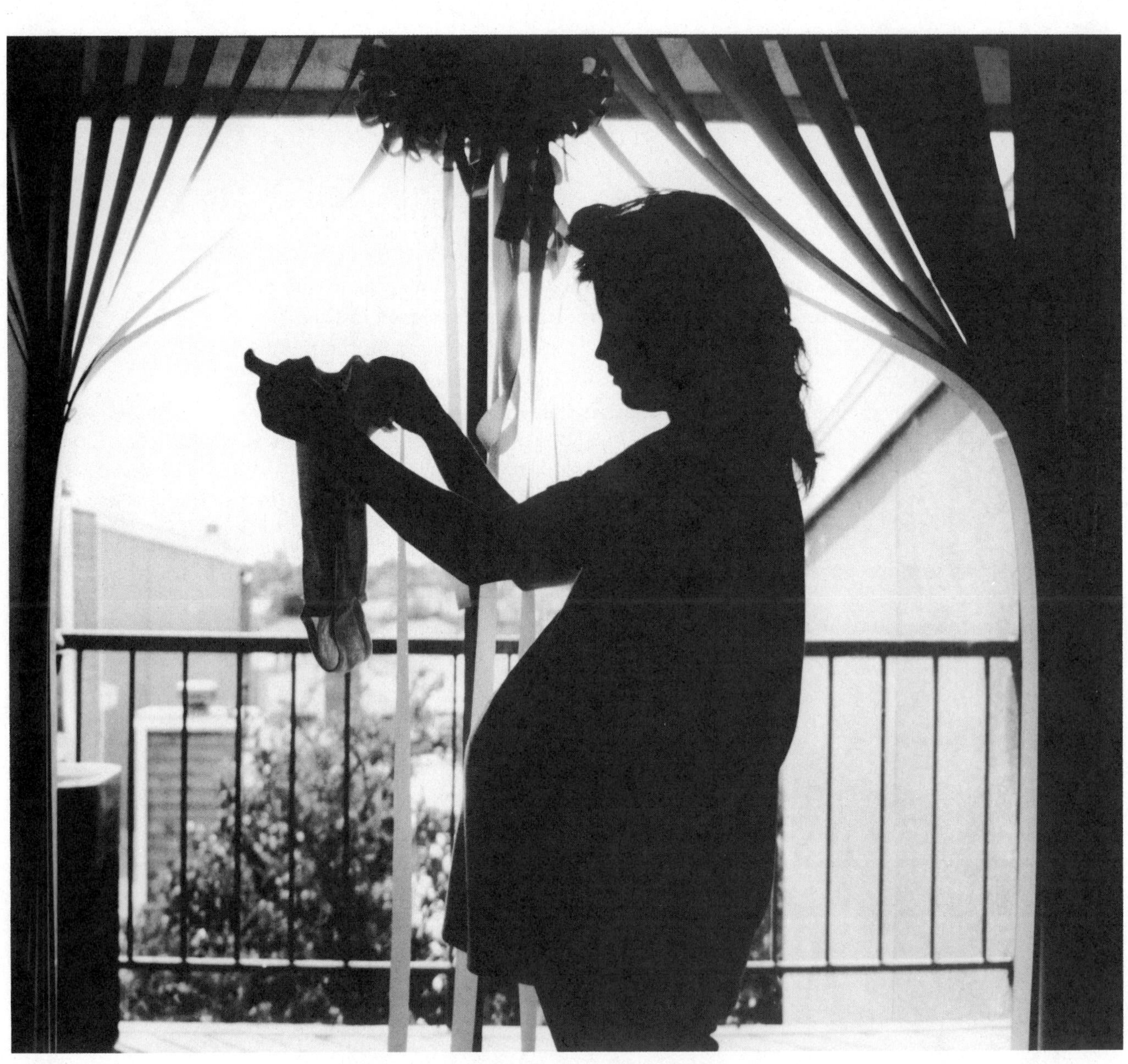

Nutritional Considerations for the Adult Woman: Pregnancy, Lactation, and Other Nutritional Factors

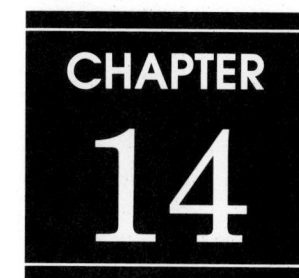

OUTLINE

I. HEALTHY PREGNANCY
  A. Nutritional Status
  B. Unusual Dietary Patterns
  C. Health Care
  D. Age
  E. Weight
  F. Drugs and Medications
II. METABOLIC CHANGES
  Nursing Applications
III. NUTRITIONAL REQUIREMENTS
  A. Energy/Kilocalories
  B. Protein
  C. Vitamin D and Calcium
  D. B Vitamins
    1. Folate/Folacin
  E. Iron
  F. Zinc
IV. VITAMIN-MINERAL SUPPLEMENTS
  Nursing Applications
V. NUTRITIONAL ASSESSMENT
  A. Weight Management
  B. Clinical Laboratory Values
  C. Dietary Intake and Counseling
  Nursing Applications
VI. COMMON CONDITIONS DURING PREGNANCY
  A. Nausea and Vomiting
  Nursing Applications
  B. Gastrointestinal Problems
  Nursing Applications
  C. Edema
  Nursing Applications
VII. DISORDERS OF PREGNANCY
  A. Pregnancy-Induced Hypertension
  Nursing Applications
  B. Anemia
  Nursing Applications
  C. Gestational Diabetes
  Nursing Applications
VIII. LACTATION

OBJECTIVES

THE STUDENT WILL BE ABLE TO:

- Define the dietary measures applicable to PIH.
- List nutrients (with the amounts) that are usually supplemented during pregnancy.
- Describe fetal alcohol syndrome.
- Plan food intake during pregnancy.
- List high-risk factors for pregnancy.
- Evaluate the symptoms of a PMS sufferer and counsel her regarding dietary changes that may be beneficial.
- Apply nursing application principles for clients experiencing pregnancy, breast-feeding, or PMS.
- Identify client education needs for the above clients.

TEST YOUR NQ (True/False)

1. All efforts should be made to satisfy the pregnant woman's food cravings because this is a natural instinct for needed nutrients.
2. The fetus is nourished from the mother's nutrient stores.
3. When a pregnant woman has constipation caused by the pressure of the fetus, self-medication with laxatives is not recommended.
4. A woman should eat twice as much food when she is pregnant because she is eating for 2.
5. During pregnancy, women should gain 22 to 27 lbs.
6. Iron is the only nutrient that warrants global supplementation during pregnancy.
7. Virtually all women can produce enough milk.
8. Breast milk that is too thin must be nutritionally inadequate.

9. If breast milk supply is inadequate, omit a feeding to have more milk available later.
10. PMS sufferers are encouraged to follow the Dietary Guidelines for Americans.

HEALTHY PREGNANCY

Although there is no specific definition of a healthy pregnancy, the health of both mother and infant is important. In addition to continued preservation of the mother's physical health, emotional and psychological welfare is important. The goals for an infant are that he or she is full-term (born between the 39th week and 41st week of gestation) and mature (weighing more than 6 lbs) (IM, 1990). Approximately 1 in 14 infants in the US is born weighing less than 5½ lbs, and more than 1 in 10 infants is born before 37 weeks of gestation (Wegman, 1989). **Low birth weight (LBW)** and **premature infants** have more abnormalities as well as increased morbidity (infections and illnesses) and mortality and decreased mental performance. In all cases, primary factors for success are the previous nutritional status, appropriate weight gain, and adequate intake of essential nutrients during pregnancy. Studies have shown that mothers of small babies consume less of virtually all nutrients than mothers of larger babies (Doyle et al, 1991). Apparently if the mother's nutritional status is poor, the placenta does not perform its function well.

Low birth weight–newborn weighing less than 5½ lbs (2500 gm).

Premature infant—born before the state of maturity, occurring with a gestational age of less than 37 weeks.

A classic report published in 1970 by the National Academy of Sciences (NAS, 1970) established a basis for increased nutritional requirements during pregnancy. This has been more recently followed with further recommendations published in *Nutrition During Pregnancy* (IM, 1990) regarding weight gain and nutrient supplements. This information was compiled by separate subcommittees that evaluated available scientific information to establish guidelines for optimal outcomes.

What are the goals for an infant? What are the 3 primary factors for success?

Nutritional Status

Not only is the outcome affected by nutrient intake during the pregnancy, but also preconception nutrient status exerts an important influence on maternal health and fetal growth and development. A recent history of oral contraceptive use indicates an increased need for vitamins C, B_6, B_{12}, and folate. As a result of rapid development of body parts and organs during the first trimester, birth defects are likely to occur if usual dietary habits are poor or if drug use occurs during this critical period. However, infant birth weights are affected more by nutrient intake during the second and third trimesters (Worthington-Roberts et al, 1989).

During which trimester is nutrient intake critical to prevent birth defects? When are fetal parts and organs formed? When is birth weight affected most?

Although poor nutrient intake can produce an LBW infant, it is commonly believed that the fetus is protected at the expense of the mother (Whitehead, 1988). In some instances, higher requirements are met by increased nutrient absorption; for other nutrients, such as iron and calcium, the mother's stores may be depleted if intake is inadequate.

Pica is the abnormal consumption of specific food and nonfood substances, such as dirt, clay, starch, or ice.

Women who are considered to be at high risk of having premature or LBW infants are from lower socioeconomic status or low educational level; are in poor nutritional status; are having clinical problems, such as pregnancy-induced hypertension; or are affected by behavioral/environmental factors, such as alcohol or substance abuse.

Unusual Dietary Patterns

Pica affects about 20% of **high-risk women.** Pica is more likely to be practiced by black women living in rural areas with a positive childhood and family history of pica. Pica is associated with iron deficiency and has been associated with maternal and perinatal mortality (Horner et al, 1991).

Beliefs about cravings and folklore that could influence dietary selections are regional (Carruth & Skinner, 1991). Most of these beliefs are not supported by scientific information and may be detrimental. Familiarity with local beliefs is needed to counsel **gravidas** about beliefs that are potentially detrimental to good nutrition during pregnancy.

Gravida—pregnant woman.

Special dietary restrictions may be practiced based on a food fad or ethnic, cultural, or religious customs. In addition to assessing the effects of these on nutritional status, an awareness of these practices allows the nurse to provide guidance about desirable food choices that are within these constraints.

What are some dietary practices that may affect outcome?

Health Care

The availability and use of health services are related to problems in pregnancy. Inadequate prenatal care leads to more problems for both mother and fetus. Prenatal care is also important to prevent chronic health problems such as diabetes and hypertension from affecting the embryo.

Age

Primigravida—first pregnancy.

Maternal age can lead to increased LBW infants of **primigravidas** under age 18 or over the age of 35. Most females have not completed linear growth and achieved gynecological maturity until the age of 17. Not only are many of these young girls still growing and storing nutrients in their own bodies, but also the majority have an inadequate intake of calcium, iron, vitamin A, niacin, and kilocalories. The socioeconomic disadvantages of these young mothers may affect their diet as a result of the amount of food available and their uninformed selections.

Many couples today are choosing to postpone parenthood. Pregnancy after the age of 35 is influenced by the individual's overall health. Maternal risks involve medical conditions, such as diabetes, hypertension, cardiovascular problems, and **leiomyoma uteri.** These conditions are closely supervised to lessen their impact on the fetus. A woman needs to be particularly aware of maintaining her nutritional health if a later pregnancy is anticipated. As the mother's age increases, her baby is more likely to be premature and smaller than average.

Leiomyoma uteri—fibrous tumors that may interfere with the enlarging uterus and cause spontaneous abortion.

How can age affect outcomes?

Weight

Successful pregnancies depend on ideal preconception weight plus appropriate weight gain during gestation. Weight gain during pregnancy influences birth weight more than the prepregnancy weight. The subcommittee (IM, 1990) determined body mass index (BMI) to be a better indicator of maternal nutritional status than weight alone. (BMI is discussed in Chapter 11.)

Gravidas with a BMI more than 26 are at particular risk of gaining too little weight, resulting in smaller than average or LBW infants. If the expectant mother's weight is 10% below ideal or 20% or more above the norm for her height and age group, both the gravida and the infant are at nutritional risk, with the delivery of more LBW premature infants (Naeye, 1990; Mitchell & Lerner, 1989). Women with a BMI below 19.8 frequently give birth to smaller infants than heavier women, even with the same weight gain. Ideally, weight adjustments of overweight or underweight women should be made before conception.

What are possible consequences of a gravida with BMI more than 26; weight 10% below ideal, or 20% or more above the norm; a BMI below 19.8?

Drugs and Medications

The use of tobacco, alcohol, caffeine, some medications, and illegal drugs may affect the fetus. Alcohol can cross the placenta, with alcohol abuse resulting in fetal alcohol syndrome, discussed in Nutrition Update 14–1.

Smoking appears to affect the growth of the embryo, resulting in LBW infants and prematurity. This may be related to impaired oxygen transport. Despite increased energy intakes, smoking results in lighter and shorter infants having smaller head and arm circumferences.

Pregnant women who consume large quantities of coffee (caffeine) have an increased incidence of spontaneous abortions, premature labor, and small for gestational age infants. Not only is caffeine found in coffee, tea, chocolate, cocoa, and some soft drinks, but also it is present in numerous OTC drugs. The caffeine content of various foods and beverages is listed in Appendix A-4. A specific limitation on caffeine consumption has not been established, but limited consumption of caffeine-containing products is sensible.

Numerous OTC drugs have potential adverse effects, even aspirin and antihistamines. Acetylsalicylate (ASA), a common ingredient in aspirin, may prolong pregnancy and cause excessive bleeding at delivery. The physician should be consulted before any medication is taken.

The use of tobacco, alcohol, caffeine, marijuana, and cocaine may affect maternal nutrition by increasing nutrient excretion or undesirably affecting intake.

How can alcohol, smoking, coffee, and acetylsalicylate affect the fetus?

METABOLIC CHANGES

Hormonal changes in the gravida lead to alterations in carbohydrate, fat, and protein utilization. Increased levels of estrogen and progesterone during the first trimester result in an anabolic state, increasing glycogen and fat stores. This fat storage of approximately 3.5 kg provides additional energy needed later in the pregnancy and for lactation (Whitehead, 1988).

Plasma glucose levels decline, insulin secretion increases, and tissues become less sensitive to insulin action. In addition to the fetus's requirement for glucose, the mother needs additional glucose for the increased RBCs. To meet the extra fetal glucose requirements, maternal use of glucose decreases secondary to **increased insulin resistance.** The reduction in plasma glucose is gradual and is lowest during the third trimester (Winick, 1989).

Increased insulin resistance—less glucose is allowed to enter the body cells.

During the third trimester, reductions in urea production and excretion contribute to nitrogen retention for tissue synthesis. Elevated plasma insulin may alter uptake of some amino acids to provide a large proportion of the amino acids needed by the fetus.

Plasma volume increases approximately 40% during pregnancy. Normal serum albumin in women is slightly over 4 gm/dl. By the end of the first trimester, mean albumin concentration is approximately 3 gm/dl because of expanded plasma volume and altered rates of protein synthesis (King & Weininger, 1990). This reduced albumin results in proportional decreases in plasma colloid osmotic pressure and possibly contributes to increased interstitial fluid during late gestation.

What are some metabolic changes that occur during pregnancy?

NURSING APPLICATIONS

Assessment

Physical—for recent intake of OCAs, level of education, income status, culture, religion, location of residence, prenatal care, age, weight (preconception and serial weights during pregnancy), types of drugs taken.

Dietary—for health and nutritional knowledge and skills, food budget, cravings, aversions, fad diets, beliefs about nutrition during pregnancy, pica, alcohol and caffeine intake.

Laboratory—for iron, RBCs, Hgb, Hct; glucose, insulin; BUN, albumin.

Continued

Interventions

1. Become familiar with local nutritional practices and beliefs about pregnancy since these beliefs are regional.
2. Monitor weight changes.

Client Education

- Alterations in food choices do not reflect natural instincts for required nutrients. Nutrient needs must be met by deliberate preplanning and knowledgeable food choices.
- Illegal drugs are especially harmful to the fetus, resulting in the birth of addicted infants.

NUTRITIONAL REQUIREMENTS

What nutrients may be low in pregnant women's diets for vegetarians?

The RDAs for pregnancy (Table 14–1) indicate advisable nutrient intake for optimum health of mother and fetus. In view of the increased growth and metabolism, most nutrient requirements are increased to some extent. Each vitamin and mineral will not be separately discussed; Table 14–1 shows the increased amounts recommended for each of the nutrients as established by the National Research Council (1989). According to the subcommittee report (IM, 1990), the following mean nutrient intakes are below the 1989 RDAs for pregnant women: kilocalories; vitamins D, E, folate, and B_6; and the minerals iron, zinc, calcium, and magnesium. In addition to low intake of these nutrients, gravidas on vegan diets frequently consume inadequate amounts of vitamin B_{12} and sometimes vitamin D (Dwyer, 1991).

TABLE 14–1

VITAMIN-MINERAL RECOMMENDED DIETARY ALLOWANCES AND SUPPLEMENTS

	Recommended Dietary Allowance (1)			
Nutrient	***Nonpregnant Women***	***Pregnant Women***	***Percent Increase****	**Amount of Supplement Recommended (2)**
Vitamin A	800 mcg RE	800 mcg RE	None	None
Vitamin D	5 mcg	10 mcg	100	5 mcg
Vitamin E	8α-TE	10 α-TE	25	None
Vitamin K	65 mcg	65 mcg	None	None
Vitamin C	60 mg	70 mg	16	50 mg
Thiamin	1.1 mg	1.5 mg	36	None
Riboflavin	1.3 mg	1.6 mg	23	None
Niacin	15 mg NE	17 mg NE	13	None
Vitamin B_6	1.6 mg	2.2 mg	38	2 mg
Folate	180 mcg	400 mcg	122	300 mcg
Vitamin B_{12}	2 mcg	2.2 mcg	10	None
Calcium	800 mg	1200 mg	50	250 mg
Phosphorus	800 mg	1200 mg	50	None
Magnesium	280 mg	320 mg	14	None
Iron	15 mg	30 mg	100	30 mg
Zinc	12 mg	15 mg	25	15 mg
Iodine	150 mcg	175 mcg	17	None
Selenium	55 mcg	65 mcg	18	None
Copper	1.5–3 mg	None	None	2 mg

* Percent increase for pregnant women above nonpregnancy recommendation.

Data from (1) National Research Council. *Recommended Dietary Allowances.* 10th ed. Washington, D.C., National Academy Press, 1989. (2) Institute of Medicine. *Nutrition During Pregnancy.* Washington, D.C., National Academy Press, 1990.

Energy/Kilocalories

During pregnancy, kilocalorie requirement increases to ensure nutrient and energy needs. The RDAs allow an additional 300 kcal or 36 kcal/kg body weight/day during the second and third trimesters. This additional energy is needed to (1) build new tissues (including added maternal tissues and growth of the fetus and placenta), (2) support increased metabolic expenditure, and (3) move the additional weight. Unless the gravida is significantly underweight before conception, additional kilocalories are probably not needed during the first trimester. Appropriate weight gain reflects the adequacy of energy intake. Although she is "eating for 2," normal energy requirements are not double. Since requirements of other nutrients are also increased, it is more important that foods be chosen wisely, using principally nutrient-dense foods (Fig. 14–1).

Energy requirements reflect changes in normal physical activities. Kilocaloric needs are slightly less for an older pregnant woman as a result of a lower resting BMR and activity level. Although the pregnant woman may gradually slow her pace, moderate exercise is usually encouraged.

What is the recommended kilocalorie or kcal/kg/day intake during the second and third trimester? What are the 3 reasons for this additional energy?

Protein

Protein is the basic nutrient for growth; therefore, an additional 10 to 14 gm protein or a total of 60 gm daily is recommended. This could be accomplished by an increase of 2 cups of milk (16 gm protein), 2 additional ounces of meat or meat substitute (14 gm protein), or a combination of the two. However, most clients usually consume more than 60 gm protein daily, and additional amounts are not required.

How much protein is recommended, and how could this increase be accomplished?

Vitamin D and Calcium

Vitamin D and the mineral calcium work hand-in-hand in formation of skeletal tissue. Inadequate vitamin D intake during pregnancy is associated with infant disorders of calcium metabolism—neonatal hypocalcemia and defective tooth formation. Deficiency is not likely unless the mother has a low intake of both calcium and vitamin D and insufficient exposure to sunlight. Use of vitamin D–fortified milk products is more important in winter since they are the main dietary source of vitamin D.

Early in pregnancy, hormonal and physiological adjustments promote increased calcium absorption and retention. This extra calcium is thought to be stored in maternal bone for fetal availability in the third trimester when fetal bone growth is rapid. Additional calcium (400 mg increase) is recommended beginning early during pregnancy to protect the maternal skeleton from depletion.

The RDA of 1200 mg/day of calcium is easily met by 4 servings of milk or milk products. Milk may be incorporated into cooking or used in different forms such as cheese, ice cream, or yogurt for variety (see Chapter 9, Table 9–3).

What is the recommendation for calcium? How can this additional calcium be supplied? Why is the source of vitamin D different for different seasons?

B Vitamins

Several of the B vitamin requirements are based on energy intake; usually, their intake increases automatically with additional kilocalories. Adequate intake of several B vitamins is difficult to achieve without careful selection of foods or supplementation.

Sample Menu

Breakfast
1 cup orange juice
1 bagel with 1 oz cream cheese and 1 packet raisins
1 cup 1% milk
coffee with creamer

Lunch
Tuna salad sandwich (1 oz tuna with 2 tbsp mayonnaise, 2 slices tomato, lettuce slices, on 2 slices whole wheat bread)
1 apple
2 fig bar cookies
1 cup 1% milk

Dinner
4 oz lean roast beef with 1/4 cup gravy
1/2 cup brown rice
1/2 cup spinach
1/2 cup three bean salad
2 whole wheat rolls
2 tbsp light tub margarine
1 cup strawberries
1 cup 1% milk
tea

Evening Snack
12 oz diet cola beverage
2 oz peanuts

Nutrient	RDA–Pregnant Third Trimester	Actual	% RDA
Kcal	==================*	2504 kcal	100
Protein	==================*=================	114 gm	190
Carbohydrate	=================	294 gm	94
Fat	==================*=====	107 gm	129
Cholesterol	===========	181 mg	60
Fiber–dietary	==================*===========	35.635 gm	162
Vitamin A	==================*================	1458 RE	182
Thiamin	==================*====	1.9 mg	123
Riboflavin	==================*===========	2.6 mg	161
Niacin	==================*=========	26 mg	154
Vitamin B_6	================	1.9 mg	88
Folate	==================*===	468 mcg	117
Vitamin B_{12}	==================*===================	6.8 mcg	310
Pantothenic acid	==================*==	6.2 mg	113
Biotin	=================	58.9 mcg	91
Vitamin C	==================*===================	220 mg	314
Vitamin D	===============	7.9 mcg	79
Vitamin K	==================*===================	269 mcg	414
Sodium	==================*	2807 mg	103
Potassium	==================*===================	4537 mg	227
Calcium	==================*===	1434 mg	120
Phosphorus	==================*==============	2085 mg	174
Magnesium	==================*================	591 mg	185
Iron	===========	18.3 mg	61
Zinc	==================*====	18.7 mg	125
Copper	==================	2.2 mg	97
Manganese	==================	3.3 mg	95
Selenium	==================*===================	0.18 mg	280
	+--------------------------------------		
	^0 ^50 ^100 ^150 ^200		

Carbohydrate, Protein, and Fat Distribution

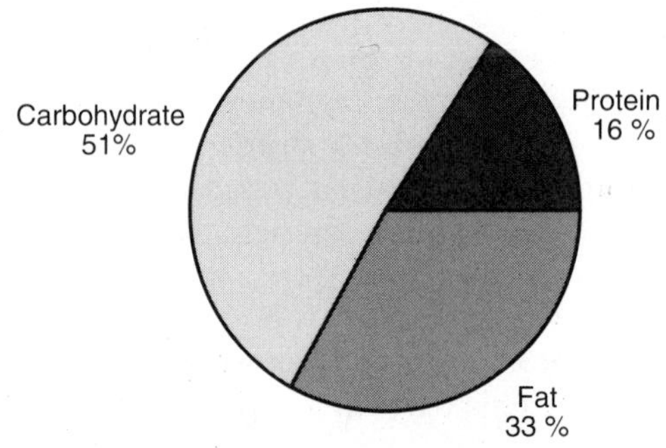

Kcal, 2504; protein, 114 gm; carbohydrate, 294 gm; fat 107 gm

Figure 14–1 Sample menu for pregnancy (3rd trimester). RDA, Recommended dietary allowance; RE, Retinol equivalents. (Nutrient data from Nutritionist III, Version 7.0, Salem, Oregon.)

Folate/Folacin

The RDA for folate (400 mcg) during pregnancy is more than double the nonpregnant allowance. Neural tube defects such as spina bifida have been attributed to periconceptional nutrient intake and especially folate in some research studies. The role of folate as coenzyme is essential for nucleic acid synthesis. Therefore, a folate deficiency might impair cell growth and replication, causing fetal anomalies. Several studies have concluded that periconceptional supplemental vitamins, especially folate, reduce the incidence of neural-tube deficits (Czeizel & Dudás, 1992; MRC, 1991). Folate is also required for increased RBC formation. Although folate intake is essential, some women take supplements providing as much as 8 times the RDA. These high intakes are reflected in cord folate levels with unknown effects on other nutrients (Huber et al, 1988).

The requirement for folate is difficult for most women to meet with food intake alone. Conscientious daily selections of raw fruits and vegetables, especially green leafy vegetables, can help ensure adequate intake. Whole-grain and folacin-fortified cereals may also supply significant amounts (see Chapter 7, Table 7–7).

What are the recommendations for folate? How can this intake be achieved?

Iron

A common problem among nonpregnant women is iron deficiency anemia, so many women commence pregnancy with diminished iron stores. The gestational requirement of iron is needed for production of RBCs, placenta, and cord and blood loss at delivery (Hallberg, 1988).

The fetus acts as a parasite; fetal **erythropoiesis** occurs at the expense of maternal iron stores. Therefore, iron deficiency anemia is seldom seen in full-term infants. Fetal accumulation of iron occurs principally in the last trimester. Premature infants, with a shortened gestation, have insufficient time to acquire adequate iron and may be born with iron deficiency anemia.

Erythropoiesis—the formation of RBCs.

Maternal iron deficiency means that cardiac output must increase to maintain adequate oxygen for the maternal and fetal cells. Iron deficiency anemia therefore places the mother at risk of cardiac arrest and poor prognosis if hemorrhage occurs at delivery. Maternal iron deficiency results in reduced fetal iron storage, increasing the risk of anemia during infancy.

Initially, plasma volume increases with resultant hemodilution and depressed hemoglobin and serum iron concentration. During the last half of pregnancy, iron absorption increases from the normal 10 to 20% to approximately 50% if adequate iron is available. Hemoglobin levels increase to about 12 mg/dl.

Approximately 18 to 21 mg of iron are needed daily. Since the average American diet does not provide this amount within the normal kilocaloric requirements, daily iron supplements are usually recommended (IM, 1990; NRC, 1989). Initiation of supplements before gestation week 24 prevents iron deficiency. If iron supplements are not provided, it may take 2 years after delivery before serum ferritin levels are normal (IM, 1990).

What is the requirement for iron? How is this additional iron supplied? What are some complications of low iron in the mother?

Zinc

Zinc is critical early in pregnancy during the formation of fetal organs, but requirements are highest in late pregnancy for fetal growth and development. The RDA for zinc is 15 mg during pregnancy. An increase in protein foods, especially meats, improves zinc intake.

What is the requirement for zinc? How can this requirement be met?

VITAMIN-MINERAL SUPPLEMENTS

Vitamin-mineral supplementation is common during pregnancy in the US. Supplementation should be based on evidence of a benefit as well as a lack of harmful effects. Excessive amounts of many nutrients may have detrimental effects on the fetus (Table 14–2). Food is considered to be the optimal vehicle for providing nutrients; supplements are not routinely recommended and should be used only after dietary evaluation indicates an intake deficit that cannot be corrected by altering food intake. The conclusion of the subcommittee (IM, 1990) was that iron is the only known nutrient warranting global supplementation. Consequently, 30 mg

TABLE 14–2

NUTRIENT SUPPLEMENTATION ASSOCIATED WITH DELETERIOUS FETAL OUTCOMES

Vitamin A	Pharmacological use of vitamin A analogues has resulted in major congenital defects (malformation of the cranium, face, heart, thymus, and CNS) and spontaneous abortion, especially during the first trimester
Vitamin D	Excessive intake of vitamin D can result in hyperabsorption of calcium, hypercalcemia, calcification of soft tissues, and mental retardation
Vitamin E	Associated with higher incidence of spontaneous abortions
Vitamin K	Menadione administered parenterally has been associated with hemolytic anemia, hyperbilirubinemia, and kernicterus in the newborn
Vitamin C	Megadoses of vitamin C have been reported to cause vitamin C dependency with symptoms of conditional scurvy observed postpartum
Iodine	Large amounts of iodides have resulted in infants with congenital goiter, hypothyroidism, and mental retardation
Zinc	Large amounts of zinc supplements during the third trimester were implicated in premature delivery and stillbirth
Fluoride	Well water containing 12 to 18 ppm fluoride produced offspring with significant mottling of the deciduous teeth

Data from Worthington-Roberts B. Nutrition deficiencies and excesses: Impact on pregnancy, Part 2. *J Perinatol* 1985 Fall; 5(4):12.

of ferrous iron is recommended to provide adequate amounts of iron during the second and third trimesters of pregnancy.

Although folate intake does not usually meet the RDA recommendations, deficiency appears to be rare among pregnant women in the US. Requirements can be met with proper food choices; low amounts of a folate supplement may be prudent if intake is questionable.

What is the recommendation of the subcommittee regarding supplementation? What types of clients may warrant multivitamin-mineral supplements?

The increased risks of adolescent pregnancies; women carrying more than one fetus; and those who use cigarettes, alcohol, or other drugs may warrant nutritional supplements. The specific nutrient amounts for a daily multivitamin-mineral preparation if supplementation is warranted are shown in Table 14–1.

NURSING APPLICATIONS

Assessment

Dietary—for kilocalories, protein, vitamin D, calcium, folate, iron, zinc; vegetarianism.

Laboratory—for albumin, protein, calcium, iron, MCV.

Interventions

1. Emphasize consumption of a well-balanced diet to ensure optimal intake of trace elements. This is preferred over routine prenatal supplements.
2. Encourage adding 1 to 2 cups of milk and/or 1 to 2 oz of meat daily. This provides the additional amounts of kilocalories (300 kcal), protein, and calcium recommended (1 cup milk provides 80 to 170 kcal, 8 gm protein, 300 mg calcium; 1 oz meat provides about 75 kcal and 7 gm protein).
3. Encourage foods high in calcium. Low calcium intake may impair bone mineral deposition, especially in women under 25 years of age. The use of dietary calcium is preferred because these foods also provide other valuable nutrients—protein, riboflavin, and vitamin D.
4. If gravida is lactose intolerant, stress eating yogurt and aged cheeses. Women who are lactose intolerant should be encouraged to increase calcium intake through the use of low-lactose, calcium-rich foods before supplementation is considered (IM, 1990).
5. If iron supplement exceeds 30 mg, give zinc and copper as prescribed. Because of interference with their absorption by iron, 15 mg zinc and 2 mg of copper are recommended.

Evaluation

* Desired outcomes include clients planning nutritious meals with their favorite foods to meet the added nutrients and kilocalories needed during pregnancy.

Client Education

- Moderate increases in whole grains, milk, and legumes can provide additional protein requirements as well as other important nutrients (IM, 1990).
- Specially formulated protein supplements are not recommended during pregnancy (IM, 1990).
- Vegetarian diets can provide reasonable amounts of trace elements; however, additional amounts in a more readily absorbable form provided by meats are advantageous during pregnancy (IM, 1990). If meats are omitted, emphasize the importance of consuming vitamin C along with nonheme sources of iron to increase absorption (see Chapter 9).
- Vitamin B_{12} (2 mcg daily) and vitamin D (10 mcg) supplements are advisable for strict vegetarians (vegans) who exclude all animal products.
- For vegan clients, emphasize the importance of eating adequate kilocalories for weight gain.
- Vitamin D may be a special concern for clients with minimal exposure to sunlight. Regular exposure to sunlight and foods fortified with vitamin D (such as milk and cheese) are recommended.
- Calcium supplements for leg cramps are not recommended (IM, 1990).
- If the gravida has an aversion to milk, suggest the addition of ⅓ cup of powdered milk to soups, cooked cereals, mashed potatoes, or casseroles.
- Nutritional reserves may be depleted with numerous pregnancies with less than a year between pregnancies.
- Iron absorption appears to be greater when given separately as an iron salt rather than as part of multivitamin-mineral supplement (IM, 1990).

Adverse symptoms, i.e., nausea or constipation, frequently occur from iron supplementation. Rather than discontinue the supplement, take with meals.

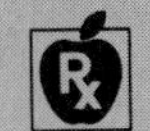

Absorption of iron supplements is enhanced if taken between meals with liquids other than milk, tea, or coffee.

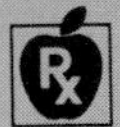

When calcium supplementation is indicated, absorption is enhanced if taken at mealtime.

NUTRITIONAL ASSESSMENT

Weight Management

The only anthropometric measurements with documented implications for assessment of gestational weight gain are prepregnancy weight-for-height and serial weight measurements. A major goal of the Institute of Medicine subcommittee (1990) was to establish optimal gestational weight gain in relation to clinical care and maternal and infant outcomes, especially birth weight. Increases in lean and fat tissue of the mother and fetus and water retention contribute to the weight gain.

Following the first trimester, weight gain should be steady and gradual. Major deviations in the rate of gain (excluding deviations related to errors in measurement or recording or to common shifts in weight related to fluid changes, bladder and bowel contents, and clothing and time of day) may signal problems and warrant further assessment.

A weight gain of 1 to 2 kg (2 to 4 lbs) is recommended during the first trimes-

TABLE 14–3

RECOMMENDED TOTAL WEIGHT GAIN RANGES FOR PREGNANT WOMEN,* BY PREPREGNANCY BODY MASS INDEX†

Weight-for-Height Category	Recommended Total Gain	
	kg	*lb*
Low (BMI <19.8)	12.5–18	28–40
Normal (BMI of 19.8 to 26)	11.5–16	25–35
High‡ (BMI >26 to 29)	7–11.5	15–25

* Young adolescents and black women should strive for gains at the upper end of the recommended range. Short women (<157 cm, or 62 in.) should strive for gains at the lower end of the range.
† Body mass index (BMI) is calculated using metric units.
‡The recommended target weight gain for obese women (BMI >29) is at least 6 kg (15 lbs).
Reprinted with permission from *Nutrition During Pregnancy.* Copyright 1990 by the National Academy of Sciences. Published by the National Academy Press, Washington, D.C.

ter of pregnancy, with a weight gain of 0.45 kg (about 1 lb) weekly during the remainder of the pregnancy for the gravida of average weight. Total recommended weight gain as determined by prepregnancy weight is shown in Table 14–3.

Gravidas are encouraged to achieve at least the lower limit of weight specified for their BMI pregestational weight. (To reduce the risk of delivering an LBW infant, black women and adolescents should target weight gain at the upper end of the target range.) Guidelines established by the subcommittee (IM, 1990) for accurate weight measurements and progress are shown in Table 14–4.

Clinical Laboratory Values

Because of the many biochemical and physiological changes occurring during pregnancy, normal female values are not valid. Electrolytes, proteins, glucose, vitamin B_{12}, folate, and vitamin B_6 are reduced, whereas triglycerides and cholesterol

TABLE 14–4

GUIDELINES FOR GESTATIONAL WEIGHT GAIN

1. Before conception, use consistent and reliable procedures to measure accurately and record in the medical record the woman's weight and height without shoes
2. Determine the woman's prepregnancy BMI (see Appendix C-2)
3. Measure height and weight at the first prenatal visit carefully by procedures that have been rigorously standardized at the site of prenatal care
4. Use consistent, reliable procedures to measure weight at each subsequent visit
5. Estimate the woman's gestational age from the onset of her last menstruation
6. Record weight and plot it on a chart included in the obstetric record
7. Set a weight gain goal together with the pregnant woman, preferably beginning at the comprehensive initial prenatal examination, and explain why weight gain is important
8. Base the recommended range of total weight gain and pattern of gain mainly on prepregnancy weight for height (see Table 14–3)
9. For women with a normal prepregnancy BMI, recommend gain at the rate of approximately 0.4 kg (1 lb) per week in the second and third trimesters of pregnancy
10. Monitor the prenatal course to identify any abnormal pattern of gain that may indicate a need to intervene. Assess the pattern of gain at each visit relative to the established weight gain goal and course leading to that goal
11. When abnormal gain appears to be real, rather than a result of an error in measurement or recording, try to determine the cause and then develop and implement corrective actions jointly with the woman

Reprinted with permission from *Nutrition During Pregnancy.* Copyright 1990 by the National Academy of Sciences. Published by the National Academy Press, Washington, D.C.

TABLE 14–5

NUTRITIONAL ASSESSMENT IN PREGNANCY: LABORATORY TESTS

Laboratory Tests	Normal Range	
	Nonpregnant	*Pregnant*
Serum protein, total	6.5–8.5 gm/dl	6–8
Serum albumin	3.5–5 gm/dl	3–4.5
Blood urea nitrogen	10–25 mg/dl	5–15
Fasting blood sugar	70–110 mg/dl	65–100
2-hr postprandial blood sugar	<110 mg/dl	<120
Folic acid, serum	5–21 ng/ml	3–15
Vitamin B_{12} serum	330–1025 pg/ml	Decreased
Hemoglobin/hematocrit	>12 mg/dl/36%	11/33
Serum iron/iron binding capacity	>50/250–400 mcg/dl	>40/300–450

are elevated. Despite these limitations, laboratory values indicate baseline information for assessment during the course of the pregnancy (Table 14–5).

Dietary Intake and Counseling

A review of the literature indicates that prenatal nutritional care improves outcome by saving lives, averting LBW, and decreasing costs of care as a consequence of LBW (Trouba et al, 1991). Although adequate weight gain is the most reliable measurable tool for assessing adequacy of kilocaloric intake, actual food choices can provide adequate kilocalories yet be deficient in vital nutrients. Nutrient intake actually deserves more attention than weight gain (Susser, 1991). Thus, the Institute of Medicine subcommittee (1990) has recommended routine assessment of dietary practices for all pregnant women in the US to determine the need for improved diet or vitamin-mineral supplements. Most women are highly motivated to make dietary changes at this time.

Pregnant women may have little or no nutritional knowledge. Nutrition counseling is often unavailable or ignored during pregnancy, yet knowledge is the key to wise food choices. In many cases, low-income expectant mothers have more opportunities to receive nutritional information through established programs, such as WIC, than the private sector.

Identification of both poor and desirable food habits and dietary patterns can serve as the foundation for appropriate nutrition counseling and intervention. Thus, risk of inadequate intakes of specific nutrients, possibilities for dietary improvement, and the potential need for supplementation can be determined. A food frequency or diet history questionnaire may be the most reliable tool to identify nutritionally unsound practices. Additionally, identification of other problems or risk factors may require special attention. Any unusual dietary practices, such as pica (discussed earlier) or fad diets, should be addressed. A discussion of the results and causes of these habits is more effective than telling clients to stop eating those items.

Most importantly, it is helpful to determine whether the gravida understands what foods she should be eating. This can be evaluated by allowing her to plan some daily menus that meet the RDA guidelines for pregnancy.

NURSING APPLICATIONS

Assessment

Physical—for prepregnancy BMI (weight, height), serial weights, race, age.
Dietary—for adequacy of intake, especially kilocalories.
Laboratory—for blood sugar, Hgb, Hct (see Table 14–5).

Continued

Interventions

1. Monitor weight gain or loss. Pregnancy is not an appropriate time for weight reduction because it may be accompanied by ketonuria and result in fetal neurological damage. Unfortunately, the present preoccupation with slimness may result in attempts not to gain weight during pregnancy, and discussion about the importance of appropriate weight gain is important.
2. If weight gain tends to be excessive, discuss the amount of foods high in fat and sugar that are consumed. These foods have poor nutrient value but are high in kilocalories.
3. Follow guidelines in Table 14–4.

Evaluation

* Weight gain is appropriate for client's height and BMI.
* Counseling is successful if the gravida can plan nutritionally adequate menus that incorporate her favorite foods.

Client Education

- Low-fat or skim milk may be used to control weight as well as decrease saturated fat intake.
- Limiting weight gain during pregnancy will affect the maternal fat deposits only after it has affected fetal growth.
- Use of laboratory tests to determine nutritional status for vitamins and minerals (other than iron) is impractical in routine prenatal care (IM, 1990). However, if problems develop, these tests are warranted.

COMMON CONDITIONS DURING PREGNANCY

Nausea and Vomiting

Hyperemesis gravidarum is severe prolonged vomiting that continues throughout pregnancy.

Avitaminosis—disease caused by vitamin deficiency.

Morning sickness, or mild nausea and vomiting, is prevalent during the first trimester. It may occur only in the morning or may last throughout the day. Despite reports of morning sickness, there is no association with poor birth outcomes (King & Weininger, 1990). Vitamin B_6 deficiency has been attributed to morning sickness, but studies have failed to determine a clear connection.

In a small percentage of pregnancies, **hyperemesis gravidarum** develops. If not controlled, it can become life-threatening, with dehydration, acidosis, weight loss, **avitaminosis,** and jaundice. The precise cause for nausea during pregnancy has not been determined but may be associated with hormonal changes.

NURSING APPLICATIONS

Assessment

Physical—for nausea, vomiting, hyperemesis gravidarum, dehydration, weight loss, yellow sclera and skin.
Laboratory—for ABGs.

Interventions

1. Offer small, frequent feedings. Nausea may be aggravated by hunger or an empty stomach, and small feedings are better tolerated with less pressure in an already diminished area.
2. Follow guidelines in Table 14–6 to help decrease nausea and vomiting.

3. If hyperemesis gravidarum occurs: (a) Hospitalization is necessary. (b) Dehydration is corrected with IV fluids and electrolytes. (c) If the woman is unable to eat within a few days, nutrition support is provided with enteral feedings (Boyce, 1992) or PPN providing amino acids, dextrose, fats, vitamins, and minerals. (d) As soon as oral feedings are tolerated, a tray without any liquids is given with clear liquids provided between meals. (e) The diet proceeds slowly as tolerated, providing foods as described in Table 14–6.

Evaluation

* Client's nausea and vomiting will diminish. If client experiences nausea and vomiting, she will still eat nutritious foods.

Client Education

- Attempts should be made to consume foods despite morning sickness.
- Women who suffer from morning sickness are less likely to miscarry or deliver prematurely.
- If excessive vomiting occurs, call the physician.

Gastrointestinal Problems

Increased production of hormones, especially progesterone, causes decreased tone, motility, and intestinal secretions in the GI tract. A problem resulting from this is **"heartburn."** Additionally, the gravida experiences a full feeling caused by lack of normal space in the abdomen that is due to pressure of the enlarging uterus. Heartburn occurs so frequently during pregnancy that a discussion of this subject is in order during the first prenatal visit. Further suggestions for coping with heartburn are detailed in Chapter 25.

Heartburn or indigestion is gastric reflux in the lower esophagus causing a burning sensation.

Decreased motility in the GI tract contributes to constipation. Late in the pregnancy, constipation may be caused by the pressure of the fetus. The client may need to be reminded to allow enough time for bowel movements and try to relax.

Hemorrhoids may result from the increased weight of the fetus and straining during fecal elimination. This problem is usually controlled by the same remedies as for constipation, i.e., increased fluid and fiber.

Hemorrhoids are enlarged veins in the anus that may protrude through the anal sphincter.

What causes heartburn in pregnancy? Constipation?

TABLE 14–6

NUTRITIONAL MANAGEMENT FOR MORNING SICKNESS

1. Eat dry toast, crackers, or some dry cereal about half an hour before getting out of bed. Jelly may be used, but no fat, such as butter or margarine
2. In the morning, get up slowly and avoid sudden movements
3. Eat several small snacks (even as many as 8) a day. These snacks may be better tolerated than large meals
4. Rest after a meal
5. Avoid fatty foods, spicy foods such as pizza, caffeine, and rich foods such as pastries
6. Eat fruits, cold foods, and complex carbohydrates (e.g., rice, potatoes, and noodles) because these foods are better tolerated
7. Keep the kitchen well ventilated to avoid odors during food preparation
8. Drink liquids such as weak tea or apple juice between meals, not during meals
9. Relax and stay calm

NURSING APPLICATIONS

Assessment

Physical—for heartburn, constipation.
Dietary—for intake of fluid and fiber.

Interventions

1. Reduce consumption of fatty and spicy foods if heartburn occurs. During the digestion of fat, carbon dioxide is produced with increased gas; spicy foods are hard to digest.
2. Discourage the use of antacids or baking soda for indigestion or gas; this practice can cause alkalemia or even anemia as the result of the antacid combining with iron.
3. For problems with constipation, suggest foods high in soluble and insoluble fiber and water. Fiber provides bulk, making stools easier to pass, and adequate fluid allows the stool to stay soft (see Chapter 2).

Evaluation

* Heartburn and constipation should be minimal. If heartburn occurs, client will eat smaller amounts frequently and consume less fatty and spicy foods. If constipation occurs, client will drink fluids and consume fiber.

Client Education

- Small frequent meals are advisable to avoid heartburn.
- Eight to 10 glasses of fluid are needed daily.
- In addition to increasing fiber intake, regular exercise, such as walking, is recommended.
- Self-medication with laxatives is not advised for constipation during pregnancy; the physician should be consulted.

Edema

Additional amounts of fluids are retained during pregnancy because of elevated levels of estrogens and progesterone. This is a common phenomenon as blood volume expands and additional fluids are retained in connective tissues. To relieve symptoms, elevation of the feet is recommended. If foods are salted excessively, edema may be helped by reducing the amount of salt used. Sodium restriction is an obsolete concept and no longer advisable; diuretics are not recommended during pregnancy either.

NURSING APPLICATIONS

Assessment

Physical—for edema.
Dietary—for salt intake.
Laboratory—for albumin.

Interventions

1. Monitor edema. Some complications of pregnancy (toxemia, pregnancy-induced hypertension [PIH]) and certain prepregnancy diseases (cardiac or renal problems) can cause edema. This requires medical intervention.

Evaluation

* Edema will decrease to prepregnancy level, or edema will diminish when legs are elevated. If edema does not diminish with elevation or edema becomes generalized, report it to the physician.

Client Education

- Do not restrict sodium unless prescribed by the physician. However, curtailing salt added to foods can be helpful.
- Do not use diuretics to reduce edema unless prescribed by the physician.
- Rapid weight gains during pregnancy usually are due to the accumulation of fluid rather than fat deposits.

DISORDERS OF PREGNANCY

Pregnancy-Induced Hypertension

The 3 symptoms of **pregnancy-induced hypertension (PIH)** are (1) edema with sudden weight gain; (2) proteinuria, which may be very low even in serious cases; and (3) hypertension. These complications increase risk of perinatal and maternal morbidity and mortality. Unless medical treatment is received, kidney failure, convulsions, and even death of the mother and fetus may occur. The formerly used term, toxemia, is a misnomer because no toxins have been found to cause this disorder. Preeclampsia usually occurs after the 20th week of conception and disappears after the pregnancy.

The hypertensive disorders of pregnancy include a mild state, preeclampsia (hypertension with proteinuria and/or edema), and the convulsive end state, eclampsia.

Clear-cut answers are not available for the cause or prevention of this serious condition. Malnutrition is generally common among these clients. Improved nutrition with protein may contribute to the decline in incidence and mortality rates of PIH. A well-balanced diet with adequate amounts of protein may prevent or lessen the disorder.

Some studies have attempted to link dietary calcium intake with PIH. A deficiency of extracellular calcium is not the primary causative factor in PIH, but it may be a compounding risk factor (Myatt, 1992). When dietary calcium intake is below 800 mg/day, calcium supplements may reduce risk of hypertensive disorders of pregnancy (Belizàn et al, 1991).

What are the 3 symptoms of PIH? Why is toxemia a misnomer? What nutrient is associated with PIH?

NURSING APPLICATIONS

Assessment

Physical—for edema, rapid weight gain, BP, convulsions.
Dietary—for calcium, protein intake.
Laboratory—for urine protein; calcium, albumin.

Interventions

1. Discuss the food pyramid or the US Dietary Guidelines to ensure client is able to plan a well-balanced menu she can afford.
2. Encourage moderate salt restriction; discuss decreasing the amount of salt added to foods in cooking and at the table and limiting the amount of highly processed foods with salt added (see Chapter 8, Table 8-3). This may help lower BP by decreasing fluid retention.

Evaluation

* PIH does not occur. If it does, convulsions and death are averted because the condition was identified and reported to the physician early.

Client Education

- Routine calcium supplements to prevent PIH are not recommended (IM, 1990).
- Excessive weight gain during pregnancy does not cause the development of PIH.

Anemia

Anemia is defined as a depressed Hgb concentration more than 2 standard deviations below the mean for healthy women of the same age, sex, and stage of pregnancy.

Three different types of **anemia** may appear during pregnancy; correct diagnosis by the physician indicates the appropriate therapy. Iron deficiency is the most common cause of anemia in pregnancy (see Chapter 18). It is most commonly associated with Hispanics and blacks, low socioeconomic status, multiple gestations, chronic use of aspirin, and limited education. Since iron requirement after the first trimester exceeds amounts commonly provided by foods, supplementation is recommended.

Abnormal complications due to ruptured tubal pregnancy or abortion may precede hemorrhaging and necessitate transfusions. Iron supplementation is required to reestablish normal blood values.

Megaloblastic anemia is extra large RBCs, caused by folate or vitamin B_{12} deficiency.

Megaloblastic anemia is occasionally seen as a result of increased folate requirement during pregnancy. Erythrocyte and serum folate levels are used to indicate folate status.

NURSING APPLICATIONS

Assessment

Physical—for fatigue, race, socioeconomic status, use of aspirin, education level.

Dietary—for iron and folate intake.

Laboratory—for RBC, folate level, MCV, Hgb, Hct, transferrin, ferritin, iron.

Interventions

1. For iron deficiency anemia, give iron supplements as prescribed and encourage basic nutrition principles to enhance iron absorption (see Chapter 9). This will enhance iron bioavailability needed to synthesize Hgb.
2. Discuss intake of foods high in folate and the effect of heat and processing on folate content. Folate is essential for RBC maturation.

Evaluation

* Anemia is prevented because foods high in iron and folate are ingested by the client; supplements are taken as ordered by the physician.

Client Education

- Choose whole-grain cereal products since folate is lost in processing.
- The use of fresh fruits and vegetables is advantageous, as these generally contain more vitamin C and folate than their counterparts that have been cooked or processed.

Gestational Diabetes

Routine screening for gestational diabetes has become commonplace, especially for the obese pregnant woman. A diagnosis of gestational diabetes mellitus is prevalent during pregnancy because of hormones synthesized by the placenta that counteract the action of insulin. An elevated glucose level for a prolonged time can result in large infants, early delivery, and increased risk of birth trauma and malformations. A strict diet is indicated. This condition is discussed in further detail in Chapter 27.

NURSING APPLICATIONS

Assessment

Dietary—for intake of concentrated sugars.
Laboratory—for urinary glucose and protein, serum glucose, Hgb A_{1c}.

Interventions

1. If client is diabetic, refer to dietitian. Dietitians are more knowledgeable about the modified diet needed. Strict adherence to a diet for diabetic clients ensures optimum fetal growth and stabilizes blood glucose levels.
2. If client is diabetic, encourage 5 to 6 meals per day to stabilize blood glucose levels.

Evaluation

* Client and fetus experience no complications from the diabetes mellitus, and serum glucose levels are controlled.

Client Education

- Teach signs, symptoms, and treatment for high and low blood glucose levels (see Chapter 27).

LACTATION

One of the goals established by the federal government for a healthier America by the year 2000 was to "increase to at least 75% the proportion of mothers who breast-feed their babies in the early postpartum period and to at least 50% the proportion who continue breast-feeding until their babies are 5 to 6 months old" (USDHHS, 1990). In 1989, 52% of mothers initiated breast-feeding in the hospital, with only 19% still breast-feeding 6 months later (IM, 1991). White mothers are more likely to initiate breast-feeding (61%) than Mexican-Americans (50%) or black mothers (25%) (Ryan et al, 1991). The Subcommittee on Nutrition during Lactation published *Nutrition During Lactation* (IM, 1991) to help health care providers understand how nutrition relates to the outcomes of lactation and aid in formulating guidelines for clinical application in the US. The subcommittee concluded that virtually all women are able to produce adequate amounts of milk to provide essential nutrients to support the growth and health of infants.

Since the decision to feed the newborn by bottle or breast is generally made during pregnancy, an informative discussion with the gravida is appropriate to help her make the best decision for herself and infant. However, she should not feel pressured in her decision. Even though breast-feeding is physiologically natural, nearly all mothers need some assistance and guidance with their first newborn. Prenatal classes promote confidence and supply pertinent information. In the US, the primigravida may be surrounded by mothers who are bottle-feeding and may not have extended family members with previous breast-feeding experience. Breast-feeding has many advantages for the infant and mother:

- Human milk is nutritionally balanced with maximum bioavailability for infants.
- Breast milk has immunologic properties that help reduce infant morbidity (especially certain infectious GI and respiratory diseases) and mortality.
- Human milk results in reduced risk of food allergies.
- Breast-feeding promotes infant oral motor and structural development.
- Maternal hormones produced as a result of lactation facilitate contractions of the uterus and control postpartum bleeding.

List 5 advantages of breast-feeding.

- Prepregnancy weight is achieved sooner.
- Breast-feeding is generally less expensive than formula feeding.
- Mother-infant bonding is enhanced.

PHYSIOLOGY OF BREAST-FEEDING

The rooting reflex causes the infant to turn the mouth toward the stimulation when touched on the cheek. Suckling involves the lips and cheeks with little tongue movement except to propel the food back for swallowing.

What are the 2 processes of breast-feeding? What causes increased milk production?

In most cases, milk secretion is well established by the end of the first week. Basically, lactation is a 2-stage process: (1) milk production and secretion by the mammary alveolar cells and (2) milk ejection through the duct system. Milk production is most active during infant sucking. The more often an infant nurses, the more milk is produced.

In full-term infants, the **rooting,** sucking, and swallowing reflexes are usually well developed. The newborn's sucking skills are not fully developed, but **suckling** is adequate to obtain the milk. The swallow is reflexive and usually develops about the fifth month of gestation.

Mother's Reflexes

Lactation involves a complex neuroendocrine process. As the newborn sucks, sensory nerve endings in the nipple are stimulated, sending impulses to the hypothalamus in the brain (Fig. 14–2). The hypothalamus stimulates the anterior pituitary to release prolactin, causing the milk to be released.

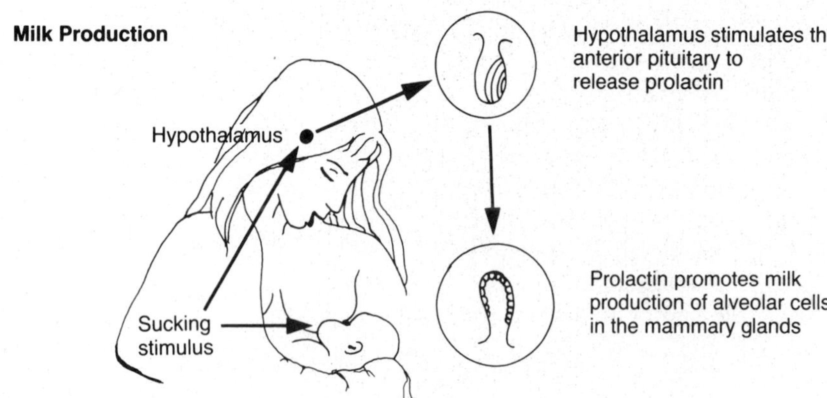
Milk Production
Hypothalamus
Hypothalamus stimulates the anterior pituitary to release prolactin
Sucking stimulus
Prolactin promotes milk production of alveolar cells in the mammary glands

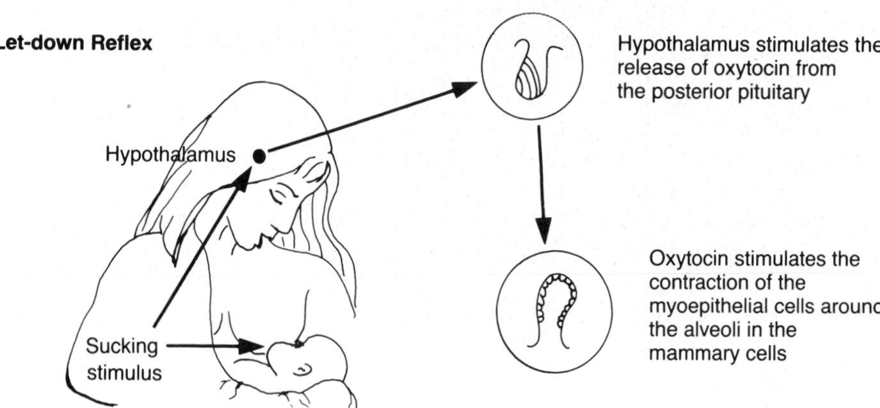
Let-down Reflex
Hypothalamus
Hypothalamus stimulates the release of oxytocin from the posterior pituitary
Sucking stimulus
Oxytocin stimulates the contraction of the myoepithelial cells around the alveoli in the mammary cells

Figure 14–2 The physiology of lactation. Sucking stimulates secretion of prolactin and oxytocin. Prolactin increases milk synthesis; oxytocin produces the let-down reflex, or ejection of the milk.

The hormone oxytocin precipitates the movement of milk into the milk ducts, where it is accessible to the suckling infant. This is called the "let-down" reflex. Milk is ejected to the infant as the sucking starts.

What are the functions of prolactin and oxytocin during breast-feeding?

COMPOSITION OF HUMAN MILK

Colostrum is relatively low in kilocalories, lactose, and fat. It is high in protein that appears to facilitate the establishment of "bifidus flora" in the digestive tract and contains immune factors to provide immunity from some diseases. Colostrum gradually changes to milk between the third and sixth day.

Colostrum is a thick, yellowish fluid secreted by the breast for the first few days after birth.

Human milk is unique in its physical structure and nutrients and contains other substances such as enzymes, hormones, and growth factors. Breast milk is normally thin with a slightly bluish color.

The overall composition of breast milk is relatively constant, regardless of the nutritional status of the mother. Compared with cow milk, human milk is high in lactose and relatively low in protein. Specific protein fractions synthesized in the breast tissue, especially lactalbumin and lactoferrin, help protect against GI infections. These amino acids are beneficial due to the infant's immature system.

The lipid content varies with the time of day and during a particular feeding. Short-chain fatty acids are produced by breast tissue, but long-chain fatty acids are influenced by the maternal diet. Breast milk contains principally unsaturated fatty acids; saturated fatty acids are lower than in cow milk. Toward the end of a feeding, the milk contains higher amounts of fat. Lipase enzyme inherent in breast milk improves fat digestion. Human milk is relatively high in cholesterol. Despite numerous studies, it is uncertain whether human milk has a beneficial or adverse effect on the development of heart disease.

The relatively low mineral content of human milk is desirable because of its low renal solute load that is appropriate for the infant's immature kidney. Although the iron content is low, approximately 50 to 75% is absorbed. Because of the high bioavailability of iron, additional sources of iron are unnecessary during the infant's first 4 to 6 months.

What are the 2 functions of colostrum; of protein fractions? Why is the relatively low mineral content of human milk beneficial for infants? What is the reason iron does not need to be supplemented during the infant's first 4 to 6 months?

Nutritional Recommendations for Breast-Feeding

For most nutrients, recommendations are similar to those recommended during pregnancy. Energy requirements are proportional to the quantity of milk produced. Approximately 85 kcal are needed for every 100 ml of milk produced (NRC, 1989), requiring approximately a 500-kcal daily increase. Although this may not be fully adequate to cover the needs for milk production, the 2- to 4-kg fat stores accumulated during pregnancy can be used to supply additional kilocalories. Thus, return to prepregnancy weight is accelerated.

Other nutrients needed in larger quantities than during pregnancy include protein; vitamins A, E, C, thiamin, riboflavin, niacin, and B_{12}; magnesium; zinc; iodine; and selenium (Fig. 14–3). Nutrients most likely to be deficient in the diet for lactating women are calcium, zinc, magnesium, vitamin B_6, and folate (IM, 1991). The subcommittee (IM, 1991) recommends, "Lactating women should be encouraged to obtain their nutrients from a well-balanced, varied diet rather than from vitamin-mineral supplements."

Dietary assessment of routine food intake is suggested, followed by counseling the woman regarding foods rich in nutrients that are deficient in the diet. When the diet is determined to be low in one or more nutrients, nutritional counseling is indicated, and if dietary changes are not feasible, nutrient supplementation may be recommended, as described by the Institute of Medicine in Table 14–7.

What is the recommendation for kilocalories during breast-feeding? What nutrients are needed in larger quantities for breast-feeding? What is the recommendation for fluid intake?

Sample Menu

Breakfast

1 cup orange juice
1 bagel with 1 oz cream cheese and 1 packet raisins
1 cup 1% milk
coffee with creamer

Lunch

Tuna salad sandwich (2 oz tuna with 3 tbsp mayonnaise, 2 slices tomato, lettuce slices, on 2 slices whole wheat bread)
1 apple
2 fig bar cookies
1 cup 1% milk

Dinner

3 oz lean roast beef with 1/4 cup gravy
1 cup brown rice
1/2 cup spinach
1/2 cup three bean salad
2 whole wheat rolls
2 tbsp light tub margarine
1 cup strawberries
1 cup 1% milk
Iced tea

Evening Snack

12 oz cola beverage
1 oz peanuts

Nutrient	RDA–Lactating, first six months	Actual	% RDA
Kcal		2688 kcal	100
Protein		109 gm	168
Carbohydrate		356 gm	105
Fat		101 gm	113
Cholesterol		178 mg	59
Fiber–dietary		34.180 gm	137
Vitamin A		1476 RE	114
Thiamin		1.9 mg	119
Riboflavin		2.4 mg	135
Niacin		24.1 mg	120
Vitamin B_6		2.1 mg	99
Folate		435 mcg	155
Vitamin B_{12}		6.6 mcg	256
Pantothenic acid		6.3 mg	114
Biotin		54 mcg	83
Vitamin C		220 mg	231
Vitamin D		8.0 mcg	81
Vitamin K		269 mcg	414
Sodium		2970 mg	97
Potassium		4366 mg	184
Calcium		1418 mg	118
Phosphorus		2018 mg	168
Magnesium		555 mg	156
Iron		18.5 mg	123
Zinc		15.3 mg	80
Copper		1.9 mg	87
Manganese		3.3 mg	93
Selenium		0.2 mg	273

^0 ^50 ^100 ^150 ^200

Carbohydrate, Protein, and Fat Distribution

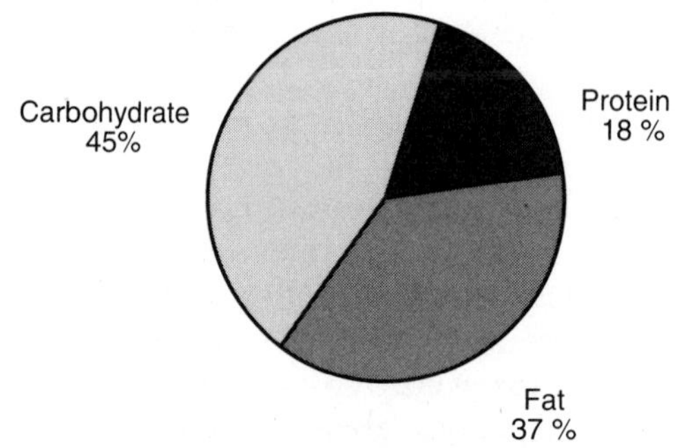

Kcal, 2688; protein, 109 gm; carbohydrate, 356 gm; fat 101 gm

Figure 14–3 Sample menu for lactation (first 6 months). RDA, Recommended dietary allowance; RE, Retinol equivalents. (Nutrient data from Nutritionist III, Version 7.0 Software, Salem, Oregon.)

The lactating woman requires additional fluids to replace that secreted in the milk. An additional 1000 ml/day (4 cups) of fluids are needed.

Effects of Maternal Nutritional Status on Breast Milk

Based on studies reviewed by the Institute of Medicine (1991), the major determinant of milk production is the infant's demand for milk, not maternal energy intake. Most women normally lose weight during lactation, but this has no apparent deleterious effects on milk production. Carbohydrate intake is important for main-

TABLE 14–7

SUGGESTED MEASURES FOR IMPROVING NUTRIENT INTAKE OF WOMEN WITH RESTRICTIVE EATING PATTERNS

Type of Restrictive Eating Pattern	Corrective Measures
Excessive restriction of food intake, i.e., ingestion of <1800 kcal of energy/day, which ordinarily leads to unsatisfactory intake of nutrients compared with the amounts needed by lactating women	Encourage increased intake of nutrient-rich foods to achieve an energy intake of at least 1800 kcal/day; if the mother insists on curbing food intake sharply, promote substitution of foods rich in vitamins, minerals, and protein for those lower in nutritive value; in individual cases, it may be advisable to recommend a balanced multivitamin-mineral supplement; discourage use of liquid weight loss diets and appetite suppressants
Complete vegetarianism, i.e., avoidance of all animal foods, including meat, fish, dairy products, and eggs	Advise intake of a regular source of vitamin B_{12}, such as special vitamin B_{12}–containing plant food products or a 2.6-mcg vitamin B_{12} supplement daily
Avoidance of milk, cheese, or other calcium-rich dairy products	Encourage increased intake of other culturally appropriate dietary calcium sources, such as collard greens for blacks from the southeastern United States; provide information on the appropriate use of low-lactose dairy products if milk is being avoided because of lactose intolerance; if correction by diet cannot be achieved, it may be advisable to recommend 600 mg of elemental calcium/day taken with meals
Avoidance of vitamin D–fortified foods, such as fortified milk or cereal, combined with limited exposure to ultraviolet light	Recommend 10 mcg of supplemental vitamin D per day

Reprinted with permission from *Nutrition During Lactation.* Copyright 1991 by the National Academy of Sciences. Published by the National Academy Press, Washington, D.C.

taining lactose synthesis and milk volume. A low carbohydrate diet for weight reduction can be hazardous to the mother (Winick et al, 1988).

Certain minerals are not affected by maternal dietary intake: calcium, phosphorus, magnesium, sodium, and potassium. On the other hand, dietary intake of selenium and iodine is positively related to their concentrations in human milk. Vitamin intake is more closely affected by maternal intake than minerals, but this depends on the specific vitamin. When maternal intake of vitamins is chronically low, the milk may contain low amounts except for folate and calcium. Folate and calcium levels of breast milk are maintained at the expense of maternal stores. Breast milk reflects an increased maternal intake (above the RDA) of vitamins B_6 and D.

The milk produced by vegans varies in its vitamin D and B_{12} content (Dwyer, 1991). Vegan mothers should use supplements or calcium-rich foods to avoid diminishing their bone reserves during lactation. A supplement containing the RDA level for vitamins D and B_{12} is also encouraged. If iron stores have been depleted during pregnancy, a supplemental source may be needed (Dwyer, 1991).

What nutrients will be extracted from the mother's stores if intake is low?

Other Factors Affecting Breast Milk

Many substances consumed by the mother have been thought to affect the milk. Certain foods, especially strongly flavored items such as raw onion, garlic, curry, chili peppers, and chocolate, may cause GI distress, rash, or irritability in the infant. They need to be omitted only if the infant is affected.

Many non-nutritive substances and drugs may be secreted in milk. Alcohol may impair the let-down reflex and is transmitted in breast milk in approximately the same proportions as in the mother's blood (Jason, 1991). Intake should be limited to less than 0.5 gm/kg daily. Large amounts of coffee intake may adversely affect the iron content of human milk.

What are other factors that can affect breast milk?

Because of the risk of medications being passed into the milk, all drugs should be used cautiously and only if essential. The physician may be able to prescribe a medication that is less likely to be secreted into the milk.

NURSING APPLICATIONS

Assessment

Physical—for socioeconomic status, types of drugs used.

Dietary—for kilocalorie, nutrient, fluid intake; alcohol and caffeine intake.

Interventions

1. Encourage intake of nutrients from fruits and vegetables, whole-grain breads and cereals, calcium-rich dairy products, and protein-rich and carbohydrate-rich foods.
2. For vegan mothers who desire to breast-feed, stress the importance of a balanced diet with appropriate supplements and eating foods in sufficient quantities.

Client Education

- Breast-feeding will help with weight loss.
- Intake of coffee, other caffeine-containing beverages and medications, and decaffeinated coffee should be limited (IM, 1991).
- Infants nursed by strict vegans frequently are at risk for megaloblastic anemia, rickets, and poor growth.

CONTRAINDICATIONS FOR BREAST-FEEDING

Galactosemia is a congenital abnormality in which the enzyme necessary to metabolize galactose is lacking.

Phenylketonuria is a congenital metabolic abnormality in which phenylalanine accumulates, causing mental retardation and other abnormalities.

In a few circumstances, breast-feeding is not recommended. Infants born with **galactosemia** require a special formula. Since breast milk contains relatively low levels of phenylalanine, an infant born with **phenylketonuria** may be breast-fed but should be closely monitored by the physician.

Certain medications are contraindicated during breast-feeding. Antineoplastic agents, therapeutic radioactive medications, some antithyroid agents, and antiprotozoan medications may pose problems (Table 14–8). If possible, the physician should use the medication least likely to pass into the milk. By taking acceptable drugs immediately after nursing, the peak serum concentration occurs before the next feeding.

Since many drugs may be prescribed on a short-term basis, cessation of lactation during the time the medication is taken is appropriate. The milk can be manually expressed and discarded until threat of drug contamination is over. Use of numerous medications has precipitated concern, whereas others are administered only under close medical supervision.

Maternal life-threatening or debilitating illness or infections, such as sputum-positive tuberculosis, may preclude breast-feeding. Rarely, heavy maternal exposure to pesticides, heavy metals, or other contaminants, such as polychlorinated biphenyls (PCBs) and polybrominated biphenyls (PBBs), would contraindicate breast-feeding.

If the mother becomes pregnant again while breast-feeding, the nutritional and psychological demands are considerable. Decreased milk supply and its taste and

TABLE 14–8

MEDICATIONS AFFECTING BREAST MILK

Addictive drugs contraindicating breast-feeding because of intoxication:
- Alcohol
- Cocaine
- Amphetamine
- Heroin
- Marijuana
- Nicotine (smoking)
- Phencyclidine (PCP)

Chemotherapeutic drugs that are possibly immunosuppressive:
- Cyclophosphamide
- Cyclosporine
- Azathioprine
- Fluorouracil
- Methotrexate
- Doxorubicin

Antipsychotic medications that are found in breast milk:
- Lithium
- Haldol

Anticonvulsants that are found in breast milk, which may cause sedation/drowsiness:
- Phenytoin
- Phenobarbital
- Primidone

Antithyroid:
- Iodides

Analgesics that may affect platelet function:
- Aspirin

Other drugs that may affect the infant:
- Ergotamine (used in medications for migraine headaches)
- Metoclopramide—CNS stimulant

Medications warranting temporary cessation of lactation:
- Antibiotics: chloroquine, chloramphenicol, sulfasalazine, metronidazole, tinidazole, dapsone, ketoconazole, tetracycline
- Radioactive medications used for diagnostic studies (gallium-67, indium-111, iodine-125, iodine-131, radioactive sodium)

Lactation-suppressing medications:
- Bromocriptine
- Estrogens
- Progestogens
- Bendroflumethiazide (diuretic)

Data compiled from American Academy of Pediatric Committee on Drugs. Transfer of drugs and other chemicals into human milk. *Pediatrics* 1989 Nov; 84(5):924–932; Stockton DL, Paller AM. Drug administration to the pregnant or lactating woman: A reference guide for dermatologists. *J Am Acad Dermatol* 1990 July; 23(1):87–103.

composition may affect the infant's desire. Contractions while nursing may indicate a need to wean the infant to prevent miscarriage.

Describe 3 situations that require cessation of breast-feeding.

Breast-feeding is contraindicated if the mother has a negative attitude about breast-feeding. Lactation is usually not successful if the mother does not want to breast-feed.

EFFECT OF BREAST MILK ON INFANT NUTRITIONAL STATUS

Breast-fed infants usually have a lower energy intake as a result of less milk intake than bottle-fed infants. Therefore, breast-fed infants gain weight more slowly than formula-fed infants after the first 2 to 3 months. This slower growth rate is sometimes used as a rationale for discontinuing breast-feeding or supplementing breast milk with formula or solid foods. This should not be a cause for concern, as long-term growth status is not attributable to breast-feeding (Pomerance, 1987).

To ensure adequate nutrition for the breast-fed infant, certain measures are recommended (IM, 1991). All newborns, regardless of the method of feeding, should receive an injection of vitamin K at birth to prevent hemorrhagic bleeding. If the infant is not exposed to sunlight, a supplement of 5- to 7.5-mcg vitamin D should be provided. When the fluoride content of the household drinking water is below 0.3 ppm, fluoride supplements are recommended. If the mother is a complete vegetarian, breast-fed infants may develop vitamin B_{12} deficiency (even if the mother is not deficient) and should be provided with vitamins D and B_{12} supplements (Dwyer, 1991). Inadequate zinc intake has been documented to decrease the growth rate in infants breast-fed longer than 4 months (Walravens et al, 1992).

Why do breast-fed infants grow at a slower rate than bottle-fed infants? Which nutrient should be given at birth? Based on assessment of maternal intake, which other nutrients may need supplementation before 4 months of age?

Breast milk is adequate to meet the infant's needs for at least 4 months. Supplemental foods during that time may reduce iron absorption. Between 4 to 6 months, iron-rich foods or a daily low-dose oral iron supplement should be initiated.

SUPPORTIVE ROLE OF THE NURSE

There are 2 main factors to successful breast-feeding: believing that one can breast-feed and allowing the infant to suck enough for the milk release. Confidence is not as easy to obtain for the new mother as might be expected. Without support and valid information, she can easily become discouraged with rumors, superstitions, and questions about her ability to produce adequate milk.

Many statements are offered as reasons not to initiate or to discontinue breast-feeding: frequency of feeding; infant's crying, sleeping, and fussy behavior; breast and nipple problems; maternal fatigue; and concern about inadequate milk supply. A discussion of many factors is important for establishment of successful lactation to allay fears and concerns; the primigravida should receive counseling about nutrition during lactation and should be screened for possible nutritional problems (IM, 1991), as shown in Table 14–7. The nurse can play an important role in helping the mother thoroughly understand the benefits of breast-feeding. If the mother's breast-feeding expectations can be elicited and in-hospital feeding experiences discussed in light of these expectations, some of these disappointments or conflicts can be resolved before leaving the hospital (Kearney et al, 1990).

Nurses must be thoroughly knowledgeable, and preferably those who have breast-fed their own children are assigned to work with and support the primigravida. Bedside teaching is more effective than merely distributing manuals or announcing the availability of a call-in breast-feeding/lactation consultant.

La Leche groups provide information and teach women to breast-feed successfully. Women who belong to La Leche groups share their experiences of breast-feeding their own children. A La Leche friend can become a confidant offering emotional support and comradeship.

Successful lactation and establishment of an adequate milk supply are strongly influenced by early management. The medical facility can support the mother who chooses to breast-feed by providing rooming-in without the rigid restrictions of routine feedings. Environmental and emotional factors may influence the degree to which breast milk is provided. Initially, a relaxed, comfortable atmosphere is important.

As previously discussed, milk production is responsive to infant sucking. Beginning in the hospital, breast-feeding practices that are responsive to the infant's natural appetite should be promoted. During the first month, infants should be allowed to nurse from 10 to 12 times daily; they should not be permitted to sleep through the night.

List 3 ways the nurse can help the client for successful breast-feeding.

Nipple Conditioning

Successful breast-feeding partially depends on prenatal preparation and correct information to prevent possible difficulties. Examination of the nipple early in pregnancy is important. Nipples may be normal and protractile or inverted, flat, short, or nonprotractile. These anatomical differences interfere with breast-feeding because the infant may not be able to "latch on" to the breast. Although nipple preparation is not necessary for all women, nipple conditioning is especially helpful for clients with inverted nipples (Table 14–9). The nipple is gently rolled between the thumb and index finger repeatedly for several minutes daily during the last trimester. Some women find that the nipple areas become less sensitive if briskly rubbed with a terry towel after bathing.

Techniques of Breast-feeding

The success rate for breast-feeding is increased by allowing the newborn to nurse immediately after birth or as soon as the mother feels ready. Early sucking helps the milk to "come in," and the colostrum helps prepare the newborn's digestive tract by facilitating **meconium** removal.

Meconium, or stool produced during fetal life, are the first stools passed by the infant.

Bottle-feedings are not offered because the difference in sucking can be confusing to the newborn (Fig. 14–4). Once the newborn becomes adjusted to taking a bottle, it becomes much harder to get him or her to take the breast, although the reverse is not true.

It is unnecessary to clean the nipples before a feeding, since human milk is bacteriostatic. When bathing, only water is used; nothing should be put on the nipples that will require washing off before nursing, such as soap, lotions, or medica-

TABLE 14–9

LACTATION PROBLEMS AND THEIR MANAGEMENT

Problem	Prevention or Therapy
Flat nipples	Manipulate the nipple before offering it to the infant to make it more erect and easy to grasp. A nipple shield with a rubber tip may be used when breast-feeding
Inverted nipples	Gently roll the nipple between the thumb and index finger repeatedly for 5 min twice a day during the last trimester
Sore nipples	Offer the breasts properly to encourage proper sucking. Hold the infant in different positions to decrease continuous pressure on the same breast. Initially offer the breast that is least sore when the sucking is strongest. Expose the breast to the air. Wear breast shields to keep the nipple dry and free from brassiere friction. Short, frequent feedings are helpful
Cracked or fissured nipples	Put some of the milk on the nipple and areola and allow to dry. Expose to the air
Breast engorgement	Frequent feedings from birth are best. Manual expression of milk before initiating a feeding and when the infant is not eating well (e.g., because of sickness) is helpful. Be sure infant is "latching on" appropriately. Use a breast pump to prevent entrapment of the milk
Mastitis or infection	Place hot washcloths on the breast, cover with thin plastic wrap, and lie down. Maintain heat with a heating pad or hot-water bottle. Nurse frequently. Take analgesics if necessary
Leakage	Cross the arms against the breasts and press firmly. Breast pads with an outside plastic coating may be worn inside the brassiere. These should be changed frequently

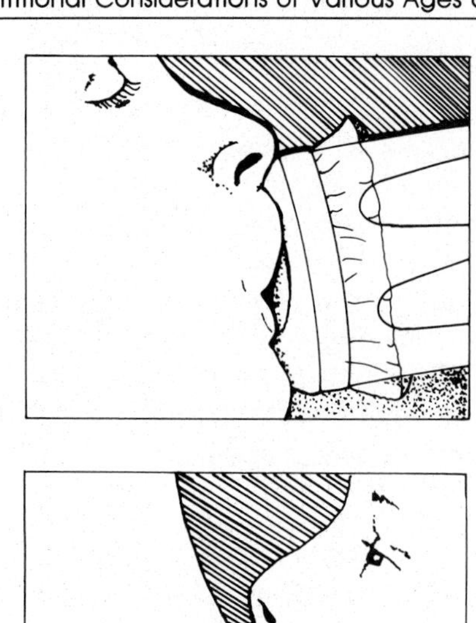

Bottle feeding elicits a different sucking action and position of the infant's lips, making a transition from bottle feeding to breast-feeding more difficult if the bottle is introduced first.

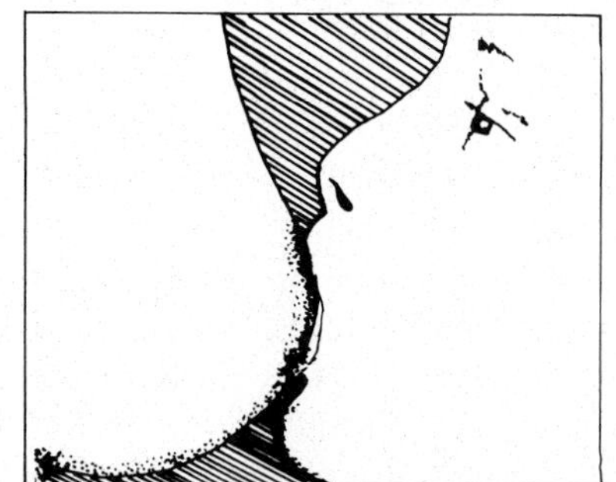

Incorrect position: With only the nipple in the infant's mouth, less milk is ejected to the infant and breast soreness will occur.

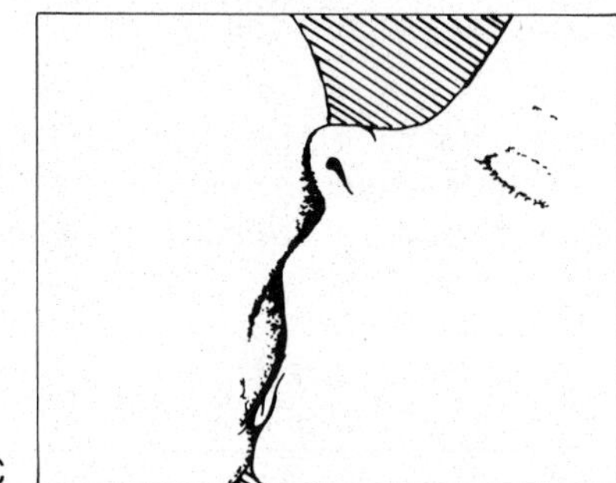

Correct position: The infant's lips should almost completely encompass the areola, and the head is positioned very close to the nipple.

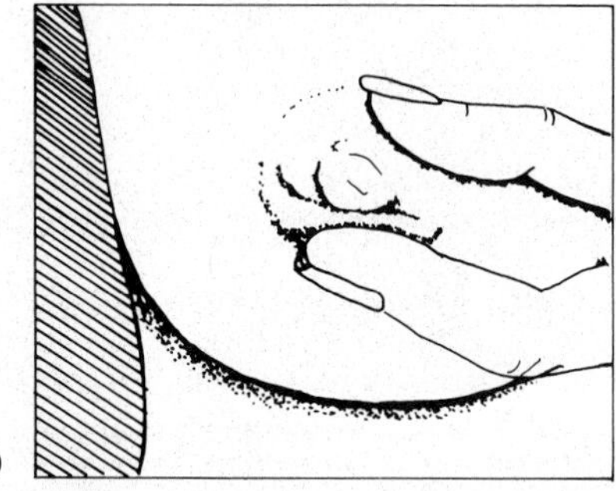

Incorrect position: Only the nipple is being offered to the infant.

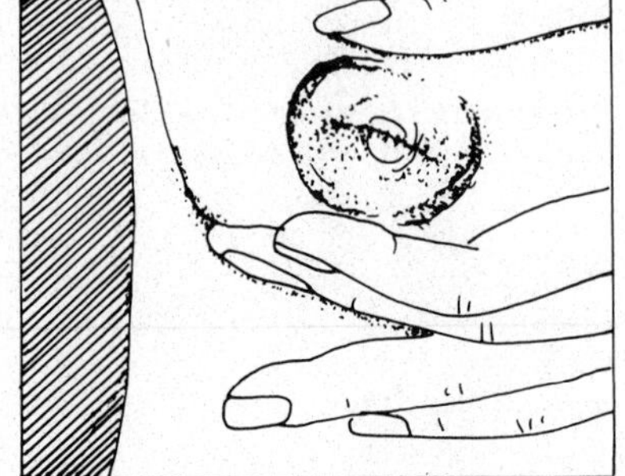

Correct position: The thumb and 1 to 2 fingers are used to offer the nipple and areola to the infant.

Figure 14–4 ***A* through *E*. Positioning of infant's mouth during breast-feeding.**

tion. The skin should be thoroughly dried to prevent moisture from making the skin softer and weaker.

In breast-feeding, the nipple plus the areola must be offered instead of only the nipple. Failure to do this results in reduced milk production. The breast can be offered using the following procedures: (1) The mother's hand is placed on her chest underneath the breast. (2) Slide 1 to 2 fingers onto the breast without touching the areola. (3) Place the thumb above the fingers to control placement of the nipple and areola into the infant's mouth. (4) Turn the infant's body toward the mother and brush the infant's cheek to elicit the rooting reflex. In addition to the mother being in a comfortable position, the infant's position should facilitate the swallowing process. Pillows or other props are needed initially to facilitate positioning.

Most infants take 80 to 90% of the milk from each breast in the first 4 minutes. If a newborn sucks longer than 10 to 20 minutes, the position should be checked because the infant may be sucking incorrectly. Feedings of 1 to 2 minutes are too brief and leave the breasts engorged. Infants are allowed to nurse on each breast for about 10 to 20 minutes, with a total nursing period of 20 to 40 minutes. Consistent nursing lasting more than 25 to 30 minutes per breast may indicate inadequate milk production or inappropriate "latch on."

To terminate a feeding, the free hand is used to insert a finger into the corner of the infant's mouth and between the gums. Unless this procedure is used to release the suction, the nipple will be pulled, causing pain and possible nipple damage.

When should the newborn be nursed? Why is bottle-feeding not offered? Describe breast care. How long should an infant nurse?

Problems Encountered During Lactation

Frequently encountered problems with lactation include flat or inverted nipples, soreness, engorgement, and **mastitis.** Management approaches to these problems are presented in Table 14–9.

Mastitis—breast infection.

Sore nipples can be extremely painful. Initially, soreness can occur at the beginning of breast-feeding and may be caused by faulty sucking technique, engorged breasts, flat nipples, or a thrush infection in the infant. Short, frequent nursing promotes speedy healing.

When the let-down reflex does not function, the milk-producing cells produce fewer fatty globules, and the kilocaloric content of the milk is decreased. Infants receiving this milk are frequently hungry. This is a frustrating situation for the mother and infant. The let-down reflex can be facilitated by taking a warm shower or drinking warm milk or tea before nursing and nursing in a darkened, quiet room in a comfortable chair. The adequacy of the infant's intake can be determined by the rate of growth and the number of wet diapers (6 to 12 diapers/day).

Continuous failure of the let-down reflex ends with engorgement or a breast infection in the mother and possible infant weight loss or termination of breast-feedings. Early breast engorgement may occur when the milk is first produced (Fig. 14–5), but this can be avoided by frequent feedings from birth. Not only is milk production stimulated, but also excess milk is removed, which otherwise becomes trapped. In engorgement, milk-producing cells are compressed and traumatized from the back pressure of the milk, so the mother produces less. Additionally, the cells that contract to cause let-down may be injured. Because the milk-ejection is easily inhibited, the nursing mother needs empathy, support, and guidance to prevent anxiety and fears and to give her confidence. "Drying-up" may occur easily with embarrassment, anger, fear, or getting chilled.

The milk-ejection reflex may cause sexual sensations during nursing, or vice versa (sexual activities may cause milk flow). To prevent women from feeling guilty about these sensations, they should know that this is nature's way of making nursing enjoyable. It is normal and quite acceptable.

Weaning is contraindicated for mastitis because it will produce engorgement, stasis, cracked nipples, and more infection. Early use of hot packs and frequent

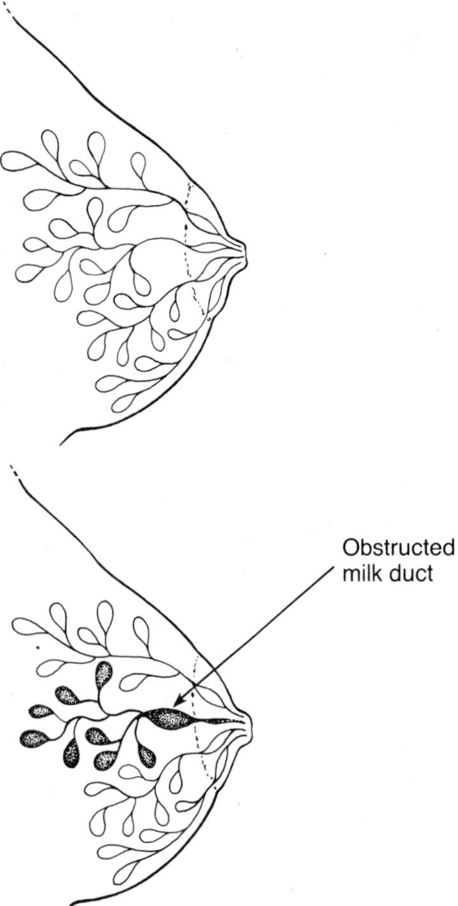

Figure 14–5 Breast engorgement caused by poor drainage from obstructed milk duct.

nursing can prevent the need for antibiotics. Neither the bacteria of the breast infection nor the antibiotics used to treat the infection have been shown to harm the infant.

Sometimes the milk may come so fast that it can choke the infant. If this is anticipated, the mother may express her breast slightly before offering it to the infant. A tense or prickling sensation in the nipples may be felt as this starts.

Describe 3 problems and treatments for each problem.

Infants will have appetite spurts that can be managed best by increasing the nursing frequency. This increases milk production. If the increased appetite persists for more than 3 to 4 days or if weight gain is inadequate, further evaluation of nursing practices and the infant's clinical status is indicated.

Manual Expression of Milk

Manual expression of milk is especially useful for women who plan to return to work. When the gravida wishes to leave her infant during a feeding period, she may prepare a bottle earlier. If an infant is born prematurely, the gravida may wish to express milk for her newborn until the infant is strong enough to suck and/or able to come home from the hospital.

With both hands around the breast against the chest wall, move the hands (not just the fingers) toward the edges of the areola, massaging the whole surface of the breast. Gently press the edges of the areola between fingers and thumb of the hand from the opposite side of the body, with the other hand supporting the breast.

Several types of breast pumps are available. Syringe-type and battery pumps that are easily sterilized are recommended.

NURSING APPLICATIONS

Assessment

Physical—for disease, types of drugs taken, psychological status of new mother, type of nipple.
Dietary—for beliefs about breast-feeding and diet.

Interventions

1. If possible, allow infant to suck immediately after birth and to remain in the room with the mother.
2. Follow guidelines in Table 14–9 if complications arise.

Evaluation

* Client can verbalize nutritional needs for lactation, how to breast-feed properly and how to care for complications.

Client Education

- Refer to prenatal classes and La Leche groups.
- Demonstrate how to express milk manually.
- Rest is essential for the mother and infant.
- Some infants reject the breast for a day or so when menstruation begins but then return to normal.

ORAL CONTRACEPTIVE AGENTS

Many nutrients (especially folate, vitamin B_6, zinc, and magnesium) are affected by OCAs. The low estrogen preparations now being used precipitate fewer changes in vitamin status than earlier preparations. Lower levels of the water-soluble vitamins are due to decreased intestinal absorption and increased metabolism. However, vitamin deficiencies have been identified only when the diet was marginal.

Increased amounts of pyridoxine may be indicated because estrogen increases the production of tryptophan, which uses pyridoxine in its metabolism. Depression and impaired glucose tolerance attributed to OCAs may be alleviated with pyridoxine supplementation (10 mg/day) (Dickey, 1991).

Megaloblastic anemia reported in women on OCAs is related to decreased folate absorption. Supplements are not necessary except for high-risk clients in whom other factors, such as deficient diet or disease, could increase chances for a deficiency to develop. To decrease risk of neural tubal defects resultant of folate deficiency, clients on OCAs who are planning a pregnancy in the near future may warrant supplementation of folate for 3 months before becoming pregnant, or they should discontinue the use of OCAs for at least 6 months before conception.

Progestins can cause weight gain related to increased appetite and altered carbohydrate metabolism, and estrogens may lead to an increase in subcutaneous fat and fluid retention.

Use of OCAs is associated with increased risk of heart disease due to changes in serum lipids. The amount and type of progestin and estrogen in the OCA can affect these changes. In general, there is a decrease in HDL cholesterol, which is an undesirable affect, since HDL is a protective factor. Increased total cholesterol, triglyceride, and LDL cholesterol levels are undesirable factors. Progestin appears to cause a decrease in HDL cholesterol levels and elevate LDL and total cholesterol levels. Since estrogens may increase HDL levels, the net effect on serum lipids is dependent on the ratio of progestin and estrogens. OCAs containing both progestin and estrogen have been shown to have little or no effect on HDL cholesterol levels but may increase fasting triglyceride levels (Godsland et al, 1990).

Describe 3 effects of OCA on nutrition.

Progestins reduce cholesterol excretion, resulting in cholesterol precipitation in the gallbladder; this may cause the formation of gallstones.

NURSING APPLICATIONS

Assessment

Dietary—for consumption of foods containing folate, vitamin B_6, and fat.
Laboratory—for HDL, LDL, cholesterol, triglycerides.

Interventions

1. Review the Food pyramid/US Dietary Guidelines so the client is aware of foods to consume to assure dietary adequacy.
2. Encourage decreased intake of fat and cholesterol-containing foods (see Chapter 1, Table 1–6).
3. Discuss the possibility of weight gain and its possible causes and prevention by decreasing kilocalorie and/or salt intake.

Evaluation

* Nutritional deficiencies from OCA use are prevented.

Client Education

- Clients on the pill for extended periods may become depleted of B vitamins, especially folate and vitamin B_6.
- OCAs may be contraindicated in clients with gestational diabetes, hypertension, family history of diabetes or heart disease.
- Routine use of multivitamins is usually unnecessary for OCA users.

PREMENSTRUAL SYNDROME

Premenstrual syndrome (PMS) may affect some women from the onset of menses until menopause, or it may not begin until later. Estimates of the prevalence of PMS among menstruating women in the US range from about 60 to 90%, with approximately 10 to 15% experiencing severe or disabling symptoms.

Individuals suffering from PMS report a wide range of symptoms. The common denominator is that the symptoms are cyclic, appearing 3 to 7 days before menses and dramatically disappearing after menstruation. One of the most common symptoms of PMS is nervous tension, exhibited by irritability, anxiety, crying, loneliness, restlessness, mood swings, and depression. Premenstrual cravings for sweets, increased appetite, and symptoms similar to hypoglycemia are often present.

Therapeutic interventions have included hormones, psychotropic medications, psychotherapy, and nutritional supplements. Nutritional factors linked with PMS include hypoglycemia; abnormal fatty acid metabolism; caffeine sensitivity; water retention; and deficiencies of vitamin B_6, magnesium, and vitamin E. Nutritional elements theorized to be the culprit, treatment, and findings are summarized in Table 14–10. The evidence that PMS is caused by any of these dietary substances is weak.

Currently, "there is no evidence that PMS is caused by a poor diet or vitamin/mineral deficiency or that it can be prevented or cured by dietary therapy" (Casey & Dwyer, 1987). As a result of the undesirable side effects of vitamin B_6 and magnesium, megadoses are not advisable. Nutrient intake (or consumption of the RDA levels) appears to be adequate. Restriction of and satisfying cravings for carbohydrate or other foods do not appear to affect other PMS symptoms.

TABLE 14–10

NUTRITIONAL THEORIES AND TREATMENT OF PMS

Theories Regarding Causes of PMS	Treatment	Evidence and Possible Adverse Effects
Vitamin B_6 deficiency	50–200 mg/day—used to treat depression and mood swings possibly caused by changes in estrogen levels related to subclinical vitamin B_6 deficiency	Evidence for the theory is weak; double blind studies reported inconsistent results. Larger doses (2–3 gm) have resulted in a reversible peripheral neuropathy
Subclinical hypoglycemia induced by deficiencies of vitamin B_6 and magnesium, which causes carbohydrate cravings	Carbohydrate intake is curtailed and distributed throughout the day to maintain blood sugar levels and affect neurotransmitter levels to decrease depression	Evidence of this theory is weak; studies have been poorly controlled; symptoms of PMS are not relieved by eating as they are with hypoglycemia
Unsaturated fatty acids	Evening primrose oil or certain vegetable oils that contain EFA are precursors of prostaglandins that stimulate ovarian progesterone synthesis	No deficiencies of EFA have been demonstrated during PMS. Studies showing positive effects were not well controlled. Primrose oil is expensive and may cause stomach irritation. Evidence is weak for both theory and treatment results
Magnesium	Magnesium supplements are used to relieve an unrecognized magnesium deficiency caused by overconsumption of high calcium and sugar	Magnesium deficiency in the US is rare. Serum magnesium levels are no lower than those of non-PMS sufferers. Increasing magnesium decreases calcium absorption. Effectiveness has not been demonstrated
Vitamin E deficiency	Vitamin E supplements at doses of 150–300 mg daily to relieve tender/sore breasts associated with PMS	One double blind study indicated vitamin E was more effective in relieving symptoms than placebo. Further research is needed. Evidence for vitamin E deficiency and the treatment is weak
Caffeine sensitivity	Abstinence from caffeine	Although the basis for the effect of caffeine is unclear, individuals vary greatly in their response to caffeine; some women benefit from withdrawal, and others are treated with caffeine
Water retention	Low-sodium diet and diuretics are used to prevent water retention and weight gain	Low-sodium diets are relatively ineffective in altering fluid balance; few studies substantiate that diuretics are more effective than placebos. The use of spironolactone (diuretic) may be more effective in treating PMS because of its antidepressant effects. However, it is very potent; dehydration and electrolyte depletion may result. Little evidence exists to support theory or treatment

NURSING APPLICATIONS

Assessment

Physical—for timing of symptoms in relation to menses, hypoglycemic symptoms (weakness, damp skin, confusion), psychological status, nervous tension.
Dietary—for cravings for sweets, increased appetite.
Laboratory—for hypoglycemia.

Interventions

1. Stress eating small meals and restricting sugar and alcohol because these may minimize PMS discomforts.

Evaluation

* Desired outcomes include client planning menus to decrease PMS symptoms and verbalizing nutritional myths of PMS.

Client Education

- Emphasize (1) following the dietary guidelines, (2) exercising regularly, and (3) reducing stress.
- Caffeine and sodium restriction does not appear to alleviate PMS symptoms in most clients.
- Nonprescription PMS supplements are available, but they may or may not contain the desired nutrients. For example, magnesium may be a component of the supplement, which is desirable; if calcium is also present, however, the absorption of magnesium would be decreased.
- Many of the PMS supplements are megadoses of vitamins; they should be taken cautiously under a physician's care.

NUTRITION UPDATE 14–1: FETAL ALCOHOL SYNDROME

As little as 2 oz/day of alcohol can cause fetal alcohol syndrome (FAS), a condition characterized by irreversible brain damage and mental retardation. Approximately 10,000 US infants are born with FAS each year (Streissguth et al, 1991). The first trimester is the most vulnerable time for the fetus, yet the woman may not even be aware of the pregnancy, especially during the first crucial month. Four to 5 drinks a day, or at least 45 drinks per month, can produce the full FAS syndrome (Table 14–11), whereas smaller amounts may be associated with adverse effects such as spontaneous abortion, growth retardation, and subtle behavioral effects without the physical anomalies (IM, 1990).

The FAS child has specific physiological deformities (Fig. 14–6). Alcohol increases urinary zinc losses, and infants with FAS have been reported to have low plasma zinc levels. It has been hypothesized that zinc deficiency may play a role in the abnormal facial features (IM, 1990). The mental and physical abnormalities cannot be reversed.

Even with adequate nutrition, normal development of fetal organs is jeopardized. Other proclivities that usually accompany alcohol consumption (e.g., smoking, excessive amounts of coffee the morning after, poor eating habits with little attention to needed nutrients, and perhaps use of tranquilizers) may also adversely affect the unborn child. Ethanol is a source of energy; thus, chronic alcoholics may have a relatively low intake of protein, essential fats, vitamins, and minerals. Alcohol may impair placental transport of amino acids, calcium, and some vitamins.

Because the brain has a special affinity for alcohol, it is one of the first organs

TABLE 14–11

FETAL ALCOHOL SYNDROME

1. Irreversible mental retardation
2. Head too small (microcephaly)
3. Irritability in infancy and hyperactivity in childhood
4. Less growth in height and weight with more discrepancy in height prenatally and throughout life
5. Eyes
   a. Too close together
   b. Mongolian look; a fold of skin starting at the root of the nose goes to the point where the eyebrow starts and may cover the inner corner of the eye (epicanthus)
   c. Drooping of upper eye lid (ptosis)
   d. Uncontrollable squinting (strabismus)
   e. Nearsightedness (myopia)
6. Nose
   a. Undefined, short, and upturned, remains too short for life
   b. No bridge from the forehead to the nose
   c. Normal pair of ridges with an indentation between them from the bottom of the nose to the upper lip is not seen
7. Ears are poorly formed and incorrectly placed
8. Mouth
   a. Prominent ridges in palate
   b. Cleft lip
   c. Cleft palate
   d. Small teeth with faulty enamel
   e. Small jaws
9. Poor coordination
10. Weak skeletal muscles seen as weakness and floppiness in infants with less ability and strength later in life (hypotonia)
11. Bones and joints underdeveloped
12. Heart—atrial and ventricular membrane wall defects

From FL Iber. The fetal alcohol syndrome. *Nutrition Today* 1980; 15(4):4–11. © by Williams & Wilkins, 1980.

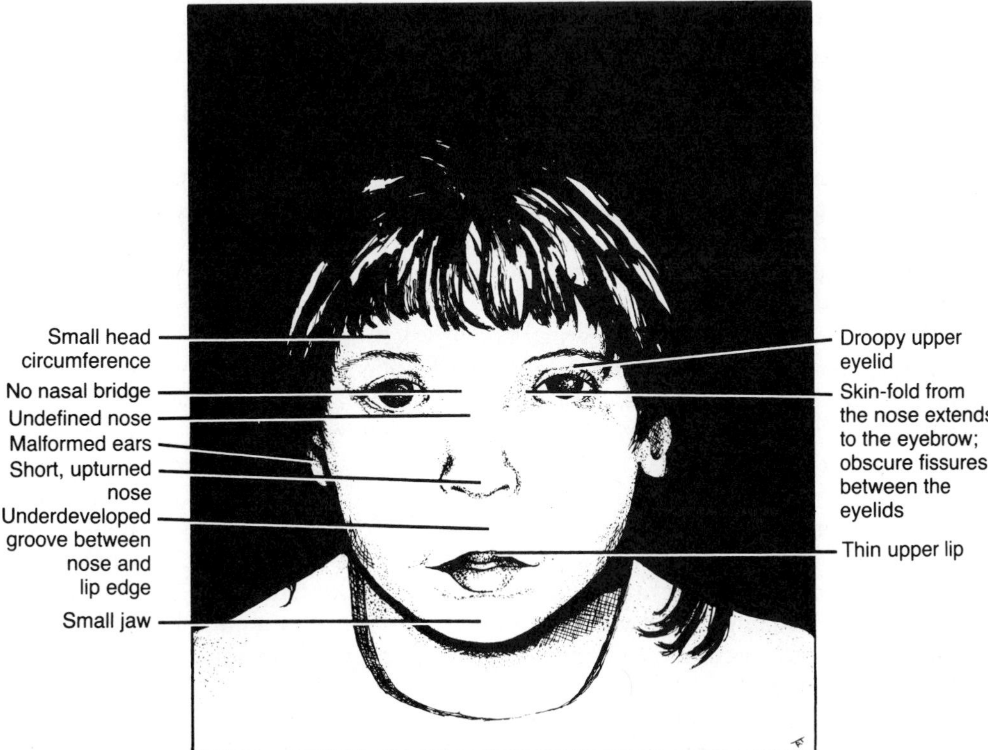

Figure 14–6 Facial anomalies of a child with fetal alcohol syndrome.

affected. Intellectual impairment is frequently reported for children with FAS. Even at birth, the circumference of the head is small (microcephaly), indicating abnormal brain capacity (i.e., 140 gm in an FAS infant compared with a normal brain weighing 400 gm). Fewer brain cells exist, with damaged cells preventing normal functioning; fewer neurons result in disorganized thought. The thinking ability of the brain is permanently disturbed; the average IQ is 68 (Streissguth et al, 1991). Maladaptive behaviors, such as poor judgment, distractability, and social interaction problems are common. Additionally, as a result of fewer total body cells, abnormal weight gain adversely affects normal cell development and growth.

Because of the global adverse effects of alcohol intake, efforts to decrease or stop intake are appropriate. Diet counseling and other efforts to improve food intake, such as referral to a social worker for food or monetary resources, are warranted. The subcommittee has recommended the use of multivitamin-mineral supplements for heavy substance abusers who have difficulty changing their habits to improve nutrient intake (IM, 1990).

NUTRITION UPDATE 14–2: ADOLESCENT PREGNANCY

Pregnancy in females under 18 presents challenges to health care professionals. Basic problems include health and social factors, which are usually complicated by psychological, educational, nutritional, and vocational difficulties. A pregnant adolescent is generally viewed as a high-risk client because of the frequency of premature or LBW infants. In 1985, 467,000 teenagers between 15 and 19 years old gave birth, with 10,000 infants born to girls under 15 years of age in the US (NCHS, 1987).

GA is the difference between chronological age and age at onset of menses.

Nutritional status is considered to be one of the most important environmental factors affecting the outcome of the fetus and the teenage mother. **Gynecological age (GA)** is an indirect measure of physiological maturity and growth potential. Teenagers with a GA of less than 4 years are still experiencing growth and physiological maturity. If the adolescent is still growing, the mother and fetus may compete for the available nutrients.

Energy and nutrient needs during adolescent pregnancy are influenced by GA, activity level, and prepregnancy nutritional status. Nutritional requirements are quite high to meet the growth needs for the adolescent and the fetus. Estimates for kilocaloric requirements are made by combining the RDA for nonpregnant females of the appropriate age with the allowance for pregnancy. Additional allowance is made for teenagers with a low pregestational weight. Increased energy requirements are usually met without concentrated effort as a result of increased appetite. However, teenagers are frequently concerned about weight gain.

Ketosis—the accumulation of ketone (acidic by-products of lipid metabolism) that occurs when inadequate amounts of glucose are available.

A pregnant teenager requires more thiamin, riboflavin, niacin, vitamin D, calcium, and phosphorus than the adult woman. Intake of kilocalorie-dense foods and erratic eating may preclude adequate intake of required nutrients. Meal skipping may increase the risk of **ketosis,** which is associated with high rates of perinatal mortality.

Since many of these adolescents are from economically deprived populations, adequate food resources may not be available. Lack of knowledge about nutrition, food cravings, and aversions are frequently causes of poor food choices.

Calcium, phosphorus, and vitamin D are essential for optimal bone growth, and larger amounts are needed during adolescence. Inadequate calcium intake may deplete maternal stores.

Teenagers may have an increased risk of iron deficiency because of increased iron requirements that are due to growth. If the adolescent is from a poor socioeconomic background, she is at risk for prepregnancy iron deficiency. Adolescents who are anemic and underweight are more likely to deliver an LBW infant.

As compared with an older woman, young adolescents with similar pregnancy weight gain and prepregnancy weight frequently deliver a smaller infant. Inadequate weight gain is more likely to occur in adolescents who (1) desire to be thin, (2) may attempt to conceal their pregnancy, (3) have inadequate food resources, or (4) use illicit drugs.

Counseling is needed to assess dietary patterns and promote changes so the adolescent will have a healthy infant. A positive approach in nutrition counseling is important to promote compliance. Adherence to suggestions or negotiated changes in food habits is related to her understanding of the role of food intake in promoting growth and health for herself and the baby. As a rule, these clients have never been responsible for their own nutritional well-being, much less another person's. One of the main objectives of nutritional counseling is to help the client to understand and carry out this responsibility.

Basic points for discussion include issues that interfere with nourishment, defining the role of foods and health, food resources, guidance in kilocaloric intake to permit appropriate weight gain, and information regarding nutrient-rich foods (ADA, 1989). Nutritional supplements are usually indicated; regular use of the appropriate prenatal vitamin-mineral supplement should be reinforced.

Active listening and empathy for the client's concerns and needs are vital. Effective counseling can elicit nutritional choices compatible with the adolescent's lifestyle and her pregnancy state.

SUMMARY

Primary factors for a successful pregnancy are the previous nutritional status, adequate weight gain, and appropriate intake of essential nutrients during pregnancy.

Both kilocalorie and protein requirements are increased during pregnancy and lactation. Other nutrient requirements, especially calcium, iron, and folate, are also increased. These increased nutrient requirements can be achieved by moderate increases in whole grains, milk, legumes, and raw fruits and vegetables. An iron supplement (30 mg) is recommended during the second and third trimesters of pregnancy. Other supplements are encouraged if dietary assessment indicates inadequacy of the diet, and dietary changes are not feasible.

Weight gain is the most reliable tool for assessing nutrient adequacy. Ideal weight gain is 25 to 35 lbs for gravidas with a desirable weight for height before the pregnancy. Nutrient intake is actually more important than weight gain. Assessment of dietary practices is encouraged, followed by other steps in the nutritional nursing process.

Breast-feeding has many advantages for infant and mother. Virtually all women are able to produce milk that provides adequate nutrients for optimal growth and health of the infant. The nurse's support and knowledge are crucial for mothers attempting and continuing breast-feeding.

NURSING PROCESS IN ACTION

Mary is a first-time mother and wants to succeed at breast-feeding. She does not think the baby will get enough milk and is afraid the infant won't "latch on." Her husband is supportive of her decision.

Nutritional Assessment

- Beliefs about breast-feeding.
- Kilocalorie, calcium, vitamin, fluid, and carbohydrate intake.
- Any prescribed medications.
- Breast and nipple conditioning.
- Role models for breast-feeding.
- Knowledge of support groups.

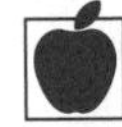

Dietary Nursing Diagnosis

High risk for ineffective breast-feeding RT inexperience with breast-feeding.

Nutritional Goals

Mother will state satisfaction with breast-feeding and verbalize activities that hinder or promote effective breast-feeding.

Nutritional Implementation 

Intervention: Clarify misconceptions by offering written material, providing video to watch or audiotapes.

Rationale: Knowledge will decrease anxiety and enhance the let-down reflex.

Intervention: Allow infant to suck immediately after birth in the birthing room if possible and then on demand rather than following a rigid schedule.

Rationale: The infant who is allowed to breast-feed immediately usually "latches on" more easily. The more the infant nurses, the more milk is produced.

Intervention: Review different positions: sitting or side lying. Use pillows for positioning and comfort.

Rationale: Correct positions facilitate breast-feeding, and comfort promotes relaxation, thus enhancing the let-down process.

Intervention: Demonstrate how to assist infant to "latch on."

Rationale: The grasp allows mother to point nipple directly into infant's mouth and does not constrict milk flow as the scissor hold does. Touching the infant's cheek stimulates the "rooting reflex" that helps infant latch on. Insertion of the areola decreases the chance of complications occurring (let-down inhibited, bruising, engorgement). Since the client is worried infant will not latch on, this will help allay fears.

Intervention: Recommend increasing feeding times, gradually building up to 40 minutes (20 minutes on each breast) per feeding; offering both breasts at each feeding; alternating the beginning side each time; inserting finger in infant's mouth to break suction; not burping infant unless infant grunts or seems full.

Rationale: Gradually building up decreases chance for sore nipples. Offering both breasts decreases chance of engorgement. Inserting finger allows nipple to be removed freely, thus decreasing chance of pain and cracks. Burping is not necessary for breast-fed infants since less air is ingested.

Intervention: Reassure client that this is a learning time for her and the baby, and they will develop together (Carpenito, 1992).

Rationale: Even though breast-feeding is physiologically natural, it does not come naturally. Education is needed.

Intervention: Encourage husband to change infant and to bring to mother for nursing.

Rationale: Since the husband is supportive, this will involve him in the infant's care and not make him feel excluded.

Intervention: Refer to La Leche League.
Rationale: This group can provide support and knowledge to the new mother.

Intervention: Encourage an additional 500 kcal daily.
Rationale: Approximately 85 kcal are needed for every 100 ml of milk produced (NRC, 1989).

Intervention: Offer foods high in vitamin B_6, magnesium, zinc, calcium, and folate.
Rationale: These are the nutrients most likely to be deficient.

Intervention: Encourage an additional 1000 ml/day of fluids.
Rationale: The lactating woman requires additional fluids to replace that secreted in milk.

Intervention: Suggest foods high in carbohydrate and avoidance of alcohol.
Rationale: Carbohydrate intake is important for maintaining lactose synthesis and milk volume. Alcohol inhibits the let-down reflex.

Evaluation

Goals have been achieved if mother states that she enjoys breast-feeding and she is glad she chose to breast-feed. She would also verbalize that inserting the whole areola rather than just the nipple is advantageous for feeding, as is a comfortable position. She will avoid alcohol.

STUDENT READINESS

1. Plan the food intake for 1 day for a pregnant woman and discuss your decisions.
2. Describe nutritional care for adolescent pregnancy.
3. Discuss FAS and explain how alcohol affects the fetus.
4. Which nutrients may be needed if dietary assessment indicates deficient intake that cannot be corrected by changing eating habits?
5. Discuss advantages and disadvantages as well as interventions for breast-feeding.
6. Describe nutritional care for PMS.
7. Outline nutrient adjustments and food modifications for vegetarian pregnant women.

CASE STUDY

Mrs. M. A. is a 30-year-old primigravida. She is now in the first trimester. Before her pregnancy, she weighed 55 kg; she is 166 cm tall. She has always been weight conscious and carefully guards against weight gain. She and her husband drink 2 to 3 cocktails each week and occasionally have wine with dinner. Although she is excited about her pregnancy, she expresses concern to the nutritionist about gaining weight. Her Hgb, Hct, and serum albumin are within normal limits.

1. How much weight should she gain in the first trimester? The second trimester? The third trimester?
2. Mrs. M. A. does not care for milk. How much milk should she drink each day? What would you suggest to her to increase her calcium intake?
3. How would you counsel her about the alcohol usually consumed?
4. Mrs. M. A. asks if she should reduce her salt intake. What would you tell her?
5. What are some helpful hints for dealing with morning sickness?

CASE STUDY

Cindy, 14 years old, is 3 months pregnant. Diet history reveals she is weight conscious and has used several fad diets to lose weight. She has a habit of skipping breakfast and usually eats only fruit and yogurt for lunch. She snacks on chips, soda pop, and nuts. Supper involves hamburgers or pizza and ice cream for dessert. She is medium frame, weighs 45 kg, and height is 5′4″. Her Hgb was 11 gm/dl with no protein or glucose in the urine. Cindy does not want an abortion and does not want to marry the father. Her family does not know because she is afraid to tell them. She does want to continue school. Cindy's menses started when she was 12 years old.

1. What is Cindy's GA? Is she in the high-risk category?
2. What are the strengths and weaknesses about Cindy's diet?
3. From the above-mentioned diet, how would you counsel Cindy?
4. Since she is a teenager, what nutrients are likely to be insufficient?
5. What are the requirements for the following: kilocalories, protein, and weight?
6. Why is a vitamin and mineral supplement ordered for Cindy?
7. What are some resources/referrals for Cindy?
8. What psychological factors could affect her eating patterns?
9. What are some nursing diagnosis/goals and interventions for Cindy?
10. How is Cindy's pregnancy different from a 26-year-old's?

REFERENCES

Abel EL, Sokol RJ. Incidence of fetal alcohol syndrome and economic impact of FAS-related anomalies. *Drug Alcohol Depend* 1987 Jan; 19(1):51–70.

American Dietetic Association (ADA). Nutrition management of adolescent pregnancy. *J Am Diet Assoc* 1989 Jan; 89(1):104–108.

Belizàn JM, et al. Calcium supplementation to prevent hypertensive disorders of pregnancy. *N Engl J Med* 1991 Nov 14; 325(20):1399–1405.

Boyce RA. Enteral nutrition in hyperemesis gravidarum: A new development. *J Am Diet Assoc* 1992 June; 92(6):733–736.

Campbell DM. Trace element needs in human pregnancy. *Proc Nutr Soc* 1988 Feb; 47(1):45–53.

Carpenito LD. *Nursing Diagnosis: Application to Clinical Practice.* 4th ed. Philadelphia, JB Lippincott, 1992.

Carruth BR, Skinner JD. Practitioners beware: Regional differences in beliefs about nutrition during pregnancy. *J Am Diet Assoc* 1991 Apr; 91(4):435–440.

Casey V, Dwyer JT. Premenstrual syndrome: Theories and evidence. *Nutr Today* 1987 Nov-Dec; 22(6):4–12.

Czeizel AE, Dudás I. Prevention of the first occurrence of neural-tube deficit by periconceptional vitamin supplementation. *N Engl J Med* 1992 Dec 24; 337(26): 1832–5.

Dickey RD. *Managing Contraceptive Pill Patients.* 6th ed. Durant OK, CIP, Inc, 1991.

Doyle W, et al. Low birth weight and maternal diet. *Midwife Health Visitor & Community Nurse* 1991 Feb; 27(2): 44, 46.

Dwyer JT. Nutritional consequences of vegetarianism. *Annu Rev Nutr* 1991; 11:61–91.

Godsland IF, et al. The effect of different formulations of oral contraceptive agents on lipid and carbohydrate metabolism. *N Engl J Med* 1990 Nov 15; 323(20):1375–1380.

Hallberg L. Iron balance in pregnancy. *In* Berger H (ed): *Vitamins and Minerals in Pregnancy and Lactation.* New York, Raven Press, 1988.

Horner RD, et al. Pica practices of pregnant women. *J Am Diet Assoc* 1991 Jan; 91(1):34–38.

Huber AM, et al. Folate nutriture in pregnancy. *J Am Diet Assoc* 1988 July; 88(7):791–795.

Institute of Medicine (IM) Subcommittee on Nutritional Status and Weight Gain During Pregnancy. *Nutrition During Lactation.* Washington, D.C., National Academy Press, 1991.

Institute of Medicine (IM) Subcommittee on Nutritional Status and Weight Gain During Pregnancy. *Nutrition During Pregnancy.* Washington, D.C., National Academy Press, 1990.

Jason J. Breast feeding in 1991. *N Engl J Med* 1991 Oct 3; 325(14):1036–1037.

Kearney NH, et al. Breast-feeding problems in the first week postpartum. *Nurs Res* 1990 March-Apr; 39(2):90–95.

King JC, Weininger J. Pregnancy and lactation. *In* Brown ML (ed): *Present Knowledge in Nutrition.* 6th ed. Washington, D.C., Nutrition Foundation, 1990: 314–319.

Medical Research Council (MRC) Vitamin Study Research Group. Prevention of neural tube defects. *Lancet* 1991 July 20; 338(8160):131–136.

Mitchell MC, Lerner E. Weight gain and pregnancy outcome in underweight and normal weight women. *J Am Diet Assoc* 1989 May; 89(5):634–641.

Myatt L. The association of calcium with hypertension of pregnancy and preterm labor. *Nutr & the MD* 1992 Feb; 18(2):13.

Naeye RL. Maternal body weight and pregnancy outcome. *Am J Clin Nutr* 1990 Aug; 52(2):273–279.

National Academy of Sciences (NAS). *Maternal Nutrition and the Course of Pregnancy.* Report of the Committee on Maternal Nutrition, Food and Nutrition Board. Washington, D.C., National Academy of Sciences, 1970.

National Center for Health Statistics (NCHS). Advance report of final natality statistics, 1985. Monthly Vital Statistics Report 36, No 4, July 17, 1987.

National Research Council (NRC). *Recommended Dietary Allowances.* 10th ed. Washington, D.C., National Academy Press, 1989.

Pomerance HH. Growth in breast-fed children. *Hum Biol* 1987 Aug; 59(4):687–693.

Ryan AS, et al. A comparison of breast feeding data from the National Surveys of Family Growth and the Ross laboratories mother's surveys. *Am J Public Health* 1991 Aug; 81(8): 1049–1051.

Streissguth AP, et al. Fetal alcohol syndrome in adolescents and adults. *JAMA* 1991 Apr 17; 265(15):1961–1967.

Susser M. Maternal weight gain, infant birth weight, and diet: Causal sequences. *Am J Clin Nutr* 1991 June; 53(6):1384–1396.

Trouba PH, et al. Summary document of nutrition intervention in prenatal care. *J Am Diet Assoc* 1991 Sept; 91(suppl 9):S21–S26.

US Department of Health and Human Services (USDHHS), Public Health Service. *Healthy People 2000.* Washington, D.C., Government Printing Office, 1990.

Walravens PA, et al. Zinc supplements in breast-fed infants. *Lancet* 1992 Sept; 340(8821):683–685.

Wegman M. Annual summary of vital statistics —1988. *Pediatrics* 1989 Dec; 84(6):943–956.

Whitehead RG. Pregnancy and lactation. *In* Shils ME, Young VR (eds): *Modern Nutrition in Health and Disease.* 7th ed. Philadelphia, Lea & Febiger, 1988: 931–943.

Winick M. *Nutrition, Pregnancy, and Early Infancy.* Baltimore, Williams & Wilkins, 1989.

Winick M, et al. Pregnancy and lactation. *In* Kinney JM, et al. *Nutrition and Metabolism in Patient Care.* Philadelphia, WB Saunders, 1988: 131–144.

Worthington-Roberts B, et al. *Nutrition in Pregnancy and Lactation.* St Louis, CV Mosby, 1989.

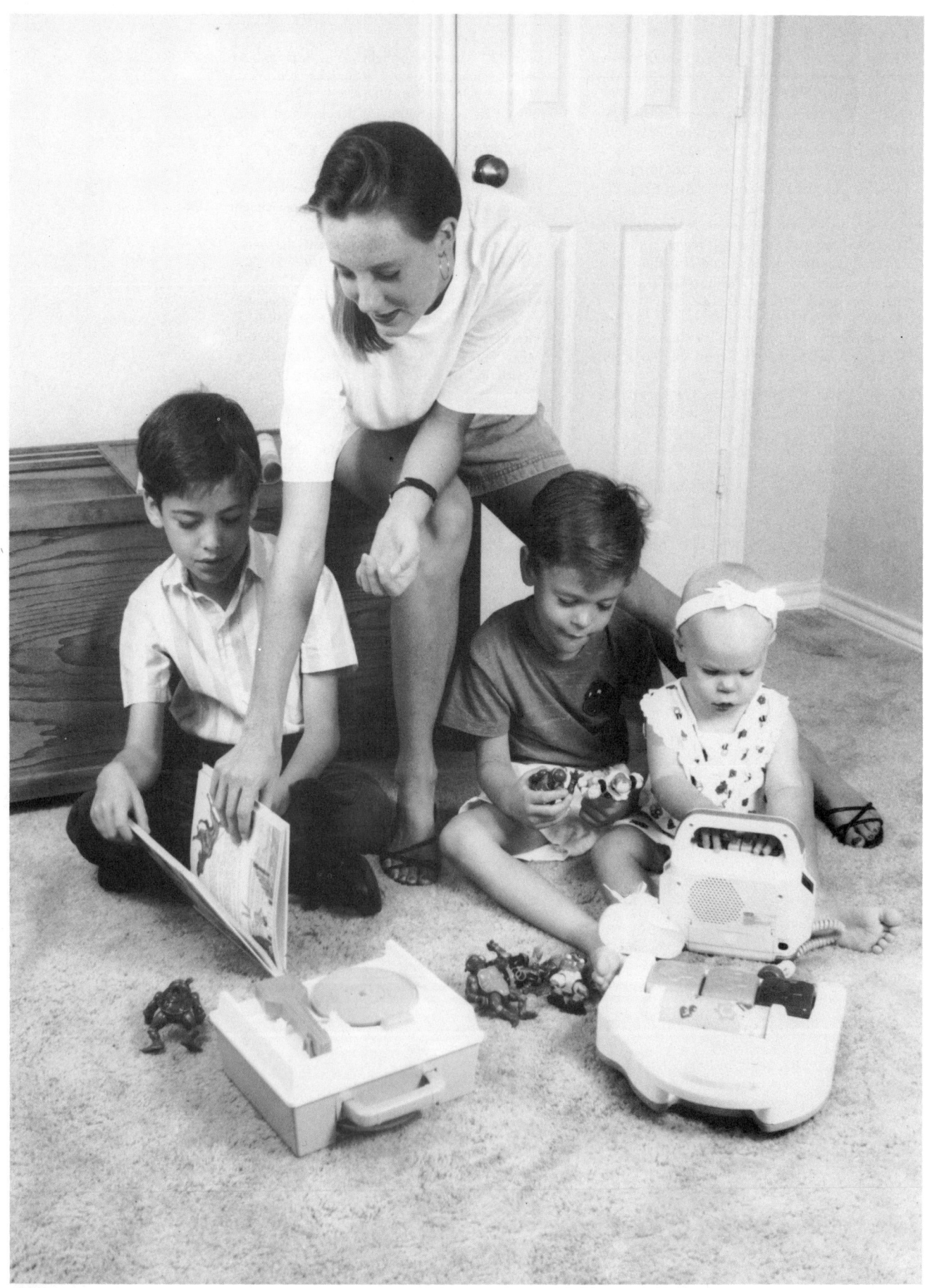

Nutritional Considerations of Infancy, Childhood, and Adolescence

CHAPTER 15

OUTLINE

IX. TODDLER AND PRESCHOOL CHILDREN
  A. Feeding Toddlers (1 to 3 Years Old)
  B. Preschool Children (4 to 6 Years Old)
  Nursing Applications
X. TODDLER/PRESCHOOL PROBLEMS RELATED TO NUTRITION
  A. Asphyxiation by Food
  Nursing Applications
  B. Dental Caries
  Nursing Applications
  C. Attention Deficit Hyperactivity Disorder
  Nursing Applications
  D. Lead Toxicity
  Nursing Applications
XI. SCHOOL-AGE CHILDREN (7 TO 12 YEARS OLD)
  Nursing Applications
XII. ADOLESCENTS
  A. Growth and Nutrient Requirements
  B. Influential Factors on Eating Habits
  C. Nutrition Counseling
  Nursing Applications
XIII. FACTORS RELATED TO SCHOOL-AGE CHILDREN'S NUTRITION
  A. Breakfast
  B. School Lunch
  Nursing Applications
XIV. ILLNESS
  Nursing Applications

OBJECTIVES

THE STUDENT WILL BE ABLE TO:

- Describe the procedure for adding infant foods after the initial stage of feeding by bottle or breast.
- Plan meals with adequate nutrients for school-age children and adolescent boys and girls according to the RDAs.
- Discuss ways to handle typical nutritional problems in infancy, childhood, and adolescence.
- Apply nursing principles to nutritional needs during infancy, childhood, and adolescence.
- Identify client education for infancy, childhood, and adolescent nutrition.

TEST YOUR NQ (True/False)

1. Commercial formulas are fairly standardized in their nutrient content.
2. Goat milk should be given to infants who are allergic to formula.
3. Solid foods should be introduced at 6 weeks of age.
4. Orange juice is the first fruit juice to offer an infant.
5. Food should be withheld from an infant with diarrhea to allow the digestive tract to rest.
6. Toddlers may refuse to eat anything except for 1 food for several days.
7. Preschool children generally dislike mixed dishes such as casseroles and stews.
8. The goal for obese children is allowing them to grow into their weight.
9. Supper is the most likely meal to be skipped by all school-age children.
10. During adolescence, more nutrients are required than for any other stage of life.

"We will tomorrow be dependent on the very children who today are dependent on us" (Select Panel, 1981). Yet nearly 55 million children in the US under the age of 12, or 1 in 8, suffer from hunger. Children at risk of undernutrition and inadequate food intake are from low-income families, have special health care needs, or have a primary caregiver who is mentally ill or chemically dependent (Splet & Story, 1991).

Several goals of the US Public Health Services' Year 2000 Health Objectives (USDHHS, 1990) particularly target improved infant and child nutrition (in addition to the breast-feeding goal addressed in Chapter 14):

1. Reduce growth retardation of low-income children age 5 and younger.
2. Reduce iron deficiency among children from 1 to 4 years of age.
3. Increase the proportion of parents and caregivers who use feeding practices that prevent baby bottle tooth decay.
4. Increase the proportion of school lunch and breakfast programs that provide menus consistent with nutrition principles in the Dietary Guidelines for Americans.
5. Increase the proportion of schools that provide nutrition education from preschool through 12th grade.
6. Increase calcium intake so at least 50% of youth, age 12 through 24, consume 3 or more servings of foods rich in calcium daily.
7. Reduce overweight to a prevalence of no more than 15% among adolescents age 12 through 19.
8. Increase to at least 50% the proportion of overweight people age 12 and older who have adopted sound dietary practices combined with regular physical activity to attain an appropriate body weight.

Achievement of these goals will be a major milestone for the optimal health of infants and children and their future.

Name 4 goals for optimal health of infants and children.

GROWTH

Growth is the definitive test of health and is used as the single most sensitive and specific indicator of nutritional status. It is important that nurses who work with infants and children be familiar with normal growth and developmental patterns that reflect the adequacy of nutrition intake. The birth weight of an infant doubles in 4 months (from 7½ to 14 lbs), and by 1 year, it has usually tripled. The growth spurt then slows down, and the infant gains only another 4 to 6 lbs until 2 years old.

The weight gain tapers off during the second year, with the weight increment slightly less than the birth weight. Weight usually proceeds at this constant rate until age 9 or 10. With the beginning of puberty, a growth spurt starts that may continue through adolescence. This growth spurt contributes about 50% to final adult weight (Gong & Heald, 1988).

Length or height is increased by 50% by 1 year of age and doubles by age 4. (Since the infant is unable to stand, recumbent length is measured.) One half of adult height is achieved by age 2½ to 3 years of age. Height increases parallel that of weight with rapid increases during adolescence. The rapid spurt in height for a girl precedes that of the boy by about 2 years (11 to 15 years in girls; 12 to 17 years in boys). The adolescent growth spurt varies in age of onset, intensity, and duration. The end of this adolescent growth spurt is signaled by slowing of growth, completion of sexual maturation, and closure of the epiphyses of long bones.

Increases in weight and height are accompanied by changes in component tissues, or lean body mass, and adiposity. Total body water decreases from approximately 70% at birth to 60% by age 1. This reduction is principally extracellular, as a result of increases in adipose tissue and lean body mass. Adipose tissue or fat storage shows more variability between different clients than any other component tissue. Until the infant is approximately 9 months of age, fat accumulates rapidly. In teenagers, lean body mass increases significantly in boys, whereas female hormones promote greater fat deposition. By about 18 years of age, body fat in girls is approximately 28%, whereas in boys, it is approximately 15%.

The period most critical to growth of the brain begins 9 months before birth and continues into the second year. During this time, the actual number of cells and the size of the head (cell mass) depend on optimum nutrients. Head circumference achieves two-thirds of its postnatal growth by 24 months of age.

Height, weight, and head circumferences are measured and compared with standard growth charts. The most commonly used growth charts in the US were prepared by the National Center for Health Statistics (NCHS). Growth charts for each sex are available for (1) height for age (assesses linear growth), (2) weight for age (assesses rate of weight gain), (3) weight for height (assesses weight status based on height—similar to BMI measurement), and (4) head circumference for age (also a measure of growth). Separate charts are available from 0 to 36 months and 2 to 18 years of age. The head circumference chart is for children under 3 years of age. These charts are provided in Appendix C–8.

Percentile measures on a scale of 100, representing the client's status in relation to 100 other age-matched and gender-matched children.

What is the desired weight gain of a child at 4 months old, 1 year old, and between 1 to 2 years old? Describe gains in height from birth through adolescence. When does the most critical growth period of the brain occur? Name the 4 charts available to assess growth.

Using these charts, the child is ranked by **percentile** division. A client at the 75th percentile is considered above average, with 75 out of 100 children being shorter/lighter and 25 being taller/heavier. If the child is not growing as expected, the adequacy of nutrient intake is investigated. Before concluding malnutrition is responsible for growth stunting, nurses must consider other possibilities. When a child is below the 50th percentile for height but weight is proportionally below the 50th percentile, genetic factors or endocrine deficiency may be responsible. Chronic disease status usually inhibits growth. Weight is more sensitive to nutritional status than height but can be influenced by hydration status.

NURSING APPLICATIONS

Assessment

Physical—for weight, length, head circumference, percentile on growth chart.

Interventions

1. Monitor serial weights and heights. If abnormality in rate of growth is detected, caution the mother to adjust feedings accordingly. If this is ineffective, refer to the physician or registered dietitian.

Client Education

- A newborn infant will lose weight for the first few days but should not lose more than 10% of the birth weight or take longer than 10 to 14 days to regain it.
- Nutritional requirements parallel rate of growth, with increased needs of all nutrients during rapid growth periods to achieve optimal height.
- Increasing size results in greater nutritional requirements, but the need for kilocalories per kilogram decreases.
- Differences in physical activity affect nutrient requirements.

NEWBORNS

Not only the present health, but also the future lifelong health for the newborn depends on the loving care and feeding from the mother or caretaker. The infant is normally able to thrive on human milk or commercially available formulas, but many of the physiological systems are immature at birth. Because of the small stomach capacity, frequent feedings are needed. Digestion and absorption of fats are inefficient, possibly related to low pancreatic lipase activity and reduced bile acid pool. Lactase levels at birth are normal, but low levels of pancreatic amylase result in an inability to handle large amounts of starches.

The newborn's immature kidneys require a low **renal solute load** because of inability to concentrate the urine. Thus, infants are vulnerable to water imbalance.

Renal solute load is the amount of solute, or nonmetabolizable dietary components, especially excess electrolytes and nitrogenous compounds (from protein metabolism), that must be excreted by the kidney.

Because of limited transplacental transfer of vitamin K, very low concentrations of vitamin K, and possibly vitamin K malabsorption, newborn infants are at risk of hemorrhagic disease (Von Kries, 1991). Oral vitamin K at birth is effective in preventing classic hemorrhagic disease, but parenteral prophylaxis is effective in preventing intracranial hemorrhage that occurs between the second and 26th weeks of life, especially in exclusively breast-fed infants (McNinch & Tripp, 1991).

Why are frequent feedings needed? Why are fats inefficiently absorbed? Why are infants unable to handle large amounts of starches? Describe possible reasons for newborn's risk of hemorrhagic diseases.

Premature and Low Birth Weight Infants

As discussed in Chapter 14, premature and LBW infants are at high risk for many complications. They are slow to catch up to normal growth rates. Their bodies contain more water and less protein and fat, bones are poorly calcified, normal sucking reflexes are poorly developed, and the GI tract and renal functions are less well developed. Immunological abnormalities persist for several months with increased susceptibility to infection for the first year. Additionally, the liver is immature in its enzyme system and iron stores. For these reasons, feedings for the premature infant are specially tailored to the infant's problems.

What are some physical problems in premature and LBW infants?

INFANT NUTRITIONAL REQUIREMENTS

Adequate nutrition is more important during infancy and childhood than for any other stage of the life cycle. Even after allowing for social and environmental factors, intake of animal products is an important predictor of cognitive performance in school, stunting or retardation of linear growth, and behavioral development (Allen, 1991). Zinc deficiency leads to growth stunting; iron deficiency anemia impairs cognitive function and school achievement (Simeon & Grantham-McGregor, 1990). Lowered resistance to infections and disease, increased apathy, and reduced activity levels are also consequences of undernutrition. Overnutrition may result in such conditions as obesity, atherosclerosis, and hypertension in adult years (Splet & Story, 1991).

What is an important predictor of cognitive performance? What do iron and zinc deficiency lead to?

Full-Term Infants

As might be expected from the rapid growth rate, energy requirements are much higher than for an adult—90 to 120 kcal/kg/day versus 30 to 40 kcal/kg/day. Additionally, infants have a higher resting metabolic rate, and intestinal absorption is relatively inefficient.

The RDA for protein is 13 gm daily. This translates to about 1.6 to 2.2 gm/kg body weight. As a result of immature renal function, total protein should not exceed 20% of the kilocalories. Both breast milk and commercial formulas provide about 50% of the kilocalories from fat to supply the high kilocaloric needs. A minimum of 0.5 to 1 gm linoleic acid per kilogram is necessary daily to prevent EFA deficiency (Walker & Hendricks, 1985).

What are the kilocaloric requirements for a full-term infant; for protein; for fat?

Premature and Low Birth Weight Infants

Premature infants, especially LBW infants, may require tube feedings or TPN because of the poorly developed sucking reflex and immature digestive system. However, if the infant is able to suck and digest foods, bottle-feeding or breast-feeding is initiated. Increased levels of nutrients are needed; feedings are cautiously administered to avoid overloading the tiny immature digestive tract. The LBW infant weighing more than 1750 gm (almost 4 lbs) can usually be fed as a term infant.

Although nutrient requirements are higher than for full-term infants, the organ systems are usually unable to handle these requirements efficiently. Protein is the primary nutrient needed. However, the digestive system is not able to digest the higher protein intake, and the renal system is unable to excrete the higher nitrogen load. Higher levels of calcium in cow's milk lead to malabsorption of saturated fatty acids and may lower calcium absorption; high lipid intake appears to lower calcium absorption.

Breast milk from mothers delivering prematurely is higher in protein and lower in lactose than full-term breast milk, but neither breast milk nor special formulas are able to sustain growth at the intrauterine rate. Fats from breast milk are better digested and absorbed than from commercial formulas. The immune substances present in mother's milk may be more advantageous than the faster growth rate established on special formulas (Winick, 1989).

When can an LBW infant be fed as a term infant? What are the energy needs of LBW infants?

Energy needs are increased from 100 kcal/kg/day for a normal infant to 140 kcal/kg/day for the LBW infant. Adequate kilocaloric intake in these infants to sustain an appropriate rate of growth requires more than 20 kcal/oz. As a result of poor body stores and physiological immaturity, premature infants require larger amounts of many of the vitamins and minerals than full-term infants.

COMMERCIAL FORMULAS

In Chapter 14, the advantages of breast milk and its nutritional adequacy were discussed. The numerous problems associated with commercial formulas in the past

TABLE 15–1

RECOMMENDED DIETARY ALLOWANCES FOR INFANTS COMPARED WITH NUTRIENT CONTENT OF HUMAN MILK, COW MILK, AND INFANT FORMULA

Nutrient	Recommended Dietary Allowances* 0 to 6 Months	6 to 12 Months	Human Milk+ (per liter)	Cow Milk‡ (per liter)	Average Commercial Formula
Kilocalories	108/kg	98/kg	750	670	680
Protein (gm)	2.2/kg	1.6/kg	11	20	15
Fat (gm)			45	36	36
Cholesterol (mg)			238	119	160
Calcium (mg)	400	600	295	1220	500
Phosphorus (mg)	300	500	143	935	300
Iron (mg)	6	10	0.2	0.5	12/1.4§
Sodium (mEq)	5	8.7	6.6	21	10
Potassium (mEq)	12.8	17.9	13	11	20
Renal solute load (mOsm/L)			79	221	150

* Data from National Research Council. Recommended Dietary Allowances. Washington, D.C., National Academy Press, 1989.
+ Data from Souci SW, et al. Food Composition and Nutrition Tables 1986/87. 3rd ed. Stuttgart, Wissenschaftliche Verlagsgesellschaft, 1986.
‡ Whole milk (3.5% fat content).
§ Level depends on whether iron fortified or not.

have been resolved (Table 15–1). If the mother elects to bottle-feed, the nurse should support this decision and provide advice about which type of formula to use and how to use it.

Although nutrients differ slightly for various brands, all commercial formulas comply with standards set by the Infant Formula Act established in 1980. Adequate nutrients are provided in an appropriate kilocaloric concentration (about 20 kcal/oz) with a desirable solute load for full-term infants. Table 15–2 lists various commercial formulas with their nutrient values and indications for their use.

Nonfat cow milk is the basis for most infant formulas with modifications to resemble human milk. Most formulas contain principally casein from cow milk as the protein source; others are whey based, which more closely simulates breast milk. However, whey-based formulas have not been shown to support growth and development any better than casein-based formulas (Winick, 1989). Lactose is generally the source of carbohydrate, but sucrose may be used. The saturated fats of cow milk are poorly digested and absorbed, so combinations of unsaturated vegetable and/or MCT oils are added to provide the EFA and fat-soluble vitamins.

As established by the American Academy of Pediatrics guidelines, the electrolyte, mineral, and vitamin contents are similar. Adequate amounts of these nutrients (except for fluoride and iron) are furnished if the infant receives 150 to 180 ml/kg/day. Fluoride is not added to formulas due to high variability of fluoride in the water supply.

Infant formulas are so well balanced that the main supplement of concern is iron. Iron deficiency is highest in infants fed commercial formulas without added iron, intermediate in infants fed human milk, and much lower in those fed iron-fortified formula (Pizarro et al, 1991). Iron-fortified formulas are recommended after 2 to 3 months of age (AAP, 1989).

Commercial formulas are more appropriate for infants than cow or goat milk. Because of its high solute load, cow milk is not appropriate for the newborn. GI problems from unpasteurized milk may result from bacterial and viral contamination. Skim milk is not appropriate for children under 2 years of age because of its higher proportion of protein and minerals and lack of essential fatty acids. Goat milk is inadequate in folate and vitamin B_{12}; additionally, its higher sodium, potassium, and protein content increases the solute load.

Malnutrition has been reported in infants fed home-recipe formulas. This may be related to variations in nutrient composition or unsanitary handling practices that may result in frequent infection or GI disorders.

What is the protein source in most formulas; for carbohydrate; for fat? Why is fluoride not added to formulas? What infants have the highest incidence of iron deficiency? Describe reasons cow and goat milk and home-recipe formulas may be harmful to infants.

Premature and Low Birth Weight Formulas

Standards for premature infants are not clearly defined. However, special formulas are available such as Preemie SMA (Wyeth), Premature Enfamil (Mead Johnson), and Similac Special Care (Ross). Special commercial formulas for premature and LBW infants are relatively high in kilocalories and protein and contain a high percentage of MCT fats that do not require lipase for digestion. They also contain higher amounts of cholesterol than standard infant formulas. Other nutrients of concern include calcium, phosphorus, sodium, iron, vitamin D, vitamin E, and folic acid. The special premature formulas ordinarily contain increased amounts of these nutrients except for iron. Formulas for preterm infants contain generous amounts of vitamin E because iron and linoleic acid content increases the vitamin E requirements by interfering with its absorption and utilization.

Name 2 formulas for premature infants. How do these formulas differ from formulas for term infants?

TABLE 15–2

INDICATIONS FOR COMMERCIAL INFANT FORMULAS (FOR INFANTS UNDER 1 YEAR OF AGE)

Formulas Appropriate for Full-Term Infants	
Products listed are suitable for the full-term infant when a cow milk formula of normal dilution or a calorically concentrated formula is desired. Nutrient distribution is essentially the same as human milk and there is little difference in composition among these products	
Normal Dilution (20 kcal/oz)	
Enfamil, without iron	Available as ready-to-feed, concentrate, or powder
Enfamil, with iron	Available as ready-to-feed, concentrate, or powder
Similac, without iron	Available as ready-to-feed, concentrate, or powder
Similac, with iron	Available as ready-to-feed, concentrate, or powder
Similac, with whey, with iron	Available as ready-to-feed, concentrate, or powder
Concentrated Kilocaloric Density	
Enfamil, with iron (24 kcal/oz)	Available as ready-to-feed; can be made from powder or concentrate by adjusting amount of water added
Enfamil, without iron (24 kcal/oz)	Available as ready-to-feed; can be made from powder or concentrate by adjusting amount of water added
Similac, without iron (24 kcal/oz)	Available as ready-to-feed; can be made from powder or concentrate by adjusting amount of water added
Similac, with iron (24 kcal/oz)	Available as ready-to-feed; can be made from powder or concentrate by adjusting amount of water added
Similac, without iron only (27 kcal/oz)	Available as ready-to-feed; can be made from powder or concentrate by adjusting amounts of water added
Formulas Specially Designed for Premature Infants with an Immature Gastrointestinal Tract	
Formulas designed for the premature infant necessitate manipulation of all three major nutrients. Lactose is found in human milk and may therefore have special significance; however, the LBW infant's lactase activity does not reach that of the full-term infant until the 9th month of gestation. Therefore, in these formulas only 40 to 50% of the carbohydrate is available as lactose. This mixture of carbohydrates facilitates utilization because multiple digestive and absorptive pathways are involved. The whey-to-casein ratio (60:40) of human milk is incorporated in these formulas because whey (1) forms smaller, more digestible curds, avoiding lactobezoar formation; (2) offers a more appropriate amino acid composition that is higher in cystine (may be essential to the LBW infant), and lower in tyrosine, an amino acid that an LBW infant may not have the metabolic pathways to handle. LBW infants frequently are unable to digest long-chain saturated fats that form insoluble calcium–fatty acid complexes, resulting in impaired absorption of fats, calcium, and other minerals. This poor digestion is thought to be related to low bile acid pools and poor reabsorption of the bile acids; thus, MCT oil has been used. The LBW infant still requires supplementation with a multivitamin preparation with these products	
Similac Special Care 20 kcal/oz	60% lactalbumin and lactoglobulin, 40% casein
Similac Special Care 24 kcal/oz	Now available with or without iron, contains 15 mg of ferrous sulfate/L
Premature Enfamil 20 kcal/oz	60% lactalbumin, 48% casein
Premature Enfamil 24 kcal/oz	60% lactalbumin, 40% casein
"Preemie" SMA	60% lactalbumin, 40% casein

TABLE 15–2

INDICATIONS FOR COMMERCIAL INFANT FORMULAS (FOR INFANTS UNDER 1 YEAR OF AGE) *Continued*

Indications for Commercial Infant Formulas (For Infants under 1 Year of Age) Composition per 100 mL

kcal (oz)	Carbohydrate	Protein	Fat	Protein (gm)	Vit. D (IU)	mg Ca/ mg PO_4	Folic Acid (µg)	mg Fe/ mg Zn	Vit. E (IU)	Na (mg/ mEq)	K (mg/ mEq)	mOsm kg H_2O
20	41% (lactose)	9% (reduced mineral whey and nonfat milk)	50% (coconut and soy oil)	1.5	42	46/31	10	0.1/0.5	2	18/.79	72/1.8	300
20	41% (lactose)	9% (reduced mineral whey and nonfat milk)	50% (coconut and soy oil)	1.5	42	46/31	10	1.3/0.5	2	18/.79	72/1.8	300
20	43% (lactose)	9% (cow milk)	48% (soy and coconut oil)	1.5	41	51/39	10	0.15/0.5	2	22/.94	81/2	290
20	43% (lactose)	9% (cow milk)	48% (soy and coconut oil)	1.5	41	51/39	10	1.2/0.5	2	22/.94	81/2	290
20	43% (lactose)	9% (cow milk and whey)	48% (soy and coconut oil)	1.5	41	41/30	10	1.2/0.5	2	22.9/.99	74/1.9	300
24	41% (lactose)	9% (reduced mineral whey and nonfat milk)	50% (coconut and soy oil)	1.8	50	56/38	13	1.5/0.6	2.5	22/.95	87/2.2	360
24	41% (lactose)	9% (reduced mineral whey and nonfat milk)	50% (coconut and soy oil)	1.8	50	56/38	13	0.13/0.6	2.5	22/.95	87/2.2	360
24	42% (lactose)	11% (cow milk)	47% (soy and coconut oil)	2.2	48	73/56	12	0.2/0.6	2.4	35/1.5	109/2.8	360
24	42% (lactose)	11% (cow milk)	47% (soy and coconut oil)	2.2	48	73/56	12	1.5/0.6	2.4	35/1.5	109/2.8	360
27	42% (lactose)	11% (cow milk)	47% (soy and coconut oil)	2.5	55	82/64	14	0.2/0.7	2.4	39/1.7	150/3.15	410
20	42% (lactose, 50%; corn solids, 50%)	11% (nonfat milk, whey protein concentrate)	47% (MCT oil, 50%; soy oil; coconut oil)	1.8	101	122/61	25	0.25/1	2.7	34/1.5	95/2.4	250
24	42% (lactose, 50%; corn solids, 50%)	11% (nonfat milk, whey protein concentrate)	47% (MCT oil, 50%; soy oil; coconut oil)	2.2	121	145/73	30	0.3/1.2	3.2	40/1.75	113/2.9	260
20	44% (corn syrup solids, 60%; lactose, 50%)	12% (demineralized whey, nonfat milk solids)	44% (MCT oil, 40%; soy oil; coconut oil)	2	223	79/40	24	0.17/ 0.68	3.1	26/1.1	75/1.9	244
24	44% (corn syrup solids, 60%; lactose, 50%)	12% (demineralized whey, nonfat milk solids)	44% (MCT oil, 40%; soy oil; coconut oil)	2.4	266	94/48	28	0.2/0.8	3.7	31/1.4	90/2.3	300
24	41.9% (lactose, 50%; maltodextrins, 50%)	9.6%	48.5% (MCT oil, 13%)	2	48	73/40	10	0.3/0.8	1.5	32/1.4	73/1.9	280

From Rombeau JL, Caldwell MD. *Clinical Nutrition: Enteral and Tube Feeding*. 2nd ed. Philadelphia, WB Saunders, 1990.

Special Problems and Intolerance to Formulas

Galactosemia is a genetic disorder that is due to lack of an enzyme to metabolize the sugar galactose produced from the hydrolysis of lactose.

Atopic—an inherited allergy manifested by eczema, wheezing, rhinitis, colic, and diarrhea.

Name 2 formulas for special metabolic problems or intolerance problems.

Numerous specialized formulas are available for infants with special metabolic problems or intolerance problems, e.g., Lofenalac (Mead Johnson) for phenylketonuria or Meat Base Formula (Gerber) for cow milk intolerance. Soy-based formulas are probably the most frequently used specialized formula for infants unable to tolerate normal formulas. They contain a different type of protein and carbohydrate. They are so unique from human milk that they are not recommended as an initial feeding formula. However, they are popularly used for infants recovering from severe diarrhea resulting in temporary lactose intolerance and for those with congenital lactase deficiency or **galactosemia.**

Breast milk, whey-based formulas, or casein hydrolysate formulas result in fewer problems of **atopic** disease than soy protein formulas (Sampson et al, 1991; Chandra et al, 1989; Miskelly, 1988).

Supplements

If iron-fortified formula is not used, iron supplementation is recommended for formula-fed infants after 4 months of age, breast-fed infants 4 to 6 months of age, and preterm infants after 2 months of age. Iron supplementation (usually ferrous sulfate or ferric ammonium citrate) is ordinarily given as liquid drops or fortified cereals.

When is iron supplementation recommended? When should fluoride supplements be given?

Fluoride supplementation is recommended for infants and children to increase the strength of teeth. Thus, fluoride supplements are encouraged if a ready-to-feed formula or formula prepared from a liquid concentrate is used. Infants receiving formulas reconstituted from a powder should be given fluoride supplements if the water supply is not fluoridated. Vitamin supplements containing fluoride may be provided as follows: 0.25 mg fluoride from birth to age 2, 0.5 mg between ages 2 and 3, and 1 mg after age 3.

FORMULA PREPARATION

Most commercial formulas are available as ready-to-feed liquids or concentrated preparations (liquid or powder) to be diluted with water. Careful dilution with a clean, sterile water supply; sterile bottles; and careful refrigeration after the formula is diluted need to be stressed. Washing hands before preparing formula is advocated to decrease the chance of contamination.

Errors in dilution are serious and can be hazardous for the infant; ready-to-feed formulas are not diluted. Dilution errors may be caused by lack of understanding of the proper preparation method, improper measurements, or by clients feeling that the infant needs more or less formula. Improper dilution of formula is reported most frequently with powdered formulas.

Necrotizing enterocolitis—acute inflammation of the bowel mucosa.

Increasing or decreasing the recommended amount of formula is not advised because of the risk of abdominal distention, diarrhea, vomiting, and **necrotizing enterocolitis** from the hyperosmolar solution or suboptimal growth from inadequate nutrients. Infants fed formulas too concentrated especially have problems (fever or infection) when fluid requirements are increased. Such infants may become thirsty and demand more to drink or refuse to consume more liquid because of anorexia related to the illness. On the other hand, water intoxication from overdiluting the formula results in hyponatremia, irritability, and coma.

Formula is an excellent medium for bacterial growth; formula not taken during a feeding should be discarded since it will be contaminated by saliva enzymes and bacteria. Heating infant formulas or food in a microwave oven can result in severe burns to the infant's mouth and throat that are due to the buildup of heat after removal from the microwave. Shaking formula and stirring food immediately after removal from the microwave can help dissipate heat; however, the temperature must be checked before feeding.

Describe complications associated with overdiluting or underdiluting formulas.

Generally, ready-to-feed formulas are the most expensive, with formulas reconstituted from a powder being the cheapest commercial formula.

TECHNIQUES FOR BOTTLE-FEEDING

Contrary to rigid feeding schedules enforced in the past, infants today are generally fed on demand, when they are hungry. Within about 2 weeks, a pattern usually develops, with the infant eating 6 times daily at 4-hour intervals. Gradually a pattern of feeding will evolve allowing parents to sleep through the night.

The position for bottle-feeding is as much like breast-feeding as possible. Touching helps to strengthen feelings of love, security, and trust and is as important as the nutrients in the formula (Fig. 15–1). The infant should never be left alone with the bottle propped during feedings.

The bottle is held at an angle with the nipple full of milk, and the infant is held with the head at breast level. The hole in the nipple should be large enough to permit the milk to drip out of the bottle without shaking. Smaller holes make the infant swallow too much air, which may lead to vomiting.

The temptation and opportunity to overfeed with a bottle is greater than with breast-feeding. Since the formula is bottled in predetermined amounts, clients are tempted to encourage the infant to consume the whole amount. Forcing the infant to finish the bottle is inappropriate, but if he or she cries after finishing the bottle, more formula may be needed. A constant weight gain according to growth charts is a wise guide to follow.

The infant should be placed over the shoulder or knees and patted gently on the back to expel air about half-way through and at the end of each feeding. Another method of burping is supporting the infant in a sitting position tilted slightly forward and gently rubbing the back with the free hand.

Describe 3 guidelines for bottle-feeding.

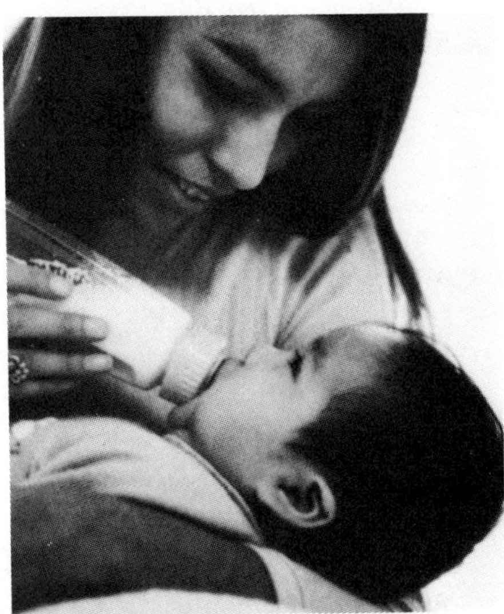

Figure 15–1 Mother feeding her infant with a bottle. (Courtesy of Gerber Products Company.)

NURSING APPLICATIONS

Assessment

Physical—for length, weight, growth rate, percentile on growth charts.

Dietary—for parent's knowledge of bottle feeding, source of iron, fluoride, and use of other supplements.

Laboratory—for sodium, calcium, especially in LBW infants.

Interventions

1. If parents are vegetarian, offer soy-based formula. These will meet the infant's needs as well as the parents' needs for following their nutritional beliefs.
2. Offer sterilized water. Fluid requirements may not be met with formula.
3. Provide LBW or premature infants with formulas that contain more than 20 kcal/oz to sustain an appropriate rate of growth.
4. Administer multivitamin supplements as prescribed. Preterm infants have high requirements for vitamins, and their intake is so small that this need cannot be met by formula alone.

Client Education

- For the first months of life, 26 to 32 oz/day of formula satisfy full-term infants.
- Avoid the practice of bottle propping.
- If using well water, boil before using to sterilize it, and have it analyzed for nitrate. High nitrate levels could result in anemia.
- The infant may indicate he or she is full by turning the head away, inattention, falling asleep, or becoming playful.
- The rate of growth is faster during infancy than at any other stage of life. Fats, a concentrated source of energy, are needed to support this rapid growth (40 to 50% of the total kilocalories is recommended).
- Despite growing concerns over heart disease, cholesterol intake may be important during the early developmental stages of infancy. There is little basis for recommending changes in fat intake before age 1 to 2.
- Mothers who have chosen to bottle-feed need to decrease their own kilocaloric intake to ensure weight loss of fat deposits accumulated during the pregnancy in anticipation of the breast-feeding process. Severe kilocaloric restriction is not advisable, and exercise and resumption of an active lifestyle as soon as possible are encouraged to help promote weight loss.
- Infants fed a soy-based formula will have stools that are darker in color and have a distinctive odor.
- Store all vitamin/mineral supplements in a safe place from children; 11 deaths from iron overdose were reported in 1991 (Litovitz & Manoguerra, 1992).

PROGRESSION OF INFANT FEEDING (TO 12 MONTHS OLD)

Consideration of the developmental stage of the infant is necessary for a successful feeding regimen. Nutrition is related to neuromuscular maturation, especially for infants (Table 15–3).

Neuromuscular Maturation

Stroking the infant's cheek elicits the rooting reflex, and the infant turns the head in that direction.

An orderly fashion of development begins with the **rooting reflex**. This reflex depends on being hungry; when the infant is full, it is not as strong.

TABLE 15–3

DEVELOPMENTAL MILESTONES IN FEEDING

Stage/Age	**Reflexes and Developmental Landmarks**	**Appropriate Nourishment**
Newborn (Birth to 10 days)	Rooting reflex Sucking Puts hand or thumb in mouth	Colostrum or infant formula
Infant 2 weeks to 3 months	Tonic neck reflex present Head control poor Bite reflex (stimulation to gums elicits a bite and release pattern) Recognizes feeding position and begins sucking and mouthing when placed in position	Breast milk or formula Begin fluoride supplement unless water contains fluoride
3 to 4 months	Development of mature suck and head control Rooting and bite reflex fade Suckle-swallow interferes with taking solid food	Breast milk or formula
4 to 6 months	Helps hold bottle Munching pattern begins Development of palmar grasp Able to bring objects to mouth and bite them Drooling (due to teething)	Semisolid or pureed foods; add 1 food at a time, beginning with rice cereal, strained vegetables, thin strained meats and fruits Provide at least 32 oz formula Begin iron supplement or fortified formula
6 to 9 months	Strong sucking pattern (less jaw movement) Gag reflex fades Holds bottle alone Develops inferior pincer grasp Able to self-feed by securing large pieces with a palmar grasp Lateral jaw movements Rotary chewing begins Cup drinking begins Can voluntarily release and resecure objects	Finger foods such as arrowroot biscuits, oven-dried toast, zwieback (foods should be soluble) Increase variety of textures (junior type for diced foods) Breast milk or fortified infant formula Fluoride supplement
9 to 12 months	Bites foods Grasps bottle and foods and brings them to the mouth Able to drink from a cup that is held Finger feeds with pincer grip Rotary chewing pattern Reaches for spoon	Same as above Fluoride supplement Breast milk or fortified infant formula (if homogenized milk is used, not > 65% of total kilocalorie intake)
12 to 15 months	Messily attempts to use cup and spoon	Provide foods that adhere to spoon when scooped (mashed potatoes, applesauce, cooked cereal and cottage cheese) Homogenized milk

Table continued on following page

TABLE 15–3

DEVELOPMENTAL MILESTONES IN FEEDING *Continued*

Stage/Age	Reflexes and Developmental Landmarks	Appropriate Nourishment
15 to 24 months	Walks alone May seek and get food independently Uses spoon to self-feed Holds glass with both hands More skilled at cup and spoon feeding Names food, expresses preferences; prefers unmixed foods Experiences food jags Appetite appears to decrease	Chopped fibrous meats, e.g., a roast or steak Solid foods Introduce raw vegetables and fruits gradually Foods of high nutrient value should be available Balanced food intake should be offered, but the child should be allowed to develop transitory food preferences Homogenized milk

Suckling, discussed in Chapter 14, is replaced with sucking by 4 months of age when the orofacial muscles are used with the mouth more pursed, and the tongue moving back and forth. This backward movement of the tongue makes the smacking noises that occur.

A forward motion of the tongue on dropping the lower jaw is typical during the first 3 months. If semisolid foods are offered at this time, the tongue will force the food out. No discriminating taste is occurring, however, just reflex action.

The sucking motion becomes developed enough to eat and handle semisolid foods from a spoon around 4 to 6 months of age. This correlates with development of fine, gross, and oral motor skills to consume appropriately the foods added to provide kilocaloric and nutrient intake (Table 15–3). If foods are not added by 6 months of age, growth may drop below the growth curves.

Describe the neuromuscular maturation of the infant.

About 6 to 8 months of age, infants develop the ability to receive food and pass it between the gums in a chewing motion. By 7 months, infants can chew, so pureed foods are not required; some variety of texture is mandatory if infants are going to accept unfamiliar foods later in life.

Introduction of Foods

Numerous false assumptions are associated with introduction of solid foods. Despite the fact that many clients introduce solid foods during the first month, no

TABLE 15–4

GUIDELINES FOR PREPARING BABY FOODS

1. Use high-quality fresh fruits, vegetables, and meats
2. Maintain safe sanitation standards; utensils and hands should be thoroughly clean
3. Follow the principles in Chapter 18 to maintain nutrient content of the food. (Do not overcook; use minimal amounts of water)
4. Omit seasonings and spices, especially salt, and use minimal amounts of sugar
5. Avoid using processed foods with a high salt content, such as ham, bacon, and hot dogs
6. Avoid spinach and beets or use sparingly. (Commercial food manufacturers use only fresh products that have been tested for nitrate content)
7. Do not use honey* for infants under 1 year of age
8. Use a blender, food processor, or baby food grinder to puree the food; add sufficient water for a smooth consistency
9. Divide the pureed food into individual-sized portions and store them in the freezer
10. Thaw only the amount for a single feeding before serving
11. Throw away leftover portions because the food may be contaminated with bacteria. Preheating results in the loss of some nutrients

* Honey frequently contains botulism spores; the immune systems of young infants do not have the capacity to resist botulism.

nutritional advantage is associated with this practice. The most common reason given for early feeding is to help the infant sleep through the night. This will naturally occur between 1 to 3 months of age with girls sleeping through the night earlier than boys. This is a developmental milestone not related to what is fed (Barness, 1985).

Disadvantages in starting semisolid foods too early are (1) unnecessary costs, (2) high probability of overfeeding, (3) effects on immature digestive system, (4) increased risk of development of food allergies, (5) reduction of milk intake in lieu of a less nutritionally complete/adequate food (Winick, 1989), (6) decreased iron absorption, and (7) decreased absorption of energy and nitrogen (Shulman et al, 1991).

Following the introduction of foods between 4 and 6 months, formula intake should remain around 32 oz daily. Foods should be presented to the infant with a spoon, never in a bottle.

Semisolids are offered before milk at feeding time, yet the amounts are limited to reserve some appetite for milk. Standard infant formulas continue to be appropriate through the first year but should be taken from a cup rather than a bottle (Foman et al, 1990; Ziegler, 1990). (The infant will need assistance with the cup.) Mixed foods should not be introduced until tolerance of each component ingredient has been determined.

Following the introduction of a new food, a waiting period of at least 7 days is recommended to observe for allergic reactions. When breast-feeding mothers switch to formula, no new foods should be introduced until tolerance of the formula is established. Foods most commonly causing allergies include milk, soy, peanuts, egg whites (including ice cream), wheat, and chocolate (Arshad et al, 1992). Early exposure to allergens in food and in breast milk may increase the frequency of allergic disorders in infants (Arshad et al, 1992). Therefore, it is advisable to not introduce these foods until after 9 to 12 months of age. Food allergies are usually outgrown if the food is eliminated from the diet for a period of time (Block, 1987).

Initially, 1 tsp of iron-fortified dry cereal is mixed with 1 to 2 tbsp of formula or breast milk daily. Rice cereal is initiated first because it is less allergenic than other cereal products. After this is well accepted, a small amount of another pureed food may be introduced.

The order of introduction for vegetables, meats, and fruits varies among pediatricians. Some prefer the introduction of vegetables after cereals, then meats followed by fruits. Because sweet flavors are well accepted, other foods are offered first. Preference for sweet foods is an innate desire.

Gradually, junior-type foods with a few lumps are introduced to initiate some chewing. The presence of a few teeth does not mean the infant is ready to actually pulverize foods. Certain vegetables are more difficult to digest and are introduced after 1 year of age: Cucumbers, onions, cabbage, and broccoli. Nitrite is naturally present in spinach and beets; their quantities should be limited.

Buying separate baby foods is not necessary. Selected foods from the family menu can be pureed for use. Guidelines for preparing baby food at home are shown in Table 15–4.

When semisolid foods are introduced, the goal should be to include all food groups as soon as possible to assure a well-balanced diet (Table 15–5). Guidelines for feeding infants to provide a balance of nutrients are similar to the Dietary Guidelines for Americans, with a few exceptions. Gradually incorporate a variety of foods, using sodium and sugar in moderation. Fat and cholesterol are not severely restricted for infants and young children. Large amounts of fiber may not be well tolerated. Proportionally, infants require more iron than do adults. Above all, offer adequate amounts of food but avoid overfeeding by observing the infant's appetite.

Jars of baby food contain more than the very young infant should have at a feeding; once a jar is opened, refrigeration is necessary, and food should be discarded after 24 hours. If the infant is fed directly from the jar, any leftover food should be discarded immediately because it is contaminated with saliva. Saliva in

List 4 disadvantages to starting semisolid foods too early. When is additional food recommended? How should this food be presented to the infant? How long is the waiting period before introducing another new food? What foods most commonly cause allergies, and when should they be introduced? What food is initially offered to infants and why? What vegetables are introduced after 1 year of age? What 2 vegetables should be limited?

TABLE 15–5

RECOMMENDED FOOD INTAKE FOR GOOD NUTRITION ACCORDING TO FOOD GROUPS AND THE AVERAGE SIZE OF SERVINGS AT DIFFERENT AGE LEVELS

		Average Size of Servings					
Food Group	**Servings/Day**	**1 Year**	**2–3 Years**	**4–5 Years**	**6–9 Years**	**10–12 Years**	**13–15 Years**
Protein foods	≥2						
meats, poultry, fish*		½–1 oz	1–2 oz	2–3 oz	3 oz	3 oz	3 oz
dry beans and peas		1–2 tbsp	2–3 tbsp	2–4 tbsp	½ cup†	½ cup†	½ cup†
eggs		1	1	1	1†	1†	1†
Milk, yogurt, cheese‡§	3–4 for ages 1–5; ≥2 over 5 years	4 oz	6 oz	4–6 oz	6–8 oz	8 oz	8 oz
Grain products	≥6						
breads		¼–½ slice	½ slice	1 slice	1–2 slices	2 slices	2 slices
cooked cereals, including rice, pasta, others		¼ cup	⅓ cup	½ cup	½ cup	¾ cup	1 cup
ready-to-eat cereal		½ oz	¾ oz	1 oz	1 oz	1 oz	1 oz
crackers		2–3	2–3	4	4–6	4–6	4–6
Vitamin-C rich food	≥1 for ages 1–5	¼–½ cup	¼–½ cup	½ cup	½ cup	½ cup	½ cup
cooked or canned fruit or vegetable juice	≥2 for those over 5 years of age	2–3 oz	4 oz	4 oz	4 oz	6 oz	6 oz
fresh citrus fruit				1 medium-size	1 medium-size	1 medium-size	1 medium-size
Vitamin-A rich dark green/orange fruits and vegetables cooked or raw (for older children)	1 for children 1–5 years; ≥2 for those over 5 years of age	2 tbsp	3 tbsp	¼–½ cup	½ cup	½ cup	½ cup
Other fruits and vegetables	≥2	¼ cup	¼–½ cup	½ cup	½ cup	½ cup	½ cup or ½ piece
Fats and oils margarine, butter, oil	3–4	1 tsp	1 tsp	1 tsp	1 tsp	1 tsp	1 tsp

Adapted from Behrman RE, Vaughan VC: *Nelson Textbook of Pediatrics,* 14th ed. Philadelphia, WB Saunders, 1992, and American Dietetic Association. *Manual of Clinical Dietetics,* 4th ed. Chicago, American Dietetic Association, 1992.
* Meat, poultry, and fish serving sizes are based on cooked product, without fat or bone.
† 1 egg, ½ cup cooked dried beans or peas, or 2 tbsp peanut butter count as 1 oz of lean meat.
‡ Children under age 2 should be given whole milk and whole milk products.
§ 4 oz milk = ½ oz cheese; 6 oz milk = 1 oz cheese; 8 oz milk = 1½ oz cheese.

The food will digest the starches, making it watery; bacteria from the mouth can multiply in the food.

Food Additives

No salt is added to baby food. Infant foods should not be salted until at least after the first year of life. The taste for salt is an acquired habit and not related to enjoyment of food unless one is accustomed to it.

Infant cereals are fortified with niacin, thiamin, riboflavin, calcium, phosphorus, and iron. Sugar and modified corn or tapioca starch may be added to desserts. Vitamin C is added to fruits and fruit juices.

List nutritive additives in baby food.

NURSING APPLICATIONS

Assessment

Physical—for infant's developmental stage, neuromuscular development, age.
Dietary—for parents' knowledge of feeding solid foods.

Interventions

1. Offer semisolid foods before breast milk or formula. By introducing new foods when hunger level is high, acceptance of new items is more likely.
2. Do not offer orange juice. Orange juice has a high frequency of allergies, so it is one of the last fruit juices introduced.
3. Avoid foods with sorbitol. This sugar substitute is a known cause of diarrhea in infants and children.
4. Increase fluid intake. When solid food is added, the solute load is increased, thereby necessitating increased fluid needs.

Evaluation

* Parents should be able to describe which foods to introduce first to the child, foods most frequently associated with allergies, and what foods to avoid until 1 year of age.

Client Education

- If cow milk is introduced during the second 6 months, solid foods should provide good sources of the iron and vitamins deficient in cow milk. No more than 65% of the kilocalories should be provided by milk (AAP, 1989).
- Pasteurized milk that has a reduced fat content is inappropriate for children under age 2.
- Honey is not appropriate for children under 1 year of age because botulism may occur.
- Try not to show any dislike of the new food being served.
- Toddlers learn about food by touching/playing with it. Allow this to occur. (Wear an apron or raincoat if necessary!)

INFANT PROBLEMS RELATED TO NUTRITION

Regurgitation

During the first 6 months, regurgitation (spitting up) is common but gradually diminishes. Regurgitation of a small amount of any milk or food eaten may cause concern to parents; however, infant growth does not appear to be affected. This problem generally resolves by 4 months.

Persistent regurgitation is frequently caused by GI reflux. The infant needs to be evaluated by a physician to determine if corrective surgery is needed. Reflux can be minimized by holding the infant at a 45- to 60-degree angle for feedings.

NURSING APPLICATIONS

Assessment

Physical—for spitting up.
Dietary—for feeding, burping practices.

Interventions

1. Burp the infant about half-way through and after the feeding. If regurgitation continues to occur, burp the infant more frequently.

Evaluation

* Parents should be able to tell the difference between vomiting and regurgitation and not be alarmed when spitting up occurs; infant's rate of growth is appropriate.

Client Education

- Regurgitation is normal.
- If vomiting ensues, notify physician.

Diarrhea

Diarrhea refers to unformed, watery stools that are unlike the usual ones.

Ketoacidosis—acidosis related to the accumulation of ketone bodies.

When **diarrhea** is accompanied by a fever over 101°F or by vomiting that lasts more than 24 hours or if diarrhea is severe (stools more than 10 times/day with a large volume of water lost), immediate attention must be given to correct the condition. Infants receiving breast milk, nonmilk formulas (soy protein or hydrolysates), and soft foods are generally able to tolerate their normal diet and benefit nutritionally from continued feeding (Lifschitz, 1991). Complete oral rehydration solutions are available that contain sodium, glucose, potassium, chloride, and base to replace that lost in stools. The American Academy of Pediatrics recommends the use of the glucose-electrolyte solution and that feeding be reintroduced in the first 24 hours of a mild diarrheal episode (Snyder, 1991). Carbohydrate intake is needed at this time to prevent **ketoacidosis.** General guidelines for dietary management of mild diarrhea are in Chapter 25. Lactose intolerance in infants (or children) can be treated with soy protein or hydrolysate formulas (Sinden & Sutphen, 1991).

NURSING APPLICATIONS

Assessment

Physical—for infant's weight percentile rank, weight loss, condition of oral cavity, skin turgor, tear formation on crying, number of wet or diarrhea diapers, depressed fontanels.
Dietary—for recent intake to determine diet-related causes of diarrhea, initiation of cow milk, fluid and nutrient intake, especially iron, formula, and other supplemental foods used; feeding practices.
Laboratory—for sodium, potassium.

Interventions

1. Replace fluid, sodium, and potassium. Acute diarrhea of 1 to 4 days results in loss of these nutrients requiring replacement.
2. Monitor I&O. This will help detect dehydration.
3. Avoid offering fatty foods. Fatty foods are not absorbed because of the rapid transit time, so diarrhea is worsened.

Evaluation

* Diarrhea should resolve, hydration status returns to normal, and laboratory results return to WNL.

Client Education

- Apple juice may cause diarrhea as a result of carbohydrate malabsorption.
- Contact the physician if diarrhea persists or is accompanied by fever to ensure that nutrients and electrolytes are replaced.
- Electrolyte solutions (Pedialyte or Lytren) are frequently prescribed by the physician.
- Sugar-sweetened beverages (in contrast to artificially sweetened beverages) prevent ketoacidosis (Lewis, 1991).
- Most soft drinks and commercial fruit drinks are hypertonic and can worsen diarrhea.
- Lactose-containing products may need to be withheld if diarrhea is severe. (Soy protein formulas may be used.)
- Reintroduce diluted milk-based products gradually.
- Pectin-containing foods such as applesauce can be used to help solidify stools.

Constipation

Difficulty in passing stools and indications of pain during bowel movements are frequent concerns of parents. Constipation, or decreased frequency or hard stool consistency, is often bothersome but clinically insignificant. It is a more frequent complaint of formula-fed infants than breast-fed infants. Constipation in children under the age of 2½ may be caused by insufficient fluid intake, allowing too much milk and not providing additional foods, anal fissures, or mild illness.

Iron-fortified formulas are blamed for numerous GI problems, especially constipation. However, studies have not found undesirable GI side effects associated with iron-fortified formulas (Anonymous, 1988; Nelson et al, 1988). If an infant receiving a formula with iron is constipated, the same formula without iron could be substituted. If the constipation resolves, iron drops can be provided at a different time of day than the feeding.

NURSING APPLICATIONS

Assessment

Physical—for weight gain; last bowel movement, history of frequency; vomiting.

Dietary—for refusal to eat, type of formula used, amount of milk given, use of supplemental foods, fluid intake.

Interventions

1. Offer fluids the infant will accept.
2. If weight gain is low, infant is refusing to eat, and/or vomiting is occurring, assess for impacted stool. If positive, remove as prescribed by the physician (lactulose, oral glycerol, or enema).

Evaluation

* Parents offer additional fluids, increase fiber-containing foods, if appropriate.

Continued

Client Education

- Increase fluid intake by offering water several times daily.
- When weaning from breast milk to formula, constipation frequently occurs.
- If supplemental foods have been added, provide a list of foods appropriate for the child's age and developmental level that are high in fiber. Prune juice, pureed prunes, and apricots should be encouraged; bananas and rice, or binding foods, should be curtailed.

Milk Anemia

What can cause iron deficiency anemia? What are the results of this anemia?

The infant's rapid growth may result in iron deficiency and anemia due to depletion of iron reserves. This occurs more frequently in infants given principally milk without iron supplementation or inadequate intake of iron-rich foods. Iron deficiency anemia in infancy increases risk for long-lasting developmental disabilities. Despite laboratory values WNL in children 5 years of age, those who had severe iron deficiency anemia as infants scored lower on mental and motor functioning tests than other children enrolling in school (Lozoff et al, 1991). However, studies have not proven that iron deficiency is the cause.

NURSING APPLICATIONS

Assessment

Physical—for mental and motor function, fatigue, paleness, socioeconomic background, birth weight.
Dietary—for milk without iron/supplements, inadequate intake of iron-rich foods.
Laboratory—for Hgb, Hct, RBC, iron, transferrin.

Interventions

1. Offer iron-rich food (such as iron-fortified cereals and meats) before milk. Intake of iron is increased since the infant is hungry.
2. When needed, add iron supplement per physician order.

Evaluation

* Laboratory results should return to WNL.

Client Education

- Cow milk should not be used until the infant has passed the 1 year mark. Cow milk contains very little iron, and microscopic bleeding may occur when the immature GI tract is exposed to milk (Ziegler et al, 1990).
- Provide a vitamin C–rich food with iron-fortified cereal to enhance iron absorption.
- Inform about WIC program.

Baby Bottle Tooth Decay

BBTD is a rampant form of caries that occurs before the age of 2.

Baby bottle tooth decay (BBTD) is a nutrition-related disorder resulting in carious teeth (Fig. 15–2). When an infant is put in bed with a baby bottle, he or she may fall asleep with milk or juice in the mouth. The erupting teeth can be detrimentally affected by the constant presence of any feeding containing carbohydrate, particularly disaccharides and monosaccharides (from milk or fruit juice). BBTD continues to be a serious problem in lower socioeconomic populations.

What causes BBTD and why?

NURSING APPLICATIONS

Assessment

Physical—for cavities in teeth, easily bleeding gums.
Dietary—for parents' knowledge of BBTD and what causes it; use of bottle propping, especially at night.

Interventions

1. When feeding an infant, hold the child and bottle; avoid bottle propping.

Evaluation

* Parents do not prop the bottle or allow infant to fall asleep with bottle in mouth. Caries do not develop.

Client Education

- Terminate nighttime bottles.
- Do not let infant suck bottle unattended.

Colic

Colic develops in 20 to 30% of all infants during the first week of life and resolves by 3 to 4 months of age. The term is derived from the impression that the pain is due to spasms of the colon, since relief sometimes follows the passage of feces or flatus. The stomach is tense with legs drawn up toward the body. A thorough physical examination of the infant is in order to be sure nothing is wrong that can be treated.

Colic is a syndrome characterized by excessive crying and increased motor activity, excessive flatus, and erratic sleeping and feeding patterns.

If an infant is allowed to suck from an empty bottle or if the nipple holes are too small (requires more sucking) or too large (forces the infant to gulp to keep up with the flow of milk), the infant swallows too much air. The simplest cause may be the infant's nursing position, which allows too much air to be swallowed. Air in the intestines may cause distention, which can cause spasms. Infants fed in a more upright position and limited to 10 minutes of sucking will minimize the amount of swallowed air.

Colic is frequently blamed on the formula, and parents may request changes.

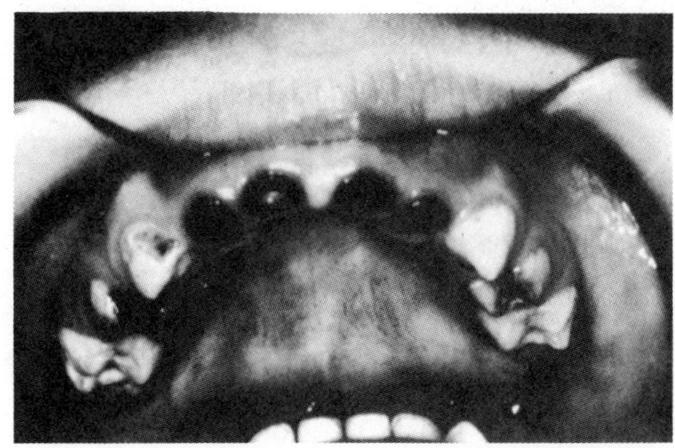

Figure 15–2 Rampant caries owing to use of nursing bottle with sugar-sweetened beverage as a pacifier. (From Nizel AE, Papas AS. *Nutrition in Clinical Dentistry.* 3rd ed. Philadelphia, WB Saunders, 1989.)

Recent studies suggest that hypersensitivity to cow milk is not the reason for colic in most healthy infants (Forsyth, 1989; Taubman, 1988).

What ar some possible causes of colic?

In the breast-fed infant, gas can be produced by foods that the mother eats, causing colic in the infant. Suspect foods include garlic, onion, broccoli, cabbage, sauerkraut, and pickles.

NURSING APPLICATIONS

Assessment

Physical—for excessive crying, increased motor activity, excessive flatus, erratic sleeping.
Dietary—for erratic feeding patterns, feeding and holding technique, nipple hole size.

Interventions

1. Demonstrate how to hold child while feeding.
2. Massage the infant's stomach.
3. Emphasize this will go away (usually in 10 to 12 weeks); this disorder is self-limiting; it does not mean they are incompetent or bad parents.

Evaluation

* Since this disorder resolves on its own, provide support and empathy to the infant and parents.

Client Education

- Although colic causes short-term stress in the mother and family, there are no long-term effects on the infant.
- Provide lukewarm formula and burp the infant frequently.
- Relaxation of the infant and mother may be a useful goal to reduce colic.
- An overtired or overstimulated infant cries more.

Cleft Palate

Cleft describes a split where parts of the upper lip or palate fail to grow together.

In the US, 1 infant out of every 700 (approximately 5000 children) is born with a **cleft** lip or palate each year. Scientists believe that any number of factors such as malnutrition, drugs, disease, or heredity may cause this condition.

Feeding the infant with a cleft palate, with or without a cleft lip, presents unique problems. The length of time needed for feedings to provide adequate nutrients can be exhaustive for both mother and infant. Because of the opening between the roof of the mouth and the floor of the nasal cavity, negative pressure cannot be created for sucking (Fig. 15–3). However, breast-feeding can usually be successful; the infant adapts by squeezing or chewing the nipple (Fisher, 1991).

What are some possible causes of cleft palate? Describe the reason feeding an infant with cleft palate is so unique. What are some techniques to help feed an infant with cleft palate?

Special devices are available if necessary. These are recommended when more than 1 to 1½ hours are required per feeding. The infant is held in a sitting position to prevent the formula from entering the nose. As soon as possible, spoon feeding is introduced.

Patience is required, and extra time for feeding must be allowed to provide needed nutrients. Table 15–6 offers some suggestions for feeding techniques to provide nutrients while minimizing risks.

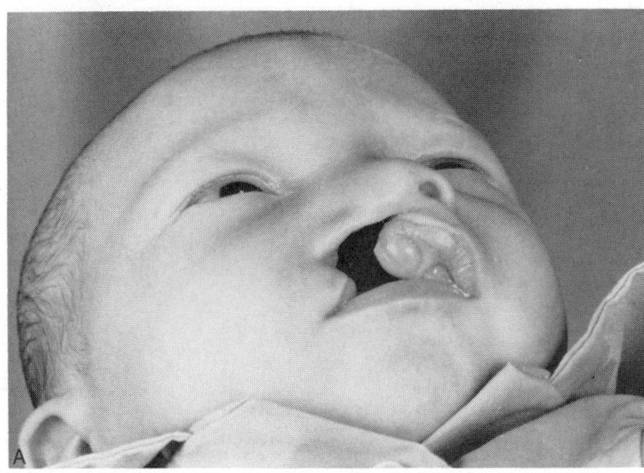

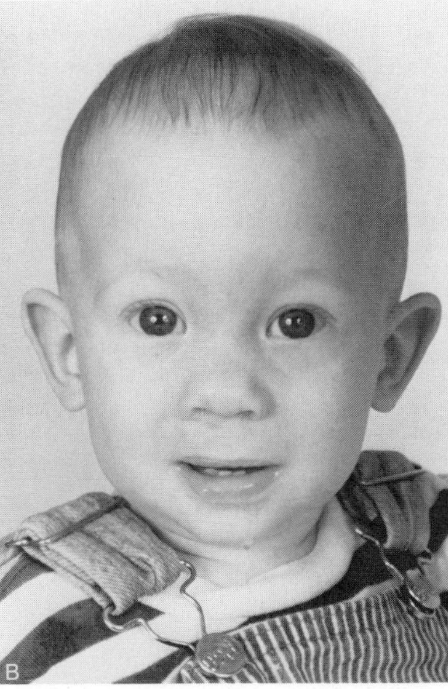

Figure 15–3 Cleft palate. *A*, Infant born with cleft lip and cleft palate; *B*, surgical repair allows a normal lifestyle—not only by repairing facial abnormalities but by permitting the consumption of food in a safe and normal manner.

NURSING APPLICATIONS

Assessment

Physical—for cleft palate/lip; aspiration; growth rate; height/weight on percentile charts.

Dietary—for feeding technique and past experiences in feeding infants.

Interventions

1. Explain that the principal problem is a lack of normal suction, but by using some different feeding techniques, the infant can obtain adequate nutrients.
2. Feed these infants slowly and at a 60 to 80 degree angle following guidelines in Table 15–6.

Evaluation

* The infant consumes 75 to 100% of needed nutrients without aspiration.

Client Education

- Introduce spoon feeding as soon as possible.
- Oral skills develop after surgery to correct the problem.
- Acidic and spicy foods may irritate the delicate tissue in the cleft area (Brooks, 1988).
- Young children with cleft palate are at increased risk for choking on foods that may slip into the trachea (see section on asphyxiation by food).
- Refer parents to the American Cleft Palate Association for literature and to local support groups.

Failure to Thrive

FTT or growth failure is defined as a weight for age less than the third percentile on the growth chart or a failure to maintain an established growth curve.

Failure to thrive (FTT) is a complex condition that may be caused by organic and/or psychosocial factors; a multidisciplinary team approach is essential. Organic FTT, constituting 20 to 40% of FTT infants, is attributed to physical

TABLE 15–6

SUGGESTIONS FOR FEEDING AN INFANT WITH CLEFT PALATE

Enlarging the hole in the nipple of the infant's bottle enables him or her to get milk more easily
Boiling new nipples before use softens them
Mixing pureed foods (fruits, vegetables, meats) with milk or broth makes a thinner consistency so they may be fed from a bottle with an enlarged hole in the nipple
Frequent burping aids in releasing excessive air intake
To prevent regurgitation, the older child should be taught to eat slowly and to take small bites
Using a straw helps some children to take liquids more easily
Feeding the child with a cleft palate takes longer than feeding a normal child; the mother needs to allow the necessary time. Fatigue on the part of the parent may interfere with the child's receiving adequate nourishment

Adapted from Nizel AE. *Nutrition in Preventive Dentistry Science and Practice.* 2nd ed. Philadelphia, WB Saunders, 1981.

causes such as diarrhea, cerebral palsy, cystic fibrosis, or oral motor problems. Most cases are classified as nonorganic FTT with the problem unrelated to disease. Most cases have elements of nutritional and emotional factors, involving the parent, infant, and environment. Nurturing is a requirement just as much as nutrients from food.

Most mothers of these infants live in suboptimal environments, have distorted perceptions of how much food their infant needs, have low self-esteem, and are stressed, with no family or peer support. Mothers report infants are in poor health, are irritable, or lack interest in eating (Smith & Lifschitz, 1990). It is unknown whether the infant's behavior affects growth directly through nutrition or independently of nutrition.

Despite the fact that few studies have actually documented inadequate intake, when infants are placed in another environment, they eat well and usually exhibit catch-up growth. However, not all infants immediately gain weight when given adequate kilocalories (Powell, 1988). Catch-up growth is dependent on providing kilocalories and protein in excess of normal need to promote a daily weight gain of 30 gm in infants and 60 to 90 gm in older children. An infant may require 150 kcal/kg of body weight; protein intake of 8% of total kilocaloric intake is recommended (Powell, 1988; Endert & Wooldridge, 1987). Half-strength formula is used initially, gradually progressing to full strength. This does not overload the infant's system and allows tolerance to occur.

Routine serial weights provide more dependable information about progress than randomly timed weights. Weight gain will also be a positive reinforcement for parents.

NURSING APPLICATIONS

Assessment

Physical—for infant's height, weight, percentile rank.
Dietary—for nutrient/food/fluid intake, kilocalories, and protein intake; formula preparation, type of milk; parental attitude and beliefs regarding diet and health.
Laboratory—for serum iron, TIBC, CBC, ferritin, transferrin; albumin, prealbumin; thyroid function tests.

Interventions

1. Feed the infant. This determines if technical feeding problems are apparent.
2. If necessary, administer IV feedings as ordered. These replace needed nutrients.

3. Monitor weight daily.
4. Empathize with the mother; point out appropriate procedures she practices when feeding the infant.

Evaluation

* Infant should gain weight to up to 50th percentile and mother should enjoy feeding and holding infant.

Client Education

- Touch is essential for well-being, fostering feelings of love, security, and trust.
- Inform about support groups.

TODDLER AND PRESCHOOL CHILDREN

Poor nutritional status (as measured by growth rate and biochemical indices) is generally more prevalent in lower socioeconomic groups, in which the amounts and variety of foods may be limited. Approximately 10% of all children, regardless of socioeconomic background, may be iron deficient. Vitamin C, vitamin B_6, and calcium are also frequently deficient in the diet.

The kilocaloric requirement is relatively high, or roughly 1000 kcal plus 100 kcal per year of life, as a result of high activity level, BMR, and growth. The high calcium requirements are generally met with formula through age 1 and homogenized milk from age 1 to 2; skim milk may be introduced after the second birthday. The RDAs for major nutrients are listed in Table 15–7.

During the preschool years, habits and food attitudes are formed that will to some extent affect health throughout life. A variety of foods should be available that provide the needed nutrients (see Table 15–5). A basic understanding of the nutrient content of foods, the role of foods in health, and food-related behaviors for these age groups is important for parents to promote food habits that are conducive to adequate nutrient intake. Foods are not only important for their relationships to health, but also contribute to social and personal pleasures.

Parental attitudes, eating habits, and food choices are the most influential factors of the child's food preferences. Foods that are disliked by one or both parents are not served often or may not be served at all. Additionally, children model their parents and tend to enjoy foods the parents like. When planning menus, the child's food preferences must be considered, but parents can control the options. Without appropriate guidance, young children will not independently make healthy food choices; therefore, the parent's role is to offer nutritious foods. The children can choose how much or even whether they will eat the food that has been provided. More food is eaten by the child when the family eats together, rather than just offering food for the child to eat alone.

TABLE 15–7

RECOMMENDED DIETARY ALLOWANCES FOR SELECTED NUTRIENTS FOR CHILDREN THROUGH ADOLESCENCE

Nutrient	Children 1–3	Children 4–6	Children 7–10	Boys 11–14	Girls 11–14	Boys 15–18	Girls 15–18
Kilocalories	1300	1800	2000	2500	2200	3000	2200
Protein (gm)	16	24	28	45	46	59	44
Vitamin C (mg)	40	45	45	50	50	60	60
Calcium (mg)	800	800	800	1200	1200	1200	1200
Iron (mg)	10	10	10	12	15	12	15

Data from National Research Council Subcommittee on the 10th edition of the RDAs. *Recommended Dietary Allowances,* 10th ed. Washington, D.C., National Academy Press, 1989.

Healthy Start is an information and educational campaign sponsored by the Food Marketing Institute, American Association of Pediatrics, and American Dietetic Association to promote healthy food choices and good eating habits as part of an overall healthful lifestyle. Materials are targeted to help parents avoid hassles in feeding children 2 to 6 years old and to be able to respond to their child's changing developmental and physiological needs (Healthy Start, 1991). Common concerns about meal planning for children, sugar, pesticide safety, healthy snacks, and fat are addressed in brochures and newsletters distributed through supermarkets.

Food jags—refusing to eat anything except one food for several days.

What nutrients are deficient in toddlers' and preschool children's diets? Explain the rationale for the high kilocaloric requirement. What is the kilocaloric requirement? What are food jags, and how can parents handle this occurrence? How do parents affect the child's intake? Describe the Healthy Start program.

Food jags are common. This is a way to assert independence. This typical developmental stage is temporary. The food obsession may cause parental concern, but overreaction may prolong rather than correct such behaviors.

Feeding Toddlers (1 to 3 Years Old)

During the second year of life, development of fine motor skills results in toddlers learning to feed themselves. Although this is a messy learning process, it is a transitional period that will stabilize by age 2. Finger-feeding may be preferred to spoon feeding; some finger-foods should be provided at every meal. A cup can be manipulated by the toddler by about 18 months of age.

Rotary chewing skills will develop in the second year. Until then, finely chopped meats are more popular. Cooked dried beans are suitable for part of the protein intake, but poor digestibility is a limiting factor for infants and small children.

Toddlers prefer regularity, so eating at the same time is desirable and helps control appetite. Regular meals also help to avoid fatigue, which can interfere with emotions as well as appetite. Children who are tired will not eat well. If the child has been very active, allow a short rest period before the meal.

Refusing to eat is a way to attract attention. Appetites are erratic and unpredictable. Parents should not force the child to eat when he or she is not hungry. Birch et al (1991) found that when well-balanced meals were provided, kilocaloric intake at any given meal varied greatly, but compensation at subsequent meals results in little variability in total energy intake. Shea and colleagues (1992) also found that energy consumption over a 24-hour period is relatively stable. If sufficient amounts are not eaten at the meal, parents may limit snacking or provide nutrient-dense snacks. Snacks can contribute significantly to adequate nutrient intake.

Describe 3 methods to help toddlers eat nutritiously.

One tart, one mild, and one crisp food is a good rule. Strong-flavored vegetables are more popular if eaten raw, e.g., turnips. Color is especially appealing to children. A tiny sprig of parsley, a carrot stick, or a slice of tomato is appreciated. Bright colors, such as green, yellow, red, and orange, are all liked.

Preschool Children (4 to 6 Years Old)

Preschoolers are relatively independent at the table as far as feeding themselves. Certain factors need to be considered to make the mealtime pleasant rather than an ordeal. By allowing children to eat with adults, they imitate others in both manners and food habits. Parental insistence on proper utensil usage, manners, and other demands that are inappropriate for this age group may result in less food intake. Parents need to ignore some inappropriate mealtime behaviors and focus on positive non-mealtime activities. Conversation and role modeling can reinforce appropriate eating behavior and promote food intake.

Although sturdy child-size tables and chairs may be used, booster chairs allow the family to eat together. Nonbreakable dishes should be heavy enough to resist spilling. Beverages presented in small squatty containers about ½ to ¾ filled result in fewer disruptive accidents.

Small amounts of food are offered several times a day. Serving sizes should be based on appetite, but initially about 1 tbsp can be offered for each year of age

(Table 15–5). Snacks can contribute significantly to the nutrient intake. Some wholesome snacks enjoyed by this age group include cheese cubes, fresh fruit, raw vegetable sticks, milk, and fruit juices.

Strong-flavored vegetables (overcooked cabbage and onions) are generally disliked. Crisp, raw vegetables are well accepted. Tough stringy fibers, such as those in celery or string beans, should be removed. Since these children still enjoy eating with their fingers, cutting fruits and vegetables into small pieces increases their acceptance. Preschoolers generally prefer their foods separate; casseroles and stews are not well liked. Foods that can be easily chewed are more readily accepted.

Describe 3 methods to assist preschool children to eat.

NURSING APPLICATIONS

Assessment

Physical—for socioeconomic level, child's age, developmental level, height, weight.
Dietary—for eating environment, frequency of meals and snacks, quantity of foods consumed, adequacy of intake, parental beliefs/preferences about food.
Laboratory—for iron, vitamin C, vitamin B_6, calcium.

Interventions

1. Encourage eating meals at regular times.
2. Monitor I&O. If sufficient amounts are not eaten, limit snacking or provide nutrient-dense snacks; offer cheese cubes, fresh fruit, raw vegetable sticks, milk, and fruit juices.

Evaluation

* Parents should be able to plan a nutritious menu and handle common food problems.

Client Education

- Offer new foods frequently; introduce 1 new food at a time with a familiar food to get more acceptance. The child is expected to taste each food that is prepared and served; but the taste may be very small.
- It is believed that atherosclerosis begins in childhood and that a reduction of fats and cholesterol in the diet after the second birthday decreases the risk of this disease.
- If the child is allowed to snack too frequently, he or she may not ever become hungry.
- Food should not be used as a bribe or reward.
- Children should not be made to clean their plates.
- Present disliked foods in a matter-of-fact manner, serving small portions (1 to 2 tsp); discard without comment if the child does not eat them.
- Successful feeding of children may be best accomplished by providing a variety of healthful foods and allowing them to eat without coercion. Without some guidance, however, children may fill up on kilocalorie-dense foods that do not provide adequate amounts of other nutrients.

TODDLER/PRESCHOOL PROBLEMS RELATED TO NUTRITION

Asphyxiation by Food

One death occurs approximately every 5 days from food-related asphyxiation in infants and children up to 9 years of age. A common cause is choking on bones, seeds, or regurgitated formula or juice. As the infant begins cutting teeth, great care should be taken to omit foods conducive to choking. Introduction of foods with texture is important from 6 months to 1 year, but the food must be easily dissolved, e.g., crackers or zwieback. When chewing has fully developed, soft raw vegetables such as peeled zucchini may be offered.

Several characteristics influence the chance of food penetrating the defenses of the mouth and pharynx. Food that is small, thin, smooth, or slick when wet may inadvertently slip through and enter the pharynx. Hard or tough foods resist mastication and may enter the pharynx prematurely without being properly chewed and mixed with saliva. Then the cough or gag reflex may be triggered after a deep inhalation that causes food to lodge in the trachea. Highly viscous foods, such as peanut butter, mold to the airway. Round or cylindrical and pliable or compressible foods can easily plug the airway. Hot dogs cause the most deaths. Other foods most often listed as causing asphyxia include apples, cookies, beans, carrots, bread, nuts, chewing gum, hard candy, and grapes.

Distractions during eating or poor caretaker supervision can play a role not only by failing to prevent asphyxiation initially, but also in averting proper rescue attempts. Information regarding choking risks in children should be disseminated not only to parents and caretakers, but also to the food industry and health professionals. When children are encouraged to eat in a relaxed atmosphere without being rushed or distracted or allowed to engage in horseplay during the meal, risks of aspiration are reduced.

List 5 foods associated with asphyxiation. What can parents/nurses do to prevent aspiration?

NURSING APPLICATIONS

Assessment

Physical—for choking, not being able to speak, child grabbing throat.
Dietary—for types of food eaten, eating habits.

Interventions

1. Perform the Heimlich maneuver if airway becomes obstructed.

Evaluation

* Client should not aspirate, or if aspiration occurs, appropriate measures were taken (Heimlich).

Client Education

- Encourage adequate chewing.
- Cut hot dogs lengthwise.
- Young children should always be supervised and seated while eating to prevent choking on foods.
- Do not allow young children to eat in a moving vehicle.
- Do not give young children hard candies.
- Asphyxiation may occur if laughing while eating.

Dental Caries

Since tooth formation begins before birth and is not completed until about 12 years of age, the actual structure of the tooth is affected by food intake during this time. Poorly developed teeth are more susceptible to decay later in life.

A clear relationship has been shown between nutritional deficiency during tooth development and tooth size, tooth formation, time of tooth eruption, and susceptibility to caries. Calcium with vitamin D must be present for proper calcification of the dentin and normal enamel. Vitamin D is critical to tooth development; later deficiency can promote tooth decay.

Teeth are more dense and hard when 1 part fluoride per million parts of drinking water is added during their formation. Excessive fluoride in water can cause permanent mottling of teeth. A 60% reduction of caries is gained by using fluoridated water during earlier growth periods. The topical administration of fluoride to teeth can also result in reduction of tooth decay.

Sealants act as a barrier protecting the decay-prone areas of the teeth from plaque and acid. It is a clear or shaded plastic material that is applied to the biting or chewing surfaces of permanent teeth.

Food selection and patterns of consumption influence dental health. Use of a toothbrush with dental floss, fluoride toothpaste, and sealants cannot completely control caries formation. Cariogenicity of food is influenced by its carbohydrate content, physical properties, and the frequency of consumption (see Chapter 4).

NURSING APPLICATIONS

Assessment

Physical—condition of oral cavity, presence of dental caries.

Dietary—for intake of sugar, frequency of snacking, calcium and vitamin D intake, source of fluoride.

Interventions

1. Provide nutritious snacks such as cheese cubes or raw vegetables.
2. Provide an opportunity to brush the teeth after eating; if not possible, rinse mouth with water.

Evaluation

* Parent can identify appropriate snacks; child does not develop caries.

Client Education

- Vitamin D-fortified milk and cheeses not only provide nutrients needed for healthy teeth, but also are noncariogenic.
- If the water supply is not fluoridated, a fluoride supplement should be provided as described earlier in the chapter.
- Avoid sticky carbohydrate foods such as candies, cookies, crackers, pastries, and raisins between meals. These contribute to dental caries by their carbohydrate content, physical properties, and frequency of consumption.

Attention Deficit Hyperactivity Disorder

Attention deficit hyperactivity disorder (ADHD) is the latest term for hyperkinetic behavior syndrome, hyperactivity, learning disabilities, or minimal brain dysfunction. The specific cause is unknown. For a diagnosis of ADHD, the child must exhibit specific symptoms before age 7. Problems seem to lessen or disappear as adolescence approaches, but some clients continue to exhibit symptoms of ADHD later in life.

ADHD is a specific behavior disorder characterized by chronic age-inappropriate behaviors with attention, impulsiveness, hyperactivity, or restlessness.

In the 1970s, the late Dr. Benjamin Feingold suggested a diet for ADHD free of all foods containing artificial colorings, flavorings, and naturally occurring salicylates. However, numerous controlled studies failed to reproduce the dramatic behavioral improvement Feingold reported. Although a minority of children may be helped by this diet, benefits may be associated with increased family involvement and expectations rather than the diet per se.

The belief that high sugar intake causes ADHD is in direct opposition to the

Does sugar cause ADHD? What effect do large amounts of carbohydrate have on the body?

results of many research studies (Gans, 1991). Sugar intake of normal boys and ADHD boys is similar, averaging 15% of the kilocaloric intake (Wolraich et al, 1986). Numerous studies have shown that carbohydrate intake has a sedative effect on the nervous system (Kruesi, 1986; Spring et al, 1986). Large amounts of carbohydrate cause drowsiness as a result of increased serotonin levels that cause decreased activity and food intake (Leprohon-Greenwood & Anderson, 1986).

NURSING APPLICATIONS

Assessment

Physical—for weight, height, growth rate, percentile rank, activity level, attention span.

Dietary—for nutrient intake, eating habits.

Interventions

1. Do not severely restrict the diet. There is little evidence to indicate that ADHD is affected by megavitamins, sugar intake, caffeine, food allergens, or food dyes (Myers et al, 1989).

Evaluation

* Child's diet is not severely restricted for management of ADHD.

Client Education

- There are no validated tests for food-related behavioral problems.
- The overwhelming conclusion of scientific information is that neither sugar nor food additives cause ADHD.
- External cues, such as parties or celebrations, possibly associated with sugar intake will cause hyperactivity.

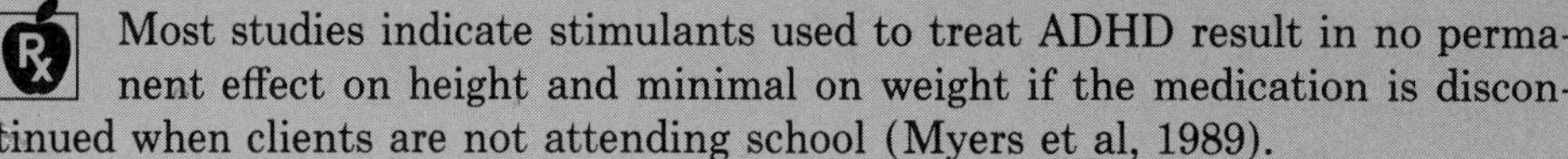

Most studies indicate stimulants used to treat ADHD result in no permanent effect on height and minimal on weight if the medication is discontinued when clients are not attending school (Myers et al, 1989).

Lead Toxicity

Lead is more readily absorbed from the GI tract during infancy and early childhood than in adulthood; thus, children are more susceptible to lead exposure. Nutritional status can influence susceptibility to lead toxicity. A federal initiative is to reduce environmental lead exposure from major sources such as paint, urban soil, dust, and drinking water. To decrease lead exposure, several preventive measures have been implemented. Lead solder is used in fewer food cans, and glass and plastic containers are replacing cans. New national standards established by the Environmental Protection Agency will reduce the allowable lead in drinking water from 50 parts per billion (ppb) to 5 ppb.

Lead is ingested from toddlers' normal hand-to-mouth activities; in older children, playing with dirt or lead-contaminated objects may result in lead ingestion.

Various nutritional factors can reduce absorption and tissue accumulation of lead in children at high risk of elevated lead exposure: (1) A diet providing at least the RDA for calcium (include 4 cups milk) decreases lead absorption. (2) A well-balanced diet is not a cure for lead poisoning, but deficiencies in calcium, iron, zinc, protein, and fat enhance lead toxicity. (3) Although adequate amounts of minerals are important, high levels may be toxic.

The effects of lead toxicity are most pronounced in children and fetuses because it can damage the CNS and kidneys. Lead also decreases normal production of RBCs. Screening for lead toxicity can prevent irreversible physiological damage and fatality. Even low levels of lead exposure may impair intellectual performance (Needleman & Gatsonis, 1990). As serum lead levels rise, general cognitive, verbal, and perceptual abilities are increasingly affected by slower learning aptitudes, which appear to be irreversible (Brown et al, 1990).

What are some ways to decrease lead in the environment; in the diet? What are the effects of lead poisoning?

NURSING APPLICATIONS

Assessment

Physical—for living conditions, vomiting, irritability, weight loss, malaise, headache, and insomnia.

Dietary—for pica, type of water ingested, calcium, iron, zinc, protein, and fat intake.

Laboratory—for lead levels (>25 mcg/100 ml is toxic) and by testing for aminolevulinic acid-delta (an enzyme that increases in lead toxicity) and free erythrocyte protoporphyrin, RBC, Hgb, Hct.

Interventions

1. Give edetate calcium disodium (EDTA) as ordered, which allows calcium to be displaced by lead, and the lead-EDTA combination is excreted via the urine.

Evaluation

* The child's serum lead level should return to below 25 mcg/100 ml.

Client Education

- Some bone meal sold in health food stores for calcium supplementation contains dangerous amounts of lead.
- Children should consume a well-balanced diet, with 4 cups of milk.
- Parents who are preparing infant formula should follow these guidelines (Shannon & Graef, 1992): (1) Allow cold water to run for 2 minutes to flush the water system before using tap water to make formula or use bottled water; (2) do not boil water for formula preparation.

SCHOOL-AGE CHILDREN (7 TO 12 YEARS OLD)

These middle childhood years are the result of early growth and development; reserves are laid down for upcoming rapid adolescent growth. New activities and new friends begin to influence choices and broaden one's horizons. The child will be exposed to different foods and food patterns. These new ideas may affect food choices at home.

Although food preferences are established early, children begin to accept more foods. Almost all foods are liked; vegetables are the least favorite. Planning menus around food groups is important to include all the necessary nutrients. Foods containing mostly sugars or fats are not eliminated, but they should not replace recommended amounts from the food groups. The appetite is usually good; but food habits and intake may suffer because children do not take time for meals. A specific amount of time (15 to 20 min) at the table may prevent the child from forming the habit of gulping down food. Poor appetite may be caused by stresses, such as schoolwork and emotional difficulties.

Good manners can and should be learned at this age; however, punishment or continuous correction at the table is not appropriate. Children learn by imitating adults at family mealtime.

Students are ravenous after school. Although bakery products, soft drinks, candy, and chips are favorites, nutritious snacks are preferable. More access to money may result in expenditures at fast food restaurants and from vending machines. These foods are usually high in fat, salt, and sugar.

At this stage of life, it is also important for children to form good exercise habits. Sports interests should be cultivated while the child is young. Although team sports are important, activities that rely more on individual participation such as swimming can be maintained throughout life. Even at this early age, weight control is a balance between physical activity and food intake. Good exercise habits need to be cultivated early in life.

Weight loss or gain reflects inadequate or excessive intake, which should be balanced with an appropriate amount of exercise. The goal for obese children is weight maintenance or reduction in the rate of weight gain while height increases. By "growing into their weight," body fat decreases without compromising lean body mass and growth.

Describe 4 ways to help school-age children eat nutritiously and stay healthy.

NURSING APPLICATIONS

Assessment

Physical—for schoolwork or emotional difficulties, height, weight, serial weights, activity level, sports interests.

Dietary—for nutrient/fluid intake, appetite, food preferences, child's/parent's beliefs about nutrition.

Interventions

1. Have nutritious snacks readily available.
2. Do not recommend weight reduction diets for overweight children.

Client Education

- Children involved in meal preparation are more likely to eat the food prepared and to be aware of what is in the food.
- Have nutritious foods available for snacks such as dried fruits, yogurt, popcorn, low-fat cheese, or dry roasted seeds or nuts.

ADOLESCENTS

Major biological, social, psychological, and cognitive changes occur during adolescence. Because of these changes, 17% of US teenagers are considered to be at nutritional risk (AAP, 1985). It is not surprising that many adolescents consume less than adequate amounts of nutrients, and fitness levels are declining (AMA, ADA, 1991). Rapid growth rates cause them to be particularly susceptible to nutrient deficiencies. Many of their eating practices place them at risk for developing chronic diseases later in life.

Growth and Nutrient Requirements

Growth of long bones, secondary sexual maturation, and fat and muscle deposition create an increased nutrient requirement. Although the RDAs provide recommended nutrient intakes by chronological age, nutrient needs closely parallel physical development. For instance, adolescent girls need to increase their energy intake sooner and decrease it more quickly than boys because of earlier onset of puberty and lower total body weight once adulthood is reached. Adolescent boys have greater nutritional needs than adolescent girls because of growth rates and body composition changes (see Table 15–7). A 15-year-old boy requires 3000 kcal as compared with 2200 kcal for a 15-year-old girl.

The need for calcium and iron is of particular importance. As a result of the dramatic increase in skeletal mass, calcium needs are greater than at any other time of life (NRC, 1989). Calcium intake during adolescence promotes calcium retention and bone mineral density. Adequate calcium intake is important for achievement of peak bone mass.

What 3 factors increase nutrient requirements? Explain why calcium and iron requirements are increased.

The expansion of blood volume and increase in red cell mass and muscle mass, especially in boys, and the need to replace iron losses associated with menstruation in girls require increased iron. Participation in sports activities leads to RBC destruction. Poor dietary habits result in inadequate folate; riboflavin; vitamins B_6, A, and C; iron; and calcium intake.

Influential Factors on Eating Habits

Complex external factors, such as family, peers, mass media, and economic and sociocultural factors, and internal factors, such as physiological needs, body image, self-concept, food preferences, and personal values/beliefs toward health and nutrition, all influence food choices. Probably the strongest influential factor among teenagers is peer pressure. Not only are food choices affected, but also the times available to eat may be determined by group activities. As adolescents move toward independence, they begin to spend more time with their friends; eating is an important form of socialization.

Teens who eat with their families on a regular basis usually have more nutritious diets. If parents have been authoritarian, teenagers may use food to express rebellion against parental authority. On the other hand, permissive parents leave teens on their own, which fosters poor eating habits.

Most adolescents are stressed because of continual changes. Sexuality, body image, scholastic and athletic pressures, relationships with friends and relatives, finances, career plans, and ideological beliefs may cause conflicts as adolescents try to understand their identity. The presence of stress can decrease the utilization of several nutrients, particularly vitamin C and calcium.

Adolescents, especially girls, are often obsessed about their body image and a desire to be thin. They are eager to try fad diets, which may be inadequate in nutrients. This is unfortunate because nutrients during this period are necessary to build the basic strength of their bodies to last a lifetime. Obesity, anorexia nervosa, and bulimia are serious health concerns amenable to early treatment. These problems are discussed in Chapters 19 and 20. Prevention may be the only successful treatment in some cases.

In addition to body shape and size, the age-old problem of acne vulgaris affects the teenager's self-image. The increased hormone secretions, especially testosterone, during this period affect the **sebaceous glands** of the skin. Copious amounts of **sebum** are produced. Contrary to popular opinion, scientific studies do not show any correlation between diet, or eating chocolate, carbonated beverages, or fatty foods, and acne. The oral or topical use of retinoic acid (a vitamin A acid) appears to decrease production of sebum and thereby reduces acne lesions. This medication appears to be more effective than tetracycline but still requires close medical supervision to prevent toxicity symptoms. A well-balanced diet along with good skin care helps lessen the severity of acne.

Sebaceous glands present in the skin around the hair follicles produce sebum, which is an oily secretion.

Favorite food choices are carbonated beverages, milk, steak, hamburgers, pizza, spaghetti, chicken, french fries, ice cream, oranges, orange juice, apples, and bread. Vegetables are not popular. Milk consumption is being replaced by carbonated beverages, especially in adolescent girls. In one study, approximately 20% of adolescent boys and 40% of girls omitted milk on the day they were surveyed (Ritchko, 1991).

About 25% of an adolescent's kilocalories come from tasty, high-kilocalorie, low nutrient dense foods, making overeating easy (Dwyer, 1991). Such problems as excessive intake of sodium, sugar, and fat; frequent snacking; skipping meals; eating on the run; and reliance on convenience and fast foods are accentuated during this time.

Busy schedules cause clients to miss meals, especially breakfast and lunch. Girls skip meals more often than boys. Girls who scored high on personal adjustment, emotional stability, family relations, and conformity missed fewer meals and had better diets than other girls. Skipping meals may make weight control more difficult.

What is the strongest influential factor affecting teenagers' nutrition habits? What nutrients are affected by stress? Describe food myths about acne.

Fast food restaurants, vending machines, and convenience stores fit adolescents' busy, active lifestyles. The nutrient value of fast foods is provided in Appendix A-3. Fast foods are acceptable nutritionally when consumed in moderation as a part of a well-balanced diet. Lower kilocalorie items and a wider variety of selections, such as salad and low-fat milkshakes, now on the menu can contribute to nutrient requirements without providing excessive kilocalories.

Snacking is often essential for meeting daily energy and nutrient needs, especially when the adolescent is physically active or in a growth period. Adolescents who do not snack between meals or eat 3 meals daily have poorer diets than those who eat more frequently. These snacks can offer significant nutrients and can be improved with the substitution of a shake for a cola or by adding orange juice.

Nutrition Counseling

The best tactic for nutrition counseling among adolescents is to appeal to their physical image or their muscular development for sports. The earlier information is presented, the more likely it is to be accepted and used later in life. In helping adolescents improve their eating patterns, the best approach is to praise good food choices, ignore those that are neutral, and discourage harmful practices (Farthing, 1991).

Identify 2 ways to approach adolescents to improve eating patterns.

NURSING APPLICATIONS

Assessment

Physical—for activity level, weight, height, growth spurt, use of illicit drugs, body image, self-concept, influence of peer pressure, stress level.

Dietary—for nutrient intake (especially of iron; folate; riboflavin; vitamins B_6, A, and C; calcium); energy and protein intake; use of fast foods, convenience foods, or vending machines; food preferences; personal values/beliefs toward health and nutrition; alcohol intake.

Laboratory—for calcium, iron, RBC, Hgb, Hct.

Interventions

1. Individualize dietary recommendations and approaches (Carruth, 1990).
2. Encourage calcium-containing foods.
3. Praise good eating patterns.
3. Even if special diets are necessary (as in juvenile diabetes), allow teenagers to assume responsibility for food choices.
4. Monitor drug and alcohol intake. Money may be used to purchase drugs and alcohol rather than food, thus resulting in decreased nutrient intake.

If client is taking tetracyline, discourage taking the medication with milk, as tetracycline complexes with the calcium in milk, resulting in poor absorption of both. However, total abstention from milk and milk products during tetracycline therapy is unnecessary. Milk can be consumed 2 to 3 hours before or after taking tetracycline.

Client Education

- Teenagers should be aware of the long-term risks and benefits of good nutrition, but the best approach is to focus on the short-term benefits of eating well.
- Restriction of kilocalorie intake during the rapid growth period will compromise lean body mass accumulation despite a seemingly adequate protein intake (which is used for energy instead of growth) (Pipes, 1989).
- Intense physical activity can cause increased urinary loss of calcium and RBC destruction.
- Snacking can have a positive influence on the overall nutritional status of the teenager. Parents can stock the kitchen with nutritious snack foods, e.g., cooked meats, raw vegetables, milk, cheese, fruit, nuts, peanut butter, and popcorn to encourage good eating habits.
- Use of dietary supplements by most adolescents is not needed.

FACTORS RELATED TO SCHOOL-AGE CHILDREN'S NUTRITION

Breakfast

Name 3 reasons breakfast is important.

The meal most likely to be skipped by all school-age children is breakfast. Numerous excuses are given. This meal, which breaks the 10- to 14-hour fast, provides nutrients and energy that are necessary to fuel the morning's activities. The morning meal may help to improve attitude, increase work output, and result in a better attention span. Children who omit breakfast are more likely to be careless and listless in the late morning hours. The detrimental effect on mental status is more pronounced in undernourished children (Simeon & Grantham-McGregor, 1987).

Breakfast should furnish at least one-fourth to one-third of the nutrients for the day. Foods do not have to be the traditional breakfast items; most children prefer choices that are readily available, quick to prepare, and good tasting.

Breakfasts are offered by some schools. The federal School Breakfast Program requires 3 food components to provide children with a good start toward meeting their daily nutritional needs. Children from low-income families may receive free or reduced-price breakfasts. An average of 4.4 million children participated in this program in 1991 (Matsumoto, 1991). Minimal requirements are established, as shown in Table 15–8.

School Lunch

Lunch may be provided by the school or brought from home. The federal government requires participants of the National School Lunch Program to provide approximately one-third of the RDAs for children. The school lunch program is one of the most successful anti-hunger and nutrition programs developed by the government. New, different, and disliked foods are introduced to children in a setting where they are anxious to conform. Free or reduced price meals are served to an average of 24.2 million children from low-income families yearly (Matsumoto, 1991). Schools are encouraged to follow the Dietary Guidelines for Americans by lowering fat, sugar, and salt of the foods served.

Many changes have been implemented in the school lunch program to increase participation and provide healthier meals. Popular items, such as pizza or burritos, may appear on the menu; skim or low-fat milk or cultured buttermilk must be offered; fresh fruits are provided rather than desserts such as cake (Table 15–9).

"Offer versus serve" was designed to reduce plate waste and food costs in the lunch program without sacrificing the nutritional integrity of meals. It allows students to refuse 1 or 2 items that they do not intend to consume. In other words, of the 5 items on the menu, the student must take only 3 or 4.

What percentage of the RDAs is provided by the National School Lunch Program? What 3 nutrients are lowered in these meals? What other changes have been made?

The School Lunch Program is usually more nutritious, not because it is a hot meal, but because box lunches generally contain less variety. Normally, only favorite foods are carried. Packed lunches are also limited to foods that travel well and do not need heating or refrigeration.

NURSING APPLICATIONS

Assessment

Physical—for height, weight; socioeconomic status.
Dietary—for breakfast habits, where lunch is taken.

Interventions

1. Offer nontraditional foods such as cold pizza or breakfast burritos.
2. Stress how breakfast will help with sports and schoolwork.

Evaluation

* Child eats breakfast regularly and consumes a nutritious lunch; clients who qualify for free or reduced-price meals participate.

Client Education

- Routine breakfast consumption is one of the key habits linked to better health.
- Skipping meals may make weight control more difficult.
- Children who eat breakfast have higher intakes of nutrients than children who omit this meal.
- Children who omit breakfast are more likely to be obese.
- Organize breakfast foods the night before to expedite the rush in the morning; choose foods that are quick to prepare.
- Plan foods that can be eaten en route to school, i.e., bagels, toast, or biscuit sandwiches.

TABLE 15–8

MINIMAL REQUIREMENTS OF THE FEDERAL SCHOOL BREAKFAST PROGRAM

1. Milk—½ pint pasteurized fluid, whole, skim, low-fat milk or cultured buttermilk served as a beverage or on cereal
2. Vegetables and fruit—½ cup of fruit or vegetables or ½ cup of full-strength fruit or vegetable juice
3. Bread or cereal—a serving of bread or ¾ cup or 1 oz of cereal, or an equivalent combination. (The variation in serving size for cereal allows for a smaller serving of the high-density granola-type cereals)

The following is encouraged but not mandatory:

A meat or meat alternate—1 oz (edible portion as served) of meat, poultry, or fish; or 1 oz of cheese, or 1 egg, or 2 tbsp of peanut butter; or an equivalent amount of any combination of these foods

TABLE 15–9 **SCHOOL LUNCH PATTERNS FOR VARIOUS AGE/GRADE GROUPS**

Components	Minimum Quantities				Recommended Quantities†	Specific Requirements
	Preschool ages 1–2 **(Group I)**	***Preschool ages 3–4*** **(Group II)**	***Grades K–3 ages 5–8*** **(Group III)**	***Grades 4–12 age 9 and over*** **(Group IV)***	**Grades 7–12 age 12 and over (Group V)**	
Meat or meat alternate						Must be served in the main dish or the main dish and one other menu item
A serving of one of the following or a combination to give an equivalent quantity:						Vegetable protein products, cheese alternate products, and enriched macaroni with fortified protein may be used to meet part of the meat/meat alternate requirement. Fact sheets on each of these alternate foods give detailed instructions for use
Lean meat, poultry, or fish (edible portion as served)	1 oz	1½ oz	1½ oz	2 oz	3 oz	
Cheese	1 oz	1½ oz	1½ oz	2 oz	3 oz	
Large egg(s)	½	¾	¾	1	1½	
Cooked dry beans or peas	¼ cup	⅜ cup	⅜ cup	½ cup	¾ cup	
Peanut butter	2 Tbsp	3 Tbsp	3 Tbsp	4 Tbsp	6 Tbsp	
Vegetable and/or fruit	½ cup	½ cup	½ cup	¾ cup	¾ cup	No more than one-half of the total requirement may be met with full-strength fruit or vegetable juice
Two or more servings of vegetable or fruit or both to total						Cooked dry beans or peas may be used as a meat alternate or as a vegetable but not as both in the same meal
Bread or bread alternate	5 per week	8 per week	8 per week	8 per week	10 per week	At least ½ serving of bread or an equivalent quantity of bread alternate for group I, and 1 serving for groups II–V, must be served daily
Servings of bread or bread alternate						Enriched macaroni with fortified protein may be used as a meat alternate or as a bread alternate but not as both in the same meal
A serving is:						*Note: Food Buying Guide for Child Nutrition Programs,* PA-1331 (1983) provides the information for the minimum weight of a serving
1 slice of whole-grain or enriched bread						
A whole-grain or enriched biscuit, roll, muffin, etc						
½ cup of cooked whole-grain or enriched rice, macaroni, noodles, whole-grain or enriched pasta products, or other cereal grains such as bulgur or corn grits						
A combination of any of the above						
Milk	¾ cup (6 fl oz)	¾ cup (6 fl oz)	½ pint (8 fl oz)	½ pint (8 fl oz)	½ pint (8 fl oz)	At least one of the following forms of milk must be offered: Unflavored low-fat milk; Unflavored skim milk; Unflavored buttermilk
A serving of fluid milk						*Note:* This requirement does not prohibit offering other milks, such as whole milk or flavored milk, along with one or more of the above

US Department of Agriculture, National School Lunch Program. USDA recommends, but does not require, that you adjust portions by age/grade group to better meet the food and nutritional needs of children according to their ages. If you adjust portions, groups I–IV are minimum requirements for the age/grade groups specified. If you do *not* adjust portions, the group IV portions are the portions to serve all children.

* Group IV is highlighted because it is the one meal pattern that will satisfy all requirements if no portion size adjustments are made.

† Group V specifies recommended, not required, quantities for students 12 years and older. These students may request smaller portions, but not smaller than those specified in group IV.

ILLNESS

Children who are ill at home or in the hospital require special treatment to meet their nutritional needs while their appetite is poor. A temporary decrease in food intake during short periods of illness does not pose any major problem. Parents need not try to force food during this time. Children with chronic or severe illnesses or injuries must be watched more closely.

A hospitalized child who understands some of the conditions and problems may be more cooperative; understanding the environment will ease the fears and frustrations and make it seem more familiar. By explaining procedures and the reasons for various treatments, the child will better understand what is occurring. Most of all, the presence of a parent is of utmost importance to help allay fears. Although food intake is encouraged, too much coaxing and attention will cause children to rebel and become manipulative.

Dehydration can occur rapidly in young children and infants when body fluids are lost and not adequately replaced (fever, vomiting, and diarrhea). To insure against dehydration, offer the child small amounts of favorite beverages at least hourly, expecting him or her to take some. Water or diluted fruit juices may be given. Beverages sweetened with sugar, rather than artificially, are preferred because they offer some kilocalories as well as fluid. Foods that have a high water content, e.g., congealed gelatin, Popsicles, or sherbet, are offered frequently.

Plain foods low in fat and delicately seasoned are better tolerated and have more appeal to the sick child. Frequent small meals, rather than 3 larger ones, also increase intake.

What foods are offered to the child to insure against dehydration? What foods are offered to the sick child? How can the environment be manipulated to increase intake?

Manipulation of the environment can encourage the sick child to eat. Colorful and cleverly designed straws, napkins, and plates can induce children to eat. Food intake can also be increased by socialization during the meal. Children who are hospitalized can be allowed to eat together. When possible, someone should sit and talk with the child during mealtime. Including parents in planning the care and having them readily available to encourage the child help provide security and support.

NURSING APPLICATIONS

Assessment

Physical—for hydration level, vomiting, diarrhea, reason for illness, weight, height, apprehension.
Dietary—for food preferences, actual food and fluid intake.
Laboratory—for sodium, potassium, calcium.

Interventions

1. Address the child's questions.
2. Explain all procedures according to the child's developmental level.
3. Allow parents to assist as much as possible.
4. Monitor I&O.
5. Involve the child (if old enough) in altering his or her fluid intake.

Evaluation

* The illness is resolved with minimal or no weight loss, and parents contributed to the care.

Client Education

• Teach client or family how to monitor intake. Provide pencil and paper.

SUMMARY

From infancy to adolescence, adequate nutrition is essential to support the rapid growth and development during the different stages of life. The nutritional needs of infants are best met by breast milk; however, formula feedings simulate breast milk and are suitable alternatives.

Growth by height and weight are key techniques to assess the health status of children. Nutrient intake influences the physical, emotional, and mental abilities of each client. Nutrient needs for all stages of growth can be met by providing a well-balanced diet based on all the food groups.

Regardless of the growth rate or state of health, the critical need for nutritional education is constantly present. All nurses can teach good practices for optimal nutrition.

Several disorders that can affect nutritional status were discussed. Sensitive nursing care may help minimize these nutritional interruptions.

NURSING PROCESS IN ACTION

Cathy, who is 16 years old, approaches the school nurse about her weight. Cathy is concerned about gaining too much weight and skips breakfast frequently because it takes too much time. She does not like milk, but fruit juices are "okay." She likes swimming, but does this only in the summer. Her current weight is 126 lbs and height is 5′6″.

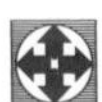

Nutritional Assessment

- Food preferences; adequacy of kilocalorie/fluid/nutrient intake, especially folic acid, riboflavin, vitamin B_6, vitamin A, vitamin C, iron, and calcium; alcohol intake.
- Menses history.
- Peer influence, family support.
- Her peers' and family's beliefs/values about nutrition, weight, and health.
- Body image, self-concept.
- Stress and activity level.
- Use of fad diets, illicit drugs, convenience foods, or vending machines.

Dietary Nursing Diagnosis

High risk for altered health maintenance RT insufficient knowledge about healthy nutrition habits.

Nutritional Goals

Client will maintain weight of 126 lbs and verbalize good nutritional principles.

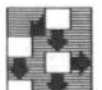

Nutritional Implementation

Intervention: Suggest eating foods high in calcium and iron (chicken, cheeseburger, orange juice with calcium).

Rationale: As a result of dramatic increases in skeletal mass, calcium needs are greater than at any other time of life. Iron replaces losses associated with menstruation in girls. Foods listed are favorites of typical adolescents and contain calcium and iron. Since she likes fruit juices better than milk, orange juice with calcium will help meet her calcium needs.

Intervention: Explain that people who skip breakfast are more likely to have problems with weight control, i.e., obesity.
Rationale: Since she is concerned about gaining weight, this may motivate her to try nutritionally good eating patterns.

Intervention: Offer suggestions such as cold pizza, bagels, or breakfast burritos for breakfast.
Rationale: She says she does not have time for breakfast, and these suggestions are fast to prepare and can be eaten en route to school.

Intervention: Discourage the use of fad diets.
Rationale: Adolescent girls are eager to try fad diets, which are inadequate in nutrients. Nutrients are needed during this period to build the basic body strength to last a lifetime.

Intervention: Relate how good intake can help improve swimming.
Rationale: Cathy likes swimming, so this may be an appropriate motivator.

Intervention: Suggest going to an indoor swimming facility during winter months or joining a swim club or swim team.
Rationale: Weight control is a balance between physical activity and food intake. Only exercise habits that are appealing to the client will be continued.

Intervention: Allow her to make the final choices for meals/foods eaten.
Rationale: The developmental stage during adolescence is finding their identity; permitting choices allows independence to achieve identity rather than role confusion.

Intervention: Show her on a weight chart that her weight is acceptable for 5′6″.
Rationale: Cathy is concerned that she is overweight. Concrete evidence may help lessen this fear.

Evaluation

Cathy should still weigh 126 lbs and state, "skipping breakfast does not help me lose weight, swimming is good for me, but I should not overdo it, and cheeseburgers are good for me since they provide calcium and iron."

STUDENT READINESS

1. Plan meals for a family for 1 day with a 2-year-old toddler, a 10-year-old boy, and a 15-year-old girl.
2. What is the treatment for an infant with diarrhea?
3. What are the differences between LBW and premature infants, and how do these differences affect their food intake?
4. Discuss feeding a newborn infant from birth to age 1.
5. What is considered normal weight for a newborn infant?
6. A mother wants to know about nutrition for her preschooler. What would you tell her?
7. A mother tells you that since her child is hyperkinetic she is going to stop all sugar. How would you respond?

CASE STUDY

Jennifer C. is brought to the physician's office for a 6-month checkup. She weighed 3.2 kg at birth and now weighs 6.9 kg. She was bottle-fed from birth. At 3 months, she was started on cereals but has resisted all attempts to increase her solid food intake. She is allowed to go to sleep with a bottle and is often propped up in her crib with a bottle at the day care center.

1. What additional assessment data would you need?
2. Is Jennifer's weight gain within the expected range?
3. How much should she gain in the next 6 months?
4. What tentative nursing diagnosis could you derive?
5. The nurse encourages Jennifer's mother to discontinue the habit of allowing her to go to sleep with a bottle and to request that the day care center do the same. Why?
6. The physician recommends that solid foods be introduced gradually to Jennifer. What foods should be introduced first?
7. If Jennifer's mother decides to prepare the food at home, what procedures should she use?
8. When will Jennifer be old enough for finger-foods?
9. Why should egg whites be withheld until 1 year of age?

REFERENCES

Allen LH. Child nutrition and growth. *Food & Nutrition News* 1991 63(3):15–18. (A publication of National Life Stock & Meat Board.)

American Academy of Pediatrics (AAP) Committee on Nutrition. Follow-up or weaning formulas. *Pediatrics* 1989 June; 83(6):1067.

American Academy of Pediatrics (AAP) Committee on Nutrition. *Pediatric Nutrition Handbook.* 2nd ed. Elk Grove Village, IL, American Academy of Pediatrics, 1985.

American Medical Association (AMA) and the American Dietetic Association (ADA). *Targets for Adolescent Health: Adolescent Nutrition and Physical Fitness.* Chicago, AMA and ADA, 1991.

Anonymous. Is colic associated with diet? *Nutr Reviews* 1988 Nov; 46(11):374–379.

Arshad SH, et al. Effect of allergen avoidance on development of allergic disorders in infancy. *Lancet* 1992 June 20; 339(8808):1493–1497.

Barness LA. Infant feeding: Formula, solids. *Pediatr Clin North Am* 1985 Apr; 32(2):355–362.

Birch LL, et al. The variability of young children's energy intake. *N Engl J Med* 1991 Jan 24; 324(4):232–235.

Block SA. Prospective appraisal of complaints of adverse reactions to foods in children during the first 3 years of life. *Pediatrics* 1987 May; 79(5):683–688.

Brooks MD. Nutrition overview of cleft lip and palate. *Topics Clin Nutr* 1988 July; 3:9.

Brown MJ, et al. Lead poisoning in children of different ages. *N Engl J Med* 1990 July 12; 323(2):135–136.

Carruth BR. Adolescence. *In* Brown ML (ed): *Present Knowledge in Nutrition.* 6th ed. Washington, D.C., Nutrition Foundation, 1990: 325–332.

Chandra R, et al. Effect of feeding whey hydrolysate, soy and conventional cow milk formulas on incidence of atopic disease in high risk infants. *Ann Allergy* 1989 Aug; 63(2):102–106.

Dwyer J. Teenagers' diets: Hazards, virtues, problems, solutions. *Nutr & the M.D.* 1991 Nov; 17(11):1–3.

Endert CM, Wooldridge NH. Nonorganic failure to thrive. *Dietetic Currents* 1987; 14(1):1–6. (A publication of Ross Laboratories.)

Farthing MC. Current eating patterns of adolescents in the United States. *Nutr Today* 1991 March/Apr; 26(2):35–39.

Fisher JC. Feeding children who have cleft lip or palate. *West J Med* 1991 Feb; 154(2):207.

Foman SJ, et al. Formula for older infants. *J Pediatr* 1990 May; 116(5):690–696.

Forsyth BW. Colic and the effect of changing formulas: A double blind, multiple crossover study. *J Pediatr* 1989 Oct; 115(4):521–526.

Gans DA. Sucrose and unusual behavior. *Nutr Today* 1991 May–June; 26(3):8–14.

Gong EJ, Heald FP. Diet, nutrition, and adolescence. *In* Shils ME, Young VR (ed): *Modern Nutrition in Health and Disease.* Philadelphia, Lea & Febiger, 1988: 969–982.

Healthy Start campaign launched at Food Marketing Institute Convention. *ADA Courier* 1991 June; 30(6):1,6.

Kruesi MFP. Carbohydrate intake and children's behavior. *Food Technology* 1986 Jan; 40(1):150–152.

Leprohon-Greenwood CE, Anderson GH. An overview of the mechanisms by which diet affects brain function. *Food Technology* 1986 Jan; 40(1):132–138.

Lewis P. Starvation ketosis after rehydration with diet soda. *Pediatrics* 1991 Oct; 88(10):806–807.

Lifschitz F. Management of acute diarrheal disease. Proceedings of a symposium, May 18–19, 1990. *J Pediatr* 1991 Apr; 118 (suppl 4):S25–S138.

Litovitz T, Manoguerra A. Comparison of pediatric poisoning hazards: An analysis of 3.8 million exposure incidents. *Pediatrics* 1992 June; 89(6):999–1006.

Lozoff B, et al. Long-term developmental outcome of infants with iron deficiency. *N Engl J Med* 1991 Sept 5; 325(10):687–694.

Matsumoto M. Domestic food assistance costs are rising. *Food Rev* 1991 Oct-Dec; 14(6):40–42.

McNinch A, Tripp JH. Haemorrhagic disease of the newborn in the British Isles: A two year prospective study. *Br Med J* 1991 Nov 2; 303(6810):1105–1109.

Miskelly FG. Infant feeding and allergy. *Arch Dis Child* 1988 Apr; 63(4):388–393.

Myers DA, et al. The hyperactive child: An update. *Tex Med* 1989 March; 85(3):25–31.

National Research Council (NRC). *Recommended Dietary Allowances.* 10th ed. Washington, D.C., National Academy Press, 1989.

Needleman HL, Gatsonis CA. Low-level lead exposure and the IQ of children. *JAMA* 1990 Feb 2; 263(5):673–678.

Nelson SE, et al. Lack of adverse reactions to iron-fortified formula. *Pediatrics* 1988 March; 81(3):360–364.

Pipes P. *Nutrition in Infancy and Childhood.* 4th ed. St Louis, Times Mirror/Mosby College Publishing, 1989.

Pizarro F, et al. Iron status with different infant feeding regimens: Relevancy to screening and prevention of iron deficiency. *J Pediatr* 1991 May; 118(5):687–692.

Powell GF. Nonorganic failure to thrive in infancy: An update on nutrition, behavior, and growth. *J Am Coll Nutr* 1988 May; 7(5):345–353.

Ritchko SA. What are children eating? Results from USDA's 1987–88 Nationwide Food Consumption Survey. Presentation at the Public Voice for Food and Health Policy Conference on Children and Nutrition: Building our Nation's Health. Washington, D.C., Jan 14, 1991.

Sampson HA, et al. Safety of casein hydrolysate formula in children with cow milk allergy. *J Pediatr* 1991 Apr; 118(4, Pt 1):520–525.

Select Panel for the Promotion of Child Health, Better Health for our Children: A National Strategy. Rockville, MD, U.S. Department of Health & Human Service, Public Health Service, Office of Maternal and Child Health, 1981.

Shannon M, Graef J. Hazard of lead in infant formula (Letter). *New Engl J Med* 1992 Jan 9; 326(2):137.

Shea S, et al. Variability and self-regulation of energy intake in young children in their everyday environment. *Pediatrics* 1992 Oct; 90(4): 542–546.

Shulman RJ, et al. Impact of dietary cereal on nutrient absorption and fecal nitrogen loss in formula-fed infants. *J Pediatr* 1991 Jan; 118(1):39–43.

Simeon DT, Grantham-McGregor S. Nutritional deficiencies and children's behavior and mental development. *Nutr Res Rev* 1990; 3:1–24.

Simeon D, Grantham-McGregor S. Cognitive function, undernutrition, and missed breakfast. *Lancet* 1987 Sept 26; 2(8561):737–738.

Sinden AA, Sutphen JL. Dietary treatment of lactose intolerance in infants and children. *J Am Diet Assoc* 1991 Dec; 91(12):1567–1571.

Smith MM, Lifschitz F. Failure to thrive. *Contemporary Nutrition* 1990; 15 (5). (A publication of General Mills.)

Snyder JD. Use and misuse of oral therapy for diarrhea: Comparison of U.S. practices with American Academy of Pediatrics recommendations. *Pediatrics* 1991 Jan; 87(1):28–33.

Splet PL, Story M. Child nutrition: Objectives for the decade. *J Am Diet Assoc* 1991 June; 91(6):685–688.

Spring BJ, et al. Effects of carbohydrates on mood and behavior. *Nutr Rev* 1986 May; 44(suppl):51–60.

Taubman B. Parental counseling compared with elimination of cow's milk or soy milk protein for the treatment of infant colic syndrome: A randomized trial. *Pediatrics* 1988 June; 81(6):745–761.

US Department of Health and Human Services (USDHHS). *Healthy People 2000.* National Health Promotion and Disease Prevention Objectives. Washington, D.C., Superintendent of Documents, 1990.

Von Kries R. Neonatal vitamin K. Prophylaxis for all. *Br Med J* 1991 Nov 2; 303(6810):1083–1084.

Walker W, Hendricks KM. *Manual of Pediatric Nutrition.* Philadelphia, WB Saunders, 1985.

Winick M. *Nutrition, Pregnancy, and Early Infancy.* Baltimore, Williams & Wilkins, 1989.

Wolraich ML, et al. Dietary characteristics of hyperactive and control boys. *J Am Diet Assoc*

1986 Apr; 86(4):500–504.

Ziegler EE. Milks and formulas for older infants. *J Pediatr* 1990 Aug; 117(2 Pt 2):S76–S79.

Ziegler EE, et al. Cow milk feeding in infancy: Further observations on blood loss from the gastrointestinal tract. *J Pediatr* 1990 Jan; 116(1):11–18.

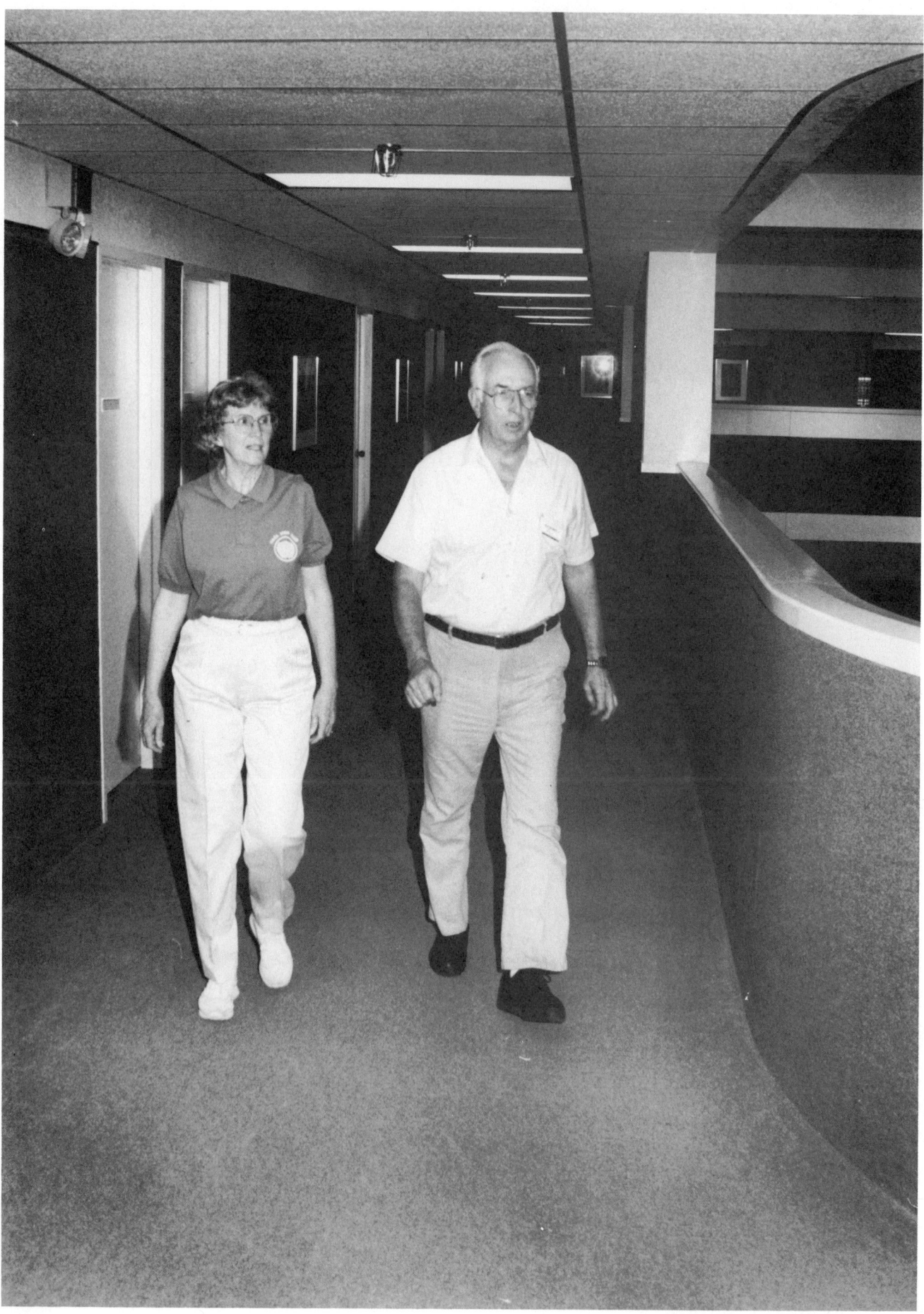

CHAPTER 16

Nutritional Considerations of the Older Adult

OUTLINE

C. Supplements
D. Adaptive Equipment
Nursing Applications
V. PHARMACEUTICALS
Nursing Applications
VI. NUTRITIONAL ASSESSMENT
A. Anthropometric Measurements
B. Biochemical Measurements
VII. LONG-TERM CARE FACILITIES
VIII. COMMUNITY SERVICES
A. Federal Programs
Nursing Applications
IX. CONDITIONS THAT AFFECT NUTRITIONAL STATUS
A. Alzheimer's Disease
Nursing Applications
B. Multi-Infarct Dementia
Nursing Applications
C. Other Causes of Dementia
Nursing Applications

OBJECTIVES

THE STUDENT WILL BE ABLE TO:

- Discuss physiological changes that alter the elderly client's nutritional status.
- Discuss differences in amounts of nutrients needed by elderly clients as compared with younger adults.
- Describe factors that influence the food intake of older clients.
- Explain dietary procedures for maintaining the individual's ego and self-integrity.
- Discuss dietary changes that could be made to provide optimum nutrient intake.
- Apply nursing application principles for nutritional needs of the elderly client.
- Identify client education for elderly clients.

TEST YOUR NQ (True/False)

1. New denture wearers should introduce meats first, followed by beverages or liquid intake.
2. Nutritional needs for a 51-year-old client are different than those for an 81-year-old.
3. Healthy elderly women require increased amounts of iron.
4. Energy requirements decrease with age.
5. Self-medication with vitamins is a healthy practice for the elderly.
6. Elderly clients need 2 servings of vitamin C–rich foods daily.
7. Mineral oil is a good inexpensive laxative.
8. Laetrile (ground nutmeat of apricot kernels) can slow down the process of aging.
9. Antioxidants increase the life span.
10. During the initial stages of Alzheimer's disease, clients frequently forget to eat some meals or may eat meals twice.

Major shifts in the age of the population are affecting American health care needs. Compared with 30 million people aged 65 years and older (10% of the population) in 1988, this population is expected to increase to approximately 39 million people (16%) by 2010 (US Bureau of the Census, 1990; 1989). Improved medical care and good nutrition have helped us increase our life span; it is now important to increase the quality of that life.

NUTRITION SCREENING INITIATIVE

Malnutrition in the elderly usually occurs gradually. By the time it is recognized, full-blown medical problems are present that must be addressed rather than correcting a lifestyle issue with simple measures. Up to 65% of clients admitted to acute care hospitals and 50% of nursing home clients are at risk of malnutrition (Silver, 1991). Approximately 85% of our geriatric population have chronic diseases and conditions that increase their risk of poor nutritional status (Committee, 1986).

A multidisciplinary project of the American Dietetic Association, the American

DETERMINE YOUR NUTRITIONAL HEALTH

The warning signs of poor nutritional health are often overlooked. Use this checklist to find out if you or someone you know is at nutritional risk.

Read the statements below. Circle the number in the yes column for those that apply to you or someone you know. For each *yes* answer, score the number in the box. Total your nutritional score.

	YES
I have an illness or condition that made me change the kind and/or amount of food I eat.	2
I eat fewer than 2 meals per day.	3
I eat few fruits or vegetables, or milk products.	2
I have 3 or more drinks of beer, liquor or wine almost every day.	2
I have tooth or mouth problems that make it hard for me to eat.	2
I don't always have enough money to buy the food I need.	4
I eat alone most of the time.	1
I take 3 or more different prescribed or over-the-counter drugs a day.	1
Without wanting to, I have lost or gained 10 pounds in the last 6 months.	2
I am not always physically able to shop, cook and/or feed myself.	2
TOTAL	

Total Your Nutritional Score. If it's—

0–2 *Good!* Recheck your nutritional score in 6 months.

3–5 *You are at moderate nutritional risk.* See what can be done to improve your eating habits and lifestyle. Your office on aging, senior nutrition program, senior citizens center or health department can help. Recheck your nutritional score in 3 months.

6 or more *You are at high nutritional risk.* Bring this checklist the next time you see your doctor, dietitian, or other qualified health or social service professional. Talk with them about any problems you may have. Ask for help to improve your nutritional health.

Figure 16–1 Checklist for the "warning signs" of poor nutritional health. (Reprinted with permission from the Nutrition Screening Initiative, a project of American Academy of Family Physicians, American Dietetic Association, and National Council on the Aging and funded in part by a grant from Ross Laboratories, a Division of Abbott Laboratories.)

Academy of Family Physicians, and the National Council on Aging has launched a Nutrition Screening Initiative (NSI) to identify people at nutritional risk before significant deterioration of health. Key **risk factors** have been identified as potential indicators of poor nutritional status in persons over age 65 (Fig. 16–1). The simple check list, requiring only a few minutes to complete, is accompanied by a discussion of warning signs. These risk factors are used by clients to help determine whether a professional should be consulted. If so, the professional can further assess whether nutritional well-being is indeed impaired and to what extent and what measures should be implemented before the situation becomes severe (Fig. 16–2). Level 1 screening is designed to be administered in community settings by nurses or trained health workers. If indicated, these clients are referred to a physician, dietitian, or other preventive interventions (economic assistance, shopping, transportation assistance, and so forth). Level 2 screening is the most comprehensive of the NSI tools and is designed for health professional use generally requiring physician and dietetic or health care team involvement (White et al, 1992).

A risk factor is a major identifiable biological or environmental circumstance or event that increases the risk of malnutrition, suggesting special care and attention.

The general consensus is that "prevention of malnutrition is better than treatment during a crisis" (Davies, 1988). Most elderly clients are easily motivated to make changes that will affect their health if the information is presented with an understandable rationale.

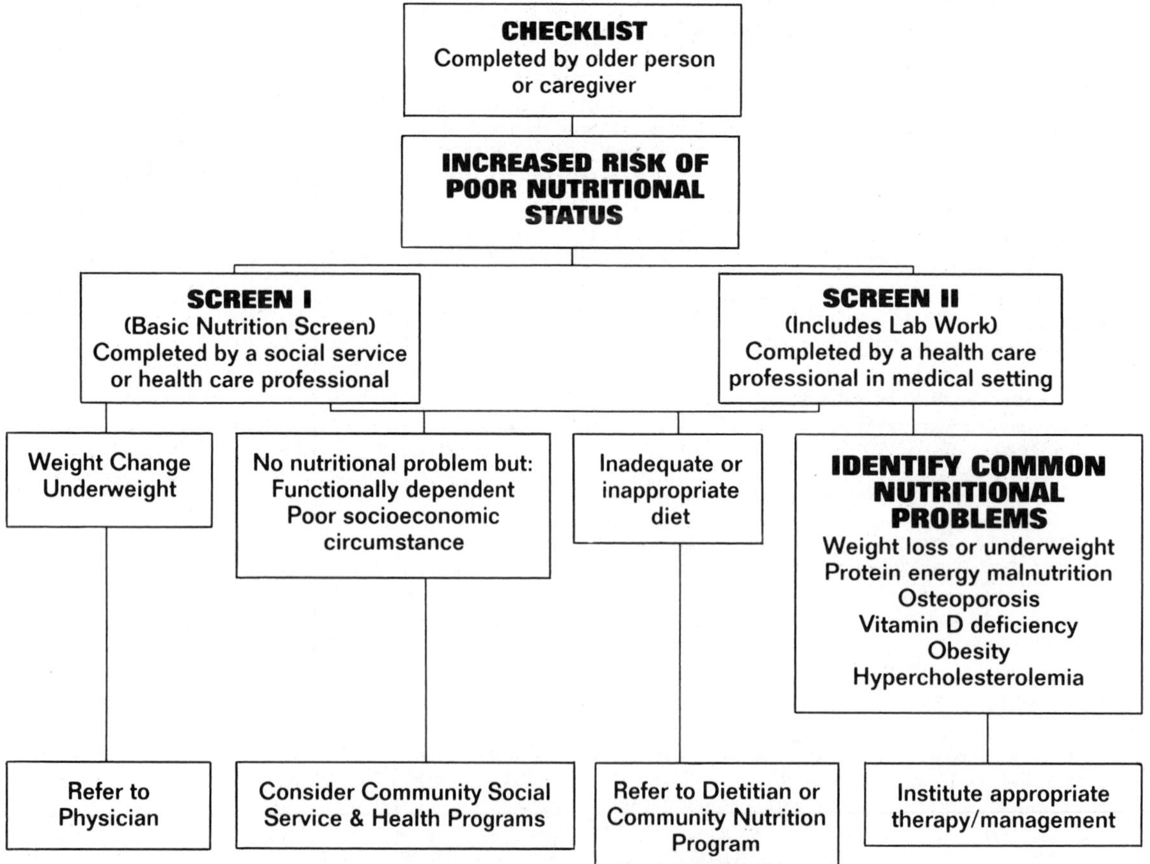

Figure 16–2 A practical approach to nutritional screening. (Reprinted with permission from the Nutrition Screening Initiative, a project of American Academy of Family Physicians, American Dietetic Association, and National Council on the Aging and funded in part by a grant from Ross Laboratories, a Division of Abbott Laboratories.)

FACTORS INFLUENCING NUTRITIONAL NEEDS AND STATUS

Physiological Factors

Many organ functions begin to decline by age 30, and so a number of physiological changes may significantly influence nutritional requirements of elderly people. **Homeostatic mechanisms** decline with age, and the precarious physiological balance may be upset by disease; physical and/or mental disabilities; and environmental, economic, and social disabilities (Davies & Knutson, 1991). Yet chronological age and functional capacity do not always correlate.

Homeostatic mechanism—the body's ability to correct for nutritional imbalances, i.e., decreased nutrient intake accompanied by an increase in absorption or efficiency of use.

In addition to the functional decline of many body organs, which may affect absorption, transportation, metabolism, or excretion of nutrients, food intake may be affected by other age-related physiological changes. Visual, auditory, and olfactory sensory organs may be impaired. Poor vision makes food preparation not only difficult, but also hazardous. Poor hearing increases isolation and decreases socialization.

How may functional decline of body organs affect nutrients?

Cardiopulmonary System

Cardiac stroke volume at higher work loads is decreased as well as oxygen transport being reduced to the tissues because of changes in the respiratory system (Roe, 1987). Increased peripheral resistance caused by loss of arterial elasticity and atherosclerotic deposition increases the work load of the heart. Hypertension, affecting about two-thirds of the elderly, is a significant medical and nutritional problem (Sowers, 1987). Normal physical changes, such as decreased strength and shortness of breath on exertion, may lead clients mistakenly to believe they are "anemic."

Oral Cavity and Gastrointestinal Tract

Several physiological changes in the oral cavity and GI tract are significant factors in nutritional status. Many of these GI conditions are further discussed in Chapter 25. A progressive decline in taste and smell sensitivity affects food choices and quantity since "nothing tastes good." Renal failure also leads to deterioration of taste sensitivity. **Taste thresholds** are high for the basic sensations of sweet, salty, sour, and bitter (Schiffman, 1991). Elderly clients may confuse taste sensations, describing sour foods as metallic and salty foods as tasteless. Foods may be overly seasoned with salt or sugar as a consequence of **anosmia** and **hypogeusia.** Losses in salt or sugar perception make it difficult for clients to comply with a low sodium or diabetic diet. Other seasonings can be used to help replace the taste of salt or sugar.

Taste threshold is the lowest concentration at which taste can be detected.

Anosmia—loss of smell; hypogeusia—loss of taste.

By age 65, 50% of Americans are edentulous (Bidlack, 1986). Generally, clients who wear dentures have reduced masticatory efficiency—75 to 85% less than with natural teeth (Martin, 1991). Clients with seriously compromised natural dentition or ill-fitting dentures tend to alter their food choices to reduce chewing. Figure 16–3 compares improperly fitted dentures with correctly fitting ones in the same client. Even though clients have dentures, they may not wear them, or they may not be able to chew because of sore gums. Therefore, consumption of some meat and fresh fruits and vegetables may decrease, which results in reduced energy, iron, and vitamin C intakes.

Many commonly used medications, especially diuretics, antidepressants, and hypnotics, cause **xerostomia,** which compromises oral processing of foods and utilization of nutrients. Xerostomia affects more than 75% of the elderly and has significant detrimental effects on nutrient intake (Rhodus & Brown, 1990).

Xerostomia—dry mouth or lack of salivation.

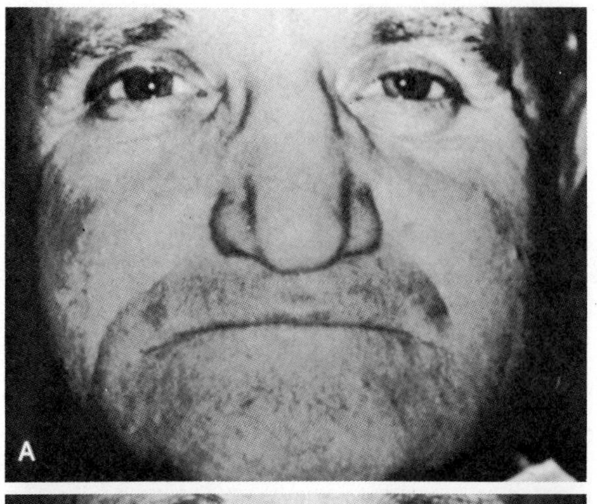

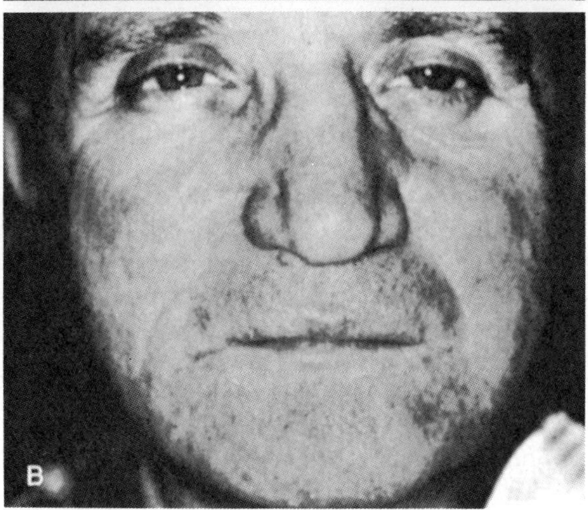

Figure 16–3 *A*, Geriatric client wearing dentures with incorrect occlusal vertical dimension; note overclosure. *B*, Same client with correct occlusal vertical dimension; note improvement in facial appearance. (From Nizel AE. *Nutrition in Preventive Dentistry: Science and Practice.* 2nd ed. Philadelphia, WB Saunders, 1980.)

Dysphagia—difficulty with swallowing.

Atrophic gastritis—chronic stomach inflammation with atrophy of the mucous membrane and glands, and diminished HCl secretion.
Achlorhydria—complete lack of gastric acid production.

How is taste affected in the elderly? How can ill-fitting dentures affect intake? What can cause xerostomia, and how does it affect nutrition? What nutrients are affected with diminished HCl secretion? What can achlorhydria cause? What can cause constipation?

Changes in esophageal motility and deterioration of nerve function may cause **dysphagia.** This frequently observed disorder increases risk of aspiration pneumonia and morbidity from inadequate nutrition. Clients with swallowing problems eat slowly and may not be able to consume adequate amounts.

Diminished HCl secretion may affect absorption of calcium, iron, and vitamin B_{12}. **Atrophic gastritis** and **achlorhydria** (frequently observed in elderly clients) result in pernicious anemia because vitamin B_{12} cannot be separated from the food protein (Russell, 1990). Additionally, the lack of acid permits overgrowth of bacteria that use much of the available vitamin B_{12}. Decreased secretion of digestive enzymes does not appear to impair nutrient absorption in healthy older clients except for decreased calcium and zinc absorption (Bowman et al, 1992).

Constipation may be a consequence of altered GI motility, along with loss of bowel muscle tone, inadequate food and fluid intake, low-fiber diets, and inactivity. Additional causes include chronic laxative use and some medications, especially analgesics and antihypertensives. Constipation can be corrected by increasing fiber-containing foods, fluid intake, and activity level. Irritant laxatives should be avoided. A serious consequence of constipation is fecal impaction that may result from impairment of rectal sensation and abnormalities of motor function related to medications or disease (Wrenn, 1989).

Renal System

As a consequence of aging and certain chronic conditions (diabetes, hypertension, and atherosclerosis), renal function progressively declines. Reduced numbers of nephrons and diminished cardiac output result in less blood flow through the kidneys. Thus, drug and metabolic waste excretion and urine concentration are decreased. Reabsorption of glucose, amino acids, ascorbic acid, and plasma protein is reduced. Nitrogenous compounds from excessive protein intake may present problems for clients with compromised renal function.

What happens to the nephrons because of aging? Which nutrient reabsorption is reduced? What can happen to sodium and potassium with impaired kidney function? What can cause dehydration in the elderly?

Impaired kidney function is sluggish in response to dietary sodium reduction; an elderly client requires a longer period to conserve sodium to maintain salt balance (Lindeman, 1991). Impaired renal function can sometimes result in hyperkalemia.

Thirst Mechanisms

Decreased thirst sensations are associated with aging. Therefore, fluid intake may not increase automatically to offset increased water losses from the compromised kidney. Thus, elderly clients are prone to dehydration.

Fever, which can lead to mild dehydration in a healthy client, may result in severe dehydration in elderly clients. Increased water intake can aid impaired renal functions by reducing the osmotic concentration of fluids being filtered by the kidneys.

Musculoskeletal System

Bone **resorption** progresses rapidly in elderly clients. Bone loss may be associated with physical inactivity, unavailability of calcium (inadequate dietary intake, imbalance in calcium to phosphorus ratio, and decreased calcium absorption), changes in hormones affecting calcium metabolism, and altered vitamin D metabolism associated with impaired renal function. Bone loss increases susceptibility to fractures and possible disability. Osteoporosis or shortening and outward bowing of the spine may develop.

Resorption—reabsorbed.

Lean body mass declines, whereas adipose tissue increases. Losses occur in particular in muscle tissue, **visceral** compartments and other protein tissues such as connective tissue and collagen, and immune bodies (Roe, 1987). Clients with decreased lean body mass may have fragile esophageal tissues and are at increased risk of problems associated with passing a feeding tube (tearing or perforation leading to hemorrhage, peritonitis, and so on) (Chernoff, 1990). Decreases in visceral protein result in an inability to respond to a physiological injury or insult and declining function of many organ systems. Muscle mass can be preserved by increasing physical activity (Steen, 1988).

Visceral compartments are body proteins (internal organs and blood) other than muscle tissue. Decreased levels are reflected in lowered serum albumin levels.

What is bone loss associated with? Where do lean body mass losses occur? Why does BMR decrease? Where does body fat accumulate?

BMR decreases with less muscle mass (Fig. 16–4). In older clients, the BMR may be as much as 10 to 12% below the level of 20-year-olds (see Chapter 10). Body

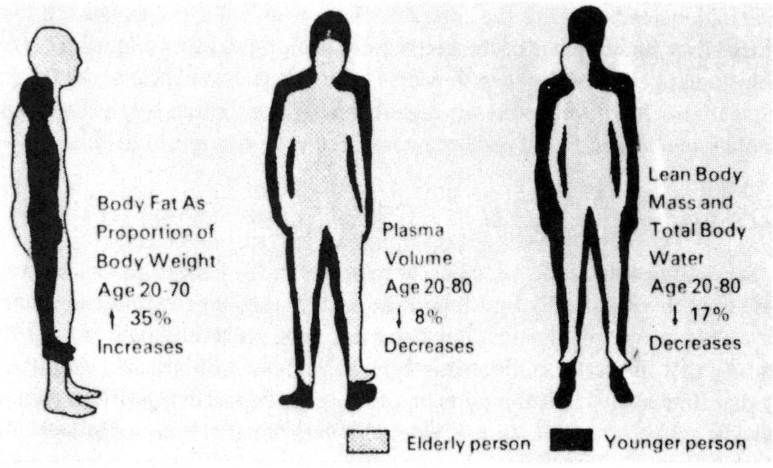

Figure 16–4 Changes in the body with aging. (From Vestal RE. *Drugs and the Elderly*. NIH Pub. No. 79-1449. Washington, D.C., U.S. Department of Health, Education and Welfare, 1979.)

fat increases slowly with aging, resulting in more truncal and internal fat as opposed to subcutaneous fat.

Immune Function

T cells are thymus-derived lymphocytes of cell-mediated immune system.

Involution—natural gradual degeneration that occurs with increasing age. Vestigial—remaining structure that at one time was a functioning entity.

Why is the immune response compromised in the elderly? What nutrients can improve immune response?

Compromise of immune function is common in the elderly. A decline in **T lymphocyte cell** function results in reduction of cell-mediated immune mechanisms. During adulthood, thymic **involution** occurs, and by age 60, the remaining thymus is **vestigial.** Fewer circulating lymphocytes, especially T helper cells (James et al, 1990), explain the high rate of bacterial infections in elderly clients. Adequate intake of kilocalories; protein; iron; zinc; vitamins A, C, and E; and B complex vitamins is associated with improved immune responses (Penn et al, 1991; Chandra, 1990).

NURSING APPLICATIONS

Assessment

Physical—for height, weight, TSF, chronic disease, dentures, swallowing process, xerostomia, condition of mouth and gums, fever.
Dietary—for adequacy of nutrient and fluid intake.
Laboratory—for WBC with differential, especially lymphocytes, vitamin B_{12}, Hgb, Hct, calcium, sodium, potassium.

Interventions

1. Encourage new denture wearers to swallow liquids with the dentures first, then chew soft foods, and, last, bite and pulverize regular foods. It is easier to master the complex masticatory movements in this order and protects the mouth from becoming sore.
2. Monitor denture wearers because they may be more prone to accidental choking from improper mastication.
3. Closely monitor food and fluid intake of clients with constipation, diarrhea, or urinary or fecal incontinence. When elderly clients experience these problems, they frequently become apprehensive about eating or drinking.
4. For edentulous clients, inquire about the preferred texture of food. Do not assume edentulous clients require pureed foods. The lack of visual appeal and flavor of these foods may cause the appetite to become depressed.

Client Education

- Less muscle tissue and lower activity level result in a reduced kilocaloric requirement.
- Physical training enhances muscle strength and preserves muscle mass; muscle repletion is unlikely (Davies, 1988).
- If xerostomia is present, use artificial salivas, gum, or hard, sugarless candies; practice frequent oral hygiene care; and drink adequate fluids (Rhodus & Brown, 1990).
- Decreased sodium with high potassium intake (from foods) has been successful in lowering blood pressure (Hallfrisch, 1991). Before advising a client to increase potassium-rich foods, be sure a potassium-sparing diuretic is not prescribed or a renal condition present.
- Frequency of bowel movements is individualized; daily bowel movements are unnecessary for health in some elderly clients.
- Explain to clients with achlorhydria the role of oral vitamin B_{12} supplements to maintain their feeling of well-being.

Socioeconomic and Psychological Factors

Economic Factors

Most retired people live on fixed incomes that are significantly lower than when they were employed. Poverty is estimated to be double the rate in younger adults; 25% of those living independently have an annual income under $10,000 (Nutrition Screening, 1990). Inflation, failing health, and medical bills can have a devastating effect on fixed incomes. The food budget frequently suffers and is a risk factor for inadequate nutrition. For example, fresh fruit and vegetable choices may be curtailed because of their high cost.

What are economic factors that can affect nutrition in these clients?

Social Factors

An inability to drive or access to transportation affects utilization of health services and availability of food. Approximately one-third of noninstitutionalized clients over 65 live alone (Nutrition Screening, 1990). As a rule, clients who live with a spouse consume better diets. Women who live alone are at greater risk (Murphy et al, 1990); men living with their spouses have the least risk. Although clients who live alone consume fewer kilocalories, it may not be less nutritious (Davis et al, 1990). Clients who live with another person and are socially active tend to consume a larger variety of foods. An inactive client who lives alone may lack motivation to prepare well-balanced meals, especially if appetite is poor.

As a rule, which clients consume a better diet? Who is at greatest risk; least risk? Which elderly clients consume a larger variety of foods?

Psychological Factors

Apathy and depression can predispose elderly clients to decreased appetite and interest in food. Loss of a spouse frequently leads to anorexia and depression. Depression is difficult to distinguish from symptoms related to the stresses of later life—illness and changes in lifestyle. Depression may mistakenly be considered by some as a natural and inevitable component of aging; therefore, treatment may not be obtained. Loneliness is related to dietary inadequacies (Walker & Beauchene, 1991).

What psychological factors can affect nutrition?

NURSING APPLICATIONS

Assessment

Physical—for living arrangements, socioeconomic status, source of income, allocation of funds, marital status, mental status.
Dietary—for motivation to eat and drink.

Interventions

1. Allow more time to eat and, if possible, visit with the client while eating. An older client usually eats slowly, and lack of socialization during meals has been implicated in the anorexia of aging.
2. Frequently monitor the client's nutritional status. Chronic disease and financial burdens imposed by limited income are among the most important factors influencing nutritional status.
3. Monitor menus and food supply periodically to determine the adequacy of food intake. Nutrient-dense foods are especially important for clients who have a low-kilocalorie intake.

Client Education

- Nutrition counseling can provide information on consuming adequate amounts of high-quality protein to help clients living on a limited budget.

Continued

- Discuss economical fruit, vegetable, and meat selections (see Chapter 18).
- Make wise selections of convenience foods. Explain how to read food labels to make selections that are appropriate for restricted diets or to provide a well-balanced diet.

NUTRIENT REQUIREMENTS

Recommended Dietary Allowances

Which nutrients are different from the RDAs of adults 23 to 50 years of age?

Metabolism to maintain body functions requires all the same nutrients, but nutrient amounts may be influenced by stress and diseases of aging. Current RDAs provide guidelines for nutrient requirements of adults over 51. Elderly clients differ from one another more than any other group. The general consensus is that dietary needs of clients between 50 and 60 years of age are different from those over 70, but inadequate information was available for the NRC to establish a different RDA. Per the RDA, nutrient allowances are the same as for adults 23 to 50 years of age except for kilocaloric requirements, the B vitamins closely associated with energy intake (thiamin, riboflavin, and niacin), and a lower iron allowance for women because of menopause (Table 16–1).

Fluids

Fluid intake is of particular concern because elderly clients are susceptible to fluid imbalances secondary to physiological changes previously discussed. Certain

TABLE 16–1

NATIONAL ACADEMY OF SCIENCES–NATIONAL RESEARCH COUNCIL RECOMMENDED DIETARY ALLOWANCES, REVISED 1989

	Men	Women
Age (yr)	51+	51+
Weight (kg)	77 (170 lb)	65 (143 lb)
Height (cm)	173 (68 in.)	160 (63 in.)
Energy (kcal)	2300	1900
Protein (gm)	63	50
Fat-Soluble Vitamins		
Vitamin A (mcg retinol equivalents)	1000	800
Vitamin E (mg α-tocopherol equivalents)	10	8
Vitamin D (mcg cholecalciferol)	5	5
Water-Soluble Vitamins		
Ascorbic acid (mg)	60	60
Folacin (mcg)	200	180
Niacin (mg)	15	13
Riboflavin (mg)	1.4	1.2
Thiamin (mg)	1.2	1
Vitamin B_6 (mg)	2	1.6
Vitamin B_{12} (mcg)	2	2
Vitamin K (mcg)	80	65
Minerals		
Calcium (mg)	800	800
Phosphorus (mg)	800	800
Iodine (mcg)	150	150
Iron (mg)	10	10
Magnesium (mg)	350	280
Zinc (mg)	15	12
Selenium (mcg)	70	55

Adapted from National Research Council Subcommittee on the Tenth Edition of the RDAs: *Recommended Dietary Allowances,* 10th ed. Washington, DC, National Academy Press, 1989.

chronic illnesses (heart and kidney disease) lead to impairment of various homeostatic mechanisms controlling water balance. Seemingly mild stresses—such as imposed fluid restriction in preparation for some laboratory procedures; the presence of fever, infection, or diarrhea; or the use of diuretics—can upset the normal homeostasis. In hospital settings, such minor disturbances are cumulative, often occurring too frequently to permit the sluggish corrective responses of the elderly until profound and even potentially fatal derangements have occurred. Dehydration is probably the primary cause of confusion in elderly hospitalized clients (Chernoff & Lipschitz, 1988). In normal situations, 6 to 8 glasses of fluids per day (roughly 30 ml fluid/kg body weight) are recommended.

Adequate fluids must be provided for both normal and abnormal fluid losses. An elderly client may intentionally restrict fluids because of nocturia, incontinence, or having to request assistance to be toileted. Offering soups, juices, milk products, soft drinks, tea, and coffee can enhance fluid intake since plain water is not highly favored by elderly clients.

What may cause an elderly client to restrict fluids intentionally? What types of fluid could nurses offer elderly clients?

NURSING APPLICATIONS

Assessment

Physical—for skin turgor, weight, dry mucous membranes.
Dietary—for fluid intake, RDA intake.
Laboratory—for sodium, potassium, BUN, urine specific gravity.

Interventions

1. Monitor I&O.
2. If the client is confined to bed or paralyzed, ensure a minimum of 2 to 2.5 L/day if not contraindicated by renal or heart problems. This prevents kidney stones by naturally flushing the kidneys.

Client Education

- Do not let beverages interfere with food intake.
- Adequate fluid intake is beneficial in preventing and treating constipation.

Energy

Recommended energy intake reflects average requirements of groups of people and actually varies significantly with clients, depending on the amount of lean body mass and activity level. The RDA for clients over 51 has been lowered to 2300 for men and 1900 for women (or 30 kcal/kg). Generalized use of kilocaloric estimates ignores activity level and the role it plays in kilocaloric balance. This decrease of kilocalories from the younger age group is related to lower BMR and physical activity.

Protein

An intake of 12 to 14% or more of the energy needs should come from protein foods, or a minimum of 50 gm in a 1900-kcal diet. An allowance of 0.8 to 1.0 gm/kg appears to be adequate despite some studies that indicate higher needs because of decreased protein utilization and chronic diseases and other studies that indicate decreased requirements related to diminished muscle mass. Added stress from surgery, infection, injury, GI disease, or routine drug usage increases catabolism, thereby increasing dietary protein levels required to maintain nitrogen balance. Inadequate monetary resources to purchase meat products is a principal reason elderly clients consume less protein.

Negative nitrogen balance is observed in immobilized clients. There is no evidence that providing excess protein will reverse this process in the immobilized client unless exercise is provided to prevent the rate of body protein loss and preserve muscle mass. Excess protein intake should be monitored to prevent dehydration and further damage to compromised kidneys.

What is the requirement for protein?

Carbohydrate

Since carbohydrates have not been identified as essential nutrients, there is no RDA for simple or complex carbohydrates. Currently, approximately 45% of the kilocalories are from carbohydrate. A larger amount of complex carbohydrates is advisable since tolerance of simple sugars diminishes with aging. This also increases vitamin and mineral intake as well as dietary fiber, which contributes to enhanced bowel motility.

Fat

The upward adjustment of carbohydrate is balanced with less dietary fat. According to US Dietary Guidelines, less than 30% of the energy requirement should come from fat (USDA, USDHHS, 1990). However, the benefit of decreasing cholesterol and fat intake to lower serum cholesterol levels in clients over 70 is not established (Garber et al, 1989; Henderson, 1989). If kilocalories need to be increased to maintain a client's weight, emulsified fats are well absorbed (Simko & Michael, 1989). Decreased fat absorption has been related to drug therapy, GI surgery, or disease. Curtailing dietary fat to as little as 15 to 25 gm daily provides adequate levels of EFA without compromising other necessary nutrients if intake is good.

What is the recommended level for fat intake?

Minerals

Dietary mineral intake may need to be adjusted, based on assessment of the client's nutritional status. Excess or even normal dietary levels can have deleterious consequences in certain diseases, particularly chronic illness such as hypertension or congestive heart failure. On the other hand, rigid and severe restrictions may seriously affect food acceptance. Thus, individualization is crucial.

Calcium

Elderly clients (especially women) usually have a negative calcium balance and lose bone mass, leading to spontaneous fractures. Inadequate calcium intake is possibly one reason for this, but genetic, hormonal, and environmental factors are also important. Decreased physical activity contributes to calcium loss over the years. The combined use of alcohol, antacids, and drugs also disturbs calcium reserves (see Chapter 9).

Milk provides needed calcium. However, regular consumption of milk is unpopular because of its expense and the frequent trips needed to purchase it. The use of dry milk is also unpopular but can be incorporated into many foods without deleterious effects on taste.

Why do elderly clients have negative calcium balance? How can calcium intake be increased?

Iron

The mean iron intake of older healthy clients is generally adequate until age 75. No differences have been found between young adults and active older clients in their ability to absorb iron, but disease conditions are major contributors to iron deficiency. Many GI diseases can significantly reduce dietary iron absorption, and GI bleeding increases iron losses. Therapeutic drug use can markedly alter dietary iron utilization.

Zinc

Dietary zinc appears to be closely related to energy intake and can be adequate with careful food selection on a modest kilocalorie intake. Older adults seem to consume only marginal amounts of zinc (less than 45% of the RDA) because of lower protein consumption. In addition, intestinal absorption is decreased in those over 65 years of age. Lower serum levels of zinc may be the result of chronic, long-term marginal zinc intake (Chandra, 1990). Numerous health problems are associated with zinc deficiency—hypogeusia, poor appetite, delayed wound healing, and depressed immune function. Even though zinc supplementation is popular, self-medication with amounts of zinc above the RDA (15 mg) may be harmful, as discussed in chapter 9. A physician's diagnosis and recommendation should be obtained.

What can happen with zinc deficiency?

Fat-Soluble Vitamins

A literature search (Suter & Russell, 1989) indicated vitamin A requirements were higher than the 1989 RDA, with vitamin D recommendation being lower than needed, especially for the large number of elderly who are not exposed to sunshine (Gloth et al, 1991).

Vitamin A

Absorption of vitamin A is increased with age, but intake is usually below the RDAs. Vitamin A stores may become depleted in elderly clients stressed by disease and malnutrition (Black et al, 1988) and with cirrhosis, alcoholism, and chronic GI disorders.

What may cause vitamin A stores to become depleted?

Vitamin D

Vitamin D status may be compromised in the elderly, especially if chronically ill and/or institutionalized. A deficiency may be the result of several causes: dietary insufficiency, malabsorption, kidney disease, and inadequate exposure to sunlight. Vitamin D stores decline with age, particularly in those unable to go outdoors. Additionally, aging appears to reduce the conversion of the precursors to the active form both in the skin and by the kidneys. Since adequate vitamin D nutriture is required for optimal absorption of calcium, inadequate intake affects bone mineralization.

Impaired bone mineralization in the absence of vitamin D is referred to as senile osteomalacia, the adult counterpart of rickets. Progressive decalcification of the bone results in symptomatic pain in sites such as the ribs, lower lumbar vertebrae, pelvis, and legs. Osteomalacia and osteoporosis are similar in some of their pathological problems, e.g., hip fractures. Table 16–2 compares these 2 conditions.

What may cause low vitamin D levels in the elderly? What is a complication of inadequate vitamin D intake?

Water-Soluble Vitamins

Suter and Russell (1989) concluded the current RDA for folate was higher than required; those established for vitamins B_6 and B_{12} were potentially lower than needed (Ribaya-Mercado et al, 1991). The recommended amounts for other vitamins appeared appropriate.

TABLE 16–2

SKELETAL CHANGES OF AGING

Imbalance	Causes	Effects
Osteoporosis or excessive bone resorption	Immobilization Hyperparathyroidism Decreased hormone secretion Chronic inadequate calcium intake	Decreased stature Kyphosis Spontaneous fractures Low back pain
Rickets/osteomalacia or low levels of minerals in bones	Dietary deficiency of calcium and/or vitamin D Deficiency of calcium and/or vitamin D due to fat malabsorption, medications, or chronic renal disease	Soft, flexible bones and skeletal deformities Bone pain and generalized weakness Fractures (in adults)

Ascorbic Acid

What may cause low vitamin C levels? What condition may be delayed in elderly clients with higher intakes of vitamin C?

Many elderly clients have low plasma and tissue levels of ascorbic acid. This is generally considered to be a consequence of inadequate intakes or increased requirements related to routine medications. Several epidemiological studies have shown that cataract formation is delayed in clients with higher intakes of vitamin C (Rosenberg, 1988).

B Complex

Neurological symptoms similar to dementia may result from deficiencies of vitamin B_6, B_{12}, and folate. Diets are reported to be marginal. Normal folate nutriture can be maintained despite low folate intake (Suter & Russell, 1989) and malabsorption (secondary to atrophic gastritis), possibly as a result of increased bacterial folate synthesis in the upper GI tract (Russell et al, 1986).

With increasing age, serum pyridoxal phosphate decreases. Clinical evidence (such as an increased prevalence of carpal tunnel syndrome) and biochemical indices suggest an altered vitamin B_6 metabolism that could result in a higher requirement (Suter & Russell, 1989; Munro et al, 1987). Economical factors and chewing problems may negatively affect meat consumption, thus negatively affecting vitamin B_6 and B_{12} intake.

What may contribute to normal folate nutriture with low folate intake? What symptoms may be treated with vitamin B_{12}?

Cobalamin may be less available in elderly clients because of atrophic gastritis and bacterial overgrowth. Clients with psychotic depression have been reported to have lower cobalamin levels (Bell et al, 1991). Although studies have reported decreased symptoms (confusion, disorientation, and neurological problems) in clients treated with vitamin B_{12}, there are insufficient data to suggest a change in the RDA (Suter & Russell, 1989).

Nutrient Supplements

Approximately half of the clients in this age group routinely take vitamin–mineral supplements; this is usually unrelated to their needs. The AMA (1987) has concluded that vitamin/mineral supplements are unnecessary for clients who consume a nutritionally balanced diet with a variety of foods. There is evidence of potential toxicity of some supplements, but studies have not directly investigated the effects of high doses in the elderly. However, the AMA has stated that supplements containing 50 to 150% of the RDIs may be appropriate if a client consumes inadequate amounts of food (AMA, 1987).

NURSING APPLICATIONS

Assessment

Physical—for activity level, chronic diseases.
Dietary—for intake of previously discussed nutrients.
Laboratory—for albumin, calcium, magnesium, potassium, nitrogen balance, iron.

Interventions

1. If immobilized, provide moderate amounts of protein.
2. If on limited income, suggest enriched breakfast cereals to increase intake of iron and other nutrients.
3. Offer milk frequently or incorporate dry milk into foods.
4. In making recommendations to change life-long dietary patterns in clients over 70 years of age, use a rational approach. Overzealous dietary manipulation may lead to failure to eat adequate amounts and subsequent malnutrition (Morley et al, 1986).

Evaluation

* Client should consume at least two-thirds of the suggested RDA for nutrients discussed.

Client Education

- Women require fewer kilocalories than men, but other nutrient requirements are similar to those of men.
- If energy intake is not appropriately decreased, overweight or obesity may develop.
- If dietary intake appears inappropriate (excessive amounts of salt, sugar, or fat), recommend modest changes in intake that appear to be in line with the client's preferences.
- Vitamin supplements over 100% of the RDIs should be taken only if there is a specific need or if recommended by a physician.
- Use of vitamin/mineral supplements does not eliminate the need to consume a nutritionally balanced diet, nor do they protect against the development of chronic diseases associated with inappropriate food intake.
- Consume a vitamin C–rich food daily.
- Review economical sources of folate and cooking practices to retain folate.

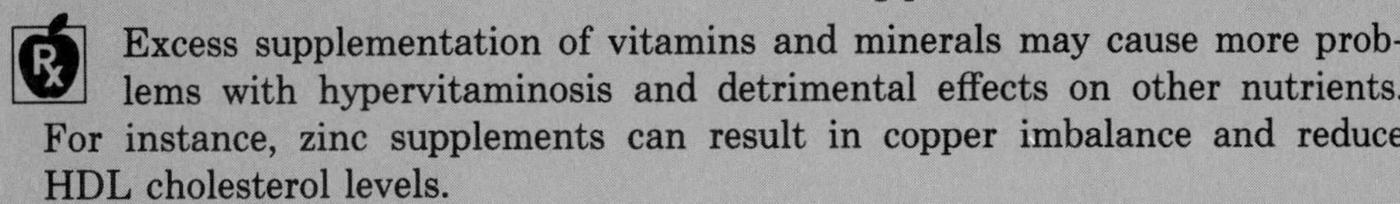

Excess supplementation of vitamins and minerals may cause more problems with hypervitaminosis and detrimental effects on other nutrients. For instance, zinc supplements can result in copper imbalance and reduce HDL cholesterol levels.

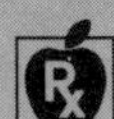

Fat-soluble vitamins are not absorbed when mineral oil is taken, which may be a frequent practice among clients with constipation.

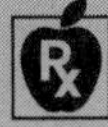

Vitamin B_{12} deficiency may result from ascorbic acid supplementation.

EATING PATTERNS

Deficiencies

Numerous surveys, including the 10-State Nutrition Survey, the Health and Nutrition Examination Survey (HANES), and USDA food consumption studies, have clearly shown that persons 50 years of age and older consume less food than younger adults. Inadequate amounts of water and nutrients are consumed both in the community and in institutions. Nutrients usually reported to be deficient in the community include thiamin, riboflavin, folacin; vitamins D, B_6, and B_{12}; and the minerals iron, copper, zinc, magnesium, and calcium (Ahmed, 1992). This has also been confirmed by biochemical measures. Despite nutrient adequacy of a hospital diet, 38% of elderly clients ingested less than 65% of their nutritional requirements. This was most frequently true in clients over 65 years old and weighing less than 80% of their IBW (Rammohan et al, 1989). Deficiencies of calcium, iron, zinc, thiamin, and folate may be related to specific diseases or disorders frequently observed in older clients.

Surveys have indicated improvement in choices with more low-fat meats and milk and whole-grain bread. However, intake of high-fiber foods (fruits, vegetables, high-fiber cereals) changed little between 1977 and 1987 (Popkin et al, 1992).

Dairy products, fruits, and vegetables are frequently lacking in the diet, especially for those living alone. In general, elderly clients choose softer foods with a decrease in protein and fatty foods and more carbohydrate foods.

Describe what elderly people choose to eat and types of foods that are decreased. Which clients are at risk of developing malnutrition?

Clients with recent drastic lifestyle changes, e.g., moving from their home to an apartment or institution, are at nutritional risk. In general, clients with less education and income; housebound clients, especially those living alone; those with physical disabilities, depression, and other mental disorders; and those who do not have regularly cooked meals are considered to be at risk of developing malnutrition.

Snacks

Snacks are popular, averaging 2 per day (afternoon and evening). These may provide important additional energy, but they are often high only in carbohydrate, particularly sucrose.

Supplements

Milk-based food supplements, such as an instant breakfast mix, are economical and can help prevent nutrient deficiencies. A tasty supplement augments overall nutrient intake to maintain nutritional status. On the other hand, commercial liquid nutrition supplements, such as Ensure (Ross) or Sustacal (Mead Johnson), are more convenient and may be preferred.

Adaptive Equipment

One of the most basic of all self-care skills is that of feeding oneself. Although disabled clients have used adaptive equipment to feed themselves, little attention has been given to the elderly with functional disabilities that may result from a stroke or arthritis. Physical limitations such as strength, grasp, or range of motion to hold a utensil or get the utensil or to maneuver it to the mouth have significant impact on nutrition. These physical limitations can be dealt with by teaching new techniques to compensate for limitations and by using adaptive equipment. Once a client is dependent on others for eating, continued reliance frequently develops, rather than attempting to regain independent abilities.

What can be a result of loss of independence in eating? What are some positive effects of independence in eating?

Independence in eating results in several other rewards. Obviously, increased personal pride, self-respect, and dignity are important. Normally, morale improves when clients are able to join others in the dining room and leave the facility to visit relatives and friends in their homes. Another benefit is increased intake. Adaptive equipment offers elderly clients with limited mobility as much potential as any other disabled group (Figs. 16–5 through 16–8).

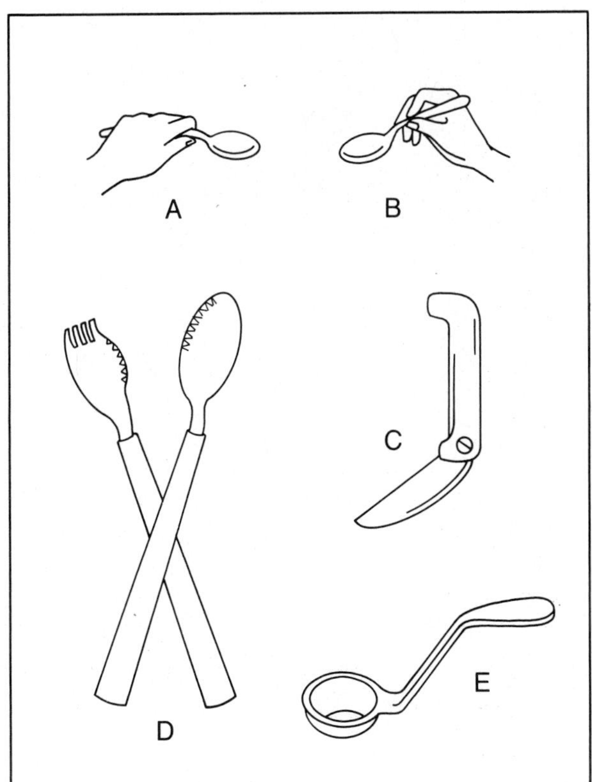

Figure 16–5 Hand position on silverware. *A*, Palmer grasp. *B*, Conventional grasp. *C*, Angled knife. *D*, Combination cutlery. *E*, Bent handle.

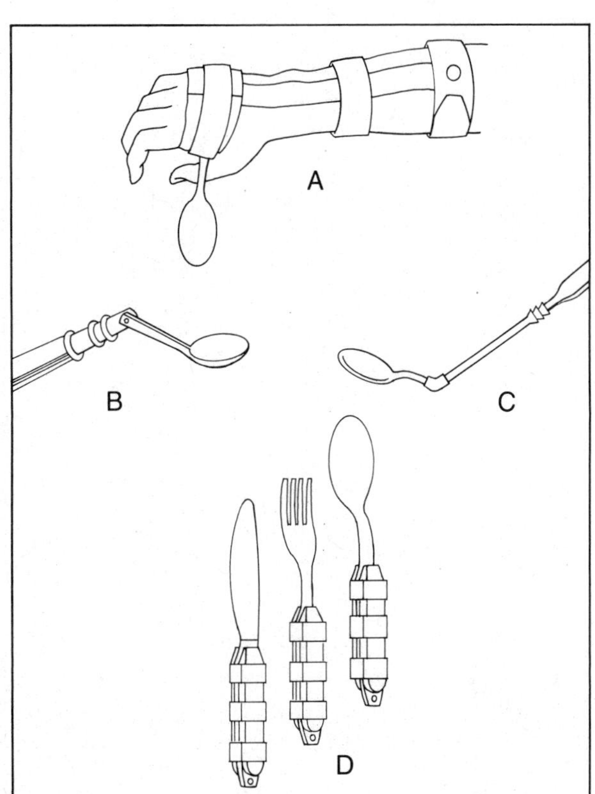

Figure 16–6 Variations on silverware. *A*, Wrist support. *B*, Swivel spoon. *C*, Spoon extension. *D*, Built-up handles.

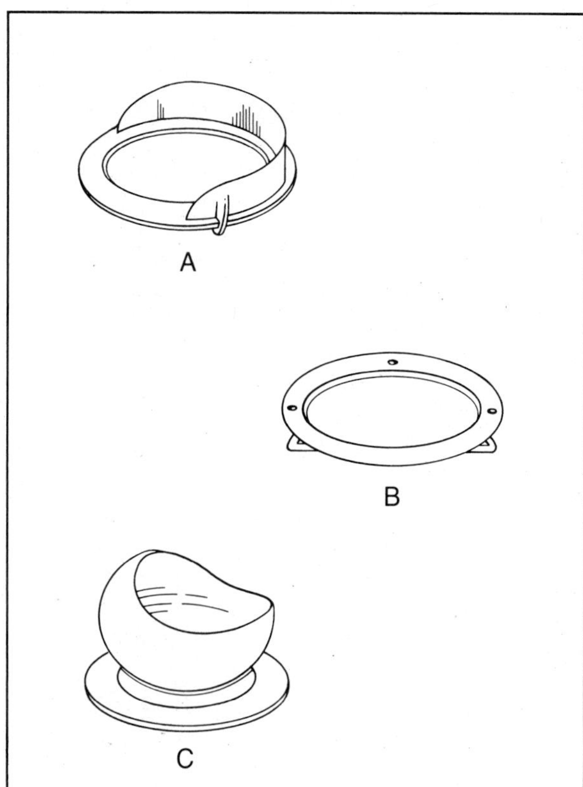

Figure 16–7 Bowls and plates for easier eating. *A*, Plate guard. *B*, Suction plate. *C*, Scooper bowl.

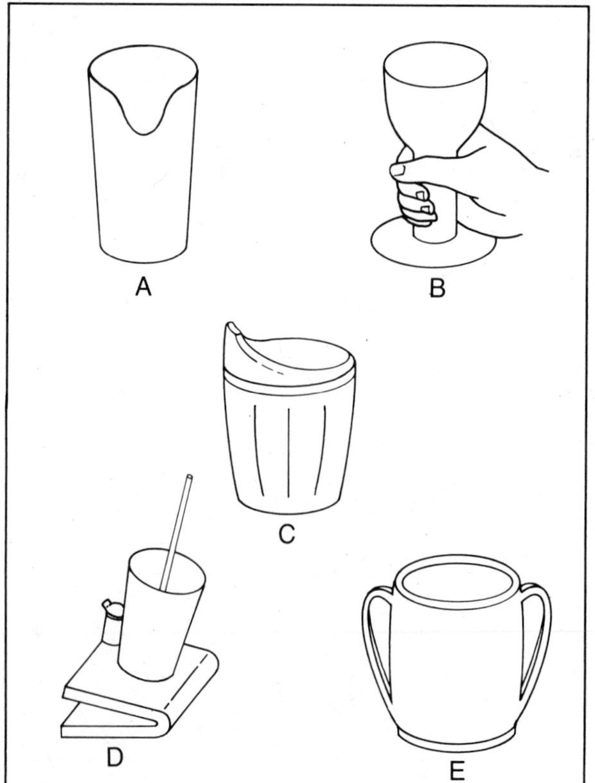

Figure 16–8 Cups and glasses for special drinking problems. *A*, Nose cutout glass. *B*, Easy grip cup. *C*, Snorkel lid. *D*, Tilting glass holder. *E*, Two-handled mug.

NURSING APPLICATIONS

Assessment

Physical—for chronic diseases, financial status, drastic lifestyle changes, educational level, psychological status, use of adaptive equipment, living arrangements.
Dietary—for nutrient intake, use of snacks, supplements.

Interventions

1. Offer a milk-based food supplement, i.e., an instant breakfast mix combined with either liquid or dry milk or a commercial liquid or pudding nutrition supplement.
2. For malnourished hospitalized clients or clients with dysphagia, 60 ml of 2 kcal/ml nutrition supplements provided concurrently with medications may result in increased kilocaloric acceptance and desirable weight gain (Raymond, 1991).
3. Monitor I&O.
4. Consult with occupational therapist for adaptive equipment.

Client Education

- Rather than 3 meals a day, frequent feedings of smaller amounts as well as nutrition supplements are beneficial.
- Teach clients how to plan and prepare meals that are in line with current diet and health recommendations (Popkin et al, 1992).

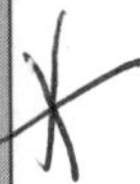

PHARMACEUTICALS

Approximately 45% of elderly clients living independently take multiple prescription drugs that can interfere with appetite and nutrient absorption (Nutrition Screening, 1990). Clients in long-term care facilities generally take more drugs than those living independently. Medications are more likely to be used excessively or misused (Table 16–3).

Although drug-nutrient interactions can compromise anyone's nutritional status, these problems are accentuated in the elderly. Physiological and pathophysiological changes, such as decreased hepatic and renal clearance, result in greater variability and less predictability in the drug's effects.

TABLE 16–3

REASONS FOR DRUG ABUSE

Client Factors
Giving incomplete drug history to all the physicians consulted
Altering dosages—larger amounts taken to relieve symptoms
Being overly concerned about health (conviction that he or she is suffering from a serious ailment or preoccupied with daily bowel movements)
Mismanaging drugs—not taken as scheduled, leading to increased or decreased frequency (increases with number of drugs taken concurrently)
Sharing drugs with others
Being influenced by advertisements
Health Care Provider Factors
Prescribing medicines by several physicians
Improperly prescribing dosage in relation to client's current weight and renal function
Failing to correlate current drug usage to symptoms
Inappropriately using drugs to control client behaviors (sedatives and tranquilizers)
Inadequately reviewing care plans by nurses

Adapted from Roe DA. *Geriatric Nutrition.* 2nd ed. Englewood Cliffs, NJ, Prentice-Hall, 1987.

Because older clients are more likely to have chronic diseases, they are more vulnerable to adverse nutrient-drug interactions and the effects of altered absorption and utilization. Nutrient reserves are gradually depleted. Drug-induced nutritional deficiencies occur more frequently in clients with marginal dietary intake and chronic diseases (Chernoff & Lipschitz, 1988). Nutrient-drug interactions more common to this group are vitamin B_6 deficiency in cancer victims; decreases in magnesium, phosphate, calcium, and potassium caused by diuretics; and decreased folate and iron levels caused by chronic aspirin intake. The routine use of aspirin for arthritis or to prevent heart disease causes gastritis and bleeding and may result in iron deficiency anemia.

The heavy use of antacids, laxatives, and analgesics may cause side effects that are undetected for long periods because of subclinical effects until stress results in their discovery. The possibility of folate deficiency anemia should be included in examinations of elderly hospitalized clients on anticonvulsants and sulfasalazine. Other factors to consider are chronic drug use (cimetidine, phenytoin, and antacids), alcohol consumption, and prior GI surgery, which have a negative influence on folate status. Corticosteroids increase urinary excretion of vitamin C. Anti-inflammatory drugs such as aspirin, indomethacin, and phenylbutazone inhibit ascorbic acid metabolism. High doses of digoxin (for body weight) cause serious anorexia with or without nausea and vomiting. Chronic PEM may result from **"digitalis cachexia."**

Digitalis is a known cause of cachexia, or state of malnutrition and ill health characterized by marked anorexia, early satiety, weight loss, tissue wasting, anemia, organ dysfunction, and, ultimately, death.

Additionally, drugs are sold to delay aging. Free radicals produced during normal metabolism lead to cellular damage. Therefore, vitamins A, C, and E and selenium are marketed to delay aging. Scientific evidence does not substantiate this theory, and most nutritionists caution against large doses of selective vitamins and minerals (Schneider & Reed, 1985). Superoxide dismutase (SOD) tablets, which are marketed to prolong life, have not been shown to produce consistent effects on aging. In fact, this enzyme is hydrolyzed in the GI tract, so blood serum shows no increase over normal amounts after its ingestion.

Lethal amounts of cyanide are found in oils extracted from American apricot (Laetrile) or peach kernels. Whether the oil from apricot kernels in other parts of the world is beneficial has not been investigated. To date, no specific nutrient or medication has been found to be effective in slowing the aging process.

Describe 3 drug-nutrient interactions in the elderly.

NURSING APPLICATIONS

Assessment

Physical—for types of drugs taken, including OTC drugs and aspirin use.
Dietary—for beliefs and attitudes about foods delaying the aging process; multivitamin/mineral use.
Laboratory—for folate, vitamin B_{12}, Hgb, Hct.

Interventions

1. Discourage use of large amounts of antioxidants (vitamins A, C, and E and selenium) and superoxide dismutase and Laetrile (ground nutmeg of apricot kernels).
2. Encourage bedridden clients to take medications with a full cup of water to prevent kidney stones.

Evaluation

* Desired outcome is client verbalizing beneficial and harmful nutrient/drug combinations.

Client Education

- Compare the cost of laxatives and stool softeners versus cost of whole-wheat bread.

- Add bran to foods to decrease use of laxatives.
- A well-balanced diet following the Dietary Guidelines for Americans may delay the symptomatic aging process.
- Factors that slow the aging process include regular exercise, abstinence from smoking, and reducing stress.

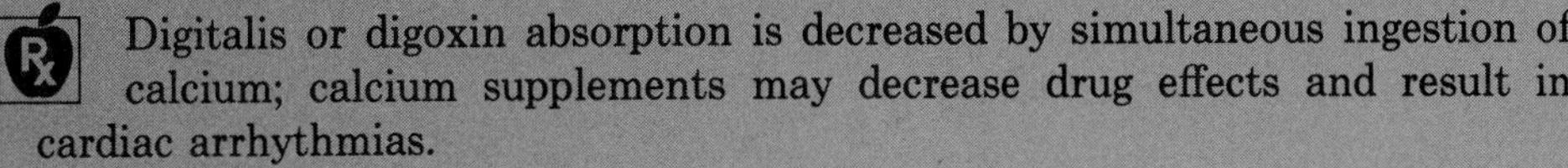

Digitalis or digoxin absorption is decreased by simultaneous ingestion of calcium; calcium supplements may decrease drug effects and result in cardiac arrhythmias.

NUTRITIONAL ASSESSMENT

Overlapping symptoms caused by aging, dietary deficiencies, and disease obviously complicate treatment of the elderly. Because malnutrition, or loss of lean body mass, is similar to aging symptoms, without appropriate screening and assessment, PEM may be overlooked. Assessing food intake becomes a basic priority that can alleviate unnecessary suffering and possibly malnutrition from chronic inadequate protein intake. Functional status, mobility, strength, mental status, and neurological impairment can be assessed by watching a client walking and performing a simple task such as obtaining and drinking a glass of water.

Anthropometric Measurements

Anthropometric measures are significantly affected by the aging process. Clients are notably unreliable regarding height and weight. Yet accurate data of these nutritional indicators are important. Height decreases with age as a result of thinning of the vertebrae, **kyphosis,** and osteoporosis. For clients who are unable to stand erect, recumbent length may be obtained or ankle-knee height measured to extrapolate height.

Kyphosis—abnormally increased curvature of the spine, also called hunchback.

Weight is an important indicator of nutritional status. Although weight fluctuations are indicative of changing clinical status, weight gradually decreases after age 60 or 70 related to changes in body composition. Serial weights are important to assess for changes or undesirable trends to prevent nutrient depletion and/or deterioration of health status. A BMI less than 24 indicates nutritional deficiency, and values greater than 27 suggest obesity.

It is a well-established fact that obesity increases risk of death from heart disease and other chronic illnesses, increases disabilities, and decreases mobility (Harris et al, 1988; Rudman, 1989). Less well recognized is the fact that above age 60, the mortality risk of being underweight becomes greater; mild overweight is associated with the least mortality (Andres, 1990).

Weight loss may be related to numerous factors, including anorexia, physiological problems (acute and chronic diseases), socioeconomic status, social isolation, and/or psychiatric disease (dementia or depression). Aggressive nutrition support is more successful and economical than recovery of lost status. A combination of low body weight and rapid unintentional weight loss is predictive of mortality and morbidity in elderly clients (Fischer & Johnson, 1990).

What does obesity increase risks for? What may weight loss be related to?

Biochemical Measurements

Serum albumin is a fairly reliable indicator of protein nutriture, ruling out effects of hydration status, medications, and chronic and current diseases or conditions. A low cholesterol level may also be important in identifying clients at risk and is significantly correlated with the presence of decubiti and WBC count (Verdery & Goldberg, 1991; Rudman et al, 1987). Cholesterol levels below 131 mg/dl were associated with a tenfold increase in relative risk of mortality in a study conducted by Verdery and Goldberg (1991) in nursing home clients. The least risk was 154 to 193 mg/dl. A combination of depressed albumin and cholesterol values may be compounding risk factors (Kaiser & Morley, 1990).

Describe frequent correlatations associated with low cholesterol levels on the elderly's health. What is the best laboratory value for identifying iron deficiency anemia in the elderly?

Since tissue iron stores increase with age, serum transferrin levels are depressed; therefore, assessment of serum transferrin levels may be falsely misleading. Serum ferritin levels may be the best laboratory value for identifying geriatric clients with iron deficiency anemia (Josten et al, 1991). Most other biochemical measures are similar to those found in other age groups.

LONG-TERM CARE FACILITIES

Approximately 5% of the elderly live in long-term care facilities; from 23 to 85% of these clients may be malnourished (Drinka & Goodwin, 1991; Thomas et al, 1991). Because of early hospital discharges, nursing home clients are more likely to be acutely ill. Malnutrition and hypovitaminosis are prevalent among nursing home residents; Drinka and Goodwin (1991) recommend an inexpensive multiple vitamin supplement containing 100% of the RDIs for all clients. Malnutrition is usually due to inadequate intake (related to client's inability or unwillingness to eat) and increased nutritional needs.

The trend for menus in long-term care facilities is to restrict dietary fat and cholesterol. This may be appropriate for overweight clients, but a majority of long-term care clients have difficulty maintaining their weight, so restrictions may be undesirable. The use of 6 small feedings daily and/or nutritional supplements, or more aggressive support such as enteral feedings may be required. A dining room should be adequately staffed to encourage eating. Additionally, such measures as allowing more time for clients to eat, better positioning, and adaptive equipment may help clients feed themselves and enhance their intake (Smiciklas-Wright, 1990).

How many clients are malnourished in long-term facilities? What can nurses in these facilities do to enhance intake?

COMMUNITY SERVICES

One of the main goals for senior citizens is to maintain their independence and health as long as possible. The government has taken a giant step forward with nutrition programs and provision of home health services for this purpose.

Federal Programs

In 1972, Congress created a comprehensive nutrition program for elderly clients designed to relieve social as well as nutritional problems by providing meals predominantly in congregate settings. The Nutrition Program for the Elderly (Title VII) has become the largest program in promoting better health among senior citizens by providing food and nutrition education through federal funding. Other supportive services provided include transportation, primary health care services, and light housekeeping assistance.

These programs provide food that meets a significant amount of the RDAs for one day at minimal or no cost. This alleviates some of the problems for those with fixed income, no transportation, and little incentive to cook for themselves. This nutrition program helps reduce isolation of older clients by offering them an opportunity to participate in leisure time and recreational activities and to combine food with friendship.

Although the primary thrust of the nutrition program is to provide meals in a group setting, meals may also be delivered to clients who are homebound because of illness, incapacitating disability, or extreme transportation problems. These programs operate on weekdays with a hot meal provided at noon and sometimes a cold meal for later. Spouses of the homebound participants may also receive a home-delivered meal, regardless of age or condition. In such cases, food is often delivered by senior volunteers who visit with the shut-ins while they eat. This program has been shown to reduce hospital stays (Weiss et al, 1991).

Participants are given an opportunity to contribute to all or part of the meal cost, but no one may be turned away for inability to pay. Participants determine if and how much they will pay. In most cases, participants pay something for their meals, even those who are employed by the project or who assist as volunteers. Contributions are handled in strict confidence. These funds are used to increase the number of meals served.

Food stamps are another useful nutrition support system. However, many elderly clients are hesitant to ask for any financial help. Transportation may also be a problem.

Federal programs are estimated to reach only 20% of the elderly who need them. Many of the low-income elderly survive by whatever free shelters and food may be found. It is hoped that the nation's goals and objectives for healthy older adults will help improve quality of life for elderly Americans.

Describe community resources for the elderly.

NURSING APPLICATIONS

Assessment

Physical—for independence and support, transportation, ability to drive.
Dietary—for knowledge of dietary community resources.

Interventions

1. Assist client to contact resources. Additional input from a caring person can motivate a client to achieve desired outcomes of obtaining assistance successfully.

Evaluation

* Client uses community resources available.

Client Education

- Explain the availability of these resources.
- Problem solve/suggest alternatives for transportation, e.g., church, family, significant others and so forth.

CONDITIONS THAT AFFECT NUTRITIONAL STATUS

The prevalence of **dementia** in clients over age 80 is between 20 and 36% (Weiler, 1987).

Dementia—impairment of memory and other cognitive functions.

Alzheimer's Disease

Alzheimer's disease is the major cause of dementia in the elderly. It is a slow progressive disease, characterized by deterioration of judgment, orientation, memory, personality, and intellectual capability with a usual duration of 6 to 10 years between onset and death.

Although much has been learned about the disease, a specific cause has not been elucidated. Aluminum toxicity was thought to be a factor at one time, but it is currently believed that aluminum accumulates secondary to a neurochemical defect. Nutritional deficiencies have been shown to cause changes in the brain similar to those found in Alzheimer's disease. But clients with Alzheimer's disease are typically well nourished initially, and eating patterns appear better than in clients without the disease (Root & Longenecker, 1988).

Numerous nutritional therapies have been studied without effective results. Trials of lecithin and choline have not shown any improvement in cognitive function or slowing the rate of progression of the disease (Dysken, 1987). However, lecithin or choline along with medications that act on the **cholinergic** system have shown some improvement in Alzheimer's clients.

Cholinergic—activation of parasympathetic fibers by acetylcholine.

Alzheimer's disease has significant effects on nutritional status. Initially, clients may have problems with food purchasing and preparation. Appetite and food intake fluctuate with mood swings and increasing confusion (Claggett, 1989). They may forget when they last ate, skipping some meals and sometimes eating meals twice. Food preferences change that may be tied into decreases in olfactory functions. Sweet and salty foods are preferred.

During the middle phase of the illness, clients become agitated and may pace all night, increasing kilocaloric expenditure. Weight loss is common (Franklin & Karkeck, 1989). Energy requirements may increase as much as 1600 kcal/day (Rheaume et al, 1987). In clients with abnormal sleep patterns, caffeine may be withheld since caffeine is a CNS stimulant.

Appetites are usually good, but kilocaloric intake is usually inadequate to maintain body weight unless snacks and/or liquid nutrition supplements are provided. Clients may hoard food or fail to chew it sufficiently, increasing the risk of choking. Ability to use utensils deteriorates. Finger foods may be more appropriate to allow clients to continue self-feeding (Seltzer et al, 1988). Foods requiring a knife to be eaten should be presented already cut. Serving foods one at a time helps decrease confusion. A larger mid-day meal is recommended when cognitive abilities are at their peak (Suski & Nielsen, 1989).

Describe what happens to nutritional status in the initial, middle, and late stages of Alzheimer's disease.

During the final stage, which is characterized by severe intellectual impairment, clients may not recognize food or refuse to eat. Enteral feedings are usually indicated to maintain nutritional status resulting from impaired cognition.

NURSING APPLICATIONS

Assessment

Physical—for food purchasing and preparation; height, weight, IBW, weight loss; disease stage; chewing and swallowing status.

Dietary—for adequacy of food and fluid intake; food preferences, intake of vitamins and minerals.

Interventions

1. During the middle stage, offer frequent feedings with nutritional supplements, fortified beverages and/or puddings.
2. Present foods in a ready-to-eat form.
3. Use nonverbal cues while eating, i.e., picking up food with fork or spoon. These cues help clients associate thoughts with behavior.

Evaluation

* Desired outcomes include client eating 75 to 100% of meals and maintaining body weight.

Client Education

- Use simple 3 to 5 word explanations.
- Inform of community groups, Alzheimer's support group for significant others.

Multi-Infarct Dementia

Multiple strokes may result in dementia and, depending on their location in the brain, may cause sensory and motor abnormalities. The risk of a stroke is increased by hypertension, diabetes, hypercholesterolemia, impaired cardiac function, and excessive alcohol intake (Gray, 1989). Since nutrition intervention is advisable for many of the previously mentioned conditions, food choices may decrease the incidence of stroke.

Frequently a client's abilities to self-feed or swallow are affected. Facial and tongue movements may be affected, thus increasing chance of aspiration. Nutrition support is provided on an individual basis, from enteral feedings for those with dysphagia to texture modifications for affected oral-motor functions. Adequate protein intake requires specific planning and attention. Pureed diets are less expensive than enteral feedings.

NURSING APPLICATIONS

Assessment

Physical—for location of stroke in the brain, physical disabilities, high BP, dementia.
Dietary—for food choices, especially sodium, sugar, cholesterol, and alcohol.
Laboratory—for glucose, cholesterol, triglycerides, LDL, HDL.

Interventions

1. Raise head of bed to 45- to 90-degree angle while feeding and keep head of bed raised 30 minutes after eating to decrease chance of aspiration.
2. Individualize nutrition support. Consult dietitian and/or speech-language pathologists as needed.

Evaluation

* Client consumes 75 to 100% of diet without aspiration.

Client Education

- Use soft foods that are easier to swallow.
- Reinforce individualized guidelines provided by the speech-language pathologist.

Other Causes of Dementia

Thiamin, folate, and vitamin B_{12} deficiencies have been associated with dementia. The association between vitamin B_{12} and dementia is somewhat controversial, but low serum vitamin B_{12} levels in approximately one-third of elderly clients with dementia without other symptoms of deficiency have shown complete recovery with vitamin B_{12} injections (Lindenbaum et al, 1988). Elderly clients with dementia frequently have subnormal folate levels. Whether dementia precipitates inadequate food intake or poor food selection, thus resulting in folate deficiency, or vice versa is unclear. Therefore, a trial of folate supplementation is justified if serum folate levels are low. Thiamin deficiency resulting in memory deficits is generally associated with Wernicke-Korsakoff syndrome or alcoholism, which is addressed in Chapter 20. In general, dementia associated with vitamin deficiencies may be reversible, but nutrition therapy is not always successful because of irreversible brain changes.

NURSING APPLICATIONS

Assessment

Physical—for dementia, malnutrition.
Dietary—for thiamin, folate, and vitamin B_{12} intake.

Interventions

1. Give vitamin B_{12} and/or folate as ordered.

Evaluation

* Client consumes two-thirds of the RDAs for thiamin, folate, and vitamin B_{12}.

Client Education

- Use simple 3- to 5-word explanations.

SUMMARY

Little has changed since the days of Ponce de Leόn. Everyone would like to know the secrets of longevity. Although the following suggestions may sound simple, present-day nutritional knowledge suggest that longevity is affected by (1) choosing a variety of foods from basic food groups, (2) planning menus to provide desirable nutrients, and (3) avoiding overindulgence and overweight. Moderate exercise and frequent medical and dental check-ups are also important.

Age affects the older client's nutritional requirements in many ways. Physiological changes in body organs, rates of absorption, medications, illnesses or abnormal physical conditions, availability of food, and attitude toward life all play intricate parts in this complex nutritional regimen. In fact, good nutrition throughout life may make the difference between older clients who are active and productive and those who need frequent medical care, hospital admission, and even institutionalization for physical or emotional disabilities. Therefore, consideration of nutritional status and potential problems during nursing care helps maintain independence for these clients.

NURSING PROCESS IN ACTION

A 75-year-old client is not eating because he states he is not hungry and food does not taste good. He has lost 14 lbs (usual weight, 170 lbs) and does not like a lot of red meat or milk.

Nutritional Assessment

- Height, weight, IBW, % weight loss.
- Nutrient/fluid intake in relation to RDAs.
- Alterations in taste or smell.
- Support group, significant others, living arrangements, social support.
- Psychological status.
- Albumin, protein, Hgb, ferritin, calcium.

Dietary Nursing Diagnosis

Altered nutrition: Less than body requirements RT anorexia secondary to taste changes.

Nutritional Goals

Client will consume at least 66% of the RDAs and gain 1 lb/week to IBW and verbalize ways to increase protein and calcium intake.

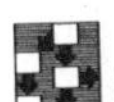

Nutritional Implementation 

Intervention: Offer small, frequent meals.
Rationale: This helps the elderly client consume adequate amounts of nutrients by decreasing fatigue and feelings of fullness that may occur with larger meals.

Intervention: Suggest use of spices such as lemon juice, thyme, and basil.
Rationale: These spices may improve the taste of foods since an elderly client's taste thresholds are altered.

Intervention: Emphasize use of eggs, turkey, chicken, fish, meats marinated in wine or vinegar, soy products, e.g., tofu and bacon bits (Carpenito, 1992).
Rationale: Since he does not like red meats, client may obtain needed protein in a more acceptable manner.

Intervention: Emphasize the use of yogurt, cream cheese, cheese, or ice cream.
Rationale: Since he does not like milk, these foods are alternatives to supply the needed calcium.

Intervention: Encourage adding powdered milk to soups, sauces, cereals, and casseroles.
Rationale: These are methods to increase both protein and calcium consumption.

Intervention: Encourage the client to walk outdoors for daily.
Rationale: Exercise is important to maintain bone densit tion, dependent on vitamin D, can be obtained through sunshin

Intervention: Suggest mixing meat with vegetables.
Rationale: Since he enjoys vegetables, this form may b him and enhance protein intake.

Intervention: Refer to Meals on Wheels or other fede (food stamps), community meal centers, churches.
Rationale: Anorexia may be due to lack of socialization

 Evaluation

Client should be eating more than 66% of the RDAs and gaining 1 lb/week until desired body weight is achieved. Other behaviors such as consuming yogurt, eggs, fish, and dry milk added to foods increase calcium and protein intake should also be observed.

STUDENT READINESS

1. Plan a day's menus for an elderly client without dentures.
2. What are some of the nutrients that might be harmful because of excessive intake?
3. What are some vitamins and minerals that might influence mental attitudes because of their deficiencies?
4. Discuss the reasons elderly clients might not eat adequately.
5. Visit a group meal program. Review the menu and discuss beneficial effects of the program's various activities.
6. List nutritional interventions to assist a healthy elderly client and an Alzheimer's client to eat.

CASE STUDY

A 75-year-old man widowed for 2 years is seen in the health care clinic for decreased intake. He states that nothing tastes good. He is on a limited, fixed income from Social Security. He has lost 6 lbs within the last year. His current weight is 130 lbs; height is 5′7″.

He fixes a bologna sandwich occasionally but mostly eats frozen food suppers. He thinks meats and fruits are too expensive to buy and "they spoil before I can eat them." He will eat vegetables in the summer because a neighbor shares products from his garden. He does not want to use any community resources because he does not "want a handout."

1. Explain why "food does not taste good."
2. What psychological and social factors may influence his dietary patterns?
3. What are some practical ways to increase protein and calcium in his diet?
4. How could you address his attitude of not wanting to accept "a handout"?
5. What physical data should you assess on this man to determine nutritional status? What laboratory data?
6. List 5 nutritional interventions to perform for this client.
7. What are the strengths and weaknesses of his diet?
8. What behaviors would indicate this client is meeting his nutritional needs?

REFERENCES

Ahmed FE. Effect of restriction on the health of the elderly. *J Am Diet Assoc* 1992 Sept; 92(9):1102–1104.

American Medical Association (AMA) Council on Scientific Affairs. Vitamin preparations as dietary supplements and as therapeutic agents. *JAMA* 1987 Apr 10; 257(14):1929–1936.

Andres R. Mortality and obesity: The rationale for age-specific height-weight tables. *In* Hazzard WR, et al, eds. *Principles of Geriatric Medicine and Gerontology.* 2nd ed. New York, McGraw-Hill, 1990: 759–765.

Bell IT, et al. B complex vitamin patterns in geriatric and young adult inpatients with major depression. *J Am Geriatr Soc* 1991 March; 39(3):252–257.

Bidlack WR, et al. Nutritional requirements of the elderly. *Food Technology* 1986 Feb; 40(2):61–70.

Black DA, et al. Hepatic stores of retinol and retinyl esters in elderly people. *Age Aging* 1988 Sept; 17(5):337–342.

Bowman BA, et al. Gastrointestinal function in the elderly. *In Nutrition of the Elderly.* New York, Raven Press, 1992: 43–50.

Carpenito LJ. *Nursing Diagnosis: Application to Clinical Practice.* 4th ed. Philadelphia, JB Lippincott, 1992.

Chandra RK. The relation between immunology nutrition and disease in elderly people. *Age Aging* 1990 July; 19(4):S25–S31.

Chernoff R. Physiologic aging and nutritional status. *Nutr Clin Practice* 1990 Jan; 5(1):8–13.

Chernoff R, Lipschitz DA. Nutrition and aging. *In* Shils ME, Young VR, ed. *Modern Nutrition in Health and Disease.* Philadelphia, Lea & Febiger, 1988: 982–1000.

Claggett MS. Nutritional factors relevant to Alzheimer's disease. *J Am Diet Assoc* 1989 March; 89(3):392–396.

Committee on Education and Labor. Compilation of the Older Americans Act of 1965 and related provisions as amended through December 29, 1981. Washington, D.C., 97th Congress, 1986.

Davies L. Practical nutrition for the elderly. *Nutr Rev* 1988 Feb; 46(2):83–108.

Davies L, Knutson KC. Warning signals for malnutrition in the elderly. *J Am Diet Assoc* 1991 Nov; 91(11):1413–1417.

Davis MA, et al. Living arrangements and dietary quality of older U.S. adults. *J Am Diet Assoc* 1990 Dec; 90(12):1667–1672.

Drinka PJ, Goodwin JS. Prevalence and consequences of vitamin deficiency in the nursing home: A critical review. *J Am Geriatr Soc* 1991 Oct; 39(10):1008–1017.

Dysken M. A review of recent clinical trials in the treatment of Alzheimer's dementia. *Psych Ann* 1987 March; 17(3):178–191.

Fischer J, Johnson MA. Low body weight and weight loss in the aged. *J Am Diet Assoc* 1990 Dec; 90(12):1697–1704.

Franklin CA, Karkeck J. Weight loss and senile dementia in an institutionalized elderly population. *J Am Diet Assoc* 1989 June; 89(6):790–799.

Garber AM, et al. Screening asymptomatic adults for cardiac risk factors: The serum cholesterol level. *Ann Intern Med* 1989 Apr; 110(8):622–639.

Gloth FM 3rd, et al. Is the recommended daily allowance for vitamin D too low for the homebound elderly? *J Am Geriatr Soc* 1991 Feb; 29(2):137–141.

Gray GE. Nutrition and dementia. *J Am Diet Assoc* 1989 Dec; 89(12):1795–1802.

Hallfrisch J. Dietary needs of older people. *Nutr & the MD* 1991 July; 17(7):1–2.

Harris T, et al. Body mass index and mortality among nonsmoking older persons. *JAMA* 1988 March 11; 259(10):1520–1524.

Henderson CT. Approaches to nutritional care in the elderly. *Comp Therapy* 1989 June; 15(6):25–30.

James SJ, et al. Modulation of age-associated immune dysfunction by nutritional intervention. *In* Morley JE, et al. *Geriatric Nutrition: A Comprehensive Review.* New York, Raven Press, 1990: 203–224.

Josten E, et al. Diagnosis of iron-deficiency anemia in a hospitalized geriatric population. *Am J Med* 1991 May; 90(5):553–554.

Kaiser FE, Morley JE. Cholesterol can be lowered in older persons. Should we care? *J Am Geriatr Soc* 1990 Jan; 38(1):84–85.

Lindeman RD. The aging renal system. *In* Chernoff R, ed. *Geriatric Nutrition: The Health Professional's Handbook.* Gaithersburg, MD, Aspen, 1991: 253–269.

Lindenbaum J, et al. Neuropsychiatric disorders caused by cobalamin deficiency in the absence of anemia or macrocytosis. *N Engl J Med* 1988 June 30; 318(26):1720–1728.

Lowik MRH, et al. Dose-response relationships regarding vitamin B_6 in elderly people. *Am J Clin Nutr* 1989 Aug; 50(2):391–399.

Martin W. Oral health in the elderly. *In* Chernoff R, ed. *Geriatric Nutrition: The Health Professional's Handbook.* Gaithersburg, MD, Aspen, 1991: 107–182.

Morley JE, et al. UCLA Ground Rounds: Nutrition and the elderly. *J Am Geriatr Soc* 1986 Nov; 34(11):823–832.

adequacy and energy intake of older Americans. *J Nutr Ed* 1990 Nov/Dec; 22(6):284–291.

Munro HN, et al. Nutritional requirements of the elderly. *Ann Rev Nutr* 1987; 7:23–49.

Murphy SP, et al. Factors influencing the dietary *Nutrition Screening Initiative Survey.* Washington, D.C., Peter D Hart Research Associates; February 1990.

Penn ND, et al. The effect of dietary supplementation with vitamins A, C, and E on cell-mediated immune function in elderly long-stay patients: A randomized controlled trial. *Age Aging* 1991 May; 20(3):169–174.

Popkin BM, et al. Dietary changes in older Americans, 1977–87. *Am J Clin Nutr* 1992 Apr; 55(4):823–830.

Rammohan M, et al. Hypophagia among hospitalized elderly. *J Am Diet Assoc* 1989 Dec; 89(12):1774–1779.

Raymond JL. Calorie-dense feedings given during medication pass improves supplement intake in senile nursing home patients (poster session). *J Am Diet Assoc* 1991 Sept; 91(Suppl 9):A26.

Rheaume Y, et al. Meeting nutritional needs of Alzheimer's patients who pace constantly. *J Nutr Elderly* 1987; 7(1):43–52.

Rhodus NL, Brown J. The association of xerostomia and inadequate intake in older adults. *J Am Diet Assoc* 1990 Dec; 90(12):1688–1692.

Ribaya-Mercado JD, et al. Vitamin B_6 requirements of elderly men and women. *J Nutr* 1991 July; 121(7):1012–1074.

Roe DA. *Geriatric Nutrition.* 2nd ed. Englewood Cliffs, NJ, Prentice-Hall, 1987.

Root EJ, Longenecker JB. Nutrition, the brain and Alzheimer's disease. *Nutr Today* 1988 July-Aug; 23(4):11–18.

Rosenberg IH. Scientific basis for changing the RDAs for the elderly. *Nutr Today* 1988 Sept-Oct; 23(5):36–37.

Rudman D. Nutrition and fitness in elderly people. *Am J Clin Nutr* 1989 May; 49(Suppl 5):1090–1098.

Rudman JD, et al. Antecedents of death in the men of a Veterans Administration nursing home. *J Am Geriatr Soc* 1987 June; 35(6):496–502.

Russell RM. Gastrointestinal function and aging. *In* Morley JE, et al. *Geriatric Nutrition: A Comprehensive Review.* New York, Raven Press, 1990: 231–238.

Russell RM, et al. Folic acid malabsorption in atrophic gastritis: Possible compensation by bacterial folate synthesis. *Gastroenterology* 1986 Dec; 91(6):1476–1482.

Schiffman SS. Taste and smell losses with age. *Contemp Nutr* 1991; 16(2):1.

Schneider EL, Reed JD. Life extension. *N Engl J Med* 1985 May 2; 312(18):213–222.

Seltzer B, et al. Management of the outpatient with Alzheimer's disease: An interdisciplinary team approach. *In* Volciet L, et al, eds. *Clinical Management of Alzheimer's Disease.* Rockville, MD, Aspen, 1988: 13–28.

Silver AJ. Assessing the nutritional status of the elderly. *J Am Diet Assoc* 1991 Sept; 91(Suppl 9):A156.

Simko V, Michael S. Absorptive capacity for dietary fat in elderly patients with debilitating disorders. *Arch Intern Med* 1989 Sept; 149(9):557–560.

Smiciklas-Wright H. Aging. *In* Brown ML, ed. *Present Knowledge in Nutrition.* 6th ed. Washington, D.C., Nutrition Foundation, 1990: 333–340.

Sowers JR. Hypertension in the elderly. *Am J Med* 1987 Jan; 82(1B):1–8.

Steen B. Body composition and aging. *Nutr Rev* 1988 Feb; 46(2):45–51.

Suski NS, Nielsen CC. Factors affecting food intake of women with Alzheimer's type dementia in long-term care. *J Am Diet Assoc* 1989 Dec; 89(12):1770–1773.

Suter PM, Russell RM. Vitamin nutriture and requirements of the elderly. *In* Munro HN, Danford DE, eds. *Nutrition, Aging, and the Elderly.* New York, Plenum Press, 1989: 245–291.

Thomas DR. A prospective study of outcome from protein-energy malnutrition in nursing home residents. *JPEN* 1991 July-Aug; 15(4):400–404.

US Bureau of the Census. *Statistical Abstract of the United States: 1990.* 110th ed. Washington, D.C., US Government Printing Office, 1990.

US Bureau of the Census. *Projections for the Population of the United States by Age, Sex and Race, 1989 to 2080.* Current Population Report Series. P-25, No. 1018, Washington, D.C., 1989.

US Department of Agriculture (USDA), US Department of Health and Human Services (USDHHS). *Dietary Guidelines for Americans.* 3rd ed. Home and Garden Bulletin No. 232. Washington D.C., US Government Printing Office, 1990.

Verdery RB, Goldberg AP. Hypocholesterolemia as a predictor of death: A prospective study of 224 nursing home residents. *J Gerontol* 1991 May; 46(5):M84–M90.

Walker D, Beauchene RE. The relationship of loneliness, social isolation, and physical health to dietary adequacy of independently living elderly. *J Am Diet Assoc* 1991 March; 91(3):300–304.

Weiler PG. The public health impact of Alzheimer's disease. *Am J Public Health* 1987 Sept; 77(9):1157–1158.

Weiss EH, et al. Meals on wheels, malnutrition and hospital stay (poster session). *J Am Diet Assoc* 1991 Sept; 91(suppl)(9):A112.

White JV, et al. Nutrition Screening Initiative: Development and implementation of the public awareness checklist and screening tools. *J Am Diet Assoc* 1992 Feb; 92(2):163–167.

Wrenn K. Fecal impaction. *N Engl J Med* 1989 Sept 7; 321(10):658–662.

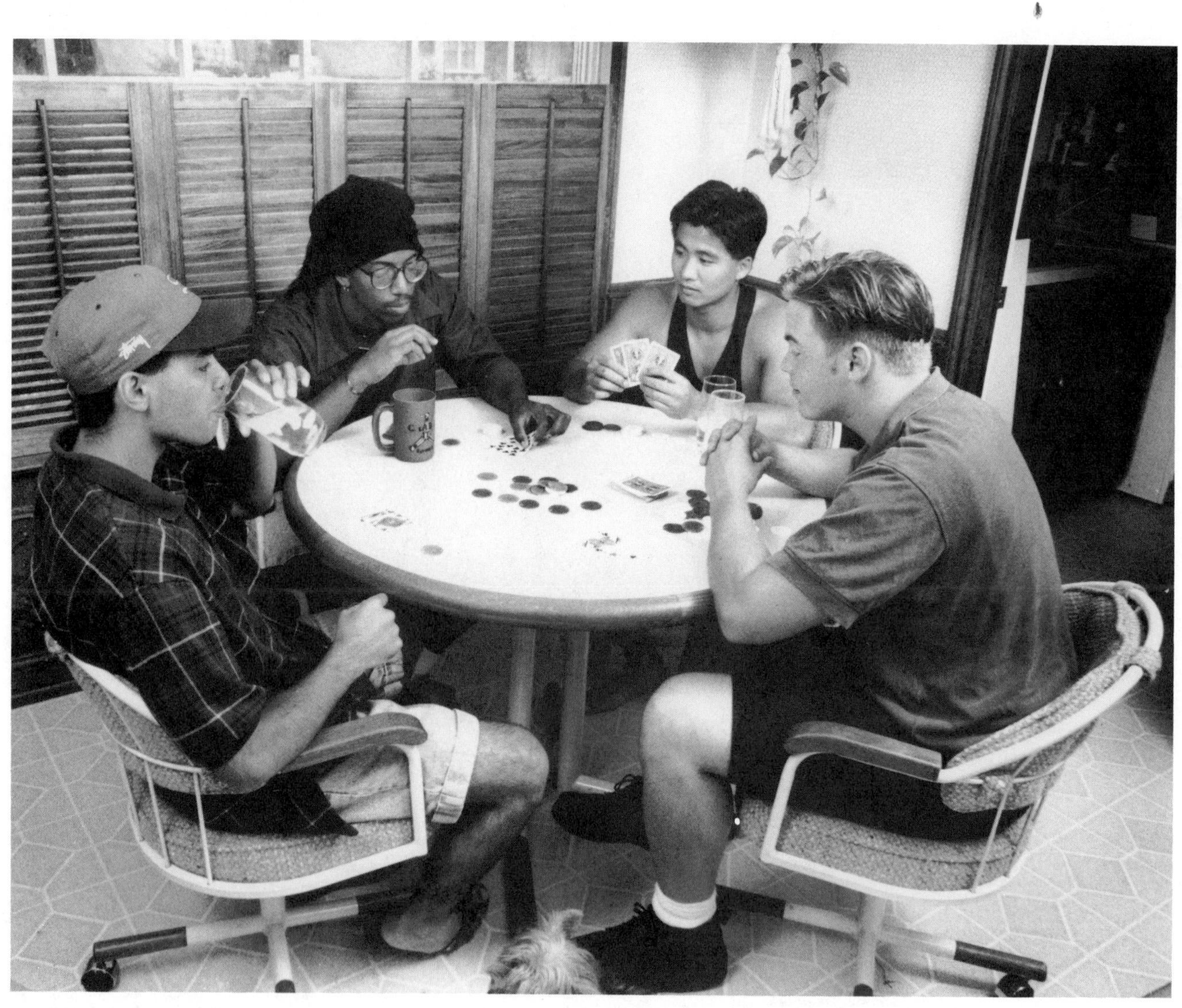

Nutritional Considerations for Ethnic and Religious Influences

CHAPTER 17

OUTLINE

I. HABITS OR PATTERNS
   A. Cultural Factors
   B. Economic Factors
   C. Status and Symbolic Influences
II. WORKING WITH CLIENTS WITH DIFFERENT FOOD PATTERNS
   A. Respect for Other Eating Patterns
   B. Effecting Change
III. BLACK AMERICAN PRACTICES
   Nursing Applications
IV. HISPANIC AMERICAN PRACTICES
   A. Mexican Practices
   B. Puerto Rican Practices
   C. Cuban Practices
   Nursing Applications
V. NATIVE AMERICAN PRACTICES
   Nursing Applications
VI. ASIAN PRACTICES
   A. Chinese Practices
   B. Japanese Practices
   C. Vietnamese Practices
   D. Korean Practices
   Nursing Applications
VII. ITALIAN PRACTICES
   Nursing Applications
VIII. MIDDLE EASTERN PRACTICES
   Nursing Applications
IX. RELIGIOUS FOOD RESTRICTIONS
   A. Jewish Restrictions
   Nursing Applications
   B. Other Religions

OBJECTIVES

THE STUDENT WILL BE ABLE TO:

- Identify reasons for food patterns.
- Discuss each culture's unique and beneficial food traditions.
- Relate individual feeding problems within an institution to cultural influences.
- Discuss ways to adapt a menu to suit particular cultural patterns.

- Adapt a hospital menu to comply with strict Jewish dietary laws.
- Apply the nursing process to improve nutritional intake of different cultures.
- Identify client education information for the various cultures.

TEST YOUR NQ (True/False)

1. Culture can affect food patterns.
2. Black Americans eat soul foods.
3. Hispanic Americans believe in the yin-yang theory of food balance.
4. Mexicans eat tacos at every meal.
5. Native Americans have a high incidence of NIDDM.
6. Chinese people may become constipated in the hospital.
7. Italians consume a large breakfast.
8. Jewish people avoid pork.
9. Japanese people consume a food called kimchi.
10. Religion can affect food patterns.

HABITS OR PATTERNS

In terms of food choices, people are creatures of habit. Patterns throughout societies are quite evident; however, the term "habit" connotes inflexibility. Clients change their habits for numerous reasons; hence, the term "food patterns" is more descriptive of food choices. Many factors are associated with the formation of food patterns and preferences. Food patterns are generally developed during childhood and reflect the family's lifestyle as well as its ethnic or cultural, social, religious, geographic, economic, and psychological components. All of these influence a client's attitudes, feelings, and beliefs about food. However, the factors that seem to predominate food choices are cultural and economic.

What are the 2 predominant factors that affect food choices?

Cultural Factors

One of the most interesting and visible ways cultural differences are expressed is through the foods a client eats or does not eat. Although milk is the only food used by everybody worldwide, many cultures consider it appropriate only for infants and children.

Children of different cultures, exposed to what adults eat, do not question whether this is what they should be eating. Cultural food patterns establish the foundation for a child's lifelong eating customs regarding time and number of meals per day, foods acceptable for specific meals, preparation methods, likes and dislikes, foods suitable for specific members of a group, table manners, the social role of foods and eating, and attitudes toward eating and health. Patterns and attitudes internalized during childhood promote a sense of stability and security for the older client (Fig. 17–1).

Not only do many ethnic groups coexist in the US, but also the development of literally thousands of localized patterns has resulted in distinct and discrete patterns of consuming foods in different combinations that have remained quite consistent over the past decade. For example, few clients in the northern US would

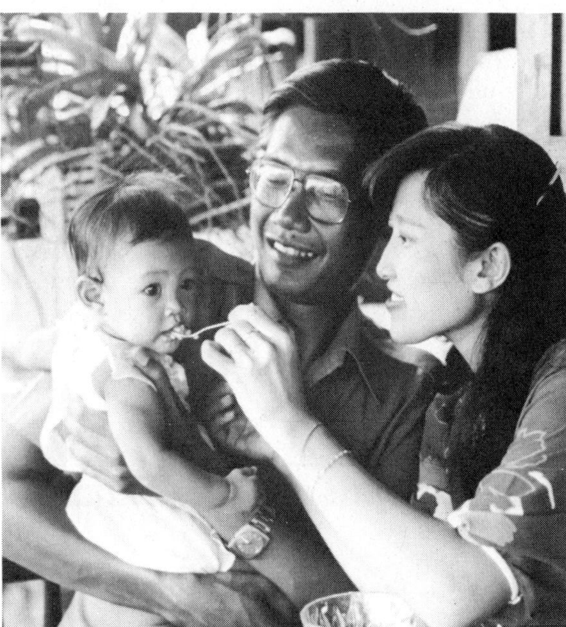

Figure 17–1 Eating habits are established at a very young age. (WHO photo by T. Kelly.)

routinely choose grits, and many Southerners would not recognize lentils. Although American diets are diversified, they have become more homogeneous because of transportation, advertising, mobility, new methods of production, changes in income distribution, and appreciation of one another's heritage.

No culture has ever been known to make food choices solely on the basis of nutritional and health values of food. For example, broccoli is one of the most nutritious vegetables (based on nutrient density) available in the US but is a less popular vegetable; whereas the tomato, the most commonly eaten vegetable, rates sixteenth as a source of vitamins and minerals.

Individual food preferences do not ordinarily influence nutritional adequacy of the diet. Insufficient quantities of basic food groups (milk, fruits and vegetables, cereals, and meats) have the greatest effect on nutritional adequacy rather than specific aversions, such as to turnips or rye bread.

Economic Factors

When clients relocate, established food patterns are carried to the new location; however, these patterns are retained only if the foods are available at an affordable price. Therefore, problems arising within various cultural groups are economic rather than the fault of traditional food patterns. Foods from the "old country," which were cheapest at "home," may be expensive or possibly not available in their new location. Gradually, the diet conforms to the food resources of the new location. Evidence of malnutrition increases as income level decreases.

What are some economic factors that can affect food patterns?

Status and Symbolic Influences

Nutritional value is secondary, especially if a food has established social, religious, or economic status (Parraga, 1990). A food in various cultures will have a different prestige or status within the society. For example, beef is regarded as a high status food among some people in the US, but Hindus from India consider cows sacred and do not eat beef. Foods may obtain their status rating from religious beliefs, availability, cost, cultural values, and traditions or even because a highly respected person has endorsed it.

Even today in many cultures, men are more highly valued than women. Thus, male members of the household may be fed first, with the women and children being allowed to eat only after the men are filled. Consequently, women and children may receive insufficient quantities and less variety of foods.

Because of symbolic meanings of food, eating becomes associated with sentiments and assumptions about oneself and the world. Foods sometimes become symbolic to clients not only because of religious connotations but because foods are often used as rewards. After a child has fallen, a mother may give the child candy to help forget the pain and stop the crying. How many times has a mother been overheard to say, "Just behave yourself, and I'll buy you an ice cream cone when I finish this"? Frequently food is withheld for bad behavior.

How may foods obtain status?

WORKING WITH CLIENTS WITH DIFFERENT FOOD PATTERNS

Respect for Other Eating Patterns

Nurses must be prepared to meet the unexpected. Recognizing that eating habits and patterns vary with clients and that characteristic cultural patterns are usually observed among different nationalities and religious groups is important. Of course, clients are partial to their own food pattern; however, too many clients, including nurses, are convinced that their own beliefs, attitudes, and practices are the best way and assume that everyone should follow them. Nurses who evaluate their own beliefs about foods and are aware of their own cultural heritage are more effective in helping clients improve intake. It is important when working with clients who have strong cultural ties to be sensitive to their preferences and to avoid being judgmental. Only by the nurse avoiding cultural biases will clients open up to reveal crucial information that will allow the nurse to help them.

Even when cultural food patterns are known, an analysis of the situation may be clouded because of unique individual habits. Information should be obtained regarding food habits by open-ended questions rather than questions that put words into a client's mouth. For example, "Did you have anything to eat this morning?" might elicit a different response than, "What did you have for breakfast this morning?"

Clients sometimes refuse to eat a particular food or to comply with a diet regimen because of cultural or religious beliefs. Generally, if these preferences/beliefs are known, an adequate diet can be planned around them, and the client is more receptive to minor changes in the diet pattern.

Effecting Change

Food preferences and attitudes are more important factors for effecting change (Parraga, 1990). Several basic facts help in approaching clients from various ethnic groups to promote sound nutritional practices:

1. One can find advantages and faults in each cultural food pattern. These patterns have contributed to the survival of the group in a particular environment. Clients have a remarkable ability to obtain a nutritious diet out of available foodstuffs. Some eating patterns that appear strange may actually be adaptive by enhancing or preserving nutritional value.
2. Other food patterns are nutritionally superior or at least comparable to "ordinary" American traditions.

3. Each food, food behavior, and tradition can be categorized as **beneficial, neutral,** or **potentially harmful.** Tofu, used in Asian cooking, is beneficial because it increases the protein and calcium content of the diet. Efforts should be made to alter only the patterns that affect the nutritional value undesirably. For example, since many water-soluble vitamins are destroyed by heat, the practice of cooking foods (especially vegetables) for long periods of time is discouraged unless the liquids are consumed and/or iron cookware is used. An understanding of ethnic food habits can be used by the nurse to encourage beneficial practices or to incorporate beneficial practices into the client's diet.
4. Food patterns are generally deeply ingrained, contribute to psychological stability, and are hard to change. If it is necessary to change the diet for health or medical reasons, suggest minimal alterations to traditional foods and present the information with options to the whole family. Additionally, compliance is improved when the client has some control over food choices, understands the meal plan, and feels responsible for following the suggestions.
5. Cultural patterns tend to be used more consistently by older family members. The unique characteristics of several of the more prevalent ethnic and religious groups are presented in this chapter to provide some understanding of a few practices that might affect clients' acceptance of food and their ability to adjust to a special diet.

A food that is beneficial promotes health by contributing necessary nutrients. Neutral foods are not especially beneficial but are not harmful to health. Foods are not usually harmful, but customs that affect the nutritional content of the food may be potentially harmful.

It is not possible to cover the dietary practices of all cultures and religions. Clients from any culture have different tastes and preferences; therefore, it is important not to stereotype cultural groups. It is especially important for the nurse to become familiar with patterns common in the local area. Table 17–1 categorizes foods of different cultures and regions with a brief description to help introduce some unique and interesting foods.

Name 3 methods to promote sound nutritional practices in various ethnic groups.

TABLE 17–1

CULTURAL AND REGIONAL FOODS

Name of Food	Culture/Region	Type of Food	Description
Adobo	Filipino	Meat	Meat with soy sauce
Ajinomoto	Japanese	Grain	Wheat germ
Anadama	New England	Grain	Cornmeal-molasses yeast bread
Arroz blanco	Puerto Rican	Grain	Enriched white rice
Bacalao	Puerto Rican	Meat	Salted codfish
Bagels	Jewish	Grain	Bread dough, doughnut-shaped, boiled in water and baked
Baklava	Greek	Dessert	Layered pastry made with honey
Bok choy	Asian	Vegetable	Green leafy, stalk-like vegetable
Brioche	French	Grain	Egg-rich cake bread, used as sweet roll or shell for entrees
Bulgur	Middle Eastern	Grain	Granular wheat product with nut-like flavor
Burrito	Mexican	Combination	Sandwich; tortilla filled with beef-bean mixture and fried or baked
Café con leche	Latin American	Beverage	Coffee with milk
Cape Cod turkey	New England	Meat	Codfish balls
Challah	Jewish	Grain	Sabbath or holiday twisted egg-bread
Chayote	Mexican	Vegetable	Squash-like vegetable
Chitterlings	Southern US	Meat	Intestine of young pigs, soaked, boiled, and fried
Chorizo	Mexican	Meat	Sausage
Cilantro	Mexican	Seasoning	Coriander, similar to parsley

Table continued on following page

TABLE 17–1

CULTURAL AND REGIONAL FOODS
Continued

Name of Food	Culture/Region	Type of Food	Description
Crackling	Southern US	Snack	Crispy pieces of fried pork fat
Croissants	French	Grain	Buttery, flaky, crescent-shaped rolls
Crumpets	English	Grain	Muffin-like product cooked on griddle then toasted
Cush	Montana	Grain	Cornbread mixed with butter and water and fried
Dandelion greens	Southern US	Vegetable	Leaves from dandelion plant
Dolmathes	Greek	Combination	Grape leaves stuffed with beef
Enchiladas	Mexican	Combination	Tortilla filled with meat and cheese
Escargots	French	Meat	Snails
Falafel	Middle Eastern	"Meat"	Vegetarian-type meatball
Fatback	Southern US	Fat	Fat from loin of pig
Feijoada	Brazilian	Meat	Black beans with meat
Feta	Greek	Milk	Soft, salty white cheese from sheep or goat milk
Finnan haddie	Scottish	Milk	Salted, smoked haddock
Frijoles fritos	Mexican	"Meat"	Refried pinto beans
Gazpacho	Spanish	Soup	Cold soup with chopped tomatoes, green peppers, and cucumbers
Gefilte fish	Jewish	Meat	Seasoned fish ground and shaped into balls
Goulash	Hungarian	Meat	Stew seasoned with paprika
Grits	Southern US	Grain	Hulled and coarsely ground corn
Guava	Cuban	Fruit	Small, yellow or red sweet tropical fruit
Gumbo	Creole	Combination	Well-seasoned okra stew with meat or seafood
Hangtown fry	California	Meat	Fried oysters and eggs
Hoe cake	Southeast US	Grain	Thin corn cake
Hog maw	Southern US	Meat	Stomach of pig
Hoppin' John	Southern US	Combination	Blackeyed peas and rice
Hushpuppies	Southern US	Grain	Fried cornbread
Jalapeños	Latin American	Vegetable	Hot peppers
Jambalaya	Creole	Combination	Well-seasoned combination of seafoods, tomatoes, and rice
Kale	Southern US	Vegetable	Dark green leafy vegetable, similar to spinach
Kasha	Jewish	Grain	Coarsely ground buckwheat, toasted before cooking in liquid
Kelp	Asian	Vegetable	Seaweed
Kibbeh	Middle Eastern	Meat	Fresh raw lamb, ground and seasoned, similar to meat loaf
Kielbasa	Polish	Meat	Sausage
Kimchi	Korean	Vegetable	Peppery fermented combination of pickled cabbage, turnips, radishes, and other vegetables
Kuchen	German	Dessert	Yeast cake
Latkes	Jewish	Grain	Pancakes, sometimes from potatoes
Lard	—	Fat	Shortening-like product from pork
Limpa	Swedish	Grain	Rye bread
Lox	Jewish	Meat	Smoked salmon
Matzo	Jewish	Grain	Unleavened bread
Menudo	Mexican	Meat	Stew made with tripe (cow's stomach)
Minestrone	Italian	Soup	Vegetable soup
Miso	Asian	"Meat"	Fermented soybean paste
Moussaka	Greek	Combination	Meat and eggplant casserole
Mush	Southwest US	Grain	Cooked cereal, usually cornmeal
Pan Dowdy	New England	Dessert	Dumplings and fruit
Papaya	—	Fruit	Large, yellow melon-like tropical fruit
Pasta	Italian	Grain	Macaroni, spaghetti, and noodles in various shapes made from wheat

TABLE 17–1

CULTURAL AND REGIONAL FOODS
Continued

Name of Food	Culture/Region	Type of Food	Description
Pepperoni	Italian	Meat	Hot sausage
Phyllo	Greek	Grain	Paper-thin pastry for making meat, vegetables, cheese and egg dishes, and sweet pastries
Pilaf	Middle Eastern	Grain	Rice enriched with fat and sometimes vegetables, bits of meat, and spices
Poi	Polynesian	Vegetable	Root vegetable, especially taro, cooked and pounded, mixed with water, and sometimes fermented
Polenta	Italian	Grain	Cornmeal or cornmeal mush
Poke	Southern US	Vegetable	Dark green leafy vegetable
Potato latkes	Jewish	Vegetable	Potato pancakes
Pot liquor (likker)	Southern US	Vegetable	Liquid from cooking green vegetables or bones
Proscuitto	Italian	Meat	Ready-to-eat, cured, smoked ham
Prickly pear	Native American	Fruit	Fruit of cactus
Pumpernickel	—	Grain	Yeast bread with wheat, corn, rye, and potatoes
Ratatouille	French	Vegetable	Well-seasoned casserole of eggplant, zucchini, tomato, and green pepper
Red-eye gravy	Southern US	Gravy	Fried ham gravy
Safrito	Puerto Rican	Seasoning	Specially seasoned tomato sauce
Sake	Asian	Beverage	Rice wine
Salt pork	Southern US	Fat	Salted pork fat from the belly
Sancocho	Puerto Rican	Combination	Soup with meat and viandas
Sashimi	Japanese	Meat	Raw fish
Sauerbrauten	German	Meat	Pot roast in spicy, aromatic, sweet-and-sour marinade
Scones	English	Grain	Round, flat, unleavened sweetened bread
Scrapple	Pennsylvania Dutch	Combination	Solid mush from cornmeal and the by-products of hog butchering
Shoofly pie	Pennsylvania Dutch	Dessert	Molasses pie
Shoyu	Japanese	Seasoning	Soy sauce
Sopapillos	Mexican	Grain	Rich fried bread
Spatzle	German	Grain	Small dumplings
Spoonbread	Virginia	Grain	Baked dish with cornmeal
Spumoni	Italian	Dessert	Fruited ice cream
Stollen	German	Dessert	Christmas fruitcake
Strickle sheets	Pennsylvania Dutch	Dessert	Coffee cake
Strudel	German	Dessert	Light pastry, filled with fruit or cheese
Tacos	Mexican	Combination	Fried tortillas, filled with meat, vegetables, and hot sauce
Tempura	Japanese	Combination	Deep-fried seafood or vegetables
Teriyaki sauce	Hawaiian	Seasoning	Sweetened soy sauce
Tofu	Asian	"Meat"	Soybean curd
Tortillas	Mexican	Grain	Pancake-like leathery bread
Trotters	Southern US	Meat	Pig's feet
Viandas	Puerto Rican	Vegetable	Starchy tropical vegetables, including plantain, green bananas, and sweet potatoes

BLACK AMERICAN PRACTICES

Food of black Americans is not significantly different from other clients living in the same area. Distinct differences exist between those living and raised in the North compared with those in the South. As a cultural group, many blacks are in

"Soul food" is both a food preparation method (fried, barbecued meats) and specific foods (chitterlings, ham hocks, grits, black-eyed peas).

lower socioeconomic groups which of itself may precipitate nutritional problems. Well-seasoned **"soul foods"** are preferred. Most of these foods are economical. Poke salad, collards, and many other greens and vegetables are combined with fatback and cooked for long periods.

Their relatively high intake of yellow and dark green leafy vegetables, fish, and poultry are desirable patterns. On the other hand, extensive use of frying, overcooking of vegetables, low intake of milk and dairy products, and use of high-sodium foods may lead to nutritional problems. Nutrients that are often inadequate for black women include calcium, magnesium, iron, zinc, vitamin B_6, vitamin E, and folacin; these nutrients plus vitamin A and riboflavin are frequently lacking in the diets of black men (NFCS, 1986; 1985).

Geophagia, or eating earthy substances such as dirt or clay, occurs mainly in lower socioeconomic groups.

Pica was originally a cultural pattern among pregnant black women resulting from nutritional needs. **Geophagia** is most common among children under 3 years of age and pregnant women but may be practiced by some men. In many African societies, the biological need for calcium, iron, and other minerals by pregnant and lactating women is partially met by eating clays from nutrient-rich sources. This practice continued after arrival in the US. Clay eggs are still sold in some areas of the South and shipped to relatives in the North. Geophagia leads to iron deficiency because the clay inhibits the absorption of iron and perhaps also potassium and zinc. It is therefore believed that geophagia is both a cause and consequence of anemia. When clay is not available, laundry starch is sometimes substituted, which can irritate the stomach and is almost entirely lacking in minerals.

Black Americans tend to have medical problems somewhat different from white Americans. The high rate of obesity, especially in women, may be a contributing factor to diabetes and hypertension. Hypertension, twice as great among blacks than whites, is the most prevalent chronic disease. The cause of hypertension may be related to genetic, environmental, and dietary factors. Salt sensitivity or low intakes of potassium or calcium have been implicated (Falkner, 1990; Sowers et al, 1989). Blacks demonstrate a greater increase in BP and retain more sodium with functional changes in peripheral vascular resistance in response to sodium intake than whites (Falkner & Kushner, 1990). The rate of NIDDM in blacks is 50 to 60% higher than in whites (Bertorelli, 1990). Other health risks include infant mortality, baby bottle tooth decay, iron deficiency anemia, osteoporosis, and lactose intolerance.

What are desirable food patterns in the black culture? What nutrients are often inadequate for black women? How does geophagia affect intake?

NURSING APPLICATIONS

Assessment

Physical—for BP, weight, nausea, vomiting, flatus, diarrhea after ingesting milk or dairy products, soft bones, fatigue.

Dietary—for use of soul foods, pica or geophagia practices, salt and salt-cured foods; sufficient nutrient intake.

Laboratory—for blood glucose; serum iron, Hgb, Hct, MCV.

Interventions

1. Offer buttermilk, yogurt, and fermented cheese or sometimes small quantities of milk to provide calcium to blacks who are lactose intolerant.
2. Encourage the practice of yellow and dark green leafy vegetables, fish, and poultry.
3. Monitor for muscle weakness, as this is a common sign of low potassium from geophagia.

Client Education

- Geophagia can be a cause or a symptom of anemia.
- Ingestion of both clay and laundry starch is not advisable and may be harmful.

- Obesity may lead to diabetes or hypertension.
- Explain methods of food preparation that conserve nutrient content of food (see Chapter 18).

HISPANIC AMERICAN PRACTICES

Mexican Practices

Throughout Latin America, foods and illnesses are believed to possess varying degrees of **"hot"** and **"cold."** The classification is not rigidly defined, and foods placed in these different categories vary from person to person. The hot-cold theory is not based on the temperature of food. Hot foods are believed to be more easily digested than cold foods. A balanced intake of the contrasting hot-cold foods is supposed to maintain health. Contrasting foods eaten simultaneously blend in the stomach, tempering each other. The concept of "hot-cold" may have an important effect on food choices during an illness or condition, but it is difficult to predict which foods the client will avoid because of inconsistency in classifications. Folk remedies may be used to cure diseases.

Hot foods include chili peppers, onion, garlic, cereal, beef, and most oils. Cold foods include most fresh vegetables, staples, corn, beans and squash, most tropical fruits, and low-prestige meats (goat, fish, and chicken).

Mexican food is a fascinating combination of both Spanish and Indian influences, using many foods native to America. The basically vegetarian diet combines maize (corn) and beans, which provide a high-quality protein mixture. Fresh vegetables, including tomatoes, corn, avocados, onions, squash, cabbage, and lettuce, are used in various dishes but are not served separately (Table 17–2). Many flavors and seasonings are creatively combined. For example, nutmeg, chocolate, cinnamon, red pepper, and onions plus other seasonings may be combined in a recipe. There seems to be no limitation as to what seasonings can be combined.

The most typical dishes are the native Mexican ones, made with **masa.** These include tortillas (Mexican bread), tamales, tacos, enchiladas, tostadas, and many others. Tortillas prepared from corn treated with lime water significantly increase dietary calcium. Flour tortillas are nutritionally comparable to white bread when enriched flour is used. Yeast breads are increasingly replacing the tortilla.

Masa—corn kernels soaked in lime water, then ground to a meal.

TABLE 17–2

TYPICAL MEXICAN AMERICAN MENU

Breakfast
Fried eggs
Mexican sausage
Tortillas
Coffee with milk
Lunch
Chicken soup with noodles
Rice
Refried beans
Jalapeño peppers
Tortillas
Soda
Dinner
Beef stew with vegetables
Refried beans
Tortillas
Lettuce and tomato salad
Soda

Milk is usually limited in the diet, but some cheeses, especially Monterey Jack, are used in meal preparation. Dried beans, either pinto or calico, staples of the Mexican diet, are eaten at every meal. They are usually cooked, mashed, and refried and provide a good source of protein, iron, and calcium. With acculturation, the use of animal proteins is increasing, especially in regard to use of beef (Borrud et al, 1989). Meats, especially poultry, pork chops, wieners, and cold cuts, are used. Eggs are served frequently.

Chili peppers, used as a seasoning, are a valuable source of vitamin A and supply some vitamin C. Chili peppers contain capsaicin, which lowers the body temperature by causing sweating. Hot peppers have other attributes: (1) They facilitate the digestion of starches, (2) increase gastric secretions, (3) stimulate the appetite by adding variety and increasing fluid intake, and (4) inhibit the growth of some bacteria, including *Staphylococcus* and *Salmonella.* Most vegetables in the Mexican home are cooked so long that much of the original nutritive value is lost. Mexican Americans generally consume few fruits, but bananas and melons are popular. Most foods, including meat, beans, tortillas, and rice are fried using lard, salt pork, and bacon fat.

Although native Mexicans eat 3 large meals a day, families in the US usually serve a main meal with leftovers or easily prepared snacks for the other meals. Candy and soft drinks are common snacks.

The traditional Mexican American diet has several desirable aspects. The fiber content is high with a large amount of complex carbohydrates. The amount of animal fat is less than the typical American diet. Processed foods are not used often.

On the other hand, most cooking procedures require added fat, using principally saturated fats. The diet is frequently low in calcium, iron, and vitamins A and C because of inadequate amounts of milk products and green leafy vegetables and fruits.

Several nutrition-related health problems are of concern. In families of low socioeconomic status, including immigrant and migrant workers, growth stunting has been reported in children over 2 years of age (NDC, 1988). Obesity is common in Hispanic American children, and the rate of obesity in adults is 2 to 4 times the rate of white adults. The prevalence of diabetes is also twice as high in Mexican American men and women (Bertorelli, 1990). Cultural factors appear to influence obesity and diabetes more than socioeconomic factors (Hazuda et al, 1988). Studies support the fact that Hispanic immigrants from Mexico have a better health profile than those who have been in the US for a long time (Marwich, 1991).

Describe the hot-cold concept of food balance. What are the advantages of hot peppers? What are the desirable aspects of the Mexican diet?

Puerto Rican Practices

Many Puerto Ricans also subscribe to the hot-cold theory of health and disease. However, diseases are classified as hot or cold, and food and medications are hot, cold, or cool.

As in other Latin American countries, both Indian and Spanish influences are reflected in the popular Puerto Rican national dishes. Rice (cooked grainy) and red kidney or white beans stewed with bacon or olive oil, garlic, onions, and often peppers are consumed daily. **Safrito** is used as a relish to season foods.

Safrito is a mixture of tomatoes, green peppers, sweet chili peppers, onions, garlic, oregano, and fresh coriander cooked together in lard or vegetable oil.

A variety of fruits and vegetables—**viandas,** acerola, mango, avocado, corn, okra, chayotes, tubers, and citrus fruits—are eaten regularly in Puerto Rico. The acerola (also called the West Indian or Barbados cherry) is the highest known natural source of vitamin C (1000 mg/100 gm portion). However, many of these items are very expensive in the US. Fruits, especially banana and guava, are eaten as snacks. Very few dark green leafy vegetables are used.

Viandas—starchy vegetables including plantains, sweet potatoes, green bananas, cassava, and breadfruit.

Chicken, pork, and beef are normally fried but are usually limited in the diet because they are expensive. Salted dried codfish (bacalao) is a popular dish. Eggs are frequently used as the main dish in the form of an omelet.

Even though milk is well liked, it is seldom drunk as a beverage. Intake may be low because of its cost. Café con leche (coffee with milk) contains 2 to 5 oz of milk and constitutes the largest part of milk intake. Native white cheese is popular but expensive.

Most foods are cooked a long time or fried. Lard and salt pork are used to flavor many dishes. **Malt beer** has an exaggerated reputation for being nutritious and may be given to children and lactating women.

Malt beer uses germinated barley extract added to liquid, which is then allowed to ferment. Although this provides more nutrients than ordinary beer, the alcohol content is undesirable for the fetus and young children.

A typical breakfast might consist of café con leche with or without bread; if income permits, butter, eggs, oatmeal, and fruit may be added. Lunch is usually a light meal that may consist of rice and/or beans and sometimes bacalao. In the US, the lunch meal has been modified most, with a traditional American meal of soup and/or sandwich. Dinner is the larger meal and may include rice, beans, viandas, and a little meat if income permits. Dessert is not an essential part of the meal. In the US, Puerto Ricans have a less balanced diet than other Hispanic groups (Trevino, 1990).

What is eaten daily in the Puerto Rican diet? Describe typical meals for the Puerto Ricans.

Cuban Practices

Cubans enjoy many cut-up vegetables, fine stews, and casseroles flavored with sage, parsley, bay leaves, thyme, cinnamon, curry powder, capers, onions, cloves, garlic, and saffron. Saffron is such an integral part of Cuban foods that some dishes are considered anemic-looking and unpalatable unless they have a deep golden saffron hue.

Cubans serve soup daily. Chicken, fish, or a meat soup is served before each major meal. A bowl of salad is always brought to the table, whether it is eaten or not. Fried foods, especially fish, poultry, and eggs, are popular.

Everyone eats rice and beans of many kinds. Fruits and vegetables are plentiful; however, they are not consumed on a regular basis. Cubans use a lot of plantains. A sample main meal, generally served at noon, is shown in Table 17–3.

Normally, breakfast is coffee and bread. Adults drink a lot of strong coffee and rum; milk and carbonated beverages are given to children.

What is served daily in the Cuban diet? What are the typical beverages of Cubans?

NURSING APPLICATIONS

Assessment

Physical—for height/weight, IBW; BP, scurvy, night blindness.

Dietary—for home remedies, which foods/diseases belong in either the "hot" or "cold" category; folk remedies used; nutrient intake, especially calcium, iron, vitamin C; food intake, especially milk, candy, soft drinks, malt beer.

Laboratory—for blood glucose.

Interventions

1. Encourage the practice of using different seasonings.
2. Encourage regular consumption of fruits and vegetables, especially those typically used in their culture.
3. Incorporate some cheese and milk into the diet daily to boost calcium intake, which is normally low.
4. To lower saturated fat, encourage alternate food preparation methods (boiling, baking, broiling, and microwave cooking).

Client Education

- Candy and carbonated beverages should be consumed in moderation.
- Vegetable oil may replace lard in cooking. This keeps saturated fat intake lower.

Continued

- For Puerto Rican children and lactating women, explain that foods are a better source of nutrients than malt beer.
- Corn tortillas may be a good source of calcium, whereas flour tortillas contain 1 to 2 tsp of lard.
- Beans are a good source of protein and can be used as a meat substitute.

NATIVE AMERICAN PRACTICES

In the Native American or Indian culture, food has great religious and social significance. Health is perceived as a state in which the entire being is in balance; illness indicates disharmony or imbalance. A complex set of rules may be followed to maintain harmony, whereas chants or healing ceremonies are used to treat illness based on its perceived cause, not its symptoms.

Traditional foods vary among tribes, but the basic Native American diet consists of corn, beans, and squashes. Corn is a status food for most tribes. Food scarcity and a lack of variety are still problems for Native Americans living on reservations. Stage of acculturation determines use of traditional foods, modern processed foods, and federally donated commodity foods (NDC, 1988).

Diets on some reservations are considered to be poor, supplying less than two-thirds of the RDAs for kilocalories, calcium, iron, iodine, riboflavin, and vitamins A and C. As a rule, diets are high in carbohydrate, saturated fat, sodium, and sugar.

Fresh fruits, vegetables, and meats are expensive, if available at all. Chili peppers add spice to the diet and are a good source of vitamins C and A. Relatively small amounts of dairy products are consumed, so that calcium intake is often low. The principal source of calcium is bread dough or tortillas to which commodity nonfat dry milk has been added (Wolfe & Sanjur, 1988). Mutton and wild game are preferred meats.

Several leading causes of death among Indians, especially tuberculosis and high maternal and infant death rates, are attributable to poverty and isolated living conditions. An exceptionally high prevalence of baby bottle tooth decay (50 to 80%) has resulted in extensive campaigns to educate parents (Broderick et al, 1989; Phillips & Stubbs, 1987).

Poor nutrition is directly related to several leading causes of death. Heart disease and cirrhosis of the liver are common. The most significant nutrition-related health problem is obesity and obesity-related diabetes. Pima Indians have the highest known rate for NIDDM of all population groups, with a prevalence of nearly 50% of those over 35 years of age (Lillioja et al, 1988). Hyperinsulinemia in the Pima tribe reflects a resistance to insulin action. Low hemoglobin values have been well documented, and mild thyroid deficiency is also frequent.

What is a status food for most tribes? What are reservation diets like?

TABLE 17–3

TYPICAL CUBAN DINNER

Rum
Guacamole salad (avocados and pineapple)
Bean soup
Bacalao (salted dried codfish)
Rice or black beans
Boiled sweet potatoes
Guava paste and cheese
Coffee

NURSING APPLICATIONS

Assessment

Physical—weight, IBW; stage of acculturation, adequacy of cooking facilities, living location; soft bones, scurvy, night blindness.

Dietary—for nutritional beliefs, types of food eaten, alcohol intake, nutrient intake.

Laboratory—for tuberculosis test, blood glucose, insulin, Hgb, thyroid function tests (T_3, T_4).

Interventions

1. Offer buttermilk, yogurt, and fermented cheese since lactose deficiency is prevalent.
2. Incorporate tribal customs as much as possible.

Client Education

- When teaching, involve the extended family. Counsel client/family regarding economical food purchases and sanitary food practices (see Chapter 18).

ASIAN PRACTICES

Although food patterns have changed drastically in the US, Asian clients have maintained strong ties to their native foods. Rice remains the staple food in their diet. Although most adults prefer their native foods, children prefer both American and native foods (Story & Harris, 1989).

The prevalence of diabetes in Asians increases following relocation into Western societies. This may be related to acculturation and differences in nutrient intake, which usually lead to increased consumption of total fat, animal fat, animal protein, and simple carbohydrates and a lower intake of total and complex carbohydrates (Bertorelli, 1990). Clients may also be at risk of chronic diseases such as hypertension and stroke as a result of their traditional high-sodium diets (NDC, 1988).

As a general rule, Asian pregnant women have good dietary habits that need to be reinforced. Improvement in the practice of consuming calcium-containing foods is suggested (Newman et al, 1991).

Chinese Practices

The Chinese believe that eating is truly one of the joys of life. Nourishment of the body for a happier and longer life is considered most important, thereby leading to the development of hygienic food and the belief in a harmonious mixture of foods.

The **yin-yang concept** reflects these beliefs. Foods and diseases are categorized as yin or yang, relating to the reaction a food has within the body and not its temperature or seasoning. Yang foods, used frequently for blood building, are excellent nutrient sources needed for erythropoiesis (Ludman et al, 1989).

Yin is a passive feminine force that complements the active, masculine yang. Yin foods are generally bland, such as grains and vegetables. Yang foods are very spicy, take a long time to prepare, contain a lot of fat, and are necessary for health and strength. Most meats, alcoholic beverages, and deep-fried dishes are considered yang.

Nutritionally, the yin-yang system has been beneficial, creating variety in the diet and balancing the amounts of animal protein, grains, and vegetables. The Chinese favor moderation in diet and would reject extreme diets (such as one allowing only raw fruits and vegetables). If a proposed diet is not balanced in terms of yin and yang foods, it may not be followed. Overeating or obesity is not prevalent because of the belief that one should leave the table only 70% full (Newman, 1986).

China is a very large country, and regional differences in eating patterns exist, reflecting food availability and styles of cooking. In the northern areas (especially around Peking), the staple food is wheat flour made into noodles, steamed bread, and dumplings. Foods are generally light and delicately seasoned, frequently with wine stock, garlic, and scallions.

Throughout southern regions of China, rice is not only a staple, but also symbolizes life and fertility. Cuisine in southern regions (especially around Canton) offers the most varied menu. Cantonese cooking is subtle and the least greasy of all the regional styles. Stir-frying techniques are superior. Szechwan cooking (southwestern China) is highly seasoned with fagara pepper, which is very strong and hot. Cooks from the coastal region in southeast China use more soy sauce and sugar and specialize in salty and gravy-laden dishes.

In general, the preparation of Chinese food takes longer than the actual cooking. The cutting technique is of prime importance. A properly planned dinner has small portions of several dishes. Although it may not have a main course, the meal presents a variety of colors, textures, and flavors.

Pork is the primary meat, eaten almost daily. Variety of flavor is also important, and small portions of chicken, duck, and lamb are purchased by the ounce to garnish rice or to add to vegetable dishes.

Soybean products are abundant and cheap; hence, they are used in many ways in Asian cuisine. Soybeans yield tofu (soybean curd), soy sauce, oil, and bean sprouts. Tofu is a good source of protein and iron, is easily digested, and is popular. It can also be a good source of calcium if calcium salts are used to precipitate the curd. Sweet-and-sour spareribs are frequently chosen by expectant Chinese mothers. The preparation is nutritively adaptive since added vinegar leaches calcium from the bones into the meat, making it available to the body.

Describe the yin-yang concept. Compare northern and southern differences in eating patterns; southeastern and southwestern differences.

The Chinese use many different vegetables in cooking—bean sprouts, bamboo shoots, water chestnuts, gourds, and others. These are normally stir-fried or briefly cooked in hot water. A Chinese broth may cook for hours, but vegetables are not added until a short time before the soup is served. However, raw vegetables are rarely served. Popular seasonings are ginger, soy sauce, and garlic. Although soybean oil, peanut oil, and lard are the most frequently used fats, the diet is relatively low in fat.

Japanese Practices

Many Japanese dishes are ideally suited to American life, most being very economical and nutritious. The Japanese take great pride in the visual effects of foods they use. The arrangement of food, color contrast, and even shape are as important as cooking and seasoning. The rules for picking up chopsticks, holding bowls and teacups, and eating soups are well established.

Much of the food is cooked on a hibachi (a small grill) by broiling, steaming, boiling, and stir-frying. Stir-fry cooking preserves vitamins because the food is cooked only briefly.

Because meat is expensive in Japan, it is stretched with vegetables. Fish is used in many fascinating ways. Soybean products are an important source of protein. Tofu (soybean curd) is used extensively.

Many vegetables, usually steamed and served with soy sauce, are included. Seaweed, bamboo shoots, and bean sprouts are common vegetables. Few salads are served. Rice or noodles are staples and take the place of bread.

Fruit is the usual dessert, especially melons, berries, and tangerines. Other Japanese sweets are made of bean paste.

The use of extraordinary flavors is typical of Japanese cuisine; their wheat

TABLE 17–4

TYPICAL JAPANESE MENU

Breakfast
Rice Miso shiru (bean paste soup) Egg (usually raw) Tsukudami (fish cooked in shoyu) Umeboshi (salted plum) Green tea
Lunch
Rice or noodles Boiled vegetables Broiled fish Green tea
Dinner
Rice Suimono (clear soup) Sashimi (raw fish) Teriyaki (fish) Chawani mushi (steamed custard) Tsukemono (pickles) Tempura Green tea

germ powder, called ajinomoto, enhances flavors. Soy sauce is also an important seasoning.

Unsweetened green tea is the national beverage, but beer and **sake** are popular and served with the meal. Milk is included in the children's diet but rarely used by adults (Table 17–4).

Sake—rice wine.

What is the benefit of stir-frying? What is the usual dessert for Japanese?

Vietnamese Practices

A blending of Chinese and French cuisines has resulted in the light and subtle tastes of the Vietnamese culture. White rice and other foods are served separately rather than mixing them together; vegetables are stir-fried. As in other Asian cultures, rice is a staple and may be eaten at every meal. Because of the use of chopsticks, all items are cut in bite-size pieces before cooking.

Nuoc mam is a salty condiment added to almost every cooked dish. Other condiments may be added to nuoc mam, such as chili, garlic, and sugar, to vary the taste for blending with different foods. Compared with northern Vietnamese, those from southern areas prefer spicier food and use a lot of chili peppers. They also use a lot of coconut. Black pepper and ginger are popular northern spices. Lemons and limes are also a preferred flavoring.

One of the most popular dishes is a delicate beef-and-noodle soup called **pho.** Chicken soups, quite different from the Western type, are equally popular.

A wide variety of vegetables, such as bamboo shoots, bok choy, broccoli, carrots, cauliflower, cabbage, sweet potatoes, squash, watercress, and spinach are generally stir-fried or steamed. Many fruits are eaten raw. Sugar cane is plentiful.

Very little fresh milk is available but may be given to the children. Sweetened condensed milk is available for coffee. Lactose intolerance is common.

Vietnamese do not use a lot of fats in preparation but prefer lard as the cooking medium when available or affordable. Otherwise vegetable oil is used for frying. Tea is the most popular beverage.

Nuoc mam is the liquid drained from wooden casks in which alternating layers of fresh fish and salt have been tightly packed and allowed to ferment.

Pho is a combination of beef, beef bones, onions, ginger, and cinnamon that are simmered all day with water being added when necessary. Just before serving, freshly cut scallions, onions, more thinly sliced beef, bean sprouts, and thin white rice noodles are added and cooked briefly.

What may be eaten at every Vietnamese meal? Compare the differences between North and South Vietnamese diets.

Korean Practices

The main staple of the Korean diet is rice mixed with other grains since a diet consisting only of white rice is nutritionally unbalanced and causes health problems. White rice is often mixed with barley, millet, and red beans.

The Koreans eat 3 hearty meals daily, all about the same proportion (Table 17–5). The use of chopsticks makes it important to serve food cut into small pieces. Many foodstuffs are grilled. Soups, containing seaweed, meat, or fish, are always served.

A status food in Korea is ginseng, whose root is said to resemble the human fetus. It is believed to be a panacea for curing illnesses regardless of age or sex and is considered an aphrodisiac.

Since Korea is a peninsula, fish products abound and account for 85% of the nation's animal protein intake. Every conceivable kind of fish is served, either raw, freshly steamed, or salted and dried. Eggs are scarce and, therefore, expensive. Beef is the preferred meat. Meat marinades contain a lot of sugar and provide a crispy coating.

Kimchi is a combination of chopped vegetables that are highly seasoned, salted, and fermented underground or in special earthenware containers. Kimchi must ferment without being disturbed for at least a month and is best after 2 or 3 months.

Kimchi is one of the most nutritious preservation processes available not requiring refrigeration. Kimchi can be made from naturally grown vegetables, such as cabbage, turnips, cucumbers, and other seasonable vegetables. At least one variety is served at each meal.

Many vegetables grow in Korea, and both fresh and à la kimchi ones are preferred staples. Vegetables are never overcooked. Vegetable dishes are seasoned with red and black pepper, garlic, sesame seed oil, and soy sauce. Many types of seaweed are available and are highly prized for their nutritive value; seaweed soup is a must for expectant mothers. Noodles, made from rice flour, are popular.

Many fresh fruits are available (apples, peaches, strawberries, pears, watermelon, blackberries, pomegranates, currants, cherries, and pears) and are served with each meal and as snacks. Although cakes and pastries are not usually served with meals, many small shops specialize in such goodies.

TABLE 17–5

TYPICAL KOREAN MENU

Breakfast
Cream of corn soup
Rice
Kimchi
Barley tea
Lunch
Bean curd soup with brown sauce
Hot turnip slices
Kimchi (two or more types)
Toasted seaweed
Rice
Pears
Barley tea
Dinner
Hot vegetable soup
Spinach salad seasoned with sugar, vinegar, and sesame oil
Kimchi (two or more types)
Dried fish
Rice
Pomegranates
Barley tea

A number of products essential to the Korean diet are made from soybeans: soy sauce, soybean pastes, bean sprouts, bean curd, and soy milk. Bean curd and soy milk are the "dairy products" of Korea. Since there is no room for a dairy industry in this densely populated country, only children are given milk, which may be purchased daily in very small (about 90 ml) containers. Because of the scarcity of milk, babies are often breast-fed until they are 2 years of age.

The basic seasonings of Korean cooking consist of soy sauce, bean paste, and red pepper paste. Other important ingredients that make the taste distinct are sesame seed, sesame oil, garlic, green onion, red pepper, vinegar, sugar, rice wine, mustard, and red pepper. Vegetable fats, such as sesame oil and bean oil (made from brown beans), are used for cooking.

Korea has never been a tea-drinking nation. Ginseng is made into a very popular drink. The beverage that usually accompanies a Korean meal is barley water, served cold in summer and warm in winter. Instead of wasting any grains stuck to the pan after the rice for the meal has been removed, some water is added. This rice water simmers slowly while the meal is being eaten and is then served after the meal.

What is a status food in Korea? What 2 items are seen at every Korean meal?

NURSING APPLICATIONS

Assessment

Physical—for degree of acculturation, native location.
Dietary—for nutrient intake, especially protein, calcium, vitamin C, and sodium; cultural beliefs, such as yin-yang or use of ginseng.
Laboratory—for protein, albumin.

Interventions

1. Encourage many of their nutritional cultural patterns except for the use of high-sodium items.
2. Encourage the use of tofu and milk in the form of cheese, custards, or ice creams since lactose intolerance is prevalent.
3. Since rice in the US is not mixed with other grains (as practiced in Korea) to increase its nutritive value, encourage whole-grain or enriched rice.
4. For Koreans unable to purchase seaweed, suggest stronger tasting greens (turnip greens, kale, and mustard greens) similar in taste.
5. Ask whether or not Chinese clients prefer ice in their beverages because ice is believed to be harmful since it may shock the system.
6. If client is on sodium-restricted diet, monitor intake of Asian condiments such as soy sauce, pickles, nuoc mam, or kimchi.
7. Monitor for constipation because during hospitalization, fiber content of the diet may be less than normal, resulting in constipation.

Client Education

- Rinsing rice decreases nutrient value.
- Tofu is an excellent source of protein and iron and can also be a good source of calcium.
- Explain food purchasing and storage principles (see Chapter 18).
- The intake of raw fish has been implicated in stomach cancer, carries a risk of infestation with fish tapeworms, and has been associated with outbreaks of gastroenteritis (Schantz, 1989; Eastaugh & Sheperd, 1989).
- The medicinal properties of ginseng are poorly researched.
- Long-term abuse of ginseng may be associated with hypertension. Other adverse reactions (less frequently seen) can include nervousness, sleeplessness, skin eruptions, morning diarrhea, edema, and irregularities in blood glucose level.

Continued

- When sugar intake must be limited (as in diabetes) for a Korean, sugar substitute can be dissolved in hot water and poured over the meat, which is broiled until the crispy texture is achieved.
- Kimchi provides a zesty accompaniment to plain boiled foods, but because it is not readily available in the US, a Mexican salsa may be an acceptable substitute.

ITALIAN PRACTICES

Italians have preserved their cultural heritage partly because of the importance they place on sharing food with families and friends. Mealtime is leisurely and associated with warmth and fellowship. Normally, breakfast is light, and the largest meal is at noon with a smaller evening meal (Table 17–6).

The Italians, with their fertile imagination, have developed 2 simple ingredients, flour and water, into numerous pastas that are deliciously filling and "budget stretchers" for expensive meats. Parmesan cheese is used as an accompaniment for flavoring many dishes. The native cheese is freshly grated into a wooden bowl before each meal and added to spaghetti, soup, or whatever the main course may be.

A healthy Italian food pattern is the eating of many greens. Salads are served whenever possible, at lunches and dinners. Popular vegetables include broccoli, escarole, asparagus, cauliflower, eggplant, and mushrooms.

Veal, fish (fresh, dried, and pickled), highly seasoned cold cuts (salami, coppa, and prosciutto), and chicken are frequently used meats. Bread is essential to every meal. Heavy desserts are not desired; the meal may be complimented with fresh fruit and cheese. Garlic, wine, olive oil, tomato puree, and a mixture of herbs (thyme, basil, oregano) are used to season foods.

What is a healthy eating pattern in this culture? Describe the types of beverages ingested and why.

Wine and black coffee are the beverages most frequently chosen. Milk is generally avoided because of milk-borne epidemics common in Italy in the past. Italians generally believe wine is good for adults to drink with a meal, and even a small amount for children is good.

NURSING APPLICATIONS

Assessment

Physical—for BP, height/weight, IBW.
Dietary—for nutrient intake, especially calcium; overall food intake and quantity; alcohol intake.
Laboratory—for calcium.

Interventions

1. Encourage the use of whole-grain or enriched breads.
2. Encourage the use of cheeses, especially skim milk cheese, for their calcium content.

Client Education

- Domestic oils, such as soybean, cottonseed, and corn, are less expensive for cooking and seasoning foods than olive oil.

TABLE 17–6

TYPICAL ITALIAN LUNCH AND DINNER

Lunch
Mixed green salad with olive oil–vinegar based salad dressing
Risotto alla Milanese (Rice, Milan style)
Zucchini e pepperoni fritti (summer squash with green peppers)
Italian bread sticks
Fruit
Wine
Dinner
Olives and insalata
Minestrone
Paticcio di polenta (cornmeal dish with mushroom filling)
Hard rolls
Wine

MIDDLE EASTERN PRACTICES

Nine separate countries around the eastern Mediterranean Sea (Greece, Turkey, Lebanon, Syria, Iraq, Iran, Israel, Jordan, and Egypt) have similar eating patterns and certain attitudes toward food.

Lamb and goat are staple meats of the Middle East. Neither pasturage nor climate is suitable for cattle, and beef is not a status food. A very popular meat dish is **dolma.** The eastern Mediterranean countries enjoy all varieties of saltwater and fresh-water fish, shellfish, and **roe.** Many Muslims avoid pork and wild birds. Vegetables and legumes are frequently the main dish.

Dolma is made of ground meat mixed with rice, herbs, and spices and wrapped in leaves or stuffed into vegetables.

Roe—fish eggs.

Bread is the staple of life; each mouthful of food is eaten with a bite of bread. A meal without bread is unthinkable, and the bread is usually homemade, fresh, and warm. The more compact dark bread is preferred to refined white bread.

Pilaf is a festive dish for the entire Near East. Beans and lentils rank just behind bread and rice in popularity. Boiled beans are served cold at breakfast with a dressing of olive oil and lemon juice and perhaps a bit of garlic for extra taste.

A variety of vegetables, both cooked and raw, are served. In the Middle East, there are more than 120 ways of preparing eggplant. The most frequent seasonings used in vegetable preparation are onions, fresh tomatoes or tomato paste, olive oil, and parsley.

The best-known sweet is **baklava.** However, sweets are served mostly on holidays or social calls. A bowl of fresh fruit is the usual dessert. This may consist of cucumbers, guavas, mangos, citrus fruits, dates, figs, pomegranates, or bananas. No meal is ended without coffee or tea, but coffee takes precedence most of the time. In Iran, the favorite drink is tea, hot and sweet.

Baklava—layered pastry made with honey.

Cooking fats used in Middle Eastern cooking include olive and sesame oil, butter, and ghee (clarified butter from goat, sheep, or camel milk). Animal fat is used when the dish is to be eaten hot and oil is used when it is likely to be eaten cold. A meal is not regarded as tasteful and well prepared unless a large quantity of fat has been added. Mint, oregano, and cinnamon are popular spices; the most popular herb is garlic (except in Iran, where it is considered vulgar). Olives in dozens of shapes and colors are popular.

Milk is not normally consumed as a beverage by adults; however, it is given to children. Many Middle Easterners believe that yogurt is the supreme health food, curing many ills, conferring long life and good looks, prolonging youth, and fortifying the soul. Yogurt is used in many ways: mixed with diced cucumber as an appetizer; as a topping on rice, fried vegetables, and desserts; or eaten plain. Thin yogurt (diluted with water) is safer and less perishable than milk and very thirst quenching. A Greek specialty cheese is feta, a white cheese from sheep or goat milk.

If any modified diet is ordered, consult with a dietitian since eating patterns may have to be altered in the following ways: (1) In planning carbohydrate-limited diets, one of the difficulties is to decrease bread consumption; (2) the amount of fat in the diet could pose problems for low-kilocalorie, diabetic, or low-fat diets; (3) the traditional feta cheese and olives, 2 favorite foods, are high in sodium and would have to be eliminated from a sodium-restricted diet.

What is the staple of life for the Middle East? In the Middle East, what is the supreme health food?

The Muslim faith forbids wine, and many clients in the Near East do not drink alcoholic beverages. Christians and Jews, of course, follow a different tradition.

NURSING APPLICATIONS

Assessment

Physical—for original area of residence, height, weight, IBW.
Dietary—for nutrient intake, especially calcium, sodium, and fat; food intake, especially feta and olives.
Laboratory—cholesterol, triglycerides.

Interventions

1. Encourage continued intake of yogurt and white cheese to increase the protein and calcium content of the diet since milk is not usually consumed by adults.
2. Do not force men and women to eat together, as this is taboo in some Middle Eastern cultures.

Client Education

- Use low-fat cheeses to decrease fat intake.

RELIGIOUS FOOD RESTRICTIONS

Religious beliefs affect eating patterns, attaching symbolic meanings to food and drink. Some examples of this are the bread and wine served during the Christian communion service and the Hindu reverence for the cow. These patterns do not usually result in any nutritional problems but could affect clients' food intake during a hospital stay or make them reluctant to follow a dietary prescription.

Jewish Restrictions

Jewish dietary laws are adhered to in varying degrees because of the differences in interpretation and importance placed by the 3 basic groups: (1) Orthodox—strict observance, (2) conservative—nominal observance, and (3) reform—less ceremonial emphasis and minimum observance of the general dietary laws. It is important for the nurse to remember that not all Jews follow a kosher diet and that some are more strict about their diet than others.

Regulations about the types of food that may or may not be eaten are derived from biblical laws. Jewish clients observe many holidays and holy days that are associated with fasting and specific food traditions. Foods that are permitted are

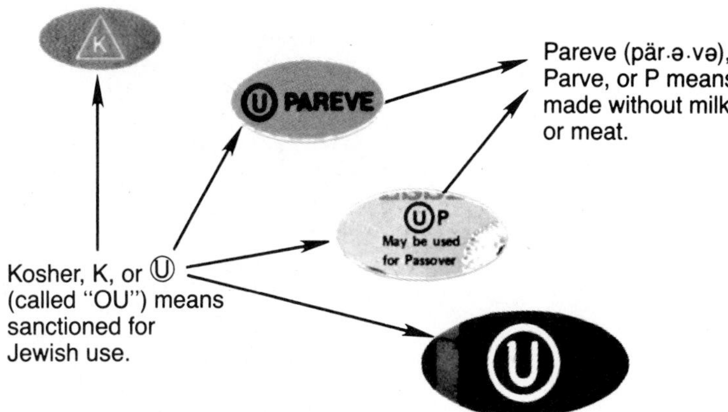

Figure 17–2 Kosher food labeling: All designations mean kosher; the Ⓤ signifies the endorsement of the Union of Orthodox Rabbis, which honors the strictest Jewish laws. Other designations, such as "K," are usually local sanctions.

called kosher, which means fitting or proper. An example of labels identifying kosher foods is shown in Figure 17–2. Some of the regulations with regard to foods and their preparation are described in Table 17–7.

Jewish dietary laws present no problem in providing nutritionally adequate diets in the home. (The amount of calcium needed can be obtained at breakfast and the one "dairy" meal ordinarily consumed.)

Other than food restrictions, Jewish cookery is influenced by the country or locale in which the Jews are living and the country from which they migrated (e.g., France, Germany). The diet is rich in pastries, cakes, preserves, and relishes. Fish and dairy products are used abundantly.

Because of a high incidence of diabetes, obesity, and coronary heart disease, therapeutic diets are often necessary. To insure compliance with a diet, it is important to take a careful dietary history. Diabetic and weight reduction diets can be planned to provide variety within compliance of the restrictions and to include some favorite foods, such as bagels or **matzo.**

Matzo—unleavened bread.

Notification of the dietary department is crucial if the client is Jewish. The dietary department can make appropriate alterations in the diet so acceptance is enhanced in the following ways: (1) Kosher meats can be purchased from wholesale distributors; (2) foods can be cooked in foil-lined pans and served on disposable plates; (3) crackers, margarine, bread, some brands of gelatin, and broth-type soups can be omitted from trays because these foods may not be kosher; (4) special attention can be given to the insulin-requiring diabetic for special holiday traditions, especially those requiring fasting and serving wine in religious celebrations; (5) soaking beef or veal in a large amount of water removes some of the added salt. Many favorite Jewish foods are highly salted and must be noted if client is on a sodium-restricted diet.

What nutrients are usually high in the kosher diet? What are some ways to increase acceptance of hospital diets for Jewish clients?

NURSING APPLICATIONS

Assessment

Physical—for weight, IBW; BP; original country of residence.
Dietary—for adherence to Jewish dietary laws.
Laboratory—for blood glucose, cholesterol, triglycerides.

Interventions

1. Allow family to bring food if not contraindicated.

Client Education

- Use low-fat cheeses and low-cholesterol egg substitutes to decrease fat intake.
- Foods eaten on holy days, especially Passover foods, are especially high in cholesterol and/or fat.

TABLE 17–7

JEWISH FOOD RESTRICTIONS

1. Only meat from cloven-hoofed animals that chew cud (cattle, sheep, goat, or deer) is allowed. The animals must have been killed observing rigid rules that result in minimal pain to the animal and maximal blood drainage. Preparations of koshered meats may be by 1 of 2 methods:
   a. The meat is soaked in cold water for ½ hr, salted with coarse salt, and drained to deplete blood content. It is then thoroughly washed under cold running water and drained again before cooking
   b. The meat is first prepared by quick searing or cooking over an open flame, which permits liver to be eaten since it cannot be prepared by the above method
2. Meat and dairy products cannot be served at the same meal, nor can they be cooked or served in the same set of dishes. Milk or milk products may be consumed just before a meal but not until 6 hr after eating a meal with meat products. Fish or eggs can be eaten with dairy products or meat meals. Eggs that have a blood spot are not allowed
3. Only fish with fins and scales are allowed: no shellfish or scavenger fish (catfish, shrimp, escargot, lobster) may be eaten

Other Religions

Table 17–8 lists food restrictions and practices of several religious groups. These restrictions need consideration only in institutional settings and sometimes when the client is on a modified diet.

TABLE 17–8

FOOD RESTRICTIONS OF VARIOUS RELIGIONS

Religious Group and Food Restrictions	Clinical Implications with Institutional Situations or with Modified Diets
Catholic	
Abstinence from meat, meat soups, or gravy on Ash Wednesday and Fridays during Lent	Fish or other meat substitutes are generally offered on these days
Mormon	
No alcoholic beverages No stimulants	Substitutes should be given to clients for regular coffee, tea, and most carbonated beverages, especially if the client is on a liquid diet
Muslim	
No pork or pork products; no animal shortenings	Hospitalized clients may need assistance in selecting from hospital menus to see that vegetables are not cooked with any animal shortenings or pork seasonings
Only kosher meats allowed*	Although institutional meats are not normally kosher, they may be purchased
Regular gelatin made with pork, marshmallow, and other confections made with pork are not allowed No alcoholic products or beverages (including extracts such as vanilla or lemon)	Nurses should assist the client in selecting from the hospital menu to be certain he or she receives adequate food considering these restrictions
Fasting is common (mandatory for 1 mo each year)	Fasting can be precarious with some medical problems, especially diabetes and hypoglycemia
Recommended foods: honey, milk, dates, meat, seafood, and vegetable and olive oil	Some of these foods may be contraindicated on a special diet (honey on a diabetic diet) and should be noted
Seventh-Day Adventist	
Optional vegetarianism: (1) strict vegetarianism, (2) ovolactovegetarianism, (3) no pork or pork products, shellfish, or blood	If sodium is restricted, the use of soy-based meat analogues should be noted because they are high in sodium. Strict vegetarians need assistance to select a well-balanced menu from the regular hos-

TABLE 17–8

FOOD RESTRICTIONS OF VARIOUS RELIGIONS
Continued

Religious Group and Food Restrictions	Clinical Implications with Institutional Situations or with Modified Diets
	pital diet. Assist clients in choosing from hospital menu to receive foods not seasoned with pork
No alcoholic beverages No beverages containing caffeine	Substitutes should be made for the regular coffee, tea, and some carbonated beverages ordinarily given, especially if the client is on a liquid diet
Snacking between meals is discouraged (mealtimes are at intervals of 5 to 6 hr)	Some diabetic, hypoglycemia, and ulcer-type diets require more frequent feedings

* Kosher means the food is blessed by a Muslim and pertains to 4-footed animals only.

SUMMARY

Once again, we are reminded of the basic concept of nutrition whereby the body needs nutrients, not specific foods. Nutritionally, clients have traits reflecting their culture and heritage, their religion, and their social or economic status. Various cultural food patterns have resulted in the survival of that culture; nutritional deficiencies resulting from these patterns are generally due to extenuating circumstances, such as economic problems. When nutritional problems are manifest, it is the nurse's responsibility to assist clients to make compromises or subtle changes, not by trying to change their whole diet. A knowledge of the nutrients in many foods enables nurses to assist clients in altering their dietary intake in deficient areas. Consideration of client cultural and personal food preferences may improve compliance with suggested nutritional changes.

NURSING PROCESS IN ACTION

A Native American is admitted to the unit. From the dietary history, the diet is low in protein, calcium, and vitamins C and A. The client likes chili peppers.

Nutritional Assessment

- Weight, height, scurvy (decreased vitamin C), and night blindness (vitamin A).
- Food intake, especially fruits, vegetables, meat, and alcohol; types of food eaten (processed, reservation).
- Cooking and food storage, facilities.
- Tribal affiliation.
- Blood glucose, sodium, cholesterol, triglycerides.

Dietary Nursing Diagnosis

High risk for altered health maintenance RT low intake of protein, calcium, and vitamins C and A.

Nutritional Goals

Client will consume foods high in protein, calcium, and vitamins C and A while still retaining some input of cultural values and food preferences.

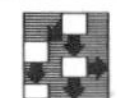 Nutritional Implementation 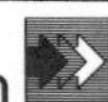

Intervention: Offer buttermilk, yogurt, and fermented cheese.
Rationale: Since lactase deficiency is prevalent among Native Americans, calcium can be obtained from sources other than milk.

Intervention: Offer corn at meals.
Rationale: This will show acceptance of tribal values, as corn is a status food.

Intervention: Encourage use of chili peppers.
Rationale: These are high in vitamin A and are a good source of vitamin C. Additionally, client likes this food so consumption is enhanced.

Intervention: Incorporate tribal customs as much as possible.
Rationale: This indicates to the client that his beliefs and values are respected.

Intervention: When teaching, involve the extended family/tribe.
Rationale: This values the Native American concept of need for tribal decision making and the importance of the extended family.

Intervention: Eat with client in silence.
Rationale: Native Americans are comfortable with silence, so this would display respect for his customs.

Intervention: Demonstrate how to combine beans and tortillas.
Rationale: This is an economical method to increase protein intake because the basic Native American diet consists of beans.

Intervention: Offer sweet potatoes.
Rationale: This is high in vitamin A content and is acceptable to his cultural beliefs.

 Evaluation

The client should eat the following foods after discharge: buttermilk, yogurt, fermented cheeses, corn, and sweet potatoes. The use of chili peppers is also desirable because this provides vitamin C and incorporates the client's cultural beliefs and preferences. Additionally, scurvy and night blindness should be prevented (from a lack of vitamins C and A, respectively).

STUDENT READINESS

1. What ethnic groups are most prevalent in your area?
   a. List dietary problems and some suggestions for altering the diet.
   b. Plan a 2-day menu that would fulfill the RDAs and use many of their favorite foods or patterns.
   c. Would a client have any problem being able to follow that menu, such as economic hardship or the local availability of special foods?
2. Other than good foods to eat, what other lifelong eating customs are learned as a child?
3. State some reasons why all whites in the US do not have the same eating patterns.
4. You notice on the chart that a new client is Jewish. Discuss the consequences of each of the following actions:
   a. Call in the regular diet order written by the physician, ignoring the fact that the client is Jewish.
   b. Call the dietitian to come talk to the client immediately.
   c. Check with the client to determine food preferences that would necessitate special foods.
5. Why is it important to be especially

sensitive to clients' eating patterns when they are ill?

6. Define geophagia and pica. Are these practices helpful or harmful and why?
7. Name the cultures associated with the following terms:
   a. Soul food
   b. Hot-cold foods
   c. Pasta
   d. Yin and yang

CASE STUDY

A community health nurse is assigned to an area of the city that has a concentration of Southeast Asians. In assessing the nutritional status of clients, she makes the following observations:

- Many of the new immigrants are at nutritional risk because they may have lived in areas with decreased availability of food or have been in prison camps for up to 5 years.
- Pregnant women often restrict their food intake during the last trimester to ensure small babies and easier deliveries. Little emphasis is placed on the pregnant woman's diet.
- Fruits and vegetables are often restricted in the first month postpartum.
- There is minimal intake of dairy products.
- Infants are usually bottle-fed.
- Bottles filled with milk or sweetened liquids are used as pacifiers.

1. What nutritional problems can you identify from these data?
2. How can the nurse help to eliminate these problems?

REFERENCES

Bertorelli AM. Nutrition counseling: Meeting the needs of ethnic clients with diabetes. *Diab Ed* 1990 July-Aug; 11(4):285–286, 289.

Borrud LG, et al. Food group contributions to nutrient intake in whites, blacks, and Mexican Americans in Texas. *J Am Diet Assoc* 1989 Aug; 89(8):1061–1069.

Broderick E, et al. Baby bottle tooth decay in Native American children in Head Start centers. *Public Health Reports* 1989 Jan-Feb; 104:50–57.

Eastaugh J, Sheperd S. Infectious and toxic syndromes from fish and shellfish consumption. A review. *Arch Intern Med* 1989 Aug; 149(7): 1735–1740.

Falkner B. Differences in blacks and whites with essential hypertension: Biochemistry and endocrine. *Hypertension* 1990 June; 15(6 Pt 2):681–686.

Falkner B, Kushner H. Effect of chronic sodium loading on cardiovascular response in young blacks and whites. *Hypertension* 1990 Jan; 15(1):36–43.

Hazuda HP, et al. Effects of acculturation and socioeconomic status on obesity and diabetes in Mexican Americans. *Am J Epidemiol* 1988 Dec; 128(12):1289–1301.

Lillioja S, et al. Impaired glucose tolerance as a disorder of insulin action. Longitudinal and cross-sectional studies in Pima Indians. *N Engl J Med* 1988 May 12; 318(19);1217–1225.

Ludman EK, et al. Blood-building foods in contemporary Chinese populations. *J Am Diet Assoc* 1989 Aug; 89(Aug):1122–1124.

Marwich C. Hispanic HANES takes long look at Latino health. *JAMA* 1991 Jan 2; 265(2):177, 181.

National Dairy Council (NDC). Diet and nutrition-related concerns of blacks and other ethnic minorities. *Dairy Council Digest* 1988 Nov-Dec; 59(6):31–36. (A publication of National Dairy Council.)

Nationwide Food Consumption Survey (NFCS). Continuing Survey of Food Intakes by Individuals. Women 19–50 and their Children 1–5 Years, 1 day, 1986. NFCA, CSFII, Report No. 86-1. US Department of Agriculture, 1986.

Nationwide Food Consumption Survey (NFCS). Continuing Survey of Foods Intakes by Individuals, Men 19–50 Years, 1 day, 1985. NFCS, CSFII, Report No. 85-3. US Department of Agriculture, 1985.

Newman JM. *Melting Pot.* New York, Garland Publishing, 1986.

Newman V, et al. Nutrient intake of low-income Southeast Asian pregnant women. *J Am Diet Assoc* 1991 July; 91(7):793–799.

Parraga IM. Determinants of food consumption. *J Am Diet Assoc* 1990 May; 90(5):661–663.

Phillips MG, Stubbs PE. Head Start combats baby bottle tooth decay among Native American families. *Children Today* 1987 Sept-Oct; 16(5):25–28.

Schantz PM. The dangers of eating raw fish. *N*

Engl J Med 1989 Apr 27; 320(17):1143–1145.

Sowers JR, et al. Calcium and hypertension. *J Lab Clin Med* 1989 Oct; 114(4):338–348.

Story M, Harris LJ. Food habits and dietary change of Southeast Asian refugee families living in the United States. *J Am Diet Assoc* 1989 June; 89(6):800–803.

Trevino FM, ed. Hispanic Health and Nutrition Examination Survey 1982–84: Findings on health status and health care needs. *Am J Public Health* 1990 Dec; 80(suppl):1–72.

Wolfe WS, Sanjur D. Contemporary diet and body weight of Navajo women receiving food assistance: An ethnographic and nutritional investigation. *J Am Diet Assoc* 1988 July; 88(7):822–827.

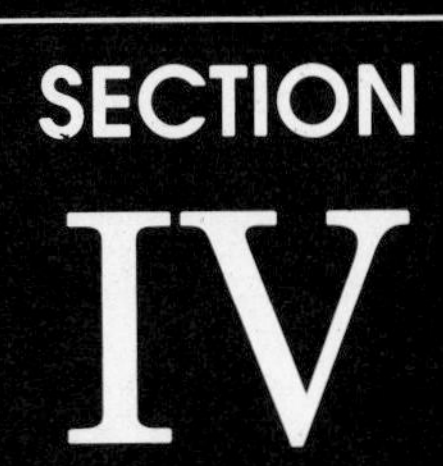

Nutrition Support for Vulnerable Populations

Many clients are at risk of malnutrition (overnutrition or undernutrition). This section will provide you with information regarding clients who need assistance in improving their food choices, whether this means adding specific foods (to correct for nutritional deficiencies or food intolerances), providing additional nutrients (to allow for increased metabolic needs), or helping clients to lose or gain weight (to prevent health problems). As you work with these clients, you will constantly be referring back to information you learned about the nutrients and integrating this information with the age, culture, and gender of the client to individualize nutritional care.

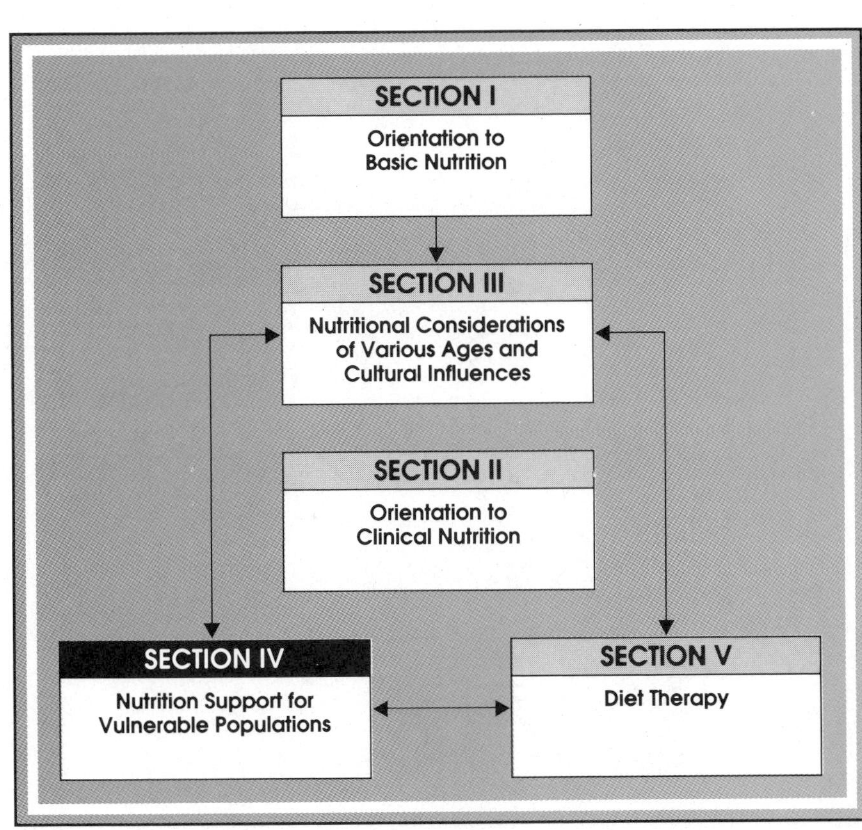

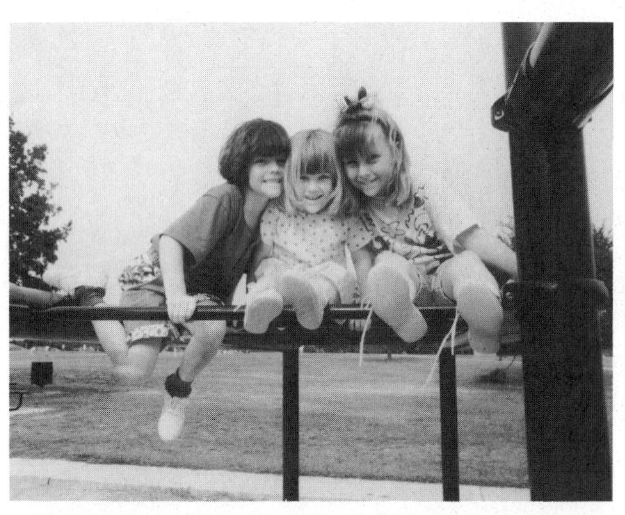

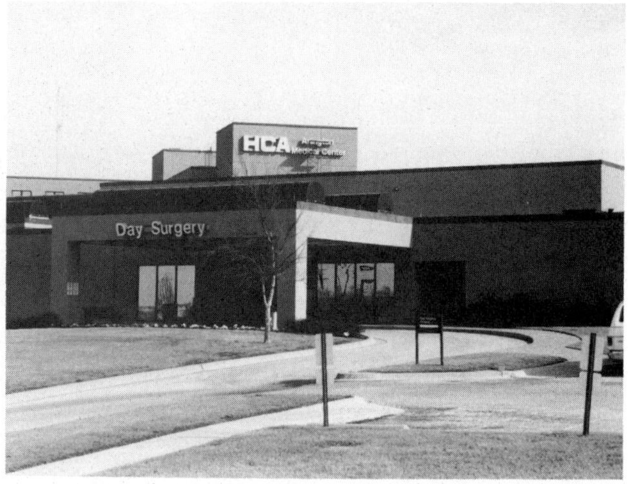
HCA
Day Surgery

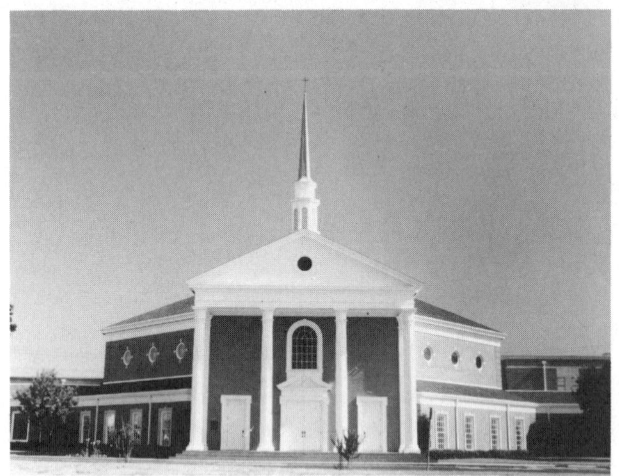

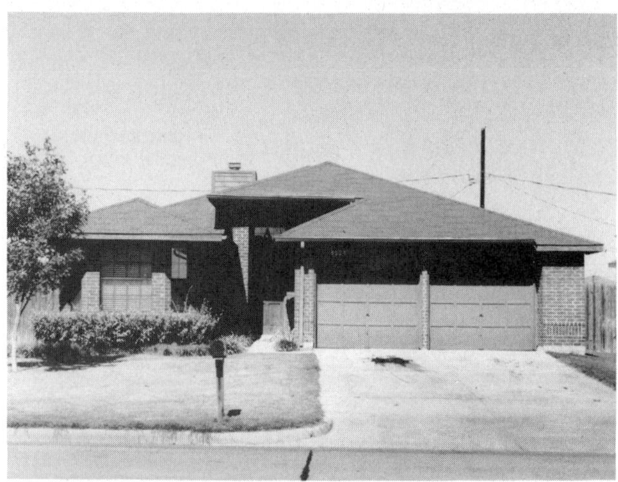

CHAPTER 18

Community Challenges

OUTLINE

Nursing Applications

III. COMMON NUTRITION-RELATED DISEASES
- A. Osteoporosis
  1. Risk Factors
  2. Causes and Physical Consequences
  3. Therapies
  4. Nutritional Care

Nursing Applications
- B. Rheumatoid Arthritis
  1. Causes and Physical Consequences
  2. Therapies
  3. Nutritional Care

Nursing Applications
- C. Osteoarthritis
  1. Causes and Physical Consequences
  2. Nutritional Care

Nursing Applications

OBJECTIVES

THE STUDENT WILL BE ABLE TO:
- Cite economical buys in each food group.
- Describe food preparation and storage techniques to retain nutrient value.
- List differences in marasmus and kwashiorkor.
- Describe various types of nutritional anemias.
- Distinguish the difference between folate deficiency and pernicious anemia.
- Identify laboratory values to help detect possible nutritional problems.
- Apply nursing application principles to each of the following: economical food purchasing, food preparation, hunger, malnutrition, nutritional anemias, osteoporosis, rheumatoid arthritis, and osteoarthritis.
- Identify client education necessary for economical food purchases, nutritious and sanitary food preparation, hunger, malnutrition, nutritional anemias, osteoporosis, rheumatoid arthritis, and osteoarthritis.

TEST YOUR NQ (True/False)

1. Americans spend one-third of their income on food.
2. An example of a manufactured convenience food is a carbonated beverage.
3. Frequently it is difficult for malnourished clients to eat adequate amounts.
4. Kwashiorkor and marasmus are the same thing.
5. An excess of iron can cause iron deficiency anemia.
6. Alcohol-dependent clients are prone to megaloblastic anemia.
7. Strict vegetarians are at risk of developing vitamin B_{12} anemia.
8. Excessive caffeine intake may decrease calcium loss.
9. Zinc intake is often below the RDA in clients with rheumatoid arthritis.
10. In osteoarthritis of weight-bearing joints, weight gain is an especially effective treatment.

Over the past 30 years, holism, consumerism, and cost containment have had a profound impact on all health care disciplines. These forces have shifted the client role from recipient to active participant and pushed health care into communities. The ultimate goal is no longer cure but prevention and health promotion.

GENERAL NUTRITION CONCERNS OF CLIENTS

Economical Food Purchases

Despite increasing concern about optimal nutrition, Americans are also anxious about food prices and try to conserve their food dollars. Most clients spend only about 20% of their income on food. Of the amount allocated to food, less than 25% of expenditures pays raw food cost (Fig. 18–1). Selecting the most nutritious products within one's available money is a common problem, and a general knowledge of food costs can be used to assist clients in stretching their food dollar. High-priced foods may not be the most nutritious; palatable, nutritious foods can be provided on a low-cost budget (Table 18–1).

If the amount of kilocalories is not of concern, foods supplying the most nutrients per dollar include beef, fresh potatoes, brown rice, wheat germ, milk, eggs, and peanut butter. On the basis of **nutrient density,** the best buys are spinach, liver, tomatoes, canned tuna, nonfat and low-fat milk, tofu, dry-roasted peanuts, eggs, and fresh carrots (Schaus & Briggs, 1983). As shown in Fig. 18–2, more of the food dollar should be spent for fruits, vegetables, grain products, milk, and dry beans; less is needed for meats and fats, sweets, and beverages.

Nutrient density is determined by dividing the amount of a specific nutrient of a food by the number of kilocarlories it provides.

The average dollar value of food stamps per household (family of 4) is $182 per month (FRAC, 1991). In many instances, food stamp allotments, based on USDA's Thrifty Food Plan, fall from 4 to 17% short of amounts needed to purchase minimal foodstuffs for adequate nutrition (Crockett et al, 1992). Thus, clients receive less than adequate nutrition, miss meals, and experience hunger. Prices tend to be higher in small, independent stores. Without transportation, low-income consumers are often limited to small independent stores more common in inner city areas or to spending more money for travel or delivery services.

Families on food stamps or on a very low food budget need to learn skills in buying and storing foods. By using every penny to its fullest, adequate nutrition can be provided on fairly limited budgets. To stretch the food dollar, it is necessary to (1) purchase the least expensive items in each of the basic food groups; (2) rely on minimum servings of meats; (3) use meat substitutes frequently (e.g., legumes and

If kilocalories are not of concern, what are the best food buys? What are the best buys for nutrient density? What changes should be made in how Americans spend their money on food? Name 4 things families on limited food budgets can do to minimize expenditures on food.

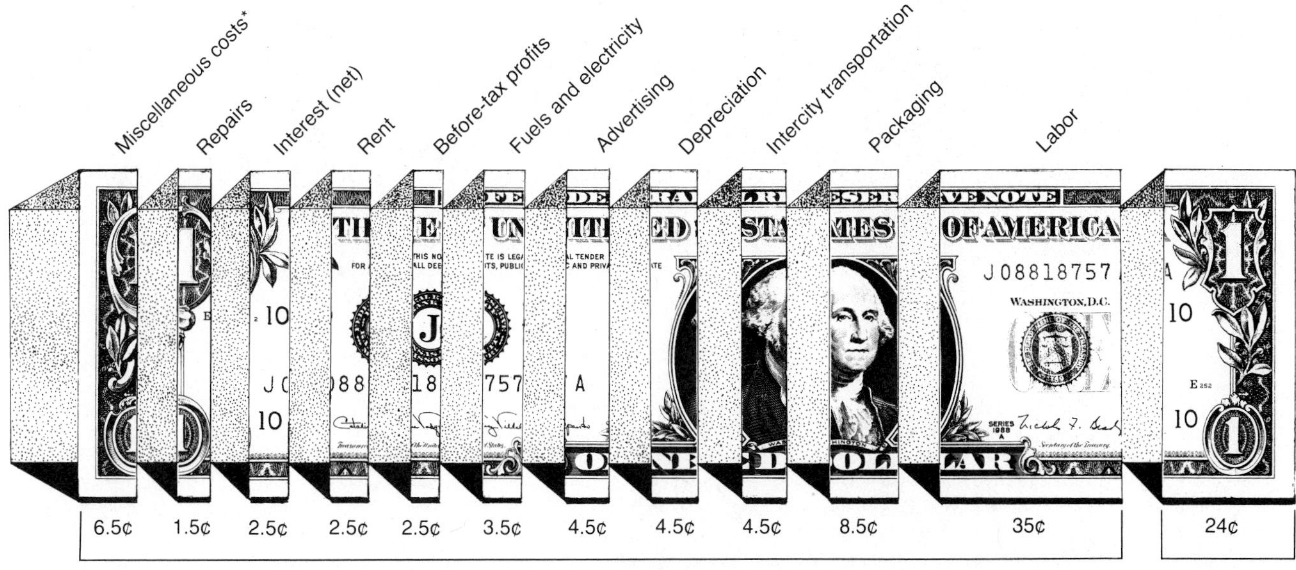

Figure 18–1 Dividing up the American food dollar (1989 data). Includes food eaten at home and away from home. *Other costs include property taxes and insurance, accounting and professional services, promotion, bad debts, and many miscellaneous items. (From *Food Cost Review, 1989.* July 1990. Contact: Howard Elitzak (202) 786-1870. Agriculture Economic Report 636, pg 41.)

TABLE 18–1

NUTRITIONAL BARGAINS FROM THE BASIC FOOD GROUPS

Food Group	More Economical	More Expensive
Milk	Skim and 2% milk	Whole milk
	Nonfat dry milk	Whole milk
	Evaporated milk	
Cheese	Cheese in bulk	Grated, sliced, or individually-wrapped slices
	Cheese food	Cheese spreads
Ice cream	Ice milk or imitation ice cream	Ice cream or sherbet
Meat	Home-prepared meat	Luncheon meat, hot dogs, canned meat
	Regular hot dogs	All-beef or all-meat hot dogs
	Less tender cuts	More tender cuts
	US Good and Standard grades	US Prime and Choice grades
	Bulk sausage	Sausage patties or links
	Pork or beef liver	Calves liver
	Heart, kidney, tongue	
	Bologna	Specialty luncheon meats
Poultry	Large turkeys	Small turkeys
	Whole chickens	Cut-up chickens or individual parts
Eggs	Grade A eggs	Grade AA eggs
	Grade B eggs for cooking	
Fish	Fresh fish	Shellfish
	Chunk, flaked, or grated tuna	Fancy-pack or solid-pack tuna
	Coho, pink, or chum salmon (lighter in color)	Chinook, king, and sockeye salmon (deeper red in color)
Fruits and vegetables	Locally grown fruits and vegetables in season	Out-of-season fruits and vegetables or those in short supply and exotic vegetables and fruits
	Grades B or C	Grade A or Fancy
	Cut up, pieces, or sliced	Whole
	Diced or short cut	Fancy-cut
	Mixed sizes	All the same size
	Fresh or canned	Frozen
	Plain vegetables	Mixed vegetables or vegetables in sauces
Fresh fruits	Apples	Cantaloupe
	Bananas	Grapes
	Oranges	Honeydew melon
	Tangerines	Peaches
		Plums
Fresh vegetables	Cabbage	Asparagus
	Carrots	Brussels sprouts
	Celery	Cauliflower
	Collard Greens	Corn on the cob
	Kale	Mustard greens
	Lettuce	Spinach
	Onions	
	Potatoes	
	Sweet potatoes	
Canned fruits	Applesauce	Berries
	Peaches	Cherries
	Citrus juices	
	Other juices	
Canned vegetables	Beans	Asparagus
	Beets	Mushrooms
	Carrots	
	Collard greens	
	Corn	
	Kale	
	Mixed vegetables	

TABLE 18–1

NUTRITIONAL BARGAINS FROM THE BASIC FOOD GROUPS *Continued*

Food Group	More Economical	More Expensive
	Peas	
	Potatoes	
	Pumpkin	
	Sauerkraut	
	Spinach	
	Tomatoes	
	Turnip greens	
Frozen fruit	Concentrated citrus juices	Cherries
	Other juices	Citrus sections
		Strawberries
		Other berries
Frozen vegetables	Beans	Asparagus
	Carrots	Corn on the cob
	Collard greens	Vegetables, in pouch
	Corn	Vegetables, in cheese and other sauces
	Kale	
	Mixed vegetables	
	Peas	
	Peas and carrots	
	Potatoes	
	Spinach	
	Turnip greens	
Dried fruits and vegetables	Potatoes	Apricots
		Dates
		Peaches
Breads and cereals	Day-old bread	Fresh bread
	White enriched bread	Rolls, buns
	Cooked cereal	Whole grain
	Regular cooking oatmeal	Ready to eat cereals
	Plain rice	Quick cooking or instant oatmeal
	Long-cooking rice	Seasoned rice
		Parboiled or instant rice
	Graham or soda crackers	Specialty crackers

From Green ML, Harry J. *Nutrition in Contemporary Nursing Practice*. New York, John Wiley & Sons, 1981.

peanut butter); (4) serve larger quantities of grains, cereals, and pasta products; (5) prepare most foods from scratch rather than buying convenience foods; and (6) eliminate most highly processed foods that are expensive or have poor nutrient content (e.g., carbonated beverages and potato chips).

Convenience Foods

Convenience foods are usually popular because they save time in meal preparation, planning, purchasing, and clean-up. Variety of food served is also expanded. However, convenience foods prepared by food manufacturers may cost more because of extra handling and packaging. Convenience foods also require more preservatives.

Basic convenience foods include peanut butter, pasteurized processed cheese, instant coffee, and frozen orange juice. In general, basic convenience foods, especially vegetables, cost less than fresh ones cooked at home, although this varies with seasonal availability. **Complex** convenience products generally cost more than foods prepared at home. **Manufactured** convenience foods offer many kilocalories but few nutrients and are considered expensive. When items can be purchased in more than one form, such as pizza, those with more convenience usually cost more.

Basic convenience foods have been processed using techniques such as canning, freezing, or drying.

Complex convenience foods include soups or jellies and jams.

Manufactured convenience foods cannot be prepared at home, such as dry cereals and carbonated beverages.

What are benefits/drawbacks of convenience foods? Give examples of basic, complex, and manufactured convenience foods.

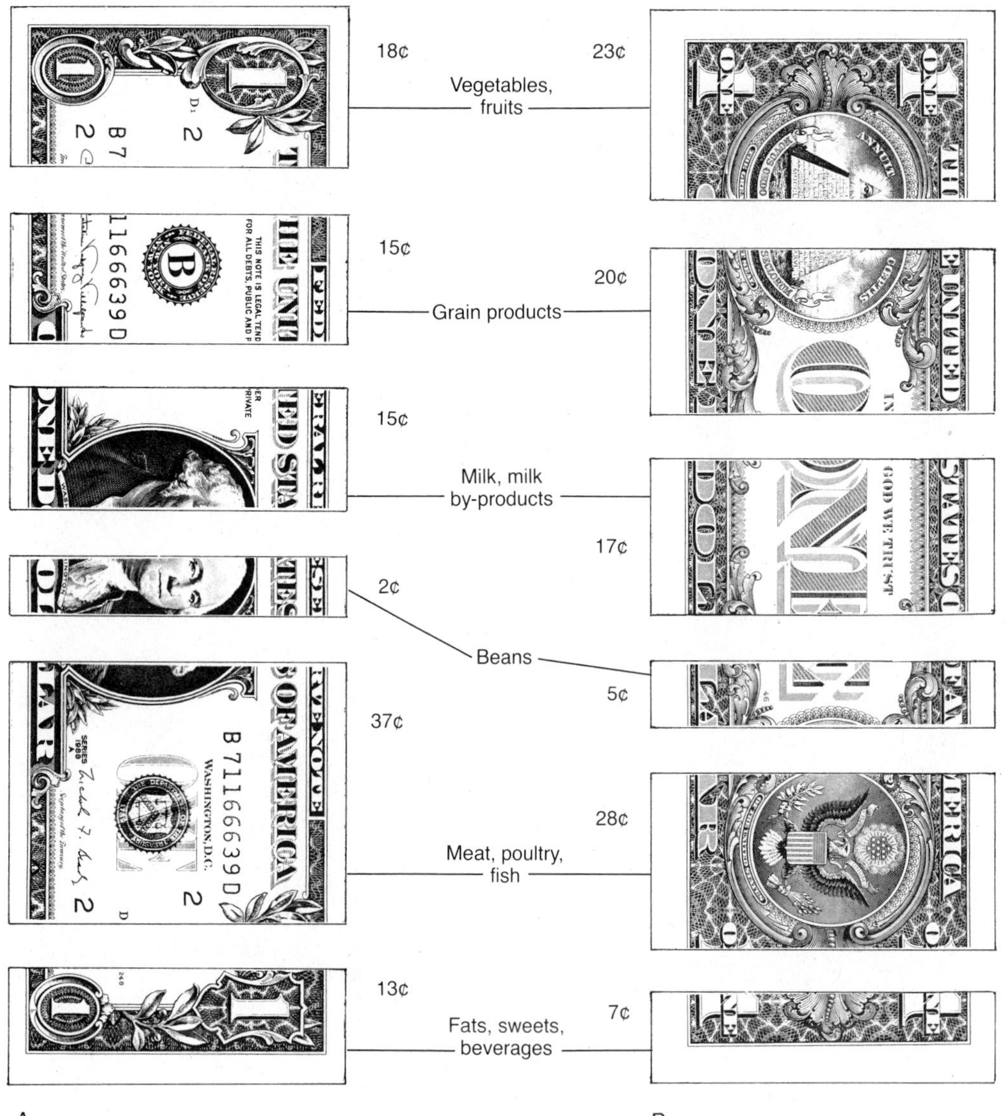

Figure 18–2 **The food dollar. *A*, How it was spent by survey households. *B*, How it might be spent for better nutritional balance. (From Peterkin BB. Making food dollars count. *Family Economics Review* 1983; 4:23.)**

Fast Foods

Fast-food sales have increased dramatically, becoming an integral part of our fast-paced lifestyle. Spending for meals and snacks away from home has risen substantially from 1965, more than double the at-home rate. Clients are eating out more as incomes rise and even more women enter the work force.

Although some believe that fast food is junk food, this is not always true. Nutritional analysis by fast-food chains and independent studies reveal that their menu items contain rich sources of protein (30 to 50% of the RDAs). Additionally, items are available that (if selected) provide 20 to 30% of the RDAs for thiamin, riboflavin, ascorbic acid, and calcium. When a hamburger or roast beef sandwich is selected, substantial amounts of iron are supplied by the beef.

Most fast-food menus lack a rich source of vitamin A. In many cases, salads have been an added selection because of consumer demand. This provides a source of vitamins A and C as well as dietary fiber; however, the cost may be 2 to 7 times higher than if purchased at supermarkets. Shortages of other nutrients, specifically biotin, folate, pantothenic acid, iron, and copper, are also reported.

Several other problems with fast foods have been of concern. (1) Kilocalorie count of a meal is generally between 900 to 1800 kcal (33 to 66% of the RDA for young men or 45 to 90% for young women); (2) sodium content is very high, ranging from 1000 to 2515 mg; and (3) fat content of some fast-food meals can be as high as 51% of kcal consumed. The impact of fast foods on nutritional status depends on how frequently a client consumes them, composition of each item selected, and what other foods are eaten during the day. Wise choices are possible when clients know their own nutritional needs and nutrient content of menu items. Nutritional analysis of many items offered by fast-food chains is shown in Appendix A–3.

What are the benefits/drawbacks of fast foods?

NURSING APPLICATIONS

Assessment

Physical—for income, food budget, number and age of family members.

Dietary—for use of convenience foods, fast foods, number of meals eaten out, special dietary needs.

Interventions

1. Assist the client in planning a week's menu and grocery shopping list. Menus can be assessed for nutrient adequacy and food costs, followed by discussion of good points and recommendations.
2. If kilocalories, sodium, and fat should be restricted, discourage fast-food chains and/or provide suggestions for appropriate selections (for example, salads or broiled chicken).

Evaluation

* Client/family eats nutritious meals within their budget and makes nutritious food choices when eating at fast-food chains.

Client Education

- Protein sources are generally the most expensive budget items; however, it is unnecessary to buy choice quality grades for good nutrition. Table 18–2 shows the relative cost of 20 gm of protein from various sources.
- Discuss guidelines presented in Table 18–3 to help client adjust food purchases.

Food Processing

Active, mobile lifestyles and an increasing number of women working full-time or part-time outside the home have led to a continued rise in the consumption of processed foods. Although foods "homegrown" and made from "scratch" can give clients control over how it is handled and what is added, this is not feasible for most Americans.

Effect of Processing on Nutrients

Nutrient content of foods can be affected by the way food is handled—type of processing to which the food is subjected (milling, cooking, freezing, and so forth) as well as how it is stored. In general, most minerals, carbohydrates, lipids, and proteins as well as vitamin K and niacin are nutritionally **stable.** Thiamin, folate, riboflavin, and ascorbic acid are most likely to be seriously depleted by processing

Stable nutrients are those with more than 85% retention during processing and storage.

TABLE 18–2

MEATS AND MEAT ALTERNATES: COST OF 20 GRAMS PROTEIN FROM VARIOUS MEATS AND MEAT ALTERNATIVES*

Food	Cost/Market Unit	A.P.† Amount to Provide 20 gm Protein	E.P.‡ Amount to Provide 20 gm Protein	Cost/20 gm Protein (Dollars)
Dry beans	0.29/lb	⅓ cup	1½ cup	0.07
Whole fryer	0.59/lb	3½ oz	2½ oz	0.14
Ready-to-cook turkey	0.79/lb	3⅓ oz	2⅓ oz	0.17
Bread, white enriched	0.50/24 oz	10 slices	10 slices	0.18
Eggs (large)	0.69/dozen	3.3 count	3.3 count	0.19
Beef liver	0.89/lb	3½ oz	3 oz	0.19
Whole milk	1.99/gal	2½ cup	2½ cup	0.19
Cured picnic ham, bone-in	0.89/lb	3 oz	3 oz	0.26
Regular ground beef	0.96/lb	4 oz	2⅔ oz	0.26
Peanut butter	1.48/lb	5 tbsp	5 tbsp	0.27
Tuna, canned	0.56/6.5 oz	3⅓ oz	3⅓ oz	0.28
Pork and beans, canned	0.35/lb	1½ cup	1½ cup	0.35
Frankfurters	0.99/lb	3 count	3 count	0.37
Rump roast, bone-in	1.79/lb	3½ oz	2¼ oz	0.40
Processed American cheese	2.12/lb	3¼ oz	3¼ oz	0.43
Beef, round steak bone-in	1.89/lb	3⅔ oz	3 oz	0.45
Ham, boneless	2.69/lb	3 oz	3 oz	0.50
Beef, chuck roast, bone-in	1.99/lb	4 oz	3 oz	0.54
Split chicken breasts with bone and skin	2.28/lb	4 oz	2½ oz	0.60
Perch fillet, frozen	2.59/lb	3⅓ oz	3 oz	0.59
Sliced bologna	2.29/lb	5¾ oz	5¾ oz	0.82
Sliced bacon	1.69/lb	10 slices	10 slices	0.86
Center-cut pork chops	2.99/lb	4½ oz	2½ oz	0.88
Beef, porterhouse steak	4.99/lb	4⅔ oz	3 oz	1.53
Breaded fish fillets, frozen	4.20/lb	2 count	2 count	1.53

* Prices in Arlington, TX, July 1992.
† A.P.—as purchased, including weight of bone, skin, fat lost in cooking, and so forth.
‡ E.P.—edible portion, cooked.

TABLE 18–3

BASIC PRINCIPLES FOR ECONOMICAL FOOD PURCHASES

1. Purchase the least expensive items in each basic food group
2. Rely on minimal servings of meats
3. Use meat substitutes (e.g., legumes, nuts, peanut butter, and cheese) several times each week
4. Serve larger quantities of grains, cereals, and pasta products
5. Prepare most foods from scratch rather than buying convenience items
6. Eliminate most highly processed foods that are expensive or have low nutrient content (e.g., carbonated beverages and potato chips)
7. Plan weekly menus, using the food pyramid as a guideline
8. Plan menus around seasonal foods or weekly specials advertised in newspapers
9. Buy store brands. They are almost always a good buy for the money
10. Prepare a shopping list and stick to it. Avoid impulse buying, but be prepared to make substitutions if a similar item is a better buy
11. Read labels to determine if similar products are comparable in nutritive value
12. Compare unit prices. Generally, the price per ounce is stated, which makes it easier to compare various sizes
13. Buy larger sizes (which are usually cheaper) if the food will be eaten before it spoils
14. Shop at large supermarkets rather than small operations or convenience stores
15. Avoid purchasing snack foods and many sugar-coated breakfast cereals. They are not wise food purchases because of their low nutritive values. The price per ounce is often astonishing.

and storage and method of preparation. Nutritional value of home-cooked foods is frequently about the same as processed foods. However, highly processed foods, such as potato chips, are not as nutritious as the fresh form, such as a baked potato.

Food processing attempts to maintain optimum qualities of color, flavor, texture, and nutritive value. Not everything done to foods by industrial processing has been good; however, not all processing is detrimental. The milling process removes the bran coat of grains. This bran coat contains lipids that are removed, producing grain that is more stable to deterioration, and thereby increases its shelf-life. Nutritionally, this results in a reduction of fiber and a loss of 70 to 80% of thiamin, riboflavin, vitamin B_6, and other nutrients. Enrichment replaces some nutrients lost in processing but not all of them.

Fresh fruits and vegetables have a higher nutritive value and better taste immediately after harvest but rapidly deteriorate if transported long distances or improperly stored. Frozen foods that are packed immediately after harvesting may be higher in nutritive value than their fresh counterparts available in the supermarket.

What nutrients are lost in processing? Which vitamins are most likely to be seriously depleted by processing and storage?

Sanitation Principles

Food carefully chosen for its nutritional value may be adversely affected by how it is handled and prepared before its consumption. Edibles must be handled with care to prevent contamination with food-borne organisms and sometimes must be properly cooked to kill any organisms naturally present. Certain foods, such as pork and eggs, require sufficiently high temperatures to destroy microorganisms. Tips related to nurses' and clients' handling foods that affect food safety are listed in Table 18–4.

Methods of Preparation

In many instances, cooking foods enhances their palatability, increases their digestibility, and destroys pathogenic organisms. Cooking affects acceptability as well as nutritional value. Following a few guidelines can help preserve nutrients during cooking (Table 18–5).

Adding large amounts of fats during the cooking process, such as frying food, is discouraged. Specific methods of preparing meats are recommended to lessen natural fat content. Meats cooked to the well-done stage contain less fat. To remove fats during cooking, meats can be boiled, microwaved in a colander or on paper towels, or roasted or broiled on a rack. Cooking increases digestibility of protein in meats.

Cellulose in fresh produce is generally softened by cooking; total volume and

TABLE 18–4

FOOD SANITATION QUALITY ASSURANCE

In home:

1. Hot foods should be kept above 140°F until served; cold foods should be kept below 40°F until served. Food should not be allowed to stand at room temperature longer than 1 hr, as the bacterial count can double every 15 to 30 min in cooked foods that are allowed to cool
2. Always wash hands before and after working with food
3. Handle foods as little as possible. Do not touch utensils in areas that will come into contact with the mouth
4. Cover mouth and nose for a cough or sneeze, and wash hands before handling food

In hospital:

5. Keep food covered in clients' rooms until served to prevent contamination
6. Stock refrigerator with sufficient food for 24 hr only. Date all foods when received and discard perishable foods after 48 hr
7. Food brought from outside the facility to clients by relatives and friends should be monitored
8. Do not allow anyone other than the client to eat from the client's tray

TABLE 18–5

GUIDELINES TO PRESERVE NUTRIENTS DURING PREPARATION

1. Prepare fresh produce as near to serving time as possible since exposure to air results in deterioration of many nutrients
2. Do not soak fruits and vegetables that have been cut. Water-soluble vitamins and some minerals (especially potassium) are leached into the water
3. Scrub outer portions of fruits and vegetables rather than pare them. When necessary, pare as thin as possible
4. Use parings and portions of vegetables not generally consumable to make soup stock; these are a very rich source of potassium and water-soluble vitamins
5. Leave produce whole or in large pieces so less surface area is available for oxidation of nutrients
6. Store any fruits or vegetables that have been cut or otherwise processed, such as fruit juice, in air-tight containers. Container size should be appropriate for the amount to be stored to prevent excessive oxidation from air inside the container
7. Cook foods just until tender or for shortest time possible. A covered pan minimizes cooking time because steam increases the temperature inside
8. Use the least amount of liquid possible in cooking. Cover the pan to minimize the amount of water necessary. Use leftover liquid, which contains water-soluble vitamins, in gravies and soups
9. Serve vegetables as soon as they are cooked
10. Do not add baking soda while cooking vegetables

bulk of the food is decreased so that a greater quantity of these low-kilocalorie foods can be eaten.

A relatively new method of cooking to most Americans is stir-frying, which is an old Asian technique. This method is highly recommended and has an added benefit of being speedy. Foods are cut in small pieces and cooked very briefly over high heat with or without a small amount of vegetable oil. Vegetables retain their nutrient value, color, and crispness.

What 2 cooking methods are time-savers and retain nutrient content of food? What methods can be used to decrease fat content of meats?

A microwave oven is another time-saver. Because of shorter cooking time and smaller quantity of water added, this method is believed to conserve nutrients. However, nutrient content of foods cooked in a home microwave oven contain about the same vitamin levels as those prepared conventionally (Love & Prusa, 1992; Klein, 1989).

NURSING APPLICATIONS

Assessment

Physical—for kitchen, storage facilities, skill and educational level of person who cooks.

Dietary—for use of processed foods, food handling procedures, food preparation techniques.

Interventions

1. Stress following guidelines in Table 18–5.

Evaluation

* Successful outcomes include client demonstration of nutritionally prepared foods; healthy food preparation techniques are used at home.

Client Education

- Products that can be stored at room temperature should be kept in cool, dry areas in airtight containers.
- Regular ground beef is more economical than ground round and total fat content can be significantly reduced by using a low-fat cooking method and by rinsing crumbled ground beef after cooking (Harris, 1992; Love & Prusa, 1992).

Food Additives

Purposes

The use of food additives makes many foods available by preventing spoilage and keeping food wholesome and appealing. Many clients are apprehensive about additives because of chemical names on the label. Even the names of vitamins on labels are unfamiliar, i.e., thiamin mononitrate. Food additives can be beneficial for several reasons.

1. Improve nutritional value. Enrichment and fortification have helped reduce malnutrition in the US.
2. Prevent oxidation and spoilage. Preservatives retard spoilage caused by mold, air, bacteria, fungi, or yeast and preserve natural color and flavor. Antioxidants prevent oxidation of fats and oils, fruits, and vegetables.
3. Maintain product consistency. Emulsifiers enable particles to mix and prevent separation. Stabilizers and thickeners contribute to a smooth uniform texture.
4. Provide leavening or control pH. Leavening agents, such as yeast and baking powder, are used to make foods light in texture and baked goods rise.
5. Enhance flavor and appearance. These substances are the most widely used and controversial additives. Included in this category are coloring agents, natural and synthetic flavors, spices, flavor enhancers, and sweeteners. Sugar, corn syrup, and salt are used in the largest amounts. Without these products, foods are less appealing, a factor that influences selections and controls nutrient intake.

Safety

During the 1950s, the Delaney committee investigated food additives. The Delaney clause prohibits the use of any food additive if it is found to be carcinogenic in humans or animals. Additives deemed to be harmless were labeled "generally recognized as safe" (GRAS). These substances met certain specifications of safety under what might be called a "grandfather clause"—in other words, they are generally recognized by experts as safe, based on their use in foods for years without any known occurrence of health problems.

In 1960, similar legislation was passed for color additives. Colors currently in use were required to undergo further testing to continue being marketed. Since then, approximately 90 of the original 200 color additives have been classified as safe and continue to be added to foods.

The use of additives is regulated by law. Before a newly proposed additive can be marketed, it must undergo strict testing to establish its safety for the intended purpose. Safety levels of additives have been established by the FDA, limiting both the quantity and how the additive can be used. Currently, additives are specific, well-known substances that meet specifications for purity and have been shown as convincingly as possible to be free from harmful effects in the amounts commonly used.

Almost all food additives (99%) are derived from natural sources or are synthetically produced to be identical to the natural chemical substance. In many instances, the effects of chemicals naturally present in a food are observed, and this chemical is then added to other foods to achieve a similar effect. For instance, calcium propionate in Swiss cheese was observed to retard mold. It was then added to bread to inhibit mold growth.

Currently, additives are as safe as science can make them. They are designed not to be toxic, and most of them would have to be ingested in very large amounts to produce acute symptoms. Of course, allergic reactions to food additives can be experienced by some clients, just as allergies to specific foods can occur. Nurses need to be concerned and aware of progress and changes that may have beneficial health effects for consumers. Local, state, and federal legislation is necessary to assure a healthy food supply.

NURSING APPLICATIONS

Assessment

Physical—for possible allergic reaction (wheezing, rash, and itching).
Dietary—for intake of additives.

Interventions

1. Stay abreast of local, state, and federal food additive laws.
2. Allay client's fears concerning food additives.

Evaluation

* Client verbalizes benefits of food additives.

Client Education

- Food additives are tested before use. They are considered safe but, as is true for everything eaten, should be consumed in moderation.

NUTRITIONAL RISKS OF COMMUNITY CLIENTS

Hunger

Hunger has been defined as a "recurrent, involuntary lack of access to food" (Dietz & Trowbridge, 1990), or "discomfort, weakness, or pain caused by lack of food" (ADA, 1990).

Poverty was defined as a yearly income below $12,700 for a family of 4 in 1990.

How can hunger hurt the society?

Most Americans are unaware of the prevalence of **hunger** in the US. The homeless constitute a large percentage of the hungry. A 1987 survey indicated some 600,000 people are homeless (Saal & Douglas, 1992). However, many of the hungry are behind closed doors. Approximately 32 million people in the nation maintain a home but live below **poverty** level.

In the long run, hunger hurts everyone as a result of health problems, increased education costs, and less than optimal productivity. Yet this serious health problem is treatable with a simple cure of providing food.

Causes

Poverty is a root cause of hunger. Approximately one-third of the monthly income of poverty-level families is spent on food; an average meal costs $0.68 (FRAC, 1991). Meals are often skimpy, and when grocery money runs out, families go to bed without dinner.

The proportion of income spent on shelter is 3 times greater for a poor family than for a typical middle-class American family (FRAC, 1991). Approximately 56% of all poor family renters spend at least 55% of their income on shelter (A Place to Call Home, 1991). Affordable housing for low-income households has been defined as costing less than 30% of income. Thus, to maintain a home, these families give up food.

The homeless are at even greater risk of hunger. Nearly 6 times as many homeless children as children from poverty-level homes stated their families frequently ran out of food and that they were fairly often or always hungry (FRAC, 1991).

Employment-related problems, such as unemployment, low wages, lack of marketable skills, and inflationary costs, are also contributing factors. Mental illness and substance abuse are other causes for hunger. To add to these problems, affordable mental health and substance abuse services are limited.

Cuts in the federal, state, and local budgets have resulted in less financial assistance available, placing more people at a greater risk of hunger. Millions of eligible families are unaware of options for obtaining assistance or are declared ineligible for food stamps by onerous regulations.

What are some causes of hunger?

Prevalence

In 1985, the Physician Task Force (1985) estimated that hunger afflicted 20 million Americans, or 1 out of 12. As evidenced by the numbers of people requesting emergency food assistance, the level of hungry people has increased dramatically (FRAC, 1991). FRAC's Community Childhood Hunger Identification Project found that 1 in 8 American children under age 12 suffers from hunger (some 11.5 million children); millions of other children are at risk of going hungry. It is estimated that some 32,000 children are homeless (Saal & Douglas, 1992) and constitute the fastest growing segment of the homeless population.

Impact

Most of the attention has been focused on hunger in children; pregnant women, infants, and the elderly are also vulnerable to adverse effects of hunger. Acute and chronic effects on health and behavior have been observed. Insufficient food intake affects clients' mental and physical conditions. Growth stunting without muscle wasting is characteristic of homeless children who experience moderate chronic nutritional stress (Fierman et al, 1991). Hungry children are more likely to suffer from unwanted weight loss, fatigue, irritability, concentration problems, and dizziness as well as frequent headaches, ear infections, and colds. These problems also result in more absenteeism from school (FRAC, 1991).

Missing a meal such as breakfast can reduce a child's ability to respond to the environment, thereby negatively affecting learning. Apathy, disinterest, irritability, and a low tolerance for frustration are common behaviors in hungry children. These hungry children are unable to concentrate in school and are less likely to reach their potential to become fully productive adults.

Prolonged hunger can increase the risk of malnutrition and reduce immune response (ADA, 1990). Pregnant women are at risk of delivering LBW infants and developing iron deficiency anemia; children are at risk of iron deficiency anemia and reduced growth rate.

How can prolonged hunger affect different population groups?

Solutions

As the late Mayer (1986) stated, "The goal of nutrition is to apply scientific knowledge to feed people, feed them adequately, and feed them all. By its very nature, nutrition is a set of scientific disciplines whose end is action." Aggressive action is needed to solve the hunger problem in a timely manner (ADA, 1990).

Federal assistance programs, discussed in Chapter 11, are already available to address hunger in the US. Many of these programs are not being fully used. Full use of these programs, with increased availability and benefits, and increased awareness of programs are good starts for eliminating hunger. Of 2000 families eligible for food stamps, 37% were not participating (FRAC, 1991). Reasons given for nonparticipation were (1) bureaucratic barriers, (2) uninformed/misinformed about eligibility, and (3) embarrassed to use food stamps. Benefits for those who are eligible are currently inadequate to alleviate hunger. Food banks, food pantries, and other community resource agencies are also available to provide food and meals to hungry persons.

The WIC program has proved to be cost-effective in improving participants' health and nutritional intake. Currently, slightly over 50% of those eligible participate.

School breakfast and lunch programs have also proved to be cost-effective. Children participating in both the breakfast and the lunch program were significantly less likely to suffer from the problems (already discussed) associated with hunger. Children who receive breakfast at school have fewer absences. Despite increasing numbers of school districts participating in the breakfast program, less than 50% of schools offer this program.

NURSING APPLICATIONS

Assessment

Physical—for income, percentage of income spent on home or whether homeless, employment-related problems, mental illness, substance abuse, weight loss, growth rate in infants/children.

Dietary—for use of food stamps, beliefs/knowledge about federal, state, and local food resources.

Laboratory—for CBC with differential.

Interventions

1. Let client ventilate feelings/beliefs about "handouts" of food. Discuss embarrassment issues matter of factly. Help client to recognize that inadequate funds for food is not a sign of failure, but asking for help takes strength/courage and wisdom. In due time, the client may be able to help someone else.
2. Refer to social worker for assistance in filling out forms.
3. Emphasize use of WIC, school breakfast and lunch programs, food banks, food pantries.
4. Offer to help serve at community food resource centers or food donation drives.
5. Stay abreast of federal, state, and local food resources. Let your voice be heard by federal, state, and local legislatures.

Evaluation

* Client/family receives adequate amounts of food to prevent hunger and uses federal, state, and local food resources.

Client Education

- Inform of federal, state, and local food resources. Present information in a positive manner stating how it will benefit client/family. Most parents desire the best for their children; therefore, stress benefits children will receive (increased growth, learning, productivity, and so forth) by participating.
- Proper nutrition can decrease money spent on health problems.

Malnutrition

With increasing levels of homeless people and migrant workers, and implementation of diagnosis-related groups (DRGs), malnutrition has become more prevalent in the community as well as within the hospital. Serious nutritional deficiencies, as evidenced by weight loss, pressure sores, dehydration, hepatic failure, and chronic infections, are observed in 65% of the elderly (Hunger and the Elderly, 1986) and 25 to 50% of all admissions to acute care facilities (Roubenoff et al, 1987).

Clients may become malnourished in the hospital or community as a result of inability to absorb nutrients, refusal to eat foods provided, difficulty in purchasing and preparing food, financial constraints, or poor cooking facilities.

Illness, stress, and trauma have catabolic effects increasing nutritional requirements, while oral intake is minimal. Certain conditions — cancer, AIDS, GI disorders, chronic heart failure, chronic pulmonary disease, renal and hepatic failure, alcoholism, and conditions with high metabolic needs — are more frequently associated with a diagnosis of malnutrition (Weddle et al, 1991). Additionally, a number of institutional practices (Table 18–6) are contrary to optimal nutritional care, resulting in deterioration of a client's nutritional status. Deficiencies of several nutrients are more prevalent than an isolated nutrient deficiency.

What percentage of elderly clients and acute care admissions have nutritional deficiencies?

Causes and Physical Consequences

When a client's intake is inadequate to meet physiological requirements over an extended period of time, the body is virtually starved, as endogenous energy stores are used to maintain body functions. The degree of starvation and presence of stress determine the extent and type of malnutrition.

After the onset of starvation, glycogen stores are the predominant fuel. With fasting, these glycogen stores are rapidly depleted within 12 to 24 hours. Initially, glucose is the obligatory fuel for brain cells and RBCs; the body is unable to convert significant amounts of fatty acids into glucose. With continued starvation, hepatic **gluconeogenesis** is enhanced.

Gluconeogenesis — glucose synthesis from noncarbohydrate sources.

The body contains no reserve protein deposits that can be used when exogenous protein is not available. When exogenous protein is not available for basic maintenance, protein from lean muscle tissue and, to some extent, **visceral** protein may be used. Protein present in visceral organs is necessary; even mild protein losses from these areas can impair normal metabolic processes and immune responses. Protein deficits compounded with acute stress have a profound impact on many body functions.

Visceral proteins are protein within the soft organs, i.e., heart, lungs, and GI tract.

Fortunately, with prolonged starvation, the body adapts to conserve vital proteins. **Ketones** are used rather than glucose, thereby decreasing the rate of protein catabolism because fatty acids are now being used for energy. Decreased insulin secretion promotes **lipolysis.** Normal amounts of fat stores can provide more than 150,000 kcal, representing the largest energy resource. Use of fat as fuel results in less protein and nitrogen losses (urinary urea nitrogen decreases). Additionally, the BMR also drops as the body attempts to conserve its available fuel (Fig. 18–3).

Ketones are normal metabolic products of lipid oxidation.

Lipolysis is fat mobilization from adipose tissue to metabolize for energy.

Marasmus is caused principally by inadequate kilocalorie intake and is characterized by an emaciated appearance that is due to muscle and fat stores being used for energy.

Malnutrition affects the whole body, especially metabolic systems, with (1) reduced synthesis of enzymes and plasma proteins, (2) increased susceptibility to in-

TABLE 18–6

UNDESIRABLE PRACTICES AFFECTING THE NUTRITIONAL HEALTH OF HOSPITAL CLIENTS

Failure to record height and weight
Rotation of staff at frequent intervals
Diffusion of responsibility for client care
Prolonged use of glucose and saline intravenous feedings
Failure to observe client's food intake
Withholding meals because of diagnostic tests
Use of tube feedings in inadequate amounts, of uncertain composition, and under unsanitary conditions
Ignorance of the composition of vitamin mixtures and other nutritional products
Failure to recognize increased nutritional needs due to injury or illness
Performance of surgical procedures without first making certain that the client is optimally nourished, and failure to give the body nutritional support after surgery
Failure to appreciate the role of nutrition in the prevention of and recovery from infection; unwarranted reliance on antibiotics
Lack of communication and interaction between physician and dietitian. As staff professionals, dietitians should be concerned with the nutritional health of *every* hospital client
Delay of nutrition support until the client is in an advanced state of depletion, which is sometimes irreversible
Limited availability of laboratory tests to assess nutritional status; failure to use those that are available

From Butterworth CE. The skeleton in the hospital closet. *Nutrition Today* 9(2):4, 1974. © by Williams & Wilkins, 1974.

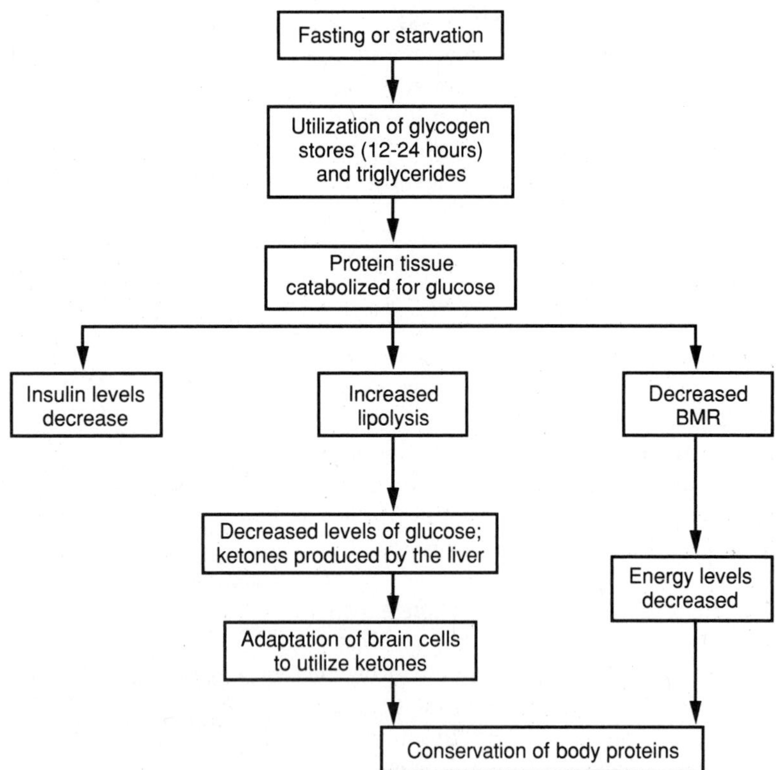

Figure 18–3 Physiological responses to starvation. BMR, Basal metabolic rate.

Kwashiorkor, generally defined as protein deficiency, appears in the US as a result of stress from major surgery, injury, or infection, when nutrient requirements are high but intake is curtailed.

Describe the body's response to starvation.

Cachexia is a severe stage of malnutrition, with weight loss, muscle wasting, weakness, anorexia, and early satiety.

fection, (3) poor wound healing, and (4) mental lassitude. In other words, it contributes to client morbidity and mortality. PEM involves 2 distinct deficiency states: **marasmus** and **kwashiorkor** (Table 18–7). The combination of protein and kilocalorie deficiency is called marasmic kwashiorkor.

Marasmus or Energy Deficiency

Marasmus is a chronic illness with gradual wasting (underweight) leading to severe **cachexia.** These clients are emaciated (skin and bones). If kilocaloric intake is inadequate, available body fat stores and, to some extent, muscles are depleted as a result of starvation. Weight loss is due to loss of muscle and fat; TSF reflects loss of fat stores; reduced MAMC reflects use of skeletal muscle for energy (Fig. 18–4). Muscle wasting, evident in extremities and trunk, also occurs in intestines, heart, and other organs. Visceral protein measurements (serum albumin and transferrin) may be within normal limits or slightly reduced (usually not below 2.8 gm/dl). Thus, immunocompetence and wound healing are reasonably good.

What are the effects of marasmus on a body? Why is it important to implement nutrition support?

Although marasmus is not particularly life-threatening, nutrition support should be initiated to prevent the development of hypoalbuminemia (kwashiorkor) if stress or trauma is incurred. Response and cure are slow; appropriate planning is vital to ensure long-term improvements in nutritional status and changes in eating patterns.

Kwashiorkor or Protein Deficiency

Hypermetabolism caused by an acute life-threatening illness results in a catabolic state, increasing risk of developing kwashiorkor if nutritional intake is inadequate. McClave et al (1992) determined that stress-induced hypoalbuminemia increased length of hospitalization by 29%, mortality fourfold, and development of nosocomial infection and sepsis almost 2.5 times above that seen with marasmic PEM. Typical cases are clients under acute stress who have been on standard dex-

TABLE 18–7

COMPARISON OF MARASMUS AND KWASHIORKOR

Disease	Clinical Setting	Time Course to Develop	Clinical Features	Laboratory Findings	Clinical Course	Mortality
Marasmus	↓ kilocalorie intake	Months or years	Starved appearance Weight <80% standard for height Triceps skinfold <3 mm Midarm muscle circumference <15 cm	Not severely affected	Reasonably preserved responsiveness to short-term stress	Low, unless related to underlying disease
Kwashiorkor	↓ protein intake during stress state	Weeks	Well-nourished appearance Easy hair pluckability Edema	Serum albumin <2.8 g/dl Total iron binding capacity <200 mcg/dl Lymphocytes <1500/mm³ Anergy	Infections Poor wound healing, decubitus ulcers, skin breakdown	High

From Weinsier RL, et al. *Handbook of Clinical Nutrition.* 2nd ed. St. Louis, CV Mosby, 1989.

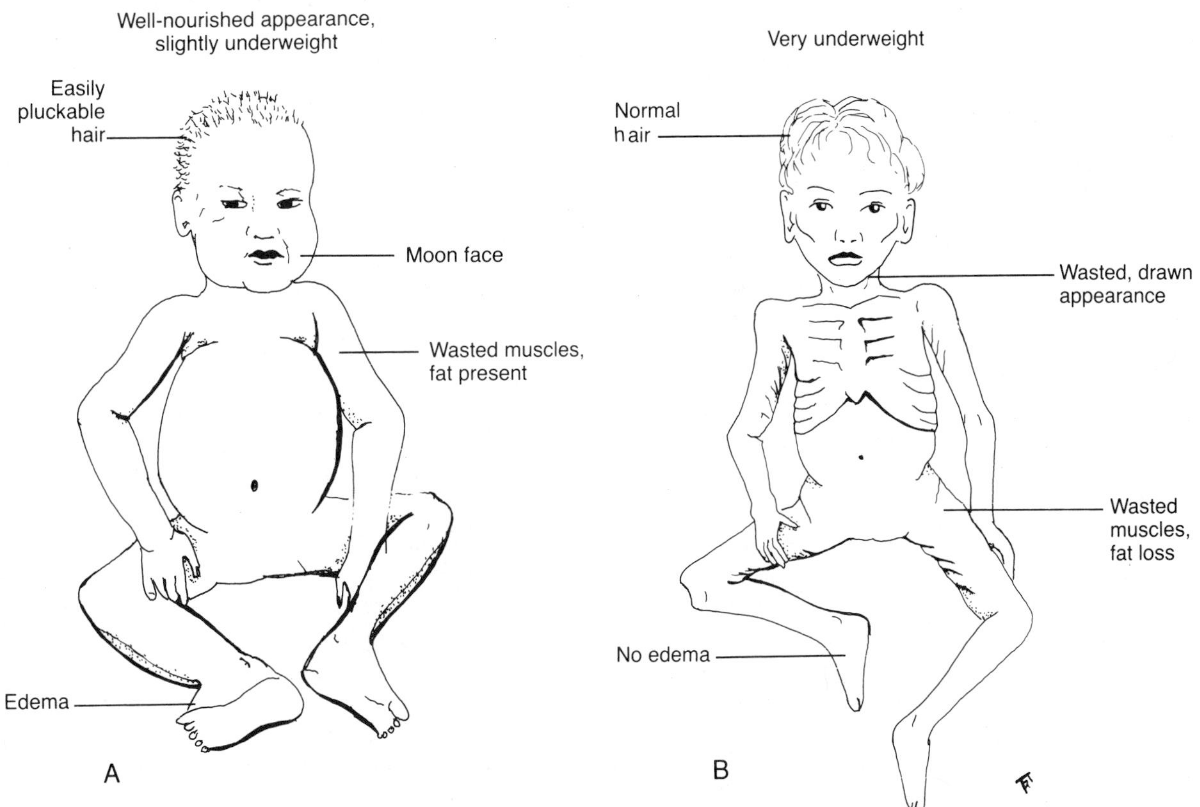

Figure 18–4 **Physical changes of the two principal forms of protein-energy malnutrition: Kwashiorkor (*A*) contrasted with marasmus (*B*).**

Despite adequate amounts of insulin, hyperglycemia is present, presenting what is called insulin resistance or inability of the available insulin to allow glucose to enter a cell.

trose solutions for an extended period of time (2 weeks or more). The continuous carbohydrate supply interferes with normal physiological adaptive functions during starvation, whereby increased amounts of fats are catabolized for energy. In other words, increased amounts of fat are catabolized with starvation; when IV solutions are given, this does not occur. Additionally, elevated levels of epinephrine, glucagon, and cortisol cause hyperglycemia, whereas tissues are **insulin resistant.**

As opposed to relatively normal laboratory findings with marasmus, kwashiorkor can be diagnosed principally using laboratory results (see Table 18–7). It is distinguished by a gradual protein loss that is due to inadequate hepatic synthesis. Visceral organ functions are impaired, as exhibited by the presence of decreased immune competence (low TLC) and low protein levels (albumin, transferrin, and prealbumin). Body weight, skinfold thickness, and MAMC may remain stable because somatic proteins are relatively stable. In some cases, classic symptoms of kwashiorkor, i.e., skin breakdown, poor wound healing, edema, and easily pluckable hair, are present (see Fig. 18–4). Fatty liver may develop, but serum cholesterol and triglyceride levels are low.

What are the classic signs of kwashiorkor?

Nutritional Care

With both marasmus and kwashiorkor, a goal of nutritional care is to reverse the downward trend. When initiating nutrition support for a marasmic client, kilocalories and protein are gradually increased to allow for readaptation of metabolic and intestinal functions. Aggressive repletion can result in metabolic imbalances such as hypophosphatemia and cardiorespiratory failure. If enteral or parenteral nutrition is necessary because of inadequate oral intake or compromised GI function, initiate at a slow rate with gradual increases.

On the other hand, aggressive nutrition support is necessary for kwashiorkor due to high kilocalorie and protein requirements. Enteral or parenteral feedings are usually required to provide adequate nutrients. Gastroparesis and diarrhea often accompany enteral feedings.

For both marasmus and kwashiorkor, oral feeding is preferable, as it is least expensive, most enjoyable, and less invasive for clients. For severely anorectic clients, sweets may be the only intake for a while, but if these are enjoyed and provided, appetite gradually improves with inclusion of other foods (Winograd & Brown, 1990). If allowed, preferred foods brought in by families/significant others may improve intake. Thus, compliance and kilocalorie intake are enhanced when clients are offered foods they enjoy.

Early satiety is a frequent complaint of clients with marasmus or kwashiorkor. Large meals may seem overwhelming for these clients, who may tire easily during mealtimes; therefore, smaller, more frequent meals are desirable. Adding fats, such as gravies, butter, cream, creamed soups, and whole milk, provides a concentrated source of kilocalories and reduces the volume of food needed.

Liquid supplements may be indicated for either marasmic or kwashiorkor clients. These supplements are more nutrient dense than most foods and provide protein, vitamins, and minerals that enhance oral intake. If several nutritional supplements are available, allow clients to choose formulas they prefer to ensure compliance; the dissimilar tastes appeal to different clients. Supplements served cold over ice are more palatable. Small sips help prevent weakness, abdominal cramps, and diarrhea. If liquid intake is adequate, supplements such as Magnacal (Sherwood), Two-Cal HN (Ross), and Sustacal HC (Mead Johnson) can be used; at 1.5 to 2 kcal/ml (rather than the usual 1 kcal/ml), more kilocalories are consumed in a smaller volume (Beare & Myers, 1990).

Why is nutritional care of marasmus initiated gradually? Describe nutritional care for marasmus; kwashiorkor.

Glucose polymers, such as Polycose (Ross) or Moducal (Mead Johnson), provide needed kilocalories and spare protein. Since they have a mild sweetening effect, food taste is not significantly altered. However, these supplements may cause carbonated drinks to taste "flat" (Beare & Myers, 1990). Microlipid (Sherwood Medical), a fat supplement, provides kilocalories in a concentrated form (9 kcal). Protein supplements, such as ProMod (Ross) or Propac (Sherwood Medical), are added to textured foods to promote anabolism.

NURSING APPLICATIONS

Assessment

Physical—for body weight, weight gain (edema); percent weight loss, TSF, MAMC, skinfold measurements; taste or smell alterations; stressors.
Dietary—for appetite, food intake.
Laboratory—for albumin, transferrin, prealbumin; glucose, TLC ($<1200/mm^3$); cholesterol, triglycerides; phosphate, magnesium.

Interventions

1. Monitor length of time clients are receiving standard dextrose solutions only. If time is 2 weeks or longer, notify physician.
2. Monitor I&O.
3. Refer to dietitian or social worker.

Evaluation

* Desired outcomes include client gains weight, TSF and MAMC increase, and abnormal laboratory values return to WNL.

Client Education

- Inform of community resources such as WIC, food stamps, and Meals on Wheels.
- Emphasize the importance of good nutrition, stressing economical sources of nutrient dense foods.
- Use evaporated milk, half-and-half, or cream rather than milk in drinks or food preparation to increase kilocalories provided.
- Increase intake of high fat breads such as muffins, biscuits, and croissants.
- Eat snacks such as ice cream, puddings, cheese, and dried fruit.
- Add croutons, bacon bits, sunflower seeds, Chinese noodles, and cheese to salads. Use large amounts of dressing.
- Avoid artificial sweeteners; instead use sugar, honey, or corn syrup.

Microcytic Anemia or Iron Deficiency Anemia

Despite an abundance of iron in our food supply, iron deficiency is a common chronic deficiency observed in clients either in communities or hospitals. Target populations at risk for anemia include infants, especially premature infants (no iron reserve); young children 5 to 8 years of age and pregnant women (increased need); and young women (low kilocalorie intake and menses). At least 30% of the US population is estimated to be iron deficient.

What clients are at risk for anemia?

Causes and Physical Consequences

Iron deficiency anemia is a gradual progession with depletion of storage iron followed by iron deficiency then iron deficiency anemia. Initially, iron is mobilized from body stores to maintain hemoglobin synthesis (reflected by depressed **ferritin** level).

During the second stage, iron stores become depleted, and less iron available to the bone marrow results in a state of iron-deficient **erythropoiesis** (Fig. 18–5). Transferrin saturation is decreased. Hemoglobin may or may not be depressed, and numbers of **microcytic** cells are increased.

Iron deficiency anemia indicates that the amount of iron in the body is inadequate to maintain hemoglobin levels and other functioning iron compounds.

Iron is stored in all cells as ferritin; 60% of ferritin is in the liver.

Erythrocytes are mature RBCs. Erythropoiesis or RBC development begins in the bone marrow.

Microcytic—small in size.

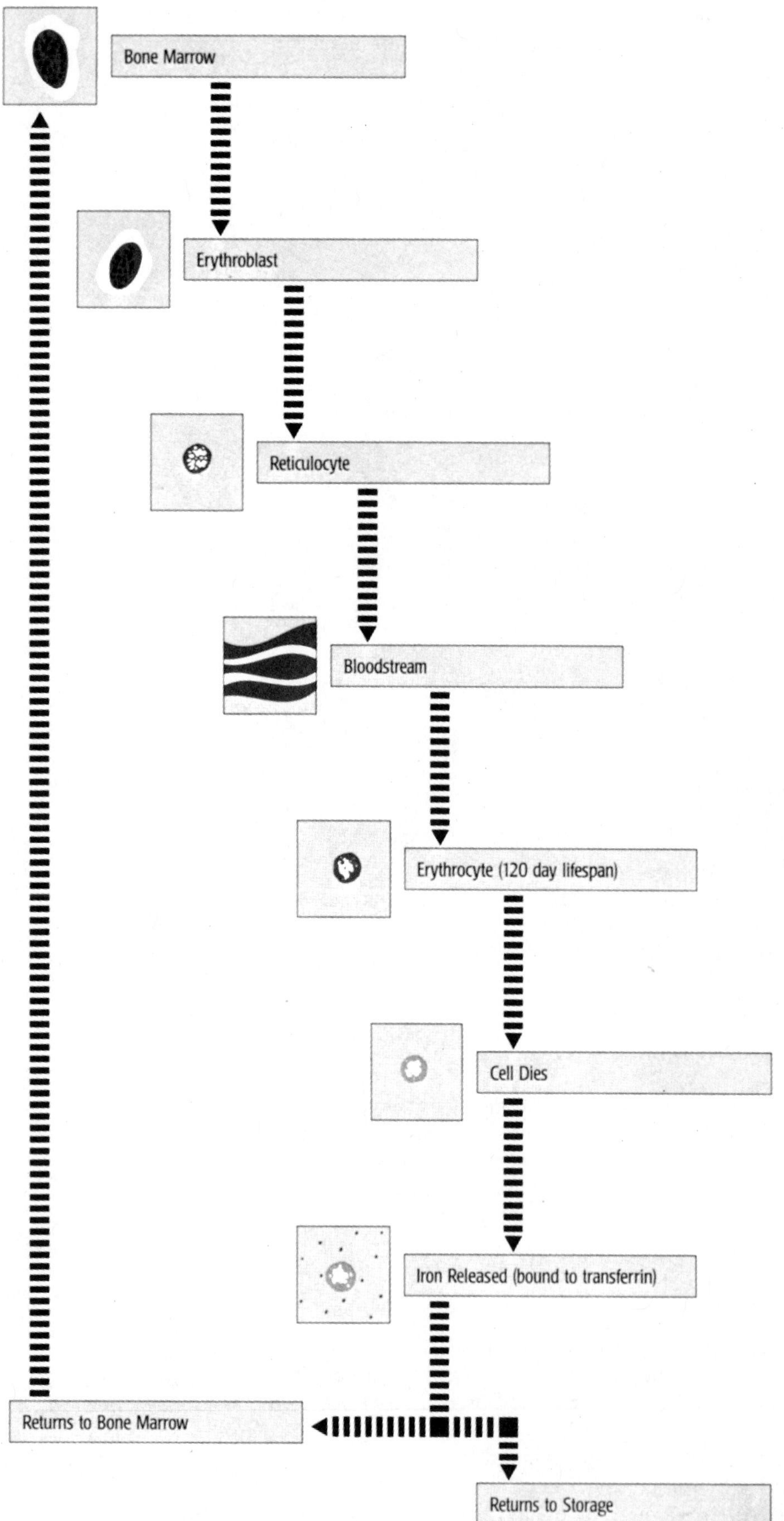

Figure 18–5 The life span of one blood cell. (From National Live Stock and Meat Board. *Iron in Human Nutrition.* Chicago, National Live Stock and Meat Board, 1990.)

Microcytic and **hypochromic** cells replace normal cells during the third stage of iron depletion (Fig. 18–6). Hemoglobin, **hematocrit,** and **mean corpuscular volume** are decreased. Thus, following a depressed hemoglobin finding, other tests are needed to determine the stage of iron deficiency and correctly diagnose this type of anemia (Table 18–8).

Blood loss (less evident in the GI tract), decreased gastric acidity, and decreased intake or bioavailability may cause iron deficiency anemia, especially in the elderly. Since anemia develops slowly, many clients continue with activities but gradually slow down without recognizing this condition.

Hypochromic—abnormally pale erythrocytes because of lack of hemoglobin.

Hematocrit (Hct) measures the percentage of red cells. Mean corpuscular volume (MCV) indicates individual red cell size, describing the ratio of volume of packed cells to total red cell count.

Describe the 3 stages of iron deficiency anemia. What 3 factors may cause iron deficiency anemia?

Pica is consumption of nonfood items.

Nutritional Assessment

Assessment should include knowledge about a client's diet, **pica,** environment, use of drugs, fever, fatigability, bleeding episodes (particularly of the GI tract), susceptibility to bruising, and infections. Frequently, clients have unintentionally curtailed their iron intake in an attempt to decrease cholesterol intake. They may not be anemic, but they have depleted stores. Thus, when blood losses occur, iron stores are low, precipitating iron deficiency anemia. Many women routinely consume in-

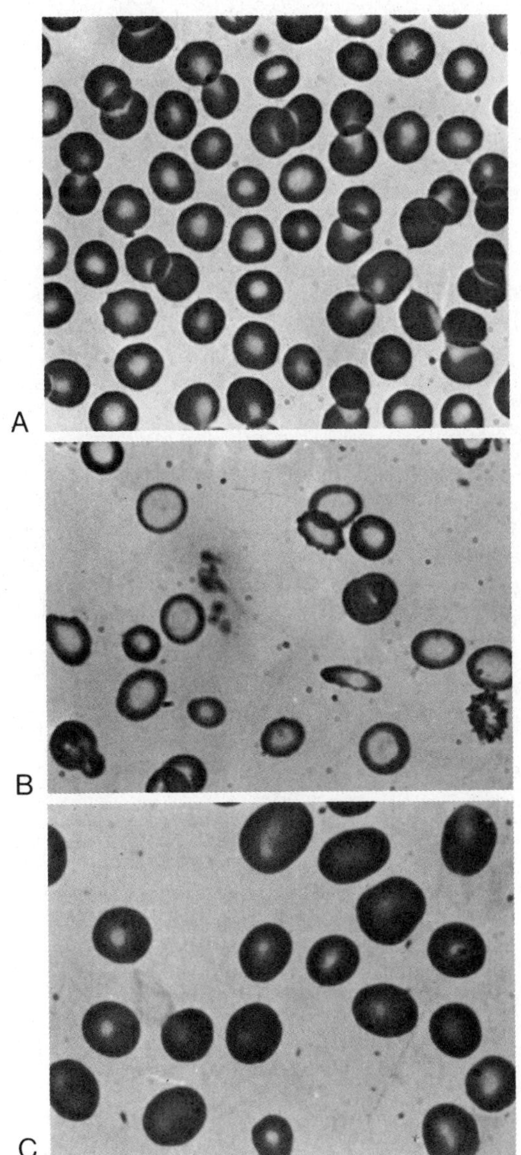

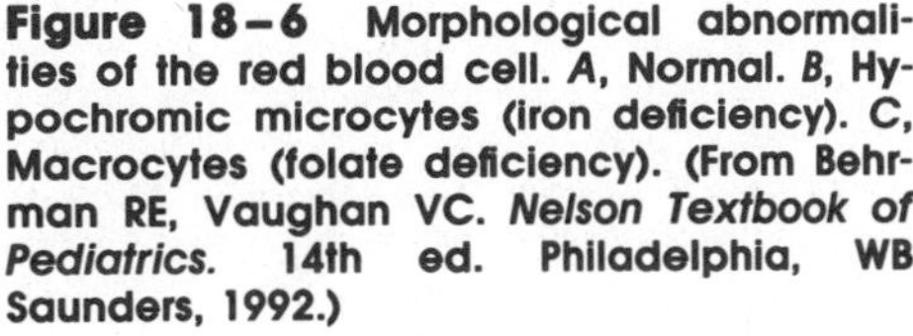

Figure 18–6 Morphological abnormalities of the red blood cell. *A,* Normal. *B,* Hypochromic microcytes (iron deficiency). *C,* Macrocytes (folate deficiency). (From Behrman RE, Vaughan VC. *Nelson Textbook of Pediatrics.* 14th ed. Philadelphia, WB Saunders, 1992.)

TABLE 18–8

NORMAL VALUES FOR COMMON LABORATORY TESTS

Laboratory Component	Normal Value	Purpose	Iron Deficiency Anemia	Megaloblastic Anemia	Anemia Secondary to Chronic Disease
Erythrocyte count (RBC)		Amount of RBC in blood; supports other tests to diagnose anemia	Normal or depressed	Depressed	Depressed
Men	4.2–6.2 million/mm^3				
Women	3.6–5.4 million/mm^3				
Children	4.6–4.8 million/mm^3				
Hemoglobin (Hgb)		Carries oxygen; measures severity of anemia, response to therapy	Depressed	Depressed	Depressed
Men	14–18 gm/dl				
Women	12–16 gm/dl				
Children	11–13 gm/dl				
Hematocrit (Hct)		Concentration of RBC in 100 ml blood; aids in diagnosing anemia and hydration	Depressed	Depressed	Depressed
Men	40–54%				
Women	38–46%				
Children	36–40%				
Mean corpuscular volume (MCV)		Indicates size of cell; aids in diagnosing and classifying type of anemia	Depressed (<80)	Elevated (>94)	Normal
Adult	87–100 mm^3				
Child	82–92 mm^3				
Mean corpuscular hemoglobin concentration	30–36%	Determines Hgb concentration; aids in diagnosing type of anemia	Depressed (<30)	Normal (>31)	Normal
Serum iron		Estimates total body iron; helps distinguish between iron deficiency anemia and anemia of chronic disease	Depressed	Normal	Normal or depressed
Men	70–150 mcg/dl				
Women	80–150 mcg/dl				
Total iron binding capacity		Determines iron bind-capacity of transferrin	Elevated	Depressed or normal	Normal or depressed
Men	300–400 mcg/dl				
Women	300–450 mcg/dl				
Percent saturation	25–50%	Same as above	Depressed	Normal	Depressed
Reticulocyte count	60,000 reticulocytes/mm^3 (or 0.5–2% of total erythrocytes)	Measures amount of premature RBCs; helps determine response to therapy	Depressed	Depressed	Normal
Ferritin		Reflects iron stores (distinguishes between deficiency and chronic disease)	Depressed	Normal	Normal or elevated
Men	20–300 ng/ml				
Women	20–120 ng/ml				
Children	7–140 ng/ml				
Transferrin	240–400 mg/dl	Measures iron available to tissues	Normal or elevated	Normal	Depressed
Folic acid	2–14 mg/dl	Assess type of megaloblastic anemia	Normal	Depressed or normal	Normal
Vitamin B_{12}	200–1100 pg/ml	Assess type of megaloblastic anemia	Normal	Depressed or normal	Normal

adequate amounts of iron related to their low kilocalorie intake. Increased emphasis on high-fiber products has resulted in less iron absorption (Brune et al, 1989). Excessive zinc intake also decreases bioavailability of iron. Use of zinc supplements by the elderly in an effort to retard macular degeneration may result in iron deficiency anemia (Frambach & Bendel, 1991).

What factors need to be assessed? Name 6 clinical symptoms that occur with iron deficiency anemia.

Clinical symptoms include pallor (especially nail bed and palmar crease), fatigue, labored breathing, palpitations, and reduced capacity for work. Vague GI complaints (flatulence, constipation, diarrhea, and nausea) are fairly common. Iron deficiency results in impaired ability to maintain body temperature (Beard & Borel,

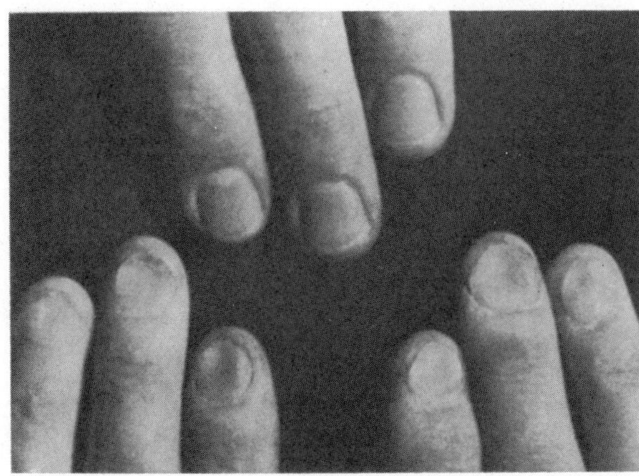

Figure 18–7 Fingernails of an iron-deficient adult *(below)* compared with those of a normal subject. (Reproduced with permission from Rosenbaum E, Leonard JW. Nutritional iron deficiency anemia in an adult male. *Ann Intern Med* 1964; 60:683.)

1988) and an inability to resist infection. As shown in Figure 18–7, fingernails may become dull, thin, brittle, flattened, and then spoon-shaped (Fairbanks & Beutler, 1988).

Nutritional Care

When anemia occurs, diet alone cannot supply adequate amounts of iron, so oral iron supplementation is necessary to replenish the "savings account." Ferrous sulfate is the preferred treatment and the least expensive iron preparation. Iron absorption is essentially equal from other ferrous salts (gluconate or fumarate). Absorption of iron from all ferric salts is poor.

Iron absorption is best when supplements are taken on an empty stomach. However, many side effects are associated with supplementation between meals, including nausea, constipation, and/or diarrhea. Tolerance of oral supplements can be increased by initiating therapy with 1 tablet daily and gradually increasing to recommended dosage. If this cannot be done, give medicine with meals. Oral therapy is necessary for 6 to 12 months to replenish iron stores completely (Beutler, 1988).

Other nutrients essential for accelerated cell repletion during anemia include folate, vitamins B_{12} and C, and zinc. Although zinc is not a structural element in hemoglobin, it is necessary for cell division. Anemia is not likely from zinc deficiency alone, but zinc deficiency usually accompanies iron deficiency anemia because of common food sources.

What is the preferred treatment for iron deficiency anemia?

NURSING APPLICATIONS

Assessment

Physical—for symptoms listed under nutrition assessment.

Dietary—for adequacy of dietary intake, especially red meats, green vegetables, enriched cereals and bread; cholesterol, fiber intake, use of vitamin/mineral supplements.

Laboratory—for Hgb, Hct, MCV, ferritin, transferrin, serum iron, free erythrocyte protoporphyrin, TIBC (see Table 18–8).

Interventions

1. Administer ferrous sulfate as ordered or instruct client/family regarding correct administration.
2. Encourage iron-rich foods (see Chapter 9, Table 9–5); if principally non-heme sources are consumed at a meal, a source of vitamin C enhances absorption of non-heme iron.

Continued

Evaluation

* Successful outcomes include client consuming iron-rich foods and taking ordered supplement to enhance erythropoiesis. Additionally, laboratory results return to normal.

Client Education

- If iron supplement is liquid, dilute with water or juice and drink with straw to prevent tooth staining.
- Stools may turn black or greenish black when iron supplements are taken.
- Iron stores are replenished slowly; therapy should be continued for at least a year (Beutler, 1988).
- Participation in competitive sports induces GI blood loss and may contribute to iron deficiency.

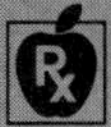
When iron supplementation is required, the presence of riboflavin and vitamin C increases absorption.

Megaloblastic (Folate) Anemia

Causes and Physical Consequences

Megaloblastic anemia refers to extra large RBC but fewer in number.

At one stage of RBC maturation, every cell requires folate. Because of altered DNA synthesis caused by lack of folate, RBCs become larger than usual with hemoglobin synthesis continuing at a normal rate (see Fig. 18–6). These macrocytes have flimsy membranes, are fragile, and are irregular in shape. Anemia results from their decreased numbers and shorter lives. Diagnosis is complicated because distinguishing between folate or vitamin B_{12} deficiency is difficult as a result of close interrelationships. Megaloblastic anemia is common in pregnant women and infants (increased demand), senior citizens (low income, improper diet), and alcohol-dependent clients (decreased intake and impaired liver storage).

Who is prone to megaloblastic anemia?

Nutritional Care

Folate replacement is necessary because diet alone is inadequate to replace lost stores. Iron supplements may also be ordered because when folate is deficient, iron usually is also.

What is the treatment for folate deficiency anemia?

NURSING APPLICATIONS

Assessment

Physical—for sex, age extremes, mouth (especially tongue, usually sore); pale skin color, shortness of breath.

Dietary—for dietary intake, especially of dark green leafy vegetables, liver, whole-grain breads; alcohol intake.

Laboratory—for Hgb, Hct, MCV, folate (see Table 18–8).

Interventions

1. Encourage rich sources of folate (see Chapter 7, Table 7–7).
2. Give folate and iron as ordered.

Evaluation

* Desired outcomes include client consuming folate-containing foods and taking ordered supplements to enhance erythropoiesis. Additionally, laboratory results return to normal.

Client Education

- Raw vegetables are a better source of folate; heat destroys this vitamin.
- Daily intake of dietary folate is necessary.

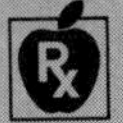
Large doses of folate can negate therapeutic effects of anticonvulsants (Cerrato, 1991).

Pernicious (Vitamin B_{12}) Anemia

Causes and Physical Consequences

Another type of megaloblastic anemia is pernicious or vitamin B_{12} anemia. This occurs when vitamin B_{12} is deficient in the diet, absorption is inadequate, or requirements are increased. Since every RBC requires vitamin B_{12} for maturation, a lack of vitamin B_{12} causes altered DNA synthesis, resulting in large, fragile RBCs. With vitamin B_{12} malabsorption or no dietary source (strict vegetarians), normal body stores are usually sufficient for 3 to 4 years. Vitamin B_{12} deficiency is most common among strict vegans.

A lack of **intrinsic factor** causes a type of vitamin B_{12} anemia called pernicious anemia. This is commonly observed in clients over 60 years secondary to gastric mucosa atrophy. It is more prevalent among women, who have longer longevity than men. Clients who have malabsorption syndromes or GI operations are prone to develop pernicious anemia months or even years later.

Intrinsic factor—a gastric protein essential for absorption of vitamin B_{12}.

What can cause vitamin B_{12} or pernicious anemia?

Nutritional Care

Clients with pernicious anemia especially need nutritional counseling since many are not eating a well-balanced diet. Giving the appropriate vitamin is essential because folate supplementation for a client who is deficient in vitamin B_{12} may produce hematological improvement, whereas neurological damage from vitamin B_{12} deficiency continues to progress. The neurological damage may be irreversible.

Intramuscular injections for treatment of pernicious anemia are not always necessary. An oral vitamin is less expensive than injections (Lederle, 1991).

Why is it important to treat vitamin B_{12} deficiency anemia correctly?

NURSING APPLICATIONS

Assessment

Physical—for yellowish skin; glazed, red, sore tongue; tingling and numbness in extremities; malabsorption; previous GI surgeries.
Dietary—for intake of animal products, alcohol intake.
Laboratory—for Hgb, Hct, MCV, vitamin B_{12} (see Table 18-8). A urine test called Schilling's test is positive in pernicious anemia.

Interventions

1. Give vitamin B_{12} as ordered.
2. If not vegetarian, encourage intake of foods high in vitamin B_{12} (see Chapter 7, Table 7-10). If vegetarian, encourage intake of eggs or dairy products. Dietary intake helps reduce depleted stores.
3. Refer to dietitian.

Evaluation

* Desired outcomes include client consuming foods high in vitamin B_{12} and taking ordered supplements to enhance erythropoiesis. Additionally, laboratory results return to normal.

Continued

Client Education

- Clients with permanent gastric or ileal damage need monthly injections or oral vitamin B_{12} for life.
- Vitamin B_{12} shots are not always indicated for "tired blood."

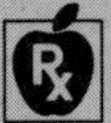 When oral vitamin B_{12} supplements are ordered, take with vitamin C to enhance absorption.

COMMON NUTRITION-RELATED DISEASES

Osteoporosis

Osteoporosis is an age-related disorder characterized by decreased bone and an increased susceptibility to fractures in the absence of other recognizable causes of bone loss.

Osteoporosis is a common and costly disease. As many as 24 million Americans are affected by osteoporotic complications, which cause 1.5 million fractures annually and incur a financial burden of $10 billion (National Osteoporosis Foundation, 1991). Fractures resulting from osteoporosis are a significant source of bone pain, disability, and disfigurement. Approximately 12 to 20% of clients hospitalized with hip fractures developed lethal respiratory complications as a result of the imposed bed rest (Wardlaw, 1988), and between 12 to 20% of these clients die within 1 year of the fracture (Consensus Development Conference, 1991).

Risk Factors

Genetic factors contribute significantly to attainment of peak bone mass. Fair-skinned, underweight white women are at greatest risk for osteoporosis. Peak bone mass is achieved at approximately 35 years of age. Men have approximately 30% more bone mass at peak than do women, and blacks have approximately 10% more bone mass than do whites. Early menopause is a strong predictor for the development of osteoporosis.

Other risk factors include calcium and vitamin D deficiency, immobilization, physical inactivity, alcoholism, cigarette smoking, and excessive exercise that produces amenorrhea (Table 18–9). A physical environment that increases risk of slipping and neuromuscular and visual problems of clients may contribute to a fall and

TABLE 18–9

FACTORS ASSOCIATED WITH BONE ACCRETION/MAINTENANCE AND BONE LOSS/OSTEOPENIA

Accretion/Maintenance	Loss/Osteopenia
Eumenorrhea	Amenorrhea
Estrogen replacement	Late menarche
Black race	Early menopause
Thiazide diuretics	Glucocorticoid use
Fluoride (1–6 mg)	Hyperparathyroidism
Physical activity*	Hyperthyroidism
Dietary calcium	Thyroid hormone replacement
	Excessive aluminum consumption
	Alcoholism
	Cigarette smoking
	Slender figure
	Bed rest (months)
	Dietary fiber*
	Extensive lactation for 3 or 4 children

* The degree of effect remains to be established.

From Wardlaw G. The effects of diet and life-style on bone mass in women. Copyright the American Dietetic Association. Reprinted from Journal of the American Dietetic Association, *J Am Diet Assoc* 1988 Jan; 88(1):17–22, 25.

consequently a fracture. Excessive protein or caffeine intake may increase calcium loss in urine and enhance osteoporotic changes (Consensus Conference, 1984). Two commonly used medications that have a documented effect on bone mineralization are thiazide diuretics, principally used for blood pressure control, and glucocorticoids, used to reduce inflammation. Diuretics positively affect bone mineralization, whereas high doses of glucocorticoids negatively affect bone mineralization. A calcium and vitamin D deficiency early in life appears to affect bone mineralization negatively more than intake after age 35.

Name 5 risk factors for osteoporosis.

Causes and Physical Consequences

There are 2 broad categories of osteoporosis, primary and secondary. Rapid, disproportionate loss of **trabecula of bone** occurs following menopause. This spongy type of bone is the predominant type found in vertebral bodies and the distal radius, making these bones at greatest risk of postmenopausal fractures. Typical age-related bone changes, seen in clients over 70 years of age, affect both cortical and trabecular bone (Fig. 18–8). The most frequently encountered fractures among

Trabecula of bone is the lattice-type structure forming a network of supportive tissue that is filled with bone marrow.

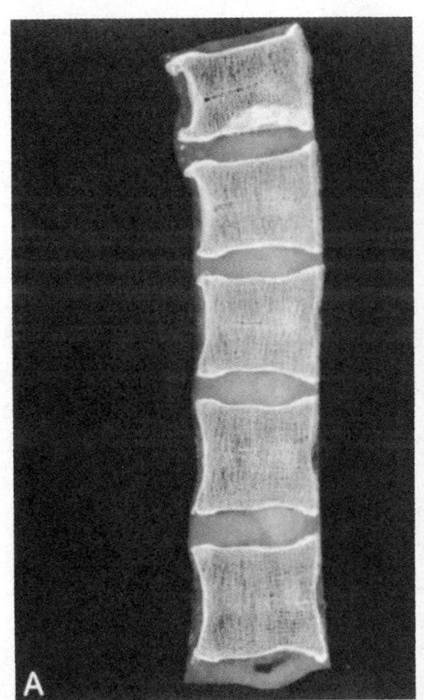

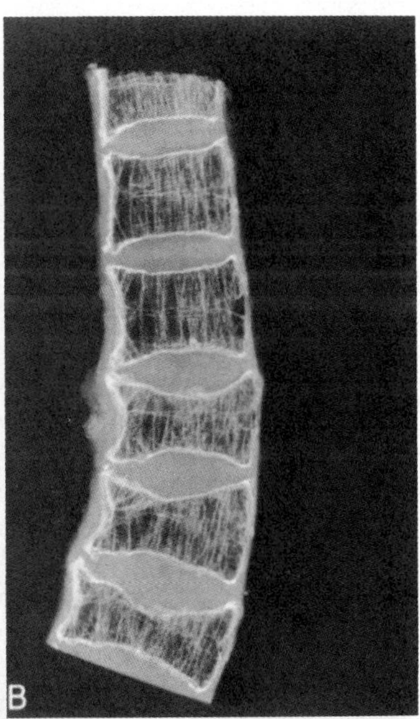

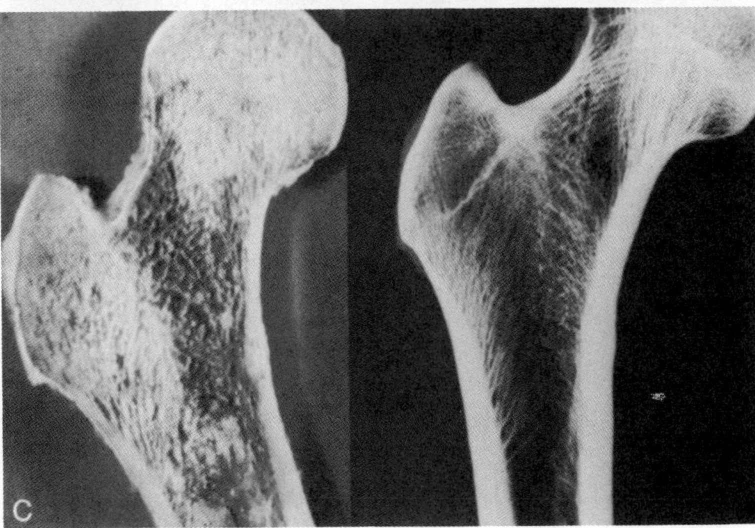

Figure 18–8 In osteoporosis, vertebrae may collapse. *A*, Radiograph of segment of the spine showing normal content of trabecular bone. *B*, Radiograph of segment of the spine showing extensive loss of trabecular bone and collapsed vertebrae. Note the "codfish" appearance. C, A section through the proximal end of the femur, seen by the naked eye and by radiography. The outer shell of cortical bone and the mesh of trabecular bone are visible; note particularly how trabecular bone is laid down along the lines of greatest horizontal and vertical stress. (From Kinney JM, et al. *Nutrition and Metabolism in Patient Care*. Philadelphia, WB Saunders, 1988. (From the collection of Dr. V. Fornasier.))

CT produces a picture of internal body images of a predetermined plane of tissue. It can measure the density of an entire bone or trabecula portion. Photodensitometry uses 2 energy levels to measure trabecula bone mass, where osteoporosis begins.

Describe what happens in osteoporosis. Where do most fractures occur?

this group are those of the hip. Secondary osteoporosis is loss of bone mass as a result of other underlying pathology.

Decreased bone mass may be seen on x-ray films; however, these are relatively insensitive unless bone loss is greater than 20 to 30%. Other more sensitive diagnostic techniques include **computed tomography** (CT), **photodensitometry,** and biopsy.

Therapies

For individuals at risk for osteoporosis, an objective of treatment is to slow or stop the disease progression before irreversible structural changes have occurred. Classically, the regimen has included estrogen for postmenopausal women, calcium, vitamin D, exercise, and nutritional adjustments. Numerous theories proposing mechanisms for the effect of estrogen in reducing rate of bone loss have been inconclusive (Lindsay, 1991). If estrogen is initiated, it should be taken for at least 10 to 15 years. Stopping earlier seems to accelerate bone loss (Urrows et al, 1991). Calcitonin and bisphosphonates (etidronate) inhibit **osteoclast** bone resorption (Reginster, 1991; Watts, 1990). Calcitonin also stimulates calcium absorption from the GI tract.

Osteoclast—bone cells associated with absorption and removal of bone.

Sodium fluoride and parathyroid hormone appear to increase bone mass. These 2 drugs could eventually result in a clinical cure for osteoporosis (Riggs, 1991).

Walking, exercise, or active lifestyle is beneficial in prevention and treatment of osteoporosis.

Nutritional Care

The relationship between diet and bone maintenance or enhanced mineral content is not clear-cut. A diet high in protein has been shown to increase urinary calcium, but the impact of this increased loss is in doubt. Studies have not demonstrated a negative effect on calcium balance by increased protein or phosphorus intake. Also, fecal calcium excretion may increase if a high-fiber diet is followed.

On the other hand, adequate calcium intake at all stages of life, with a daily intake of 800 mg for all healthy adults, continues to be emphasized. Calcium is not the cause of bone health but is necessary for healthy bones.

Calcium intake in about one-half of adult Americans is less than 500 mg/day (Heaney, 1991). Calcium intakes of 1000 mg for premenopausal women and 1500 mg/day for postmenopausal women were endorsed at the Consensus Conference in 1984 on osteoporosis and were confirmed at the 1991 osteoporosis symposium (Heaney, 1991). Increasing vitamin D intake to 500 IU can significantly reduce late wintertime bone loss and increases bone density in the spine (Preventing wintertime bone loss, 1992).

Dietary modifications for clients at risk include at least 2 servings of dairy products daily (to provide 75% of RDAs) except for those with documented urinary calculi (Walden, 1989). For clients who have inadequate intake of milk or milk products (including those who are lactose intolerant), inclusion of calcium supplements may be beneficial (Reid et al, 1993). Caffeine is used in moderation since caffeine increases calcium excretion.

A diet low in boron also increases calcium excretion (Cerrato, 1990). Thus, consumption of fresh fruits and vegetables is recommended to increase boron intake.

Clients who are trying to lower cholesterol intake may inadvertently decrease calcium intake. To reduce cholesterol and not adversely affect calcium intake, predisposing clients to osteoporosis, Hinders (1991) suggests the following guidelines: (1) substitute skim milk products and low-fat yogurts and cheeses for whole milk and cheeses; (2) increase daily intake of fruits, vegetables, and whole-grain products; (3) use unsaturated oils, i.e., safflower, sunflower, canola, corn, or olive; and (4) reduce (not eliminate) red meat.

Describe nutritional care for osteoporosis.

NURSING APPLICATIONS

Assessment

Physical—for weight, exercise habits, menopause, amenorrhea, race, sex, fractures, types of medications, cigarette smoking, home environmental factors that could lead to falls.

Dietary—for calcium, vitamin D, protein, caffeine, and fiber intake.

Laboratory—for 24-hour urinary calcium, ionized calcium, and phosphorus; alkaline phosphatase.

Interventions

1. Encourage diet high in calcium (1000 to 1500 mg) (see Chapter 9, Table 9–2) and vitamin D (100 to 500 mg/day) (see Chapter 6, Table 6–3). Calcium slows the rate of bone loss; vitamin D is needed for calcium absorption.

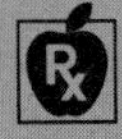 Withhold calcium-rich foods or enteral feeding formulas for 2 hours after giving etidronate disodium.

Evaluation

* Client should consume adequate calcium-containing and vitamin D-containing foods or supplements; no bone fractures will be experienced.

Client Education

- If on high-fiber diet, increase calcium intake above the RDA.
- If client is unable to tolerate estrogen therapy or elects not to use it, bone loss can be retarded with exercise plus calcium supplement (Prince et al, 1991).
- Calcium carbonate is the most readily absorbed calcium supplement.
- Calcium citrate maleate, currently used in orange drink, is well absorbed and is a good source of calcium for clients unable to tolerate milk.
- Check the home for factors that could lead to falls, i.e., throw rugs, slippery bathtubs, electrical cords, poor lighting, and other hazards (Urrows et al, 1991).
- A life-long intake of calcium is necessary for prevention of osteoporosis.
- For high-risk postmenopausal client, substituting herbal teas or noncola drinks for caffeine drinks may be beneficial (Cerrato, 1990).
- The National Osteoporosis Foundation is a valuable resource for clients.

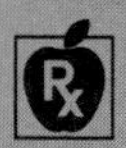 Adverse side effects of thiazide diuretics include elevated serum levels of uric acid, lipids, and glucose and low levels of potassium, magnesium, and sodium.

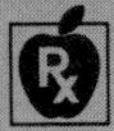 When high doses of glucocorticoids are necessary, calcium supplements with vitamin D are recommended (Mitchell & Lyles, 1990).

Rheumatoid Arthritis

Arthritis has been called "everybody's disease" because it affects everyone directly or indirectly, sooner or later. Arthritis is America's leading crippling disease, affecting 1 in 7 people, or 1 in every 3 families. A million people develop arthritis each year. Arthritis is second only to heart problems as the cause of disability payments. Over 90% of arthritis clients spend nearly $1 billion annually on unproved remedies (Panush, 1991). Of the various forms of arthritis, 2 have nutritional implications, rheumatoid arthritis and osteoarthritis.

The word arthritis literally means joint inflammation and refers to more than 100 related rheumatic diseases.

Causes and Physical Consequences

Rheumatoid arthritis is an autoimmune, systemic disease involving chronic inflammation and destruction that begins in the synovial membrane of joints and spreads to other joints (Fig. 18–9). The immune cells are localized; they remain at the affected joint, which means the chronic inflammation does not go away. Outgrowths of inflamed tissue may invade and damage cartilage and disfigure joints so they cannot return to normal.

"Anemia of chronic disease" is common in clients with inflammation and neoplasms and cannot be explained by other causes.

This chronic inflammation is a common cause of **"anemia of chronic disease"** that is subject to frequent misdiagnosis. The life span of RBCs is lessened, and erythropoiesis is depressed despite adequate available iron. Apparently iron, trapped in iron storage sites, is not released to developing erythroblasts. Treatment with iron supplements in this form of anemia is ineffective. In rheumatoid arthritis, a correct diagnosis of type of anemia is important. Iron deficiency anemia is also prevalent in this population because of increased GI bleeding related to therapeutic treatments. Serum ferritin is the most distinguishing factor for diagnosis between nondeficiency anemia and anemia of chronic disease (see Table 18–8) (Beutler, 1988).

What happens to joints in rheumatoid arthritis?

Therapies

Using adaptive equipment is especially beneficial for these clients to protect their bodies against pain and further destruction (see Chapter 16, Figs. 16–4

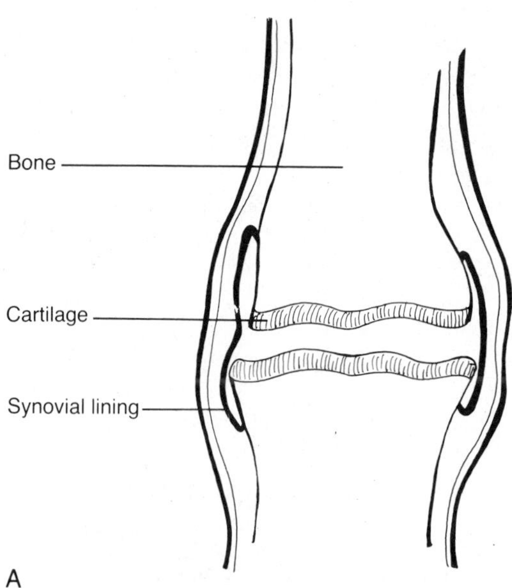

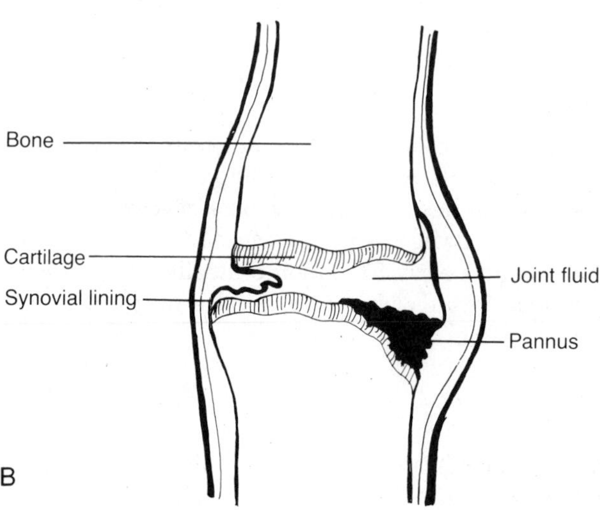

Figure 18–9 ***A,*** **Normal joint.** ***B,*** **In rheumatoid arthritis, the protective cartilage in the joint is destroyed around the inflamed area because of substances released by the cells (pannus).**

through 16–7). Other modes of therapy include medications (salicylates, nonsteroidal anti-inflammatory drugs (NSAIDS), corticosteroids, methotrexate), adequate rest, physical therapy, and diet.

What are some therapies for this condition?

Nutritional Care

Interest in dietary factors affecting arthritis has been renewed because of reports that symptoms have been alleviated by means of diet. The role of food in the management of rheumatoid arthritis is controversial and has not been defined at this time, pending further investigation. Significant improvement, e.g., a reduced number of tender joints and shorter duration of morning stiffness, appears among many clients who are able to lose weight.

One of the most popular theories is that foods trigger allergic reactions, which in turn aggravates arthritis. Immunological sensitivity to certain foods is believed to aggravate rheumatoid arthritis in less than 5% of clients (Buchanan et al, 1991; Panush, 1991). When food allergies are suspected, foods most likely to cause allergies are withheld and introduced one at a time for observation. Foods implicated include milk and milk products, corn, and cereals (Panush, 1990). Citrus fruits and tomatoes have also been suggested (Darlington et al, 1990).

Universally, subjects have significantly improved during fasting periods. This improvement appears to be related to less production of chemical mediators of inflammation rather than elimination of a dietary allergen (Buchanan et al, 1991).

Some clients have reported improvement (duration of early morning stiffness and less joint tenderness and swelling) on diets supplemented with eicosapentaenoic acid (Kremer et al, 1990; Tulleken et al, 1990; van der Tempel et al, 1990). The hypothesis is that production of prostaglandins or leukotrienes is decreased, producing less inflammatory activity. Since symptoms are only modestly lessened, the use of omega-3 fatty acids (or fish oils) has not been endorsed by the American College of Rheumatology (Panush, 1991).

Based on findings that fatty acids can modulate the inflammatory process in rheumatoid arthritis, a study was undertaken in which clients fasted for 7 to 10 days, followed by a gluten-free vegan diet for 3 to 5 months, and gradually changed to a lactovegetarian diet for a year. Symptoms (i.e., swelling in joints, morning stiffness) significantly improved and were maintained for the entire year (Kjeldsen-Kragh et al, 1991). Since the vegan gluten-free diet requires extensive planning to meet vitamin and mineral requirements, it should not be undertaken without the help of a dietitian.

At this time, there is no specific valid diet for clients with rheumatoid arthritis, but goals are to (1) maintain IBW to decrease limitations, (2) consume balanced diets for the best quality of life, and (3) preserve the integrity of immune responses. Vitamin E and zinc are of primary importance in maintaining immune function, yet they are often below the RDAs in clients with rheumatoid arthritis (Panush et al, 1983). Disabilities and chronic diseases of these clients probably interfere with their nutritional status because of physical limitations and emotional depression.

What foods have been implicated in rheumatoid arthritis? List the nutritional goals for clients with rheumatoid arthritis.

NURSING APPLICATIONS

Assessment

Physical—for height, weight/weight changes, IBW; ability to purchase and prepare food, need for adaptive equipment; emotional state, income.

Dietary—for diet/nutrient (especially zinc and vitamin E) intake, feeding skills, special or fad diets, vitamin/mineral supplements, food sensitivities.

Interventions

1. Refer to OT and PT for adaptive devices for eating and food preparation.

Continued

2. Offer a balanced diet and foods high in vitamin E and zinc (see Chapters 6 and 10, respectively).

Evaluation

* Client should maintain IBW, have decreased joint tenderness and swelling, avoid use of fad diets, and consume a balanced diet.

Client Education

- The Arthritis Foundation can provide valid up-to-date information to clients.
- Follow balanced and healthy diets, be skeptical of "miraculous" claims, and avoid diets or fad nutritional practices that may jeopardize nutritional status (Panush, 1991).

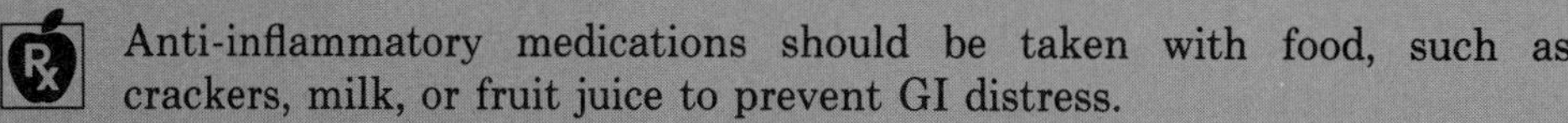
Anti-inflammatory medications should be taken with food, such as crackers, milk, or fruit juice to prevent GI distress.

Low doses of methotrexate are frequently effective in treating rheumatoid arthritis. However, toxic manifestations (hair loss, nausea and vomiting, stomatitis, leukopenia, anemia, and thrombocytopenia) are frequently observed (Alarcón et al, 1989).

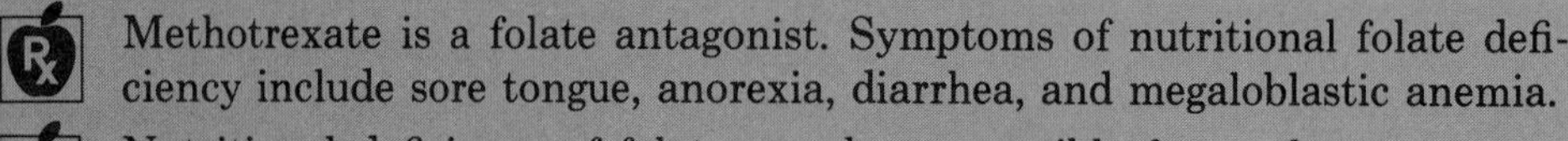
Methotrexate is a folate antagonist. Symptoms of nutritional folate deficiency include sore tongue, anorexia, diarrhea, and megaloblastic anemia.

Nutritional deficiency of folate may be responsible for methotrexate toxicity; 1 mg of folate daily significantly lessens toxicity of methotrexate without altering efficacy (Morgan et al, 1990; 1987).

High doses of corticosteroids cause nitrogen wasting in clients despite an anti-inflammatory and appetite-stimulatory benefit (Roubenoff et al, 1990).

Osteoarthritis

Causes and Physical Consequences

Injury to a joint may precipitate painful bony growths, which are a common sign of osteoarthritis or degenerative arthritis (Fig. 18–10). After the pain subsides, the growth remains. The inflammation around the cartilage and underlying bone is very painful.

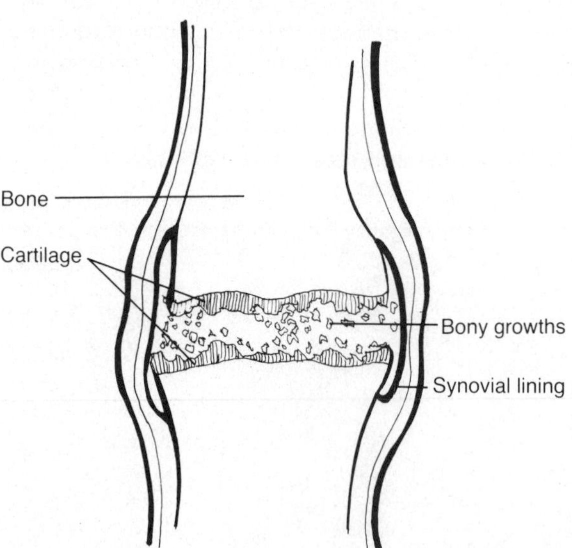

Figure 18–10 Osteoarthritis, characterized by degeneration of the cartilage and bony growths of the joint.

Osteoarthritis appears more frequently in older clients and may develop from ordinary stresses or "wear and tear" on joints. Studies indicate that 3 to 5 times the body weight is loaded across a joint surface during weight bearing (Liang & Fortin, 1991).

Nutritional Care

In osteoarthritis of the weight-bearing joints, weight loss is especially effective. Changing dietary habits or increasing physical activity is especially difficult for these clients because of pain and stiffness. A planned supervised program combining dietary and behavioral approaches with low-impact exercise will be more successful than just advising clients to lose weight.

NURSING APPLICATIONS

Assessment

Physical—for mobility to eat and prepare food, weight, height, IBW, emotional state, pain.
Dietary—for anorexia, reason for eating, calcium and vitamin D intake.
Laboratory—for calcium.

Interventions

1. Refer to OT, PT for assistive devices for cooking and eating.
2. Praise for maintenance of IBW or weight loss.
3. Encourage independence in activities of daily living (ADLs).

Evaluation

* Client lost weight and maintained the new body weight.

Client Education

- Refer to Arthritis Foundation.
- Refer to weight control programs that integrate behavior modification, diet, and exercise.

SUMMARY

Community nutrition involves not only health prevention, but also health restoration if illness occurs. A knowledge of basic nutritional principles is vital to assist clients to purchase economical food choices and prepare nutritious foods. In the community, several nutritional illnesses or nutrition-related diseases will be observed by nurses employed in physician's offices or community health settings. Nurses must be knowledgeable to care for these clients and possibly avert a hospital admission or make a hospital stay shorter.

NURSING PROCESS IN ACTION

A 17-year-old girl comes into the clinic and is diagnosed with iron deficiency anemia. She has clinical symptoms typical of this anemia. Ferrous sulfate and zinc are ordered. She takes tetracycline for acne.

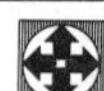

Nutritional Assessment

- Pica.
- Dietary intake, especially red meats, green vegetables, enriched foods, cholesterol, fiber intake.
- Drug use.
- Hgb, Hct, MCV, ferritin, TIBC, iron, transferrin saturation.
- Menses history.

Dietary Nursing Diagnosis

Altered nutrition: Less than body requirements RT increased need for iron.

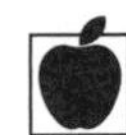

Nutritional Goals

Client will consume iron-rich foods and iron supplement; laboratory results will return to normal.

Nutritional Implementation

Intervention: Give ferrous sulfate as ordered. Do not give iron supplement with tetracycline (allow at least 2-hour intervals).
Rationale: Ferrous sulfate elevates serum iron concentrations and is either converted to hemoglobin or stored as ferritin until it is needed for erythropoiesis. Tetracycline can significantly reduce iron absorption (Corbett, 1992).

Intervention: Give zinc as ordered.
Rationale: Zinc is necessary for RBC division, and zinc deficiency usually accompanies iron deficiency anemia because of common food sources.

Intervention: Stress the importance of heme versus non-heme iron and consuming vitamin C–containing foods with non-heme iron.
Rationale: Heme iron is from animal products and absorbed well by the body, whereas non-heme iron is from plant and other sources. To increase absorption of non-heme iron, vitamin C is needed.

Intervention: Inform client of foods high in iron: egg yolks, meats, green leafy vegetables.
Rationale: These foods help replace lost stores.

Intervention: Discuss the effects of cholesterol and fiber intake on iron levels.
Rationale: If cholesterol intake is decreased, iron consumption may also be lowered because of common food sources. High fiber intake may interfere with iron absorption.

Intervention: Monitor Hct level with the client; explain that it will take at least 6 months for this to reach desirable level.
Rationale: This may act as a motivating factor to comply with diet and supplements; seeing the Hct level rise may be a positive reinforcer.

Intervention: Offer fluids every 2 hours and inform her that stools will turn black or greenish black.
Rationale: Iron is constipating. Appropriate information will decrease fear of the unknown and not cause her to become alarmed when this occurs.

Evaluation

Client consumed iron-rich foods and supplements to promote erythropoiesis; laboratory results returned to normal.

STUDENT READINESS

1. Plan an inexpensive menu for 1 day, using low-cost foods.
2. A client wants to know about convenience and fast foods. What would you tell him or her?
3. Compare marasmus and kwashiorkor in terms of dietary deficiencies, clinical findings, laboratory data, and nutritional rehabilitation.
4. List nursing interventions for iron deficiency anemia.
5. Why must pernicious anemia be identified and treated before folate treatment is started?
6. A client asks you why he has to take zinc when his iron stores are depressed. How would you respond?
7. What recommendations could you offer to a client to ensure the availability of folate?
8. List nutritional interventions you could do for clients with osteoporosis, rheumatoid arthritis, and osteoarthritis.

CASE STUDY

Mr. S. R., a 75-year-old retired farmer, has been living alone since his wife died 12 years ago. He has been progressively withdrawn over the past months and increasingly despondent over his failing health. His son found him unconscious on the kitchen floor. On admission, he is extremely thin (height, 70 inches; weight, 110 lbs); there are multiple bruises present and several small open lesions on his arms and legs. He is admitted to the hospital for malnutrition.

1. What diagnostic studies would you anticipate for Mr. S. R.?
2. Assuming a medium frame, determine Mr. S. R.'s IBW.
3. Why is the TLC an important aspect of nutritional assessment?
4. List possible nursing diagnoses for Mr. S. R. and some nutritional interventions.

CASE STUDY

Mrs. I. H. is a 74-year-old widow. She has lived alone since her husband's death 12 years ago. She has complained of fatigue for the past 2 years. Her Hgb is 8.6 gm/dl and Hct 25.8%. On questioning by the nurse, Mrs. I. H. states, "Cooking isn't any fun anymore." Although she lives close to the market, she buys mostly prepackaged meals. She also has dentures that "never did fit right" and so chooses foods that are soft and require minimal chewing.

1. What additional data do you need?
2. What lifestyle factors must you take into consideration?
3. The desirable level of Mrs. I. H.'s hemoglobin is ________.
4. What interventions could you perform to increase iron, folate, and vitamin B_{12} intake, especially since she eats soft foods that require minimal chewing?
5. What are some ways to evaluate nursing care of Mrs. I. H.?

REFERENCES

Alarcón GS, et al. Methotrexate in rheumatoid arthritis. Toxic effects as the major factor in limiting long-term treatment. *Arthritis Rheum* 1989 June; 32(6):671–676.

American Dietetic Association (ADA). Position of the American Dietetic Association: Domestic hunger and inadequate access to food. *J Am Diet Assoc* 1990 Oct; 90(10):1437–1441.

Beard J, Borel M. Iron deficiency and thermoregulation. *Nutr Today* 1988 Sept-Oct; 24(5):41–45.

Beare P, Myers J. *Principles and Practice of Adult Health Nursing.* St. Louis, CV Mosby, 1990.

Beutler E. The common anemias. *JAMA* 1988 Apr 22/29; 259(16):2433–2437.

Blaylock J. Elitzak H: Food expenditures. *Nat Food Review* 1990 July-Sept; 13(3):17–24.

Brune M, et al. Iron absorption: No intestinal adaptation to a high phytate diet. *Am J Clin Nutr* 1989 March; 49(3):542–545.

Buchanan HM, et al. Is diet important in rheumatoid arthritis? *Br J Rheumatol* 1991 Apr; 30(2):125–134.

Cerrato P. Your patient's anemia—but the problem isn't iron. *RN* 1991 July; 54(7):61–64.

Cerrato P. Piecing together the osteoporosis puzzle. *RN* 1990 Apr; 53(4):77–82.

Consensus Conference. Osteoporosis. *JAMA* 1984 Aug 10; 252(6):799–802.

Consensus Development Conference. Prophylaxis and treatment of osteoporosis. *Am J Med* 1991 Jan; 90(1):107–119.

Corbett JV. *Laboratory Tests and Diagnostic Procedures with Nursing Diagnosis.* 3rd ed. Norwalk, CT, Appleton & Lange, 1992.

Crockett EG, et al. Comparing the cost of a thrifty food plan market basket in three areas of New York state. *J Nutr Ed* 1992; 24 (suppl):72S–79S.

Darlington G, et al. Dietary treatment of rheumatoid arthritis. *Practitioner* 1990 May 8; 234 (1488):456–460.

Dietz WH, Trowbridge FL. Symposium on the identification and prevalence of undernutrition in the United States. Introduction. *J Nutr* 1990 Aug; 120(8):917–918.

Fairbanks VF, Beutler E. Iron. *In* Shils ME, Young VR (eds). *Modern Nutrition in Health and Disease.* 7th ed. Philadelphia, Lea & Febiger, 1988:193–226.

Fierman AH, et al. Growth delay in homeless children. *Pediatrics* 1991 Nov; 88(11):918–925.

Food Research and Action Center (FRAC). *Community Childhood Hunger Identification Project. Executive Summary.* Washington, D.C., March 1991.

Frambach DA, Bendel RE. Zinc supplementation and anemia. *JAMA* 1991 Feb 20; 265(7):869.

Harris K. Which ground beef is the best buy? *J Tx State Nutr Council* 1992 Spring; 2(1):16–17.

Heaney RP. Effect of calcium on skeletal development, bone loss, and risk of fractures. *Am J Med* 1991 Nov 25; 91(suppl 5B):5B-23S–5B-27S.

Hinders S. Calcium and cholesterol: A balancing act. *Am J Nurs* 1991 Dec; 91(12):35.

Hunger and the Elderly. Joint Hearing before the Domestic Task Force of the Select Committee on Hunger and the Select Committee on Aging, House of Representatives: 99th Congress, Second Session. Serial No. 99-15. Committee Publ. No. 99-572. Washington, D.C., US Government Printing Office, 1986.

Kjeldsen-Kragh J, et al. Controlled trial of fasting and one-year vegetarian diet in rheumatoid arthritis. *Lancet* 1991 Oct 12; 338(8772):899–902.

Klein BP. Retention of nutrients in microwave-cooked foods. *Contemp Nutr* 1989; 14(2):1–2. (A General Mills publication.)

Kremer JM, et al. Dietary fish oil and olive oil supplementation in patients with rheumatoid arthritis. Clinical and immunologic effects. *Arthritis Rheum* 1990 June; 33(6):810–820.

Lederle FA. Oral cobalamin for pernicious anemia: Medicine's best kept secret? *JAMA* 1991 Jan 2; 265(1):94–95.

Liang MH, Fortin P. Management of osteoarthritis of the hip and knee (editorial). *N Engl J Med* 1991 July 11; 325(2):125–127.

Lindsay R. Estrogens, bone mass, and osteoporotic fractures. *Am J Med* 1991 Nov 25; 91(suppl 5B):5B-10S–5B-13S.

Love JA, Prusa KJ. Nutrient composition and sensory attributes of cooked ground beef: Effects of fat content, cooking method, and water rinsing. *J Am Diet Assoc* 1992 Nov; 92 (11):1367–1371.

Mayer J. Social responsibilities of nutritionists. *J Nutr* 1986 May; 116(5):714–717.

McClave SA, et al. Differentiating subtypes (hypoalbuminemia vs marasmic) of protein-calorie malnutrition: Incidence and clinical significance in a university hospital setting. *JPEN* 1992 July-Aug; 16(4):337–342.

Mitchell DR, Lyles KW. Glucocorticoid-induced osteoporosis: Mechanisms for bone loss. *J Gerontol* 1990 Sept; 45(5):M153–158.

Morgan SL, et al. The effect of folic acid supplementation on the toxicity of low-dose methotrexate treatment of rheumatoid arthritis. *Arthritis Rheum* 1990 Jan; 33(1):9–18.

Morgan SL, et al. Folate status of rheumatoid arthritis patients receiving long-term low dose methotrexate therapy. *Arthritis Rheum* 1987 Dec; 30(12):1348–1356.

National Osteoporosis Foundation. *Physician Resource Manual on Osteoporosis. A Decision Making Guide.* 2nd ed. Washington, D.C., National Osteoporosis Foundation, 1991.

Panush RS. American College of Rheumatology position statement: Diet and arthritis. *Rheum Dis Clin North Am* 1991 May; 17(2):443–444.

Panush RS. Food induced (allergic) arthritis: Clinical and serologic studies. *J Rheumatol* 1990 March; 17(3):291–294.

Panush RS, et al. Diet therapy for rheumatoid arthritis. *Arthritis rheum* 1983 Apr; 26(4):462–471.

Physician Task Force on Hunger in America. *Hunger in America—The Growing Epidemic.* Boston, Harvard University School of Public Health, 1985.

A Place to Call Home: The Low Income Housing Crisis Continues. Center on Budget and Policy Priorities and Low Income Housing Coalition. Washington, D.C., Dec 1991.

Preventing wintertime bone loss: Effects of vitamin D supplementation in healthy postmenopausal women. *Nutr Rev* 1992 Feb; 50(2):52–54.

Prince RL, et al. Prevention of postmenopausal

osteoporosis. A comparative study of exercise, calcium supplementation and hormone-replacement therapy. *New Engl J Med* 1991 Oct 24; 325(17):1189–1195.

Reginster J. Effect of calcitonin on bone mass and fracture rates. *Am J Med* 1991 Nov 25; 91(suppl 5B):5B-19S–5B-22S.

Reid IR, et al. Effect of calcium supplementation on bone loss in postmenopausal women. *N Engl J Med* 1993 Feb 18; 328(7):460–464.

Riggs BL. Treatment of osteoporosis with sodium fluoride on parathyroid hormone. *Am J Med* 1991 Nov 25; 91(suppl 5B): 5B-37S–5B-40S.

Roubenoff R, et al. Catabolic effects of high-dose corticosteroids persist despite therapeutic benefit in rheumatoid arthritis. *Am J Clin Nutr* 1990 Dec; 52(6):1113–1117.

Roubenoff R, et al. Malnutrition among hospitalized patients. *Arch Intern Med* 1987 Aug; 147(8):1462–1465.

Saal NM, Douglas PD. Teaching nutrition survival skills. *J Am Diet Assoc* 1992 May; 92(5):547.

Schaus EE, Biggs GM. Nutritionally economic foods. *J Nutr Ed* 1983; 15(4):130–131.

Tulleken JE, et al. Vitamin E status during dietary fish oil supplementation in rheumatoid arthritis. *Arthritis Rheum* 1990 Sept; 33(9):1416–1419.

Urrows ST, et al. Profiles in osteoporosis. *Am J Nurs* 1991 Dec; 91(12):32–37.

van der Tempel H, et al. Effects of fish oil supplementation in rheumatoid arthritis. *Ann Rheum Dis* 1990 Feb; 49(2):76–80.

Walden O. The relationship of dietary and supplemental calcium intake to bone loss and osteoporosis. *J Am Diet Assoc* 1989 March; 89(3):397–400.

Wardlaw G. The effects of diet and life-style on bone mass in women. *J Am Diet Assoc* 1988 Jan; 88(1):17–22, 25.

Watts NB. Cyclical etidronate. *The Osteoporosis Report* 1990 Winter; 6(4):2, 6.

Weddle DO, et al. Inpatient and post-discharge course of the malnourished patient. *J Am Diet Assoc* 1991 March; 91(3):307–311.

Winograd CH, Brown EM. Aggressive oral refeeding in hospitalized patients. *Am J Clin Nutr* 1990 Dec; 52(6):967–968.

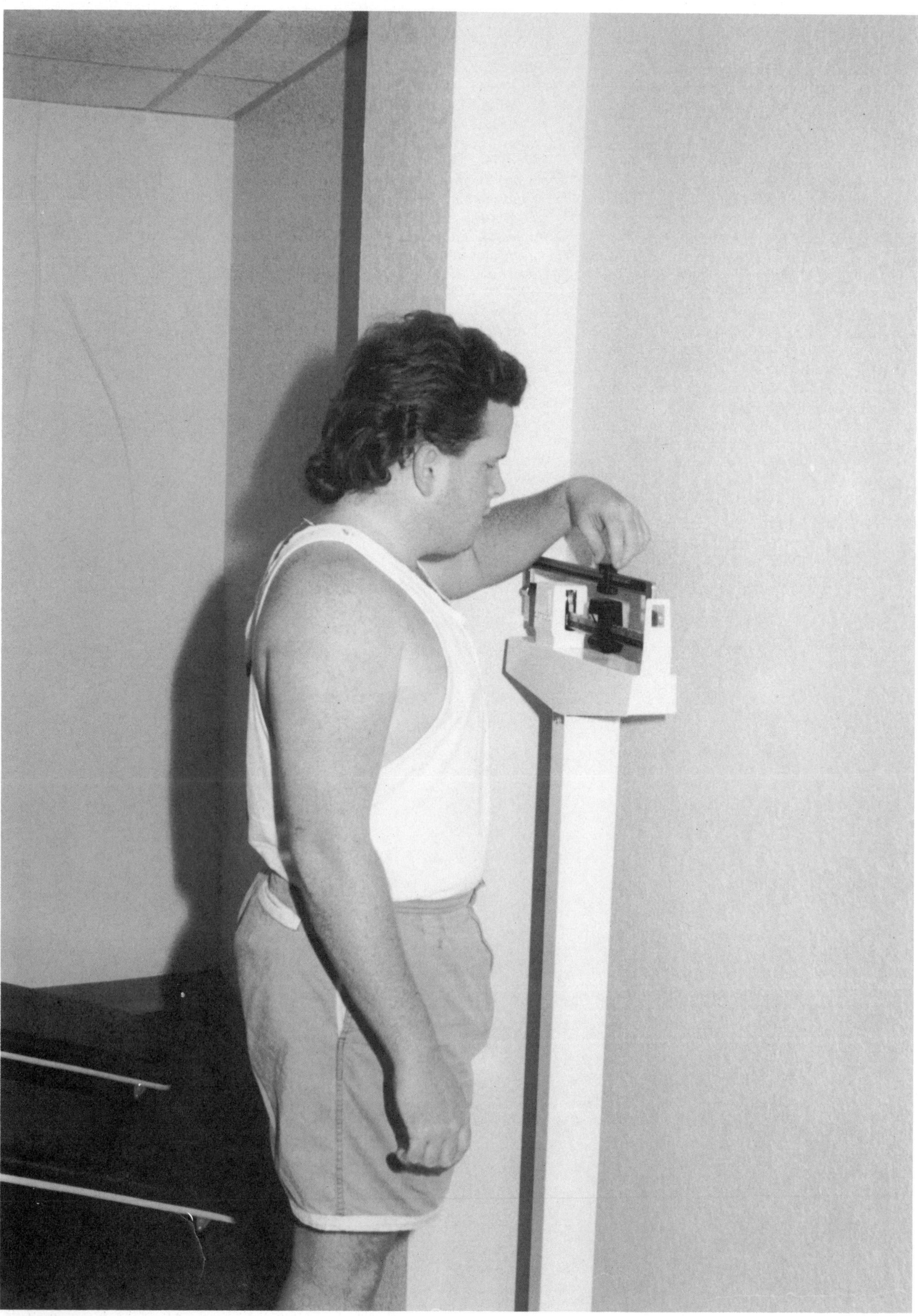

CHAPTER 19

Problems of Weight Control

OUTLINE

I. DEFINITION OF OBESITY
II. BODY FAT
  A. Weight Distribution
III. CAUSES OF OBESITY
  A. Hyperplastic Versus Hypertrophic Obesity
  B. Lipoprotein Lipase
  C. Heredity
  D. Appestat
  E. Hypothyroidism
  F. Total Energy Expenditure
IV. REALITIES FOR TREATMENT OF OBESITY
V. NUTRITIONAL ASSESSMENT
  Nursing Applications
VI. TREATMENT STRATEGIES
  A. Reduction Diets
    1. Kilocalories and Protein
    2. Fat
    3. Carbohydrate
    4. Fiber
    5. General Considerations
  Nursing Applications
  B. Fasting
  Nursing Applications
  C. Very Low Calorie Diets
  Nursing Applications
  D. Fad Diets
  Nursing Applications
  E. Exercise
  Nursing Applications
  F. Behavior Modification
  Nursing Applications
  G. Use of Drugs
    1. Appetite Suppressants
    2. Thermogenic Drugs
    3. Diuretics
    4. Gastrointestinal Tract Drugs

OBJECTIVES

THE STUDENT WILL BE ABLE TO:

- Evaluate food intake and mobility of a client to determine the future course of weight gain or loss.
- Discuss different food choices as well as activities to achieve desired weight.
- List psychological factors that influence weight control.
- Suggest alternate behavior patterns to support clients in their programs.
- Evaluate personal goals for optimum health and weight.
- Discuss ways to evaluate new and old fad diets to determine their degree of acceptability.
- Evaluate the use of surgery for the morbidly obese, and discuss problems clients may expect after surgery.
- Apply nursing principles for clients who want to gain or lose weight.
- Identify client education information for weight gain or loss.

■ TEST YOUR NQ (True/False)

1. Overweight and obesity mean the same thing.
2. Appestat is a computer program that helps clients lose weight.
3. Weight yo-yoing is dangerous.
4. On a reduction diet, carbohydrate foods are advisable and allowed.
5. Behavior modification is a technique to help clients lose weight.
6. Appetite suppressants used alone are an effective method to lose weight.
7. Liposuction is a good way to alleviate obesity.
8. If a child is obese, strict kilocalorie restriction is needed.
9. To help a client gain weight, moderate exercise is recommended.
10. Eating nuts, gravies, and homogenized milk can help clients gain weight.

According to data gathered in the Second National Health and Nutrition Examination Survey (HANES) from 1976 to 1980, approximately 34 million US adults were overweight (over 26%), with a higher percentage of these individuals being women (56%) (Kuczmarski, 1992). One of the goals of the US Public Health Services' Year 2000 Health Objectives for the nation is to reduce prevalence of obesity to less than 20%. Another health objective indirectly addresses prevention of obesity: "To increase to at least 30% the proportion of people aged 6 and older who engage regularly, preferably daily, in light to moderate physical activity for at least 30 minutes per day" (USDHHS, 1990).

Because of lack of scientific data, one's desirable weight is somewhat hypothetical and may continue to change as knowledge increases. Contrary to popular opinion, life expectancy is not inversely correlated with underweight. Slight increases in weight after age 18 are associated with a decreased risk of mortality, whereas >10 kg weight gain is associated with an increased mortality (Sjöström, 1992). However, excess body fat is associated with premature mortality and increases risk of NIDDM, hypertension, cardiovascular disease, gallbladder disease, and colon and postmenopausal breast cancer. Estimated cost of these medical conditions attributable to obesity was $39.3 billion in 1986 (Colditz, 1992). Other risks and complications of obesity are associated with pregnancy (impaired glucose tolerance); decreased fertility (menstrual and sperm abnormalities); surgery (pneumonia, wound infection, thrombophlebitis); and increased problems with sleep apnea, gout, and arthritis.

What are conditions associated with obesity?

DEFINITION OF OBESITY

The terms **overweight** and **obesity** are used interchangeably but are technically very different. Desirable body weight (DBW) or ideal body weight (IBW) can be used to denote a weight for height considered to be healthy for a client. Morbid obesity refers to more than 100 lbs over DBW. For example, a client weighing 163 lbs with a desirable weight of 130 lbs is about 25% overweight and may be called obese.

Overweight, defined as excess weight for height, is identified as 10 to 20% above DBW. Obesity, or 20% above DBW, is excess accumulation of body fat.

Many clients, although normal or below normal in weight, have excess amounts of fat stores. Athletes are usually overweight because of increased muscle mass, not fat. Being overweight is not the same as being fat or obese. Additional muscle tissue aids body functions, but excessive fat tissue interferes with normal body metabolism. A desirable weight for a client depends on the amount and location of body fat and other weight-related medical problems.

What is the difference between overweight and obesity? What is morbid obesity?

BODY FAT

Desirable body fat for women is 20 to 25% with a minimum of 12% for survival. Fat stores above 20% are needed for hormonal and reproductive functions. Men require only 2 to 3% body fat for survival; 15 to 18% is desirable. Men with more than 25% body fat and women with more than 30% are considered obese (Bray, 1989).

Assessment techniques can help confirm or discredit visual appraisals regarding body fat. Underwater weighing, bioelectrical impedance, body mass index (BMI), and skinfold thickness measurements can be used to estimate body fat. (BMI and skinfold thickness measurements are discussed in Chapter 9.) As discussed in Chapter 5, some fat stores are essential. Adipose tissue is maintained at a relatively constant level and seems to be regulated by a sensitive feedback mechanism (Poissonnet et al, 1988).

The most reliable method of determining body fat is hydrostatic or underwater weighing (Fig. 19–1). Measuring **body density** provides information regarding body fat and fat-free mass. Although the technique is relatively simple, appropriate facilities are expensive.

Body density is determined from the weight of a submersed body as compared with out of water weight.

Determining body fat using an electrical impedance machine is becoming more popular. Total body electrical conductivity estimates lean tissue and fat based on differences in electromagnetic waves. Electrodes are applied, and impedance or resistance is measured (Fig. 19–2). Formulas estimate percentage of body fat. Results are very reliable as compared with body density technique (Segal et al, 1988).

What is desirable body fat for women; for men? What percentage is considered obese for the sexes?

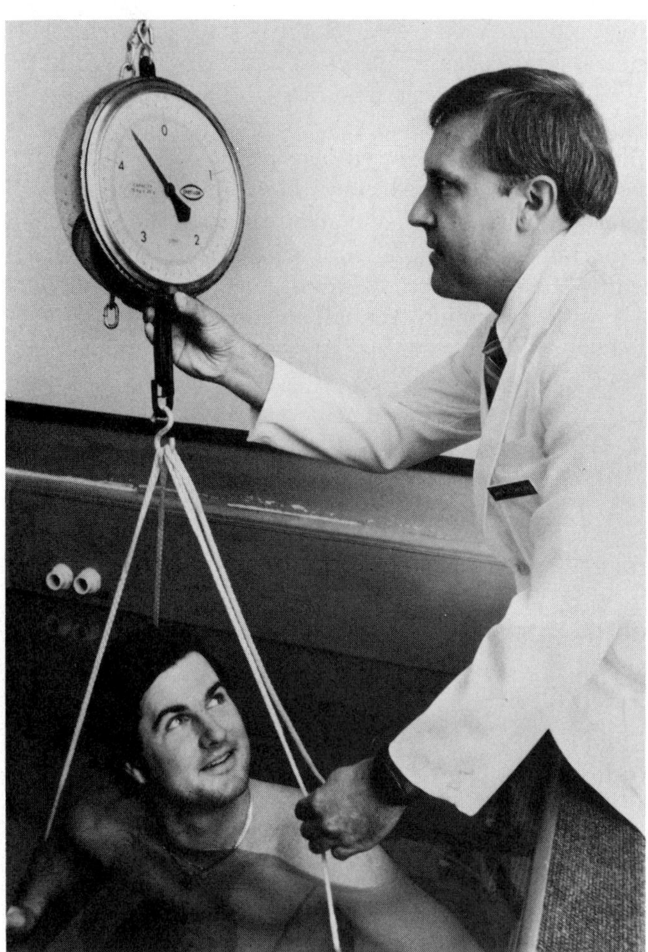

Figure 19–1 Dr. Kenneth Cooper's Aerobics Center in Dallas offers underwater weighing for determining body fat composition.

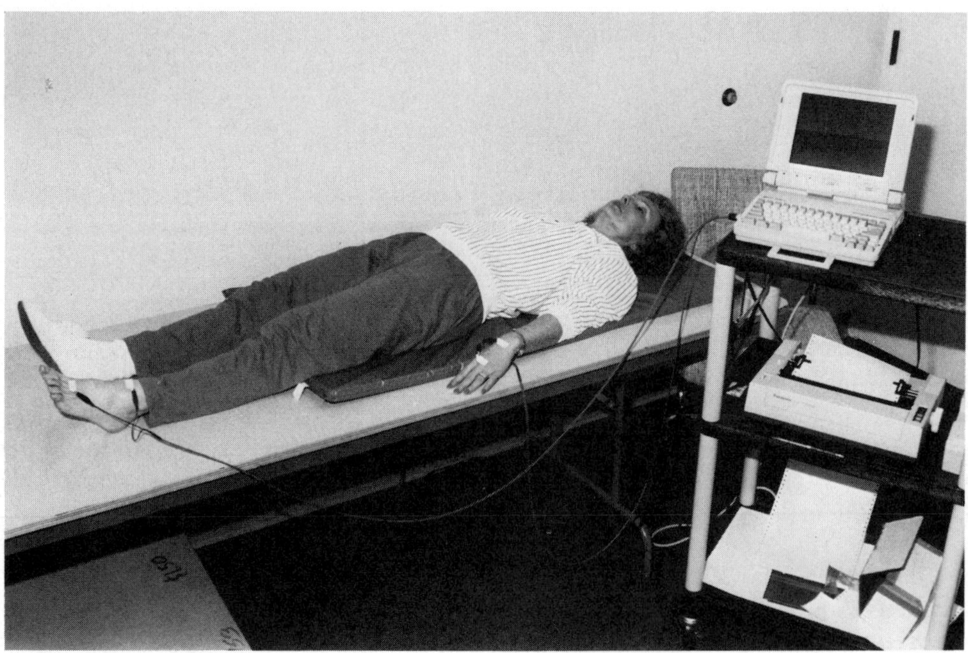

Figure 19–2 Determining body fat using a bioimpedance machine.

TABLE 19–1

DETERMINING WAIST-HIP RATIO*

To determine waist circumference:
Measure at the narrowest area above the navel
To determine hip circumference:
Measure at the maximal gluteal protrusion
Gynoid example: Waist—26"; hip—37"
26/37 or 26 ÷ 37 = 0.70 typical low-risk ratio*
Android example: Waist—45"; hip—35"
45/35 or 45 ÷ 35 = 1.28 typical high-risk ratio*

* Higher risk is associated with > 0.8 for women, > 1 for men.

Weight Distribution

Although a layer of subcutaneous fat covers the whole body, thickness of the fat differs in various anatomical regions and between clients. The location of fat accumulation has been classified as **android** or **gynoid obesity.** Data indicate that waist-hip ratios correlate best with risk factors associated with obesity (Table 19–1).

Excess fat in the abdominal area, known as android obesity, or an "apple-shaped" body is characteristic of men.

Accumulation of fat in the hips or femoral area (thigh), called gynoid obesity, or a "pear-shaped" body is typical of women.

Upper-body obesity, commonly seen in men, is associated with increased risk of coronary heart disease (Thompson et al, 1991; Bjorntorp, 1985), certain cancers (especially of the breast and endometrium) (Schapira et al, 1991; Ballard-Barbash et al, 1990), and high blood pressure (Kanai et al, 1990). Risks for these diseases increase steeply when the waist-hip ratio is above 1 in men and .8 in women, as shown in Figure 19–3. Regardless of BMI, any amount of increased abdominal fat increases health risks (Bray, 1990). In contrast, lower body or gynoid obesity is relatively benign. However, it also means clients will have more difficulty in losing weight and maintaining IBW.

What are risks associated with upper and lower body fat?

CAUSES OF OBESITY

Obesity is the result of consistent kilocaloric overconsumption in excess of energy expenditure. Control of food intake has been investigated from many different aspects: hormonal, metabolic, dietary (composition, perceived senses), social, and psychological (see Chapter 10). Precise causes of obesity are not well understood, but several influences have been identified. Obesity probably has different causes, thereby resulting in different characteristics and warranting differing treatments.

Hyperplastic Versus Hypertrophic Obesity

The size, number, and distribution of fat cells are used to classify obesity and estimate prognosis. Obesity can be divided into 2 classifications: **hyperplastic** and **hypertrophic.** Cell multiplication occurs during peak growth periods: late infancy, early childhood (up to 6 years of age), adolescence, and pregnancy. The complexity and magnitude of obesity are more easily understood if overeating has occurred during any of these periods; total number of fat cells is increased when obesity develops during childhood. Adequate nutrition for growth during these stages without excessive amounts of energy is imperative.

Hyperplasty refers to increased numbers of fat cells; hypertrophy refers to increased fat cell size.

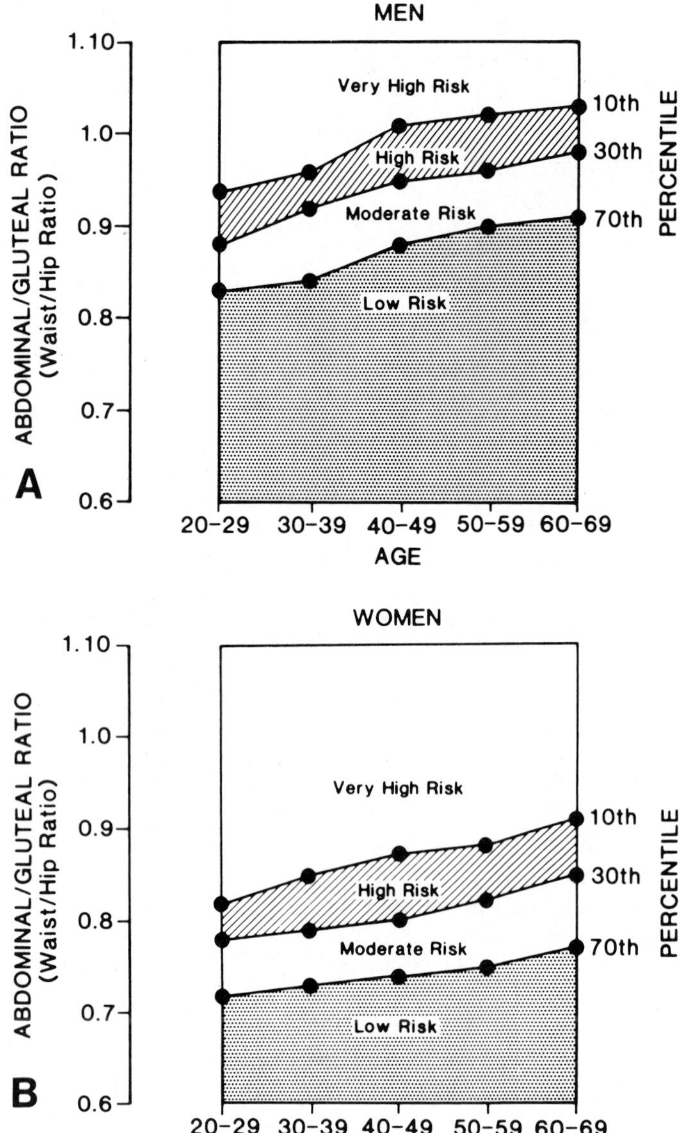

Figure 19-3 Percentiles for fat distribution. The percentiles for the ratio of abdominal circumference to gluteal circumference (ratio of waist to hips) are depicted for men (*A*) and women (*B*) by age groups. The relative risk for these percentiles is indicated based on the available information. (From Bray GA. Nutrient balance and obesity: Classification and evaluation of the obesities. *Med Clin North Am* 1989; 73(1):161–183. (Data from Canadian Standardized Tests for Fitness (15 to 16 years of age), Operations Manual. Minister of State, Fitness, and Amateur Sports, FAS 7378.))

Birth weights do not correlate with subsequent obesity in adult life. Obese infants do not necessarily become obese children. In children who are lean, fat cells decrease in size after the first year of life (Bray, 1990). Obesity may begin as early as age 2 for girls and age 3 for boys.

In hypertrophic obesity, fat cells expand to increase body weight. This type of obesity primarily occurs after puberty and tends to correlate with android distribution. Weight loss is principally reduced fat cell size, but prolonged reduction in body fat may lead to decreased numbers of fat cells.

Describe differences between hypertrophic and hyperplastic obesity.

Clients who are approximately 75% above IBW usually have hypertrophic obesity. Clients with hyperplastic obesity have trouble losing weight and following weight loss; weight is regained more rapidly in clients with hyperplastic obesity than in clients with hypertrophic obesity.

Lipoprotein Lipase

Lipoprotein lipase (LPL) is an enzyme present in adipose tissue that determines uptake of circulating plasma triglycerides by fat cells. Elevated LPL activity associated with obesity appears to preserve rather than cause obesity (Eckel, 1989).

Heredity

Genetic factors probably contribute to obesity, especially with regard to fat distribution (hips, buttocks, abdomen, thighs, or waist). Children with one or both obese parents are at high risk of becoming obese. This may be more closely linked to genetic factors than environmental factors (Bray, 1990; Stunkard et al, 1990). Several studies have suggested the existence of a genetic basis for obesity, but a specific defective gene has yet to be identified (Goldsmith, 1990).

Appestat

The **setpoint (or appestat) theory** proposes that a control system in clients dictates how much fat they will have. Deviations from this setpoint result in restorative forces functioning to return the weight to the setpoint weight (Weigle, 1990). For instance, after a holiday eating binge or fasting associated with acute illness, clients may experience pronounced satiety or hunger. This is true in both normal-weight and obese clients, indicating that the regulatory system operates independently of factors that determine the setpoint weight (Weigle, 1990).

The normal weight maintained by a client without conscious effort may be referred to as "setpoint" weight that is regulated at a predetermined level by a feedback control mechanism.

This theory explains why it is as difficult for a thin client to gain weight as it is for an obese one to lose weight. The body adjusts the appetite for kilocaloric intake to maintain its setpoint. This setpoint changes at different stages of life. Although it is not clear as to what controls the appestat, the only way to lower this setpoint is through increased physical exercise. This can apparently help maintain weight loss as well. Opponents believe this theory is an oversimplification of a complex system that regulates body weight (Harris, 1990).

Describe appestat theory.

Hypothyroidism

Obesity caused by hypothyroidism occurs in fewer than 1% of overweight clients. In hypothyroidism, BMR is lowered because of a deficiency in thyroid secretion. This results in excessive retention of kilocalories that would normally be expended in basal metabolism.

Total Energy Expenditure

A client's BMR accounts for approximately 70% of basal energy expenditure (BEE). BMR depends principally on the amount of fat-free mass (muscle tissue). After age 25, BMR decreases. Unless food intake decreases accordingly, weight is gained.

A major component of overall BEE is physical activity, which also usually decreases after the age of 25. Since many obese clients are less active, fewer kilocalories are expended, which in turn results in weight gain when the same amount of food is eaten. Additionally, the BMR begins to decrease when energy is restricted; this may in part be attributed to decreased muscle mass. Within 2 weeks of restricted intake, BMR can decrease more than 20%.

REALITIES FOR TREATMENT OF OBESITY

In some cases, understanding physiological benefits of weight loss can be motivating for some clients. As shown in Figure 19–3, weight loss is highly desirable with certain risk factors and advisable for others. Weight loss is associated with a decrease in serum glucose, cholesterol, systolic blood pressure, and uric acid. Other physical conditions that can be expected to improve with weight loss include shortness of breath, ease of tiring, fluid retention, gastric disorders, headaches, energy level, interest in sex, joint pains, muscle cramps, pulse rate, restless sleep, urinary infection, and varicose veins.

Preoccupation with weight loss has resulted in a dramatic surge in the number, variety, and cost of available weight loss programs. A survey in the Boston area revealed commercial outpatient programs can range from $108 to $2120 (for a nutritionally balanced hypokilocaloric 12-week diet program) (Spielman et al, 1992). At any particular time, as many as 40% of women and 24% of men report they are dieting (NIH, 1992). Annually approximately $35.8 billion is spent on diets and diet-related products and services in the US (Thompson, 1990).

Treatment of obesity has a high level of client noncompliance and failure. Regaining lost weight frequently occurs. Approximately 80 to 100% of those who lose significant amounts of weight regain it (Pi-Sunyer, 1988). Any treatment for weight loss should always be a serious undertaking with a high level of client motivation and long-term commitment. This approach increases chances that the plan will be followed until weight is lost and that weight loss will be maintained.

If a client wants to lose 10 lbs and is unsure he or she will be able to maintain the weight loss, it may not be a good idea to lose weight. Benefits of weight loss are greater for one who is obese than for a client 10 lbs over IBW. Losing weight can be accomplished by eating less, increasing activity, or a combination of both.

When 2 lbs (4.4 kg) per week are lost, clients are more enthusiastic about the method of loss. (One pound of fat equals 3500 kcal.) Food intake with 500 kcal less than needed per day results in a 1 lb loss per week. An additional energy expenditure of 500 kcal per day is recommended for the other pound of weight loss.

Yo-yoing—repeated cycles of weight loss and gain.

Yo-yo dieting is common among clients between ages 30 and 44; this may have adverse health consequences (Lissner et al, 1991). Individuals who have lost weight only to put it back on are frequently unable to lose weight even on 800 kcal, take longer to lose added weight, and regain weight more rapidly. Research from the weight cycling project (Brownell, 1988) indicates that weight cycling may increase the proportion of fat to lean tissue, redistribute body fat to the abdominal area, increase desire for fatty foods, and increase risk of developing heart problems. Possibly with weight cycling, people become more metabolically efficient with the body interpreting these periods of low kilocaloric intake as starvation.

Fatty tissues in reduced-obese clients are conducive for refilling; obesity recurs if energy intake increases above maintenance levels. Therefore, it is extremely important that overweight clients be taught skills to maintain weight loss. Prevention of relapse should become a central focus of weight loss programs (Lissner et al, 1991).

Name 5 benefits of weight loss. What are some results of yo-yoing? What is a recommended method to lose 2 lbs per week?

NUTRITIONAL ASSESSMENT

Treatment for obesity should be individualized; assessment of etiologic factors contributing to obesity helps ascertain whether a weight loss program should be attempted and specific components of that program. Table 19–2 indicates facts that need to be known to assess risks and assist clients in determining goals for weight loss.

NURSING APPLICATIONS

Assessment

Physical—for age, cause of obesity; body frame, weight, height, IBW/DBW; percentage of body fat (above 25% for men, 30% for women) using underwater weighing, bioelectrical impedance, TSF, or BMI; waist-hip/waist-thigh ratio (see Table 19–2); motivation level.

Dietary—for intake, focusing on fat, saturated fat, total volume; frequency of eating (see Table 19–2).

Laboratory—for any abnormalities, especially cholesterol, glucose; triiodothyronine (T_3), thyroxine (T_4).

Interventions

1. Monitor prescription medication use associated with hyperphagia (see Table 19–2) that would lessen self-control.
2. Develop an individualized comprehensive program to promote adherence and compliance to the regimen. For most clients, a program that incorporates diet, exercise, and behavior modification is more effective in long-term weight control.

Evaluation

* Client will have weekly weight loss and adhere to exercise program.

Client Education

- Explain different causes of obesity.
- Treatments are remedies, not cures.
- Predictors of successful long-term weight loss and maintenance include regular physical activity, family support, internal motivation, and ability to focus on positive changes (more energy, lower blood pressure, and so forth).
- Losing weight is relatively easy compared with maintaining weight loss.

TREATMENT STRATEGIES

Overweight and obesity have been treated with numerous strategies: diet, exercise, behavior modification, drugs, and surgery. A realistic goal regarding the rate and amount of weight loss must be established for each client. No one treatment is best for everyone; each modality varies in effectiveness, risk, and cost.

Reduction Diets

Despite the numerous diets that have been devised for weight loss, there is no easy sure fire method. The mainstay of weight loss is restriction of energy intake.

TABLE 19–2

ASSESSMENT OF ETIOLOGIC FACTORS

1. Family history of obesity
2. Age of onset of obesity
3. Presence of or family history for risk factors (hypertension, coronary heart disease, diabetes mellitus, cancer)
4. Fat distribution
5. Presence of endocrine diseases
6. Dietary intake, focusing on fat, saturated fat, total volume, and frequency of eating
7. Frequency and level of physical activity
8. Drugs associated with hyperphagia (glucocorticoids, amitriptyline, lithium, cyproheptadine, phenothiazides, birth control pills)
9. Other factors
   a. Pregnancy or number of previous pregnancies
   b. Recent changes in physical activity associated with life changes
   c. Operations
   d. Emotional factors (boredom, anger, depression, guilt, lack of self-esteem)

Failure to lose weight on less than 1200 kcal per day may be attributed to a higher energy intake than reported and overestimation of physical activity (Lichtman et al, 1992). Many problems, including deaths, have occurred from use of imbalanced diets and formulas. A weight reduction diet needs to be followed for an extended period of time; therefore, it must be appealing and flexible as well as affordable for the client. It can be balanced yet energy deficient. The diet should include foods from each food group to provide necessary nutrients.

Kilocalories and Protein

What are recommendations for kilocalories and protein?

For individuals with mild obesity, nutritionally balanced, low-energy diets composed of conventional foods are generally recommended (AMA, 1988). A 1100- to 1200-kcal diet (or slightly higher for men) can provide conventional distribution of carbohydrates, protein, and fat. Approximately 20% of the total kilocalories should be from proteins to provide an adequate amount of protein (50 to 60 gm). When energy levels are below 1200 kcal, it is difficult to obtain recommended levels of iron, calcium, magnesium, vitamin B_6, zinc, and copper (USDA, 1990).

Fat

What is the recommendation for fat intake and why?

Excessive fat intake is discouraged. However, to provide fat-soluble vitamins and EFA and their absorption, the diet should be composed of a minimum of 20% fat of total kilocaloric intake. Dietary fat increases satiety; fat restriction reduces kilocaloric density of the diet. Low-fat diets have been suggested as the most effective dietary measure for weight loss and maintenance. In 3 recent studies investigating the effect of low-fat diets on weight loss, independent conclusions were that (1) weight loss was more closely associated with the percentage of dietary fat rather than changes in total kilocaloric intake (Sheppard et al, 1991), (2) increased weight loss occurred on a low-fat diet despite overall increased kilocaloric intake (Prewitt et al, 1991), and (3) weight can be lost by reducing dietary fat without any further restrictions of food intake (Kendall et al, 1991). Additionally, a low-fat intake is beneficial to reduce risk factors for chronic diseases, such as hypercholesterolemia and cancer. A fat intake of 20 to 25% can be translated into daily fat (gm) intake for various kilocaloric levels as indicated in Table 19–3.

Carbohydrate

Ketosis—the accumulation of ketones (acidic byproducts of lipid metabolism) that occurs when inadequate amounts of glucose are available for energy.

Although large amounts of sugars are not recommended, a minimum of 20% of the kilocalories from carbohydrate prevents **ketosis.** Consumption of complex carbohydrates in meals and snacks has been advised for weight loss. Complex carbohydrates maintain glycogen stores for optimum energy levels. Also, carbohydrate ingestion triggers a significant increase in brain serotonin followed by a decrease in the hunger impulse. Low serotonin levels encourage a person to eat more carbohy-

TABLE 19–3

TOTAL DAILY FAT INTAKE FOR SPECIFIC KILOCALORIC LEVELS*

Kilocaloric Level	Gm fat/day
1200	27–33
1500	33–42
1800	40–50
2000	44–56
2200	49–61
2400	53–67

* Total fat intake limited to 20 to 25% of the total daily kilocalories.

drates and less protein. Therefore, all reduction diets should allow ample starchy foods to discourage binge eating.

What is the recommendation for carbohydrate and why?

Fiber

Another strategy to increase satiety is through high-fiber intake (0.7 gm/kg of DBW), which provides bulk with low kilocaloric density foods. Miles (1992) found that high-fiber diets may enhance weight control because of reduced digestibility of protein, carbohydrate, and fat. However, in view of several reports of intestinal obstruction from increased bran, clients should be encouraged to increase fluid intake while progressively increasing fiber intake.

General Considerations

Diets may be based on a general guide, such as the food exchange lists (Appendix D-1). A diet that totally eliminates one category (fat or carbohydrate) or specific group of foods (fruits or meats) is inadvisable because essential nutrients may be lacking. Indispensable to any weight loss program is a preplanned food allotment with specified times throughout the day to lessen deprivation syndrome and eliminate excessive food intake. Total amount of foods should be divided into 3 or more feedings. Eating only once or twice a day has been associated with increased adipose tissue and serum cholesterol and impulsive snacking (Schlundt et al, 1992). Some "free" foods or beverages may be available for snack periods, but regular mealtimes are important.

What are some general considerations for reduction diets?

NURSING APPLICATIONS

Assessment

Physical—for serial weights.
Dietary—for type of diet, percentage of protein, fat, carbohydrates, snacking and eating patterns, fiber, complex carbohydrate intake.
Laboratory—for cholesterol.

Interventions

1. Praise client for adhering to diet; do not belittle for noncompliance. Try to help the client problem solve.
2. Point out benefits and foods allowed on reduction diets, not what the client should not eat.

Evaluation

* Client loses weight by consuming a diet high in complex carbohydrates and fiber with reduced intake of fat and kilocalories.

Client Education

- A weight-reduction diet should satisfy the following criteria (Byerly et al, 1987): (1) Meet all nutrient needs except energy, (2) suit client's tastes and habits, (3) minimize hunger and fatigue, (4) be accessible and socially acceptable, (5) encourage a change in eating pattern, and (6) favor improvement in overall health.
- The mainstay of weight loss is restriction of energy intake.
- Although a 1200-kcal diet is relatively safe, success rate is poor because of slow weight loss unless accompanied by an exercise program to augment rate of weight loss.
- A diet that requires the least amount of change in dietary patterns has better long-term success.

Fasting

Hyperuricemia—elevated levels of uric acid, which increase risk of precipitating gout or renal uric acid stones.

Total fasting is extremely hazardous and is not recommended for more than 3 days unless in a hospital setting. Short-term fasting has not been effective in excessively obese clients; prolonged fasting is of temporary benefit. Total fasting may result in ketosis, **hyperuricemia,** excessive loss of lean body mass, hyponatremia, hypokalemia, hypoglycemia, and other adverse side effects.

NURSING APPLICATIONS

Assessment

Physical—for loss of muscle mass, flank pain.
Dietary—for use of fasting to lose weight.
Laboratory—for urine ketones; sodium, potassium, glucose, uric acid.

Interventions

1. Discourage clients from fasting unless under close medical supervision because of increased risks and negative effects on lean body mass.

Evaluation

* Client does not fast.

Client Education

- Fasting is not a desirable or healthy way to lose weight.
- Explain the hazards of fasting.

Very Low Calorie Diets

Very low calorie diets (VLCDs) containing less than 800 kcal daily may be recommended for severely or morbidly obese adults (>30% overweight). Current popular VLCDs contain 50 to 75 gm/day of high-quality protein, 30 to 45 gm carbohydrate, and adequate quantities of vitamins and minerals. This regimen contains minimal carbohydrate; the only fat is from lean meat, fish, and poultry. When administered with close medical supervision, current VLCDs are much safer than their liquid protein predecessors that contained collagen as the sole source of protein. Initial rapid weight loss is seen while preserving lean body mass as a result of the protein or protein/carbohydrate mixture. (The protein-sparing modified fast provides 1.5 gm protein/kg of DBW.)

Another regimen is a liquid formula that provides approximately 33 to 70 gm protein daily. This liquid diet includes approximately 30 to 45 gm carbohydrate and 2 gm fat. Both regimens require vitamin and mineral supplements; results have been comparable.

Weight loss is more rapid than with conventional diets because of lower kilocaloric intake, averaging 1.5 to 2 kg/week. Comparison of VLCD regimens containing 420 kcal, 600 kcal, and 800 kcal/day indicates no significant differences in rate of weight loss or changes in body composition (Foster et al, 1992).

Before initiation of either of these regimens, individuals should have a cardiac evaluation and remain under close medical supervision while on the diet. Weight loss–associated protein and potassium losses and metabolic consequences, including risk of gallstones and ketosis, warrant careful selection of individuals for these regimens (ADA, 1990). Changes in hormones affecting synthesis and regulation of lipoproteins lead to elevated cholesterol concentrations as weight is lost. This hypercholesterolemia is transient and resolves when weight loss ceases (Phinney et al,

1991). Hypercholesterolemia increases potential for gallstones. The decrease in BMR (23.8% decrease) is similar for clients on a 1000- to 1200-kcal diet (Burgess, 1991; Foster et al, 1990). Adding fiber to VLCDs reduces hunger and increases frequency of bowel movements (Astrup et al, 1990).

VLCDs should be administered only to clients with severe obesity (30 to 40% above DBW) while under medical supervision before and throughout the program. Hypertension, hyperlipidemia, and hyperglycemia decrease on this regimen, and maintenance of weight loss of 36% for women and 39% for men at 42 months has been reported (Anderson et al, 1991). A maintenance program for at least 12 months is vital (ADA, 1990; Wadden et al, 1990).

Describe VLCD regimen.

NURSING APPLICATIONS

Assessment

Physical—for colicky pain after meals, BP.
Dietary—for type of regimen used, kilocalories allowed.
Laboratory—for protein, potassium, urine ketones, cholesterol, triglycerides, glucose.

Interventions

1. Stress the importance of a maintenance program following the VLCD regimen to maintain weight loss.
2. Discuss foods appropriate to eat and changes in dietary patterns after the VLCD diet is discontinued.

Evaluation

* Client should lose weight and not develop gallstones.

Client Education

- Extremely restricted diets may be counterproductive unless weight loss is maintained.
- Many problems, including death, have occurred from use of imbalanced diets and formulas; do not use VLCDs unless prescribed by a physician.
- VLCDs are not advisable for clients with a history of gallbladder disease.

Fad Diets

With more than 25% of the population overweight, Americans are still looking for a magic formula to lose weight. A fad diet usually does not have a scientific basis. According to promoters of fad diets, specific foods or food combinations usually facilitate weight loss, implying that a specific food or combination of foods oxidizes body fat, increases metabolic rate, or inhibits voluntary food intake. These diets are frequently deficient in essential nutrients.

Such diets can be recognized instantly when they promise secret formulas to melt away fat without exercise while eating without limitation and, of course, immediate results of several pounds lost. Miraculous promises are a good reason to run the other way. Table 19–4 provides some questions to check out the validity of a diet.

Results of fad diets can be devastating and have even led to death. Other benefits, such as rapid weight loss, may not be long-lasting. Diets that provide adequate nutrients and changes in lifestyle behaviors are desirable and more effective.

NURSING APPLICATIONS

Assessment

Physical—for weight.
Dietary—for use of fad diets.
Laboratory—for urine ketones.

Interventions

1. Use Table 19–4 to determine the safety of weight reduction diets. Discourage use of diets that are nutritionally unbalanced.

Evaluation

* Client does not use a fad diet to lose weight.

Client Education

- Permanent weight control is achieved by changes in lifestyle behaviors, not diet per se.
- Immediate weight loss results, such as occurs with low-carbohydrate diets, disappear. Reduction in weight represents water loss instead of fat, so weight is quickly regained when normal food intake resumes.

Exercise

Treatment of obesity is improved when energy expenditure is increased along with decreased kilocaloric intake. Exercise alone produces only a modest effect on weight loss, but it can be useful for other reasons. Energy expenditure declines when energy intake is reduced, possibly attributed to loss of lean body mass (and decreased BEE), decreased cost of physical activity as a result of lower body weight, and lower thermogenic effect of food related to decreased intake (Nelson et al, 1992; Heshka et al, 1990). Plateaus observed on energy-restricted diets may result from these combined factors. Whether physical activity helps preserve lean body mass or not is unresolved, but exercise definitely affects energy metabolism.

The effect of exercise on food intake appears to differ between lean and obese individuals. In nonobese individuals, increased food intake was associated with moderate physical activity to favor weight maintenance, whereas obese individuals make little change in energy intake in response to exercise (Nieman et al, 1990; Kissileff et al, 1990).

TABLE 19–4

EVALUATING WEIGHT LOSS DIETS

Is the program preceded by careful screening to determine the degree of overweight and its contributing causes?
What is the nature of the diet program? (Are special foods, beverages, or vitamins required?)
Are individual differences considered in determining energy needs?
What is the recommended rate of weight loss?
How successful is the program?
Are advertisements and endorsements based on solid facts or testimonials?
How much does the program cost, what do the fees include, and how is payment required? (Are there costs for foods, nutrient supplements, initial membership, or weekly fees?)
What are the side effects and health risks associated with the program?
Is proper medical supervision provided?
Is an exercise and behavior modification component included?
Does the program offer a maintenance plan and, if so, at what cost?
Can you live with the program indefinitely?

Compiled from National Dairy Council. Promoting a healthy weight. *Dairy Council Digest* 1991 March-Apr; 62(2):7–12.

A prevalent misconception is that a set amount of exercise is necessary to be beneficial. The ideal goal is an exercise of adequate intensity for at least 20 minutes 3 times a week. Most persons must start below this level. On conditioning, exercise can be increased to 30 minutes 5 times a week if clients desire to increase kilocaloric expenditure. Any exercise activity, even though it is below ideal level, still offers physiological and metabolic benefits. Table 10–1 (see Chapter 10) indicates energy expenditure during various activities.

Although effects of physical activity on body composition are controversial, exercise incorporated into a weight control program offers advantages of improved cardiovascular fitness, plasma lipoprotein profile, and carbohydrate metabolism; increased energy expenditure; and enhanced psychological well-being.

The overall use of energy throughout the day is a significant factor in kilocaloric balance. Total body movement during an activity is more important than its degree of difficulty. Increasing the amount of walking and using stairs rather than elevators are practical ways to expend more kilocalories, and these habits are easy to maintain. If exercise fits into one's lifestyle, it is more likely to be repeated, whereas a formal exercise program is seldom continued.

What may cause plateaus? What is the ideal goal for exercise?

NURSING APPLICATIONS

Assessment

Physical—for type and frequency of exercise.
Dietary—for kilocaloric intake.
Laboratory—for triglycerides, cholesterol, LDL, HDL.

Interventions

1. Encourage exercise to maintain muscle mass and elevate the lower BMR associated with weight reduction.
2. Suggest practical ways of exercising, i.e., walking to the mailbox or walking to the television to change channels rather than using a remote control box.

Evaluation

* Client exercises 3 times a week.

Client Education

- Consult with physician before starting to exercise.
- Weight loss on a hypokilocaloric diet is enhanced with a regular exercise program (Keim, 1991).
- Exercise is an alternative behavior for eating, prevents boredom, and permits increased energy intake, which improves nutrient adequacy.
- Energy saved by parking the car closer to walk less or watching television an extra half hour instead of a more active pursuit can easily cause a weight gain of 10 to 20 lb/year.
- Because of differences in sex and age as well as duration and intensity, exercise can increase, decrease, or have no effect on food intake.

Behavior Modification

Behavior modification for overeating was developed approximately 20 years ago in response to drop-out rates in reduction programs and dismal results following achievement of weight loss. Data currently suggest one of the most important components of a weight control program is behavior modification through which new ways of dealing with old habits can be learned.

Behavior modification for weight control refers mainly to getting in touch with the reality of actual foods being consumed, quantity, and when and why eating occurs.

TABLE 19–5

BEHAVIOR MODIFICATION TECHNIQUES

1. Eat regularly in the same place
2. Use smaller plates and containers
3. Put down the utensils between each bite
4. Do not watch television or read while eating
5. Take at least 20 minutes to eat each meal
6. Store leftover food immediately to avoid returning for second helpings
7. Buy only appropriate food to have available
8. Arrange an attractive meal and serve it accordingly
9. Sit down to eat
10. Leave a small amount of food on the plate (1 or 2 bites)
11. Do not taste food while preparing; an alternative is to chew gum or brush teeth to help resist temptations

Behavioral interventions are more effective for mildly overweight individuals than for obese individuals. Techniques are enhanced when a comprehensive program includes diet and exercise programs tailored for clients.

The rationale is that major changes in eating and exercise behaviors are necessary for long-term weight control; changes are more effective if preceded by an analysis and understanding of eating patterns. Weight loss should be motivated by internal rather than external reasons. ("I am doing this for myself" rather than "I will lose weight for my son's wedding.")

A diary is kept recording food and emotional status as well as the environment to reveal antecedents for food intake. These records provide new insights and help clients devise strategies for dealing with eating habits. Component techniques include self-monitoring (using an intake diary), stimulus control (antecedents leading to eating), slowing rate of eating, and reinforcement (self-rewards for appropriate eating behaviors). Some techniques used are shown in Table 19–5.

Although behavior modification approaches to weight control have been helpful, maintaining weight loss still remains a problem. Newer programs are longer in duration (20 to 24 weeks) and more comprehensive (Wing et al, 1992). New approaches to maintain weight reduction have been emphasized, such as relapse prevention training, use of social support systems, and posttreatment contacts with the therapist. Clients in group settings are generally more successful at maintaining weight loss than clients seen individually by a counselor.

Describe 3 behavior modification techniques to help clients lose weight. List 3 methods to help clients maintain weight.

Support, understanding, and praise from family and friends are also emphasized. Individuals in reduction programs lose more weight when spouses attend meetings with them and understand the program and reasons for the desire to lose weight. Supportive spouses are less likely to initiate conversations pertaining to food or tempt participants with food or situations likely to induce overeating and are more likely to praise changes in eating habits.

NURSING APPLICATIONS

Assessment

Physical—for type of behavior modification techniques used.
Dietary—for food diary.

Interventions

1. Monitor for internal versus external motivation by having clients verbalize reasons for weight loss.
2. Encourage spouse to attend group sessions; spouses' participation helps them understand the program and be more supportive of the dieter's goals.
3. Explain that weight regain occurs frequently. Encourage participation in re-

lapse prevention training, use of social support systems, and posttreatment contacts with the therapist to prevent weight regain.

Evaluation

* Client adheres to behavior modification techniques and attends relapse prevention training.

Client Education

- Major behavior changes are necessary for long-term weight control; these are more effective if clients analyze and understand their own eating patterns.
- Self-control helps build self-esteem.
- In addition to desirable weight loss, behavior therapy has a decreased attrition rate and usually results in improved psychological traits.
- Change way of thinking: Consider eating as energy intake, while exercise is energy consumption, and cheating is an off-target behavior (Carpenito, 1991).

Use of Drugs

Americans, always looking for a magic pill to cure ailments, frequently use appetite suppressants to lose weight. Indeed, $80 million was spent on appetite suppressants in a 1-year period. Considerable controversy exists over drug use for obesity. Effective in early 1992, the FDA banned use of more than 100 substances in OTC weight control aids (DHHS, 1991). Caffeine, papaya enzymes, alcohol, kelp, guar gum and other bulking agents, and sugars were included in the list of active ingredients deemed ineffective for weight loss. Certain others are still being investigated. Information regarding drugs used for weight control is summarized in Table 19-6. In general, although drugs may be used for weight loss, they are not the sole answer to management of obesity.

Appetite Suppressants

Prescription appetite suppressants include amphetamines, such as Benzedrine and Ionamin, and nonamphetamines, such as fenfluramine (Pondimin). These drugs induce anorexia as a result of their effect on brain catecholamines. Amphetamines also stimulate the CNS, which results in increased motor activity. The euphoriant effect of amphetamines has led to their widespread abuse and dependency by some individuals. Amphetamines can become a crutch in a weight loss program; the FDA recommends that they should be prescribed by physicians only for a short period of time.

Fenfluramine is more effective as an appetite suppressant than amphetamines; it apparently has a depressant effect on the CNS, causing sedation rather than stimulation. However, the effects of depressing or stimulating body metabolism 24 hours a day should be considered.

Phenylpropanolamine (PPA) hydrochloride is widely available in OTC preparations marketed for weight loss, as shown in Table 19-6. Approximately 40% of college women and 6% of men indicated they have taken PPA pills and acknowledged they ignore label recommendations about dosage amounts (Diet pill ingredients, 1991). These drugs may cause **vasoconstriction,** bronchodilation, and tachycardia.

Vasoconstriction—blood vessels become smaller in diameter, leading to elevated blood pressure.

Name 2 appetite suppressants, and describe how they affect the body.

An opioid antagonist, naloxone, has been demonstrated to decrease food intake by approximately one-fourth the normal amount. With increased dosage, hepatic function is adversely affected (Weintraub & Bray, 1989).

TABLE 19–6

PHARMACEUTICAL DIET AIDS

Products	Examples	Action	Comments
Prescription			
Amphetamines and derivatives	Dexedrine Desoxyn Preludin	Pharmacological properties of neurotransmitter, norepinephrine: Stimulates central nervous system Increases motor activity, heart rate, and blood pressure Increases serum triglycerides Suppresses appetite	*Side effects:* May be abused and cause dependency. Insomnia, restlessness, irritability, tremor, excess perspiration, dry mouth, epigastric discomfort, constipation, palpitations *Contraindications:* coronary artery disease, severe hypertension, hyperthyroidism, glaucoma, history of drug abuse
Fenluramine Fluoxetine	Pondimin Prozac	Modulates serotonin metabolism: Reduces physiological activity including food intake	*Side effects:* Mild hypotensive action, dry mouth, drowsiness, lethargy, lightheadedness, diarrhea
Opioid antagonists	Naloxone	Reduces food intake in obese subjects and animals	Large dose may alter hepatic function
Thyroid	Triiodothyronine (T_3)	Prevents decline in metabolic rate that normally occurs with weight loss	Extra weight loss appears to be loss of fat free mass
Ephedrine	Mudrane Primatene	Alpha and beta antagonist; increases energy expenditure (if given orally)	*Side effects:* May increase blood pressure, heart rate, and peripheral vascular resistance; insomnia; and increased nervousness
Diuretics	Diurex	Increases fluid loss; weight loss temporary	*Side effects:* Can cause dehydration, hypokalemia
Over the Counter			
Phenylpropanolamine	Appedrine Dexatrim Dietac Codexin Prolamine	Temporary reduction of appetite	*Side effects:* High doses increase blood pressure in some clients *Contraindicated:* Pregnant and nursing mothers; clients with diabetes, hypertension, or heart, kidney, or thyroid conditions
Benzocaine	Reducets Spanhal Diet-trim	Benzocaine is a local anesthetic that deadens taste buds. May contain a sweetener, thus increasing blood glucose level before meal	Data are limited to demonstrate effectiveness in weight control; no recent safety studies

TABLE 19–6

PHARMACEUTICAL DIET AIDS
Continued

Products	Examples	Action	Comments
Prescription			
Bulking agents or fiber	Pretts Taper	Delays gastric emptying and absorption rate. Creates feeling of fullness and satiety	Clinical usefulness in weight control needed; has not been well researched. Banned by FDA for weight control

Thermogenic Drugs

Large doses of thyroid hormones induce a state of hypermetabolism that results in weight loss. Effects of this hypermetabolism are unknown. Triiodothyronine (T_3) is being used experimentally because low-carbohydrate reduction diets are accompanied by a decreased serum concentration of T_3. The use of T_3 can prevent decreased metabolic rate that accompanies low-kilocalorie diets.

Ephedrine, when administered orally, can increase energy expenditure. Although results of studies have been contradictory, weight loss of asthmatic clients being treated with ephedrine was noted. Ephedrine may mildly affect obese clients who have been unsuccessful with other attempts to lose weight (Pasquali et al, 1987).

Name 2 thermogenic drugs and how they affect the body.

Diuretics

Diuretics are often combined with anorectic agents for weight loss. This results in loss of body fluid but not body fat. Diuretics are rarely indicated physiologically for obesity; however, the rapid weight loss they cause provides a psychological lift. Loss of electrolytes can become a life-threatening situation if a client is fasting; complications occasionally occur when a low-kilocalorie diet is closely followed.

Gastrointestinal Tract Drugs

Benzocaine, long known for its ability to numb pain, is marketed in candies and gum for use before meals to reduce food intake. Appetite is suppressed because of increased blood glucose level and a decreased ability to taste and enjoy food. If the recommended dosage of 2 candies (25 kcal each) is taken before each meal, the additional kilocaloric intake from the candy is about 150 kcal/day.

What does benzocaine do?

NURSING APPLICATIONS

Assessment

Physical—for drugs used (prescribed and OTC).
Dietary—for kilocalories consumed.
Laboratory—for T_3, potassium, sodium.

Interventions

1. Because of side effects of many medications, encourage a client to consult a physician before taking them.
2. Undesirable potential side effects may result from OTC medications; emphasize the importance of following dosage recommendations on the package.

Evaluation

* Client does not use drugs for weight loss unless prescribed by a physician.

Continued

Client Education

- Use of diet pills may prevent a client from attempting lifestyle changes, such as decreasing fat intake and establishing a regular exercise program, which help to prevent relapse.
- Most appetite suppressants result in decreased appetite and weight loss; however, they seem to become less effective with time.
- The same effect could be obtained from the intake of a salad (with no-kilocalorie dressing) or a large glass of tomato juice before a meal as the use of benzocaine-containing candy or gum.

Rx Whenever appetite suppressants or any other drugs for weight loss are prescribed, they should be used in combination with a kilocalorie-restricted diet and behavior modification program for maintenance of weight loss (Stunkard, 1985).

SURGICAL TREATMENT

Gastrointestinal Surgery

Intestinal bypass—bowel is shortened to reduce absorption of ingested kilocalories; gastroplasty—stomach size is decreased to prevent overeating.

Several types of surgical treatment have been used for morbid obesity (Fig. 19–4). Two basic types of surgery have been used: (1) **bypass** and (2) **gastroplasty.** Some metabolic complications are experienced by all clients with surgery for weight loss, but gastroplasty is devoid of long-term metabolic complications (Halverson, 1992). Although the ideal technique is unknown, the surgical treatment currently preferred is vertical banded gastroplasty (VBGP). By limiting stomach capacity, weight loss is greater than with bypass surgeries. This weight loss is maintained in 50 to 60% of clients after 5 to 10 years (Sugerman et al, 1992).

Different criteria are established to determine candidates for bypass surgery. In general, clients are morbidly obese—from 100 to 300 lbs over normal weight (BMI > 40) and may have a high-risk condition such as hypertension or diabetes mellitus (Deitel & Shahi, 1992). Older clients have more difficulty in adjusting to the consequences; therefore, few surgeries are performed on clients over 50 years old. No previous history of liver dysfunction, renal disease, serious myocardial disease, or bowel disease can be present. Figure 19–5 shows a candidate before and after surgery.

Dumping syndrome—rapid emptying of the gastric contents into the intestine, resulting in nausea, weakness, and sweating after eating.

What are the 2 basic surgeries for obese clients? What is the preferred surgery? What are some requirements clients must meet before surgery is performed?

These operations induce weight loss by causing early satiety or food aversions. Some surgeries are associated with early satiety. Also, **dumping syndrome** symptoms lead to an aversion to sweets (Sugerman et al, 1992). If eating habits are not changed, the small stomach pouch or shortened intestinal tract may be stretched enough eventually to permit return to prior weight.

Most subjects benefit from some psychotherapy. Behavior modification techniques start before surgery.

Nutritional Care

For the first 2 months following gastric surgery, the diet is restricted to liquids. The staple line must be protected from disruption by controlling not only consistency, but also volume of liquid and rate of ingestion. When the stomach is reduced to a pouch that holds a volume of 10 to 30 ml with a small stoma diameter of 10 to 12 mm, clients must make drastic changes in eating behavior. A 30-ml medicine cup and a clock help clients realize how small a quantity can be eaten over a period of 30 minutes. A chemically defined formula may be used until regular liquids and pureed foods are tolerated.

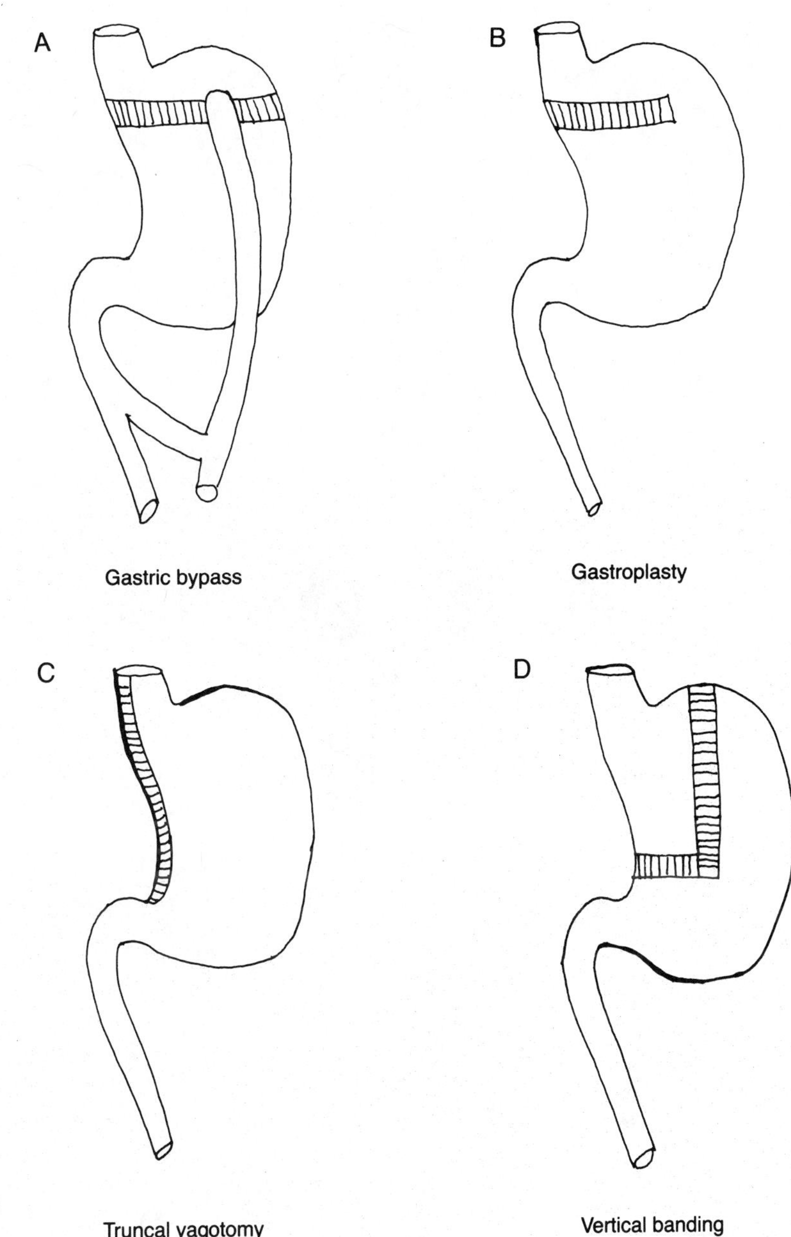

Figure 19–4 Gastric surgeries. *A*, Roux-en-Y gastric bypass. *B*, Horizontal gastroplasty. *C*, Truncal vagotomy. *D*, Vertical banded gastroplasty.

Dietary restrictions are necessary to prevent vomiting and promote weight loss (Kral, 1992). Individuals should avoid soft kilocalorie-dense foods (ice cream, cheese), easily dissolvable foods (cake and cookies), and high-kilocalorie liquids. Obstruction may result from red meat, soft bread, pasta, and citrus membranes. On the other hand, raw vegetables and high protein foods are encouraged. Because of decreased absorption, supplements such as iron, calcium, and vitamins (especially vitamin B_{12}) may be recommended (Kral, 1992). Adequate chewing is important, and foods should not be "flushed" down with liquids. A quiet, relaxed atmosphere for eating is needed.

Weight loss is well tolerated among clients who remain normally nourished (with controlled intake). By contrast, those who become malnourished experience frequent vomiting, or those who lose weight too rapidly after surgery are frequently found to be deficient in thiamin, folate, and vitamin B_{12} (Kral, 1992). Thus, special attention should be given to intakes of these nutrients.

Describe nutritional care for bypass clients.

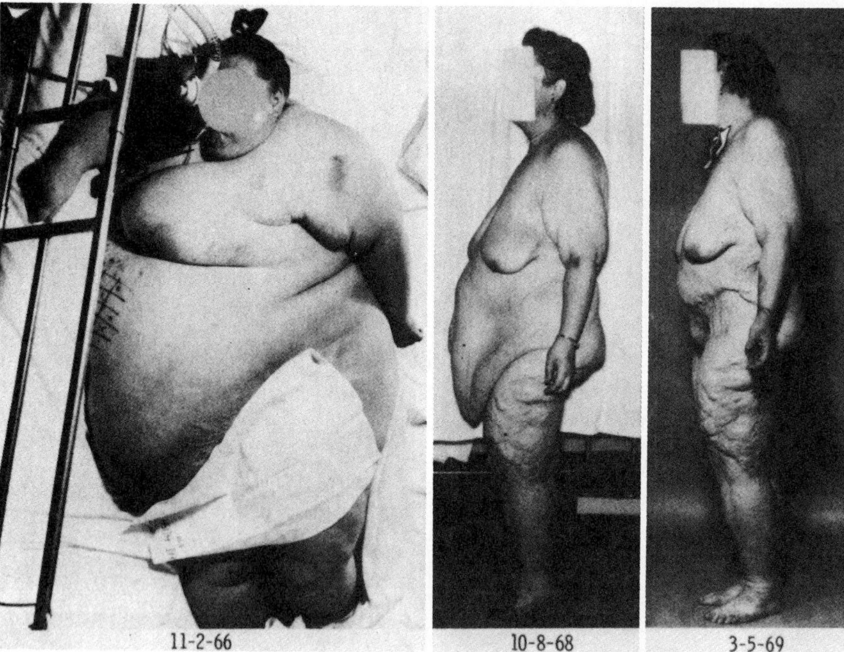

Figure 19–5 This client weighed more than 535 lbs and required respirator assistance for 3 months. Early in 1968, after her weight had been reduced to 330 lbs in the hospital, she had a gastric bypass. In 14 months, she weighed 212 lbs. Her present weight is 229 lbs, and she has had redundant skin removed from the lower abdomen, thighs, and arms. (From Asher WL. *Treating the Obese.* Copyright 1974, Peter G. Lindner, M.D.)

NURSING APPLICATIONS

Assessment

Physical—for type of surgery, vomiting, weight changes.
Dietary—for type of diet ordered; foods allowed and avoided; thiamin, folate, and vitamin B_{12} intake; amount and timing of fluid intake.
Laboratory—for glucose, RBC, Hgb, Hct, MCV, iron, protein, albumin, transferrin, calcium.

Interventions

1. Following surgery, monitor for complications, especially for wound infections and intra-abdominal abscess, incisional hernias, thrombophlebitis, hepatitis, transient gastrojejunostomy obstruction, and atelectasis, which are frequently seen.
2. Monitor for vomiting and diarrhea, which occur if speed of eating or volume eaten is too great. Occasionally these complications may require surgical revision or diet modification.

Evaluation

* Client loses weight and experiences no complications from surgery.

Client Education

- A quiet, relaxed atmosphere for eating is needed.
- Clients must be cautioned to pay attention to feeling satisfied and eating moderate amounts.
- Adequate intake of iron and calcium is necessary to prevent iron and calcium deficiency, respectively.
- Encourage clients (who are not receiving a potassium supplement or have renal disease) to eat foods and drink fluids high in potassium, such as oranges, potatoes, and bananas, to help prevent hypokalemia.
- Clients often are not hungry after the small pouch replaces their normal stomach capacity. They must be cautioned about hypoglycemia and encouraged to consume adequate amounts.
- Increased intake of insoluble fiber is not recommended because of less gastric acid secretion or decreased GI motility, which may lead to impaction.

Other Surgical Techniques

A **balloon procedure,** used to aid weight reduction without open surgery, can be performed in about 10 minutes on an outpatient basis using local anesthesia. The floating balloon in the stomach causes a full feeling when small amounts of food are consumed. This procedure can irritate stomach linings and cause perforations and stomach ulcerations and intestinal blockages. Best results are obtained when treatment is coupled with dietary modification, but energy deficient diets may result in just as much weight loss (Geliebter et al, 1991).

Balloon procedure—a deflated balloon is inserted through the client's throat into the stomach and inflated to the size of a grapefruit.

Lipectomy can remove small to modest amounts of adipose tissue, but not enough fat can be removed to affect obesity significantly. Lipectomy is best when used to remove localized unsightly adiposity. Adverse results include dimpling or wavy contour and infections and possible death. Long-term results of this procedure are unknown.

Liposuction or suction-assisted lipectomy is a relatively new procedure to remove local fat deposits.

What complications can occur with balloon procedure or lipectomy?

NURSING APPLICATIONS

Assessment

Physical—for type of surgery performed; other health conditions.
Dietary—for food/nutrient/kilocaloric intake.

Interventions

1. After liposuction, encourage iron-rich foods to promote hemoglobin synthesis since blood may be lost during the procedure.

Client Education

- Avoid coffee, alcohol, tobacco, and aspirin because the first 3 items are gastric irritants, and aspirin may cause gastric bleeding.

PREVENTION OF OBESITY (IN CHILDHOOD)

The more information gained about the effects of overweight, the more imperative preventing obesity becomes. Childhood-onset obesity is recognized as a serious disease with potential implications for morbidity and mortality in adulthood. The longer a child is obese, the greater the risk of a weight problem during adulthood. An obese preschooler has a 25% chance of being an overweight adult, whereas an obese 13-year-old has a 75% chance of remaining obese as an adult. The first step in preventing obesity is early control of excessive weight during childhood. If accelerated weight gain is arrested, hyperplasia may be controlled. Therefore, if a child has one or both obese parent(s) and is gaining weight at the 95th percentile without proportionate height, intervention at an early age may be warranted.

According to a National Health and Nutrition Examination Survey, prevalence of obesity increased by 54% among 6- to 11-year-olds and 39% among 12- to 17-year olds between 1963 and 1980 (Gortmaker et al, 1987). Not only are numbers of obese children increasing, but also children are getting fatter.

Childhood obesity has been attributed to lifestyle, with dietary intake being the major factor. As intake has increased with greater food availability, physical inactivity has increased, with more time spent in front of the television.

Prevention of obesity requires an environment that encourages individuals and families to adopt appropriate eating and exercise habits (ADA, 1989). The child or his or her problem with fat should not be singled out. The whole family should be given the same selections, not providing high kilocalorie snacks and desserts for some, with fruit being provided for the overweight child. Special attention only angers and humiliates obese children. Children should eat 3 meals and several snacks daily. At least one regular family meal daily provides an opportunity for children to learn good eating habits. Mealtime should be an enjoyable, social occasion, and parents can play an important role by setting a good example. Parents must be instigators of weight control among their children to avoid problems of obesity as these children mature.

Severely restricting kilocaloric intake is not advisable for obese children. The demand for nutrients must be met to ensure normal growth and development. Usually the goal is to maintain weight or reduce rate of weight gain. Weight maintenance during increases in height results in a decrease in percentage of body fat without compromising lean body mass and growth. Additionally, encouragement from parents for the child to be physically active as well as role modeling is important. Physical activity in childhood may help develop a lifelong commitment to physical exercise. Exercise programs are planned to expend 300 kcal per session. This may mean twice as much activity as is recommended for adults because of lower body mass. Initially activities considered to be fun are encouraged until the child gains confidence in his or her ability to exercise (Parker & Bar-Or, 1991).

What is the first step in preventing obesity? What is the goal for obese children? What type of behavioral program produced good results?

Some weight control programs are available for children using behavioral approaches to promote healthy eating and activity patterns. In a 10-year follow-up study of a behavioral, family-based treatment for obese children, Epstein et al (1990) found significantly greater decreases in percentage of overweight children in the group in which both parent and child were reinforced for behavior change and weight loss. Although obese parents regained their weight lost during treatment, their children did not. This may have been related to shorter history of habits resulting in obesity that permitted children to be more responsive to treatment than adults (Stunkard & Berkowitz, 1990).

NURSING APPLICATIONS

Assessment

Physical—for age in relation to anticipated growth spurt; percentile on growth chart; family's view of obesity.

Dietary—for client/family beliefs and knowledge of nutrition.

Interventions

1. Monitor family history; graph height and weight for children to detect abnormal growth rates so intervention may be implemented before obesity develops.
2. Stress appropriate eating and exercise habits.

Evaluation

* Child "grows" into height with no undue weight gain.

Client Education

- Offer praise or hugs instead of food for rewards.
- High-kilocalorie treats or occasional visits to fast-food restaurants should not be banned, but their frequency is limited.
- Healthy snack foods should be readily available.
- Discourage low nutrient dense foods (carbonated beverages, chips, candy).

WEIGHT GAIN

In contrast to the abundance of information regarding obesity, very little information is published for clients who need to gain weight. Acute weight loss may be a symptom of disease and should be investigated medically.

The theory of an appestat or a setpoint gains favor among naturally thin clients who experience difficulties in changing their weight no matter what they eat. Gaining and maintaining weight is as difficult for them as it is for an obese client to lose and maintain weight loss.

For thin individuals who want to gain weight, many tips for weight reduction can be reversed. However, the goal is to increase muscle mass as well as body fat. For this reason, exercise should be a vital part of the program. Nervous tension can use many kilocalories and should be minimized.

An allowance of 500 to 1000 kcal/day is gradually added to an individual's kilocaloric intake, based on current body weight and ability to tolerate increased amounts of food. Kilocalorically dense foods are provided using nuts, gravies, sauces, homogenized milk, and ice cream. Broth-type soups and large amounts of low-kilocalorie salads are held to a minimum. Portions at mealtime are increased as tolerated with supplemental feedings between meals, but so as to not interfere with mealtime appetite. Other effective tips are given in Table 19–7.

Why is exercise important for clients trying to gain weight?

NURSING APPLICATIONS

Assessment

Physical—for BMIs <20 for men or 19 for women; weight; exercise habits.
Dietary—for kilocalorie intake.

Interventions

1. Help client deal with nervous tension, which can be an inefficient drain on kilocaloric utilization.

Evaluation

* Client should gain weight to desirable body weight.

Client Education

- Eat frequently but not so much as to affect mealtime appetite.
- Incorporate kilocalorie-dense foods into meals.

TABLE 19–7

PRINCIPLES FOR WEIGHT GAIN

1. Do not drink before a meal; minimize fluid intake with meals
2. Include a large meal for supper and a snack before bedtime
3. Increase the fat portion of the diet to 30 or 35% of total kilocalories
4. Eat nutrient-dense foods first during a meal, then foods containing fewer kilocalories (e.g., soup and salad)
5. Eat quickly, but chew the food well. Do not gulp the food down, but do not loiter
6. Use sauces and gravies as well as embellishments such as nuts, olives, jams, jellies, margarine, and mayonnaise
7. Do not engage in needless nervous activities, but exercise to stimulate appetite and build body muscle
8. Snack frequently on energy-dense foods such as dried fruits and nuts. However, snacking should not interfere with meals

SUMMARY

Obesity is a complex problem that causes great pain, misery, and ill health. It must be regarded as life-threatening. Prevention of obesity begins early in life. Overfeeding young children and/or teenagers leads to increased numbers of fat cells (hyperplasia) throughout life. Excessive food intake later in life leads to increased size of fat cells (hypertrophy). The main emphasis for weight control should be prevention rather than cure.

Education is imperative to understand the relationship between energy intake from various foods and weight changes. Behavior modification is usually the key for clients making appropriate adjustments in their food choices. Exercise is imperative, not merely physical exercise, such as games and sports, but being more active throughout the day. Nurses have an important role in assisting clients to lose weight effectively and safely.

Weight gain can be just as frustrating as weight loss. Nurses can provide assistance and information to clients to help them gain weight effectively and safely.

NURSING PROCESS IN ACTION

An obese client is admitted to lose weight. He does not exercise but does want to lose weight so he will not have to have an "operation."

Nutritional Assessment

- Height, weight, IBW, BMI, waist-hip ratio.
- Previous methods used to lose weight.
- Motivation level.
- Food/nutrient/kilocalorie intake.
- Eating habits.
- Support from family, significant others.
- Cholesterol, protein, transferrin, potassium, sodium, triglycerides, glucose.

Dietary Nursing Diagnosis

Altered nutrition: More than body requirements RT excessive kilocalorie intake in relation to energy expenditure.

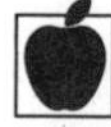

Nutritional Goals

Client will lose 2 lbs/week until DBW is attained.

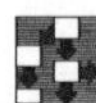

Nutritional Implementation

Intervention: Assist with food diary.

Rationale: A food diary helps client become aware of eating patterns and antecedents that precede eating.

Intervention: Offer diet that allows high intake of complex carbohydrate and fiber and reduced intake of fat and kilocalories.

Rationale: Complex carbohydrate and fiber are effective in a weight loss program by increasing satiety and discouraging binge eating. Fat reduction enhances weight loss because kilocaloric intake is closely associated with the amount of total fat intake. A deficit of 3500 kcal is needed to lose 1 lb.

Intervention: Suggest simple exercises such as walking.

Rationale: Treatment of obesity is improved when energy expenditure is increased along with decreased kilocaloric intake.

Intervention: Suggest support groups such as Weight Watchers, Overeaters Anonymous, and Take Off Pounds Sensibly (TOPS).

Rationale: Clients in group settings are generally more successful at maintaining weight loss than clients seen individually by a counselor.

Intervention: Discuss benefits of weight loss.

Rationale: Understanding physiological benefits of weight loss can be motivating for some clients.

Intervention: Refer to a dietitian.

Rationale: Dietitian's knowledge and expertise is needed to reduce weight safely and effectively.

Intervention: Discourage yo-yoing.

Rationale: Yo-yoing may contribute to more health problems.

Intervention: Collaborate with client to develop a plan incorporating diet, exercise, and behavior modification.

Rationale: This combination of therapies has proved more effective for long-term weight control.

Intervention: Indicate how his weight loss is preventing surgery.

Rationale: He does not want surgery, so this may be a motivating factor.

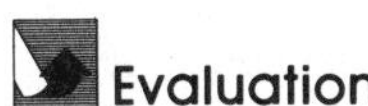

Evaluation

Client lost 2 lbs/week, and surgery was avoided.

STUDENT READINESS

1. Outline a discussion with the mother of an obese child for future guidelines to achieve normal weight.
2. List some ways that friends might sabotage your reduction program if you were trying to lose weight.
3. Offer some defenses by role playing clients can use when friends or family appear to be sabotaging efforts to lose weight.

4. Plan a 1200 kcal/day diet for a woman who works outside the home.
5. Suggest activities for clients 10, 25, 50, and 70 years old to lose 1 lb/week.
6. Using a typical restaurant menu, tell how to keep the kilocalorie count down while participating in a dinner with friends.

CASE STUDY

Mrs. J. T. is a 38-year-old homemaker who has been referred for diet counseling. Her height is 156 cm and her current weight is 127 kg. She has been overweight since childhood and has tried a variety of diets with varying degrees of success; however, weight loss has never been maintained. She states that with 4 children, 2 of whom are teenagers, it is difficult to cook low-kilocalorie meals. She enjoys cooking and seems to spend much of her time involved with meal preparation.

Over the past 2 years, she has been less active and has been snacking throughout the day. She is frustrated by her weight problem and concerned about her health after hypertension was diagnosed at her latest physical examination.

1. What should be Mrs. J. T.'s desirable body weight for a medium frame?
2. What type of data do you need to collect for a nutritional assessment of this client?
3. What nursing diagnoses can be developed for this client? Identify appropriate goals.
4. Determine Mrs. J. T.'s daily kilocaloric needs.
5. Outline a diet plan for 1 day for Mrs. J. T.
6. What complications are frequently found among clients who are chronically obese?

CASE STUDY

Shanna P. is a 13-year-old who was brought to the physician's office for a yearly physical examination. Her weight at this time is 90.7 kg and height is 174.8 cm.

Questions by the nurse indicate that Shanna has always been overweight but has gained approximately 25 lbs since starting junior high school. She is a finicky eater and refuses many meat and vegetable dishes. She does not exercise except in physical education class and spends most of her time at home watching television. All laboratory work was normal, but her blood pressure was elevated (130/88).

Exogenous obesity with hypertension is diagnosed, and the client and her family are referred for dietary counseling.

1. Why are the early adolescent years so important for weight?
2. What other times in the life cycle is excess weight a particular problem?
3. What factors may have prompted the development of this child's obesity?

4. What should she weigh?
5. What tentative nursing diagnoses could you develop?
6. List goals for this client.
7. Develop a diet plan for Shanna.
8. Plan a day's menu of low-kilocaloric foods that would be acceptable for most adolescents.

REFERENCES

American Dietetic Association (ADA). Position of the American Dietetic Association: Very-low-calorie weight loss diets. *J Am Diet Assoc* 1990 May; 90(5):722–726.

American Dietetic Association (ADA). Position of the American Dietetic Association: Optimal weight as a health promotion strategy. *J Am Diet Assoc* 1989 Dec; 89(12):1814–1817.

American Medical Association (AMA) Council on Scientific Affairs. Treatment of obesity in adults. *JAMA* 1988 Nov 4; 260(17):2547–2551.

Anderson JW, et al. Safety and effectiveness of a multidisciplinary very-low-calorie diet program for selected obese individuals. *J Am Diet Assoc* 1991 Dec; 91(12):1582–1584.

Astrup A, et al. Dietary fibre added to very-low-calorie diet reduces hunger and alleviates constipation. *Int J Obesity* 1990 Feb; 14(2):102–112.

Ballard-Barbash R, et al. Body fat distribution and breast cancer in the Framingham study. *J Natl Cancer Inst* 1990 Feb 21; 82(4):286–290.

Bjorntorp P. Regional patterns of fat distribution. *Ann Intern Med* 1985; 103(suppl 6 pt 2):994–995.

Bray GA. Obesity. *In* Brown ML, ed. *Present Knowledge in Nutrition.* Washington, DC, Nutrition Foundation, 1990: 23–38.

Bray GA. Nutrient balance and obesity: Classification and evaluation of the obesities. *Med Clin North Am* 1989 Jan; 73(1):29–45.

Brownell K. The yo-yo trap. *Am Health* 1988 March; 7(3):78–84.

Brownell KD. Obesity and weight control: The good and the bad of dieting. *Nutr Today* 1987 May–June; 22(3):4–9.

Burgess NS. Effect of a very-low-calorie diet on body composition and resting metabolic rate in obese men and women. *J Am Diet Assoc* 1991 Apr; 91(4):430–434.

Byerly L, et al. *Popular Diets—How They Rate.* 2nd ed. Santa Monica, California Dietetic Association, Los Angeles District, 1987.

Carpenito LJ. *Nursing Care Plans and Documentation: Nursing Diagnosis and Collaborative Problems.* Philadelphia, JB Lippincott, 1991.

Colditz CA. Economic costs of obesity. *Am J Clin Nutr* 1992 Feb; 55(suppl 2):503S–507S.

Deitl M, Shahi B. Morbid obesity: Selection of patients for surgery. *Am Coll Nutr* 1992 Sept—Oct; 11(4):457–462.

Department of Health and Human Services (DHHS). Weight control drug products for over-the-counter human use; certain active ingredients; final rule. *Fed Reg* (21 CFR Part 310), August 8, 1991.

Diet pill ingredients deemed losers. *Tufts University Diet and Nutrition Letter* 1991 Dec; 9(10):1–2.

Eckel RH. Lipoprotein lipase. A multifunctional enzyme relevant to common metabolic diseases. *N Engl J Med* 1989 Apr 20; 320(16):1060–1068.

Epstein LH, et al. Ten-year follow-up of behavioral, family-based treatment for obese children. *JAMA* 1990 Nov 21; 264(19):2519–2523.

Foster GD, et al. A controlled comparison of three very-low-calorie diets: Effects on weight, body composition and symptoms. *Am J Clin Nutr* 1992 Feb; 55(2):811–817.

Foster GD, et al. A controlled trial of the metabolic effects of a very-low-calorie diet: Short- and long-term effects. *Am J Clin Nutr* 1990 Feb; 51(2):167–172.

Geliebter A, et al. Clinical trial of silicone-rubber gastric balloon to treat obesity. *Int J Obesity* 1991 Apr; 15(4):259–266.

Goldsmith MF. Heart disease researchers tailor new theories—now maybe it's genes that make people fat. *JAMA* 1990 Jan 5; 263(1):17–18.

Gortmaker SL, et al. Increasing pediatric obesity in the United States. *Am J Dis Child* 1987 May; 141(5):535-540.

Halverson JD. Metabolic risk of obesity surgery and long-term follow-up. *Am J Clin Nutr* 1992 Feb; 55(suppl 2):602S-605S.

Harris RB. Role of set-point theory in regulation of body weight. *FASEB J* 1990 Dec; 4(15): 3310-3318.

Heshka S, et al. Weight loss and change in resting metabolic rate. *Am J Clin Nutr* 1990 Dec; 52(6):981-986.

Kanai H, et al. Close correlation of intra-abdominal fat accumulation to hypertension in obese women. *Hypertension* 1990 Nov; 16(5): 484-490.

Keim N. Physiological and biochemical variables associated with body fat loss in overweight women. *Int J Obesity* 1991 Apr; 15(4):283-293.

Kendall A, et al. Weight loss on a low-fat diet: Consequences of the imprecision of the control of food intake in humans. *Am J Clin Nutr* 1991 May; 53(5):1124-1129.

Kissileff HR, et al. Acute effects of exercise on food intake in obese and non-obese women. *Am J Clin Nutr* 1990 Aug; 52(2):240-245.

Kral JG. Overview of surgical techniques for treating obesity. *Am J Clin Nutr* 1992 Feb; 55(suppl 2):552S-555S.

Kuczmarski RJ. Relevance of overweight and weight gain in the United States. *Am J Clin Nutr* 1992 Feb; 55(suppl 2):495S-502S.

Lichtman SW, et al. Discrepancy between self-reported and actual caloric intake and exercise in obese subjects. *New Engl J Med* 1992 Dec 31; 327(27):1893-1898.

Lissner L, et al. Variability of body weight and health outcomes in the Framingham population. *N Engl J Med* 1991 June 27; 324(26): 1839-1844.

Miles C. The metabolizable energy of diets differing in dietary fat and fiber measured in humans. *J Nutr* 1992 Feb; 122(2):306-311.

National Institutes of Health (NIH) Technology Assessment Conference Panel. Methods for voluntary weight loss and control. *Ann Intern Med* 1992 June 1; 116(11):942-949.

Nelson KM, et al. Effect of weight reduction on resting energy expenditure, substrate utilization, and the thermic effect of food in moderately obese women. *Am J Clin Nutr* 1992 March, 55(3):924-993.

Nieman DC, et al. The effects of moderate exercise training on nutrient intake in mildly obese women. *J Am Diet Assoc* 1990 Oct; 90(11): 1557-1562.

Parker D, Bar-Or O. Juvenile obesity. The importance of exercise and getting children to do it. *Physician Sportsmed* 1991 June; 19(6):113-119, 125.

Pasquali R, et al. Does ephedrine promote weight loss in low-energy-adapted obese women? *Int J Obesity* 1987; 11(2):163-168.

Phinney SD, et al. The transient hypercholesterolemia of major weight loss. *Am J Clin Nutr* 1991 June; 53(6):1404-1410.

Pi-Sunyer FX. Obesity. *In* Shils ME et al, eds. *Modern Nutrition in Health and Disease.* Philadelphia, Lea & Febiger, 1988:795-816.

Poissonnet CM, et al. Growth and development of adipose tissue. *J Pediatr* 1988 July; 113(7):1-9.

Prewitt TE, et al. Changes in body weight, body composition, and energy intake in women fed high- and low-fat diets. *Am J Clin Nutr* 1991 Aug; 54(2):304-310.

Schapira DV, et al. Upper body fat distribution and endometrial cancer risk. *JAMA* 1991 Oct 2; 266(13):1808-1811.

Schlundt DG, et al. The role of breakfast in the treatment of obesity: A randomized clinical trial. *Am J Clin Nutr* 1992 Feb; 55(2):645-651.

Segal KR, et al. Lean body mass estimation by bioelectrical impedance analysis: A four-site cross-validation study. *Am J Clin Nutr* 1988 Jan; 47(1):7-14.

Sheppard L, et al. Weight loss in women participating in a randomized trial of low-fat diets. *Am J Clin Nutr* 1991 Nov; 54(5):821-828.

Sjöström LV. Mortality of severely obese subjects. *Am J Clin Nutr* 1992 Feb; 55(suppl 2):516S-523S.

Spielman AB, et al. The cost of losing: An analysis of commercial weight loss programs in a Metropolitan area. *Am Coll Nutr* 1992 Feb; 11(1):36-41.

Stunkard AJ. Behavioral management of obesity. *Med J Aust* 1985 Apr 1; 142(suppl 2):13S-20S.

Stunkard AJ, Berkowitz RI. Treatment of obesity in children. *JAMA* 1990 Nov 21; 264(19):2550-2551.

Stunkard AJ, et al. The body mass index of twins who have been reared apart. *N Engl J Med* 1990 May 24; 322(21):1483-1487.

Sugerman HJ, et al. Gastric bypass for treating severe obesity. *Am J Clin Nutr* 1922 Feb; 55(suppl 2):560S-566S.

Thompson CJ, et al. Central adipose distribution is related to coronary atherosclerosis. *Arteriosclerosis Thrombosis* 1991 March-Apr; 11(2): 327-333.

Thompson T. Diets shape up. *Health* 1990 May; 22(5):51-53.

United States Department of Agriculture (USDA) and United States Department of Health and Human Services (USDHHS). *Nutrition and Your Health: Dietary Guidelines for Americans.* 3rd ed. Home and Garden Bulletin No. 232, Washington, DC, Governmental Printing Office, 1990.

United States Department of Health and Human Services (USDHHS), Public Health Service. *Healthy People 2000.* National Health Promotion and Disease Prevention Objectives. Washington, DC, Superintendent of Documents, 1990.

Wadden TA, et al. Long-term effects of dieting on resting metabolic rate in obese outpatients. *JAMA* 1990 Aug. 264(6):707–711.

Weigle DS. Human obesity. Exploding the myths. *West J Med* 1990 Oct; 153(4):421–428.

Weintraub M, Bray GA. Drug treatment of obesity. *Med Clin North Am* 1989 Jan; 73(1):237–249.

Wing RR, et al. Behavioral treatment of severe obesity. *Am J Clin Nutr* 1992 Feb; 55(suppl 2):545S–551S.

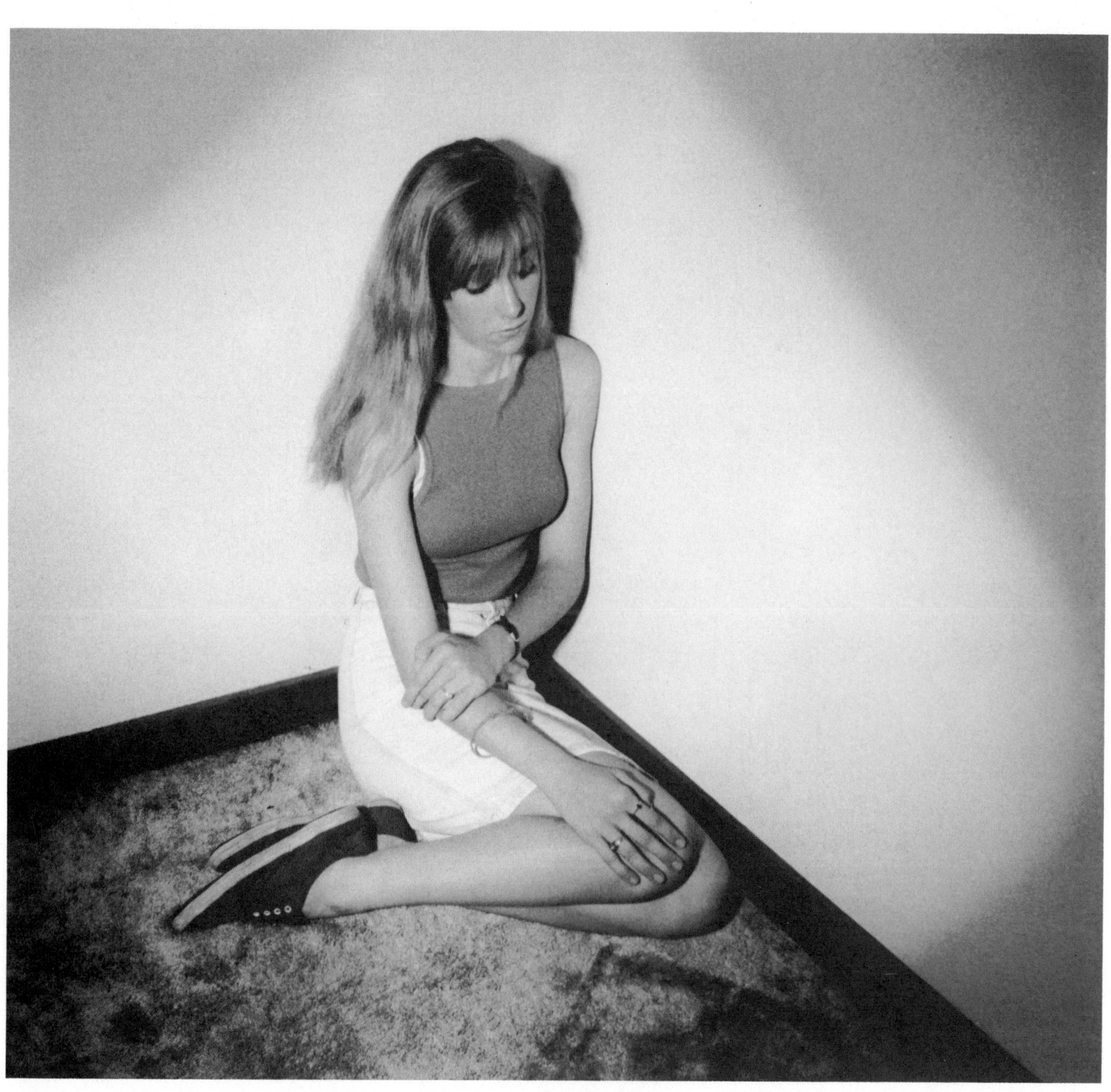

CHAPTER 20

Nutrition Support for Mental Health Alterations

OUTLINE

I. ROLE OF NUTRIENTS ON BRAIN FUNCTIONING
  A. Nutrient Precursors to Neurotransmitters
  B. Nutrient Deficiencies
II. ANOREXIA NERVOSA
  A. Theories
    1. Family Relationships
    2. Biological Factors
  B. Characteristics
  C. Nutritional Effects of Anorexia Nervosa
  D. Nutritional Effects of Therapies
  E. Nutritional Assessment
  F. Nutritional Care
    1. Goals
    2. Treatment Modalities
    3. Promoting Intake
    4. Nutritional Counseling
  Nursing Applications
III. BULIMIA
  A. Theories
    1. Family Relationships
    2. Biological Factors
  B. Characteristics
  C. Nutritional Effects of Bulimia
  D. Nutritional Effects of Therapies
  E. Nutritional Assessment
  F. Nutritional Care
    1. Goals
    2. Treatment Modalities
    3. Preventing Binging/Purging
    4. Nutritional Counseling
  Nursing Applications
IV. CHEMICAL DEPENDENCY
  A. Nutritional Effects of Chemical Dependency
    1. Alcohol
    2. Cocaine/Crack
    3. Marijuana
    4. Heroin
  B. Nutritional Effects of Therapies
  C. Nutritional Assessment

D. Nutritional Care
1. Detoxification
2. Goals
3. Promoting Normal Eating Patterns
4. Nutritional Counseling

Nursing Applications

V. SCHIZOPHRENIA
A. Theories
B. Nutritional Effects of Schizophrenia
1. Decreased Intake
2. Protein Energy Malnutrition
3. Increased Water Intake
C. Nutritional Effects of Therapy
D. Nutritional Assessment
E. Nutritional Care

Nursing Applications

VI. DEPRESSION
A. Nutritional Effects of Depression
B. Nutritional Effects of Therapies
1. Tricyclics
2. Monoamine Oxides Inhibitors
3. Atypical Antidepressants
4. Electroconvulsive Therapy
C. Nutritional Assessment
D. Nutritional Care

Nursing Applications

VII. MANIA
A. Nutritional Effects of Mania
B. Nutritional Effects of Therapy
1. Lithium
2. Tegretol
3. Depakene/Depakote
C. Nutritional Assessment
D. Nutritional Care

Nursing Applications

OBJECTIVES

THE STUDENT WILL BE ABLE TO:

- Discuss nutritional effects of various mental health alterations.
- Describe nutritional effects of pharmacological therapies used for treatment of mental health alterations.
- Discuss nutritional assessment for mental health alterations.
- Describe nutritional care for mental health alterations.
- Identify nutritional principles related to mental health alterations for client education.
- Apply nursing application principles for clients with mental health alterations.

TEST YOUR NQ (True/False)

1. A carbohydrate-rich meal increases brain levels of tryptophan.
2. The typical anorectic client is an achievement-oriented young woman.
3. Clients with anorexia are prone to hyperkalemia.
4. Folate levels are high in clients with bulimia.
5. Vitamin requirements, particularly for B complex vitamins, are higher in alcohol-dependent clients than in nonalcoholics.

6. Cocaine users may have high physiological levels of vitamin A.
7. Cough mixtures are advocated for clients taking disulfiram.
8. When caring for a schizophrenic client, the nurse should taste the food to demonstrate it is not poisoned.
9. A hypertensive crisis can occur if a client is taking monoamine oxidase inhibitors and consumes cheese.
10. If sodium intake is low or restricted, lithium excretion decreases.

ROLE OF NUTRIENTS ON BRAIN FUNCTIONING

For centuries, food intake has been thought to influence mental well-being and behavioral functioning. Indeed, malnutrition during critical periods of rapid brain growth (prenatally and postnatally) has resulted in irreversible impairment of brain growth and function as well as behavioral and emotional deficits.

Nutrient Precursors to Neurotransmitters

Three amino acids (tryptophan, tyrosine, and choline) typically found in protein foods are precursors for **neurotransmitters;** vitamins also have essential roles as enzymes in neurotransmitter formation. Foods also contain neurotransmitters; gamma-aminobutyric acid (GABA), an amino acid, is an example. Thus, diet may influence or change the amount of neurotransmitters released from neurons.

Neurotransmitters are chemical links for communication of neurons.

Tryptophan, readily available in milk, is necessary for synthesis of serotonin, a neurotransmitter that affects food selection, pain sensitivity, sleep, mood (depression), and behavior (aggression). Pyridoxine (vitamin B_6) is involved in this reaction. Surprisingly, a carbohydrate-rich meal, not a protein-rich meal, increases brain levels of tryptophan and promotes serotonin synthesis. Carbohydrate intake causes tryptophan to bind with the carbohydrate to form a carbohydrate-tryptophan combination, thereby resulting in increased transport of tryptophan into the brain because carbohydrate (glucose) is the brain's preferred source of energy. In contrast, protein-rich meals tend to diminish serotonin production because other amino acids supplied by the meal compete with tryptophan for uptake into the brain. Tryptophan therapy may have a role in treatment of depression, but thus far, trials have resulted in inconsistent results.

Tyrosine is needed for synthesis of catecholamine neurotransmitters: dopamine, epinephrine, and norepinephrine. Additionally, vitamin C and copper play key roles in this conversion. Depression or mild Parkinson's disease may benefit from tyrosine supplementation.

Choline, found in liver, oatmeal, soybeans, cauliflower, cabbage, or lecithin, is necessary for synthesis of acetylcholine, the neurotransmitter affected in Alzheimer's dementia. Thiamin is needed for acetylcholine synthesis.

An amino acid neurotransmitter called GABA has been implicated in development of anxiety. Antianxiety drugs decrease anxiety by altering GABA functioning.

Nutrient Deficiencies

Deficiencies of various minerals and vitamins have been linked to mental symptoms. Poor diets can result in a deficiency of any of these nutrients, but more frequently, more than one is in short supply.

Clinical iron deficiency alters synaptic sensitivity to dopamine and serotonin, resulting in altered cerebral function. Magnesium and zinc deficiencies have been associated with depression.

Wernicke's encephalopathy and Korsakoff's psychosis are associated with thiamin deficiency. Additionally, thiamin restriction can lead to depression, irritability, aggressive behavior, and personality changes; low thiamin levels are observed in the schizophrenic and alcohol-dependent client. Thiamin deficiency may be secondary to anorexia (Carney, 1990).

Riboflavin and pyridoxine deficiencies, which normally occur concurrently, have been associated with depression (McLaren, 1988). These deficiencies are generally associated with undernutrition rather than a particular drug or alcohol intake. Pyridoxine has been effective in relieving depression in women with pyridoxine deficiency caused by oral contraceptives.

Vitamin B_{12} deficiency is associated with mental changes, organic psychosis, peripheral neuropathy, and affective disorders.

Folate deficiency has been observed in dementia; many geriatric clients have been diagnosed with senility when the true problem was inadequate amounts of folate. Many alcohol-dependent clients have depressed folate levels, but this also occurs in clients with mania and schizophrenia (Carney, 1990). Folate deficiency is frequently found in depression (Godfrey et al, 1990). Numerous antifolate drugs (methotrexate, trimethoprim, triamterene, anticonvulsants, antituberculous drugs, alcohol, and oral contraceptives) have been reported to cause depression. Folate repletion has been effective in improving mental status secondary to depression and decreasing hospitalization.

What type of diet increases serotonin synthesis and why? What nutrients are needed for synthesis of catecholamine neurotransmitters? What can thiamin deficiency cause? How can a lack of vitamin B_{12}, folate, and vitamin C affect mental functioning?

Specific mental changes, i.e., lassitude and depression, may appear with vitamin C deficiency. Personality changes have also been reported.

The brain is sensitive to food consumption, which alters neurotransmitter levels. In general, changes in brain chemistry are observed only when meals are rich in carbohydrate-containing foods. When a meal contains a mixture of protein and carbohydrate, little or no change in brain biochemistry is anticipated. Chronic dietary choices that are deficient in vitamins and minerals affect neurotransmitters, but meal to meal variations do not.

ANOREXIA NERVOSA

Although anorexia nervosa (AN) appears primarily in adolescent girls, this disorder can affect adolescent boys and middle-aged men and women as well. Approximately 10% of AN clients are male.

What do AN clients fear?

Clients with AN have an exaggerated, intense fear of becoming fat. Thus, zealous self-imposed dieting leads to extreme weight loss. This dieting is frequently accompanied by excessive physical activity. Since these individuals deny that an illness exists, they do not seek professional or medical help on their own.

Theories

Body image—how people view their physical self.

AN is not merely an illness of weight and appetite; it is a psychological problem relating to inner doubts and lack of appropriate **body image**. There is no one known, accepted theory for the cause of AN; most health care professionals believe this disease is a multifaceted problem. Edelstein et al (1989) have proposed that anorexia may be an early stage of bulimia since as many as 50% of anorexics often develop bulimia, and 20% of bulimics began with AN.

Family Relationships

Family interrelationships are frequently significant contributing factors. Overachieving parents can influence a child's behavior in many ways. Regardless of whether the parents' goal is perfectionism in the child, a perfect child makes them look like ideal parents, which can develop into strong interdependent roles. Families are generally close-knit. A client with AN usually has conflict issues related to separation from the family. Clients whose families have a history of eating disorders or of alcohol abuse have an increased risk for developing AN (Edelstein et al, 1989). Valuable information for nurses regarding these clients and their families may be found in the book *The Golden Cage* by Hilda Bruch (1978).

What types of families may lead to AN?

Biological Factors

AN may be caused by a disturbance in the hypothalamic–anterior pituitary–gonadal axis (Fava et al, 1989). However, this disturbance may be a result of malnutrition. A self-perpetuating vicious downhill spiral develops in susceptible clients: Dieting causes weight loss, which leads to hypometabolism and further dieting.

Mood, appetite, and behavior may affect endocrine functioning, causing a disturbance that predisposes clients to AN (Williamson, 1990). Luteinizing hormone is decreased to a prepubescent level in AN clients. This low level may possibly cause the amenorrhea frequently observed. Amenorrhea that develops secondary to self-starvation disrupts hypothalamus functioning. Lack of appetite stimulation progresses to a total lack of hunger stimulation (Palmer, 1990). In other words, these clients do not eat because stimulation of hunger centers is depresssed. Increased serotonin activity could possibly be a contributing factor to the restricted eating and obsessive behaviors in this illness (Kaye & Weltzin, 1991).

Too much secretion of cortisol may lead to AN. Excess cortisol adversely affects the hypothalamus, causing a decrease in hunger stimulation. Depression, which also may be a result of excessive cortisol secretion, causes decreased appetite and weight loss (Palmer, 1990).

The GI tract itself may also cause a predisposition for AN. Previous GI disturbances in infancy and childhood are likely in AN clients. Slow gastric emptying has also been observed. These 2 irregularities may sensitize a client's awareness of gastric fullness and discomfort, thereby leading to less intake.

Describe biological theories for AN.

Characteristics

Typical clients with AN may be described as achievement-oriented perfectionists, who seek to rule their life by controlling their body through refusing to eat. These young individuals, generally surrounded with all the evidences of success, become, as Sir Richard Morton described in 1689, "skeletons only clad with skin" (Bruch, 1978), as shown in Figure 20–1.

Anorectic clients often take over the kitchen, cooking and feeding others but eating very little or nothing. Compulsive behaviors may include cutting food into tiny pieces before eating or routinely eating at the same time of day (Edelstein et al, 1989). Clients with AN may become excellent gourmet cooks, spending hours planning menus, finding special recipes, and shopping for exotic ingredients. In-depth knowledge of nutritional and kilocaloric value of foods is commonly exhibited by clients. Other behaviors are listed in Table 20–1.

Depression, difficulty in falling asleep, early morning waking, and decreased libido may also occur. Nearly 1 out of 4 AN clients attempts suicide, a signal of their disturbed condition.

Describe a typical anorectic. List criteria for a diagnosis of AN.

Criteria for a diagnosis of AN include a weight loss equal to or exceeding 15%

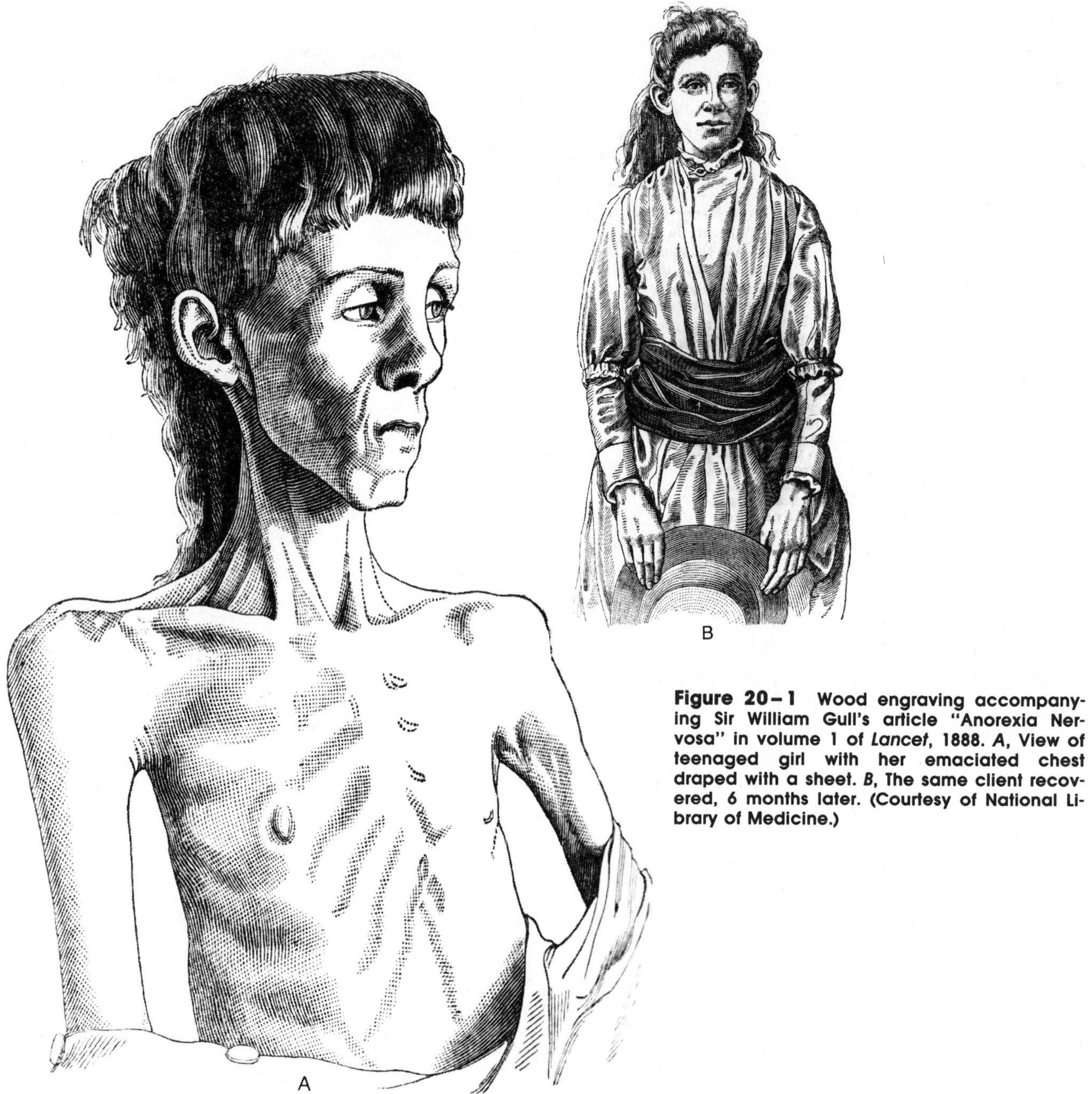

Figure 20–1 Wood engraving accompanying Sir William Gull's article "Anorexia Nervosa" in volume 1 of *Lancet*, 1888. *A*, View of teenaged girl with her emaciated chest draped with a sheet. *B*, The same client recovered, 6 months later. (Courtesy of National Library of Medicine.)

below expected or original body weight, amenorrhea (for women), and an excessive desire for slimness with a distorted body image.

Nutritional Effects of Anorexia Nervosa

Numerous nutritional effects occur in clients with AN (Table 20–2). Most of the physical symptoms (bradycardia, ECG changes, hair loss, dry skin, brittle nails, and lanugo-like hair growth) nurses observe in AN clients are related to excessive weight loss and malnutrition. These clients are literally in a state of starvation and can appear emaciated because of decreased body fat and muscle mass.

Dehydration, which causes changes in blood pressure (hypotension and ortho-

TABLE 20–1

CHARACTERISTIC TRAITS OF INDIVIDUALS WITH ANOREXIA NERVOSA

Exhibits ideal behavior
Rarely displays anger
Devoted to school/work; outstanding student/worker
Exercises compulsively, following strenuous exercise regimens
Feels inferior
Denies illness
Wears oversized clothing
Anxious about others' opinions about them
Low self-esteem
Usually from upper-class and middle-class background
Lonely

static hypotension) and blood urea nitrogen level, is attributed to decreased fluid intake (Pomeroy & Mitchell, 1989).

Clients may also experience bloating or early satiety and complain of abdominal pain. These discomforts are associated with delayed gastric emptying. Abdominal pain is usually benign but may signal gastric dilatation, which may lead to gastric rupture, requiring emergency surgery (Pomeroy & Mitchell, 1989). Another complication associated with abdominal pain is **superior mesenteric artery syndrome**.

Superior mesenteric artery syndrome—vascular compression of the distal duodenum.

Serum cholesterol and carotene levels are elevated in AN; reasons for these elevations are unclear (Pomeroy & Mitchell, 1989). Edelstein et al (1989) believe elevated serum carotene is related to increased consumption of carrots and other betacarotene-containing vegetables; yellow skin may occur. Vitamin deficiencies are usually rare (Pomeroy & Mitchell, 1989). However, minerals, such as potassium, calcium, magnesium, chloride, and sodium, may be decreased.

Bone mineral density is decreased in AN clients, predisposing clients to osteoporosis (Plehn, 1990). Onset of amenorrhea is significant in development of bone mineral loss. The younger a client, the more bone mineral is lost. When an AN client recovers, bone mineral density improves, but it is still lower than normal (Biller et al, 1989).

Describe 2 nutritional effects of AN.

Nutritional Effects of Therapies

Although the major focus of treatment is on psychotherapy and nutrition education, occasionally drugs are prescribed for AN clients. Pharmacotherapy is based on 2 principles: (1) AN is a disorder secondary to other psychiatric disorders, and

TABLE 20–2

NUTRITIONAL EFFECTS OF ANOREXIA NERVOSA

GI	Delayed gastric emptying
	Gastric dilatation and rupture
	Superior mesentery artery syndrome
	Refeeding edema
Metabolic	Growth retardation
	Delayed onset of puberty
	Osteoporosis and osteopenia
Nutrients	Trace minerals and vitamins deficiencies (rare)
	Increased serum levels of cholesterol and carotene

(2) AN affects hypothalamic control of food intake and hypothalamic-endocrine regulation (Tolstoi, 1989).

Tricyclic antidepressants and monoamine oxidase inhibitors (MAOIs) may be prescribed (see section on depression in this chapter for nutritional effects and treatment). These medications are mainly given to promote weight gain. If a client is malnourished, antidepressants may not be effective in an AN client possibly as a result of suppression of thyroid function or reduction of drug-binding sites on serum transport proteins (Slaiman, 1989; Soubrie et al, 1989).

Metoclopramide, cyproheptadine, and clomiphene citrate may also be administered. Metoclopramide (Reglan) increases gastric emptying rate, thereby negating the delayed gastric emptying time most AN clients experience. Monitoring bowel sounds and output is a necessary measure because of common GI side effects of nausea and diarrhea. Even though nausea may occur, this medicine should be given 30 minutes before meals.

The mechanism whereby cyproheptadine (Periactin) induces weight gain is unknown. Currently it is not endorsed by the FDA as an appetite stimulant. Numerous GI side effects of Periactin include epigastric distress, nausea, vomiting, dry mouth, diarrhea, and constipation; these may be avoided by administering Periactin with food. Monitoring I&O and bowel sounds is also beneficial, as is providing mouth care and lozenges.

Clomiphene citrate (Clomid) stimulates ovulation to restore menses. Clomid recipients may experience abdominal discomfort, distention, bloating, nausea, and vomiting. Taking this medicine with food or right before bedtime may alleviate these symptoms. However, this drug may not be effective until fat stores are replenished.

Describe drug therapy for AN.

Nutritional Assessment

A client's physical condition is assessed and stabilized, followed by a nutritional assessment and development of a care plan. Baseline data should include electrolyte studies, CBC, ECG, and vital signs.

To understand clients better, a thorough diet history must be obtained, noting self-medication dieting practices (OTC diet aids), exercise routines, and unusual eating rituals. Clients with AN are usually resistant to assessment and treatment; they perceive weight loss as a solution to problems. Achievement of weight loss makes them special and in control, so they are not receptive to changing this (McKenna, 1989). Nurses must develop a rapport and trust with these clients as soon as possible. A structured, not open-ended, interview is advocated since these clients initially lack insight and do not have the ability to connect feelings with behaviors (Love & Seaton, 1991; McKenna, 1989). Love & Seaton (1991) suggest that nurses periodically ask clients, "How is this interview going for you so far?" and say, "You are doing a great job. I know many of these questions are difficult for you to answer, particularly since you don't know me very well."

Determining the extent of a client's sensitivity to weight regulation is advised. Clients with AN relentlessly pursue thinness—breaking the 100 lb barrier is desirable. Inquire about how often clients weigh themselves; anorectics may weigh 20 times a day (Edelstein et al, 1989). Determine how clients react if they are unable to weigh themselves; being unable to weigh usually produces anxiety.

Clients with AN believe a few ounces of food is excessive; compensatory action for "excessive" intake may involve fasting for longer than a day or exercising more than an hour each day (Edelstein et al, 1989). Even though clients may be skin and bones (the percentage of body fat is significantly decreased), these clients still state they are fat, confirming a distorted body image. Some questions to ask include, "How do you see yourself?"; "Do others see you in the same way?"; and "Is there a particular area of your body that you dislike?" (Love & Seaton, 1991; McKenna, 1989).

Amenorrhea can be a cardinal sign of AN and may occur in 20% of clients before goal weights are attained (Plehn, 1990). Ask clients, "Are your periods regular?"; "Do you sometimes miss a period?"; "If so, for how long?"

Results of anthropometric measurements usually indicate body fat below 22%. Some clients with AN may lose up to 40% of their original body weight (Plehn, 1990). Daily monitoring may include weight, laboratory values, and mental acuity.

What parameters are assessed in an AN client?

Nutritional Care

Outpatient treatment is the preferred choice, but when clients are a danger to themselves (suicidal) or if their physical (>30% weight loss below normal weight or failure to gain weight) or psychological (complete denial) condition makes outpatient treatment ineffective, hospitalization is required. Ideally the client is an active participant in this decision about hospitalization, which should be kept to a minimum. Once clients are stabilized and nutritionally rehabilitated, outpatient therapy can be implemented as deemed necessary.

Goals

After clients have been physiologically and psychologically stabilzed, major nutritional goals are refeeding for weight gain and normalization of eating patterns. Nurses must be aware that nutritional goals are not effective unless physiological and psychological stabilization has occurred. Additional goals are healthy family interactions concerning food and maintaining weight within a safe range. Principles for dietary regimens are given in Table 20–3.

List 3 nutritional goals for AN clients.

Treatment Modalities

Successful outcomes require comprehensive treatment by a multidisciplinary team that addresses individual psychosocial, nutritional, and medical problems. This team usually comprises a psychotherapist and/or psychiatrist, registered dietitian, nurses, social worker, and physician. This pooling of specialties provides more effective treatment as well as a support system for team members when difficult decisions are necessary or progress appears slow.

If the client is extremely malnourished, the first concern is to re-establish physiological stability. Control of eating behavior occurs only after psychological care is rendered. The foundation of treatment includes psychotherapy and nutrition education using individual, family, and group modalities. All of these modalities, tailored to individual needs, promote resolution of underlying issues of identity, self-esteem, control, individuation, assertiveness, intimacy, conflict resolution, body image, and perfectionism.

Realization of body size before and after weight reduction is extremely difficult. Photographs or use of mirrors (Miller, 1991) can assist clients to get in touch with their own body images. Another technique involves having clients draw their perceived body outline on a large sheet of paper mounted on the wall. Then a client

TABLE 20–3

DIET PRINCIPLES FOR CLIENTS WITH ANOREXIA NERVOSA AND BULIMIA

1. Maintain a balanced intake of nutrients. In anorexia nervosa, gradually increase total kilocaloric intake; in bulimia, kilocaloric intake may be decreased or increased depending on client's physical status.
2. Offer a specific set of dietary guidelines (contracts) to help clients maintain a feeling of control.
3. Encourage regular eating patterns.
4. Specify appropriate quantities of food necessary for weight maintenance.
5. Use a 12-step program based on Overeater's Anonymous philosophy if advocated by hospital/clinic.

stands in front of this mounted paper while a nurse or therapist actually draws the client's body (Miller, 1991). Discussion of discrepancy ensues.

Behavior modification techniques are generally unsuccessful if they are inappropriately coercive, or if someone else's will is imposed on the client. However, when used appropriately and in conjunction with education and psychotherapy, success is enhanced. Some health care professionals advocate using a 12-step program for eating disorders similar to those used for alcohol and drug dependency (Devlin, 1991; Riley, 1991). This approach uses group therapy, peer support, honesty, and abstinence from problematic foods and other compulsive eating behaviors (Devlin, 1991).

Why is a multidisciplinary team necessary? What are the foundations of treatment?

Promoting Intake

Methods of accomplishing refeeding are individualized. During the initial recovery phase, method of intake should attempt to minimize GI disturbances by providing easily digested foods served frequently. Options for repletion of nutritional status include a regular diet, use of nutrition supplements (alone or in combination with food intake), total fluid diet, tube feedings, or TPN (used only for clients whose metabolic status is unstable). Tube feedings are used for clients whose weight is 40% below their IBW.

Goals for weight gain are established individually, usually an increase of 1 lb weekly. Initially a rapid weight gain occurs with refeeding as a consequence of fluid retention and increased glycogen stores. Weight plateaus or drops as edematous fluid is lost before a slow, continuous weight gain.

Documentation of current weight and kilocaloric intake is reinforcement in treating hospitalized AN clients. For accurate body weights, clients are weighed at the same time each day on the same scale in the same clothing. Remember that clients with AN may try to make nurses believe that weight is being gained. Therefore, have clients urinate before weighing since they may ingest fluids to elevate weight falsely. Check clothing; sometimes weights are hidden in clothes. Weighing clients so they cannot see the actual weight may be beneficial (Edelstein et al, 1989). Changes in MAC measurements can also help determine if weight gain is "truly" weight gain. Expectations of excessive weight gain or harsh punishments are ineffective.

Nursing staff or dietetic technicians maintain kilocalorie counts to monitor intake. Because these clients are controlling, close attention is necessary to determine that food is actually eaten.

The current trend in treatment is to allow clients to be in control of food eaten and subsequent weight gain. Popular foods include cereals, low fat dairy products, yogurt, bagels, fish and poultry, pound cake, and pudding. Common foods avoided are casseroles, breaded or fried foods, sauces, gravies, or rich desserts like blueberry pie (Anonymous, 1991).

Clients have a higher percentage of food dislikes, which may be related to alterations in taste function because of zinc and copper deficiencies. Normal acuity returns when eating patterns are normalized.

What are some ways to promote intake?

Nutritional Counseling

Nutritional counseling is an important part of therapy to correct nutritional beliefs and eating behaviors. Food beliefs are entrenched as a result of abnormal behaviors exercised over an extended period of time and inability to differentiate food and nutrition truths from myths. Typical myths, such as carbohydrates and dairy products are fattening; or eating breakfast makes one hungry all day, or all eating leads to weight gain, are common. Although these clients are aware of kilocaloric food values, they do not understand the relationship between kilocalories and nutrients for health and how to balance energy intake with expenditure. Their false beliefs must be challenged with factual information. Registered dietitians and nurses can facilitate clients' return to normal, healthy, eating patterns by providing counseling and education on topics such as normal nutrition and weight maintenance.

NURSING APPLICATIONS

Assessment

Physical—body image, former weight, present weight, IBW, percent weight changes, TSF; relevant medical history, menses history, heart assessment, edema; exercise habits; family attitudes about weight.

Dietary—for food preferences, detailed diet history (number and content of meals and snacks), appetite; knowledge of nutritional and kilocaloric values of food; perception of excessive intake; client/family's beliefs about food intake.

Laboratory—for low WBC, Hgb, Hct; hypokalemia, hypocalcemia; elevated BUN; albumin; acid-base balance (pH); liver enzymes.

Interventions

1. Treat each client as an individual; all have their unique set of problems and beliefs. Improvement requires trust, empathy, and collaboration from nurses.
2. Do not have prolonged discussions about food or recipes.
3. Limit mealtime to 30 minutes.
4. Help client make positive statements about body.
5. Help client to draw pictures of self.
6. Involve client in goal setting.
7. Encourage client to keep a journal for the following: time and quantity of specific food eaten, feelings, thoughts.
8. Gradually increase kilocalories provided. This reduces excessive edema. Do not proceed too quickly with numerous nutritional changes, as this may result in withdrawal.
9. Do not force feed; food rejection is part of this illness.
10. Do not make food an issue. Give choices.
11. Encourage kilocalorie-dense foods to reduce bulk of meals.
12. Gradually introduce food items client has restricted.
13. Expect anger, manipulation, belligerence, and suspiciousness. Remain matter-of-fact and nonjudgmental.

Evaluation

* Client will have met the goal for weight gain; consumed frequent, small meals a day; and begun menses.

Client Education

- Refer to American Anorexia/Bulimia Association, AN and Related Eating Disorders or the AN and Associated Disorders.
- Reframe client's negative self talk to positive. For instance, client states, "I look pregnant and fat." Change to "You are starting to put on weight, which is healthy. This is your body's way of becoming stronger."
- Reiterate that client will still be in control of his or her life and that he or she will in fact be in better control because of improvement in health and well-being.
- Use handouts, booklets, articles, and other written information about nutrition. This gives clients control over which information they accept.
- Explain how emotions and physical aspects relate to food intake and weight changes.

BULIMIA

Binges—periods of overeating.

Purging—use of laxatives, enemas, vomiting, diuretics, or exercise to negate effects of overindulgence.

Bulimia occurs more frequently than AN. All ages, even the elderly, and either gender may be affected by bulimia. Males constitute 20% of bulimic clients. As many as 8 to 19% of college-age women may experience bulimia (Mitchell, 1989).

This eating disorder by itself is not associated with significant weight loss or distorted body image; an individual might even be normal or slightly overweight and appears healthy. Bulimia is characterized by intentional, although not necessarily controllable, secret **binges** usually followed by **purging.**

Theories

Typically bulimia and AN occur for the same reason: fear of becoming fat. However, clients with bulimia try to control this fear by repeatedly restraining eating, but this backfires and leads to binging and purging (Edelstein et al, 1989). Thus, these clients feel they are at the mercy of food (McKenna, 1989).

Family Relationships

Alcohol, sexual, or physical abuse in families increases a client's chance of developing bulimia. Clients frequently report parents, especially fathers, as "distant, unapproachable, or workaholics" (Edelstein et al, 1989).

Biological Factors

Neurochemical factors are present in bulimia. Serotonin activity is reduced in clients with normal weight bulimia (Kaye & Weltzin, 1991). Since high serotonin levels correlate with satiety, a low serotonin level may precipitate binging because satiety is low (Wilson & Kneisl, 1992).

A recent theory for bulimia involves endorphins, which are natural pain killers. These endorphins overstimulate brain opiate receptors, leading to a binge/purge cycle. This concept has gained popularity because naltrexone (Trexan), an opiate antagonist, has been effective in arresting binge/purge cycles.

How do serotonin levels affect binging?

Characteristics

Clients with bulimia exhibit many of the same characteristics as anorectic clients, especially in their background and personality traits. Only differences are discussed. Bulimics are more sociable but underneath feel profoundly separated from other people (McKenna, 1989). Usually these clients appear very mature, but this is a defense mechanism to hide insecurities, maintaining the myth that dependency needs have been met. Appearance is extremely important; they are extremely well-groomed and apply makeup before making breakfast or getting their mail (Edelstein et al, 1989).

Clients with bulimia acknowledge their eating behaviors are not normal. They have strong appetites and may binge several times a day with intakes ranging from 1200 to 11,500 kcal per episode. Binges usually involve a "forbidden" food—one that clients believe to be high in kilocalories. Binges may last from 15 minutes to several hours, may be planned or spontaneous, but ordinarily are related to stress.

These binges occur most often in the late afternoon or evening and end with purging. Self-induced vomiting is the main choice of purging (for white adolescent girls); laxative and/or diuretic abuse is used more frequently by black adolescent girls (Emmons, 1992). As many as 100 laxatives a day may be taken (Edelstein et al, 1989). Vomiting may be induced by sticking a finger or other object down the throat. Some individuals apply external pressure to the neck. Eventually most bulimic clients can vomit by merely contracting their abdominal muscles.

Families may be upset with clients for eating them out of house and home. A single binge can cost from $8 to $50 since binging food consists mainly of high-carbohydrate, easily digested junk food (Plehn, 1990). Compulsive stealing, of both food and money to buy food, is another common characteristic.

Drinking while binging reduces abdominal pain and discomfort as well as guilt. Alcohol abuse is so common that all clients with bulimia should be assessed for alcohol intake. If these conditions occur concurrently, alcohol abuse must be treated before bulimia can be resolved (Edelstein et al, 1989).

Name 3 typical characteristics of clients with bulimia.

Nutritional Effects of Bulimia

Nutritional effects of bulimia stem from purging and the method employed for purging. Vomiting, laxative abuse, and diuretic abuse can have similar and dissimilar nutritional effects (Table 20–4). All 3 methods may result in hyperuricemia, hypokalemia, hyponatremia, and FVD.

Self-induced vomiting can cause oral cavity trauma; bruises and irritations in the oral cavity may be observed. Frequent vomiting causes erosion of tooth enamel and enlargement of parotid glands; these are classic signs of bulimia. Amylase levels are elevated, suggesting gland involvement. Do not falsely assume oral problems result from poor dental hygiene practices; rather these oral problems develop secondary to frequent vomiting (Hofland & Dardis, 1992). Since HCl is lost in vomitus, metabolic alkalosis may occur. Rare and severe GI complications include esophageal rupturing from frequent vomiting and gastric rupture caused by binging. Low levels of chloride and magnesium are the result of vomiting. Lastly, another classic sign of bulimia associated with self-induced vomiting is abrasions and calluses located on

TABLE 20–4

NUTRITIONAL EFFECTS OF BULIMIA

Type of Purging	Gastrointestinal	Metabolic	Nutrients
Self-induced vomiting	Enlarged parotid glands Increased serum levels of amylase Esophageal perforation and rupture Esophagitis Dental problems Oral cavity trauma Halitosis Easily bleeding, boggy gums	Metabolic alkalosis Fluid volume deficit	Decreased serum levels of chloride, magnesium, sodium, and potassium Increased serum levels of uric acid
Cathartic abuse	Cathartic colon Reflex constipation Occult bleeding Hemorrhoids Rectal discomfort Steatorrhea Laxative dependency	Metabolic acidosis Fluid volume deficit Edema	Decreased serum levels of potassium, sodium, and magnesium Increased serum levels of uric acid
Diuretic abuse		Fluid volume deficit Edema	Decreased serum levels of potassium, sodium, and chloride Increased serum levels of uric acid

Data compiled from Hofland SL, Dardis PO. Bulimia nervosa: Associated physical problems. *J Psychosocial Nurs* 1992 Feb; 30(2):23–27; Pomeroy C, Mitchell JE. Medical complications and management of eating disorders. *Psych Ann* 1989 Sept; 19(9):488–493.

dorsal surfaces of fingers and hands secondary to friction of the teeth (Hofland & Dardis, 1992; Edelstein et al, 1989; Pomeroy & Mitchell, 1989).

Laxative abuse may lead to hypomagnesemia because diarrheal loss may contain 10 to 15 mEq/L of magnesium. Hypocalcemia can also develop, along with hypomagnesemia, causing muscle spasms of hands and feet (Edelstein et al, 1989). If calcium levels drop below normal, tetany, seizures, cardiac arrhythmias, and even death can ensue. Metabolic acidosis may occur from bicarbonate loss in liquid feces. As would be expected, the GI tract is adversely affected. Frank or occult (hidden) bleeding may occur, predisposing clients to anemia. Steatorrhea and hemorrhoids are also possible. Constipation, bloating, and lower abdominal pains, sometimes called cathartic colitis, secondary to intestinal motility dysfunction may result (Hofland & Dardis, 1992). Reflex constipation is another problem. A vicious cycle develops: Laxative abuse leads to GI hypofunctioning, which causes constipation, leading to laxative dependency for bowel movements.

Diuretic abuse can lead to hypochloremia and edema. Diuretics inhibit renal tubular reabsorption of chloride, causing hypochloremia secondary to increased chloride excretion. Edema occurs when diuretics are discontinued. This appears to be related to chronic water and electrolyte loss, which results in excessive secretion of aldosterone, leading to sodium and water retention (Hofland & Dardis, 1992).

Several other complications can occur resultant of inadequate absorption regardless of purging method chosen. Riboflavin deficiency may result in glossitis. Niacin deficiency, which produces a dry mouth or burning tongue, may also occur (Edelstein et al, 1989).

What nutritional problems can occur from bulimia?

Nutritional Effects of Therapies

Just as in AN, medications used for bulimia are antidepressants (tricyclics, MAOs, and fluoxetine). Other drugs used are fenfluramine (Pondimin) and metoclopramide HCl (Reglan).

Pondimin may minimize binging and purging. This drug elicits a release of serotonin, reducing binge/purge cycles. Dry mouth, abdominal pain, and nausea are possible side effects. To minimize these effects, provide mouth care, lozenges, and ice chips; monitor for abdominal pain. If pain is present, report to physician. Although nausea may occur, this medicine should be given before meals. A life-threatening adverse reaction can occur if Pondimin is given concurrently with MAOIs; thus, do not give together, or consult the physician if these drugs are ordered simultaneously.

Reglan closes the lower esophagus; thus, it is contraindicated in bulimics unless a conscious decision is made by the client not to induce vomiting (Edelstein et al, 1989).

How does Pondimin work? What must a client do before Reglan can be given?

Nutritional Assessment

A complete physical assessment is performed because clients who abuse laxatives, emetics, and/or diuretics can have severe, life-threatening complications. If cardiac problems are present (bradycardia, hypotension), an ECG and chest x-ray film are necessary. (ECGs are required if a client abuses ipecac since this emetic can cause heart problems.) Routine laboratory tests include CBC, renal function tests, and electrolytes. Sometimes urine samples may be obtained to detect diuretic or laxative use.

Although bulimic clients are not as resistant to assessments and treatments as AN clients, secrecy is prevalent because overwhelming shame is associated with bulimia. Most clients are hesitant to open themselves up to questions (McKenna, 1989). Thus, questions should be asked matter-of-factly in a structured manner

(Love & Seaton, 1991; McKenna, 1989). Areas that should be assessed include dietary habits, bulimic tendencies, and weight history.

Physical problems related to eating include sore throat, cavities, swollen parotid glands, diarrhea, and constipation. Most bulimics have a list of "bad" or fattening (forbidden) foods and binge/purge if this food is eaten. Bulimics may consider anywhere from 5000 to 10,000 kilocalories as excessive eating. Ask how the client feels after this binge/purge cycle; this behavior often causes depression.

Clients with bulimia may have weight fluctuations of 10 lbs. Assessing body fat is not a reliable indicator in bulimia because the percentage of body fat is similar between bulimic and normal clients. However, folate and hemoglobin levels and bone mineral density are significantly lower in bulimics (Howat et al, 1989).

What areas should be assessed in a client with bulimia? Why is body fat not an indicator of bulimia? What parameters can be used instead?

Nutritional Care

Outpatient treatment is preferred because it allows clients an opportunity for self-mastery, control, and autonomy (Love & Seaton, 1991). If clients practice excessive purging tactics or have a decreased serum potassium level or other fluid and electrolyte disturbances, hospitalization is necessary. Of course, clients should be involved in this process.

Goals

Goals include normalizing eating patterns, correcting nutritional deficiencies, and reducing binge/purge cycles.

Treatment Modalities

Behavioral, cognitive, and psychological (individual and group) modalities are incorporated into treatment by a multidisciplinary team. Physiological and psychological stabilization must occur before clients can adequately control their eating behaviors. Nutrition education is provided to invoke new eating habits. Individual, family, and group modalities as well as behavior modification may be used.

Preventing Binging/Purging

Methods to reduce binging episodes are individualized, and relapses may occur. Regression can be frustrating for both the nurse and the client. Support from the multidisciplinary team decreases these frustrating times. Important elements of care for decreasing binging/purging include education, self-monitoring, and meal planning by clients. Following feedings, involvement in a social setting lasting up to 1 hour after meals reduces opportunities for purging. Also a journal recording the following information is helpful: time of binging/purging, behavior before and after binging/purging, thoughts before and after binging/purging, and money spent on food. Initially exclude high-risk binge foods then slowly reintroduce. Use a firm, direct approach for promoting normal eating patterns (Mitchell, 1989). Substituting increased fiber and fluid intake rather than using laxatives may be accepted by clients with bulimia.

Nutritional Counseling

Diet may be very restrictive. Self-imposed restrictions may cause clients to feel starved or deprived, leading to a binge/purge cycle (Edelstein et al, 1989). Nutrition education/counseling by a registered dietitian is recommended to provide information on topics such as normal nutrition and healthy eating habits. Many bulimic clients believe that purging negates effects of kilocalories consumed. Nurses and registered dietitians can dispel this myth and other misconceptions these clients have by reinforcing healthy nutrition truths and modeling acceptable eating patterns. Handouts and pamphlets are beneficial because clients are allowed to choose what information they accept.

Describe nutritional care for bulimics.

NURSING APPLICATIONS

Assessment

Physical—for weakness, lethargy; hoarseness, esophagitis, dental cavities; low self-esteem, worthlessness, guilt, shame; enlarged parotid glands, calluses or cuts on knuckles, dehydration, I&Os; menses; height, weight/weight changes, IBW.

Dietary—for frequency of binge and purge, list of forbidden foods; type of purging used, preoccupation with food, weight, diets; meaning of excessive eating; types of foods overeaten; alcohol/drug abuse, nutritional beliefs and attitudes; nutrient intake, especially folate.

Laboratory—for hypokalemia, hypochloremia; magnesium, calcium, and sodium levels; Hgb, folate; bone mineral density; ABGs; urine pH.

Interventions

1. Refer to dietitian.
2. Make a contract with client not to binge or purge.
3. Monitor up to 1 hour after meals to decrease purging.
4. Assist with journal.
5. When the cause of binging is revealed, suggest alternate methods of dealing with stress, e.g., writing, talking, painting.
6. Suggest rinsing mouth with an alkaline solution (sodium bicarbonate and water) rather than brushing after vomiting. Brushing has shown to increase enamel loss on teeth.

Evaluation

* Desired outcomes include client does not binge and purge, eats well-balanced meals, consumes "forbidden food" without guilt, employs different coping mechanisms other than binging/purging, and verbalizes correct nutritional information.

Client Education

- When food is eaten out of the original container rather than on a serving utensil (plate or bowl), the temptation to overeat is enhanced. The risk of overeating may be decreased by eating only at the dining table.
- Three meals a day with 1 or 2 snacks, providing a minimum of 1200 kcal/day, is beneficial.
- Purging does not eliminate kilocaloric value of food just eaten.
- Discuss consequences of electrolyte imbalances: muscle spasms, kidney problems, and cardiac arrest.
- Refer to American Anorexia and Bulimia Association; the AN and Bulimia Resource Center can provide valuable information.

CHEMICAL DEPENDENCY

Chemical dependency—when alcohol/drug use is uncontrollable.

Chemical dependency has a major impact on society, causing social and personal upheavals that affect the entire family and society, not just the chemically addicted individual. It is rare to find dependency on just one chemical; rather

polyabuse is more common. Since alcohol is the most common form of chemical dependency in the US, emphasis is focused on alcohol. Some clinicians think that a faulty hepatic enzyme system predisposes clients to alcohol dependency, but this has yet to be proved.

Polyabuse—more than one chemical is abused.

Nutritional Effects of Chemical Dependency

Even a well-balanced diet may be inadequate because chemical dependency accelerates nutrient metabolism, increasing nutrient requirements. Inactivated vitamins and coenzymes needed to metabolize energy, inadequate nutrient storage in the damaged liver, poor use of nutrients, increased breakdown of muscles and organs, increased losses of nutrients through diuresis and diarrhea, and increased use of nutrients to detoxify and metabolize drugs all promote nutritional problems (Beckley-Barrett & Mutch, 1990).

What factors promote nutritional problems in chemical dependency?

Alcohol

Alcohol requires no digestion. Alcohol is rapidly absorbed from an empty stomach and small intestine. Alcohol delays gastric emptying. When food and alcohol are consumed together, absorption of alcohol and food is delayed.

The body has no storage mechanism for alcohol; therefore, it must all be metabolized, predominantly by the liver. Very little alcohol is excreted in urine or through the lungs. In nonalcoholics, rate of metabolism is fairly constant, but a client with chronic alcoholism develops a supplemental system for metabolism, and the rate may double. There are no feedback controls to limit this rate. The large percentage of hydrogen from alcohol unbalances liver cell chemistry. When large quantities of ethanol must be oxidized, several metabolic problems may develop, including **hyperuricemia,** enhanced production of lipids and lipoproteins, decreased lipid oxidation resulting in **steatosis,** reduced **gluconeogenesis** leading to hypoglycemia, and inhibition of drug metabolism (Lieber, 1991). Chronic effects of alcohol dependency are not related to intoxication but rather to the amount and duration of alcohol consumption.

Hyperuricemia—elevated blood levels of uric acid. Steatosis—large amounts of fat accumulated in the liver. Gluconeogenesis—production of glucose from noncarbohydrate products.

Alcohol dependency is a major cause of nutritional deficiency secondary to reduced food intake (Figure 20–2). Since alcohol contains few nutrients other than kilocalories, nutrient intake may become insufficient and affect nutritional status in several ways. (1) Appetite is suppressed, and diet is poor. (2) Alcohol damage may compromise digestion and absorption in the stomach and intestine, frequently resulting in nausea, diarrhea, impaired water and electrolyte absorption, and ulceration. Absorption of thiamin, vitamin B_{12}, folate, magnesium, zinc, and glucose is decreased; iron absorption is increased. (3) Alcohol may damage the liver and interfere with transport, activation, catabolism, utilization, and storage of almost every nutrient in the body. (4) Vitamin requirements, particularly for the B complex, are higher in alcoholic clients than in nonalcoholics.

Nutritional deficiencies are more frequently marginal than overt. An alcohol-derived nutritional deficiency may result in suboptimal health and contribute to frequently seen conditions such as anemia, clotting problems, convulsions, and small bowel malfunction. Several neurological complications of alcohol dependency, such as polyneuropathy and Wernicke-Korsakoff syndrome, are now recognized as vitamin deficiencies resulting primarily from thiamin deficiency. Night blindness, which responds to administration of vitamin A (and sometimes zinc supplements), is commonly found in clients with chronic alcoholism. Other signs of malnutrition are reviewed in Table 20–5.

Heavy alcohol consumption results in various toxic effects with the most striking influences on the brain and liver, but the pancreas is also frequently affected.

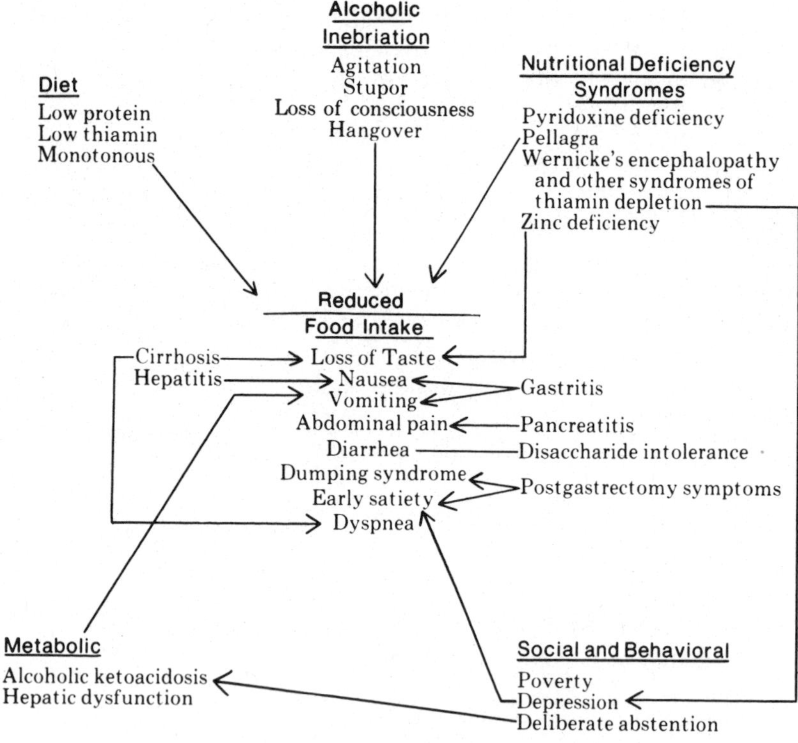

Figure 20–2 Summary of factors contributing to reduced food intake. (From Roe DA. *Alcohol and the Diet.* Westport, CT, AVI Publishing, 1979. © Van Nostrand Reinhold.)

Hepatitis and cirrhosis, discussed in Chapter 26, are the most common hepatic complications of alcohol dependency.

Despite a nutritionally adequate diet, fatty liver infiltration is a consequence of ethanol metabolism mainly caused by an increased synthesis and decreased degradation of fatty acids. If a client abstains from alcohol, fatty liver and alcoholic hepatitis are reversible, but cirrhosis is not. Once signs of portal hypertension are present, cessation of alcohol intake seems to have little impact on the progression

TABLE 20–5

CLINICAL DEFICIENCIES IN THE ALCOHOL-DEPENDENT CLIENT

Clinical Symptoms	Causes and Nutritional Implication
Wernicke-Korsakoff syndrome	Thiamin deficiency
Shuffling gait (motor weakness), polyneuropathy	Thiamin deficiency, vitamin B_{12}
Generalized weakness	Chronic blood loss; folic acid and iron deficiencies
Macrocytic anemia	Decreased folate stores
Edema, fatty liver, hypoalbuminemia, anemia	Protein deficiency; increased loss with ascitic fluid
Photosensitive dermatitis, stomatitis, gastritis, diarrhea, peripheral neuropathy	Niacin deficiency
Dermatitis, stomatitis cheilosis	Riboflavin deficiency
Alcoholic withdrawal convulsions, mild ataxia, skin lesions, irritability, insomnia	Pyridoxine deficiency
Delirium tremens	Increased magnesium excretion; decreased intake of magnesium (must be replenished parenterally)
Cardiac myopathies	Potassium deficiency due to decreased intake, poor absorption, and increased urinary losses
Night blindness	Increased zinc excretion and/or vitamin A deficiency
Osteomalacia and fractures	Vitamin D deficiency
Increased prothrombin time	Vitamin K deficiency

of cirrhosis. Alcohol dependency is also a risk factor in adverse fetal outcomes (see Chapter 14).

Usually heavy drinkers are considered more at risk of sustaining adverse health consequences, but even drinking in moderation may present problems to some clients because of genetic and other biological factors that may predispose clients to specific conditions.

What metabolic problems may develop from alcohol dependency?

Cocaine/Crack

Cocaine/crack are CNS stimulants that affect nutritional status in several ways: Clients are debilitated, underweight, and vitamin-deficient (Chychula & Okore, 1990). As can be expected, stimulant effects increase kilocaloric requirements. However, cocaine causes a decreased appetite and anorexia by inactivating the hypothalamic feeding center. Consequently, these factors induce weight loss (Addison, 1990). Because of anorexia and increased metabolism, water-soluble vitamins are decreased. Common deficiencies include vitamin B_6, thiamin, and vitamin C. Conversely, vitamin A levels may be higher in cocaine users because raw cocaine contains high levels of vitamin A (Addison, 1990). During cocaine/crack withdrawal, clients frequently binge on highly refined carbohydrate foods (Nuckols & Greeson, 1989).

Cocaine—water-soluble salt or powder used for snorting, popping (subcutaneous), or IV use. Crack—cocaine mixed with equal parts of water and sodium bicarbonate to form a solution that is then heated, cooled, and cut into cocaine "rocks." Cocaine mixed with ammonia hardens to form "crystals" of cocaine. Both crack and crystals can be smoked (House, 1992).

Cocaine users have been noted to consume more alcohol, coffee, and fatty foods as compared with nonusers (Castro et al, 1987). AN and bulimia are more prevalent among cocaine users (Gold, 1988; Killen et al, 1987).

An acute GI complication associated with cocaine use is gastritis, whereas a sore throat can develop with chronic cocaine use (House, 1992). Clients addicted to cocaine have dry mouths and halitosis.

What are the nutritional affects of cocaine?

Marijuana

Increased food intake in marijuana users results in weight gain. Although intake is increased, poor food choices, i.e., excessive high-kilocaloric, high-fat foods with few fruits and vegetables, may lead to possible nutritional deficiencies. Physical manifestations include muscle weakness, bleeding gums, fatigue and dyspnea on exertion, indigestion, and sore tongue. Low plasma zinc levels may contribute to loss of appetite. Increased thirst (dry mouth) and cravings for sweets are also reported (Wilson & Kneisl, 1992).

What are the nutritional effects of marijuana?

Heroin

One of the dangers associated with heroin use is malnutrition. Nausea and vomiting may also be experienced. On withdrawal from heroin, diarrhea, loss of appetite, and flulike symptoms may occur.

Insulin response is altered with heroin use, which leads to an exaggerated and delayed insulin response. Thus, glucose metabolism is adversely affected (Mohs et al, 1990), and glycosylated hemoglobin levels are increased.

Hyperkalemia is associated with heroin use, especially overdose. High levels of heroin can destroy skeletal muscles, releasing potassium rapidly. If renal function is compromised (frequently seen with heroin overdose), hyperkalemia is exacerbated.

What are the effects of heroin on nutrition?

Nutritional Effects of Therapies

Disulfiram (Antabuse) may be used as treatment for some alcohol-dependent clients. Antabuse works by inhibiting **acetaldehyde dehydrogenase.** Consequently, accumulation of acetaldehyde, which is toxic to the body, produces nausea, vomiting, flushing, dizziness, tachycardia, headache, palpitations, convulsions, hy-

Acetaldehyde dehydrogenase—an enzyme that metabolizes alcohol.

potension, shock, and even death. Anytime alcohol in any form is ingested, a disulfiram reaction occurs. Therefore, clients must abstain from alcohol for at least 12 hours before taking disulfiram and must be informed of consequences of any alcohol intake. Obviously, beer, wine, and liquor would be excluded, but other less obvious alcohol-containing items must also be avoided: cough mixtures, aftershave lotions, liniments, colognes, cold remedies, and sauces or foods that incorporate alcohol (wine, liqueurs) during cooking.

DTs—a severe form of alcohol withdrawal occurring 2 to 3 days after the last drink that produces memory disturbances, agitation, anorexia, and hallucinations.

Antianxiety drugs (Librium and Valium) may also be prescribed to prevent **delirium tremens (DTs).** Typical food–drug interactions with antianxiety medicines involve alcohol and caffeine. Since alcohol is not being consumed, this is not a major problem unless a client is noncompliant. If this occurs, sedation results. Conversely, caffeine may negate antianxiety effects of the medication.

During cocaine/crack withdrawal, antianxiety (Valium), tricyclic antidepressants (mainly Tofranil), anticonvulsants (phenobarbital), and antipsychotics (mainly Haldol) may be given. Antidepressants and antipsychotics are discussed in this chapter under depression and schizophrenia, respectively. Typical GI effects of phenobarbital include nausea, vomiting, constipation, diarrhea, and epigastric pain. Offering small, frequent meals and monitoring bowel sounds and bowel movements are necessary nursing interventions. If phenobarbital must be used longer than 1 year, liver damage, megaloblastic anemia, rickets, and osteomalacia can occur. (This is rare in cocaine/crack–addicted clients).

Several drugs are administered to reduce cocaine/crack cravings. Most health care professionals believe that these cravings are due to a decrease in dopamine; thus, amantadine and bromocriptine (Parlodel) are given to increase dopamine levels and to stimulate dopamine receptors. Parlodel affects nutrition in many ways: nausea, vomiting, abdominal cramps, constipation, diarrhea, anorexia, dry mouth, and GI bleeding. To minimize these effects, administer with food; monitor I&O; assess bowel sounds and bowel movements every shift; monitor CBC results; offer small, frequent meals; and provide mouth care. Side effects of amantadine include nausea, anorexia, and constipation. Offering small, frequent meals with fiber and suggesting exercise help negate adverse GI effects.

Methadone used for opioid (heroin, morphine) dependency seems to decrease cravings for opioid by stimulating CNS opioid receptors. No significant interactions occur with food. Since methadone is addictive, withdrawal symptoms may develop when it is discontinued. Clonidine (Catapres), administered to prevent withdrawal symptoms, may cause dry mouth, which can be alleviated with lozenges or ice chips. Catapres may increase sensitivity to alcohol.

What causes a disulfiram reaction, and what substances should be avoided?

Nutritional Assessment

Malnutrition is a common phenomenon with both alcohol and drug dependency. Common symptoms associated with malnutrition can be observed during an assessment, such as flaky, dry skin; muscle wasting; weight loss; and so forth. Most clients minimize how much they actually drink or use drugs.

Assessment of dietary habits is paramount. Typically poorly balanced meals lacking variety and regularity and compulsive overeating or undereating patterns are present. Eating is not a high priority when drugs are used; money is spent on obtaining the chemical rather than food. Consumption of sugar and caffeine is elevated (Dietitians, 1991), and vitamin intake, especially B complex vitamins, is usually decreased.

Since laboratory values usually indicate that most chemically dependent clients are deficient in protein, water-soluble vitamins, iron, zinc, and magnesium, a dietary assessment of these parameters determines if vitamin/mineral supplements are necessary. If the liver has been affected, liver function tests (LFTs) are elevated. Nurses need to be aware of this because compromised LFTs indicate that clients have a narrowed therapeutic window for iron or fat-soluble vitamin supplements, and supplementation may trigger toxic levels, especially iron. Low WBCs indicate a suppressed immune status and increased risk of infections, especially HIV. An inadequate diet adversely affects healing, so nutritional care is essential.

What parameters are assessed in alcohol/drug–dependent clients?

Nutritional Care

Nutritional care involves several components: (1) evaluating nutritional status on detoxification; (2) rehabilitation of nutritional status by providing palatable, nourishing meals and supplements; (3) encouraging normal eating patterns; (4) providing nutrition education and counseling to the user/family; and (5) assisting client/family in development of an eating plan supportive of stable recovery (Beckley-Barrett & Mutch, 1990; Marcus & Katz, 1990). Just as in other mental health disorders, a multidisciplinary team approach meets the needs of clients in a holistic manner.

Name 3 components of nutritional care for alcohol/drug–dependent clients.

Detoxification

During detoxification, physiological status is stabilized. Food can be used to minimize symptomatic discomfort of acute withdrawal (Dietitians, 1991). Treatments to alleviate nausea, vomiting, diarrhea, and electrolyte disturbances are instituted. The main challenge is getting clients to consume enough kilocalories. Therefore, the diet is highly individualized according to the client's needs and preferences. Nutrient requirements are dependent on the chemical abused and physical status of clients. Fluid requirements are usually 2000 ml/day.

Goals

Immediately after detoxification, nutritional goals include promoting physical healing, reducing severity of post–acute withdrawal symptoms, and decreasing drug and alcohol cravings (Dietitians, 1991). Collaborative involvement between the client and health care team to develop good nutrition habits is essential to meet these goals.

Promoting Normal Eating Patterns

Re-establishment of normal eating patterns reduces the nutritional insult of chemical dependency. Eating regularly and prudently are encouraged. Balance, variety, kilocaloric appropriateness, and increased complex carbohydrate intake with moderate amounts of protein and limited quantities of fats are desirable (Beckley-Barrett & Mutch, 1990). Ultimately clients should be able to make their own food choices. Thus, nutrition education/counseling is important.

Nutritional Counseling

Counseling about issues such as **substance substitution,** cravings, snacking, eating disorders, food-related emotional issues, and modified diet regimens is an important component for recovery (Beckley-Barrett & Mutch, 1990). These issues could compromise the quality of nutritional rehabilitation and recovery or lead to other problems, so alternatives (community nutritional resources and problem-solving techniques to prevent relapse) are discussed with clients/families (Beckley-Barrett & Mutch, 1990). This counseling process is initiated on admission or after the detoxification period, depending on a client's need.

When a client replaces sugar, caffeine, nicotine, or excessive food intake for the previously abused drug, substance substitution has occurred.

Follow-up care is beneficial to these clients. Weekly or monthly nutrition/chemical education sessions may lay the foundation for preventing relapse and enhancing recovery.

Describe education needs of chemically dependent clients.

NURSING APPLICATIONS

Assessment

Physical—for type of chemical(s) abused, blackouts, DTs, suicidal tendencies, occupation (health care workers are prone to chemical dependency); weight, height, IBW, MAMC, TSF; malnutrition (raw, beefy tongue; easily bleeding gums; cheilosis), cardiomyopathy.

Dietary—for food/nutrient intake, meal patterns, vitamin and magnesium intake, eating disorders.

Laboratory—for WBCs, iron, MCV; electrolytes, alcohol/drug levels; protein, albumin, prealbumin; elevated LFTs; hepatitis screen, uric acid, HDL cholesterol, urine drug screen.

Interventions

1. Give thiamin as ordered.
2. Encourage 3 regular meals a day.
3. If possible, use actual foods rather than supplements, but provide supplements if necessary.
4. For alcohol-dependent clients, avoid a high-protein, high-fat diet because this is associated with increased incidence of voluntary drinking (Yung et al, 1983).
5. Allow clients to make their own food choices.
6. Encourage clients to eat with others for socialization at mealtimes.
7. Be aware of the organization called NutraPro, which develops nutrition education materials for professionals working with chemically dependent clients.
8. Emphasize positive aspects of the diet such as, "This food will help you diminish and cope with drug cravings."
9. Help clients eliminate food identifications as good or bad (Dietitians, 1991).
10. Assist clients in identifying nutrition warning signs that may indicate a possible relapse, i.e., skipping meals, eating high-fat foods.
11. Become aware of possible treatments of the future: use of calcium and vitamin D to modify the withdrawal process (Mohs et al, 1990), vitamin B_6 supplements to reduce cocaine cravings (News Brief, 1992a).

Evaluation

* Successful outcomes include client eating 3 meals a day, ingesting adequate kilocalories for height and weight, abstaining from chemical use, and participating in follow-up care. Nurses need to realize that relapses are common in chemical dependency, and clients should not be condemned for this relapse nor nurses be overly anxious that proper care was not rendered. However, clients, not nurses, should assume responsibility for their behaviors that may have caused the relapse.

Client Education

- Refer to AA (Alcoholics Anonymous), NA (Narcotics Anonymous), CA (Cocaine Anonymous), Al-Anon, Alateen, Women for Sobriety, or National Council on Alcoholism and Drug Dependence.
- The liver can metabolize only 10 ml of alcohol or 1 oz of whiskey every 90 minutes.
- Drinking in moderation and with meals is better tolerated. However, in alcohol dependency, total abstinence is recommended.

SCHIZOPHRENIA

Schizophrenia is a frightening disorder not only to clients, but also to nurses. All areas of a client's life are affected: mood, perception, thinking, behavior, and communication. These alterations cause seemingly bizarre behaviors **(hallucinations, delusions)** by a schizophrenic. This disorder is chronic and affects both men and women equally (Sulliger, 1988). Age of onset is usually in the early 20s.

Hallucinations are false perceptions that may involve all 5 senses; auditory hallucinations are most frequent (hearing voices). Delusions are false beliefs ("I'm a messenger for aliens.").

Theories

Numerous theories exist for the development of schizophrenia. There is a strong correlation of family history and perinatal and prenatal complications with its development.

Clients with schizophrenia have increased levels of amino acids. Initially elevated amino acid levels compete with dopamine for transport within the brain; dopamine is decreased. Subsequently, increased numbers or sensitivity in dopamine receptors lead to elevated dopamine activity even though the dopamine is at normal levels. This increased dopamine activity is thought to cause schizophrenia (Bjerkenstedt et al, 1985). Nurses should bear in mind that further research is needed to determine whether dopamine activity is the cause or result of schizophrenia.

What is a theory for schizophrenia?

Nutritional Effects of Schizophrenia

Decreased Intake

The most prominent nutritional effect of schizophrenia is decreased food intake caused by abnormal mental functioning. Typical delusions are (1) the food is poisoned, (2) some foods hold magical powers, or (3) organs (insides) are rotting away. These delusions should not be argued or challenged. Initially modify the diet to ensure adequate intake.

Another reason for decreased intake is **catatonic stupor.** Although this is a rare occurrence, nurses need to be familiar with this type of behavior. Some clients eat food if it is placed near them, whereas others may need to be fed by a nurse. In extreme cases, tube feeding or TPN may be implemented.

Catatonic stupor is a state in which a client does not move and appears oblivious to surroundings.

Protein Energy Malnutrition

A prolonged decreased intake can lead to PEM; this occurs mainly in the homeless schizophrenic. Life on the streets results in sporadic intake: from nothing, to food from trash cans, to a free meal from a community mission (Gray & Gray, 1989). This malnutrition increases risk of infections.

Increased Water Intake

Excessive water intake leads to **psychogenic polydipsia.** Fluid intake is not based on need; water is consumed in excess of excretion capabilities of the kidneys. From 3 to 4 gallons of water may be consumed to rid or cleanse the body of something harmful, depending on the delusion. For example, clients may drink to eliminate poisons within their bodies or to cleanse themselves from sin.

Psychogenic polydipsia is water intoxication frequently encountered in some schizophrenic clients.

Any type of fluid may be consumed, including tea; juices; water from toilets, bathtubs, or drinking fountains; or even the client's own urine. These clients may spend inordinate amounts of time at drinking fountains or carry cups with them at all times in case a source of liquid is found (Stanley-Tilt, 1989).

What are nutritional effects of schizophrenia?

Nutritional Effects of Therapy

Schizophrenia is treated by administering antipsychotics. These drugs frequently cause dry mouth and constipation (Table 20–6). Weight gain may occur with all antipsychotics except molindone (Moban) and loxapine (Loxitane). It is unclear whether sedation and decreased activity or increased appetite and carbohydrate craving are the culprits (Gray & Gray, 1989), but in a study using clozapine, the unique neuropharmocologic effectiveness of the drug was associated with weight gain (Leadbetter et al, 1992). Alcohol consumption with antipsychotics increases sedation. Therefore, concomitant use is avoided.

Other nutrient interactions include vitamins. When large doses of vitamin C are given with fluphenazine (Prolixin), absorption of the drug is decreased. Chlorpromazine (Thorazine) increases riboflavin depletion and cholesterol absorption (Gray & Gray, 1989).

Describe possible nutritional effects of antipsychotics.

Incompatibilities between liquid antipsychotics and certain juices and liquids are problematic. When mixed with these juices or liquids, precipitates may be formed, resulting in a medication underdose (Table 20–7).

Nutritional Assessment

Nutritional assessment of schizophrenic clients is an integral component of the interdisciplinary treatment team. Some considerations to observe during an assessment are as follows: (1) allow the client space; (2) begin with what the client typically eats; (3) use simple, concrete words, such as "foods" as opposed to "nutrients", "eat" as opposed to "consume" or "ingest"; (4) delay usual parameters of normal nutritional assessment until trust is developed; and (5) keep the conversation reality focused, i.e., do not delve deeply into delusions, but stay focused on assessment.

Assessment of nutrient and fluid intake is necessary to determine if malnutri-

TABLE 20–6

INTERVENTIONS FOR ANTIPSYCHOTIC SIDE EFFECTS

Gastrointestinal Side Effects	Interventions
Dry mouth	Reassure client this will subside in 1–2 weeks Offer frequent sips of water or ice chips Encourage sugarless chewing gum, hard candy, Chap Stick Inspect mucous membranes Consult with physician for saliva substitute if dry mouth becomes severe Provide frequent oral care
Constipation	Offer high-fiber foods Offer favorite fluids every hour Encourage exercise Monitor bowel sounds
Increased appetite/weight gain	Offer moderately kilocalorie-restricted diet Encourage walking Provide low-kilocalorie snacks Emphasize eating less refined sugar and total fats
Hyperglycemia	Monitor blood glucose levels Assess for polyuria, polydipsia, and polyphagia Confer with physician to alter insulin dose if diabetic
Nausea	Give with meals Monitor I&O Offer small, frequent feedings Limit fatty foods

Data compiled from Haber J, et al. *Comprehensive Psychiatric Nursing*. 4th ed. St. Louis, Mosby, 1992.

TABLE 20–7 **COMPATIBILITY OF LIQUID ANTIPSYCHOTICS AND VARIOUS LIQUID**

Beverage	Thorazine	Prolixin	Haldol	Loxitane	Trilafon	Mellaril	Navane	Stelazine
Water	☺	☺	☺		☺	☹	☺	☺
Milk	☺	☺			☺	☹	☺	☺
Coffee	☺	☹	☹		☹	☹		☺
Tea	☺	☹	☹		☹	☹		☺
7-Up, Sprite	☺	☺		☺	☺	☺		☺
Apple juice/cider		☹	☺		☹	☹	☹	
Apricot nectar		☺			☺		☺	
Cranberry juice	☹					☺	☺	
Grape juice/drink						☹		
Grapefruit juice	☺	☺		☺	☺		☺	☺
Lemonade						☺+		
Orange juice	☺	☺	☺	☺		☺+	☺	☺
Pineapple juice		☺			☺	☺	☺	☺
Prune juice	☹	☺			☺		☺	☺
Tang	☹			☺				
Tomato juice	☺	☺	☺		☺	☹	☺	☺
V-8		☺			☺	☹	☺	☺
Cola	☺	☹	☺	☺	☹	☹	☹	☺

+ Canned only

☺ –Compatible

☹ –Incompatible

Blank–no information

Data from Kerr, L.E. Oral liquid neuroleptics: Administer with care. *J. Psychosoc Nurs Mental Health Services.* 1986 March; 24(3):33–38.

tion or water intoxication is present. Determination of food preference is helpful in increasing intake. However, if a client believes staff is trying to poison him or her, asking preferences causes the client anxiety because he or she will think the nurse is trying to gain information to "trick" him or her into eating. Thus, do not ask delusional clients their food preferences.

List 3 considerations to observe during nutritional assessment of schizophrenic clients.

Nutritional Care

Although the importance of adequate food intake cannot be overemphasized, measures must be taken to increase intake without making food a focal conflict point. Team members are responsible for using ingenuity and different strategies to increase food acceptance. Because of the complexity of schizophrenia, clients with the same symptoms may respond differently. Therefore, diets must be individually tailored for clients.

If clients are unable to care for themselves, nurses need to feed or assist with feeding. For clients who are partially able to care for themselves, reminding them about mealtimes ("Lunch is here") or supervising eating (sitting with clients who are eating to give specific directions) is appropriate.

Arguing about any delusions regarding food is not beneficial nor is tasting food to show it is not poisoned. Arguing and tasting food reinforces the delusion. Initially if clients want to eat in their room, make provisions for this or allow clients to eat either before or after other clients. The setting should be calm, not rushed. Allow clients to keep their tray longer if necessary. Nurses need to be matter-of-fact while serving food, or suspicious clients will continue to question caregiver's motives. A simple statement of "here is your food" is recommended.

NURSING APPLICATIONS

Assessment

Physical—for weight; appetite; infections; delusions, hallucinations; type of antipsychotic, medication side effects; psychomotor movement, water intoxication (headache, nausea, vomiting, abdominal cramps, weakness, stupor, convulsions, coma).

Dietary—for food preferences, kilocalorie, nutrient, water and alcohol intake.

Laboratory—for protein, albumin, prealbumin, transferrin; lymphocytes; sodium (low in water intoxication).

Interventions

1. Discuss treatments and goals in concrete terms; explain to the client what will happen and show equipment to be used. Do not say that blood is about to be drawn because some clients will think colors or crayons will be used.
2. Serve food in individual unopened containers for a client with delusions of poisoned food.
3. When delusions occur, state, "I know you believe the food is poisoned, but no one means to harm you."
4. Follow guidelines in Tables 20–6 and 20–7.
5. If fluid intoxication is occurring, limit water intake.

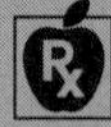 Monitor for riboflavin deficiency (cheilosis and fissures around the eyelids) if chlorpromazine (Thorazine) is given.

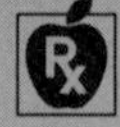 If client is taking large doses of vitamin C and fluphenazine (Prolixin), monitor for effectiveness of Prolixin. Consult the physician for a larger dose of Prolixin or decrease vitamin C.

Evaluation

* Parameters to evaluate include client not losing weight or experiencing excessive weight gain, eating 75 to 100% of diet ordered, and decreasing the number of times delusions or hallucinations occur.

Client Education

- Do not teach while the client is actively hallucinating or having delusions.
- Improvement of mental and physical status is enhanced by proper food intake.
- Use simple, concrete terms.

DEPRESSION

Nearly everyone has experienced **depression** at one time or another. This depression can range from transient to chronic, from mild to severe. Depression, a mood disorder affecting women twice as often as men, afflicts 35 million people. Therefore, it is the most common mental health problem nurses encounter. Numerous theories abound for depression, including biological, psychological, and sociological aspects. Even though there is no nutritional theory that explains the cause of depression, nutritional status may contribute to depression, as discussed previously under nutrient deficiencies.

Depression involves an unrealistic or inappropriate reaction (exaggerated sadness) to an event or internal conflict. Major depression requires antidepressant and/or psychotherapy treatment.

Nutritional Effects of Depression

Many depressed clients suffer from anorexia and weight loss. In fact, these classic signs of depression are major criteria used for diagnosis. Conversely, in limited cases, some clients overeat.

Anorexia and weight loss may occur for several reasons: loss of pleasure in eating and lack of energy or motivation to eat. Occasionally delusions may also interfere with intake. These delusions usually focus on worthlessness, such as being dead or rotting away inside, and being unworthy, rather than the persecutory delusions of schizophrenia.

Depression can increase risk of heart attack and stroke by accelerating atherosclerosis development in high-risk men. Carotid artery plaque buildup of depressed men with excess **fibrinogen** was 3.7 times greater than in nondepressed men with excess fibrinogen. Additionally, depressed men with high blood levels of LDL suffered 1.9 times as much carotid plaque buildup as nondepressed men with similar LDL levels. Nurses must note that only men were tested; thus, results may not apply to women (News Brief, 1992b).

Fibrinogen is a blood clotting factor that contributes to atherosclerosis.

What are the nutritional effects of depression?

Nutritional Effects of Therapies

Depression is treated with antidepressants and/or **electroconvulsive therapy (ECT)**. Tricyclic antidepressants, MAOIs, and atypical antidepressants (trazodone, fluoxetine, and bupropion) are the drugs of choice.

ECT is inducing a grand mal seizure in depressed clients with the use of drugs and electrical currents.

Tricyclics

Anticholinergic properties of tricyclics commonly cause constipation and dry mouth. Dental caries, mouth ulcers, gum disease, and oral thrush can develop from dry mouth (Brasfield, 1991). Rare but possible complications resulting from constipation include impaction or paralytic ileus. Since dry mouth and constipation are also observed with antipsychotics, treatment is the same. Sometimes the physician may lower the dose or move the total dose to bedtime to help decrease these anticholinergic side effects (Brasfield, 1991). Weight gain is an expected outcome with tricyclic use. If weight gain is not desired, modestly restrict kilocalories, encourage exercise, and provide low-kilocalorie snacks.

Concurrent use of alcohol with tricyclics is discouraged because of the excessive sedation that results.

Monoamine Oxidase Inhibitors

MAOIs also cause dry mouth, constipation, and weight gain. Additionally, when MAOIs are combined with tyramine-containing foods, classic hypertensive crisis may develop. Norepinephrine, a hormone, acts as a neurotransmitter; tyramine can cause release of norepinephrine. The enzyme MAO maintains normal levels of norepinephrine by inactivating norepinephrine and preventing absorption of tyramine that is present in foods. Norepinephrine accumulates in the brain when MAOIs are given, improving mood. However, when MAO is inhibited (as with MAOI medications), tyramine from consumption of certain foods may elevate blood tyramine levels, which increases blood pressure. Severe, throbbing headache, neck stiffness, nausea, sweating, chest pain, and intracranial hemorrhage are manifestations of hypertensive crisis. As shown in Table 20–8, fewer foods need to be avoided because of findings that have not convincingly linked previously suspected foods to a hypertensive crisis (Gray & Gray, 1989).

Describe why a hypertensive crisis results when certain foods are consumed. What foods should be avoided?

Atypical Antidepressants

Trazodone (Desyrel) can cause several GI side effects, including decreased/increased appetite, bad taste in the mouth, dry mouth, hypersalivation, nausea, vomiting, diarrhea, flatulence, and constipation. Giving this drug shortly after meals helps alleviate most of these side effects. Monitoring bowel sounds, I&O, and liver tests also need to be implemented. Mouth care is essential.

Fluoxetine (Prozac) does not cause weight gain; conversely, weight loss may occur. GI side effects are similar to side effects of tricyclic medications.

Bupropion (Wellbutrin) also is not associated with weight gain. Nausea and vomiting are frequent side effects of Wellbutrin. Consulting the physician to lower the dose or to give more frequent, smaller doses or giving with meals may help decrease these annoying side effects.

Electroconvulsive Therapy

Dietary restrictions occur in pre-ECT care. Clients are NPO 6 to 8 hours before ECT. After ECT, any type of food can be eaten if gag reflex is present, swallowing is coordinated, and orientation is intact. ECT has improved food intake and caused weight gain in adult clients (Tayek et al, 1988).

TABLE 20–8

GUIDELINES FOR CLIENTS ON MONOAMINE OXIDASE INHIBITORS

Foods to avoid
Cheese (except cottage and cream cheese)
Smoked or pickled fish
Liver
Italian green beans
Meats and yeast extracts
Dry sausage
Sauerkraut
Beer, ale, chianti, and vermouth
Foods to use in limited amounts
Avocados
Bananas
Soy sauce
Sour cream
Yogurt
Foods that were previously restricted but now allowed
Chocolate
Figs
Raisins
Yeast breads
Caffeine-containing beverages

Data from Gray G, Gray L. Nutritional aspects of psychiatric disorders. *J Am Diet Assoc* 1989 Oct; 89(10):1492–1498.

Nutritional Assessment

Assessment of depressed clients is performed as on any other client. Standard measurements, such as anthropometric measurements, dietary history, and laboratory values, may be used. Changes in eating patterns and appetite are frequently observed in depressed clients with resultant weight loss. Dehydration, determined by physical findings and laboratory results (decreased skin turgor, dry mucous membranes, high urine specific gravity, and possible electrolyte imbalances), may occur. Alcohol and chemical use must also be assessed. The only special consideration is to allow more time for responses to questions. Since thought and motor processes are slowed, more time is needed for clients to comprehend and respond.

Nutritional Care

Promoting adequate intake in depressed clients is a real challenge. Individualization of diets is essential and requires a multidisciplinary team effort. Collaboration with clients to identify and provide preferred foods enhances intake. Allow more time to eat since movements are sluggish. Offer small, frequent high-kilocalorie meals/feedings because large meals may seem overwhelming. Unless contraindicated, involve the family as needed either to bring client's favorite foods or to eat with the client. If family cannot dine with the client, nurses may; this may be the stimulus a client needs to eat.

Conversely, overindulgence may occur in some depressed clients. Eating is a method of coping for these clients. Nurses must provide viable options (coping mechanisms) to replace eating. Therefore, before initiating weight-control measures, determine a client's willingness and motivation.

Describe nutritional care for depressed clients?

NURSING APPLICATIONS

Assessment

Physical—for weight, IBW, weight changes; delusions, suicide risk, psychomotor retardation; type of medication prescribed and side effects, use of ECT therapy; BP.

Dietary—for anorexia; food preferences, usual eating patterns, and related problems, including loneliness or boredom; food/fluid/pica, alcohol intake.

Laboratory—for sodium, potassium, serotonin; urine specific gravity and ketones.

Interventions

1. Monitor I&O.
2. Offer foods high in complex carbohydrates and proteins to provide a balance of tryptophan, a precursor of serotonin.
3. If severely depressed, offer fluids instead of foods since consumption of fluids requires less energy.
4. Monitor for inadequate intake, which may depress serum levels of thiamin, riboflavin, niacin, and vitamins B_6 and B_{12}.
5. Consult with dietitian as needed.
6. If overconsumption is occurring, monitor for hoarding of food and taking food from others.
7. To prevent unwanted weight gain, encourage clients taking antidepressants associated with weight gain to increase exercise and avoid high-kilocaloric beverages.

Continued

Evaluation

- Client should lose or gain weight as needed, verbalize that eating is pleasurable, ask for a favorite food, and consume 3 to 6 meals a day.

Client Education

- Loss of appetite is a symptom of the disease. Intake improves as the disease abates.
- Good physical health, which is affected by nutritional status, is an adjunct to psychiatric treatment.
- If the client is on MAOIs, teach foods to avoid.
- ECT therapy requires increased kilocaloric intake.
- Emotional stress lowers nitrogen and calcium levels. Consume adequate amounts of protein-containing and calcium-containing foods.

MANIA

When a client experiences periods of mania with alternate periods of depression, this is termed bipolar disorder. A manic client exhibits hyperactivity, euphoria, elation, and ever-abounding energy. Just watching these clients may evoke certain reactions in nurses who may become swept up in the excitement, wary of all the excitement, or tired from all the excitement!

Incidence of mania is about 0.4% in the general population, with women having a slightly higher rate than men (Kaplan & Sadock, 1989). Bipolar disorder affects approximately 1 to 3 million people in the US. Alterations in neurotransmitters are suspected as a cause of mania.

Nutritional Effects of Mania

What are the nutritional effects of mania? Why do these effects occur?

Decreased intake of nutrients/fluids occurs because clients are too busy to eat, leading to weight loss. Hyperactivity, inability to concentrate, and grandiose ideas increase nutritional needs. Hyperactive clients rarely want to sit and eat; sometimes they are unable to remember when they last ate because of their inability to concentrate. If grandiose ideas are present, clients may think they do not require food like "normal" people or are superior to these mundane facts of life.

Nutritional Effects of Therapy

Lithium is the drug of choice for bipolar-manic episodes. If improvement is not seen, carbamazepine (Tegretol) or valproic acid derivatives (Depakote and Depakene) may be given.

Lithium

Administering lithium with meals may decrease common GI side effects: nausea, vomiting, anorexia, diarrhea, and abdominal pain. These side effects often develop on initiation of lithium but diminish with continued use.

Weight gain secondary to lithium intake may be related to (1) increased appetite; (2) increased thirst, thereby causing consumption of kilocalorie-containing liquids; and (3) altered carbohydrate metabolism. Glucose tolerance is impaired, and insulin sensitivity is increased (Gray & Gray, 1989).

Fluid intake is also altered. Inhibition of antidiuretic hormone occurs when lithium is taken. This results in excessive urination (polyuria). Large amounts of fluids (polydipsia) are needed to counteract this fluid loss.

Lithium excretion is greatly affected by sodium intake. Since both lithium and sodium are positive ions, they compete for renal reabsorption in the proximal tubules. Therefore, if sodium intake is low or restricted, lithium excretion decreases. Less excretion of lithium means more remains in the blood, leading to the possibility of life-threatening lithium toxicity. Conversely, if sodium intake is abnormally high, increased lithium excretion may trigger a return of manic behavior.

Caffeine intake and lithium excretion are also positively correlated. Thus, when caffeine intake is high, lithium excretion is high, promoting a return of manic symptoms resultant of decreased serum lithium levels. Lithium toxicity may develop if caffeine intake decreases.

How do fluid, sodium, and caffeine intake affect lithium levels?

Tegretol

Tegretol should be taken with food to avoid nausea, vomiting, and abdominal pain. Anorexia, dry mouth, glossitis, and stomatitis are other GI side effects of Tegretol. Hypercholesterolemia is frequently observed; hyponatremia caused by inappropriate ADH syndrome is a less frequent side effect. Monitoring oral mucous membranes and laboratory results is necessary.

Depakene/Depakote

GI disturbances of nausea, vomiting, and indigestion are usually temporary but can be minimized by administering valproic acid with food or using enteric-coated Depakote capsule (Karch & Boyd, 1989). Remind clients to swallow the drug whole to prevent mouth and throat irritation. Other side effects include diarrhea, abdominal cramps, constipation, anorexia with possible weight loss, or increased appetite and weight gain. Liver failure may be life-threatening. Therefore, monitor for anorexia, jaundice, vomiting, weakness, and facial edema. If these are observed, notify the physician immediately to discontinue the drug. Acute pancreatitis is also possible; monitor for abdominal pain and elevated amylase levels, and notify the physician if these occur.

Nutritional Assessment

Because of the hyperactive state of these clients, assessment may have to be performed "on the run." Refocusing clients to the nutritional assessment may be indicated ("You said earlier you normally eat 2 meals a day. What types of food do you eat?"). If a client cannot stand still long enough to obtain a weight, try to distract him or her by engaging in a conversation during the procedure. In extreme cases, ask clients how much they weigh and the last time they weighed themselves.

Eating and drinking patterns must be assessed. In clients with mania, eating and drinking patterns are altered from their normal patterns. Usually eating and drinking are erratic; generally, both are decreased, making clients susceptible to malnutrition and dehydration. Alcohol intake may be increased or decreased.

Nutritional Care

What types of foods are beneficial for clients with mania?

A high-kilocalorie diet is suggested for replacement of energy used during the hyperactive phase. Finger foods or foods that do not require utensils (sandwiches, hamburgers) are also offered. Foods and drinks that can be consumed easily while standing or pacing are beneficial. Beverages are needed to replace fluids lost through kidney excretion and diaphoresis. Fluid requirements are usually 3000 ml/day.

NURSING APPLICATIONS

Assessment

Physical—for weight fluctuations, hyperactivity, euphoria, pacing.
Dietary—for appetite; intake of caffeine, salt, fluid, carbohydrates, protein.
Laboratory—for lithium level (normal 0.5 to 1.5 mEq/ml), sodium, potassium; urine specific gravity.

Interventions

1. During the hyperactive phase, offer high-kilocalorie finger foods and beverages—fries, celery sticks with peanut butter, cheese and crackers, malts and fruit juices.
2. Monitor I&O to determine if polyuria, polydipsia, nausea, or vomiting are present, indicating lithium toxicity.

Evaluation

* Client maintains/gains weight appropriate for height, ingests 3000 to 4000 kcal/day (during periods of hyperactivity), 2000 to 3000 ml fluid/day, and consumes foods from all food groups.

Client Education

- If lithium is prescribed, explain the importance of not radically altering the diet, especially sodium, fluid, alcohol, and caffeine intake.
- If clients are on lithium and experience diarrhea and/or vomiting, omit lithium for 1 day (Haber et al, 1992).
- Refer to National Depressive and Manic Depressive Association.

SUMMARY

Treatment of mental health disorders is provided by a multidisciplinary team to assist clients in meeting nutritional needs. Team members must communicate and collaborate with the client as well as with other team members.

A nutritional assessment provides information regarding the presence/occurrence of the following: malnutrition, concurrent illnesses, medications, abuse of chemicals, abnormal or inadequate dietary habits, and food beliefs. Following this assessment, an individualized nutritional plan of care can be developed.

All mental health disorders are treated with several modalities, which can include but are not limited to cognitive, behavioral, and emotional aspects. Client education using individual, family, and group settings is essential for effective nutritional care. A primary goal involves assisting clients to normalize eating patterns.

NURSING PROCESS IN ACTION

A schizophrenic client has been admitted to the unit. He is not eating because he thinks the staff is poisoning him since he is a messenger from God. Thorazine is ordered.

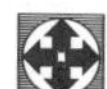

Nutritional Assessment

- Height, weight, signs of malnutrition.
- Types of food normally eaten, adequacy of nutrient/fluid/kilocalorie intake.
- Beliefs about food and nutrition, food preferences.
- Blood levels of protein, albumin, prealbumin, and transferrin.

Dietary Nursing Diagnosis

Alteration in nutrition: high risk for less than body requirements RT fear of being poisoned.

Nutritional Goals

Client will consume food from basic food groups, maintain weight, consume at least 50% of ordered diet, and drink at least 2000 ml/day.

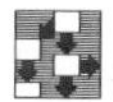

Nutritional Implementation

Intervention: Serve food in individual unopened containers such as unpeeled fresh fruit, cereal in individual boxes, and boxed fruit juices.

Rationale: This will help reduce his fear by allowing him to see that the food has not been tampered with.

Intervention: State, "I know you believe the food is poisoned, but I find that hard to believe. No one means to harm you."

Rationale: This presents reality and does not play into the delusions of the client.

Intervention: Monitor for riboflavin deficiency (cheilosis, scaly skin around nostrils).

Rationale: Since client is taking Thorazine, riboflavin deficiency is possible because riboflavin depletion is increased.

Intervention: Allow the client to eat in room if he prefers.

Rationale: Since schizophrenics have loose ego boundaries and this client is afraid of being poisoned, eating in his room initially may enhance intake by decreasing the anxiety of eating with others.

Intervention: Give directions for eating, i.e., "here is a fork to pick up your meat."

Rationale: Schizophrenic clients need concrete directions because they are incapable of abstract thinking.

Intervention: Offer favorite beverage.
Rationale: Clients are more apt to consume favorite drink and maintain fluid intake.

Intervention: Weigh weekly.
Rationale: This will help determine if client is maintaining weight.

Intervention: Do not taste the food.
Rationale: This reinforces the delusion of being poisoned.

 Evaluation

Client ate food from the basic food groups, ate two-thirds of the diet ordered, ate in his room but progressed to eating in the dining room with other clients, did not lose weight, and drank 2500 ml/day. Additionally, he stopped believing that the staff was trying to poison him. Thus, goals were achieved.

STUDENT READINESS

1. Discuss techniques and behaviors used by nurses while dealing with clients who have AN.
2. What are differences between anorexic and bulimic clients?
3. What are the similarities and differences in nutritional care of anorexic and bulimic clients?
4. Describe dietary interventions for chemically dependent clients.
5. How can a nurse help minimize nutritional effects of schizophrenia?
6. What are some strategies to promote nutrient intake in depressed clients?
7. A client taking Parnate wants to eat pizza. What would you tell this client?
8. Suggest finger foods that may be provided for manic clients.
9. A client taking lithium is on a low-sodium diet. What should you teach this client? What is the normal blood level for lithium?

CASE STUDY

Sally T. has been brought to the physician's office by her parents. She is 18 years old and attends a private school. Her parents are concerned about her weight loss over the past 15 months. She has lost 12 kg and has been progressively preoccupied with weight loss and food.

On examination, the nurse notes brittle nails, dry skin and hair, and muscle wasting. She has experienced amenorrhea for the past 5 months. Her current height is 163 cm and her weight is 42 kg. Sally states that she does not understand why everyone is so concerned about her weight because she still needs to lose a few more pounds.

1. Sally has a medium body frame. What is her ideal weight?
2. What signs of malnutrition are present?

3. What nursing diagnoses can you develop from this situation? List goals appropriate for each diagnosis.
4. What type of treatment modalities would be beneficial for Sally and her family?
5. List referrals you could recommend for Sally and her family.
6. What are some nutritional interventions for Sally?

CASE STUDY

Mr. O. C. is a 63-year-old man whose wife died 8 months ago. Since then, he has been depressed and talks about his own death. As his children become concerned, they convince him to see a physician, who prescribes Parnate, a MOAI. He is then referred for nutrition counseling.

1. What foods need to be eliminated from Mr. O. C.'s diet?
2. What is the rationale for their elimination?
3. What is the possible result of a combination of the medication and the foods to be restricted?
4. List possible nursing diagnoses and goals for this client.

REFERENCES

Addison K. Cocaine: Effects on nutrient levels (Poster Session). *J Am Diet Assoc* 1990 Sept; 90 (suppl, 9):A-65.

American Dietetic Association (ADA): Nutrition intervention in the treatment of anorexia nervosa and bulimia nervosa (Position Paper). *J Am Diet Assoc* 1988 Jan; 88(1):68–70.

Anonymous. Dominion Hospital: Eating disorders program for adolescents and adults. *Food Management* 1991 Apr; 26(4):143–144.

Beckley-Barrett L, Mutch P. Position of the American Dietetic Association: Nutrition intervention in treatment and recovery from chemical dependency. *J Am Diet Assoc* 1990 Sept; 90(9):1274–1277.

Biller B, et al. Mechanisms of osteoporosis in adult and adolescent women with anorexia nervosa. *J Clin Endocrinol Metab* 1989; 68:548–554.

Bjerkenstedt L, et al. Plasma amino acids in relation to cerebrospinal fluid monoamine metabolites in schizophrenia patients and healthy controls. *Br J Psychiatry* 1985 Sept; 147:276–282.

Brasfield KH. Practical psychopharmacologic considerations in depression. *Nurs Clin North Am* 1991 Sept; 26(3):651–663.

Bruch H. *The Golden Cage: The Enigma of Anorexia Nervosa.* New York, Vintage Books, 1978.

Carney MWP. Vitamin deficiency and mental symptoms. *Br J Psychiatry* 1990 June; 156:878–882.

Castro FG, et al. Lifestyle differences between young adult cocaine users and their nonuser peers. *J Drug Educ* 1987; 17(2):89–111.

Chychula NM, Okore C. The cocaine epidemic: Treatment options for cocaine dependence. *Nurse Pract* 1990 Aug; 15(8):33–40.

Devlin CL. Twelve step intervention in compulsive eating. *J Am Diet Assoc* 1991 Sept; 91(suppl 9):A-136.

Dietitians teach chemically dependent patients the importance of nutrition in recovery. *ADA Courier* 1991 Oct; 30(10):3–4.

Edelstein CK, et al. Early clues to anorexia and bulimia. *Patient Care* 1989 Aug 15; 23(13)155–175.

Emmons L. Dieting and purging behavior in black and white high school students. *J Am Diet Assoc* 1992 March; 92(3):306–311.

Fava M, et al. Neurochemical abnormalities of anorexia nervosa and bulimia nervosa. *Am J Psychiatry* 1989 Aug; 146(8):963–971.

Godfrey P, et al. Enhancement of recovery from psychiatric illness by methylfolate. *Lancet* 1990 Aug 18; 336(8712):392–395.

Gold M. Eating disorders are linked to chemical dependency. *Alcoholism Addiction* 1988 May-June; 8:13.

Gray G, Gray L. Nutritional aspects of psychiatric disorders. *J Am Diet Assoc* 1989 Oct; 89(10):1492–1498.

Haber J, et al. *Comprehensive Psychiatric Nursing.* 4th ed. St. Louis, Mosby, 1992.

Hofland SL, Dardis PO. Bulimia nervosa: Associated physical problems. *J Psychosoc Nurs* 1992 Feb; 30(2):23–27.

House MA. Cardiovascular effects of cocaine. *J Cardiovasc Nurs* 1992 Jan; 6(2):1–11.

Howat P, et al. The effect of bulimia upon diet, body fat, bone density and blood components. *J Am Diet Assoc* 1989 July; 89(7):929–930.

Kaplan H, Sadock B. *Comprehensive Textbook of Psychiatry.* 5th ed. Baltimore, Williams & Williams, 1989.

Karch AM, Boyd EH. *Handbook of Drugs and the Nursing Process.* Philadelphia, JB Lippincott, 1989.

Kaye WH, Weltzin TE. Serotonin activity in anorexia and bulimia nervosa: Relationship to the modulation of feeding and mood. *J Clin Psychiatry* 1991 Dec; 52(suppl):41–48.

Killen J, et al. Depressive symptoms and substance use among adolescent binge eaters and purgers: A defined population study. *Am J Pub Health* 1987 Dec; 77(12):1539–1540.

Leadbetter R, et al. Clozapine-induced weight gain prevalence and clinical relevance. *Am J Psychiatry* 1992 Jan; 149(1):68–72.

Lieber C. Hepatic, metabolic and toxic effects of ethanol: 1991 update. *Alcohol Clin Exp Res* 1991 July/Aug; 15(4):573–592.

Love CC, Seaton H. Eating disorders: Highlights of nursing assessment and therapeutics. *Nurs Clin North Am* 1991 Sept; 26(3):677–697.

Marcus RN, Katz JL. Inpatient care of the substance-abusing patient with a concomitant eating disorder. *Hosp Community Psychiatry* 1990 Jan; 41(1):59–63.

McKenna MS. Assessment of the eating disordered patient. *Psych Ann* 1989 Sept; 19(9):467–472.

McLaren D. Clinical manifestations of nutritional disorders. *In* Shils M, Young V, eds. *Modern Nutrition in Health and Disease.* 7th ed. Philadelphia, Lea & Febiger, 1988:733–745.

Miller KD. Body-image therapy. *Nurs Clin North Am* 1991 Sept; 26(3):727–736.

Mitchell J. Bulimia nervosa. *Contemp Nutrition* 1989; 14(10):1–2. (A publication of General Mills.)

Mohs M, et al. Nutritional effects of marijuana, heroin, cocaine, and nicotine. *J Am Diet Assoc* 1990 Sept; 90(9):1261–1267.

News Brief. Study seeks means to ease cocaine withdrawal. *Focus* 1992a Jan; 13(1):7.

News Brief. Depression can boost the risk of heart attack and stroke. *Health Scene* 1992b Sum;6.

Nuckols CC, Greeson J. Cocaine addiction; Assessment and intervention. *Nurse Clin North Am* 1989 March; 24(1):33–43.

Palmer TA. Anorexia nervosa, bulimia nervosa: Causal theories and treatment. *Nurse Pract* 1990 Apr; 15(4):12–21.

Plehn KW. Anorexia nervosa and bulimia: Incidence and diagnosis. *Nurse Pract* 1990 Apr; 15(4):22–31.

Pomeroy C, Mitchell JE. Medical complications and management of eating disorders. *Psych Ann* 1989 Sept; 19(9):488–493.

Riley EA. Eating disorders as addictive behavior: Integrating 12-step programs into treatment planning. *Nurs Clin North Am* 1991 Sept; 26(3):715–726.

Slaiman S. Restricted diets restrict antidepressant efficacy. *Practitioner* 1989 July 8; 333(1472):972, 975.

Soubrie P, et al. Alterations of response to antidepressants in animals induced by reduction of food intake. *Psych Res* 1989; 27:149–159.

Stanley-Tilt C. Recognizing the psychiatric water intoxicator. *Am J Nurs* 1989 Dec; 89(12):1636–1637.

Sulliger N. Relapse. *J Psychosoc Nurs* 1988; 26(6):20–23.

Tayek J, et al. Improved food intake and weight gain in adult patients following electroconvulsive therapy for depression. *J Am Diet Assoc* 1988 Jan; 88(1):63–65.

Tolstoi L. The role of pharmacotherapy in anorexia nervosa and bulimia. *J Am Diet Assoc* 1989 Nov; 89(11):1640–1646.

Williamson D. *Assessment and Diagnosis of Eating Disorders: Obesity, Anorexia, and Bulimia Nervosa.* New York, Pergamon Press, 1990.

Wilson H, Kneisl C. *Psychiatric Nursing*. 4th ed. Redwood City, CA, Addison-Welsey, 1992.

Yung L, et al. Dietary choices and likelihood of abstinence among alcoholic patients on an outpatient clinic. *Drug Alcohol Depend* 1983 Dec; 12(4):355–362.

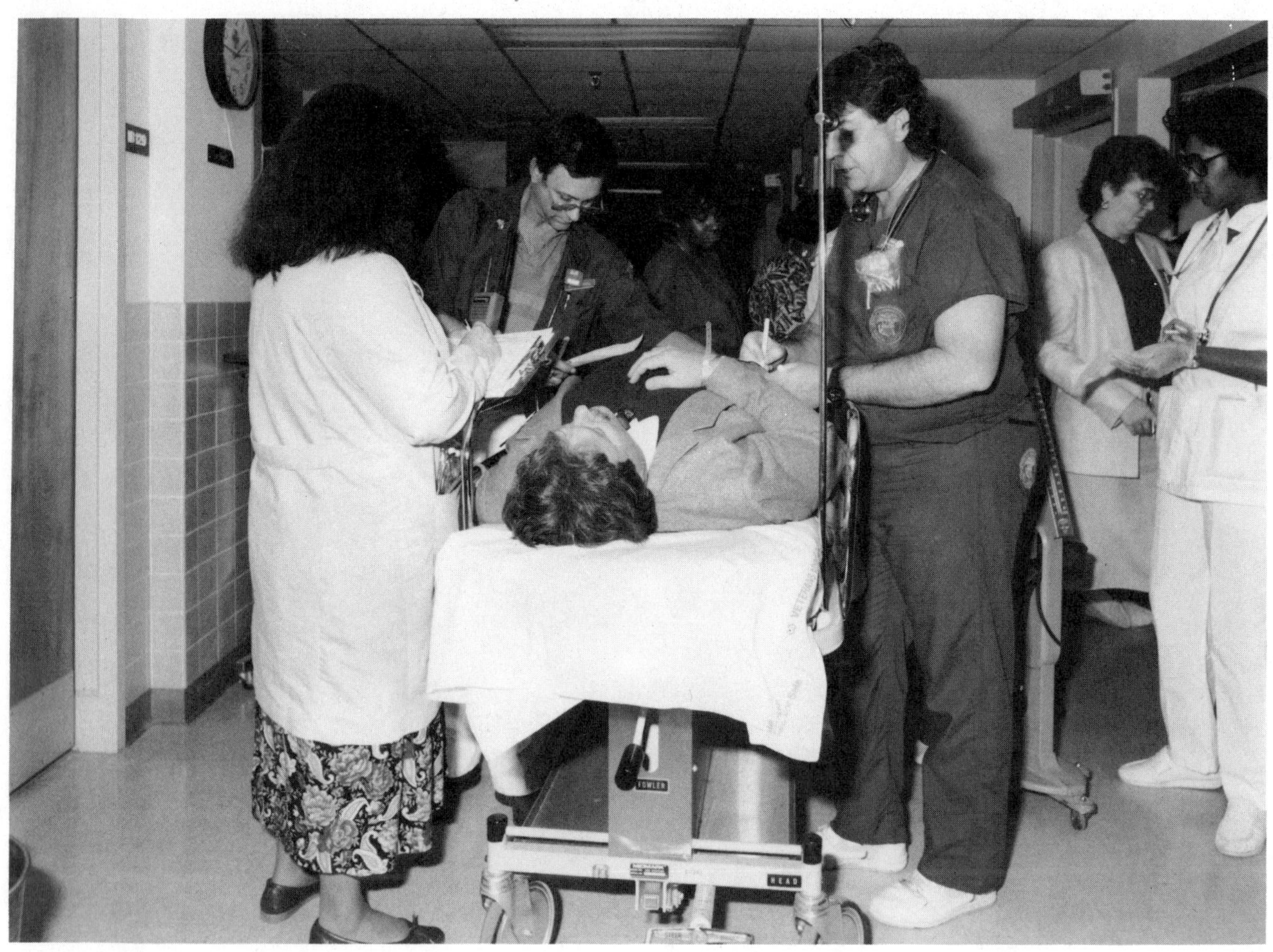

Courtesy of Eugene Davies, Medical Media, Veterans Administration Hospital, Dallas, Texas.

CHAPTER

21

Nutrition Support for Clients with Physiological Stress

OUTLINE

OBJECTIVES

THE STUDENT WILL BE ABLE TO:

- List metabolic changes caused by stress that affect nutritional status.
- Discuss dietary nutrients affected by physiological stress.
- State the usual diet order for physiologically stressed clients.
- Identify clients and types of surgical interventions that may result in malnutrition.
- Discuss nutritional care for surgical and burn clients.
- Explain effects of fever and infection on nutritional requirements.
- Apply nursing principles for nutritional care of clients with physiological stress.
- Discuss educational principles for the above conditions with clients.

TEST YOUR NQ (True/False)

1. Glucose is the major fuel used by injured tissues.
2. Vitamin C is retained by the body during stressful periods.
3. Hypermetabolism and hypercatabolism are the same thing.
4. In a malnourished client, surgery may be delayed until nutrient stores are replenished.
5. A weight gain of more than ½ lb per day is beneficial for postoperative clients.
6. Available iron in the blood stream is decreased during an infection.
7. Sepsis is a fever.
8. Two to 3 months posttrauma, obesity may become a problem in some clients.
9. For COPD clients with a high Pco_2 level, it is recommended that dietary fat intake be increased.
10. Burn clients lose protein in exudate and through the burned surface.

Physiological stress is a general term that includes surgical procedures and anesthesia (even though they are life-saving and under controlled circumstances), burns, trauma, fever, and infections.

Physiological stress can be identified as any condition or stimulus that threatens body homeostasis or a client's well-being. Effects of stressful events on metabolism and nutrient needs vary among clients. Fear and anxiety, as experienced during illness or hospitalization, are simple stress factors. A stressful event that elicits anger, fear, sorrow, or pain may have little effect on metabolism if it is of short duration.

Injury, surgery, and infection all cause similar **hypermetabolic** and **hypercatabolic** responses to re-establish body homeostasis. Treatments are slightly different depending on type, duration, and severity of the condition. As a result of hormonal secretions, a body's response to physiological stress differs from the response to starvation.

Hypermetabolism indicates an increased expenditure of resting energy and oxygen utilization that occur in direct proportion to the extent and severity of an injury or infection.

Hypercatabolism is characterized by a marked loss of protein and fat.

METABOLIC RESPONSES TO STRESS

Ebb Phase

Post-traumatic responses can be divided into 2 distinct periods: an early "ebb phase" followed by a "flow phase". After an injury, the shock or ebb phase lasts approximately 12 to 24 hours and is marked by reduced blood pressure, cardiac and renal output, body temperature, and oxygen consumption. **Glycogenolysis** in response to catecholamines and glucagon results in hyperglycemia for increased availability of glucose. The goal during this phase is to restore perfusion, maintain oxygenation, and arrest hemorrhage.

Glycogenolysis—the breakdown of glycogen in the liver to glucose.

What client symptoms are observed during the ebb phase? What are the goals?

Flow Phase

In the flow phase, hypercatabolism is being resisted, even though hypermetabolism, which peaks in 3 to 4 days, continues in response to the stress (Table 21–1). Three major hormones (glucocorticoids, catecholamines, and glucagon) that are counterregulatory to insulin are increased. This leads to hypermetabolism, altered glucose response, and accelerated nitrogen loss (tissue catabolism). The extent of these responses is generally related to severity of the injury. Although the metabolic response is systemic, localized area of injury produces an energy drain with inefficient glucose utilization due to **anaerobic glycolysis**.

Anaerobic glycolysis—the process of producing lactic acid or pyruvic acid from glucose or glycogen without oxygen.

Hyperglycemia persists during the flow phase despite normal or elevated insulin levels secondary to hepatic gluconeogenesis. As a result of glucocorticoid and catecholamine secretion, amino acids from muscle are used for gluconeogenesis. Hyperglycemia consistent with the flow phase contributes to decreased appetite. Skeletal muscle uses very little glucose because of insulin resistance. Available glucose is shunted to obligate users, i.e., injured tissues, CNS, and RBCs.

TABLE 21–1

PHYSIOLOGICAL RESPONSES TO TRAUMA

	Ebb Phase	Flow Phase
Dominant factors	Inadequate circulation due to loss of plasma volume	Increased levels of catecholamines, glucocorticoids, and glucagon
	Decreased insulin levels	Normal or elevated insulin levels
Clinical findings		Catabolic
	Hyperglycemia	Hyperglycemia
	Decreased oxygen consumption	Increased oxygen consumption and respiration rate
	Hypothermia	Hyperthermia
		Hypermetabolism
		Increased insulin resistance
	Hypovolemia; decreased cardiac output	Increased cardiac output
	Hypotension	

BCAA leucine, isoleucine, and valine.

Increased nitrogen excretion reflects losses from skeletal muscle mass. **Branched-chain amino acids (BCAA)** are used by muscles for energy. Initially skeletal muscle is catabolized, but if this continues, visceral proteins are used.

An important feature in this phase is that the body uses fatty acids and ketone bodies for energy so less skeletal protein is catabolized. Sympathetic nerve stimulation increases digestive juices and decreases peristalsis. If organ failure begins to occur, the liver is unable to synthesize proteins needed. These increased requirements accelerate development of malnutrition.

Release of aldosterone and antidiuretic hormone due to the stress causes sodium and fluid retention. Tissue catabolization from the trauma and stress hormones results in loss of potassium, phosphate, magnesium, sulfur, and zinc from cells.

To summarize, stress response protects and defends the body by attempting to maintain circulating energy substrates. The body reacts this way even though muscle wasting and weakness occur. Despite an occurrence of some anabolic processes, the overall effect initially is significant losses of both protein and fat. Although some clients may perceive this as a good opportunity to lose weight, the body does not use abundant fat stores or spare lean body mass. During stress, obese clients mobilize more protein and less fat than those within an appropriate weight range (Jeevanandam et al, 1991).

Adequacy of metabolic responses to stress is affected by the body's ability to satisfy energy requirements imposed by the catabolism without excessively depleting its protein reserves. Following the acute phase of the flow response, survival is dependent on an adaptive phase in which the stress hormone response subsides so anabolism is predominant. Recovery is dependent on anabolism for tissue repair, replacement of RBCs, and immune response to infection. If the body is unable to make this adaptation, it becomes overwhelmed and may reach a state of exhaustion; death may occur.

What happens in the flow phase? What happens in the adaptive phase?

NURSING APPLICATIONS

Assessment

Physical—for stress response, abdominal distention, constipation, infections, fluid overload, renal function.
Dietary—for anorexia.
Laboratory—for potassium, sodium, magnesium, zinc, phosphate; glucose.

Interventions

1. Monitor for problems associated with increased digestive juices, i.e., gastric discomfort sometimes precipitates an ulcer, and decreased peristalsis may cause constipation or impaction.
2. Since gluconeogenesis occurs in the liver, clients with hepatic disease may have problems coping with stressful conditions, so monitor closely for possible complications and slow rate of healing.
3. Monitor dietary intake and blood glucose response of diabetic clients closely; stressful conditions impose higher risks in these clients because of their inability to increase insulin production in response to hyperglycemia.
4. A cachectic or malnourished client has a poor tolerance for stressful situations. Close monitoring is important to prevent further complications.
5. Monitor fluids being given because increased glucocorticoids and ADH increase fluid and sodium retention and increase potassium excretion. Before giving high potassium foods, monitor renal function (urine output).

Evaluation

* Client progresses through the stress phases with minimal complications.

Client Education

- Explain to clients that this is not an appropriate time to lose weight.
- When the body is stressed, increased amounts of nutrients are needed even though clients are inactive or anorexic.

NUTRITIONAL CONCERNS FOR HYPERMETABOLIC CLIENTS

Nutritional Assessment

Nutritional assessments are important to determine (1) current nutritional status and baseline data, (2) fluid requirements, and (3) nutritional requirements (kilocalories, protein, vitamins, minerals). As discussed in Chapter 11, a careful history and physical examination, anthropometric measurements, and laboratory tests are important. Severity and an estimate of possible duration of the stress are important parameters to consider when developing a nutritional care plan.

Where feasible, nutritional assessments performed before a stressful situation (i.e., surgery) may reveal potential problems. For instance, it is sometimes appropriate to implement nutrition support before scheduled surgery to correct some problems and prevent occurrence of major ones.

Assessment for energy and protein requirements is important to prevent further harm to clients. Too many kilocalories can result in hyperglycemia, hepatic abnormalities, fatty liver infiltration, ventilator dependence (because of increased carbon dioxide production), and elevated waste products for excretion. Excess glucose may further increase metabolic rate.

An accurate weight is the cornerstone for assessing nutritional status and evaluating response to nutrition support. During stress, weight loss is likely to be principally from muscle mass and fluid losses as opposed to fat stores. Weight loss of more than 10% of premorbid weight can seriously compromise ability to combat infection or heal wounds; it increases morbidity and mortality risks. More than 40% weight loss can be lethal (Weinsier et al, 1989). Serial weights, 2 to 3 times weekly, are recommended.

Anthropometric measurements may not be as reliable as biochemical indices in determining nutritional status of clients who have undergone some form of trauma. In particular, TSF and MAMC are unreliable if severe edema is present.

Because of protein catabolism and decreased synthesis, serum levels of proteins, such as albumin and transferrin, are usually low. Low serum protein levels are not always indicative of malnutrition, but they reflect a physiological response to severity of stress or inflammation. Hypoproteinemia may result in reduced wound healing, wound dehiscence, pressure sore formation, reduced immune responsiveness, delayed gastric emptying, and reduced small intestinal mobility and absorption (Weinsier et al, 1989). Serum proteins are indicators of the amount of nutrition support that may be needed.

Besides protein, RBC indices, plasma glucose, BUN, electrolytes, and liver function tests are important to monitor frequently.

When can weight loss compromise healing? What percentage weight loss is lethal? What can hypoproteinemia cause?

Nutritional Care

Nutrition support is of primary importance during hypermetabolic stress. Metabolic response to stress can be minimized by nutrition; additionally, nutrient intake must be adequate to offset losses.

Lipogenesis is fat synthesis.

Initiating aggressive nutrition support before the flow phase is detrimental because metabolism of large amounts of protein results in increased urea synthesis, or excessive kilocalories result in **lipogenesis.** Nutrition support should be initiated when the body moves into the flow phase (see Table 21–1) and strong catabolic effects of hormones and catecholamines have subsided. A fall in blood glucose level is the most significant factor to identify transition into the flow phase. In contrast, when IV dextrose solutions are being given, identification of this phase is not as apparent. Other biochemical changes include a normal BUN, ketosis, ketonuria, and less excretion of urea nitrogen. As a general rule, nutrition support of clients in stressful situations—be it surgery, trauma, infection, burns, or fractures—should be implemented within 5 days to prevent an excessive amount of body proteins being used for energy. Oral or tube feedings protect mucosal integrity and may reduce the hypermetabolic response by decreasing production of stress hormones (Bower, 1990; Saito et al, 1987).

When should nutrition support be initiated, and how is this phase identified? What is the preferred method of nutrition support and why?

Requirements to attain positive nitrogen balance may influence the method of nutrition support. In anticipation of or following a hypermetabolic condition, the mode of nutrition support can be oral feedings with nutrition supplements or enteral or parenteral feedings as appropriate (see Chapter 13). When intake is inadequate to meet elevated requirements, a combination of oral feeding, enteral feeding, or parenteral nutrition may be required. Enteral feedings are currently the preferred method of nutrition support due to improved nitrogen balance and less septic morbidity than TPN (Moore & Moore, 1991).

Energy Requirements

Primary goals for nutrition support are to decrease amount of weight loss and restore anabolism by furnishing nutrients to meet increased demands and replace lost tissue protein. During anabolism, adequate nonprotein kilocalories (carbohydrates and fats) must be supplied for energy to reserve protein for tissue rebuilding. As shown in Table 21–2, energy requirements for most of these clients secondary to surgery, trauma, or infections are in the range of 1.2 to 1.5 times the BEE, or 35 to 45 kcal/kg daily. If a client is suffering from more than one of the catabolic conditions (for instance, both sepsis and multiple fractures), energy requirements are additive; energy requirement may increase to 1.7 to 2 times the BEE. The use of portable indirect calorimetry machines that measure oxygen consumption and carbon dioxide production provides the most accurate determination of individual energy requirements (see Chapter 10). Providing more than double the BEE to produce weight gain cannot be justified, and adjustments in weight should be attempted only after resolution of the stress. For most clients, 2000 to 3000 kcal meets these maintenance requirements; however, burn clients may need 4000 to 7000 kcal daily.

What are general energy requirements of clients with physiological stress?

Protein Requirements

A disproportionately high ratio of protein to kilocalories is necessary to provide sufficient amounts for increased requirements and to maintain optimal immunological response (Fig. 21–1). If protein intake is inadequate, as much as 1 lb tissue protein may be catabolized daily. Additional protein losses from tissue breakdown (caused by sepsis, fever, infection, or trauma), exudates, discharges, or hemorrhaging can cause nitrogen losses. Depletion of body protein can result in serious complications, since it is important for many physiological functions related to stress (Table 21–3). When formation of transport proteins is inhibited, impaired tissue perfusion and pulmonary function as well as decreased nutrient absorption occur.

To attain nitrogen balance requires adequate protein and kilocalories supplied by carbohydrates and fats. Nitrogen equilibrium can be achieved and at times positive nitrogen balance obtained in otherwise catabolic clients given adequate energy

TABLE 21–2

FORMULAS FOR DETERMINATIONS OF TOTAL ENERGY REQUIREMENTS

Daily energy requirement for weight maintenance =
normal BMR[1] × stress factor[2] × 1.25[3]
Daily energy requirement for weight gain =
maintenance energy + 1000 kcal[4]

1. Normal BMR (usually 1500 to 1800 kcal/day) can be determined using standard nomograms or formulas. The approximate values of the basal metabolic rate for adults of average size are given below:

Body Weight (kg)	50	55	60	65	70	75	80
Normal BMR (kcal/day)	1316	1411	1509	1602	1694	1784	1872

2. Stress factor is the term used to correct the normal BMR for the effects of a disease process:

Condition	**Stress Factor**
Mild starvation	0.85–1.00
Postoperative recovery (no complications)	1.00–1.05
Cancer*	1.10–1.45
Long-bone fracture	1.25–1.30
Peritonitis	1.05–1.25
Severe infection of multiple trauma*	1.30–1.55
Burns >40% body surface area	2.00

3. The basal kilocaloric requirements of the stressed client are adjusted upward an additional 20 to 25% for hospital activity and the stress associated with treatment. This adjustment is unnecessary for clients receiving artificial ventilation who are paralyzed or are heavily sedated.
4. If anabolism and weight gain are the goals, an additional 1000 kcal/day may be added to maintenance requirements to provide for a weight gain of approximately 1 kg (2 lb)/week. Weight maintenance, not weight gain, should be the primary objective in most critically ill clients.

Example: Weight maintenance for burn client weighing 65 kg:

1602 × 2.00 × 1.25 = 4005 kcal

* Proportional to the extent of the disease.
From ME Shils, VR Young, eds. *Modern Nutrition in Health and Disease.* 7th ed. Philadelphia, Lea & Febiger, 1988. Reprinted with permission.

and protein. Protein can be synthesized only if kilocalorie requirements have been met.

Protein requirements can be calculated as follows:

Moderate stress = 1 to 1.5 gm/kg body weight

Severe stress = 1.5 to 2 gm/kg body weight

Therefore, for a stressed client weighing 70 kg, 100 to 140 gm of protein may be needed. To determine protein adequacy, nitrogen balance is assessed in critically ill clients with UUN (see Chapter 3).

Arginine is normally a NEAA for normal unstressed clients. Endogenous production of arginine may not be adequate for positive nitrogen balance during trauma or stress. Adequate arginine has been shown to diminish protein catabolism, improve immune function, and accelerate wound healing (Gottschlich et al, 1990a).

Describe protein requirements.

Fluid Requirements

In addition to normal fluid losses, stressed clients may have increased fluid requirements because of losses from exudates, hemorrhage, vomiting, diuresis, and fever. Initially adequate replacement of fluid loss is of paramount importance. When clients are unable to consume enough fluids, IV infusions maintain hydration and correct electrolyte imbalances. However, stress may lead to renal shutdown.

How may stressed clients lose fluids? Why must I&O be monitored?

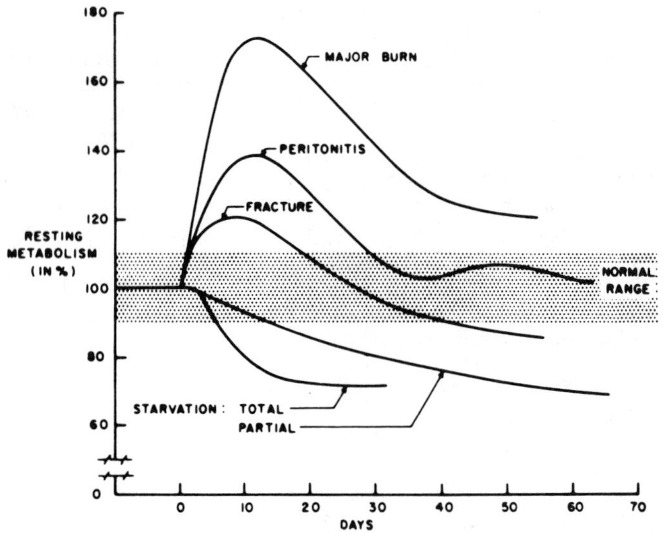

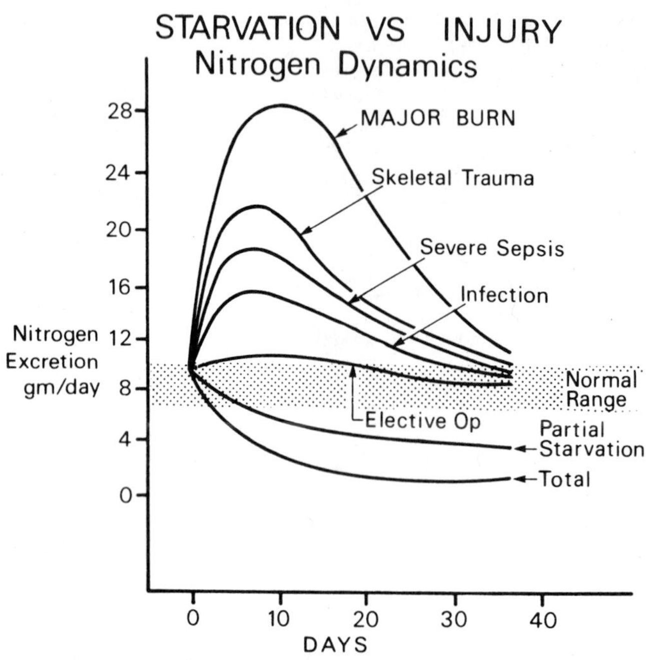

Figure 21–1 Changes in metabolic rate and nitrogen excretion as a result of physiologic stress. Shaded areas indicate normal ranges. (From Long CL, et al. Metabolic response to injury and illness: Estimation of energy and protein needs from indirect calorimetry and nitrogen balance. *JPEN* 1979; 3:452.)

TABLE 21–3

PHYSIOLOGICAL FUNCTIONS OF PROTEIN AS RELATED TO STRESS

Enhances	Prevents
Tissue synthesis for wound healing	Hypovolemia shock
Bone healing	Edema
Resistance to infection	Fatty deposits in the liver
Replenish hemoglobin due to blood loss	Loss of muscular strength

Renal function must be monitored by fluid output as well as intake. Oral intake should begin as soon as possible.

Vitamin Requirements

Although all vitamin requirements are increased during stress, a few play vital roles in the recovery (Table 21–4). If possible, adequate amounts of vitamins should be obtained from foods. Reliance on multivitamin supplements can be risky since only 10 to 12 nutrients may be provided instead of the 40 or more needed. Minor surgery does not necessitate supplementation; however, clients fasting longer than 4 days or on routine IV infusions or parenteral therapy require a therapeutic source of vitamins. Many B vitamins are required for antibody formation and white blood cell function.

Ascorbic acid has long been recognized for its role in wound healing and collagen formation. Urinary excretion of ascorbic acid is increased during stress. Oral or parenteral supplements may be prescribed for extensive tissue regeneration.

Tissue regeneration is dependent on vitamin A. Low plasma retinol levels usually correspond with decreased zinc levels. It is believed that increased hormone secretions can also precipitate low vitamin A levels.

TABLE 21–4

ROLE OF NUTRIENTS DURING STRESS

Nutrient	Physiological Role in Stress
Protein	Necessary for protein and collagen synthesis and production of histamine. Deficiency results in depressed cell-mediated immunity, macrophages, and neutrophils
Arginine	Conditionally essential amino acid under special circumstances. Increases thymic size and production of lymphocytes and decreases incidence of infection
Linoleic acid	Essential component of cell membranes, metabolized to biologically active compounds including prostaglandins. Deficiency results in impaired wound healing. Excessive amounts are immunosuppressive
Omega-3 fatty acids	Components of cell membranes, used by cells to produce prostaglandins. Deficiency results in immunological changes. Increased amounts improve cell-mediated immune response
Vitamin A	Required for tissue integrity and collagen formation; maintains immune function (lymphocytes, macrophages, and lysozymes)
Vitamin C	Enhances capillary formation, collagen synthesis, tissue integrity, and antibody production (phagocytes, neutrophils, and macrophages)
Folic acid	Needed for nucleic acid metabolism and protein synthesis; maintains immune function (lymphocytes and macrophages)
Vitamin B_{12}	Required for protein synthesis; maintains immune function (lymphocytes and macrophages)
Thiamin	Necessary for energy metabolism; maintains immune function (lymphocytes and macrophages)
Vitamin K	Needed for coagulation
Biotin	Required for antibody production
Vitamin B_6	Necessary for amino acid metabolism; maintains immune function (lymphocytes and macrophages), white blood cells, and antibody formation
Riboflavin	Necessary for energy metabolism; maintains immune function (lymphocytes and macrophages)
Niacin	Necessary for energy metabolism; maintains immune function (lymphocytes and macrophages) and tissue integrity
Zinc	Necessary in lymphocyte and phagocyte response; needed for cell division and proliferation and collagen strengths
Iron	Necessary for proper function and proliferation of neutrophils and lymphocytes and for Hgb
Copper	Necessary for collagen formation

Electrolyte/Mineral Requirements

Calcium, magnesium, manganese, copper, and especially zinc have important roles in tissue repair. Although their exact role in wound healing is not known, wounds in clients with clinical deficiencies return to normal healing rates with dietary supplementation. As a result of increased losses during stress and weight loss, zinc is frequently depleted in clients with chronic malnutrition, metabolic stress, or diarrhea (Goodson & Hunt, 1988). However, clients with renal dysfunction must be monitored to prevent high plasma concentrations of zinc.

What vitamins are needed in increased amounts during times of stress and why? What minerals are affected by stress?

Oral Intake

As soon as possible, nutrition support should be implemented. If a client is able to consume foods orally, the diet order may read "high-kilocalorie, high-protein." Although the order may not state increased minerals and vitamins, it is generally assumed that larger amounts also accompany protein and kilocalories (Fig. 21–2).

Communication is vital when ordering a high-kilocalorie, high-protein diet. By stating the purpose of the diet, confusion can be minimized. Occasionally a specific number of kilocalories and grams of protein is ordered to ensure adequacy of energy and protein. A diet specifying 3000 kcal and 150 gm of protein could be interpreted as a diabetic diet, and 3 or 4 slices of bread may be provided instead of pie à la mode. By prescribing the same diet and specifying that it is for a burn client, the intention is clear. A dietitian should be notified for prompt consultation.

Anorexia is frequently present in stressed clients, significantly decreasing food intake. Nurses are challenged to persuade clients to consume sufficient quantities of food to supply required nutrients.

List reasons why oral intake frequently decreases in stressed clients.

Some clients are unable to consume adequate amounts of food orally because of elevated requirements. Polymeric formulas left in a chilled container and accessible to clients can be taken over a period of time; their nutrient content is substantial.

Tube and Parenteral Feedings

Specialized formulas have been designed for altered requirements of stressed clients. Individual nutrients exert variable influence on different aspects of immunocompetence. Polymeric formulas, i.e., Replete (Clintec), Traumacal (Mead Johnson), Impact (Sandoz), and Promote (Ross), are formulated with variations in composition of proteins and amino acids (such as arginine and glutamine), nucleotides, micronutrients, and type of fats to boost immune function and promote wound healing. Elemental formulas for stressed clients include Alitraq (Ross), Reabilan (O'Brien/KMI), and Peptamen (Clintec).

Elemental formulas and parenteral protein solutions enriched with branched-chain amino acids (BCAA) have been advocated for use in hypercatabolic clients since serum BCAA levels are decreased. The theory is that these amino acids, which are not readily used by the liver for glucose production, may be metabolized by skeletal muscle. Presently 20 to 25% BCAA is recommended; this is the amount found in normal proteins. Studies using BCAA have not shown any difference in outcome or length of hospital stay even though positive nitrogen balance was achieved earlier. If clients can tolerate high-protein intakes (1.5 to 2 gm/day/kg), BCAA-enriched formulas should not be necessary. BCAA are currently recommended when positive nitrogen balance has not been achieved within a reasonable period of time after receiving standard feeding or formulas supplying adequate protein and energy (Bower, 1990). Travasorb Hepatic (Clintec) and Hepatic-Aid (Kendall-McGraw) contain approximately 45% BCAA.

Parenteral feedings normally consist of glucose for energy, amino acids to replace protein, and vitamins and minerals. Lipids are advocated in these feedings to

Sample Menu

Breakfast
1/2 banana
1 cup bran flakes
1 cup fruit-flavored yogurt
1 cup whole milk
coffee with non-dairy creamer and sugar

Mid-morning snack
8 oz pineapple juice
1 slice whole wheat toast
1 tsp margarine
1 packet jelly

Lunch
2.5 oz lean broiled pork chop
1/2 cup scalloped potatoes
1/2 cup cooked carrots
1/2 slice whole wheat bread
2 tsp margarine
1 baked apple

Mid-afternoon snack
2 oz cheddar cheese cubes
2 canned pear halves
4 saltines

Dinner
1/2 cup beef stroganoff
1/2 cup cooked noodles
1/2 cup cooked broccoli
1/2 cup cheese sauce
1/2 slice whole wheat bread
1 tsp margarine
1 slice cream pie with blueberry sauce
tea

Evening snack
High-kcal, high-protein milkshake with 8 oz nutrition supplement and 1/2 cup ice cream

Nutrient	RDA: Male–25 to 50 years	Actual	% RDA
Kcal		3349 kcal	115
Protein		144 gm	228
Carbohydrate		412 gm	114
Fat		136 gm	140
Cholesterol		394 mg	131
Fiber–dietary		33 gm	131
Vitamin A		3670 RE	367
Thiamin		4.1 mg	272
Riboflavin		4.4 mg	258
Niacin		32.4 mg	171
Vitamin B_6		3.6 mg	183
Folate		516 mcg	258
Vitamin B_{12}		8.9 mcg	445
Pantothenic acid		10. mg	182
Biotin		107 mcg	165
Vitamin C		153 mg	255
Vitamin D		10.5 mcg	212
Vitamin K		298 mcg	373
Sodium		4026 mg	168
Potassium		5243 mg	262
Calcium		1971 mg	246
Phosphorus		2348 mg	293
Magnesium		499 mg	143
Iron		39.5 mg	395
Zinc		22.7 mg	152
Copper		2.3 mg	104
	^ 0 ^ 50 ^ 100 ^ 150 ^ 200		

Carbohydrate, Protein, and Fat Distribution

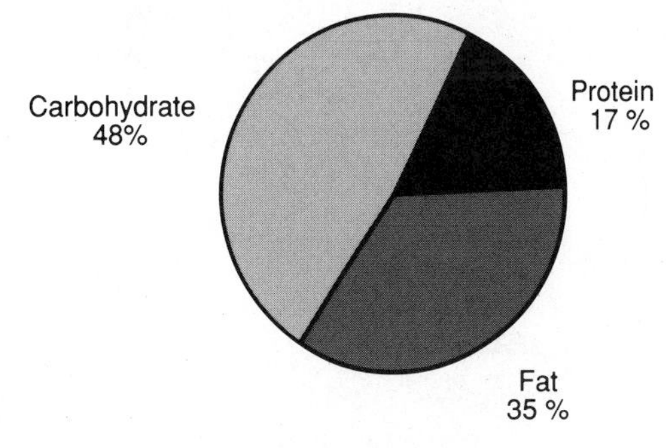

Figure 21–2 High-energy, high-protein diet. RDA, Recommended dietary allowance; RE, Retinal equivalents. (Nutrient data from Nutritionist III, Version 7.0 Software, Salem, OR.)

supply EFA and prevent side effects frequently observed when large amounts of IV glucose are used. Stress-related hypermetabolic hormones stimulate lipid catabolism. Lipids provided in IV feedings result in reduced amounts of plasma insulin, allowing amino acids to be used for synthesis of critically needed visceral proteins.

NURSING APPLICATIONS

Assessment

Physical—for weight, infections, wound healing or dehiscence, pressure sores, drainage, hemorrhaging, fatigue.

Dietary—for nutrient intake, energy and protein requirements, vitamins C and A intake, diet ordered, anorexia.

Laboratory—for potassium, sodium, phosphorus, magnesium, zinc; albumin, transferrin, prealbumin, protein; RBC, MCV, glucose, BUN, LFTs, urine ketones, UUN.

Interventions

1. Monitor weights frequently. A rapid weight gain (more than 1 lb per day) indicates water retention; weight loss suggests inadequate energy intake.
2. If edema is present, use weight as an indicator of hydration status.
3. If a client with an initial weight of 150 lbs loses more than 15 lbs (10% of premorbid weight), notify the physician immediately and consult the dietitian to prevent further weight/tissue losses.
4. If a client is NPO for longer than 4 days or receiving only parenteral intake, consult with dietitian and physician for inclusion of vitamin supplement.
5. Do not panic or automatically assume malnutrition if serum protein is low. This is a natural physiological response to the stressful situation.
6. Notify the dietitian concerning the diet ordered and client's acceptance.
7. Provide food the client normally enjoys; it is more likely to be eaten. Regardless of the diet prescription, nurses can encourage clients to maintain a well-balanced intake consisting of selections from all food groups. Foods should be served appetizingly.
8. Offer 6 feedings daily to increase intake and minimize discomfort.

Evaluation

* If client weighed 150 lbs, weight loss should be less than 15 lbs. No infections and well-approximated edges of wounds should occur.
* Monitor circulating proteins at least weekly to assist in evaluating adequacy of nutrition support. If they do not begin to rise within 10 days after initiation of nutrition support, suspect another disease condition (infection) or inadequate nutritional intake.
* Clients receive adequate kilocalories and protein and maintain body weight.

Client Education

- Adequate intake is important to avoid complications of infections and promote anabolism (healing).
- Oral intake of nutrients by using foods is better than taking a vitamin/mineral supplement.
- Because of physiological stress, greater quantities of nutrients are needed to promote anabolism. Nutrient-dense foods are recommended.
- Foods rich in vitamin A (see Chapter 6, Table 6–2), vitamin C (see Chapter 7, Table 7–2), and zinc (see Chapter 9, Table 9–6) are all important for wound healing.

SPECIAL NUTRITIONAL CONCERNS OF SURGERY

Despite the fact that surgical procedures are usually "planned" or "induced" trauma, they produce an extraordinary stress on the body. Nutritional needs are increased by this stress, yet they are often ignored.

Preoperative Nutritional Care

Good nutritional status before surgery enables a client to withstand postoperative catabolic stresses of negative nitrogen balance and several days of "starvation" without seriously hampering recovery. Wound healing and ability to resist infections at this time are also improved by adequate nutritional stores.

Preoperative nutrition therapy may be implemented to lessen possible risks. In considering preoperative nutrition support, the following factors must be considered: (1) current nutritional status, (2) extensiveness of surgery, and (3) anticipated response to nutritional therapy (Hill, 1988).

Problems are more prevalent in certain types of clients. Children and clients over 40 years old generally experience preoperative apprehension and anxiety or stressful preoperative preparation. Clients may have become depleted secondary to their condition or disease (anorexia, vomiting, diarrhea, or bleeding), especially if it is a chronic GI tract disease (fistulas, short bowel syndrome, inflammatory bowel disease). NPO status for laboratory tests and other hospital procedures may also compromise nutritional status. Long-term inadequate intake from chronic or neoplastic disease may have precipitated significant weight loss or PEM. Clients with more than 10% weight loss or with laboratory indications of poor nutritional status (decreased albumin, transferrin, prealbumin, TLC) should be considered for preoperative nutrition support. At least 500 kcal more than estimated total energy requirements should be provided for depleted clients along with 1.5 gm protein/kg body weight. Clients should receive nutrition support if starvation in excess of 5 to 7 days is expected for well-nourished clients or 1 to 3 days for malnourished clients (Buzby, 1990).

For elective surgery, nutritional repletion can be made over a period of time. Obesity increases risk for delayed wound healing, infection, and difficulty weaning from a respirator. Therefore, weight reduction is usually advisable if protein intake is adequate to maintain lean body mass.

A minimum of 7 to 10 days of nutritional repletion is needed to reduce postoperative complications and mortality significantly (Meguid et al, 1990). This therapy may benefit at-risk clients by repleting hepatic glycogen stores and amino acid pool and thus aid in liver function. Plasma transferrin and prealbumin levels may show positive responses if the client is in positive nitrogen balance, but albumin levels show little effect. Two to 3 weeks may be needed to restore debilitated clients to a satisfactory status. Oral or tube feeding nutritional repletion is cost-effective if surgical delay is not detrimental to clients.

When emergency surgery must be performed, correction of fluid and electrolyte imbalances may be required immediately before surgery. Whole blood transfusions raise hemoglobin and hematocrit levels. To prevent possible infection in an emergency situation, more aggressive treatment may be adopted, such as using antibiotics to reduce bacteria or providing exogenous albumin.

The stomach should be empty during surgery and before administering any general anesthesia; no food is allowed for at least 6 to 8 hours before surgery. Food in the stomach may be aspirated during induction of anesthesia or in recovery. The general procedure is a light dinner with fluids allowed until midnight for surgery scheduled the following morning. Surgery within the GI tract may necessitate NPO status for several days preoperatively to eliminate fecal matter. However, elemental feedings may be given.

Describe clients prone to nutritional problems preoperatively. Why is food withheld before surgery?

NURSING APPLICATIONS

Assessment

Physical—for age, vomiting, diarrhea, bleeding, weight changes, obesity, anxiety, stress.

Continued

Dietary—for protein and kilocaloric intake, medications that adversely affect food intake, time of last food and fluid intake.

Laboratory—for albumin, prealbumin, transferrin; Hgb, Hct; potassium.

Interventions

1. Whenever necessary and possible, implement a high-kilocalorie, high-protein diet to replenish body stores. An increased amount of nutrients can be ingested if 6 small feedings are offered. Liquid supplements between meals can increase kilocalorie and total nutrient content. This diet enhances nutritional status for the surgical and "starvation" period if consumed by clients.
2. Report failure to eat adequate amounts. Preoperatively the client's appetite may be diminished from psychological and/or mental stress.

Evaluation

* Nutrition support is implemented preoperatively if needed. Otherwise, client nutritional status is maintained to prevent postoperative complications.

Client Education

- GI function responds more effectively to enteral than to parenteral therapy.
- Fewer complications generally occur in clients who are well nourished but not obese.

Postoperative Nutritional Care

Malnutrition may develop postoperatively as a complication of the procedure. Resumption of adequate oral intake may be delayed because postoperative oral feedings may cause nausea, vomiting, abdominal distention, and delayed gastric emptying. This is well tolerated if a client is well nourished before surgery. If sepsis occurs, energy expenditure is elevated, and body protein stores are rapidly depleted.

Traditionally foods have been withheld postoperatively because of "post-op ileus." However, this pertains to the stomach and colon only; small intestinal motility and function are maintained (Maynard & Bihari, 1991).

Lack of intake during this period induces a starvation effect. This causes a negative nitrogen balance with increased mobilization of amino acids for energy and increased potassium excretion. IV dextrose and electrolyte solutions administered during this period provide energy for the brain and other vital organs. A minimum of 100 gm of dextrose daily prevents ketosis.

Foods are normally initiated when peristalsis returns. This function can be determined by the presence of bowel sounds or passage of flatus or stools.

Following a minor surgery, the diet is resumed as tolerated as soon as possible. For more extensive surgery, clients are first provided a clear-liquid diet and progress, as tolerated, to a regular diet or the one they had before surgery. Postoperatively a high-kilocalorie, high-protein diet that provides adequate carbohydrate and fat kilocalories can spare protein for anabolism. At least 1.5 gm protein/kg body weight is needed. In general, the diet after surgery should contain adequate kilocalories and nutrient-dense foods. If adequate amounts of nutrients and kilocalories cannot be taken, oral supplement or tube feedings may be necessary. Blood loss during surgery usually results in anemia; adequate intake of protein, iron, zinc, and folate is essential for anabolism of RBCs.

Nasojejunal—flexible weighted tube passed to the jejunum for feeding; Jejunostomy—surgically placed feeding tube into the jejunum.

Malnourished clients at high risk for complications would benefit from immediate enteral feeding, which can be provided via a **nasojejunal** tube or a feeding **jejunostomy.** Implementation of nutrition support is generally recommended to avoid excessive catabolism of muscle mass if adequate oral intake is not anticipated within 7 to 10 days. For clients who are severely catabolic or were malnourished preoperatively, if postoperative starvation is expected for 5 to 7 days, nutrition support is suggested (Buzby, 1990). An immediate goal postoperatively is nutritional maintenance with restoration of somatic and visceral proteins during the convalescent period. Enteral nutrition (if the GI tract is functional) is equally or more effective in improving or maintaining nutritional status than are parenteral feedings. (Meguid et al, 1990). Postoperative fatigue persists for months after major surgery, but it is not known if nutrition therapy affects postoperative fatigue or not.

Describe nutritional care for minor or more extensive surgery. When is nutrition support recommended?

NURSING APPLICATIONS

Assessment

Physical—for bowel sounds, flatus, stools, body weight, fatigue.
Dietary—for nutrient and kilocaloric requirement; adequacy of intake.
Laboratory—for iron, Hgb, Hct, RBCs; protein, prealbumin, albumin, transferrin.

Interventions

1. Monitor weight. During the postoperative period, in which there is a temporary inability to ingest nutrients, a weight loss of ½ lb/day reflects muscle and fat catabolism; a weight gain of more than this indicates fluid retention.
2. Following surgery, urine excretion is diminished, so do not be alarmed unless urine output falls below 30 ml/hr.
3. Keep accurate I&O records. These are essential postoperatively to determine fluid balance.
4. If postoperative ileus continues for more than 5 to 7 days, consult the physician regarding enteral feedings into the jejunum or parenteral feedings.
5. Offer vitamin C–rich foods and fluids (Chapter 7) to promote wound healing.
6. When a soft diet is prescribed, offer high-carbohydrate foods and foods with emulsified fats, such as whole milk, to provide adequate kilocalories for anabolism.
7. Following surgery, encourage overweight clients not to attempt weight loss because this will deter the anabolic process.

Evaluation

* Client should resume presurgery diet and maintain or gain weight. Additionally, no impactions should develop, and wound healing should occur.

Client Education

- Carbohydrate is the body's preferred source of energy for wound healing.
- Postoperative intestinal gas can be distressing. Ambulation is a better therapy than seltzer or carbonated beverages for intestinal gas pains.

SPECIAL NUTRITIONAL CONCERNS ASSOCIATED WITH INFECTIONS AND FEVER

One of the first parameters affected by nutrient deficiencies is immune response. Defense mechanisms needed to fight infection are highly dependent on adequate protein synthesis to support phagocytic and lymphoid cell activity and immunoglobulin production. Thus, nutritional status influences client susceptibility to infections.

Additionally, an infection can deplete nutrient stores. Infections can cause some nutrients to be lost directly via secretion or excretion, and others are lost as a result of accelerated or functionally altered metabolic processes. The extent of nutrient losses is dependent on severity of illness and the elevation and duration of temperature. Overall metabolic responses to infection can be similar despite many different types of infectious organisms. Metabolic processes and oxygen utilization are accelerated. Frequently excess body water is retained secondary to sodium retention as a result of increased secretion of aldosterone.

With the exception of iron, zinc, and vitamin A, isolated nutrient deficiencies are rare, but observations have confirmed a crucial role of several vitamins and trace elements in immunocompetence (Chandra, 1991). Low levels of zinc, iron, and many other trace elements impair resistance to infection. If serum protein levels are low, available nutrients may not be transported to where they are needed because of inadequate transport proteins (see Table 21–4). Vitamins C, A, and B complex (especially folate, B_6, and B_{12}) function within the immune system to fight off invasive organisms.

Although several researchers have postulated that vitamins, especially vitamin C, can help prevent infections, evidence does not support an enhanced immunologic effect from an excess of vitamins (Lowenstein & Parrino, 1987). Excessive intake of zinc, selenium, and vitamins A and E is associated with impaired immune responses. Monitoring the number of T lymphocytes is useful in determining both the need for supplementation and the response to therapy (Chandra, 1991).

Harmful organisms such as viruses, bacteria, and endotoxins are destroyed by leukocytes. This triggers a release of interleukin I, which in turn causes elevated body temperature by the hypothalamus. All infections decrease nutrient intake and increase nutrient losses (Scrimshaw, 1991).

A transient febrile infection has little effect on a healthy well-nourished client but has great effects if the illness persists along with inadequate food intake. Hospitalized clients may be debilitated by their primary disease and nutritional status. **Nosocomial** infections increase morbidity and mortality in malnourished clients (Scrimshaw, 1991).

Infections originating in a hospital are referred to as nosocomial.

Within hours after symptoms of an illness, iron is deposited in iron stores (hemosiderin and ferritin) leading to low plasma iron concentrations. This lasts until the infection subsides. Anemia of infection is evidenced by **hypochromic, microcytic** RBCs, low TIBC, and high ferritin levels. This appears to be an important factor in inhibiting proliferation of iron-requiring bacteria. While the infection is active, oral or parenteral doses of iron, zinc, folate, and vitamin B_{12} are ineffective in reversing anemia caused by this infection.

Hypochromic—RBCs lack color because of low Hgb. Microcytic—RBCs of small size.

The acute infectious process is characterized by increased metabolic rate, weight loss, and wasting of body protein. Anorexia accompanied by a negative nitrogen balance is closely correlated with losses of potassium, phosphorus, magnesium, sulfur, iron, and zinc.

Catabolic processes in relation to an infection are summarized in Figure 21–3. The catabolic period associated with an infectious disease is likely to last for several days or during the febrile phase of infection; the anabolic period of increased nitrogen retention is generally twice as long. The amount of energy used increases when temperature rises because of heat generated and heightened enzymatic activity. Use of antipyretic drugs reduces energy requirements produced by a fever.

Describe a body's responses to infection, especially iron. How do infections affect nutritional requirements and food intake?

Sepsis

Sepsis is the presence of pathogenic microorganisms or their toxins in the blood stream.

Describe the body's response to sepsis.

Sepsis is associated with increased levels of hormones similar to the hypermetabolic response described earlier. Elevated metabolic rate and oxygen consumption, accelerated protein breakdown and negative nitrogen balance, and altered carbohydrate metabolism are present. Weight loss, marked reduction in muscle mass, progressive hypoalbuminemia, and increased urea excretion are part of the classic metabolic effects of ongoing sepsis. Typical of the hypermetabolic response, changes in metabolism of energy nutrients are observed. Lipids appear to be the preferred fuel source (Alexander, 1988).

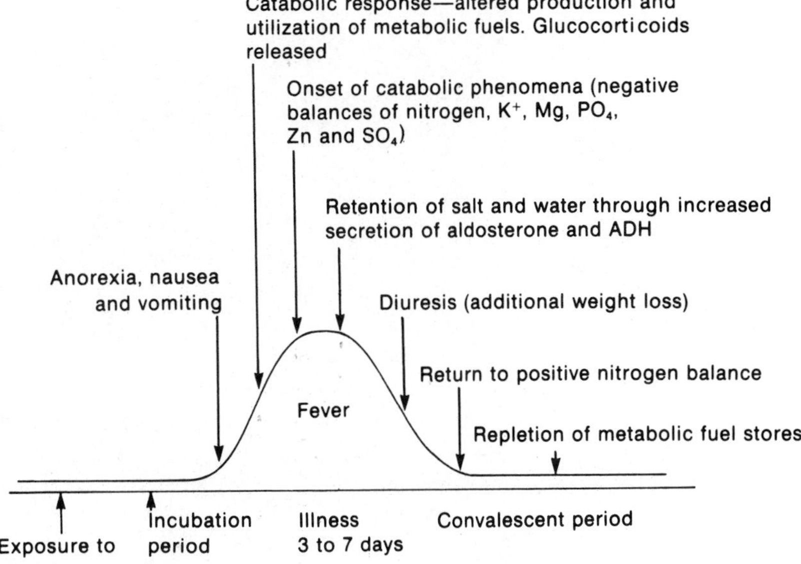

Figure 21–3 Timing of catabolic response to infection. (From Mahon LK, Arlin MT. *Food, Nutrition, and Diet Therapy.* 8th ed. Philadelphia, WB Saunders, 1992; as adapted from Beisel WR. The influence of infection or injury on nutritional requirements during adolescence. *In* McKigney JL, Munro HN (eds). *Nutritional Requirements in Adolescence.* Cambridge, MA, MIT Press, 1976, p 256.)

Nutritional Care

Each degree Fahrenheit of elevated temperature increases metabolic demands by 7% (13% for each degree Celsius). With extensive infections, such as peritonitis or cellulitis, metabolic rates may range from 25 to 50% above BMR. Energy intake should be individualized, as determined by the client's body weight and temperature.

Fluid and electrolyte balance is of concern since fluid imbalances caused by infection can range from severe overload to severe dehydration. As much as 3 to 4 L of fluids may be required to replace water lost from fever and eliminate waste products. Sodium and chloride retention are influenced more by hormones than by diet.

Since defensive mechanisms to fight infection ultimately depend on protein-synthesizing capabilities, increased protein is required for visceral protein synthesis. However, energy intake must first be adequate. Exact protein requirements have not been determined. In general, the protein allowance should be 1.5 to 2 gm/kg/day for febrile adults and 3 gm/kg/day for children. At least an equivalent of the RDAs for vitamins should be available throughout the course of an infection, or, at most, doses of many water-soluble vitamins should be doubled or tripled to replace those excreted or needed during hypermetabolism.

Recommendations regarding nutrition support of septic clients are slim. In general, 45 kcal/kg/day has been recommended with about 1.6 gm/kg/day protein (Hasselgren & Fischer, 1987). Nutrition support for clients who cannot or will not eat is imperative to offset loss of lean body mass. However, as a result of severity of the illness and frequency of malnutrition in these clients, nourishment may need to be implemented gradually. Ileus is common; thus, parenteral feedings are frequently necessary.

NURSING APPLICATIONS

Assessment

Physical—for fever (may be low grade or subnormal), weight loss, weight, percent weight change, fatigue, bowel sounds.

Dietary—for anorexia; kilocalorie and protein intake and requirements, intake of carbohydrate, fat, vitamin K, and biotin.

Continued

Laboratory—for blood cultures, albumin, BUN, creatinine; potassium, sodium; folate, iron, zinc, T lymphocytes, urea excretion.

Interventions

1. Maintain I&O records to prevent dehydration. Insufficient output may indicate fluid overload caused from cardiovascular or renal complications.
2. Allow appropriate protein/day. *Examples:*
   Adult weighing 145 lbs—
   145 lb ÷ 2.2 kg/lb = 66 kg × 1.5 gm protein/kg = 99 gm protein
   Child weighing 60 lbs—
   60 lb ÷ 2.2 kg/lb = 27 kg × 3 gm/kg = 81 gm protein
3. Allow adequate fluids [3 to 4 L of fluid (orally or IV)] daily and a 7% kilocalorie increase for every degree Fahrenheit temperature is elevated. *Example:*
   BMR is 1800 kcal; temperature 101.6°F (3°F elevated)
   3°F (temp. elevation) × 0.07 (kcal/°F of elevation) = 0.21
   0.21 × 1800 (BMR kcal) = 378 (additional kcal needed)
   1800 (BMR kcal) + 378 (kcal for temp.) = 2178 total kcal for temp. elevation
4. Question orders that treat infection-induced anemia during the active phase because certain bacterial organisms, especially *Salmonella,* proliferate rapidly in an iron-rich environment.

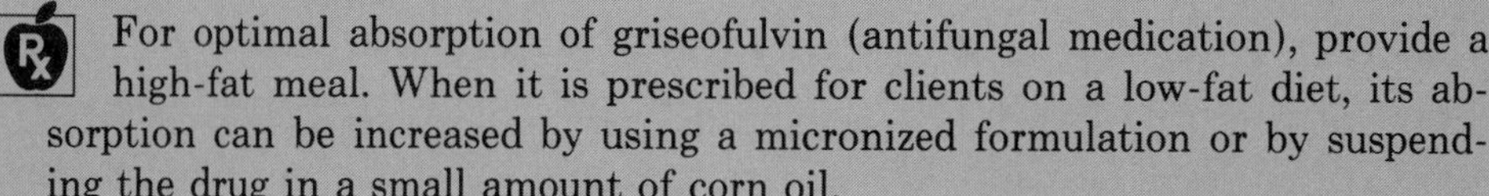
For optimal absorption of griseofulvin (antifungal medication), provide a high-fat meal. When it is prescribed for clients on a low-fat diet, its absorption can be increased by using a micronized formulation or by suspending the drug in a small amount of corn oil.

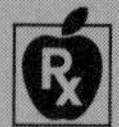
Monitor for lactose intolerance when metronidazole (Flagyl) is prescribed.

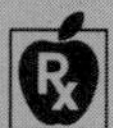
Many antibiotics inhibit bacterial synthesis of vitamins K and biotin in the GI tract; offer buttermilk or yogurt to replace GI microorganisms.

Evaluation

* When evaluating weight changes, weight loss can be masked by sodium and water retention.
* Temperature should return to normal, and malnutrition should not develop.

Client Education

* Proteins and adequate kilocaloric intake help the body fight infections.
* When bowels do not function properly, food cannot be digested and used by the body and may cause serious problems such as impactions.

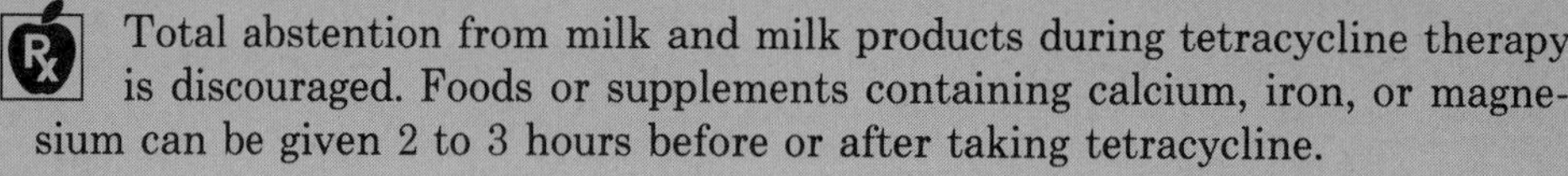
Total abstention from milk and milk products during tetracycline therapy is discouraged. Foods or supplements containing calcium, iron, or magnesium can be given 2 to 3 hours before or after taking tetracycline.

SPECIAL NUTRITIONAL CONCERNS FOR TRAUMA VICTIMS

Trauma, such as fractures, gunshot and stab wounds, and spinal cord and head injuries, causes protein losses through direct destruction of tissues. Unlike elective surgery, there is no time to replenish the body nutritionally. However, most trauma victims are young and basically healthy before the injury. Nutrition support should prevent deterioration of lean tissue and dehydration and treat any specific complications. The goal to restore a client to an active normal functioning life may involve an extended period of rehabilitation. During this time, emphasis of nutritional care changes.

Trauma imposes stress, and within moments after the event, metabolic changes (explained earlier) occur. In addition to protein catabolism caused by the stress reaction, protein-rich fluid may accumulate at the injury site, further increasing protein losses. Available energy is preferentially used to feed the healing wound. Fortunately, a client in good health before the incident has significant stores to offset initial catabolic effects.

What should nutrition therapy prevent?

Nutritional Care

Energy requirements are increased from the stress reaction and the need to reestablish metabolic processes (see Fig. 21–1). Vigorous nutrition therapy supplying elevated requirements should be implemented to achieve positive balance. In some cases, such as spinal cord and head injuries, despite provision of adequate kilocalories and protein (110% more than average actual energy expenditures), positive nitrogen balance may not be achieved for at least 3 weeks (Rodriguez et al, 1991).

Potassium losses that are due to the injury may result in metabolic alkalosis. Moderately severe hyponatremia, frequently observed especially with low sodium enteral and parenteral formulations, may be associated with autonomic dysfunction (Chin & Kearns, 1991). Calcium excretion in clients with spinal cord injury is elevated (up to 150% above normal) and may remain elevated for more than a year (Kearns et al, 1992). Pancreatitis may be secondary to peripancreatic trauma, autonomic denervation, or steroids. Because of neurological dysfunction, symptoms of pancreatitis are nausea, vomiting, and anorexia, rather than pain.

These increased requirements gradually decline, and 2 to 3 months posttrauma, obesity becomes another high-risk priority in clients with quadriplegia or paraplegia because of immobilization and decreased BMR. Decreased BMR appears to be related to the proportion of denervated muscle, i.e., the higher the lesion, the lower the energy expenditure. Energy requirement for quadriplegics is approximately 23 kcal/kg and for paraplegics 28 kcal/kg daily (Cox et al, 1985). Many of these clients were very active and able to eat everything and anything they desired without weight gain before the trauma. This can be an especially challenging task to assist clients in changing their eating patterns from high-kilocalorie, high-fat choices to low-kilocalorie, nutrient-dense foods to prevent accumulation of excessive adipose tissue.

Clients with head injuries are at risk of swallowing problems, which may necessitate enteral or parenteral feeding for nutrition support. Numerous studies have reported an average increase of 40% above predicted energy expenditure in clients with head injuries related to hypermetabolism (Ott & Young, 1991). This increase is not influenced by steroids (Moore et al, 1989) that are used to control cerebral edema and increased intracranial pressure. Barbiturates are commonly used to reduce brain metabolism, decrease cerebral blood flow, and suppress responses to stimulation (Varella, 1991). Nitrogen balance is improved with barbiturate therapy. Their effect as a CNS depressant results in decreased GI tone and motility. This may necessitate TPN (Varella, 1991). During rehabilitation, head-injured clients are likely to be hyperphagic and gain weight above their preinjury weight.

What are energy requirements for quadriplegics/paraplegics?

NURSING APPLICATIONS

Assessment

Physical—for type of trauma, height, serial weights, anorexia, nausea and vomiting, hypothermia.

Dietary—for nutrient/kilocaloric intake.

Laboratory—for protein, albumin, prealbumin, nitrogen balance; arterial

Continued

blood gases, sodium, potassium imbalances; glucose; LFTs, serum osmolarity, urea, creatinine.

Interventions

1. Monitor oral kilocaloric and protein intake closely. Injured clients rarely take adequate amounts of nutrients spontaneously. If inadequate, notify the physician or dietitian for implementation of other methods of nutrition support or combinations thereof.
2. Monitor weight closely. If weight loss continues after post-trauma diuresis, notify the physician or dietitian.
3. Refer to occupational therapy for adaptive equipment if needed.
4. For clients receiving barbiturates, monitor for bowel sounds, and if enteral feedings are being used, monitor residuals routinely.

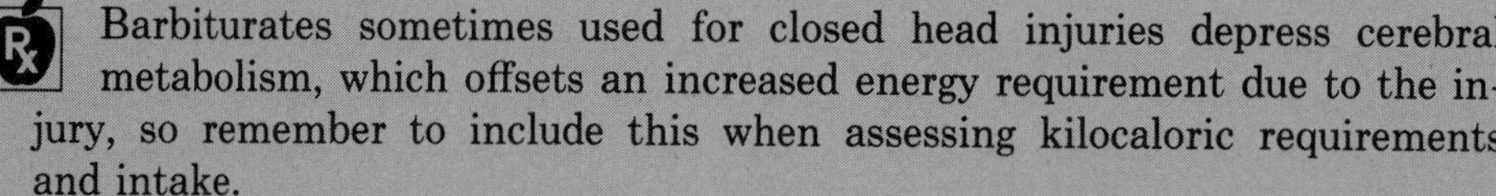

Barbiturates sometimes used for closed head injuries depress cerebral metabolism, which offsets an increased energy requirement due to the injury, so remember to include this when assessing kilocaloric requirements and intake.

Evaluation

* Client's laboratory values should return to normal; dehydration is prevented, and complications are avoided or kept to a minimum.

Client Education

- When positive nitrogen balance has been achieved and weight has stabilized within a desirable range for the condition, client needs to be instructed and encouraged to alter eating habits and to find substitutes for high-kilocaloric foods.

SPECIAL NUTRITIONAL CONCERNS FOR PULMONARY CLIENTS

COPD—obstruction of pulmonary air flow and respiratory insufficiency. Sleep apnea or failure to breathe while sleeping is a result of reduced CNS stimulation of respiration and can occur in COPD, renal failure, and cardiac failure clients as well as neonates.

Hypercapnic—excessive carbon dioxide in the blood as indicated by an elevated P_{CO_2}.

Hypoxemic—inadequate oxygen in the blood as indicated by a low P_{O_2}.

Several conditions involving the respiratory system affect nutritional status, including chronic bronchitis and emphysema, **chronic obstructive pulmonary disease (COPD), sleep apnea,** and adult respiratory distress syndrome (ARDS). Clients with chronic bronchitis are often overweight and **hypercapnic,** whereas clients with emphysema tend to be underweight and **hypoxemic.** Clients with emphysema tend to have lung deterioration that corresponds to the degree of nutritional depletion (weight loss and depletion of somatic proteins).

Physical Consequences

In contrast to healthy individuals who breathe in response to elevated carbon dioxide levels, breathing is a response to hypoxia (low O_2 levels) in clients with COPD. Respiratory muscle fatigue, hypoventilation, carbon dioxide retention, and hypoxemia are common because of a client's inability to regulate serum oxygen and carbon dioxide content.

Respiration rate may be directly influenced by nutrition because of its influence on metabolic rate, i.e., conditions that reduce metabolism reduce respiration, whereas conditions that increase metabolic rate increase respiratory rate. Malnutrition results in lower metabolism, which can be associated with poor circulation causing reduction in cardiac output and compromised respiration due to respiratory muscle weakness. Respiratory disease combined with significant weight loss leads to a hypermetabolic state that can be associated with functional deterioration or atrophy of respiratory muscles. Weight and strength of the diaphragm are reduced. This results in a reduction of respiratory response to hypoxemia. Development of malnutrition may exacerbate already existing functioning impairments.

A malnourished ventilator-dependent client can develop infections, pulmonary edema, hypophosphatemia, decreased respiratory drive, respiratory weakness, and **atelectasis** (Spector, 1989). Weaning a client from the ventilator can be difficult or impossible if the client is malnourished or develops hypophosphatemia (Spector, 1989). Hypophosphatemia impairs tissue oxygen delivery and respiratory muscle function. Acute respiratory failure is often accompanied by pneumonia and sepsis. Impairment of the immune system caused by malnutrition adversely affects recovery. Respiratory muscle fatigue can occur when the demand for energy surpasses its supply, such as during semi-starvation. BCAAs are used as energy substrate.

Atelectasis—state in which all or part of a lung is collapsed or contains no air.

Describe how malnutrition affects the respiratory system.

Nutritional Care

Clients with respiratory disease must maintain a delicate balance between obtaining adequate oxygen and eliminating carbon dioxide. Objectives of nutritional care are to (1) provide sufficient energy and protein to restore and maintain lean body mass, (2) avoid excess carbon dioxide production by limiting total energy and carbohydrate intake and increasing fat content when clinically relevant, (3) avoid stimulating excess respiration by limiting dietary protein and total energy intake to estimated metabolic requirements, (4) maintain fluid and electrolyte balance, (5) provide essential micronutrients including adequate phosphorus, and (6) maximize exercise tolerance in ambulatory clients.

List 3 goals of nutritional care for respiratory clients.

Weight

As many as 40% of clients diagnosed with COPD experience progressive weight loss; this is associated with a higher rate of mortality (Askanazi et al, 1988). A hypermetabolic state in a stable malnourished COPD client may be a factor in weight loss (Wilson et al, 1990). Additionally, nutrient requirements are increased because of infections or fever and elevated energy expenditure related to the increased effort of breathing. Kilocaloric requirement for breathing may be as high as 430 to 720 kcal/day in clients with COPD, in contrast to 36 to 72 kcal for normal individuals. The amount of weight loss generally correlates with reduction in air flow. Substrate utilization in peripheral tissues is inefficient when tissue oxygenation is poor. Thus, poor respiratory function promotes weight loss, which further hinders respiratory function. Shortness of breath from exertion results in clients becoming sedentary.

Although preventing weight loss in lung disease may not improve life expectancy, 2 to 3 weeks of refeeding improves muscle strength, endurance and exercise tolerance (Whittaker et al, 1990), and immune responses (Fuenzalida et al, 1990). Weight loss is inappropriate therapy for COPD clients of normal body weight, but weight loss for overweight clients may alleviate acute physiological abnormalities (Askanazi et al, 1988).

Despite increased kilocaloric requirements, nutrient intake is frequently decreased. Therapeutic use of bronchodilators results in an increased incidence of peptic ulcer disease. Nausea and vomiting may be related to toxic doses of theophylline. Copious amounts of chronic sputum and mucus inhibit the desire for and palatability of food. Clients are able to tolerate only small amounts at a time because a full stomach makes breathing difficult. Fatigue and shortness of breath may hamper ability to prepare meals or to eat. The mental/emotional depression associated with being ill may cause decreased food intake.

What are some effects of COPD on weight?

Distribution of Energy Nutrients

The ratio of carbon dioxide production to oxygen consumption is called the respiratory quotient (RQ).

Oxidation of carbohydrate, fat, and protein to yield energy requires oxygen. As a result, carbon dioxide and water are produced. Carbohydrates are oxidized with a higher **respiratory quotient** than lipids, i.e., more carbon dioxide is produced by oxidation of carbohydrate than fat or protein. (The overall carbon dioxide load to be expired by the lungs is greater than for oxidation of fat.)

Reducing carbon dioxide production by substituting fat kilocalories for carbohydrate can help wean clients from or avoid requiring mechanical support. Carbohydrate can provide some of the energy needs to help decrease metabolic rate. As much as 30 to 55% of the energy can be provided as fats. Excessive amounts of protein are avoided since protein may increase respiration in response to a carbon dioxide stimulus. Whether a high-fat (55%) diet is advisable on a long-term basis is controversial. In addition to the risks of hyperlipidemia, high fat intake is associated with depressed immune function.

Thus, dietary goals for a client must be individualized to establish the lowest percentage of fat that effectively lowers a client's P_{CO_2} level. A high-fat diet is particularly beneficial for clients with severe dyspnea or clients being weaned from mechanical ventilation. If clients are not hypercapnic, conventional distribution of kilocalories (50 to 60% carbohydrate, 20 to 30% fat, and 15 to 20% protein) is appropriate. For hypercapnia, 25 to 30% of kilocalories should be from carbohydrate and 50 to 55% from fat (Table 21–5).

Dyspnea—labored or difficult breathing.

An objective in sleep apnea is to increase CNS respiratory drive. Proteins, especially BCAAs, increase CNS control of respiration. Feeding a high-protein diet and BCAA supplements tends to increase **dyspnea.**

TABLE 21–5

GUIDELINES FOR HIGH-FAT, LOW-CARBOHYDRATE DIET

Guidelines	Implementation
Allow vegatables as desired	Offer favorite vegetables cooked
Allow all types of meat	Prepare as desired (broiled, boiled, baked, or fried)
Use fresh fruit or fruits without added sugar as desired	Avoid serving fruits in concentrated liquids Drain and wash fruit if sugar is added
Include milk (1–2 cups) and cheeses (1–2 oz) daily	Use whole milk and cheese products Use plain unsweetened yogurt
Increase dietary fats. Use butter, margarine (preferably PUFA), mayonnaise, gravies, sauces, sour cream, and salad dressings as desired	Mix margarine into hot foods, such as soups, vegetables, mashed protatoes, cooked cereal, and rice Add whipped cream to unsweetened fruits for dessert Add mayonnaise to salads, eggs, or sandwiches Use sour cream on vegetables, gravies, as a salad dressing for fruit, or a dip for fresh vegetables For salads, add large amounts of salad dressings, avocados, and olives
Incorporate nuts to increase protein and fat intake	Fill candy dishes with favorite nuts to promote snacking Use peanut butter in sandwiches or spread on fruits such as apple or banana, or fill celery stalks
Include 3 servings of starchy foods (bread, cereals, pasta, rice) daily	Offer a starchy food at each meal
Avoid sugar, cake, pie, honey, syrup	Substitute sugar-free custard or dietetic gelatin or pudding as desserts
Encourage frequent feedings and/or snacks	Use nutritional supplements Make milkshakes flavored with fresh un-

TABLE 21–5

GUIDELINES FOR HIGH-FAT, LOW-CARBOHYDRATE DIET
Continued

Guidelines	Implementation
	sweetened fruit in advance and freeze in 6- to 8-oz portions. Microwave to slushy consistency for snacks
Increase protein content of products	Add commercial protein powders or dry skim milk powder (1–2 tbsp) to casseroles or cereal products (or add 1–3 tsp to 1 portion)
	Substitute canned evaporated milk for milk in recipes
Conserve energy	Limit raw vegetables that require a lot of chewing and are not a nutrient-dense source of kilocalories. Nutrient-dense vegetable juices such as carrot juice or tomato juice can be consumed with less energy expenditure
	Limit meats and other foods that require a lot of chewing. When a steak is desired, it can be provided cut up in very small bite-size pieces. Ground meats can provide the same nutrients without requiring so much effort in chewing
	Limit broth-type soups. Use cream soups, using whole milk or cream, or include additional amounts of meats, dry beans, and peas in broth-based soups

Kilocalorie-Nitrogen Balance

Too many kilocalories may increase the metabolic rate and raise carbon dioxide production beyond the respiratory system's ability to eliminate carbon dioxide. A kilocaloric intake equal to or only slightly above resting energy expenditure avoids excess carbon dioxide production that is due to overfeeding and resulting lipogenesis. When kilocalories are adequate (not excessive), there is little difference between carbohydrate versus fat regimens, but a hyperkilocaloric, carbohydrate-based diet is undesirable (Talbot, 1991).

For clients with respiratory problems, BEE should be closely calculated to determine energy needs. During periods of acute pulmonary compromise or weaning from mechanical ventilation, the goal is to maintain lean muscle mass. An energy intake of 1 to 1.2 times BEE is appropriate if there is insignificant physiological stress, and no more than 1.6 times the BEE is appropriate for infected or injured clients. Protein intake should be 1.6 to 2.5 gm/kg body weight. Reduction of intake to equal BEE or less may facilitate weaning, but this should be implemented no longer than 2 days and is avoided in hypercapnic clients.

To promote weight gain, kilocaloric intake may be increased to 1.4 to 1.6 times the BEE with 1.6 to 2.5 gm protein/kg body weight if it does not impair respiratory function.

Why is a high-fat diet beneficial for hypercapnic clients? What are energy requirements for a client with respiratory problems without significant physiological stress? For a client with an infection? For the one who needs to gain weight?

Enteral Feedings

Enteral feedings are frequently used for ventilator-dependent clients with functional GI tracts. Aspiration of stomach contents is a common problem that is life-threatening to these clients. Because of compromised diaphragmatic muscles, the weakened cough reflex is not strong enough to expel the aspirate. Because customary volumes of formula are not well tolerated, tube feedings should be delivered into the small bowel at slow rates to prevent undesirable side effects.

Specialized enteral formulas such as Pulmocare (Ross) have been developed for pulmonary clients. The amount of carbohydrate is low (28%); fat content is high (55%), providing 1.5 kcal/ml since there is an increased tendency to retain fluid. Sometimes 2 kcal/ml formulas are indicated. Carbohydrate-fat ratios are more important for hypercapnic clients. Specially designed enteral formulas are not imperative (Talbot, 1991).

NURSING APPLICATIONS

Assessment

Physical—for type of respiratory disease, use of accessory muscles, lung sounds, use of bronchodilators, nausea, vomiting, sputum, depression, pulmonary edema, respiration rate, body weight/weight loss, TSF, MAMC.

Dietary—for kilocalorie and protein requirements and intake; fat and carbohydrate intake; fluid intake.

Laboratory—for albumin, arterial blood gases, especially P_{CO_2}, phosphate, theophylline level.

Interventions

1. Keep oxygen on by nasal cannula when client is eating and encourage pursed-lip breathing.
2. Prepare food (cut meat, open containers) before placing on bedside table.
3. Monitor emphysemic clients closely since they are more prone to nutritional depletion than bronchitis clients.
4. Coordinate respiratory treatments 1 to 2 hours before or after meals.
5. Avoid high-protein supplements for clients with sleep apnea.
6. Encourage high-fat, low-protein, and moderate-carbohydrate diet for hypercapnic clients.
7. Avoid hyperkilocaloric diets for clients with chronic bronchitis.
8. Provide foods high in phosphorus during the anabolic phase of nutritional repletion.
9. Restrict fluids for clients with congestive heart failure.

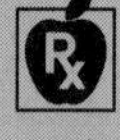
Tuberculosis is usually treated with isoniazid (INH), which interferes with metabolism of pyridoxine. Recommend pyridoxine supplements (25 to 50 mg) to physician if not ordered.

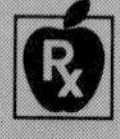
Theophylline, frequently prescribed for clients with respiratory problems, can precipitate a vitamin B_6 deficiency. Give pyridoxine supplementation (10 mg/day) to clients taking theophylline (Ubbink et al, 1990).

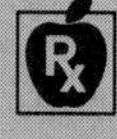
Steroids can promote protein catabolism and gluconeogenesis, which can cause negative nitrogen balance. If the client is on steroids, consult with physician or dietitian.

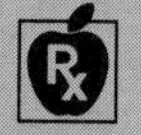
Sodium depletion in respiratory clients may result from diuretics. Low-sodium diets lead to decreased appetite. Monitor appetite, respirations, and serum sodium levels.

Evaluation

* If hypercapnic client consumes a high-fat diet and is weaned from ventilator, desired outcomes were achieved.
* If client needed to gain weight and received adequate amounts without causing respiratory difficulty, nutritional care was successful.

Client Education

- Refer to American Lung Association, Meals on Wheels, and home health care.
- For clients with dyspnea: Rest for 30 minutes before eating and avoid exercise, therapy, or treatments for 1 hour after meals.

- Six small meals a day reduce gastric distention, bloating, and oxygen requirements needed for chewing and digestion.
- Taking fluids between meals prevents excessive stomach distention and pressure on the diaphragm.
- Weight loss can improve breathing for overweight clients.

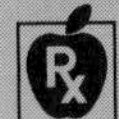
Concurrent intake of theophylline and caffeine-containing products increases risk of insomnia and cardiac problems (arrhythmias).

SPECIAL NUTRITIONAL CONCERNS FOR BURN CLIENTS

A severely burned client has all the typical hypermetabolic characteristics; nitrogen losses exceed those of any other type of stress or trauma. The amount of protein wasting and weight loss is generally proportional to the extent and severity of the injury. Although a loss of 40% of body weight is usually fatal, loss of between 10 and 40% is associated with increased debility and risk of morbidity and mortality. Hypermetabolism increases with the size of burn area; burns involving as much as 60% of the body surface may double the BMR (Deitch, 1990).

When skin surface is destroyed, the body's first line of defense against infection is lost. Loss of skin also results in increased water and heat loss; loss of water vapor and heat is directly related to burn size. Approximately 2.5 to 4 L/day of water vapor may be lost from a major burn wound. Burned surface allows leakage of protein-rich fluid, containing approximately two-thirds as much protein as plasma.

Fluid and Electrolyte Replacement

Large losses of fluids and electrolytes require replacement during the first 12 to 24 hours to maintain circulatory volume and prevent acute renal failure. IV feedings, blood transfusions, and plasma or albumin are in order.

Use of a balanced electrolyte solution, such as lactated Ringer's, may prevent electrolyte abnormalities associated with burns. Because of loss of osmotic forces, intravascular volume replacement may result in massive edema. Urine output is the most sensitive parameter for monitoring response to therapy (Bessey & Wilmore, 1988).

Insensible water loss increases as the hypermetabolic response peaks 7 to 10 days following injury and decreases as wounds begin to heal. Covering burned areas with dressings and ointments impermeable to water reduces fluid loss. Appropriate wound care is essential to prevent burn wound sepsis by controlling bacterial growth and delaying pathogen colonization.

During the flow phase, increased fluids are necessary for excretion of large amounts of waste products (such as nitrogen and potassium) by the kidney. Fluids are required to keep these wastes in solution. Because of the heavy osmotic load, urine output is not an accurate assessment parameter for adequacy of fluids after the first 48 hours. Urinary output may be significant despite clinical dehydration. At this stage, serum sodium concentration is the best parameter for monitoring hydration status (normal level, 132 to 138 mEq/L). In burns of less than 20% of the body surface area, fluids can usually be replaced orally (Ireton-Jones & Baxter, 1991). Hypotonic or sodium-free fluids may be used to replace fluid losses.

Although sodium is conserved, potassium excretion is increased if the kidneys are functioning well. Therefore, exogenous sources of potassium may be needed. Loss of other electrolytes also requires close monitoring of magnesium, calcium, phosphorus, and zinc.

What happens to fluid and electrolyte balance after a burn?

Nutritional Care

A primary goal of nutrition support is to limit weight loss to less than 10% of preburn weight. Table 21–6 summarizes nutritional care of burn clients. Following fluid resuscitation, aggressive nutrition support is implemented as clients move into the "flow" phase. This may be initiated between 12 and 48 hours postburn. Intestinal motility is commonly impaired for several days. In the past, enteral feedings have been delayed until postburn ileus resolves. If this is the practice, NG suction may be instituted with administration of parenteral feedings. This can help to reduce net nitrogen loss.

However, good results have been reported before active bowel sounds using early enteral feedings via a **transduodenal** tube with simultaneous institution of NG suction (McDonald et al, 1991). Duodenal feedings and stomach suctioning are discontinued once the ileus resolves. Early enteral feeding lessens hypermetabolic response and preserves intestinal mucosal barrier (Deitch, 1990). Delaying enteral feeding has been shown to decrease tolerance to enteral feeding (Gottschlich, 1988). Early feeding also has a dramatic positive effect on wound healing and length of care in clients with burns (Garrel et al, 1991).

Transduodenal—enteral feedings provided into the duodenum or jejunum.

What is a goal of nutritional care in burned clients? When is aggressive nutrition support implemented?

Energy and Protein

The primary concern is energy needs. On the one hand, kilocaloric requirements of clients with major burns (greater than 30% body surface) exceed those of any other injury—roughly twice the BMR may be needed to prevent significant weight loss (Cunningham et al, 1989). On the other hand, superfluous kilocalories have resulted in respiratory dysfunction, bile stasis, and liver abnormalities.

Total energy requirements may be estimated based on age, body size, and severity of burn injury. Numerous formulas are available to estimate daily kilocaloric needs, such as the one shown in Table 21–6, but using indirect calorimetry is a safer way of determining energy requirements.

TABLE 21–6

CARE OF BURN CLIENTS

Important Concerns	Implementation
Environment	Keep temperature around 32°C with 20–30% humidity
Fluids	Cover wounds to prevent fluid loss. Provide fluids in adequate amounts 2½ to 4 L/day
Energy	Calculate energy requirements using the modified Curreri formula*: (20 kcal × IBW) + (40 kcal × % of burn) when % TBSA reaches a maximum value of 50% TBSA
Protein	Provide 15–20% of energy requirements from protein or 2 to 2.5 gm/kg body weight†
Vitamins	Provide a multivitamin along with additional supplements of vitamin A (as much as 50 times the RDA is considered safe for 8 months)‡ and vitamin C (up to 10 gm/day)
Minerals	Monitor zinc, calcium, and phosphorus intake
Gastric integrity	Give antacids to maintain gastric pH >5
Mode of nutrition support	Give oral feedings with oral supplements, enteral nutrition, or parenteral nutrition to provide an adequate nutrient intake
Daily documentation	Weigh every other day until weight is stable, then weekly Record fluid I&O daily Record kilocalorie and protein intake daily

TBSA, Total burn surface area.

* Data from Allard JP, et al. Validation of a new formula for calculating the energy requirements of burn patients. *JPEN* 1990 March-Apr; 14(2):115–118.

† Data from Duke JH, et al. Contribution of protein to calorie expenditure following injury. *Surgery* 1970; 68:168–174.

‡ Data from Olson JA. Vitamin A. *In* Machlin LJ, ed. *Handbook of Vitamins. Nutritional Biochemical and Clinical Aspects.* New York, Marcel Dekker, 1990.

Hypermetabolism and protein losses in exudates greatly increase protein requirements. Provision of increased amounts of protein accelerates synthesis of visceral proteins and improves immune function, but inadequate protein results in reduced wound strength (Belcher & Ellis, 1991). Thus, approximately 20 to 25% of total kilocaloric requirement should be provided as protein (Ireton-Jones & Baxter, 1991). High protein intake is well tolerated if fluids are not restricted. Rate of protein breakdown and gluconeogenesis is reflected in UUN levels.

Feedings should also provide adequate amounts of glutamine and arginine, which stimulate the immune system, improve wound healing, and decrease morbidity and mortality in burn clients (Gottschlich et al, 1990b; Barbul, 1986). An arginine-enriched diet (9% of the protein source) has been shown to reduce hospital stay and incidence of wound infection (Gottschlich et al, 1990b).

Energy from nonprotein sources (lipids and carbohydrates) supply the remaining kilocaloric requirements. Carbohydrates are the major fuel source. Glucose is more effective than fat in promoting nitrogen retention. Since lipids may exert deleterious effects on immunologic responses and cause increased susceptibility to infection, fats are restricted to 10 to 15% (Kagan, 1991). Consequently, a high-protein, low-fat diet may be beneficial. With adequate provision of kilocalories, weight stabilization is possible and usually precedes definitive wound closure and reflects diminishing metabolic demands.

What percentage of total kilocalorie requirements should come from protein; from fat? Why are glutamine and arginine important for burn clients?

Vitamins and Minerals

All other nutrients should be supplied in adequate amounts. Because of differences in metabolism, utilization, and excretion, the RDAs are inappropriate for these clients. Although vitamin and mineral requirements are undefined, those that are involved in wound healing and immunocompetence are normally increased. This includes vitamins A and C and the mineral, zinc. Nutrients lost in urine and wound losses, especially water-soluble vitamins, are also provided in amounts above the RDA. Efficient use of nitrogen requires simultaneous availability of potassium, which is excreted heavily after a burn.

Feeding Burned Clients

The type of nutrition support used is tailored to individual factors such as age, burn size and location, GI function, fluid allowances, liver and renal function, respiratory status, and motivation. In general, a feeding tube is necessary when burns exceed 20% of total body surface. In many cases, parenteral or tube feedings used in addition to oral feedings may be lifesaving.

Burn clients do not eat well because of anorexia, pain, generalized discomfort, and emotional depression. Most are unable to consume a sufficient number of kilocalories to satisfy energy requirements. Nurses must explain the role of nutrition in the healing process and encourage these clients to eat.

When oral feedings are used solely, a minimum of 3000 kcal, 125 gm protein is provided with a high-kilocalorie, high-protein diet. Oral nutrition supplements are routinely provided. Meals can be maintained at a normal size by using protein supplements added to cream soups, milk, juices, and shakes.

If at least 75% of estimated requirements are not provided by oral intake, tube feedings may be given at night. Gastric residuals should be checked every 4 hours. Formulas providing 1.5 to 2 kcal/ml are used to provide more nutrients with smaller volumes needed. When these are used, care should be taken to provide adequate fluids. Parenteral feedings can augment enteral feedings, but TPN is not favored because of complications including catheter-related sepsis, higher cost, altered GI functioning, and inefficient utilization of nutrients.

NURSING APPLICATIONS

Assessment

Physical—for infection, dehydration, edema, urine output, weight, weight fluctuations, pain, bowel sounds, psychological state, percentage of burn.

Dietary—for anorexia; kilocaloric and protein requirements and intake.

Laboratory—for potassium, sodium, magnesium, calcium, phosphorus, zinc, UUN, prealbumin, transferrin.

Interventions

1. Monitor urine output. Initially during fluid resuscitation, urine output of 30 to 50 ml/hr in adults and 0.7 to 1 ml/kg/hr in children indicates adequate perfusion (Bessey & Wilmore, 1988).
2. Monitor for (1) resuscitation with too much hypotonic fluid, (2) excessive intake of fluids to replace evaporative water loss, or (3) use of hydrotherapy that causes sodium losses (hyponatremia) and transcutaneous absorption of water (Kokko & Tannen, 1990).
3. Weigh clients without dressings, splints, and so forth every other day until weight is stable, then weekly.
4. During the catabolic phase, monitor nitrogen balance from the UUN, not serum visceral proteins, which are poor predictors of change in nitrogen balance (Carlson et al, 1991).
5. Prealbumin reflects effects of nutrition support better than albumin. Monitor serum albumin, transferrin, and prealbumin weekly when the anabolic stage is reached.
6. Provide a warm (89.6°F [32°C]) and dry environment for burn clients to prevent further convective heat losses and increased protein catabolism associated with maintaining normal body temperature.
7. Initiate tube feedings at a rate of 30 to 50 ml/hr and increase at a rate of 20 to 25 ml/hr every 12 hours until desired volume is reached, barring complications such as gastric retention or diarrhea.
8. Schedule treatments and tests so they do not interfere with feedings; give pain medicine 30 minutes before meals if pain is preventing client from eating.
9. Provide clients with favorite foods. Family members can assist by suggesting or bringing in foods, if allowed.
10. Offer snacks frequently.
11. Provide constant emotional support and encourage clients to talk about their feelings, wants, and needs. Burn victims often experience grief and anger over body disfigurement and the many painful treatments necessary.
12. Large burns on hands or facial burns detrimentally affect client's ability to consume adequate amounts spontaneously. Feed client if necessary or refer to occupational therapist.

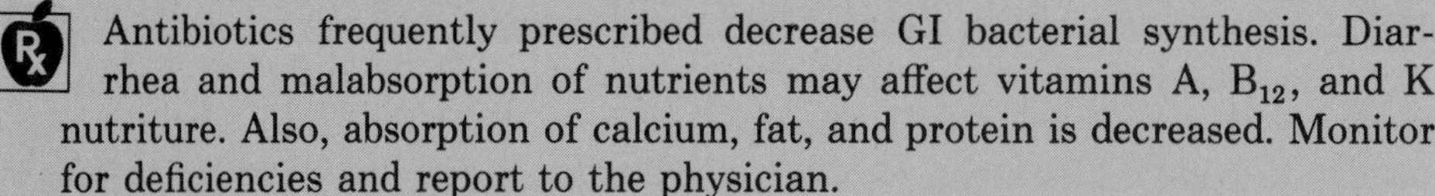
Antibiotics frequently prescribed decrease GI bacterial synthesis. Diarrhea and malabsorption of nutrients may affect vitamins A, B_{12}, and K nutriture. Also, absorption of calcium, fat, and protein is decreased. Monitor for deficiencies and report to the physician.

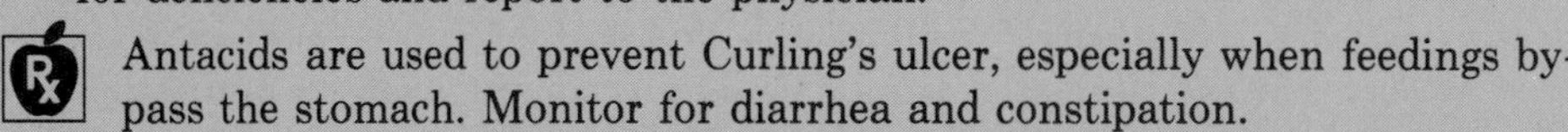
Antacids are used to prevent Curling's ulcer, especially when feedings bypass the stomach. Monitor for diarrhea and constipation.

Histamine H_2 receptor antagonists inhibit HCl secretion and may decrease iron absorption. Monitor Hgb level and suggest a vitamin C–rich food with meals.

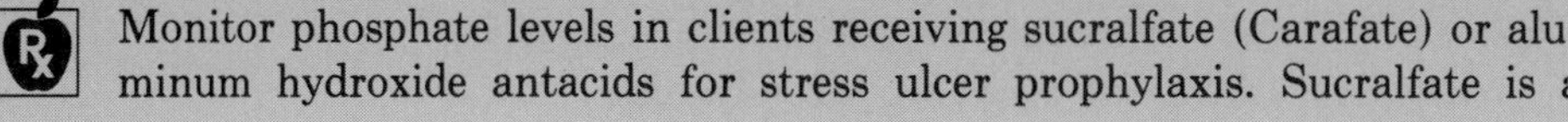
Monitor phosphate levels in clients receiving sucralfate (Carafate) or aluminum hydroxide antacids for stress ulcer prophylaxis. Sucralfate is a

complex salt of aluminum hydroxide capable of binding phosphate in the GI tract (Miller & Simpson, 1991).

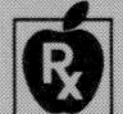
Narcotic analgesics used for pain decrease gastric motility. Monitor for constipation.

Evaluation

* If client weighs 150 lbs and lost less than 15 lbs, care was successful.
* Determine client's consumption of a high-protein, low-fat diet (100% is desirable).

Client Education

- All nutrient requirements are increased to help burns heal.
- Rest 30 minutes before and after meals.
- Consume high-carbohydrate and high-protein foods. Use glucose polymers to sweeten foods. Drink high-protein, low-fat milkshakes.
- Eat high potassium-containing foods.

COMPLICATIONS ASSOCIATED WITH PHYSIOLOGICAL STRESSES

Other complications can be caused from a prolonged period of bed rest resulting from a physiological stress. Decreases in muscle mass and bone density during immobilization are serious problems.

Immobilization

Bed rest due to fractures or paralysis results in loss of calcium, potassium, and phosphorus. Hypercalcemia is more common during periods of fluid restriction and dehydration. Immobilization causes increased bone resorption as a result of hormonal changes. Mineral losses occur to a greater extent in weight-bearing bones; this process is apparently reversible. These changes in mineral metabolism can be reversed by quiet standing for 2 or more hours daily.

Mineral losses from bone are not related to calcium intake. Although demineralization may result in osteoporosis, large amounts of dietary calcium are not wise. Serum calcium levels are elevated despite decreased GI absorption. High calcium intake or high levels of vitamin C supplements may lead to kidney stones, but restricting dietary calcium is ineffective in reducing serum calcium or urinary calcium excretion and may result in less food intake.

Pressure Sores

In 1988, the cost of pressure sores was $25,000 to 50,000 per client (Pinchcofsky-Devin, 1992). Bedridden clients frequently have poor appetites and may become nutritionally depleted because of inadequate intake. Malnutrition and hypoproteinemia have been implicated as causes of pressure sores.

Pressure sores are frequent risks because of immobilization, lack of pressure sensation, and decreased circulation. Hazards are associated with inadequate fat stores because of inadequate padding covering bony prominences or excessive fat stores because of decreased maneuverability and prolonged contact with surfaces, moisture collection between skinfolds, and impaired blood circulation.

TABLE 21–7

GUIDELINES FOR NUTRITIONAL CARE OF CLIENTS WITH PRESSURE SORES

Requirements		Normal Ranges for Treatment
Kilocalorie requirement—1.5 times the BEE		2200–3500 kcal
Protein requirement—1.5 to 2 gm/kg		75–100 gm
Vitamin C		250–500 mg
Zinc		15–25 mg
Fluids		2000–3000 ml
	Implementation	
Stage	***Tube Feeding***	***Oral Feeding***
I	No intervention	Minimum of 100 mg vitamin C from preferred food such as orange juice; vitamin supplement with zinc
II	Liquid vitamin C supplement	Minimum of 100 mg vitamin C from a preferred food; 8 oz of high-protein supplement; vitamin supplement with zinc
III	Liquid vitamin C supplement; allow 1.5–2 gm protein/kg	250 mg vitamin C twice a day; 16 oz high-protein supplement; zinc supplement
IV	Same as stage III	250 mg vitamin C (as above); double portions of protein foods; 16 oz high-protein supplement; zinc supplement

BEE, Basal energy expenditure.

Large pressure sores may lead to protein depletion because of the high protein content of the ulcer exudate. Adequate protein and kilocalories are necessary to replace protein losses and promote wound healing. A well-balanced diet, high in kilocalories (over 2000 kcal) and high-quality protein, is recommended. Small, frequent meals or nutrition supplements may be necessary to provide adequate kilocalories and protein. Clients with pressure sores are candidates for tube feedings if oral intake is inadequate.

What nutrients have been implicated in development of pressure sores? What are diet recommendations for clients with pressure sores?

Proper hydration is necessary to maintain skin elasticity. Vitamin C (250 to 500 mg) and zinc (15 to 25 mg) supplementation is recommended because of their important role in wound healing. Hemoglobin levels must be at least 10 gm/dl to provide oxygen for healing. Thus, iron supplements may be needed. Table 21–7 summarizes nutrition support of clients experiencing pressure sores, with implementation guidelines based on the method of feeding.

NURSING APPLICATIONS

Assessment

Physical—for risk of pressure sores; increased or decreased TSF.

Dietary—for appetite, protein and kilocalorie requirements.

Laboratory—for calcium, potassium, zinc, phosphorus; protein, albumin (below 3.3 mg/dl); Hgb; TLC (less than 1200).

Interventions

1. If client is not consuming adequate amounts of protein or kilocalories, attempt to determine factors compromising intake and offer support with eating (Bergstrom et al, 1992).
2. Increasing protein and kilocalorie intake of clients with pressure sores is as important as turning the client frequently and properly providing decubitus wound care. Nutritional supplements or enteral feedings may be needed.

3. Monitor plasma zinc and hemoglobin levels if pressure sore is not healing.
4. In addition to adequate nutrition, encourage range of motion (ROM) exercises and ambulation per the physician's orders to maintain dynamic equilibrium. Passive ROM is helpful in preventing contractures but is not effective in building lean body mass.
5. Offer large amounts of fluids to immobilized clients to prevent formation of renal stones from elevated serum calcium. Mobility of these clients should be attempted as soon as possible.

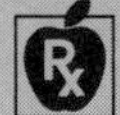 Closely monitor bedfast clients receiving corticosteroids, anticonvulsants, and barbituates for pressure sores because these medications may affect food intake or nutrient absorption (Pinchcofsky-Devin, 1992).

Evaluation

* Client with pressure sores should consume a high-kilocalorie and high-protein diet with foods high in vitamin C and zinc, and pressure sores should not increase in size and should preferably decrease.

Client Education

- For immobilized clients: Increasing calcium intake via calcium supplements or high-calcium foods is not beneficial.
- Adequate protein and kilocalorie intake is essential for healing to occur.
- Increase intake of vitamin C–rich foods, but long-term use of high levels of vitamin C supplements may precipitate renal stones.
- Consume foods that provide zinc (Chapter 9, Table 9–6).

SUMMARY

During physiological stress, the body is generally thrown into a hypermetabolic state with increased catabolism. Combined supportive treatment modalities are essential for optimal outcome; nutrition support is an important aspect of treatment. A client's well-being can be severely threatened with any stress or trauma, even a scheduled routine surgical procedure.

Recovery rate is affected by nutritional status before the stress. Extent of trauma and expected duration of recovery should be evaluated, along with consideration of a client's nutritional status. An appropriate diet then should be prescribed. In general, clients need liberal amounts of all the nutrients. Energy and protein are of primary concern; when nutrient-dense foods are ingested in sufficient quantities to provide energy and protein, increased amounts of vitamins and minerals accompany them.

Anorexia, prevalent during periods of stress, interferes with adequate intake. Inventive efforts must be made to increase nutrient intake of these clients with increased dietary needs. Between-meal feedings or nutrition supplements can be used to increase intake. In some instances, other modes of nutrition support may be implemented to avoid nutritional depletion and accompanying risks.

NURSING PROCESS IN ACTION

A client with a diagnosis of COPD is admitted to the hospital. Arterial blood gases (AGB) indicate the P_{CO_2} is 55. Dyspnea is present, so food intake has decreased. He takes theophylline.

 Nutritional Assessment

- Respiratory rate, use of accessory muscles, lung sounds.
- Type of medications used.
- Productive or nonproductive cough.
- Presence or absence of pulmonary edema or fatigue.
- Body weight and height/weight loss/TSF and MAMC.
- Protein, carbohydrate, and fat intake.
- Kilocalorie and protein requirements/BEE.
- Fluid intake.
- ABGs/pulmonary functions tests/chest X-ray.
- Phosphate, theophylline levels.
- Psychological status: depression, anxiety, anger, hopelessness, acceptance.

 Dietary Nursing Diagnosis

Altered nutrition: Less than body requirements RT anorexia and increased need for nutrients secondary to hypermetabolic state.

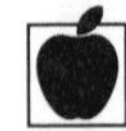 Nutritional Goals

Client will consume 85 to 100% of a high-fat diet with minimal respiratory distress.

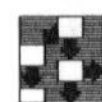 Nutritional Implementation 

Intervention: (1) Do not offer excessive kilocalories; (2) calculate the BEE.
Rationale: A kilocaloric intake equal to or slightly above BEE avoids excess carbon dioxide production caused by overfeeding and resulting lipogenesis.

Intervention: Consult with dietitian.
Rationale: Expert knowledge is needed to individualize nutritional care.

Intervention: Make sure client receives 2230 to 2520 kcal daily.
Rationale: The kilocalorie requirement for breathing is increased in a COPD client. An energy intake of 1 to 1.2 times BEE is appropriate since there is insignificant physiological stress.

Intervention: Provide a high-fat, moderate-carbohydrate, and low-protein diet. Follow guidelines in Table 21–5.
Rationale: Carbohydrates provide energy needed to decrease metabolic rate. Fat oxidation produces less carbon dioxide than carbohydrates and proteins. Protein is decreased since it may increase respiration in response to a carbon dioxide stimulus and cause dyspnea.

Intervention: Offer 6 small, frequent meals.
Rationale: Intake of large amounts of food requires more energy and oxygen to consume and can place pressure on the diaphragm, making breathing difficult.

Intervention: Provide oral care immediately before and after meals.
Rationale: Copious amounts of sputum and mucus inhibit the desire for and palatability of food.

Intervention: (1) Prepare tray for client as needed; (2) provide oxygen per nasal cannula during eating.
Rationale: Fatigue and shortness of breath may hamper ability to prepare meals or eat.

Intervention: Encourage fluid intake between meals.

Rationale: This prevents excessive stomach distention and pressure on the diaphragm. Fluids also decrease viscosity of sputum, making it easier to expectorate.

Intervention: Offer supplemental feedings as ordered.
Rationale: This ensures adequate kilocaloric intake.

Intervention: Stress avoiding caffeine.
Rationale: Caffeine is a CNS stimulant and increases metabolism.

Intervention: Teach client to use pursed-lip breathing while eating.
Rationale: Pursed-lip breathing keeps alveoli inflated longer by providing positive pressure and provides some control over dyspnea.

Intervention: Coordinate respiratory treatments 1 to 2 hours before or after meals.
Rationale: Some treatments may cause nausea or sputum production resulting in anorexia.

Intervention: (1) Monitor weight. (2) Monitor for nausea and vomiting.
Rationale: (1) Poor respiratory function promotes weight loss, which further hinders respiratory function. (2) Toxic doses of theophylline cause nausea and vomiting.

Intervention: Refer to social worker, American Lung Association, Meals on Wheels, or home health care as indicated.
Rationale: Since this is a chronic disease, psychological support is imperative.

Intervention: (1) Monitor theophylline blood level; (2) if theophylline is in a timed-release preparation, give on an empty stomach.
Rationale: (1) A high-carbohydrate, low-protein diet decreases theophylline elimination. Consequently, toxicity may occur. (2) If taken with food, toxicity may occur since this causes a rapid release of theophylline.

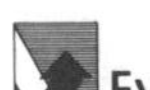

Evaluation

Evaluate the following: weight (weight is maintained), diet (consumes >85% of ordered diet), respirations (eats with nasal cannula and respirations do not increase over 24). Additionally, high-fat foods should be included in the diet, and client should be able to choose high-fat foods from menu.

STUDENT READINESS

1. What are the nutritional implications of the metabolic changes caused by stress?
2. State reasons why it is important (a) to maintain I&O records in physiologically stressed clients, (b) to provide adequate kilocalories, and (c) to provide adequate protein.
3. Why is it difficult for stressed clients to get adequate intake? List some ways of increasing their intake.
4. Why might a client with emphysema using a ventilator be given a low-carbohydrate, moderate-protein, high-fat diet or tube feeding?

CASE STUDY

Mrs. I. M. is an 85-year-old woman who has been in a nursing home following a cerebrovascular accident 6 years ago. Since the cerebrovascular accident, she has experienced difficulty with chewing and swallowing and has required increasing staff time to be fed. She has been virtually bedridden and now has pressure sores over the sacrum and greater trochanter of the left femur. Her serum Hgb is 7.4 gm/dl, Hct is 22 gm/dl, and total serum protein is 4.8 gm. An aggressive ulcer care program was implemented. Despite the care, the ulcers show no sign of healing.

1. What additional information would you need to determine why healing is not occurring?
2. List 2 nursing diagnoses for this client and a goal for each.
3. How many grams of hemoglobin are considered minimal for healing to occur?
4. What measures may be necessary to ensure that healing is possible?

CASE STUDY

Ms. J. T. is a 20-year-old college student. While returning to school after a holiday, she is involved in a multi-car accident in which her car bursts into flames. She sustains deep partial-thickness and full-thickness burns over 35% of her body surface area. One week after the original injury, her vital signs have stabilized, but her serum glucose level remains consistently above 180 mg/dl. She is placed on a high-kilocalorie, high-protein diet with vitamin and mineral supplements.

1. Before the accident, her weight was 120 lbs and her height was 5′6″. What should her daily protein allowance be at this time? Kilocaloric requirements?
2. Why does her blood glucose level remain elevated 1 week after her injury?
3. What is the rationale for a high-kilocalorie, high-protein diet for this client?
4. What vitamin and mineral supplements would you expect for the burn client?

REFERENCES

Alexander JW. Nutritional management of the infected patient. *In* Kinney JM, et al, eds. *Nutrition and Metabolism in Patient Care.* Philadelphia, WB Saunders, 1988: 625–634.

Askanazi J, et al. Respiratory diseases. *In* Kinney J, et al, eds. *Nutrition and Metabolism in Patient Care.* Philadelphia, WB Saunders, 1988: 522–530.

Barbul A. Arginine biochemistry, physiology, and therapeutic implications. *JPEN* 1986 March-Apr; 10(2):227–238.

Belcher HJ, Ellis H. An investigation of the role of diet and burn injury on wound healing. *Burns* 1991 Feb; 17(1):14–16.

Bergstrom N, et al. How to predict and prevent pressure ulcers. *Am J Nurs* 1992 July; 92(7):52–54.

Bessey PQ, Wilmore DW. The burned patient. *In* Kinney J, et al, eds. *Nutrition and Metabolism in Patient Care.* Philadelphia, WB Saunders, 1988: 672–700.

Bower RH. Nutritional and metabolic support of critically ill patients. *JPEN* 1990; 14(suppl): 257S–259S.

Buzby GP. Perioperative nutritional support. *JPEN* 1990; 14(suppl 5):197S–199S.

Carlson DE, et al. Evaluation of serum visceral protein levels as indicators of nitrogen balance in thermally injured patients. *JPEN* 1991 July-Aug; 15(4):440–444.

Chandra RK. Nutrition and immunity: Lessons from the past and new insights into the future. *Am J Clin Nutr* 1991 May; 53(5):1087–1101.

Chin DE, Kearns D. Nutrition in the spinal-injured patient. *Nutr Clin Pract* 1991 Dec; 6(6):213–222.

Cox SA, et al. Energy expenditure after SCI: Evaluation of stable rehabilitating patients. *J Trauma* 1985 May; 25(5):419–423.

Cunningham JJ, et al. Measured and predicted calorie requirements of adults during recovery from severe burn trauma. *Am J Clin Nutr* 1989 March; 49(3):404–408.

Deitch EA. The management of burns. *N Engl J Med* 1990 Nov 1; 323(18):1249–1253.

Fried RC, et al. Barbituate therapy reduces nitrogen excretion in acute head injury. *J Trauma* 1989 Nov; 29(11):1558–1564.

Fuenzalida CE, et al. The immune response to short-term nutritional intervention in advanced chronic obstructive pulmonary disease. *Am Rev Respir Dis* 1990 July; 142(1):49–56.

Garrel DR, et al. Length of care in patients with severe burns with or without early enteral nutritional support. A retrospective study. *Burn Care Rehabil* 1991 Jan-Feb; 12(1):85–90.

Goodson WH, Hunt TK. Wound healing. *In* Kinney JM, et al, eds. *Nutrition and Metabolism in Patient Care.* Philadelphia, WB Saunders, 1988: 635–642.

Gottschlich M, et al. Enteral nutrition in patients with burns or trauma. *In* Rombeau JL, Caldwell MD, eds. *Clinical Nutrition Enteral and Tube Feeding.* 2nd ed. Philadelphia, WB Saunders, 1990a: 306–324.

Gottschlich M, et al. Differential effects of three enteral dietary regimens on selected outcome variables in burn patients. *JPEN* 1990b May-June; 14(3):225–236.

Gottschlich MM. Nutritional strategies for burn patients. *RD* 1988; 8(1):6–9.

Hasselgren P, Fischer JE. Sepsis. *In* Lang CE, ed. *Nutritional Support in Critical Care.* Rockville, MD, Aspen Publishers, 1987: 345–361.

Hill GL. The perioperative patient. *In* Kinney JM, et al, eds. *Nutrition and Metabolism in Patient Care.* Philadelphia, WB Saunders, 1988: 643–655.

Ireton-Jones CS, Baxter CR. Nutrition for adult burn patients: A review. *Nutr Clin Pract* 1991 Feb; 6(1):3–7.

Jeevanandam M, et al. Obesity and the metabolic response to severe multiple trauma. *J Clin Invest* 1991 Jan; 87(1):262–269.

Kagan RJ. Metabolism and nutrition in the burned patient. *Nutr Clin Pract* 1991 Feb; 6(1):1–2.

Kearns P, et al. Nutritional and metabolic response to acute spinal-cord injury. *JPEN* 1992 Jan-Feb; 16(1):11–15.

Kokko JP, Tannen RL. *Fluids and Electrolytes.* 2nd ed. Philadelphia, WB Saunders, 1990.

Lowenstein SR, Parrino TA. Management of the common cold. *Adv Intern Med* 1987; 32:207–233.

Maynard ND, Bihari DJ. Postoperative feeding. Time to rehabilitate the gut. *Br Med J* 1991 Oct 26; 303(6809):1007–1008.

McDonald WS, et al. Immediate enteral feeding in burn patients is safe and effective. *Ann Surg* 1991 Feb; 213(2):177–183.

Meguid MM, et al. Nutritional support in surgical practice. *Am J Surg* 1990 March; 159(3):345–359.

Miller SJ, Simpson J. Medication-nutrient interactions: Hypophosphatemia associated with sucralfate in the intensive care unit. *Nutr Clin Pract* 1991 Oct; 6(5):199–201.

Moore EE, Moore FA. Immediate enteral nutrition following multisystem trauma: A decade perspective. *J Am Coll Nutr* 1991 Dec; 10(6):633–648.

Moore R, et al. Measured energy expenditure in severe head trauma. *J Trauma* 1989 Dec; 28(12):1633–1636.

Ott L, Young B. Nutrition in the neurologically injured patient. *Nutr Clin Pract* 1991 Dec; 6(6):223–229.

Pinchcofsky-Devin G. Hazards of immobility and polypharmacy. *Support Line* 1992 June; 14(3): 5–7. (A newsletter of Dietitians in Nutrition Support.)

Rodriquez DJ, et al. Obligatory negative nitrogen balance following spinal cord injury. *JPEN* 1991 May-June; 15(3):319–322.

Saito H, et al. The effect of route of nutrient administration on the nutritional state, catabolic hormone secretion and gut mucosal integrity after burn injury. *JPEN* 1987 Jan; 11(1):1–7.

Scrimshaw NS. Effect of infection on nutrient requirements. *JPEN* 1991 Nov-Dec; 15(6):589–600.

Spector N. Nutritional support of the ventilator-dependent patient. *Nurs Clin North Am* 1989 June; 24(2):407–414.

Talbot JM. Guidelines for the scientific review of enteral food products for special medical purposes. *JPEN* 1991 May-June; 15(3):99S–173S.

Ubbink JB, et al. Relationship between vitamin B_6 status and elevated pyridoxal kinase levels induced by theophylline therapy in humans. *J Nutr* 1990 Nov; 120(11):1352–1359.

Varella L. Barbituate therapy and nutrition support in head injured patients. *Nutr Clin Pract* 1991 Dec; 6(6):239–244.

Weinsier RL, et al. *Handbook of Clinical Nutrition.* 2nd ed. St. Louis, CV Mosby, 1989.

Whittaker JS, et al. The effects of refeeding on peripheral and respiratory muscle function in malnourished chronic obstructive pulmonary disease patients. *Am Rev Respir Dis* 1990 Aug. 142(2):283–288.

Wilson DO, et al. Metabolic rate and weight loss in chronic obstructive lung disease. *JPEN* 1990 Jan-Feb; 14(1):7–11.

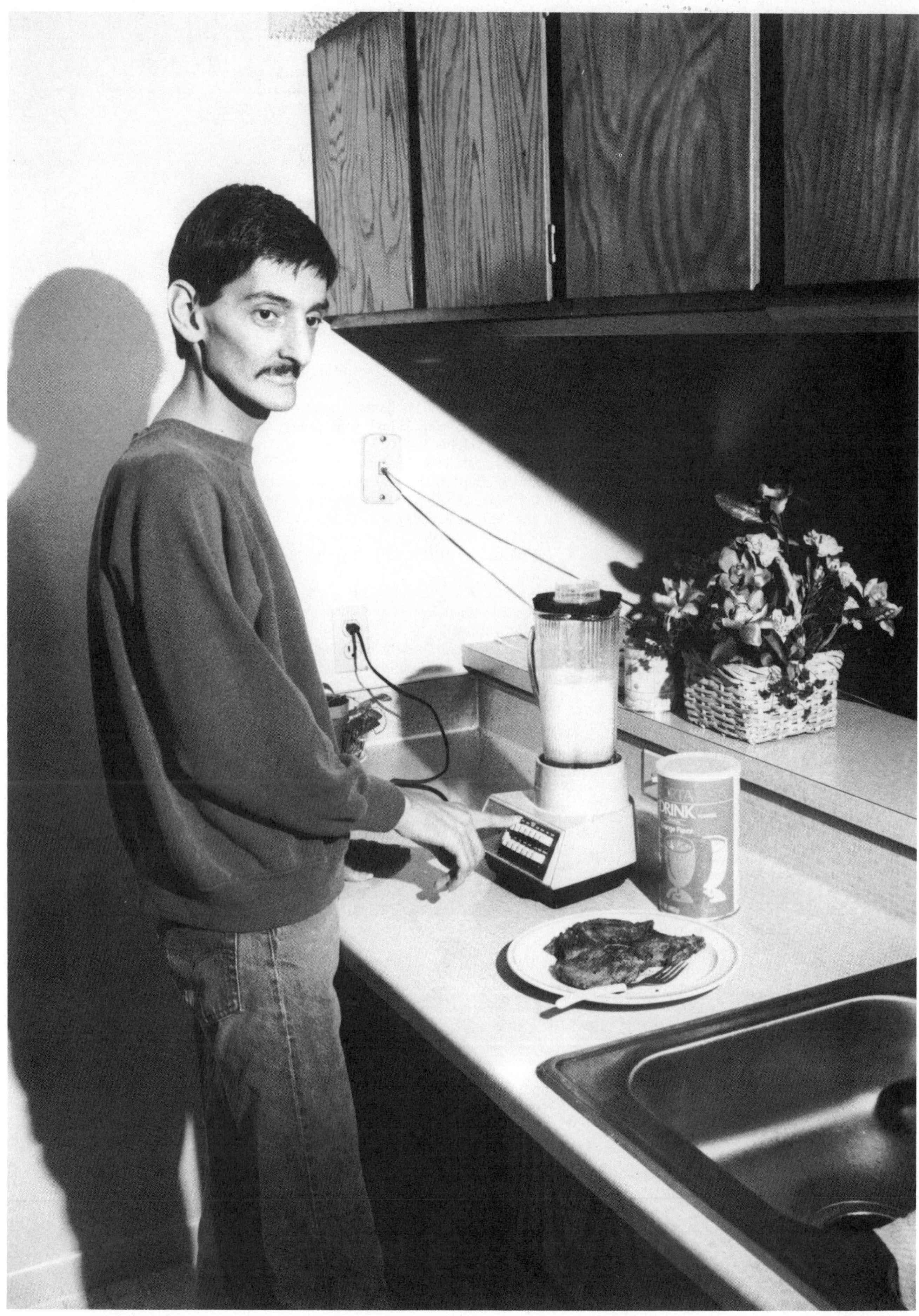

CHAPTER 22

Nutrition Support in Cancer and Immune-Suppressed Disorders

OUTLINE

I. CANCER
  A. Nutritional Effects of Cancer
    1. Anorexia
    2. Nutrient Metabolism
  Nursing Applications
  B. Nutritional Effects of Cancer Therapy
    1. Surgical Intervention
    2. Radiation
    3. Chemotherapy
  Nursing Applications
  C. Nutritional Assessment
  D. Nutritional Care
    1. Benefits
    2. Objectives
    3. Oral Intake
    4. Supplemental Feedings
  Nursing Applications
    5. Nausea, Vomiting, and Early Satiety
  Nursing Applications
    6. Dysgeusia
  Nursing Applications
    7. Diarrhea, Cramps, and Other Intestinal Upsets
  Nursing Applications
    8. Dysphagia
    9. Xerostomia
  Nursing Applications
    10. Depressed Immune Function
  Nursing Applications

II. HUMAN IMMUNODEFICIENCY VIRUS
  A. Nutritional Effects of Human Immunodeficiency Virus
    1. Anorexia
    2. Diarrhea and Malabsorption

OBJECTIVES

THE STUDENT WILL BE ABLE TO:

- Discuss the role of nutrition in the cancer client.
- List common food aversions and suggest ways to enhance food intake for clients with cancer or AIDS.
- List the effects of cancer and AIDS on nutritional status.
- Suggest ways to increase intake for clients with nausea and vomiting, early satiety, oral and esophageal lesions, dysgeusia, and xerostomia.
- Suggest possible solutions to minimize effects of diarrhea and abdominal cramps.
- Explain guidelines to prevent food-borne illnesses in the immunosuppressed client.
- Counsel clients about nontraditional nutrition therapies for cancer and AIDS and the possible benefits or detrimental effects of such.
- Apply nutritional principles when providing nursing care for cancer and AIDS clients.
- Describe client education nutrition principles for cancer and AIDS clients.

TEST YOUR NQ (True/False)

1. Cancer clients should reduce food intake to inhibit the growth of the neoplasm.
2. Aggressive nutrition support of cancer clients can decrease morbidity and mortality.
3. Jaw pain in cancer clients can be decreased by using wide-angle cups for drinking.
4. Cancer clients should be offered their favorite foods during radiation or chemotherapy to improve intake.

5. In xerostomia, a room humidifier may be useful.
6. AIDS clients are prone to diarrhea.
7. AIDS dementia has no effect on nutritional intake.
8. Total lymphocyte count is an important parameter for assessing the nutritional status of AIDS clients.
9. Pineapple juice is good for AIDS clients with oral lesions.
10. Laetrile is a recommended nutritional treatment of AIDS.

CANCER

Prevention of cancer is an important concern for most Americans. At the present rate, about 30% or 73 million Americans eventually develop cancer. Approximately 3 out of every 4 families are affected (NCI, 1989). Countless studies on epidemiology and actual food/nutrient intake have implicated dietary factors as preventing or causing various types of neoplasms. However, no individual food has been identified that specifically causes cancer, nor can any specific food prevent it. To live means we must eat. As a result of the interaction of many different dietary factors that have been implicated as the cause of tumors, guidelines for preventing cancer are generalized (Table 22–1). These guidelines are consistent with good nutrition practices.

Cancer, which is a multifaceted disease process, has no simple cause or cure. Rapidly growing cell tissue competes with the host and deprives it of needed nutrients. The malignant tumor often acts as a parasite to meet its nutrient require-

TABLE 22–1

CANCER PREVENTION

Dietary Guidelines of the National Cancer Institute*

1. Reduce fat intake to less than 30% of kilocalories
2. Increase fiber intake to 20 to 30 gm, not to exceed 35 gm
3. Include a variety of fruits and vegetables in the daily diet
4. Avoid obesity
5. Consume alcoholic beverages in moderation if at all
6. Minimize consumption of salt-cured, salt pickled, and smoked foods

The above generalized guidelines are a synopsis of information that can be divided into health habits that are either protective or risk factors for particular types of cancer†:

Protective Factors	***Food Sources***	***Reduces Cancer Risk***
Cruciferous vegetables	Broccoli, turnips, cauliflower, brussels sprouts, cabbage, kale, rutabagas	Colorectal, stomach, and respiratory cancers
High-fiber foods	Whole-grain bread and cereals; fruits and vegetables	Colon cancer
Vitamin A (beta-carotene)	Carrots, peaches, apricots, squash, broccoli	Esophagus, larynx, lung, bladder
Vitamin C	Fresh fruits and vegetables such as grapefruit, cantaloupe, oranges, strawberries, red and green peppers, broccoli, tomatoes	Esophagus, oral cavity, stomach
Maintain ideal weight	Avoid overeating; consume low-kilocalorie foods and exercise	Uterus, gallbladder, breast, and colon

Continued

TABLE 22–1

CANCER PREVENTION *Continued*

Risk Factors	*Food Sources*	*Increases Cancer Risk*
Fat	Fried foods, fatty meats, high-fat luncheon meats, sausage, full-fat dairy products	Breast, colon, uterus, prostate
Salt-cured, smoked, nitrite-cured foods	Bacon, ham, hot dogs, or salt-cured fish	Esophagus and stomach
Cigarette smoking		All, especially lung and pancreas
Alcohol		Liver
Sun		Skin

* From Butrum RR, et al. NCI dietary guidelines: Rationale. *Am J Clin Nutr* 1988 Sept; 48 (3 suppl):888–895.
† Data from Weisburger JH. Nutritional approach to cancer prevention with emphasis on vitamins, antioxidants, and carotenoids. *Am J Clin Nutr* 1991 Jan; 53(1 suppl):226S–237S.

What types of food should be increased or decreased to prevent cancer? What are prognostic indicators for survival and response to cancer therapies?

ments. Intake of a well-balanced diet provides nutrients both for the host and neoplasm or tumor. However, poor intake results in utilization of body stores to satisfy nutrient requirements of both client and tumor. Clients with deeply seated tumors (such as pancreatic or gastric) are frequently malnourished at the time of diagnosis. Progressive weight loss and malnutrition frequently observed in cancer clients are prognostic indicators for survival and for response to therapies.

Nutritional Effects of Cancer

Cachexia is characterized by marked anorexia, early satiety, weight loss, tissue wasting, anemia, organ dysfunction, and ultimately death.

Cachexia is the result of a variety of etiological factors (Fig. 22–1). Without intervention, the cycle of anorexia–weight loss–cachexia appears to be a self-perpetuating downhill spiral.

Anorexia

Anorexia associated with cancer is an important symptom of an underlying neoplasm (Fig. 22–2). Abnormalities in taste perception have been noted in some cancer clients with an elevated threshold for sweets and a reduced threshold for bitter flavors. Altered taste sensations may be secondary to deficiencies in zinc and other trace elements. Hormonal factors or neurotransmitter precursors affect the

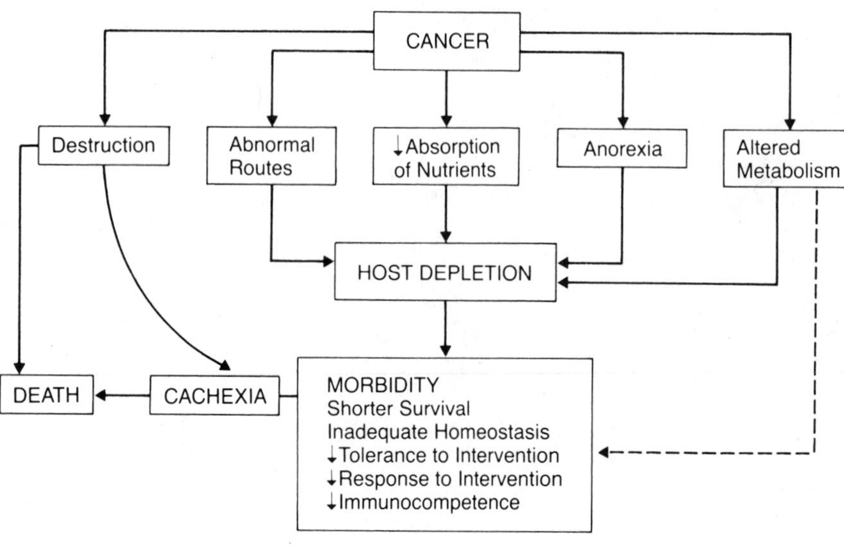

Figure 22–1 Mechanisms by which cancer disturbs host homeostasis, leading to cachexia and death. (From Daly JM, Thom AK. Neoplastic diseases. *In* Kinney JM, et al (eds). *Nutrition and Metabolism in Patient Care.* Philadelphia, WB Saunders, 1988, pp 567–587.)

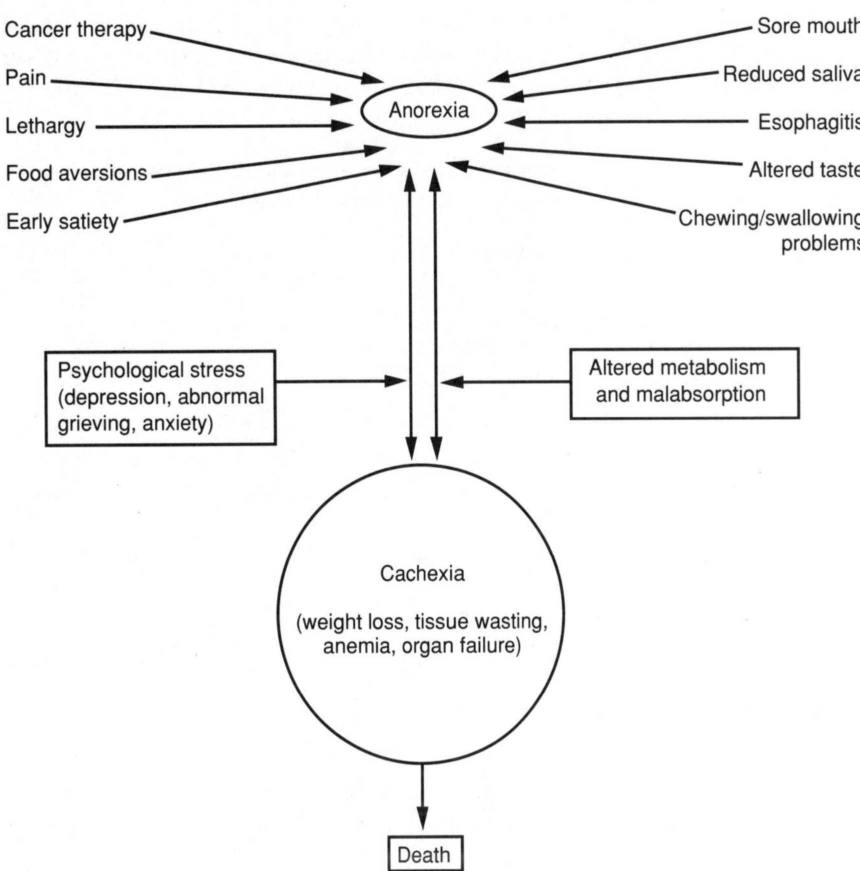

Figure 22–2 Factors precipitating anorexia.

feeding center in the hypothalamus to reduce oral intake. **Early satiety** may be related to decreased digestive secretions, mucosal atrophy, or impaired gastric emptying.

Early satiety—feelings of fullness after eating a few bites.

The location of the tumor itself may also reduce food intake, especially when the alimentary tract is affected by the tumor. Intake is reduced in clients with cancer of the oral cavity, pharynx, or esophagus because of **odynophagia** or dysphagia. Gastric cancer may lead to reduced gastric capacity or partial gastric outlet obstruction, resulting in early satiety, nausea, and vomiting. Clients with intestinal tumors often have partial obstruction or **blind-loop syndrome** that allows bacterial overgrowth and interferes with nutrient absorption.

Odynophagia—pain associated with swallowing.

Blind loop syndrome is an alteration in the anatomy of the small intestine creating a closed or partially obstructed loop into which intestinal contents may enter but are not readily evacuated.

Psychological factors undoubtedly affect appetite. Depression, grief, or anxiety resulting from the disease or its treatment may lead to poor appetite and abnormal eating behaviors. **Learned food aversions** may also contribute to a diminished or unbalanced dietary intake.

Learned aversion—dislike for a food in association with unpleasant reactions such as nausea or vomiting.

What are some contributing factors of anorexia?

Nutrient Metabolism

Since the extent of malnutrition associated with cancer is often greater than can be explained solely on the basis of diminished intake, changes in nutrient metabolism have been investigated. Extensive changes in energy, carbohydrate, lipid, and protein metabolism have been associated with neoplasms; inconsistent findings may be related to the location and type of tumor.

An elevated BMR may contribute to increased energy expenditure. Additionally, the metabolic response to starvation with the expected normal conservation of endogenous nutrient stores is inhibited. Normally during starvation, the utilization of muscle proteins for energy is gradually replaced by fatty acids to decrease glucose utilization and muscle wasting. In cancer clients, increased glucose production and

What is the cause of fat and lean body mass losses in cancer clients?

protein catabolism continue. Because of abnormalities in protein metabolism, nitrogen depletion and decreased muscle protein synthesis are observed. Thus, depletion of both fat and lean body mass is accelerated.

NURSING APPLICATIONS

Assessment

Physical—for odynophagia, dysphagia.
Dietary—for food intake, feelings of fullness, learned aversions.
Laboratory—for RBC, Hgb, Hct, albumin.

Interventions

1. Monitor for depression, grief, and anxiety, as these may decrease intake.
2. Consult the dietitian and physician concerning nutritional needs.
3. Refer client to support groups, i.e., American Cancer Society and social services.

Evaluation

* Cachexia will not occur; client will eat 50 to 75% of ordered diet; depletion of fat and lean body mass will be minimized; and client will verbalize the rationale for increasing intake.

Client Education

- Adequate intake is needed to prevent the tumor from "stealing" nutrients from the body.
- The energy to sustain body processes is increased with cancer, so additional intake is needed.
- Dietary guidelines by the National Cancer Institute (NCI) and American Cancer Society have been developed to prevent the development of cancer (see Table 22-1). Some food additives such as nitrates may increase cancer risk as well as a diet low in fiber or high in fat.
- NCI, American Cancer Society, and the American Institute of Cancer Research (AICR) have developed client literature for implementing cancer prevention guidelines.

Nutritional Effects of Cancer Therapy

Cancer can be treated by surgical procedures, radiation therapy, chemotherapy, and immunotherapy. These therapies, used individually or in combination, affect some of the normal body cells as malignant cells are destroyed. Nutritional problems result from all therapies used to treat cancer as well as from the competition of the tumor tissue for nutrients.

Surgical Intervention

The primary treatment involves surgical removal of the malignancy. Frequently the client may be subjected to numerous surgeries. This results in increased nitrogen losses and kilocaloric requirement regardless of the tumor location. The presurgical nutritional status is predictive of the client's ability to cope with the surgical stress. Aggressive nutrition support before cancer surgery can decrease morbidity and mortality for malnourished cancer clients.

In the case of tumors involving the GI tract, the ability to ingest foods orally or adequately digest and absorb nutrients may be affected. Radical surgery in the oropharyngeal area may present problems in chewing and swallowing and decreased taste sensations. Esophagectomy and vagotomy may result in poor fat absorption, gastric stasis, and diarrhea (see Chapter 25). Gastrectomy results in clinical problems proportionate to the extent of the resection. Dumping syndrome, hypoglycemia, steatorrhea, and lack of intrinsic factor are common problems necessitating nutrition intervention. When the distal ileum has been resected, vitamin B_{12} cannot be absorbed, leading to macrocytic anemia. Massive small-bowel resection presents serious long-term problems in maintaining adequate nutrition, including water and electrolyte balance (see Chapter 25).

In general, how will surgery affect nutritional status?

Radiation

Treatment of rapidly growing neoplastic cells with radiation therapy also usually affects the fast-growing normal cells (e.g., hair follicles, bone marrow, and GI mucous membranes). These effects of radiation are evident within 1 to 2 days and dissipate within about 2 weeks following treatment. Cells in the area of treatment are especially affected.

Radiation therapy especially affects the GI tract. Early transient effects include general loss of appetite, nausea and vomiting, and diarrhea caused by malabsorption secondary to mucosal damage in the GI tract. (Villi are shortened, and thickness of the mucosa is reduced, which may lead to mucosal ulcerations and reduced absorptive surfaces). Food intake is affected because of a loss of taste sensation, **xerostomia,** difficulty in swallowing, and a burning sensation in the mouth when the larynx or pharynx area is irradiated. Food aversions may be associated with upcoming therapy. Dental problems and loss of teeth may also become a dietary problem.

Xerostomia—dryness of the mouth.

Radiation damage to the small and large bowel alters intestinal function. In addition to malabsorption, obstruction (intestinal strictures) or fistulas may occur. Rapid weight loss occurs as well as vitamin deficiencies, lactose intolerance, and steatorrhea. However, these signs of radiation enteritis may not occur until 10 years after radiation exposure and can easily be confused with other entities, including tumor recurrence.

What areas of the body are affected by radiation that will influence nutritional status?

Chemotherapy

Chemotherapy has a direct effect on DNA synthesis and cell proliferation. Drugs are used to destroy malignant cells without loss of an excessive number of normal cells. Chemotherapy has more widespread effects on the body than either radiation or surgical treatment (Table 22–2).

The treatment of disease by chemical agents is known as chemotherapy.

Chemotherapy indirectly produces nausea and vomiting as a result of stimulation of chemoreceptors in the brain. Rapid cell turnover rate in the alimentary tract leads to stomatitis, oral ulcerations, and decreased absorptive capacity. As a result, changes in taste sensation and learned food aversions occur.

Additionally, production of RBCs in the bone marrow is affected with accompanying anemia, leukopenia, and thrombocytopenia. Decreased neutrophils are associated with increased incidence of sepsis. In clients receiving 5-fluorouracil, the bone marrow may produce megaloblastic cells resembling pernicious and other megaloblastic anemias. Mithramycin, an antibiotic frequently used in cancer clients, may precipitate hypocalcemia.

Adrenocortical steroids, which exert immunosuppressive activity, are a well-known cause of protein, calcium, and potassium losses. They cause increased gastric mucosal vulnerability to HCl, which can be prevented by giving antacids or histamine antagonists with the drug. Edema is a common side effect.

TABLE 22–2 **SIDE EFFECTS OF CHEMOTHERAPEUTIC AGENTS**

	Sore Mouth	**Nausea and Vomiting**	**Anorexia**	**Diarrhea**	**Esophagitis**	**Mucositis (Mouth Ulcers)**	**Abdominal Pain**	**Constipation**	**Intestinal Ulceration**	**Bone Marrow Depression**	**Weight Gain**	**Jaw Pain**
Altretamine		XX										
AMSA		XX		XX		XX						
Asparaginase		XX	XX									
Bleomycin		XX	XX	XX		XX						
Busulfan		XX										
Carmustine		XX	XX							XX		
Chlorambucil		XX	XX							XX		
Cisplatin		XX	XX							XX		
Cyclophosphamide (Cytoxin)	XX	XX	XX				XX			XX		
Cytarabine	XX	XX	XX	XX		XX	XX			XX		
Dacarbazine		XX								XX		
Dactinomycin		XX	XX			XX	XX			XX		
Daunorubicin		XX	XX			XX				XX		
Doxorubicin	XX	XX	XX			XX				XX		
Fluorouracil		XX		XX		XX				XX		
Gallium nitrate		XX										
Hydroxyurea		XX		XX		XX				XX		
Lomustine		XX								XX		
Mercaptopurine	XX	XX	XX	XX						XX		
Methotrexate		XX	XX	XX		XX	XX		XX	XX		
Methyl GAG		XX		XX	XX	XX						
Mitomycin		XX		XX								
Plicamycin		XX	XX			XX				XX		
Prednisone					XX						XX	
Procarbazine		XX	XX	XX					XX	XX		
Streptozocin		XX		XX								
Thioguanine	XX	XX								XX		
Vinblastine		XX					XX	XX				XX
Vincristine		XX	XX				XX	XX				
Vindesine		XX		XX				XX		XX		

* Data from Shils ME. Nutrition and diet in cancer. *In* Shils ME, Young VR, eds. *Modern Nutrition in Health and Disease.* 7th ed. Philadelphia, Lea & Febiger, 1988; 1380–1422; and Tabor SR. Drug chart. Amie Karen Cancer Center, Dept of Pediatrics, Cedars-Sinai Medical Center, UCLA, Los Angeles, CA 90048.

Antimetabolites, such as methotrexate, are folate antagonists. Methotrexate, 5-fluorouracil, and dactinomycin affect the GI mucosa, precipitating a malabsorption condition similar to sprue. Vincristine, vinblastine, and hydroxyurea therapy may result in constipation.

Name the common adverse side effects of chemotherapy.

NURSING APPLICATIONS

Assessment

Physical—for signs of malnutrition, location of cancer, type of therapy performed, nausea, vomiting, diarrhea, xerostomia, last treatment.
Dietary—for anorexia, medications prescribed.
Laboratory—for glucose, RBCs, MCV, WBCs, and platelets.

Interventions

1. Increase fluid and fiber intake to relieve constipation caused by medications. Monitor client closely for tolerance of fiber.
2. Offer high-protein supplements and fluids by straw when jaw pain is present.
3. Do not restrict fluids for edema caused by corticosteroids because this may be counterproductive when the cause of edema is not from cardiac or renal pathology.
4. Consult with a dietitian to determine if enteral or parenteral feedings are needed before surgery.
5. In surgeries involving the oropharyngeal area, monitor for decreased intake resultant of chewing and swallowing problems. In surgeries involving the esophagus or vagus nerve, monitor for fat-soluble vitamin deficiencies and diarrhea.
6. Monitor stools for steatorrhea and blood.

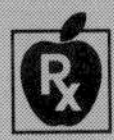
Alternate antimetabolite chemotherapy with folic acid supplements.

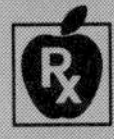
Avoid vitamin A supplements and alcohol during methotrexate therapy.

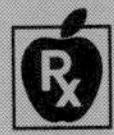
Milk products may decrease absorption of methotrexate, so do not give concurrently (Allen, 1991).

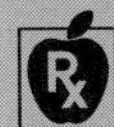
Use milk and cheese products as well as calcium supplements to offset the calcium loss encountered when mithramycin is used.

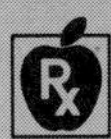
Offer a lactose-free and gluten-free diet (see Chapter 23) during dactinomycin therapy.

Evaluation

* When steroids are used, body weight is inaccurate. Do not totally rely on body weight as an indicator of treatment effectiveness or ineffectiveness.

Client Education

- Explain the type and effects of treatment to the client.
- Anorexia usually begins on the day of chemotherapy treatment and lasts for several days.
- Vincristine may cause acute jaw pain.
- If milk consumption causes abdominal cramps, gas, fatty stools, or diarrhea after consuming milk, notify the dietitian or physician.

Nutritional Assessment

Nutritional status of the cancer client is an integral component within the interdisciplinary treatment plan. Ideally the nurse and dietitian work together; the nurse reports nutritional problems observed to the dietitian and feels free to ask for assistance with these problems and/or client consultation. Malnutrition has a negative prognostic effect and can contribute to the client's morbidity and tolerance to all modalities of treatment. Severe cachexia is easily recognized, but it is vital to recognize moderate malnourishment of cancer clients so nutrition support may be implemented. As discussed in Chapter 11, nutritional assessment should include evaluation of dietary history, anthropometric measurements, and laboratory values.

Although anthropometric measures lack the precision attained by biochemical analysis of blood and urine samples, they are inexpensive, noninvasive, and easily obtained. Weight can be used to a limited extent to evaluate nutriture of the cancer client. Edema or dehydration may interfere with accurate assessments. As much as 10 lbs fluid in the lower extremities, or pedal edema, may accumulate before the condition is recognized as pitting edema. Muscle wasting is associated with peripheral edema. Since weight fluctuates more with the fluid content of the body, measurements such as MAMC (see Chapter 11) may be more accurate assessments. Muscle wastage results in progressive fatigue, weakness, and inactivity.

Weight changes are significant to assessments. Preillness weight should be compared with the current weight and evaluated at least weekly throughout the treatment period. More than a 10% weight loss within 2 to 3 weeks reflects fluid balance rather than protein or fatty tissue loss. On the one hand, weight loss indicates compromised visceral and somatic proteins including enzymatic, structural, and mechanical functions and correlates with a poor prognosis. On the other hand, weight loss is not the cause for poor prognosis.

Serum protein concentrations (albumin, prealbumin, transferrin) are used to evaluate visceral protein mass. Particularly in cancer clients, laboratory values reflect the disease state as much as the nutritional status. Total lymphocyte count is used to assess immune function. The immune system may be depressed by increasing age, trauma, anesthetics, malignancy, malnutrition, and oncological therapy. **Immunocompetence** can suggest subtle but distinct changes in immune response preceding the occurrence of frequent infections and decreased growth velocity.

Immunocompetence is an indicator of the ability to fight infection.

Elevated serum calcium occurs in a significant number of clients with malignant diseases. Hypercalcemia is usually due to secretion of parathyroid hormone–related protein by the tumor (Bilezikian, 1992). Treatment is critical because hypercalcemia often precipitates and aggravates renal failure. Since serum calcium is not a reflection of dietary calcium intake, therapy for lowering the calcium is pharmacological. Initially hypercalcemia is treated with IV saline solutions. If necessary, other medications such as calcitonin, plicamycin, biphosphonate, glucocorticoids, or loop diuretics may be prescribed to promote calcium deposition into skeletal tissue, inhibit bone resorption, or increase calcium excretion.

When does weight reflect fluid balance rather than tissue loss?

Nutritional Care

Benefits

Nutrition support can positively affect the impact of the altered nutrient metabolism, nutrition parameters, and response to therapy. It increases the well-being of the client and may permit administration of more intensive therapies. There is no conclusive evidence that adequate nutrition support preferentially feeds the tumor and increases tumor growth (Daly et al, 1990).

Research shows that high-risk cancer clients given nutrition support before surgery have fewer complications and infections, and shorter hospitalizations. Nutrition support does not cure cancer, but recovery rates are directly related to optimal nutritional status.

Objectives

Nutritional care for the oncology client may involve (1) preventive care for those capable of maintaining their weight and in good nutrition status; (2) maintenance care for those undergoing aggressive chemotherapy, radiotherapy, or combined therapy with problems of anorexia and nausea and such potential nutritional consequences as stomatitis, xerostomia, dysgeusia, dysphagia, constipation, and diarrhea; and (3) palliative care that contributes to the terminal client's comfort by providing any food tolerated.

In nutrition-depleted clients, the goal is restoration of lean tissues with concomitant restoration of fat. The objective for preventive and maintenance care is for optimal nutritional status of the client, which (1) lessens the intensity of toxicities caused by the treatment, (2) induces a more favorable tumor response to treatment, (3) increases immunocompetence with less infection, (4) lessens physical and emotional insults from treatments, and (5) improves the sense of well-being.

Various feeding techniques are used. Whenever possible, oral feedings are preferred. Progressive weight loss or the likelihood of significant weight loss if the current clinical situation persists may warrant an alternative method of feeding. Aggressive nutrition support (enteral or parenteral feedings) is indicated for the following: (1) inability to eat for a prolonged period of time (more than 5 days, depending on the client's initial nutritional status), (2) cachexia related to inadequate intake rather than tumor-induced abnormalities, and (3) malignancy that is expected to respond to therapy (Lipman, 1991). Tube feedings can be used if only intake, chewing, or swallowing is impaired. Elemental diets can be implemented if digestion is impaired, but absorption is intact.

TPN may be appropriate when the client cannot or will not eat or when the GI tract is temporarily unable to handle nutrient intake. Although TPN therapy is very expensive, it is the most effective therapy for clients who have lost a significant amount of their preillness weight. Ultimately decisions about methods of feeding depend on the client's prognosis and wishes. Involvement of the whole nutrition support team with the client and family is vital.

What are 5 objectives for nutritional care of cancer clients?

Oral Intake

The daily energy needs of cancer clients are estimated to be 35 to 42 kcal/kg to improve lean body mass and immune response; protein requirements are approximately 1.3 gm/kg (Bozzetti, 1989). The condition requires much attention to maintain body weight; a high-protein, high-kilocalorie diet is usually prescribed. Although the importance of adequate food intake cannot be overemphasized, measures must be taken to tempt clients' appetites without making food intake a focal conflict point. Even for clients with mild to moderate decreases in intake, careful evaluation of food preferences can make the difference between weight maintenance and loss. Team members are responsible for using ingenuity and different strategies to increase food acceptance. Because of the complexity of cancer, clients with the same symptoms may respond differently. The dietitian may individually tailor the diet for the client, but guidelines listed in Table 22–3 may be helpful to the nurse in increasing food acceptance.

Preparing attractive trays and providing a pleasant environment at mealtime are important to achieve the goal of increased food acceptance. The setting should be calm, not rushed. The client may need to keep the tray longer than usual.

The challenge is to identify optimal eating times. Clients should be encouraged to eat when their appetite is good. This frequently means a large breakfast with smaller feedings throughout the day. When hospitalized clients eat together, they benefit from peer support.

Because of the client's inability to consume adequate amounts during 3 meals, frequent feedings are usually indicated. As much protein and as many kilocalories as possible should be included in each snack to improve nutrient intake. Light snacks may be used, as preferred by the client. However, the popularity of nutrition supplements can be attributed to their high kilocaloric and nutrient density.

TABLE 22–3

GUIDELINES FOR ORAL FEEDING DURING ANTITUMOR THERAPY

Problem	Diet	Supplements and Aids	Poorly Tolerated Foods
Acute GI toxicity	Clear, cold liquids Light, low-fat foods	None	Milk products; cream soups; fried foods; sandwiches; sweet desserts
Stomatitits, esophagitis	Liquid and soft diet Broth-based soups; fruit ades; carbonated beverages; melons Alter texture and temperature	Glucose polymers; mild-flavored supplements; frequent oral hygiene; frequent saline rinses	Juices, especially citrus; bananas; crisp or raw foods; meats; spicy entrees; textured or granular foods; coarse bread products; extremely hot or cold foods
Viscous mucous production, xerostomia (mouth dryness)	Liquid diet. Tea with lemon; juices; fruit ades; popsicles; carbonated beverages; broth-based soups; thinned hot cereal	Glucose polymers; artificial saliva; frequent saline rinses and oral hygiene	Thick nectars and liquids; thick cream soups; thick hot cereals; bread products; gelatin; oily foods
Decreased salivation	Regular diet with high-moisture foods. Gravies; sauces; casseroles; chicken; fish; beverages with foods; citric acid–containing foods; sherbet; melons; vegetables with sauces	Artificial saliva; glucose polymers; saliva stimulants, such as sugarless lemon drops and gum; frequent saline rinses	Dry foods; bread products; meats; crackers; bananas; excessively hot foods; alcohol
Mouth blindness (hypogeusia)	Regular diet with strongly flavored foods Spicy foods with emphasis on aroma and texture	Flavored supplements; frequent saline rinses	Bland foods; plain meats; unsalted foods
Taste alterations (dysgeusia)	Regular diet with many cold foods. Milk products Emphasize experimentation	Fruit-flavored supplements	Red meats; chocolate; coffee; tea
Early satiety	High-kilocalorie diet with kilocalorically dense foods. Meat; fish; poultry; eggs; whole milk; cheese; cream soups; ice cream; whole-milk yogurt; creamed vegetables; rich desserts	Kilocalorically dense supplements; glucose polymers	Low-fat or nonfat milk products; broth soups; green salads; steamed, plain vegetables; low-kilocalorie beverages

Adapted from Aker SN, Lenssen P. A Guide to Good Nutrition During and After Chemotherapy and Radiation. 3rd ed. Seattle, WA, Fred Hutchison Cancer Research Center, 1988.

Supplemental Feedings

Suggesting a supplement is not enough. Specific directions should be given and monitored for a successful regimen. A prescription states the amount of supplement to be provided based on the client's requirements and actual intake. The actual amount of foods and beverages consumed may be recorded by the nurse or the client. Subtracting the kilocaloric intake from the estimated requirement yields the amount of the supplement prescribed.

Taste preference is the paramount factor in determining acceptance of any supplement. Many liquid and powdered supplements as well as those in the form of puddings are commercially available (see Appendix A–2). The main concern is to use types that will be consumed by the client and are economical and readily available or convenient.

What are some techniques used to increase food intake?

NURSING APPLICATIONS

Assessment

Physical—for normal and current weight (remember edema and dehydration effects), IBW, weight changes, TSF, MAMC, fatigue, weakness, anorexia, vomiting, dysphagia, mouth sores.

Dietary—for kilocalorie and nutrient intake using a 24-hour dietary recall or a 3-day diet diary or by checking the food tray; taste changes, food aversions.

Laboratory—for protein (albumin, prealbumin, transferrin); lymphocytes; calcium, electrolytes.

Interventions

1. Offer several small meals or snacks. Eating more often can compensate for reduced meal size and is preferred by some clients.
2. Use well-stocked unit kitchens to permit snacking and liberal intake.
3. Add sugar and glucose polymers to make foods more palatable and increase kilocaloric intake.
4. Provide a tasting tray containing 1 oz each of several supplements to identify client preferences.
5. Offer lactose-free supplements if the client is lactose-intolerant.
6. Use high-kilocalorie nutrition supplements. Energy value can be increased by 700 to 1000 kcal daily.
7. Leave high-kilocalorie, nutrient-dense nutrition supplements in an ice bucket in the client's room to encourage intake.
8. Serve a large breakfast to cancer clients since appetites are usually better in the morning.
9. Decrease stress at meal times by encouraging a quiet rest period before and after meals.
10. Use relaxation training to improve weight gain and arm muscle circumference in cancer clients. It can be as vital a component in the nutritional well-being of these clients as supplementation.

Evaluation

* When evaluating weight changes, if the client weighs 150 lbs, a weight change of 15 lbs within 2 to 3 weeks reflects a fluid change rather than protein or fat losses. (Remember weight × 0.10.) Also, to improve lean body mass and immune response, evaluate adequacy of kilocaloric and protein intake. This client should consume 2387 kcal and 88.7 gm protein.

Remember:

$$150 \text{ lbs} \div 2.2 \text{ lb/kg} = 68.2 \text{ kg} \times 35 \text{ kcal/kg} = 2387 \text{ kcal}$$

$$68.2 \text{ kg} \times 1.3 \text{ (protein factor)} = 88.7 \text{ gm protein}$$

Continued

* Desired outcomes include the following: MAMC would not deteriorate, laboratory work would return to near normal, and mental status would improve (no severe depression or abnormal grieving would occur). Although other factors may affect outcomes that are beyond the nurse's control, these are parameters to evaluate goal achievement.

Client Education

- Adequate intake does not increase the tumor's growth.
- Recovery is faster with nutrition support.

Nausea, Vomiting, and Early Satiety

Cancer clients may unknowingly decrease food intake because of a full feeling after eating small amounts. A diet diary can help to determine just how much is consumed. Clients may also discontinue therapy because of suboptimal control of nausea and vomiting.

Carbohydrates are digested faster; this helps in preventing early satiety and improving the ability to eat more often. Colorless, odorless foods, such as cottage cheese, applesauce, and vanilla ice cream have resulted in less nausea and vomiting and higher overall food intake for clients receiving chemotherapy (Menashian et al, 1992).

Antiemetics are most effective if started the night before chemotherapy and continued at 6-hour intervals as long as nausea persists. Foods eaten before vomiting tend to lose their popularity even though the food is not the actual culprit. Abrupt movements frequently provoke nausea; allow about 1 hour for rest after food intake. When the chemotherapeutic agent is administered monthly, the client will have several weeks without anorexia when high-protein and high-kilocalorie foods should be eaten.

Hyposmia—abnormally decreased sensitivity to odors.

Hyposmia frequently limits the appetite, too. The odor of some foods may be nonexistent or perceived as unpleasant.

NURSING APPLICATIONS

Assessment

Physical—for nausea, vomiting, early satiety.
Dietary—for food intake with diet diary.

Interventions

1. Encourage the client to eat slowly, take small bites, and chew thoroughly.
2. Encourage soft, bland foods such as rice, soft-cooked eggs, custards, nectars.
3. Provide small, frequent feedings to avoid an empty stomach and increase food intake.
4. Offer small amounts of readily digestible food frequently. Always have snacks available; waiting even for a few minutes may lessen the desire to eat.
5. Food may be tolerated better if time of treatment, especially medications, can be changed; if not, alter mealtimes to coincide with the client's appetite.
6. Provide antiemetic medications 30 minutes before meals and start the night before chemotherapy. Ondenestron (Zofran) is usually given 15 to 30 minutes before chemotherapy.
7. Avoid favorite foods when the stomach is upset to prevent learned aversions.
8. Encourage the family to suggest/provide favorite foods when the client is feeling well.

Evaluation

* Evaluate nausea as a possible side effect of drug therapy.
* If client experiences few episodes of nausea or vomiting and occasionally eats favorite foods, nursing care was effective.

Client Education

- Withhold liquids and foods until vomiting is arrested; then begin with clear liquids or crushed ice.
- Apple juice, iced tea, dry crackers or dry toast, and gelatin are especially suitable initially for nausea or vomiting. Then, other clear cold beverages or juices are followed by small quantities of easily digested foods, as tolerated.
- Limit fluids during mealtimes, including soups. Liquids may be better tolerated before or after the meal.
- Aromas from hot foods may aggravate nausea. Cold foods or foods at room temperature are better tolerated than hot ones.
- Highly spiced and acidic foods may be poorly tolerated.
- Avoid any fried, greasy, or fatty foods.
- Eat saltier foods, if permitted.
- Clients should avoid cooking foods or being in the area while food is prepared.
- Alcohol, such as a glass of wine, may be used to stimulate appetite but should be avoided during chemotherapy.
- If nauseated, remain in a sitting position. If reclining, have head 4 inches above the feet.

Dysgeusia

A common complaint of cancer clients is **dysgeusia**. Taste aversions are related more to the extent of the disease rather than the type of cancer or treatment except chemotherapy. When the tumor regresses, the dysgeusia is reversed. **Hypogeusia** and hyposmia also interfere with normal food patterns for the cancer client, but dysgeusia usually results directly in weight loss. Changes in taste acuity may be related to chemotherapeutic drugs (especially 5-fluorouracil) or decreased serum zinc or copper levels.

Dysgeusia—distorted sense of taste.

Hypogeusia—decreased taste acuity.

Often, an entire food group is eliminated from the diet when only 1 food has a distorted taste. When this occurs, serious nutrient deficiencies are likely to follow. Changes in sense of taste most frequently observed include the following: (1) sweetness is harder to taste, (2) bitter tastes become stronger, (3) salt is harder to taste, and (4) a metal taste is present in the mouth. Most high-protein foods, especially red meats, cereal products, and sweet foods, are generally less palatable. Poultry and fish are usually preferred to beef and pork. Coffee is the most commonly taste-distorted beverage.

What are the effects of dysgeusia?

NURSING APPLICATIONS

Assessment

Physical—for dysgeusia, hypogeusia, hyposmia.

Dietary—for food preferences, food groups avoided; dietary intake of zinc-containing and copper-containing foods.

Interventions

1. To achieve as much flavor as possible from foods, encourage clients to switch from 1 food to another during the meal. This minimizes sensory adaptation.

Continued

2. When tolerated, offer a variety of textures, as this may increase intake.
3. If nutrition supplements taste too sweet, add a very small amount of powdered decaffeinated coffee to counteract the sweetness.
4. If food becomes tasteless, appearance and aroma become even more important. Serve foods attractively.
5. Oral zinc sulfate has been effective in improving taste sensations, so consult the physician.
6. If clients lose their taste for coffee and tea, they may need assistance in identifying other beverages they like so their fluid intake is not decreased. Offer frozen slushes of fruits, juices, or milk.
7. Offer sugarless ginger ale, or chewing gum, or sugarless hard candies to offset cacogeusia (bad taste).
8. Offer spices and herbs to make foods more palatable.
9. If client develops an aversion to red meat, offer egg, cheese, milk-based entrees, or chilled meat salads to ensure adequate protein intake.
10. Provide unfamiliar foods or foods infrequently consumed before chemotherapy. This works as a scapegoat to reduce the likelihood of forming aversions to items in the regular diet (Andresen et al, 1990).

Evaluation

* Desired outcomes include client not eliminating any food groups but consuming all food groups, since dysgeusia, hypogeusia, and hyposmia are decreased.

Client Education

- To avoid food aversions, clients should limit intake to small amounts of 1 or 2 foods before chemotherapy.
- Eggs, cheese, and custard are good sources of protein that may have more taste appeal.
- If foods taste bitter, avoid foods cooked in metal pans. Instead, use plastic utensils and glass pots and pans.

Diarrhea, Cramps, and Other Intestinal Upsets

What type of diet might be prescribed for diarrhea?

When diarrhea is severe, food intake may have to be withheld. Beverages low in sugar are introduced first. The diarrhea may be checked by a low-residue, low-fat diet. Increased fluid intake is important. If the diarrhea is caused by resection of the ileum or if steatorrhea is present, MCT oils may be beneficial.

If diarrhea and flatulence are caused by lactose intolerance, milk and milk products have to be limited or removed completely from the diet. Lactose-free yogurt can provide calcium and protein, and replace beneficial gut bacteria that are frequently destroyed by the cancer treatment.

NURSING APPLICATIONS

Assessment

Physical—for GI disturbances.

Interventions

1. Monitor all clients for GI side effects of the medication prescribed, e.g., the frequency and characteristics of bowel movements.

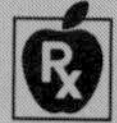

Constipation is one of the earliest signs of vincristine toxicity, so suspect toxicity if constipation develops.

Evaluation

* GI disturbances are reduced.

Client Education

- Yogurt may be well tolerated, is a source of beneficial microorganisms, and provides needed protein and calcium.
- Constipation in the cancer client may be due to medications and can be alleviated with a high-fiber diet and adequate fluids.

Dysphagia

Difficulty in swallowing may be secondary to the location of the tumor or effects of treatment. Guidelines for dealing with dysphagia problems and appropriate foods are presented in Chapters 12 and 25, respectively.

Xerostomia

Xerostomia is one of the greatest immediate complaints among clients receiving therapy. Even though water does not replace saliva, clients are encouraged to drink large amounts of fluids. Artificial salivas may be used as desired, but their effects are transitory. They buffer the acidity in the mouth and lubricate the mucous membranes.

When oral lesions are present, soft foods or foods covered with sauces, gravies, or salad dressing may be better tolerated. Cream soups and milk beverages are usually palatable.

NURSING APPLICATIONS

Assessment

Physical—for xerostomia, oral lesions, stomatitis, moistness of mucous membranes.

Interventions

1. Offer fruit nectars rather than acidic beverages when the mouth is inflamed.
2. Avoid very salty foods, hot spices, and coarse, rough foods because they are not well tolerated.
3. Encourage fluids throughout the meal to provide additional moistness (do not confuse with early satiety).
4. Use lidocaine (Xylocaine) as a mouthwash to numb the pain.

Evaluation

* Xerostomia is minimized, thereby maintaining or increasing client intake.

Client Education

- Soak foods like toast in coffee or milk.
- It may be easier to swallow liquids through a straw.
- Cold foods have a numbing effect, making them more acceptable; extremely hot foods are avoided.
- A room humidifier may be useful.
- The use of peroxide or baking soda as a mouthwash reduces pain caused by dryness and lubricates the tissues.

Depressed Immune Function

Reduced immune response makes the client more susceptible to infection. Sterile diets are unappetizing for the client. Foods that are not cooked and sanitized, such as lettuce and fresh fruits, can carry pathogens, precipitating an infection. To

Agranulocytosis—reduced leukocytes caused by depressed formation of granulocytes in bone marrow.

reduce the chances of infection, salads and fresh fruit may be eliminated, especially in clients with **agranulocytosis.** Clients who have undergone bone marrow transplants are extremely immunosuppressed. Sanitation control within the dietary department is also important.

List types of foods that should be withheld to prevent risk of infection.

NURSING APPLICATIONS

Assessment

Physical—for increased temperatures (even low grade or subnormal temperature is important).
Dietary—for use and source of uncooked fruits, vegetables, and protein foods; unpasteurized milk/milk products.
Laboratory—for WBC with differential count, blood count, other cultures.

Interventions

1. If WBC count falls below 2000/mm^3, notify the physician, use medical asepsis during client care, and monitor for life-threatening infection. Do not rely on temperature as a good indicator of severity of infection.

Evaluation

* A client free of infection is the desired result. Although excellent nursing care may not prevent a cancer client from dying, nurses can make dying as comfortable as possible for the client.

Client Education

- Wash hands before eating.
- Meats are cooked until they are well done.

HUMAN IMMUNODEFICIENCY VIRUS

Retroviruses are characterized by the presence of reverse transcriptase, which interferes with the production of DNA from RNA.

Describe why AIDS clients are prone to infection.

The human immunodeficiency virus (HIV) debilitates the body's immune system. Following the identification of HIV antibodies in the blood, a diagnosis of HIV positive is made. This **retrovirus** causes a dysfunction in the genetic core of T lymphocytes or WBCs that normally function to resist infection. Thus, the client's susceptibility to a variety of opportunistic infections (especially *Pneumocystis carinii, Cryptosporidium, Candida, Mycobacterium,* and herpes simplex) as well as certain neoplasms (Kaposi's sarcoma and non-Hodgkin's lymphoma) is increased. These infections can appear in virtually every organ system. Because of the body's inability to fight infection, acquired immunodeficiency syndrome (AIDS) develops.

Nutritional Effects of Human Immunodeficiency Virus

The course of AIDS is often complicated by profound weight loss, cachexia, multiple nutrient deficiencies, and, particularly, PEM. The cause of malnutrition is multifactorial and may involve inadequate intake, malabsorption, and/or hypermetabolism.

Anorexia

Anorexia may be attributed to respiratory and other infections, fever, dysgeusia, GI complications, cancer, adverse effects of drugs, and depression. Specific nutritional deficiencies may depress appetite and exacerbate anorectic behavior. Additionally, oral and esophageal pain during eating may decrease intake. Oral candidiasis, which produces pain and inhibits salivation, is present in 94% of people with AIDS (Barr & Torosian, 1986). Pharyngeal or esophageal lesions of Kaposi's sarcoma may cause obstruction, whereas **herpetic** or other ulcerations on the tongue and/or throat can cause difficulty in swallowing. The development of thrush may be attributed to a herpes virus, candidiasis, chemotherapy, or drugs, such as interferon.

Herpetic—related to the herpes virus.

What are some causes of anorexia in AIDS clients?

Diarrhea and Malabsorption

Over 75% of AIDS clients have chronic, long-term diarrhea (Dwyer et al, 1988). Frequently there is no diagnosable pathogen in **AIDS enteropathy.** Bowel movements clinically resemble irritable bowel syndrome. Nevertheless, a detailed workup for bacterial, viral, protozoan, and fungal causes of GI symptoms should be conducted. Nonspecific changes occur in the small bowel and colon, allowing translocation of bacteria, endotoxins, and perhaps viruses across the lumen of the gut into the lymph nodes and other organs (McQuiggan & Andrassy, 1990). Diarrhea may be affected by food intake; therefore, clients may curtail intake. Inadequate intake and decreased absorption may cause or exacerbate malnutrition (Trujillo et al, 1992). Most antidiarrheal medications are ineffective in treating AIDS enteropathy.

Chronic diarrhea and malabsorption of unknown cause in AIDS clients is called AIDS enteropathy.

Hypermetabolism

The BEE for these clients is higher than in normal healthy individuals, but this is not due to increased levels of catabolic hormones (Grunfield et al, 1992; Hommes et al, 1991). The hypermetabolic state is anticipated during active infection or when energy requirement is increased for breathing during respiratory distress.

Dementia

Approximately 60% of AIDS clients develop dementia in the later stages of AIDS (Hyman & Kaufman, 1989). Irreversible changes in mental status may be caused by *Toxoplasmosis gondii* and *Cryptococcus neoformans.* Deficiencies of trace elements have been linked to decreased cognitive functioning and peripheral neuropathies (McQuiggan & Andrassy, 1990). The client's ability to maintain adequate nutritional status is affected by conditions ranging from an inability to think clearly to severe dementia. Decreased psychomotor function increases the risk of aspiration.

What are the nutritional effects of HIV/AIDS?

Nutritional Effects of AIDS Therapies

Zidovudine (AZT or azidothymidine) initially reduces the risk for developing AIDS in HIV-infected persons who are asymptomatic or mildly symptomatic. AZT has been associated with adverse hematological findings, including reduced hemoglobin, leukopenia, neutropenia, and increased MCV. Bone marrow depression associated with AZT therapy leads to decreased vitamin B_{12} levels. The megaloblastic anemia appears to be dose related and responds only sporadically to vitamin B_{12} and/or folate supplements (McCorkindale et al, 1990; McQuiggan & Andrassy, 1990).

Another medication used to treat AIDS, dideoxycytidine (ddC), inhibits the synthesis of the viral genetic material. Its use has not been associated with megaloblastic changes.

Dideoxyinosine (ddI) also inhibits HIV replication. Similar to ddC, no megaloblastic changes are associated with its use, but the development of pancreatitis may alter food intake (nausea, vomiting) and absorption.

A variety of other drugs and therapies may be helpful in treating the various illnesses secondary to immunosuppression but do not cure the immunological problem itself. Pentamide, a medication used for *P. carinii* pneumonia, is toxic to the pancreatic beta cells. Hypoglycemia, pancreatitis, and diabetes may occur as a result of treatment with pentamidine. Pyrimethamine, used to treat toxoplasmosis, inhibits folate metabolism. Tuberculosis is treated with isoniazid (INH), which may precipitate peripheral neuropathy due to decreased absorption of pyridoxine.

NURSING APPLICATIONS

Assessment

Physical—for sore throat, diarrhea, fever, weight loss, dyspepsia.
Dietary—for anorexia, metallic taste, food preferences/diet history.
Laboratory—for RBC, Hgb, Hct, vitamin B_{12}, folate, MCV; bilirubin, glucose, amylase.

Interventions

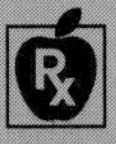
If on INH, encourage foods high in folate, niacin, vitamin B_6, and magnesium (Allen, 1991). Give vitamin B_6 tablets daily (with water).

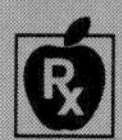
When antifolate drugs, such as pyrimethamine, are used to treat opportunistic infections, folic acid supplements may be effective during treatment (Task Force, 1989).

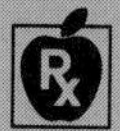
If on ddI and amylase is elevated 1½ to 2 times above normal, notify physician to discontinue the medication.

Evaluation

* Drug therapy will not adversely affect a client's intake.

Client Education

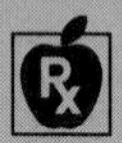
Use alcohol in moderation.

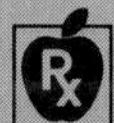
INH may produce a MAOI-like reaction if taken with certain foods. If on INH, avoid foods with histamine and tyramine, such as tuna, mackerel, sardines, aged and dry sausages and meats, imitation and hard cheeses, meat and protein extracts, Chianti and Vermouth wines, and excessive amounts of caffeine.

Nutritional Assessment

Malnutrition, a well-documented consequence of AIDS, involves weight loss, body cell mass depletion, decreased MAMC, and hypoalbuminemia. Additionally, bone marrow depression, decreased iron-binding capacity, and vitamin B_{12} and selenium deficiency are common. Body fat may be normal or elevated as a result of protein being preferentially used for energy with fat conservation (Cuff, 1990). The weight loss and malnutrition can also cause GI tract dysfunction (decreased pancreatic secretions and other enzymes), malabsorption (related to villous atrophy), and decreased absorptive surfaces. Thus, the client's nutritional status is quickly compromised. Since body reserves (fat, glycogen, and protein) are depleted, there is no energy for normal maintenance or recovery from sepsis or injury.

Currently accepted nutritional assessment parameters can be used except for TLC. TLC is not a valid assessment tool in this population because it reflects immune function, but serial measurements of TLC could be used to measure the effectiveness of nutrition support.

When diarrhea is present for long periods, assessment of protein, folic acid, and minerals may be needed. Protein, vitamins A and C, B complex, zinc, and iron deficiencies can lead to skin lesions and damage to the intestinal mucosa; additionally, pyridoxine, folic acid, and vitamin B_{12} deficiencies are associated with immunological changes. Depressed levels of vitamin B_{12} are observed early in HIV-positive clients despite adequate dietary intake (Mantero-Atienza et al, 1991). This may be reflective of impaired vitamin B_{12} absorption (Harriman et al, 1989). Frequent infections result in anemia of chronic disease despite adequate iron intake (Spence & Radcliffe, 1991).

What nutrition parameters need to be assessed and why?

Nutritional Care

Benefits

Good nutrition does not cure AIDS, but malnutrition may hasten the progression of the disease and affect outcome. At present, nutritional status is not known to affect the length of time for HIV infections to progress to AIDS.

Adequate dietary intake can help maintain strength, comfort, and level of functioning. Providing optimal nutrition has been shown to influence the functioning of lymphocytes not subject to attack by the HIV and improve resistance to opportunistic infections (Hyman & Kaufman, 1989).

A coordinated team approach is essential to provide specialized nutrition support and adequately address all the medical and psychosocial aspects affecting nutritional status. Gastroenterologists and other medical specialists, dietitians, social workers, nurses, physical therapists, and mental health professionals must all be familiar with the metabolic disturbances, GI complications, symptoms that commonly impair intake, special importance of food safety, and potential drug–nutrient interactions in the treatment of HIV.

Objectives

Nutrition intervention is important at all stages of HIV infections. During the asymptomatic period, the goal of nutrition therapy is to promote an adequate, balanced diet to minimize loss of lean body mass and prevent vitamin and mineral deficiencies. Aggressive kilocalorie replacement may help forestall the advent of diarrhea and malabsorption.

What is the goal of nutrition therapy during the asymptomatic period?

Nutritional Requirements

The appropriate diet or form of nutrition support changes throughout the course of the disease, but kilocalorie needs are very high (35 to 40 kcal/kg) indicating a high-kilocalorie, high-protein diet (Hickey, 1991). Increased nitrogen requirements during stressed states require increased amounts of high-quality protein (2 to 2.5 gm/kg) (Hickey, 1991).

The Task Force on Nutrition Support in AIDS (1989) has recommended that nutrition counseling should include the following: (1) an understanding of the value of a good diet to protect against exacerbation of nutrition complications and (2) knowledge about nutrition support options. Nutrition support can result in improved nutrition parameters (lean body mass, albumin, and iron-binding capacity) (Kotler et al, 1990).

High-fat foods are a good source of energy but may need to be restricted in the presence of malabsorption or diarrhea. Because of problems with fat malabsorption, MCT oils may be used to increase kilocalorie intake. The client may appear to be consuming adequate kilocalories but continue to lose weight because of the reduced absorptive surface of the small bowel.

When the dietary needs of any medically compromised individual cannot be met by a regular, well-balanced diet, nutrition support is appropriate (Dowling et al,

1990). Nutrition support may involve enteral or parenteral feedings or combinations thereof. Nutrition supplements with a high percentage of MCT oil such as Lipisorb (Mead Johnson) may be well tolerated. An elemental formula with less than 5% fat is indicated when ileal function is severely limited and steatorrhea is present (Task Force, 1989). The elemental formula should contain glutamine, which has been shown to be an essential substrate for the gut. Parenteral nutrition is most commonly used when (Task Force, 1989) (1) elemental formula cannot be absorbed, (2) diarrhea is caused by opportunistic infection, and (3) extensive GI lesions are present secondary to Kaposi's sarcoma.

What are recommendations for kilocalories, protein, and fat?

Some generalized guidelines are provided regarding various signs and symptoms to promote intake or lessen these effects. However, recommendations must be individualized since suggestions for one problem may be inappropriate for another (Raiten, 1991).

Anorexia, Nausea, and Vomiting

The reasons for anorexia are numerous. Early recognition of anorexia followed with nutrition intervention is essential. It is a real challenge to assist clients in promoting adequate intake to prevent weight loss.

In most cases, nausea and vomiting are temporary or intermittent, secondary to drug therapy. If the problem is persistent, organic causes need to be treated appropriately.

NURSING APPLICATIONS

Assessment

Physical—for height, preillness and current weight, MAMC, psychological state (depression, anxiety, grieving), fatigue, weakness, anorexia, nausea, vomiting.

Dietary—for kilocalorie and protein intake.

Laboratory—for protein, albumin, prealbumin, nitrogen balance; total iron-binding capacity, iron, folate, vitamin B_{12}; calcium, magnesium; liver function tests.

Interventions

1. Personal tastes are of utmost importance; individualize meal plans to stimulate intake.
2. If the client has food aversions, offer acceptable nutrient replacements.
3. Suggest small, frequent feedings, which can be less overwhelming than large meals.
4. Present foods attractively.
5. Serve meals on regular dishes. This avoids compounding the client's feelings of social isolation and provides better quality food at the appropriate temperature.
6. Encourage eating with friends or family in a pleasant environment.
7. Encourage HIV-positive clients to eat whatever they can to gain weight or prevent further losses.
8. A daily multivitamin/mineral supplement that supplies 100% of the RDA for each nutrient is advisable for clients with AIDS who have inadequate oral intake (Task Force, 1989).
9. Encourage nutrition supplements such as Lipisorb (Mead Johnson), Ensure (Ross), or Resource (Sandoz). If the supplement is used occasionally as a meal replacement, a meal is 2 to 3 cans. One can (240 ml) provides only about 250 kcal.

10. For nausea in the early morning hours, provide crackers, dry cereal, or toast. Other recommendations for nausea are provided in the cancer section.
11. If nausea is caused by medication, provide a low-fat snack or crackers/fruit before the medication.
12. Use remission periods to optimize nutrition repletion.

Evaluation

* For HIV-positive clients, weight loss will not occur. For AIDS clients, weight gain or stabilization will occur. Additionally, MAMC will remain stable or increase, and diarrhea and malabsorption will be minimal.

Client Education

- Consume favorite foods unless they precipitate diarrhea or other GI problems.
- Include high-kilocalorie, nutrient-dense snacks or nutrition supplements rather than foods that are low kilocalorie or contain minimal nutrients (salads, broth-type soups, carbonated beverages).
- Consume liquids between meals.
- Prepare meals in advance and freeze in individual servings until ready to use.
- Maintain an inventory of easy to prepare foods such as frozen dinners, eggs, and nutrition supplements.
- High-kilocalorie, high-protein milkshakes can be made in advance, frozen in individual portions, and slightly thawed in the microwave when needed.
- If tolerated, add skim milk powder or evaporated milk to dishes such as casseroles and mashed potatoes.
- Add cheese to casserole-type dishes, sandwiches, vegetables, and eggs.

Oral and Esophageal Lesions

Oral or esophageal lesions may make chewing and swallowing painful or difficult and interfere with the ability to eat. Since most of these lesions respond to therapy, only short-term modifications are needed to maintain oral food intake. If lesions are extensive or chronic, enteral or parenteral nutrition may be needed.

NURSING APPLICATIONS

Assessment

Physical—for mucosal lesions, sore gums, esophageal inflammation, dysphagia, aspiration.

Interventions

1. Offer oral care and use a topical anesthetic to improve salivation and relieve oral pain.
2. If swallowing is badly impaired and aspiration is a risk, see Chapters 12 and 25.

Evaluation

* Intake will be modified to decrease irritation of oral lesions until healing has occurred.

Client Education

- Avoid acidic beverages, i.e., citrus or pineapple, that are irritating to lesions.
- Avoid foods too cold or hot; foods at room temperature are generally more soothing.
- Consume soft, easy-to-swallow foods such as puddings, cream soups, ground meats, soft cheese, canned or cooked fruits, or bananas.

Continued

- Season foods (salt and other spices) as tolerated.
- Avoid hard dry crisp or rough textured foods such as chips, toast, English muffins. If preferred, such items can be softened in milk, gravy, sauces, coffee, or tea.
- Use a straw for drinking beverages to avoid irritating lesions or causing soreness.
- Use high-kilocalorie, nutrient-dense beverages such as nutrition supplements or milkshakes.

Dysgeusia

Changes in taste may be precipitated by medications or oral problems. Clients need encouragement to eat and advice to promote intake.

NURSING APPLICATIONS

Assessment

Physical—for altered taste sensations, especially metallic taste.

Interventions

1. Offer eggs, cottage cheese, or fish, if the taste of meats is distorted.

Evaluation

* Diet will be modified to encourage intake even though dysgeusia is present.

Client Education

- Experiment with new foods.
- Use herbs and spices to enhance flavors.
- Substitute beer and wine for some of the liquid in a recipe to improve taste.
- If mucus is a problem, use acidic foods to help break down mucus.
- Extremes in temperature and texture may be used to stimulate the appetite. (Do not confuse this with oral lesions.)

Diarrhea

Clients with GI infections and diarrhea require a higher intake of energy and nutrients. Nutrition counseling for dietary modification of such nutrients as carbohydrate, fat, and fiber may help reduce the severity of the diarrhea.

Emotional stress, some drugs, contaminated foods or formulas, and hypoalbuminemia may exacerbate diarrhea. Whatever the cause, efforts should be made to increase adequacy of intake as well as to lessen the diarrhea.

NURSING APPLICATIONS

Assessment

Physical—for emotional stress, diarrhea, type of infections present, fever, malaise, dehydration.
Dietary—for type of medications, formula used.
Laboratory—for vitamin B_{12}, albumin; stool culture.

Interventions

1. Consider using MCT oils for clients with diarrhea or malabsorption.
2. If low-volume diarrhea occurs or cryptosporidiosis or microsporidiosis are diagnosed, provide a low-fat (less than 50 gm), low-fiber, lactose-free, isotonic diet with an elemental or semi-elemental nutrition supplement. Feed-

ings provided 4 to 6 times daily are better tolerated than 3 meals (Cuff, 1990).

3. If the elemental formula does not contain glutamine and ileal functioning is severely limited or steatorrhea is present, consult the dietitian or physician to add glutamine.
4. If cytomegalovirus or *Mycobacterium avium-intracellulare* is present, use elemental feedings such as Vivonex TEN (Sandoz) or Criticare (Mead Johnson) administered via a nasogastric tube (Cuff, 1990).
5. Avoid insoluble fiber that may be irritating to the GI tract; include foods, nutrition supplements, or formulas with soluble fibers (pectins and gums) that act as a binder (Taber, 1989).
6. If bacterial overgrowth is a possible factor because of long-term antibiotic therapy, use *Lactobacillus acidophilus* cultures from fermented dairy products or pharmaceutically available cultures.

Evaluation

* Diarrhea is lessened, and intake is maintained.

Client Education

- If diarrhea is severe, replace fluids and electrolytes with water, broth, fruit juices, gelatin, commercially available electrolyte beverages, and high potassium foods such as bananas, nectars, and potatoes.
- Reduce intake of lactose-containing foods or use a lactase enzyme; try yogurt, buttermilk, and aged cheese in small amounts.
- Avoid caffeine products, e.g., coffee, tea, chocolate, and some carbonated beverages.
- Limit insoluble fiber intake such as bran, seeds, and husks of grains. Soluble fibers, as in apples, citrus fruits, legumes, oatmeal, and potatoes may be helpful. Ensure with Fiber (Ross), Sustacal with Fiber (Mead Johnson), Jevity (Ross), and Compleat Modified (Sandoz) are nutrition supplements/formulas that contain soluble fiber.
- If flatus or cramping is a problem, avoid carbonated beverages, beans, cabbage, broccoli, highly spiced foods, sorbitol-sweetened chewing gums and candy, and excessive amounts of sugar.

Depressed Immune Function

Since people with AIDS are immunocompromised, they are particularly susceptible to infection and sepsis. Food poisoning, especially salmonellosis, can lead to serious infection and death.

Exposure to food-borne pathogenic organisms can be reduced by providing a low microbial or "cooked food" or "low bacteria" diet (Moe, 1991). Foods are well cooked or excluded if they harbor gram-negative bacilli, yeasts, or molds. Diets with reduced microbial content vary widely between institutions. In addition to the uncooked fruits and vegetables commonly withheld, other items that normally contain large numbers of pathogens include fresh dairy products, spices, herbs, and nuts. The protective benefit of sterile, low microbial diets has not been well established (Moe, 1991; Aker & Cheney, 1983).

Dementia

Dementia affects nutrient intake related to behavioral changes and impaired ability to prepare foods or to self-feed. Aspiration may also be a risk factor.

NURSING APPLICATIONS

Assessment

Physical—for fever, signs and symptoms of infection.

Dietary—for use of and sources of uncooked fruits, vegetables, and protein foods, unpasteurized milk, and milk products.

Laboratory—for WBC with differential count, blood and/or other cultures.

Interventions

1. Offer a low microbial diet and avoid raw fruits and vegetables, cold cuts, and products with raw eggs because this may increase exposure to pathogenic organisms (ADA, 1989).
2. If the client has tuberculosis or hepatitis, use disposable utensils, plateware, and trays.

Evaluation

* Client does not experience food-borne illnesses.

Client Education

- Stress the importance of trace elements because many are essential for maintaining neural and immune function.
- The client should be knowledgeable about proper preparation, cleaning, and storage of food (see Chapter 18). Discuss food sanitation issues with the client to decrease the likelihood of food-borne illness.
- Herbs and spices that have not been treated with irradiation may contain harmful organisms.
- Because there are no sanitation standards for tofu, the bacterial content can be quite high. Therefore, tofu is not advocated for clients with compromised immune functions.
- Immunocompromised clients should be instructed (Griffin, 1988) (1) to cook all meats to an internal temperature of 165° F and maintain that temperature for 10 minutes; (2) never to eat raw eggs, fish, or meats such as sushi or steak tartare; (3) to avoid cross contamination of cooked foods with raw meats or vegetables; and (4) to avoid unpasteurized milk or cheese.

NURSING APPLICATIONS

Assessment

Physical—for confusion, disorientation, weakness, aspiration, ability to feed self.

Interventions

1. Refer to dietitian.
2. Pursue the cause of CNS impairments; i.e, if malnutrition is suspected, a trial period of moderate amounts of nutrients helps to determine if nutrient deficiencies are the cause.
3. If clients are unable to feed themselves, assist with the meal.
4. Demented clients who refuse to eat may require feedings via a nasogastric or preferably a PEG tube. If this appears to be needed, consult the physician to obtain an order.

Evaluation

* Dementia will not reduce dietary intake.

Client Education

- Include the family or significant others along with the client in the decision to provide nutrition support when the prognosis is poor.
- Referrals include social worker, home health, home delivery, and carry out services.

NONTRADITIONAL THERAPIES

Because of the prognosis for clients with cancer and AIDS, unproven nutrition cures for both diseases abound. It is currently estimated that over $10 billion are spent yearly on unproven remedies; approximately one-third of the money is spent for unproven cancer therapies, with a tenth of the $10 billion expenditure for AIDS (Dwyer et al, 1988). Customers are desperate and may purchase empty promises in addition to receiving conventional medical care. Those who reject good medical care will possibly be purchasing an earlier demise.

Various drugs, vitamin and herb therapy, and special diets are only a few of the many unproven therapies advocated. Some of these therapies are physiologically harmless and may offer psychological benefits (Reed et al, 1990). However, some unproven treatments may have detrimental health effects, such as vitamin and mineral toxicities or deficiencies, electrolyte imbalances, and possible exposure to contaminants. Frequently these nontraditional therapies are used without alerting the primary medical provider (Kassler et al, 1991).

Both conditions have an erratic natural course with unpredictable periods of remission. Even if no cause and effect relationship exists between a therapy and the condition, remission may occur.

Megadoses of vitamins and minerals, especially vitamins C and E and iron, selenium, and zinc, have been proposed to improve immune responses. Various diet regimens, such as Dr. Berger's Immune Power Diet and Weiner's Maximum Immune Diet, are touted to boost immune function. No scientific studies have documented these claims.

Laetrile has been proposed as a cure for cancer and AIDS with the rationale that it destroys a tumor enzyme. Laetrile, sometimes referred to as vitamin B_{17}, is extracted from the kernels of peaches, apricots, and apple seeds. Laetrile contains the chemical amygdalin, which breaks down into a toxic cyanide. There is no medical or nutritional need for vitamin B_{17}. Laetrile supporters have not been able to prove that it can control either condition; possible deficiencies of calcium, iron, riboflavin, vitamins B_{12} and D, and kilocalories and toxicities of zinc and vitamins C and A may occur (Dwyer et al, 1988).

A macrobiotic diet has been proposed to eliminate accumulated "poisons" or "impurities" in the body. This diet can only interfere with adequate nutrient intake that is critical. Eating an unbalanced diet could result in reduced protein intake and, in turn, cause rather than prevent malnutrition.

NURSING APPLICATIONS

Assessment

Physical—for malnutrition.
Dietary—for use of unconventional nutrition remedies.

Interventions

1. Empathize with these clients; avoid telling the client that nothing can be done.
2. Promote an atmosphere in which clients feel free to discuss any nonconventional therapies.

Continued

3. Include the client in therapeutic decisions; explain the risks and benefits of a therapy.
4. Discourage nontraditional dietary practices, i.e., macrobiotic and fad diets and herbal powders, in a nonjudgmental manner.

Evaluation

* Clients avoid unproven nontraditional therapies.

Client Education

- Provide correct and appropriate nutrition information.
- The client must be informed that ingesting large doses of one nutrient can affect the absorption of others and that the full effect is not known.
- Diets that do not ensure an adequate and balanced intake of nutrients may further compromise immune status.

TRANSPLANTS

Antigens are perceived as undesirable foreign substances and elicit an immune response.

Allogeneic—the use of organs from other humans having a different genetic composition.

Much progress has been made in recent years toward successfully transplanting organs to extend many clients' lives. Normally the recipient's immune system recognizes the transplanted tissue as foreign, and antibodies are produced to reject the **antigen** or foreign tissue. When surgery for any type of **allogeneic** organ transplant is performed (heart, lung, kidney, bone marrow, liver, or pancreas), the immune system is intentionally suppressed with drugs.

Before the transplant, nutritional status is evaluated based on traditional parameters. Nutrition support can help in minimizing the risk of surgery and optimizing postsurgical medical care. Enteral or parenteral feedings may be necessary to correct any nutritional deficiencies.

Gastroparesis is slight or incomplete paralysis in which the stomach is slow to empty.

Following the surgery, provision of adequate nutrients should be implemented within 48 to 72 hours. Usually 30 to 35 kcal/kg and 1.3 to 1.5 gm/kg protein are recommended to provide for the stress of surgery and wound healing. In many cases, poor appetite and **gastroparesis** often limit oral intake and can quickly contribute to deteriorating nutrition status. In the immediate postoperative period, the stress of surgery and the use of high-dose corticosteroids can result in severe protein catabolism, as evidenced by increases in protein catabolic rate and net urea generation. Oral intake usually increases gradually to meet nutritional requirements if the client is provided with supplements and counseling.

Immunosuppressive—suppressed immune system or decreased resistance to infection.

Tube feeding or TPN can be initiated postoperatively or for acute rejection and infections, which increase nutritional requirements when they occur. Medications may be **immunosuppressive;** extra precautions against food-borne illnesses must be implemented (see section on depressed immune function). As discussed in Chapter 13, casein-based enteral feedings are nucleotide free and immunosuppressive. Nucleotide-free diets used in combination with cyclosporine immunosuppression have documented desirable effects on allograft rejection and survival (Van Buren & Kahan, 1988). On this regimen, protein is provided from eggs, cheese, and milk products, with the elimination of meat, fish, and poultry and all products derived from these protein foods. Additionally, vegetables such as asparagus, spinach, mushrooms, radishes, cauliflower, celery, peas, beans, and lentils and wheat germ and bran are withheld.

Immunosuppressive and antirejection medications have side effects that can alter nutritional requirements and/or cause GI symptoms. Current immunosuppressive medications, including cyclosporine, prednisone, and azathioprine, have many nutrition-related side effects. Acute complications of azathioprine and OKT3 in-

TABLE 22-4

IMMUNOSUPPRESSIVE MEDICATION SIDE EFFECTS

Side Effect	Imuran	Prednisone	Cyclosporine	FK506*	OKT3†	RS61443*
Medication Timing	With food	With food	Mix with chocolate milk or orange juice			
Gastrointestinal						
Macrocytic anemia	X		X			
Sore mouth/throat	X					
Nausea and vomiting	X		X	X	X	X
Anorexia	X		X		X	X
Increased appetite/hunger	X	X				
Diarrhea	X				X	X
Altered tastes	X					
Gingival hypertrophy			X			
Other						
Increased protein catabolism		X				
Decreased wound healing		X				
Peptic ulcer disease (abdominal pain/gastritis)	X	X				X
Osteoporosis		X				
Metabolic						
Hypertension (sodium retention)		X	X			
Hyperkalemia			X			
Hyperlipidemia		X	X			
Hyperglycemia		X	X	X		
Hypercalciuria		X				
Hypophosphatemia		X				
Hypomagnesemia			X			

* These medications are being used experimentally in controlled trial studies at this time.
† OKT3, Orthoclone OKT3 Sterile Solution (Ortho).
Adapted from DiCecco S. Immunosuppressive medication side effects. Dietetics Department of Mayo Rochester Hospitals–Saint Marys Hospital. Rochester Methodist Hospital, Rochester MN, 1991.

clude nausea, vomiting, diarrhea, and reduced appetite. Electrolyte abnormalities such as hyperkalemia and magnesium wasting may be seen with cyclosporine therapy (Table 22-4).

Long-term nutrition support involves counseling clients regarding development of nutritional problems. These problems usually involve dietary complications resulting from the specific organ transplant and/or long-term medications prescribed. Chronic complications, including hypertension, weight control, hyperlipidemia, and osteoporosis, are often associated with long-term cyclosporine and prednisone treatment. In general, diet therapy should be individually tailored by the dietitian to meet the client's needs. Ideally, ongoing nutrition counseling is provided by a dietitian specializing in transplant nutrition.

NURSING APPLICATIONS

Assessment

Physical—for type of transplant/drugs, nausea, vomiting, diarrhea, hypertension, weight.
Dietary—for appetite, food and fluid intake, type of diet ordered.
Laboratory—for albumin, total protein, urea, CBC with differential, potassium, magnesium, hyperlipidemia.

Interventions

1. Refer to dietitian to help individualize client's therapy.

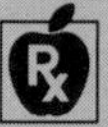 Give azathioprine with food if GI upset occurs.

Evaluation

* Diet modifications to reduce complications following transplantation are followed by the client.

Client Education

- Initially adequate intake is essential for healing, but nutritional requirements decrease following stabilization. Continued kilocalorie overconsumption results in further health problems.
- Reinforce foods allowed or to be avoided on the therapeutic diet ordered.

SUMMARY

Despite the common problems associated with cancer or AIDS, each client should be viewed as an individual with his or her own food preferences. Optimal care of both of these conditions requires a coordinated multidisciplinary team approach to address all the medical and psychosocial problems. Management of nutritional status should be an important component of the health care plan.

Adequate nutritional status is a prime goal because of its direct relationship to mortality and morbidity in cancer clients; it is related to improved survival and less relapse. Nutritional care should be optimized in the early stages of cancer, before clients become malnourished or the disease spreads. It is as significant as the treatment itself in the final balance of success. Nutrients are essential to restore immunocompetence, lessen toxicity, improve results of other therapeutic treatments, and provide optimum body weight. Recovery (if possible), reduced hospital stays, fewer infections and complications, and improved quality of life are the goals for cancer clients. Nutrition is not a cure-all for cancer, but it is a critical aspect of cancer treatment that may prolong life and improve the response to different therapies.

Several of the aforementioned goals also apply to AIDS clients: reduced hospital stays, fewer infections and complications, and improved quality of life. No one as of yet has recovered from AIDS. Proper nutrition is as important in treatment as drug therapies. Adequate nutrition support can delay the downward trend of AIDS. A broad multidisciplinary team approach is vital for individualization of nutritional care. This care should be initiated when the person is diagnosed as HIV positive. Although nutrition is not a cure-all, it is an important aspect for treating AIDS clients.

NURSING PROCESS IN ACTION

A client is admitted to the hospital with AIDS. He is having severe diarrhea and anorexia and is taking AZT. He has steadily lost weight over the last few weeks. Right now, he has no appetite, and food has no appeal, but he would rather try to eat than have a feeding tube placed.

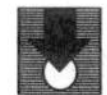

Nutritional Assessment

- Food, fluid and nutrient intake, kilocalorie and protein intake versus requirements.
- Diet history, weight, anthropometric measures.
- Ability to feed self.
- Nausea, vomiting, diarrhea, anorexia.
- Total head to toe assessment with emphasis on skin, oral mucous membranes, respiratory, abdomen, and cardiovascular systems.
- Psychological status (depression, hopelessness, anxiety, and grief).
- Types of drugs used including therapeutic, street drugs, alcohol, and tobacco.
- Laboratory studies for vitamin B_{12}, RBC, WBC with differential, Hgb, Hct, bilirubin, albumin, transferrin.

Dietary Nursing Diagnosis

Altered nutrition: Less than body requirements RT anorexia and malabsorption secondary to diarrhea.

Nutritional Goals

Client will maintain weight or gain 1 lb per week.
Client will not need a nasogastric tube for nutrition support during this hospital admission.

Nutritional Implementation 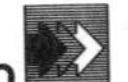

Intervention: (1) Offer small, frequent feedings. (2) Offer high-protein, high-kilocalorie meals.

Rationale: (1) These are less overwhelming than large meals. (2) Protein is needed for anabolism, and increased kilocalories are needed for hypermetabolism.

Intervention: Refer to client's dietitian and occupational therapist.

Rationale: A dietitian will supply the needed expertise in planning nutritional care, and an occupational therapist can assist client in decreasing the workload of eating.

Intervention: (1) Offer liquids between meals. (2) Offer high-protein milkshakes.

Rationale: (1) Client will not become full as quickly, so food intake may increase. (2) Milkshakes are usually well liked and provide large amounts of protein and kilocalories.

Intervention: Encourage family/friends to eat with client. If none are available, the nurse can eat with the client.

Rationale: In the US, eating is a social affair. If tradition is maintained, food intake may increase. This may also lessen the social isolation these clients experience.

Intervention: Following poor intake at a meal, give 2 to 3 cans of Ensure or Sustacal.

Rationale: To be used as a meal replacement, 2 to 3 cans is needed, not 1.

Intervention: Avoid raw fish, rare meats, and unpasteurized dairy products.

Rationale: The immune system is depressed in AIDS clients, and these foods may contain pathogenic organisms, which could increase the chance of infection.

Intervention: Praise efforts and remind him that he is meeting his goal.

Rationale: Including the client in planning will increase the likelihood of compliance.

Intervention: Offer oral hygiene before and after meals with soft toothbrush.

Rationale: Oral candidiasis, which produces pain and inhibits salivation, is present in 95% of AIDS clients.

Intervention: Give multivitamins with 100% of the RDI for each nutrient.

Rationale: This is advisable for AIDS clients who have inadequate oral intake or increased needs because of diarrhea.

Intervention: Give antidiarrheal drugs as ordered.

Rationale: These drugs help alleviate or lessen the severity of diarrhea, thereby increasing nutrient absorption.

Intervention: (1) Monitor for fever and weight changes. (2) Encourage fluid intake.

Rationale: (1) With loss of fluids from diarrhea, the body may not lose heat by evaporation, thus increasing body temperature. Weight changes tell if the goal is being met. (2) Liquids help replace fluids lost through diarrhea.

Intervention: Inform client of hospice, individual or family counselors, other local support groups, the AIDS hotline, and the availability home health agencies.

Rationale: These measures provide psychological support, a needed component of AIDS care.

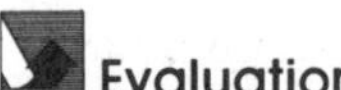

Evaluation

To determine goal achievement, the client's weight will be evaluated for increases, decreases, or maintenance (maintenance or an increase should occur).

Additionally if the client did not require a feeding tube, the goal was met.

Other considerations include the following: nutrient/kilocaloric intake is adequate, vitamin B_{12} level is stable, and diarrhea is decreased or alleviated.

STUDENT READINESS

1. How does a tumor compete with the overall nutrition of the client?
2. Differentiate between PEM and cachexia.
3. List 4 reasons why nutrition status in the cancer client is important.
4. What assessment criteria should be used to screen cancer clients?
5. Since radiation therapy affects rapidly growing cells, what normal cells are frequently affected?
6. What flavors are commonly affected by chemotherapy and radiation?
7. List ways to increase food intake in the anorectic AIDS client.
8. Why would AIDS clients feel tired? What could be done to improve these feelings?
9. What are some ways that AIDS clients can maintain optimal health?
10. How can nurses help AIDS clients feel more accepted as well as improve their general physical condition?

CASE STUDY

Elizabeth, a 35-year-old homemaker, was diagnosed with lung cancer. Height is 5′3″; weight, 130 lbs. Relatives came to be with Elizabeth and stay with her husband Michael and their 2 children, Ashley, age 13, and Jeremy, age 12.

Chemotherapy was initiated. Before Elizabeth lost her hair, her mother went to the American Cancer Society office to choose 2 free wigs.

The dietitian discussed the use of foods to provide high-kilocalorie, high-protein intake that included Elizabeth's food preferences. Each time a meal or snack would be delivered to her, the nurse explained to Elizabeth and members of her family which foods were complex carbohydrates and high-protein foods and stressed the importance of Elizabeth's eating.

1. Calculate Elizabeth's kilocaloric and protein requirements.
2. Prepare a menu with appropriate serving sizes and additional foods necessary to meet Elizabeth's nutrition needs.
3. What effect do you think that planning and shopping for foods and preparing the meals will have on each member of this family?
4. What foods might Elizabeth choose during periods of taste changes and anorexia from the chemotherapy?
5. Make a list of professionals and nonprofessionals who might help Elizabeth and her family.

REFERENCES

Aker SN, Cheney CL. The use of sterile and low microbial diets in ultraisolation environments. *JPEN* 1983 July-Aug; 7(4):390–397.

Allen AM. *Powers and Moore's Food Medication Interactions.* 7th ed. Copyright Ann Moore Allen. Pottstown, PA, 1991.

American Dietetic Association (ADA). Position of the American Dietetic Association: Nutrition intervention in the treatment of human immunodeficiency virus infection. *J Am Diet Assoc* 1989 June; 89(6):839–841.

Andresen GB, et al. The scapegoat effect on food aversions after chemotherapy. *Cancer* 1990 Oct 1; 66(7):1649–1653.

Barr CE, Torosian JP. Oral manifestations in patients with AIDS or AIDS-related complex. *Lancet* 1986 Aug 2; 2(8501):288.

Bilezikian JP. Management of acute hypercalcemia. *N Engl J Med* 1992 Apr 30; 326(18):1196–1203.

Bozzetti F. Effects of artificial nutrition on the nutritional status of cancer patient. *JPEN* 1989 July-Aug; 13(4):406–420.

Cuff PA. Acquired immunodeficiency syndrome and malnutrition: role of gastrointestinal pathology. *Nutr Clin Pract* 1990 Apr; 5(2):43–53.

Daly JM, et al. Nutritional support in the cancer patient. *JPEN* 1990 Sept-Oct; 14(5 suppl): 244S-248S.

Dowling S, et al. Nutrition in the management of HIV antibody positive patients: A longitudinal study of out-patient advice. *Eur J Clin Nutr* 1990 Nov; 44(11):823–830.

Dwyer JT, et al. Unproven nutrition therapies for AIDS: What is the evidence? *Nutr Today* 1988 March-Apr; 23(2):25–33.

Griffin P. Food counseling for patients with AIDS. *J Infect Dis* 1988 Sept; 158(3):668.

Grunfield C, et al. Resting energy expenditure, caloric intake, and short-term weight change in human immunodeficiency virus infection and the acquired immunodeficiency syndrome. *Am J Clin Nutr* 1992 Feb; 55(2):455–460.

Harriman GR, et al. Vitamin B_{12} malabsorption in patients with acquired immunodeficiency syndrome. *Arch Intern Med* 1989 Sept; 149(9):2039–2041.

Hickey MS. Nutritional support of patients with AIDS. *Surg Clin North Am* 1991 June; 71(3):645–664.

Hommes MJT, et al. Resting energy expenditure and substrate oxidation in human immunodeficiency virus (HIV)–infected asymptomatic men: HIV affects host metabolism in the early asymptomatic stage. *Am J Clin Nutr* 1991 Aug; 54(2):311–315.

Hyman C, Kaufman S. Nutritional impact of acquired immune deficiency syndrome: A unique counseling opportunity. *J Am Diet Assoc* 1989 Apr; 89(4):520–527.

Kassler WJ, et al. The use of medicinal herbs by human immunodeficiency virus-infected patients. *Arch Intern Med* 1991 Nov; 151(11): 2281–2288.

Kotler DD, et al. Enteral alimentation and repletion of body cell mass in malnourished patients with acquired immunodeficiency syndrome. *Am J Clin Nutr* 1990 Jan; 53(1):149–154.

Lipman TO. Clinical trials of nutritional support in cancer. *Hematol Oncol Clin North Am* 1991; 5(1):91–102.

Mantero-Atienza, E, et al. Vitamin B_{12} in early human immunodeficiency virus-1 infection (letter). *Arch Intern Med* 1991 May; 151(5):1019–1020.

McCorkindale C, et al. Nutritional status of HIV-infected patients during the early disease stages. *J Am Diet Assoc* 1990 Sept; 90(9):1236–1241.

McQuiggan MM, Andrassy RJ. Nutrition support of the AIDS patient. *RD* 1990; 10(3):1, 4–8.

Menashian L, et al. Improved food intake and reduced nausea and vomiting in patients given a restricted diet while receiving cisplatin chemotherapy. *J Am Diet Assoc* 1992 Jan; 92(1):58–61.

Moe G. Enteral feeding and infection in the immunocompromised patient. *Nutr Clin Pract* 1991 Apr; 6(2):55–64.

National Cancer Institute (NCI). What you need to know about cancer. Washington, D.C., USDHHS, National Institutes of Health, 1989.

Raiten, DJ. Nutrition and HIV infection: A review and evaluation of the extent of knowledge of the relationship between nutrition and HIV infection. *Nutr Clin Pract* 1991 June; 6(suppl 3):A2–A9.

Reed A, et al. Mexico. Juices, coffee, enemas, and cancer (letter). *Lancet* 1990 Sept 15; 336(8716): 677–678.

Spence R, Radcliffe J. A comparison of the iron status of HIV, ARC, and AIDS patients. Presented at the Annual American Dietetic Association Convention, Dallas, 1991.

Taber J. Nutrition in HIV infection. *Am J Nurs* 1989 Nov; 89(11):1446–1451.

Task Force on Nutrition Support in AIDS. Guidelines for nutrition support in AIDS. *Nutr Today* 1989 July-Aug; 24(4):27–32.

Trujillo EB, et al. Assessment of nutritional status, nutrient intake, and nutrition support in AIDS patients. *J Am Diet Assoc* 1992 Apr; 92(4):477–478.

Van Buren CT, Kahan BD. The renal transplant patient. *In* Kinney JM, et al, eds. *Nutrition and Metabolism in Patient Care.* Philadelphia, WB Saunders, 1988: 558–566.

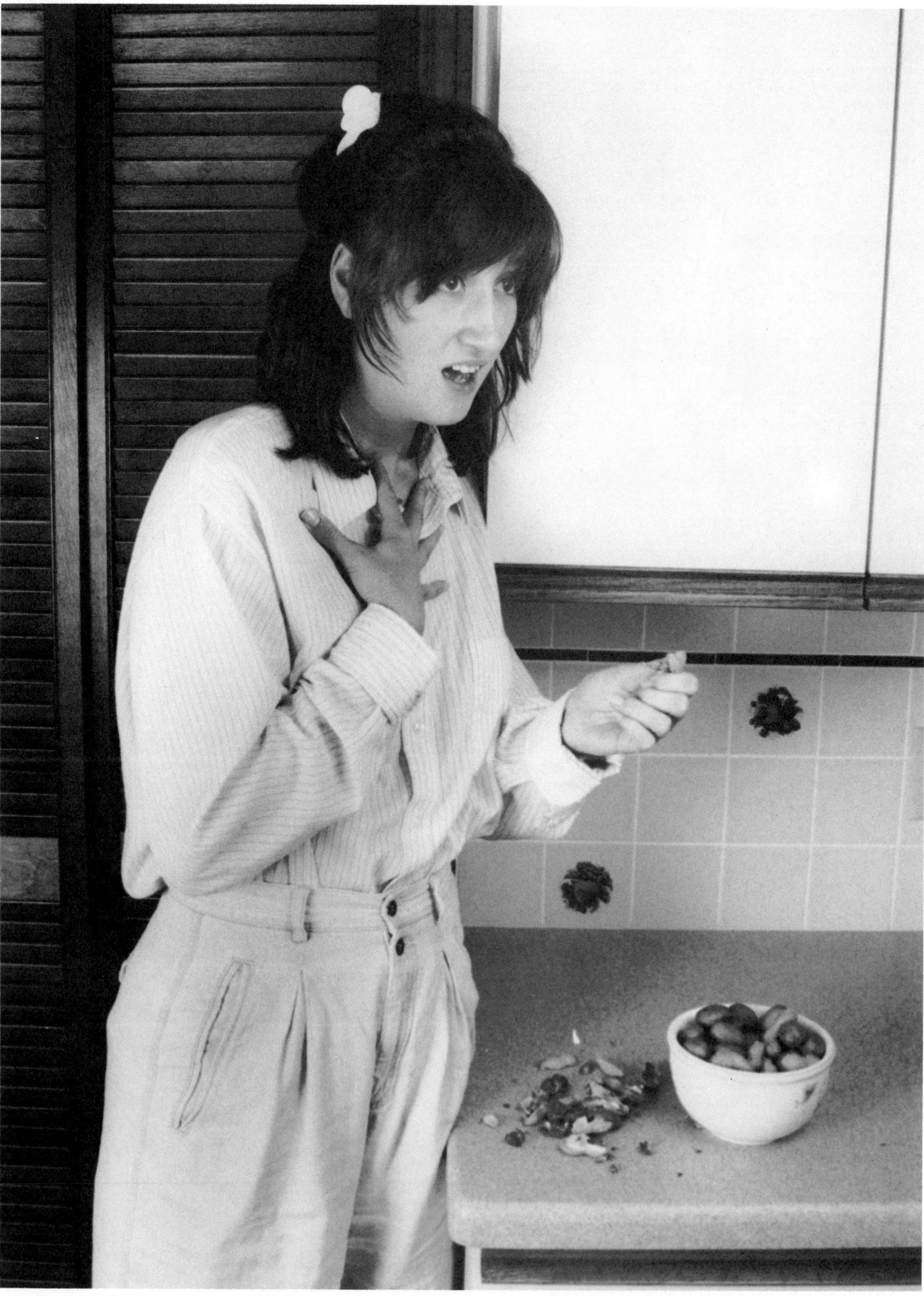

Nutrition Support for Adverse Food Reactions: Allergies and Intolerances

CHAPTER 23

OUTLINE

1. Causes and Physical Consequences
2. Nutritonal Care

Nursing Applications

VIII. PHARMACOLOGICAL FOOD INTOLERANCES
- A. Histamine
- B. Monoamines
- C. Salicylate
- D. Methylxanthines

IX. INTOLERANCE TO FOOD ADDITIVES
- A. Sulfites
- B. Monosodium Glutamate
- C. Nitrates
- D. Tartrazine (FD&C Yellow #5)

Nursing Applications

OBJECTIVES

THE STUDENT WILL BE ABLE TO:

- Define food allergy.
- Discuss the problems of identifying food allergies.
- Identify various allergic reactions.
- List foods that are most often allergenic and treatment for each allergen.
- List naturally occurring chemicals in foods and additives that may elicit an adverse food reaction.
- Apply nursing principles to food allergies/intolerances.
- Identify client teaching tips for food allergies/intolerances.

TEST YOUR NQ (True/False)

1. Over 30% of the US population suffer from food allergies.
2. Cow milk allergy is the same as lactose intolerance.
3. Corn oil can be used by clients who are allergic to corn.
4. Tofu is an alternative protein source for clients with soy allergies.
5. Yogurt may be tolerated by lactose-intolerant clients.
6. The best treatment of food allergies is to eliminate the food from the diet.
7. Blue cheese is high in histamine content.
8. Foods containing tyramine may cause migraine headaches.
9. Asthmatics may be adversely affected by nitrates.
10. Clients sensitive to aspirin are usually sensitive to tartrazine.

Adverse reaction is a general term indicating a clinically abnormal response or reaction to exposure to foods or food additives; it includes both allergic (or immunological) and nonimmunological responses to food.

Adverse reactions that involve a response of the immune system due to intake of specific foods are classified as hypersensitivity, or what is commonly known as food allergy.

As many as 8% of Americans have **adverse reactions** to particular foods (Bock, 1987). Even though 40% believe they have **food allergies,** only 1 to 2% of Americans suffer from a true food allergy (Sampson & Metcalfe, 1992), which is determined clinically by changes in the immune system. Thus, food allergy is probably overdiagnosed by laypersons and underdiagnosed by physicians. Failure to recognize and control food allergy accounts for unnecessary morbidity, invalidism, and even mortality.

The lack of standard terminology regarding "food allergies" has led to misunderstandings. Therefore, the American Academy of Allergy and Immunology Committee on Adverse Reactions to Foods adopted definitions of reactions to foods for health professionals (Anderson, 1986); diagnostic guidelines for food allergy were summarized by experts from the American College of Physicians (1989). **Food in-**

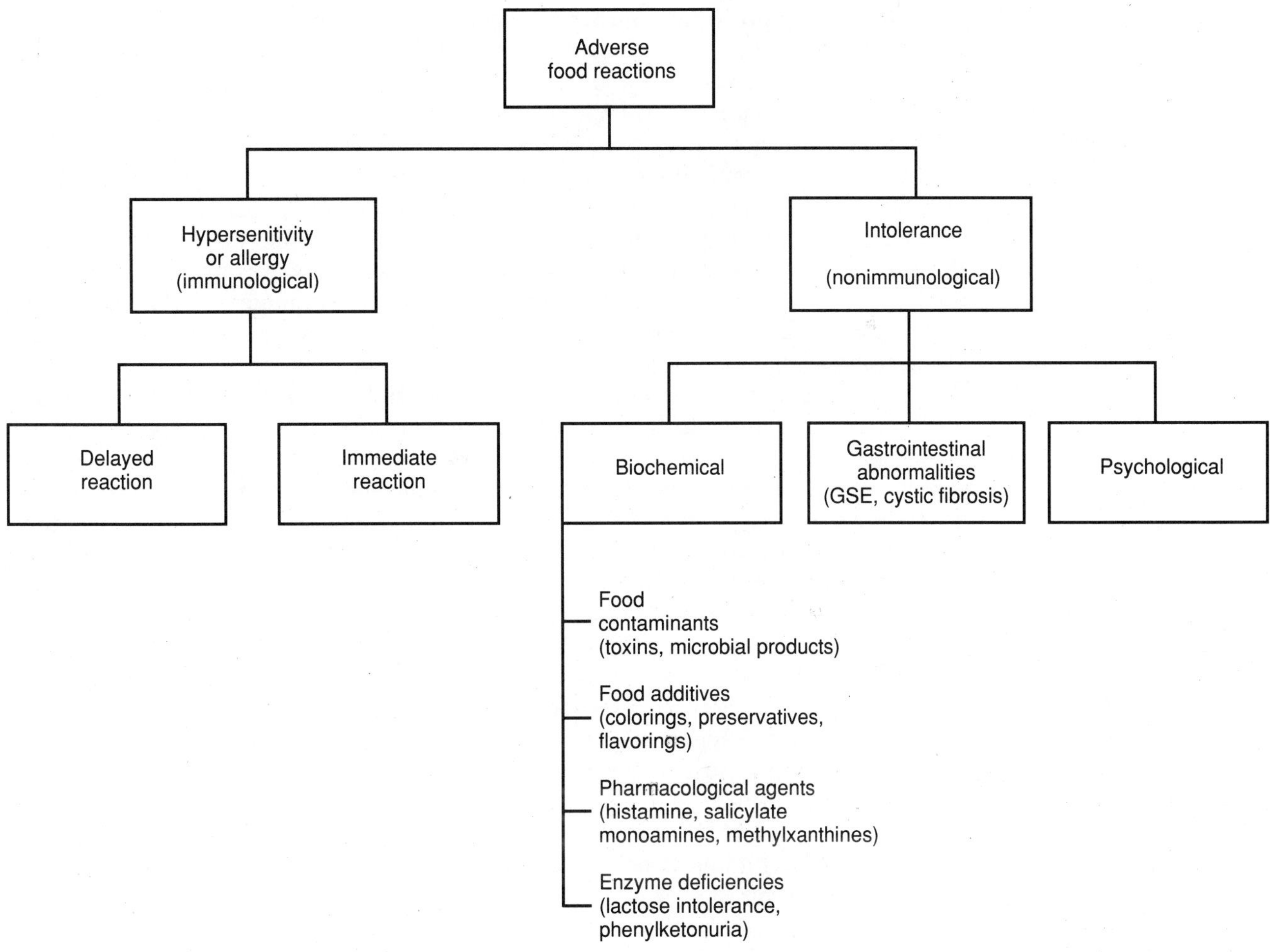

Figure 23–1 Adverse food reactions.

tolerances should not be confused with food allergies. Some examples of food intolerances include genetically determined metabolic disorders, e.g., phenylketonuria caused by an inability to metabolize phenylalanine, or lactose intolerance caused by lack of lactase enzyme (Fig. 23–1). It is important for nurses to know the correct medically accepted definitions for these terms to communicate with physicians, but when talking with clients, the term "allergy" is commonly used rather than "hypersensitivity" to prevent client confusion.

Food intolerance is a nonimmunological response to ingested food or food additives that causes an abnormal physiological response. The mechanism may be unknown or may be pharmacological, metabolic, or toxic.

An adverse food reaction may also result from **food toxicity** or **poisoning.** Toxins released from contaminated food or microorganisms or parasites in food cause food-related illnesses. Nonimmune chemical mediators are released in response to inflammation and irritation of the GI lining.

Food toxicity or poisoning is caused by the direct action of a food or food additive without immediate involvement of immune mechanisms.

Nutritional care is a primary concern in the diagnosis, treatment, and management of both immunological and nonimmunological reactions to foods. Nutritional deficiencies are unlikely to occur with avoidance of a few foods, but an allergy to staple foods such as cow milk, eggs, and wheat have far greater nutritional concerns.

Explain the difference between adverse reactions to foods, food allergy, food toxicity, and food intolerance.

CAUSES

Allergic reactions, referred to as "the great masquerader," can resemble almost any other type of physical problem or illness, e.g., ulcers, gallbladder attacks, or heart disease. Emotional factors, exercise, or stress may accentuate an allergic response by aggravating symptoms produced and by decreasing nutrient absorption.

Mechanism of the Immunological Allergic Response

Antigen—a foreign substance (usually a protein) capable of causing an immune response.

Immunoglobulins—antibodies.

Food anaphylaxis is a life-threatening allergic reaction to food or food additives that is mediated by immunological activity of IgE antibodies. Local anaphylactic reactions produce mildly irritating symptoms that can rapidly escalate into a systemic response with generalized itching, swelling, and urticaria. Urticaria (frequently referred to as hives) is a vascular reaction of the skin with slightly elevated red or pale patches (wheals). Respiration may become impaired.

An allergen is any foreign substance or antigen that induces IgE antibody production and stimulates an allergic reaction. Antigens involved in allergic reactions are called allergens.

What are some signs and symptoms of food allergies? Can food allergies be deadly? What are the most common foods that cause reactions in adults; in children?

Both nonimmunological and immunological mechanisms are present to prevent the absorption of foreign **antigens.** Approximately 98% of ingested antigens are blocked by GI barriers (Sampson & Metcalfe, 1992). Factors that increase incidence of antigen absorption include decreased stomach acidity and alcohol intake.

The immunological system, which is useful when protecting the body from disease and infection, may create an undesirable allergic reaction to natural substances that are absorbed and transported throughout the body. **Immunoglobulins** are produced by the body to combat invading antigens. Immunoglobulin A (IgA) is present in saliva and intestinal secretions; it deters antigen penetration by limiting absorption of digested antigens.

Gamma E immunoglobulin (IgE) is responsible for classic allergic reactions, causing an exaggerated antigen-antibody reaction, or allergy. Reactions occur when large molecules from food are absorbed through the GI tract and enter the blood stream. As shown in Table 23–1, food reactions may begin at the initial site exposed to an antigen (the mouth) or affect the intestine. Or these direct symptoms may be bypassed, with reactions in the skin or respiratory tract.

Responses may range from a localized reaction to a fatal systemic **anaphylactic response.** Widespread peripheral vasodilation as well as increased permeability of the capillaries and marked loss of plasma from the circulation follow. Failure to recognize the severity of anaphylactic reactions and to administer epinephrine increase the risk of a fatal outcome (Sampson et al, 1992).

Most confirmed IgE-mediated reactions are caused by a few foods: In children, milk, eggs, peanuts, soy, and wheat are the main causes; in adults, fish, shellfish (shrimp, crab, lobster), and nuts (walnuts, cashews, Brazil nuts, peanuts) are the main culprits. In controlled studies, egg, peanut, and cow milk account for 73% of food allergies in children (Bock & Atkins, 1990). Immunologically mediated food allergies usually occur almost immediately or within 2 hours after the specific food is eaten.

One of the main reasons for lack of identification of food allergies is the unlimited number of symptoms that may appear. Symptoms to a particular food **allergen** are not the same from client to client or even within the same client. An allergic client usually has a predominant condition but may experience other symptoms on different occasions.

TABLE 23–1

POSSIBLE CLINICAL MANIFESTATIONS OF FOOD ALLERGIES OR INTOLERANCES

System	Symptoms	System	Symptoms
Respiratory system	Chronic rhinitis Asthma Croup Cough Serous otitis media Bronchitis	Integumentary system	Eczema Pruritus Atopic dermatitis Rashes Urticaria
		Central nervous system	Headaches (sinus, migraine) Fatigue Drowsiness, listlessness Irritability Depression Excessive sweating
Gastrointestinal system	Swelling of lips, mouth, throat Nausea, vomiting Diarrhea Colic Protein-losing enteropathy Bloating, flatulence Constipation Gastrointestinal blood loss Malabsorption	Circulatory system	Hypotension Cardiac arrhythmias Anaphylaxis Pallor

FACTORS CONTRIBUTING TO ALLERGIC REACTIONS

Antigen Penetration

Food antigens are normally handled without unusual GI reactions. An immature GI tract is more susceptible to allergic reactions because of a lack of IgA, allowing antigen absorption. This is more likely to occur in premature infants and in infants up to 6 months of age.

GI disorders may also lead to excessive antigen uptake. In this case, GI cells are damaged and the mucus destroyed, which may cause increased permeability and permit increased antigen penetration. **Achlorhydria** inhibits normal digestion and allows larger particles to enter into the small intestine.

Achlorhydria—lack of HCl in the GI tract.

Heredity

Allergies are frequently inherited. If one parent has a food allergy, a child has a 50% chance of developing **atopic disease;** if both parents have allergies, the child has a 65% chance (Chandra, 1991). Allergies may also occur without a family history.

Atopic disease is an IgE-mediated allergic reaction with a genetic propensity.

Food Allergens

A client may be allergic to a single food or to many foods. Proteins are the most frequent penetrating antigen because of their large molecular structure. Some foods are more likely to cause specific reactions. An allergy to fish or fresh fruit results in urticaria more often than eczema, asthma, or migraine. Chocolate induces symptoms of nasal allergy or migraine headache.

Allergic Load or Tolerance Level

Several combined allergenic factors, such as stress, decreased health status, or high-pollen counts, may decrease a client's **tolerance** to a particular food. Yet at another time, without these other factors present, the same food may be acceptable. For example, avoiding milk only during ragweed season may relieve allergic symptoms. If a food is eaten often or in large quantities, the possibility of developing allergic reactions is increased.

Tolerance to a food means the amount that can be consumed without encountering an adverse reaction.

Some food families are more likely to produce allergic reactions than others. Foods within botanic families sometimes share antigenic and biological similarities. For example, a person who is allergic to peanuts may also be allergic to peas and other legumes in that family. Allergy to 1 type of fish may mean hypersensitivity to similar fish. However, allergy to shellfish generally does not imply allergy to bony fish, even though both may occur. Table 23–2 classifies different foods according to biological families.

Describe factors that contribute to allergic reactions.

TABLE 23–2

FOOD FAMILIES

Plant Kingdom	
Apple	Apple, pear, quince
Beet	Beet, spinach, chard, lamb's quarter (hay fever plants in this family are Mexican fireweed and Russian thistle)
Blueberry	Blueberry, huckleberry, cranberry
Carrot	Carrot, parsnip, celery, parsley, celeriac, anise, dill, fennel, angelica, celery seed, cumin, coriander, caraway
Cashew	Cashew, pistachio, mango
Cereal grasses	Wheat, corn, rice, oats, barley, rye, wild rice, cane sugar, millet, sorghum, bamboo sprouts (the hay fever grasses belong to this family)
Chocolate	Chocolate (cocoa) and cola
Citrus	Orange, lemon, grapefruit, lime, tangerine, kumquat, citron
Gooseberry	Currant and gooseberry
Gourd	Watermelon, cucumber, cantaloupe, pumpkin, squash, and other melons
Legume	Peanuts, peas, beans. Less important are licorice, acacia, and tragacanth
Mallow	Cottonseed and okra
Mint	Mint, peppermint, spearmint, thyme, sage, hoarhound, marjoram, basil, savory, rosemary, catnip
Mustard	Mustard, turnip, radish, horseradish, watercress, Chinese cabbage, broccoli, cauliflower, Brussels sprouts, collards, kale, kohlrabi, and rutabaga
Plum	Plum, cherry, peach, apricot, nectarine, wild cherry, almond
Potato	Potato, tomato, eggplant, peppers. This family includes all foods called "pepper" except black and white pepper, such as green pepper, chili pepper, paprika, cayene, capsicum. Belladonna, stramonium, and hyoscyamus belong to this family
Rose	Strawberry, raspberry, blackberry, dewberry, and such developed berries as loganberry, youngberry, and boysenberry
Walnut	English walnut, black walnut, pecan, hickory nut, butternut
Animal Kingdom	
Fish	All true fish, either fresh water or salt water, such as salmon, tuna, sardine, catfish, trout, crappie (fish-sensitive clients often cannot handle or otherwise come in contact with fish glue like LePage's)
Bird	All fowl and game birds: chicken, turkey, duck, goose, guinea, pigeon, quail, pheasant
Mammal	Beef, pork, lamb, rabbit, squirrel, venison. Cow milk is of the same animal origin as beef, and there is a tendency for those who are milk sensitive to be allergic to beef. Most persons allergic to cow milk cannot take the milk of other animals, such as the goat

From Van Hooser B, Crawford LV. Allergy diets for infants and children. *Compr Ther* 1989 Oct; 15(10):38–47.

DIAGNOSIS OF ADVERSE FOOD REACTIONS

When severe allergic reactions appear soon after eating, clients are able to make the obvious diagnosis and may solve their problems without medical help. Most cases of food allergies are less obvious, especially when the offending food is eaten regularly.

Suspecting that symptoms may be caused by food is a principle factor in diagnosis. If physical examinations, laboratory tests, x-ray films, and other assessments are negative and a food allergy is not considered, both the physician and the client become frustrated with finding the cause of symptoms. A medical history indicating risk factors for food allergy, such as family history of adverse food reactions and symptoms involving the GI tract, respiratory tract, and skin, requires further investigation.

Diagnostic work-up of a client with suspected adverse food reaction involves (1) confirming that the food actually causes an adverse reaction, (2) distinguishing that other causes are not the problem, and (3) determining whether or not immunological processes are involved. A detailed history and selected tests are necessary to differentiate true food allergy from a food intolerance. True food allergies have immunological processes involved.

The easiest age to evaluate food allergies is infancy. Allergic food reactions to a single food such as milk, egg, or wheat are common in the first 6 months of life. Even then, the diversity of symptoms can complicate a proper diagnosis. In infancy, food allergy is manifest in GI symptoms: colic, vomiting, diarrhea, bloody stools, nausea, malabsorption, and protein-losing enteropathy. In older infants or toddlers, dermatological problems such as eczema, urticaria, and rashes are frequently related to food allergies.

Food allergies become extremely difficult to identify in adults because so many different foods (and food additives) are consumed, which may be further complicated by OTC and prescription drugs. Allergic clients can also have clear-cut reactions to other substances, e.g., cats, dust, and mold.

How are food allergies manifested in infancy; in toddlers?

Food Diaries and Histories

One of the first steps is to correlate intake of a particular food with onset of symptoms. To do this, considerable knowledge of food content is essential. As a rule, a dietitian is the professional with the most knowledge in this field.

A diet history is an important procedure in diagnosing food allergies. This should include information regarding (1) a description of symptoms, (2) time relationship between food intake to onset of symptoms, and (3) quantity and type of food ingested (Van Hooser & Crawford, 1989). Other factors should be noted such as emotional factors, physical setting of the reaction, and exercise or temperature extremes (may aggravate symptoms) associated with the reaction.

A **food diary** can be helpful if it is used to augment a diet history, particularly when symptoms occur intermittently. By maintaining a complete list of all foods and beverages consumed, method of preparation, and resulting reactions, a food not previously suspected may be implicated. In many cases, clients are unaware of ingredients in foods, especially if the food is commercially prepared. Medications, even antihistamines, must be reported for accurate interpretations. Environmental factors, such as current pollen count, are significant to this background report. A food diary should be maintained for a long enough period to include several episodic reactions. Most clients are poorly motivated to maintain a comprehensive diary.

Food diary—a record indicating the day and time of all foods eaten and appearance of symptoms.

What information should a diet history include? Describe what is recorded in a food diary.

Food Elimination and Challenge

If a food allergy is suspected after obtaining a diet history and/or diary, elimination and rechallenge procedures are used. The "gold standard" diagnostic procedure for verifying adverse food reactions is by observing cessation of symptoms when the specific food is eliminated from the diet with return of symptoms following oral challenge. A food diary should be kept to note occurrence of symptoms.

Food Elimination

The purpose of an elimination diet is to document that removal of the suspected food results in improvement of symptoms. Suspected food(s) are eliminated for at least 2 weeks. If a client experiences relief during this period, the diagnosis is confirmed by rechallenging with the eliminated foods, adding an individual food at a time.

When milk, eggs, wheat, or other items commonly used in prepared foods are to be eliminated, clients must be counseled about prepared foods that may contain these items. Identifying specific foods in commercial products can be difficult. Not only is it imperative to read ingredient labels, but also a knowledge of other terms indicating use of the offending ingredient is necessary. (Clients may not realize that milk products include caseinate, casein, or whey and that egg products may be listed as ovomucoid or ovomucin). Ingredient labeling can be omitted if the government has established standards of product identity.

In a double-blind study, neither observer/nurse nor client knows whether a suspected or an inert substance is being given during the study.

Food elimination tests are feasible on an outpatient basis if only a few foods are suspected. These tests are simple and inexpensive. Drawbacks of food elimination tests are that the test is not **double-blind,** and subjective description of symptoms is involved. (This procedure is not recommended if a client suffers serious adverse reactions.) However, identification of food allergies is rarely this simple.

Most elimination diets require far greater restriction. When symptoms are frequent or continuous and numerous foods are suspected, a multiple-food elimination diet is recommended. During this elimination phase, diets may not be nutritionally adequate. Provision of a nutritionally balanced diet is necessary until all allergic symptoms have subsided. Nutritionally adequate hypoallergenic elemental formulas such as Vivonex (Sandoz) or Vital HN (Ross) (see Appendix A–2) can be used during this phase. Flavored formulas are necessary if consumption is to be accepted. Elemental formula with water is used for a minimum of 7 days or up to 3 weeks. When symptoms subside, foods can be reintroduced.

Describe food elimination diets.

A basic elimination diet may sometimes be used initially in the investigation (Table 23–3). Foods that are least likely to cause allergic reactions are used as the basis for this initial diet. Since milk, wheat, egg, legumes, fish, and nuts are common allergens, they are reintroduced cautiously.

Food Challenge

During the challenge phase, foods are introduced individually. If an item has been eliminated for 14 days or more, reintroduction may enhance the allergic response. For safety reasons, doses may start as low as 10 to 100 mg of the suspected food. Clients are always closely observed following testing, and those with a history of life-threatening anaphylactic reactions are never tested in this manner. Most clients with documented adverse food reactions have tested allergic to only 1 or 2 foods (Van Hooser & Crawford, 1989).

TABLE 23–3

EXTENSIVE ELIMINATION DIET: FOODS AND BEVERAGES ALLOWED

Meats and fowl	Fruit
Lamb	Cherry
Chicken	Blueberry
Turkey	Plum (prune)
Vegetables	Apple
Arrowroot	Pear
Lettuce	Banana
Asparagus	Pineapple
Artichokes	Apricot
Yams (sweet potatoes)	Grains (low allergy)
Beets	Rice
Spinach	Tapioca
Celery	Beverages
Carrots	Water
Squash	Ginger ale
Eggplant	Carbonated water
Miscellaneous	
Olive oil	
White vinegar	
Vanilla extract	

* From Van Hooser B, Crawford LV. Allergy diets for infants and children. *Compr Ther* 1989 Oct; 15(10):38–47.

Open food challenges are frequently used. Standard-sized portions of suspected foods are given, and symptoms are monitored. If symptoms appear, the food should be eliminated for 1 to 2 months and then reintroduced to confirm a reaction.

In open food challenges, a client is aware of the food being tested.

Time is allowed between challenges for symptoms to develop and disappear before trying another food (about 3 to 5 days). Foods less likely to elicit an allergic

TABLE 23–4

DIAGNOSTIC DIETARY MANAGEMENT FOR THE CLIENT WITH SUSPECTED FOOD ALLERGY

Description	Advantages	Disadvantages	Usual Use
I. Diet Diary			
Client or parent of client keeps running account of all foods eaten by client over a given period. Client or parent of client describes results and physician interprets them	Simple Cheap Can be done at home under "natural" conditions	"Fishing in the dark" Not safe if adverse reaction is serious Subjective description of signs of reaction by client or parent Subjective interpretation of results by physician	When an intermittent problem involving an unknown foodstuff is suspected
II. Random Single Food Elimination and Probability Single or Multiple Food Elimination			
On the basis of allergy history, a single food or multiple foods are eliminated from diet, generally for 3 days to 3 weeks. The food is then usually restored to diet. The process of single food elimination and rechallenge is repeated 2 or 3 times to confirm relationship between symptoms and food ingestion. Single or multiple foods may be tried in this fashion on a rotating schedule	Simple Cheap Can be done at home under "natural" conditions	"Fishing in the dark" Not safe if the adverse reaction to food is serious Trial is open, and attention is brought to the client and the problem Subjective description of signs and symptoms by client or parent of client Subjective interpretation of results by physician	
III. Elimination Diet			
Client is placed on a standard "Rowe" type of diet for 2 or more weeks at home; then foods, usually in large amounts, are added at 3- to 7-day intervals. Client or parent of client describes results and physician interprets them	Simple Cheap Can be done at home under "natural" conditions Late reactions to foods can be screened by altering intervals between individual food challenges Multiple foods and food combinations can be screened	Study is not blind nor does it involve placebo Not safe if adverse reaction is serious Subjective description of signs of reaction by client or parent of client Subjective interpretation of results by physician	When chronic, continuous, or frequent recurrent signs and symptoms are suspected of being related to an unknown foodstuff

Table continued on following page

TABLE 23–4

DIAGNOSTIC DIETARY MANAGEMENT FOR THE CLIENT WITH SUSPECTED FOOD ALLERGY *Continued*

Description	Advantages	Disadvantages	Usual Use
IV. Individual Blind Food Challenges in the Hospital			
Client is usually placed under controlled conditions for a short period of time. Results of blind challenge are compared with placebo challenge. Results of study are observed by physician	Blind placebo test Objective description of results by physician Objective interpretation of results by physician Other natural environmental factors partially controlled Safe; early treatment of adverse reaction to foods possible while client is under direct observation Client or family of client more easily convinced to eliminate suspicious food from regular diet	Complicated Expensive Challenge not done under "natural" conditions "Late" food reactions difficult to uncover because of length of time client must be under controlled conditions May involve informed consent Positive reaction does not classify cause of reaction Negative reaction does not imply that client never had or never will have an adverse reaction to specific food used as challenge	Only in clinical studies
V. Blind Food Challenge Following Fast or Synthetic Diet in Environmental Control Unit			
As in III, results are compared with placebo and objectively interpreted by physician	As in IV except that all natural environmental factors are controlled as much as possible Late food reactions and combinations can be studied because client is usually confined for longer period of time	As in IV	In chronic disease studies

From American Academy of Allergy and Immunology. *Adverse Reactions to Foods.* NIH Publication No. 84-2442, July 1984.

response are introduced first to minimize the testing period and liberalize the diet more quickly. Table 23–4 summarizes diagnostic management of food allergies along with advantages and disadvantages of each method.

In a single-blind food challenge, a client does not know the food being given, but the observer/nurse does.

Describe different types of food challenges.

Ideally a food challenge is performed in a manner that eliminates biases of the client and observer. A double-blind, placebo-controlled food challenge is best (Bock et al, 1988); however, a **single-blind food procedure** is informative and used more frequently. Disguising foods for blind testing is challenging and often impossible. Capsules may contain small amounts of the dehydrated food. Some foods can be incorporated into special recipes to mask their identity. If no symptoms appear, the dose is increased 2 to 10 times.

Cytotoxic testing—WBC, plasma, and water are placed on a slide coated with food extracts. If cells collapse, disintegrate, or change shape, an allergy exists. Provocative and neutralization testing—

Laboratory Testing

To distinguish between food allergies and intolerances, laboratory testing is performed. Elevated serum IgE levels and eosinophil counts (> 400/mm^3) are predictors of allergies. Currently available laboratory tests can greatly enhance diagnosis of allergy, but there is also a potential for misuse (Council on Scientific Affairs, 1987). Laboratory tests most commonly used with the highest degree of reliability for food allergy are skin testing and the radioallergosorbent tests (RAST). Other available tests are advocated by some devious clinicians but have not proved reliable in scientific studies (Hunter, 1991; Van Arsdel & Larson, 1988; Van Metre, 1987): **cytotoxic** or **leukocytoxic testing, provocative and neutralization testing, sublingual** or intradermal testing. Intradermal skin testing to foods is generally avoided because of a higher incidence of false-positive results and greater danger of systemic reactions (Jewett et al, 1990).

food extract is injected under the skin in amounts sufficient to elicit symptoms. A weaker or stronger injection follows to neutralize symptoms. Sublingual testing—food extract drops are placed under the tongue; documented symptoms are monitored to determine allergy.

Skin Tests

One of the more common tests for diagnosing allergies is the direct **skin test.** For a number of substances, e.g., dust, mold, and pollen, skin tests can clearly identify potential offenders, but skin testing is not as reliable for foods. A test is positive if a clinical IgE-mediated allergy exists. These tests are usually positive with immediate allergic reactions, but they may be negative with delayed-onset reactions. (Currently there is no reliable laboratory test to diagnose slow-onset food allergies). Different foods vary in their predictability. Skin test reactions to nuts, egg, milk, wheat, soy, shellfish, and fish are fairly reliable for predicting food allergy (Sampson et al, 1987). A negative skin test highly correlates with absence of allergy to foods tested.

Skin test—injection of a dilute suspension of food extract or antigen into the dermis of the skin via a scratch or prick. A wheal and flare response of 3 mm or more is considered positive for the presence of IgE antibodies/allergic reactions.

False-positive results prevent accurate diagnosis unless combined with other data. Changes in food substances that occur in cooking or the GI tract may be the reason for false-positive test results. To confirm a positive skin test, these foods are eliminated for 2 to 3 weeks. Symptomatic improvement confirms the skin test, and elimination of the food should be continued.

Which foods are fairly reliable in skin tests for allergies? What findings indicate a positive response for IgE?

Radioallergosorbent Test

The **radioallergosorbent test** detects specific antibodies against foods and indicates the presence of IgE-mediated food allergy. The RAST by itself cannot be regarded as reliable for detecting food allergies. Although no more sensitive than the skin test, it is more expensive and causes a delay in obtaining results. However, it is used for clients with extensive skin disease, which precludes appropriate skin testing, or a history of anaphylaxis or severe systemic reactions. The major advantage of this test is the lack of risk to clients.

The RAST is an in vitro test to measure levels of IgE antibodies or other immunoglobulin classes of specific antigens in the serum.

What are advantages and disadvantages of RAST?

TREATMENT

Because allergic reactions can be as varied as their sources, this mysterious puzzle requires the whole medical team, including the physician, nurse, dietitian, client, and family. Death is a very real possibility that may result directly from anaphylactic reactions or as a complication that occurs secondary to more "simple" reactions. Convulsive coughing and sneezing from allergies may cause hiatal hernias, improper food intake, malnutrition with its many ramifications, or death from choking.

Who is included in the team for treatment of allergies? What are possible complications of food allergies?

Desensitization

Subcutaneous injections of allergens are effective in desensitizing individuals for most environmental allergens. However, this technique is not useful for food allergies.

Food Avoidance

The only proven effective therapy for allergic reactions is avoidance of the offending food(s). Eliminating the allergen is the ideal way to avoid symptoms, but this is more difficult than it might seem. Food elimination is discussed in the section on nutritional care. Despite difficulties with eliminating certain foods, part of the total treatment program probably will attempt to eliminate some foods. Even minute amounts of the allergen can cause severe reactions in highly allergic clients. Rotation diets, discussed in the section on nutritional care, may offer enough relief for a client to manage a seminormal lifestyle, even though the allergy is still present.

What is the only proven effective therapy for food allergies?

Pharmacological Treatment

Antihistamines are probably the most common chemical treatment of allergic food reactions. They are most effective if taken 20 to 60 minutes before exposure to the offending food.

Cromolyn sodium (disodium cromoglycate) is a prophylactic drug used 30 to 60 minutes before food intake. Theoretically it is therapeutically effective because it reduces cellular reaction to antigen. It appears to work best when clients restrict or exclude their most highly allergenic foods (Perkin, 1990). Some studies have not found cromolyn sodium consistently effective in treatment of food allergies.

For a severe food reaction, the attending physician or allergist would meet the client at the hospital emergency room. Epinephrine is given for anaphylactic allergic reactions.

What 2 medications may be given to prevent allergic food reactions?

NUTRITIONAL CARE

Nutrient Requirements

Goals for treatment of clients with food allergies are to promote normal growth and development in infants and children or maintain body weight for adults, prevent nutrient deficiencies, and avoid allergic reactions by eliminating offending foods.

Extreme caution with close supervision must be practiced in treating infants because limited diets may be dangerously inadequate. Children with severe allergic and inflammatory reactions appear to have an increased need for nutrients. Restricted diets place strains on food intake, but even when intakes are satisfactory, some children have shown subnormal linear growth and subnormal levels of iron, prealbumin, and albumin. Losses of protein may occur with widespread eczema or a GI allergy.

The importance of replacing eliminated foods with those of similar nutrient value is critical. For example, a child who must avoid milk needs a food replacement for nutrients normally provided by milk, especially calcium, riboflavin, and protein.

What are goals of allergy treatment?

Elimination Diets

Eliminating the offending food is laborious because of difficulties in accurate identification, multiplicity of food allergens, and addition of the food into many varied products (masked identity). Counseling by a dietitian is necessary to enable clients/families to read labels and avoid inadvertently eating foods with the offending substance in a concealed form, as discussed in the following sections regarding specific food allergies. Labels must be continuously checked because food manufacturers may change ingredients without warning. Companies can be contacted for specific ingredient information and publications that provide lists of food ingredients.

After a period of elimination, a client may regain a tolerance for the food. Children especially are likely to outgrow their allergies. Most foods should be rechallenged every 1 to 2 years. Allergies to nuts and seafood appear to be longer lasting; they should be rechallenged every 3 to 6 years to determine whether allergy still persists (Sampson, 1989).

What is the normal time for foods to be rechallenged? For nuts and seafood?

Milk Allergy

The most frequently encountered food allergy is cow milk. Up to 7% of all infants and children with food allergies have adverse reactions from cow milk (van Bavel, 1988). Cow milk allergy is due to milk proteins and should not be confused with lactose intolerance, which is an adverse reaction to the sugar present in milk. Eliminating all milk products may cause dietary deficiencies of calcium, protein, vitamins A and D, and riboflavin. Calcium supplements may be warranted. Table 23–5 lists terms that indicate the presence of milk proteins and major food categories to be avoided by milk-hypersensitive clients.

TABLE 23–5

GUIDELINES FOR CLIENTS ALLERGIC TO COW MILK PROTEIN

Caution: Food Labels

Artificial butter flavor	Ghee	Rennet casein
Butter/butter solids	Half & Half	Sodium caseinate
Butter fat	Ice cream	Sour cream
Buttermilk	Lactalbumin	Sour milk solids
Casein	Lactoglobulin	Whey–demineralized whey, delactosed whey
Caseinate (magnesium, potassium, or calcium)	Lactose	Whey protein concentrate
Cheese	Milk chocolate	Yogurt
Chocolate	Milk derivative	
Cream	Milk protein	
Curd	Milk solids/dry milk solids (DMS)	
	Nonfat dry milk	

Possible Sources of Milk Protein

Caramel color
Caramel flavoring
High protein flour
Natural flavoring

Tips by Major Food Categories

Beverages	Chocolate milk; buttermilk; hot chocolate; cocoa; malted milk; milkshake; sweetened condensed milk; Ovaltine; eggnog; chocolate-flavored drink; diet drinks; such as Slender, Sego, Slim Fast; most infant formulas; General Foods International Coffees
Cereals/cereal products	Rolls, bread, pancakes, waffles, zwieback
Meats/eggs	Meats prepared with butter or milk, luncheon meats containing milk proteins, eggs or egg substitutes prepared with milk components, meat substitutes prepared with milk or milk protein components
Soups and sauces	Sauces made with milk/butter or other milk protein, white sauce, Florentine sauce, Mornay sauce, sauce mixes
Desserts	Puddings, custards, many cakes, cream pies, doughnuts, cream-filled pies
Candy	Milk chocolate, caramels, creams
Miscellaneous	Coffee-mate, Cereal Blend, Cremora, Coffee-rich, Cool Whip; all margarines and butter except margarine made with soybean; Simplesse (fat substitute); Bisquick

Imitation cheeses and soybean curd (tofu) are alternatives to milk-containing products. If not indicated on the label, cocoa products do not contain milk solids. Kosher foods that are labeled "parve" are milk-free, but clients should double check by reading the ingredient label. Milk protein added to bologna, hot dogs, tuna fish, and nondairy frozen desserts may be included as "flavoring" on the ingredient label (Gern et al, 1991). Milk-free margarines are available. Apple juice or other fruit juices, water, soy milk, and broths can be substituted for milk in recipes. Most nondairy creamers may be used but are not nutritionally equivalent to cow milk; they do not contain high-quality protein or calcium and are lower in vitamins and minerals than milk.

Infants who are sensitive to cow milk are changed to a hydrolysate formula (Nutramigen and Pregestimil [Mead Johnson]; Alimentum [Ross]) or a soy preparation (Isomil [Ross], Mull-Soy, Neo-Mull-Soy [Syntex], Nursoy [Wyeth], Prosobee [Mead Johnson]). Approximately 45% of infants placed on soy milk eventually become allergic to it too (Chandra, 1988). Meat-based formulas are also available. Spontaneous remission of cow milk allergy is frequently observed within the first 2 years of life. This may be attributed to maturity of the immune system or the GI tract. Tolerance to milk products may be reevaluated every 6 months.

What is the allergen in cow milk? What can be substituted for milk in adults/infants?

Wheat Allergy

Americans usually eat some form of wheat at every meal; therefore, this allergen is a particular challenge to live with. Wheat contains protein (gluten) and

TABLE 23–6

GUIDELINES FOR CLIENTS ALLERGIC TO WHEAT

Caution: Food Labels	
Bran	Gluten
Cereal extract	Graham flour
Cracked wheat	Malt
Durum flour	Semolina
Farina	Wheat germ
Flour—all-purpose, enriched self-rising, pastry, cake, high protein, high gluten, whole wheat	Wheat starch
Possible Sources of Wheat Protein	
Gelatinized starch	
Modified food starch	
Starch	
Vegetable gum	
Vegetable starch	
Tips by Major Food Categories	
Beverages	Malted milk, beer, gin, ale, Ovaltine, Postum, some whiskeys
Cereals/cereal products	Cream of Wheat, Shredded Wheat, Wheaties, Puffed Wheat, Grapenuts, Pablum, wheat Bran, multigrained cereals; other cereals with whole wheat or wheat starch, noodles, macaroni, spaghetti, ravioli, pastas; pancakes, waffles, bread crumbs
Meat/eggs	Meat loaf, hamburger, sausage, hot dogs and luncheon meats with wheat filler, chili, breaded meats, meat casseroles
Soups and sauces	Sauces, soups thickened with flour or containing noodles, chowder, gravy, soy sauce
Desserts	Cookies, ice cream cones, pies
Candy	None
Miscellaneous	Batters, baking mixes, salad dressings

TABLE 23–7

SUBSTITUTIONS FOR WHEAT FLOUR

Special cookbooks may be helpful. Many other recipes can be modified by the following substitutions
1 cup of wheat flour may be replaced by:
- 1 cup of wheat starch
- 1 cup of corn flour
- 1 scant cup of fine cornmeal
- ¾ cup of coarse cornmeal
- ⅝ cup (10 tbsp) of potato flour
- ⅞ cup (14 tbsp) of rice flour
- 1 cup of soy flour plus ¼ cup of potato flour
- ½ cup of soy flour plus ½ cup of potato flour

1 tablespooon of wheat flour may be replaced by (for thickening):
- ½ tbsp of cornstarch, potato flour, rice starch, or arrowroot starch
- 2 tbsp of quick-cooking tapioca

starch. Meats, fruits, vegetables, and milk products in their natural state present no problem, but when they are processed, wheat is frequently used to thicken (such as in gravy) or to coat a product (as in fish sticks). Items to be avoided are noted in Table 23–6. Rice, barley, potato, oat, or soy flour can replace wheat flour in recipes. Substitutions for wheat flour are shown in Table 23–7.

What can replace wheat in recipes? What items should be avoided in wheat allergy?

Beef and Pork Allergy

Gelatin products made from cattle or swine may cause an allergic reaction in these clients. Agar, made from seaweed, is available in pharmacies and may be substituted in preparation of salads or molded desserts.

What can be substituted in salads and molded desserts?

Corn Allergy

Corn products are used by the food industry to prepare more foods than any other edible material, making avoidance of corn almost as difficult as avoiding wheat. It is in almost every processed food on the market, from baking powders to sweeteners to luncheon meats and alcoholic beverages and medications. Fortunately few clients are allergic to corn.

Some products, such as corn oil, corn syrup, and high fructose corn syrup, contain minute quantities or no corn protein; they are usually well tolerated. Corn-free baking powder is available as well as other sugars such as honey, cane sugar, and maple syrup. Home cooking is imperative using known ingredients and reading labels closely. Guidelines are presented in Table 23–8.

What are some foods to avoid/encourage in clients with corn allergy?

Soy Allergy

Soy is a versatile legume that can be adapted for many uses. Soybean product usage has been increasing in products such as flour, oil, milk, and nuts; incidence of allergy to soy has also increased. Clients should read labels on products to avoid those containing soybeans, soy, or lecithin. Tofu, miso, and tempeh are soy products. Terms such as emulsifier, flavoring, stabilizer, lecithin, shortening, vegetable gum, vegetable oil, and textured vegetable protein (TVP) refer to nonspecific items that may contain soy. Packaged meats and fast foods often contain soy extenders or expanders that should be avoided. Cheese and meat substitutes, such as bacon bits, may be a source of soy. Soybean oil may not be a problem for soy-allergic clients (Bush et al, 1985).

What are some sources of soy?

TABLE 23–8

GUIDELINES FOR CLIENTS ALLERGIC TO CORN

Caution: Food Labels

Baking powder (with corn starch)	Dextrin	Maltodextrins
Corn alcohol	Dextrose	Modified food starch
Corn chips	Fructose	Popcorn
Corn flour	Grits	Sorbitol
Cornmeal	High-fructose corn syrup	Vinegar
Cornstarch	Hominy	
Corn sugar	Lactic acid	
Corn syrup	Maize	

Possible Sources of Corn Proteins

Food starch
Vegetable gum
Vegetable starch

Tips by Major Food Categories

Beverages	Beer, bourbon, vodka, and gin
Cereals/cereal products	Cornflakes, multigrained cereals; tortillas, tamales, cornbread
Meats/eggs	Luncheon meats and hot dogs (may contain corn syrup or dextrose)
Soups and sauces	Gravies and sauces thickened with cornstarch
Desserts	Puddings and pie fillings thickened with cornstarch, packaged pudding mixes
Candy	Some hard candy made with ingredients listed above
Miscellaneous	Canned fruits packed in heavy syrup (corn syrup); products such as English muffins are cooked in containers that are dusted with cornmeal that adheres to the baked product

Nut Allergy

Peanuts are frequently classified with legumes because they are a member of the legume family. Many persons allergic to soy may also have adverse reactions to peanuts. Peanuts contain many allergenic fractions. Pure peanut oil is nonallergenic and may be tolerated by these clients.

Other tree nuts may cause allergic reactions, including macadamia, cashews, hazelnuts (filberts), walnuts, pecans, almonds, and pistachios. These products may be contained in bread, cereals, ice cream, candy, many baked goods, salads, soups, egg rolls, and vegetarian dishes.

Egg Allergy

Egg allergy is more prevalent in infants and children than adults. Either egg whites or yolks may cause an allergic reaction, but more reactions appear to be due to egg whites. IV lipid emulsions used in TPN therapy contain egg phospholipid to emulsify fat and therefore are contraindicated in severe egg allergies.

Commercially baked products may not actually contain eggs but have been glazed with egg white. Egg whites may be used to clarify coffee or bouillon. Label ingredients that should be avoided for an egg allergy are listed in Table 23–9.

Commercial egg substitutes are available, but many low-cholesterol egg substitute products use egg white. Mayonnaise-substitute products may be acceptable, but again the label must be checked. Simplesse, a fat substitute, contains egg protein and should be avoided. Numerous vaccinations are grown on egg mediums and may be contraindicated.

TABLE 23–9

GUIDELINES FOR CLIENTS ALLERGIC TO EGGS

Caution: Food Labels

Albumin	Livetin	Ovomucoid
Dried egg yolk	Ovalbumin	Ovovitellin
Egg white	Ovoglobulin egg albumin	Simplesse®
Globulin	Ovomucin	Vitellin

Tips by Major Food Categories

Beverages	Root beer, eggnog, cocomalt, malted beverages, wine, coffee (if clarified with egg)
Cereals/cereal products	Egg noodles, some pastas (vermicelli, macaroni, spaghetti)
Meat/eggs	Breaded meats, fish and poultry; meatballs, meatloaf, croquettes, some sausages
Soups and sauces	Hollandaise sauce, tartar sauce, broth or consume clarified with egg
Desserts	Custards, puddings, meringues, ice cream, sherbet, cakes, cookies, cream-filled pies, batter, doughnuts, dessert powders, baking mixes
Candy	Fondants, marshmallows, filled candy bars, chocolate creamy nougats, divinity, fudge, cake icings
Miscellaneous	Pancake mix, mayonnaise, cooked salad dressing, fritter batter

In yeast breads and some baked goods, 1/2 tsp baking powder can be used for each egg omitted. Water or vinegar can be substituted for eggs in some recipes. Xanthan gum, baking powder, oil, cornstarch, flour, or unflavored gelatin can be used in some products with acceptable results.

Which causes more reactions—the egg white or yolk? What foods should these clients avoid?

Fish Allergy

Individuals allergic to one kind of shellfish may be hypersensitive to other members of the crustacea family (shrimp, lobster, prawn, crab, and crawfish) and the mollusk family (clams, oysters, scallops, mussels, and geoducks). However, clients allergic to shellfish are usually not hypersensitive to other forms of fish.

Rotation Diets

Rotary diversified diets are most useful for clients with numerous food allergies to reduce food allergy loads; however, their effectiveness has been controversial. A diet that rotates various food families over a period of 4 to 5 days allows potentially allergenic foods to be acceptable for some clients (Table 23–10). A 4-day rotation is used since 2 to 4 days is the approximate GI transit time. In clients who have mild to moderate allergy to several foods that cannot be completely avoided, rotation diets may be both effective and more convenient than strict elimination of these foods. The food allergy does not disappear, but the total allergenic load may be better tolerated because the immune system is not continually challenged with offending foods. Many clients have so many allergens that this is the only feasible way to handle their diets. It is a complex diet to follow.

Describe the rotation diet. What is the difference between a rotation diet and food elimination diet?

TABLE 23–10 **ROTATION DIET**

Day	Meat Related Products	Vegetables	Fruits	Beverages	Grain, Flour	Nuts	Oils, Fats	Sweetener
1	Beef Lamb Cheese	Parsley family: carrot, celery, parsnip, parsley Fungi: mushroom, yeast Spinach	Rose family: strawberry, raspberry Apple family: apple, pear, quince Mango	Milk Tea Apple juice	Oats	Brazil Cashew	Beef drippings Butter	Beet sugar (silver spoon)
2	Fish Shellfish	Sunflower family: lettuce, chicory, endive, artichokes Potato family: tomato, potato, aubergine, peppers	Citrus family: orange, lemon, grapefruit, kumquat, tangerine, lime	Orange juice Grapefruit juice Camomile tea	Buckwheat Sunflower seeds Ryvita (original) Tapioca	Filber Hazel	Olive Sunflower oil Safflower oil	100% Maple syrup 100% Maple sugar
3	Poultry Eggs	Mustard family: cabbage, broccoli, cauliflower, kale, turnip, kohlrabi, Brussels sprouts, Chinese cabbage, radish, watercress Gourd family: marrow, pumpkin, cucumber, fresh courgette, fresh gherkin	Banana Plantain Melon Pineapple Gooseberry family: gooseberry; red, black, and white currants	Pineapple juice Mint tea	Wheat Corn (maize) Rice (rice cakes) (with salt or bran only) Sago	Walnut Hickory Pecan	Corn oil	Cane sugar Molasses
4	Pork	Legume family: pea, beans, lentil, soya, chickpea Sweet potato Lily family: onion, garlic, chive, leek, asparagus	Grape family: grape, raisin, currants, sultanas Plum family: cherry, peach, apricot, plum, prune, sloe Palm family: coconut, date	Grape juice Rosehip tea White wine Soya milk (sugar-free)	Lentil Chickpea Soya Cream of tartar Carob	Peanut Almond	Peanut oil Soya oil Pork lard	

From Scadding GK, Brostoff J. The dietetic treatment of food allergy. *In* Reinhardt D, Schmidt E, eds. *Food Allergy.* New York, Raven Press, 1988.

NURSING APPLICATIONS

Assessment

Physical—for height, weight, IBW, growth pattern, recent weight changes; chronic complaints (GI distress, rashes, diarrhea, rhinitis, asthma).

Dietary—for intake of offending foods, adequacy of diet, diet history, food diaries.

Laboratory—for Hgb, Hct, albumin, histamine levels, IgE levels, skin tests, RAST results.

Interventions

1. Exclude or avoid offending allergens: read labels on foods provided to the client; check all menus served; monitor methods of food preparation.

2. Monitor onset of any reaction.
3. Ensure adequate nutritional content of a diet. If questionable, consult the physician or dietitian regarding use of elemental formulas or vitamin supplementation.
4. Assist client in maintaining an accurate food diary to determine food reactions.

Evaluation

* Desired outcomes include client verbalizing different names for the offending allergen, not experiencing adverse food reactions, avoiding the food allergen, and developing no nutritional deficiencies.

Client Education

* Inform client of Food Allergy Center, and the Food Allergy Network, which provide allergy information (does not diagnose allergies).
* Elimination diets should be used only for short periods (not more than 14 days) with careful substitution of foods with similar nutrient value.
* A warning tag or bracelet, such as Medic Alert, is advocated for severely allergic individuals.
* Clients with a history of potentially life-threatening allergic reactions are advised to carry antihistamines and an epinephrine-containing syringe at all times; they should be instructed about their appropriate use.
* Clients may react to an alcoholic beverage if they are allergic to the substance from which it is made, e.g., corn or wheat. Alcohol is not the allergen, but it hastens GI absorption, increasing adverse effects.
* For a severely allergic client, extreme caution must be used when preparing and storing foods to avoid cross contamination, e.g., foods should be tightly covered in the refrigerator and different spoons used to stir different foods.
* Parents need to inform appropriate persons at school (teachers, food service director, school nurse) about their child's food allergies.
* Calcium supplementation is recommended for children eliminating milk and milk products in their diet. However, children with atopic eczema have reacted adversely to a number of calcium supplement formulations (Devlin & David, 1990).
* Inoculation and vaccination of atopic infants should be postponed as long as possible, even 1 or 2 years, to protect the child. Combined injections of DPT (diphtheria, pertussis, and tetanus) may be given separately for reduced reactions.
* Choose seasons for vaccinations when a child is least affected by allergies.

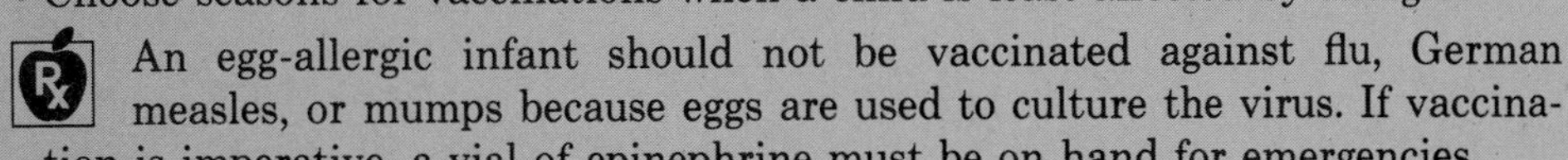
An egg-allergic infant should not be vaccinated against flu, German measles, or mumps because eggs are used to culture the virus. If vaccination is imperative, a vial of epinephrine must be on hand for emergencies.

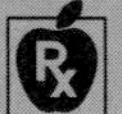
Since oral cromolyn sodium contains lactose, it may cause GI symptoms in lactose-intolerant individuals.

PREVENTION OF FOOD ALLERGIES

Prevention of food allergies is beneficial because atopic disease is the most common cause of morbidity in industrialized countries. In the 1960s, data indicated that food allergies could be prevented or delayed. Since that time, a number of studies have presented conflicting conclusions, but the general consensus is to take preventive measures to avoid the development of allergies.

Infants identified at high risk of atopic diseases include those with a positive

TABLE 23–11

INTRODUCTION OF FOODS TO PREVENT ALLERGIES IN THE HIGH-RISK INFANT

Age	Food
0–6 mo	Breast milk preferred*
	Nutramigen
	Pregestimil
	Alimentum
6 mo–1 yr	Rice cereal
1–2 yr	Cow milk†
	Wheat
	Corn
	Citrus fruits
2–3 yr	Eggs
	Tree nuts
3–4 yr	Fish
	Peanuts

* While breast-feeding, avoidance of cow milk, egg, fish, and peanut-containing foods by the mother is advised. Soy, wheat, citrus fruits, and cocoa should be used in moderation.

† Introduce foods individually and wait 3 to 5 days before adding another food.

family history of atopy, elevated cord blood IgE concentrations, and reduced T cell count at birth (Chandra, 1991; Perkin, 1990). Several strategies are strongly recommended for high-risk infants to prevent development of food allergies (Sampson, 1988; Ziegler et al, 1986). The ideal food for infants is breast milk because it is hypoallergenic. Exclusive breast-feeding is encouraged for at least 6 months. When a supplement or formula is necessary, a hydrolyzed formula, such as Nutramigen or Pregestimil (Mead Johnson) and Alimentum (Ross), is used. Cow milk and soy-based formulas are avoided for the first year. Solid foods are withheld until an infant is 6 months of age. Cow milk, wheat, corn, and citrus fruits are introduced individually and slowly after the first birthday. Eggs and tree nuts are not provided until after age 2. Introduction of fish and peanuts is delayed until 3 years of age (Table 23–11).

Avoidance of cow milk, egg, fish, and peanut-containing foods is recommended for breast-feeding mothers (Arshad et al, 1992). Proteins from these products can pass into breast milk and thereby sensitize infants. Additionally consumption of soy, wheat, citrus fruits, and cocoa should be reduced. When breast-fed infants develop an allergy to foods ingested by the mother, elimination of the food in the mother's diet alleviates an infant's symptoms. These infants can usually tolerate the offending food when it is introduced cautiously at a later age. Children usually outgrow their allergies, so restricted foods may be reintroduced after a year for further observation.

What findings identify infants as high risk for allergies? What is the ideal food for infants? What is the recommended time table for adding different foods to prevent food allergies? Why is abstinence begun early?

As a general rule, if food allergy is discovered and abstinence begun at a very young age, ability to tolerate the food returns quickly. A client who is 6 weeks old may develop a tolerance in about 3 months; if 6 months old, it takes about 6 months; if 6 years old, about 1 year; and if 15 years old, it may take as long as 2 years to develop a tolerance. Sixty to 90% of infants with early diagnosis of cow milk allergy are able to tolerate cow milk by age 2 or 3. Children whose food allergy is diagnosed at older ages have a tendency to continue experiencing problems with food allergies (Van Hooser & Crawford, 1989).

GASTROINTESTINAL FOOD INTOLERANCES

Food intolerances may be caused by abnormal chemical reactions, food contamination, GI disorders, or enzyme deficiencies. Symptoms may be any of those typical of an immunologically mediated reaction, although other responses may also be seen. Two of the more common food intolerances, lactose intolerance and **gluten-sensitive enteropathy (GSE),** have significant effects on the GI tract.

GSE and gluten-induced enteropathy are terms most often used for a variety of conditions including nontropical sprue, celiac disease, and idiopathic steatorrhea. GSE is a GI intolerance to the protein found in wheat, rye, oats, and barley.

Lactose Intolerance

Causes and Physical Consequences

Some clients are unable to digest specific carbohydrates because of insufficient amounts of disaccharide enzymes. When that carbohydrate is eaten, the disaccharide is fermented by intestinal bacteria rather than being broken down into simple sugars. This results in malabsorption of the disaccharide, accompanied by diarrhea, abdominal cramps, and flatulence.

Lactase, an intestinal enzyme responsible for lactose digestion, is the only disaccharidase whose activity is reduced in a significant proportion of older children and adults. Lactose intolerance occurs in about 92% of Asians, 79% of native Americans, 75% of blacks, 51% of Hispanics, and 21% of whites. Lactase deficiency is usually determined by indirect methods such as a lactose tolerance test by measuring blood glucose and/or breath hydrogen levels (Scrimshaw & Murray, 1988).

Three types of lactase deficiency have been identified. (1) Congenital lactase deficiency is a rare condition, which may be present at birth as a result of an inborn error of metabolism. (2) The most common problem is lactase deficiency. This is possibly an inherited problem, as evidenced by its frequency within various cultures. A normal developmental age-related decrease in lactase activity occurs. (3) Low lactase activity, called secondary lactase deficiency, may be temporary as a result of GI diseases or intestinal mucosa damage, such as in sprue, regional enteritis, and bacterial infections.

Which race has the highest percentage of lactose intolerance? What are the 3 types of lactase deficiency?

Nutritional Care

Treatment of lactase deficiency is simple—reduce lactose-containing foods. Because of the nutritional significance of milk, total elimination is not advisable (Table 23–12). Since the ability to digest lactose is not an all-or-nothing phenomenon, the amount of dairy products is reduced to a client's tolerance level. Milk is tolerated better when taken with a meal and limited to 4 oz at a time. Whole milk is tolerated better than skim milk.

TABLE 23–12

SUGGESTIONS FOR LACTOSE-INTOLERANT CLIENTS*

Milk and milk products provide the most readily available source of calcium to the body; efforts are needed to provide adequate amounts of calcium when these products are avoided. Milk/milk products are also good sources of protein, riboflavin, potassium, and magnesium. Because of different tolerance levels, each client needs to experiment to determine which method is most effective for providing necessary nutrients without discomfort

1. Consume small amounts of whole milk (4–6 oz) with meals several times a day
2. Consume fermented dairy products: yogurt,† buttermilk, aged cheese (Swiss, Colby, Longhorn), soft cheese (cream cheese, Neufchatel, cottage cheese, Farmer's, ricotta)
3. Use OTC lactase enzymes available in tablet/liquid form to hydrolyze the lactose in milk products or lactose-hydrolyzed commercially available milk
4. Increase consumption of other calcium-containing foods: salmon and sardines canned with bones, spinach, kale, broccoli, turnip and beet greens, molasses, tofu, almonds, orange, eggs, shrimp
5. Consider commercially available nutrition supplements such as Ensure (Ross), Resource (Sandoz)
6. If the above suggestions are not feasible to maintain an adequate intake of at least 600 mg calcium, consult a physician/dietitian for calcium supplements that are well absorbed. These supplements may also need to include vitamin D

* Nurses can assist in ensuring adequate calcium intake by using information in Chapter 9, Tables 9–2 and 9–3 to determine quickly calcium content of various foods the client can tolerate and enjoy.
† Unflavored yogurt is usually the best tolerated.

Fermented dairy products—especially yogurt but also buttermilk, aged cheese, and sour cream—are often better tolerated by lactase-deficient individuals. Yogurt made with the organisms *Lactobacillus bulgaricus* or *Streptococcus thermophilus* is better tolerated than nonfermented dairy products because it contains active lactase and less lactose. Yogurt buffers stomach acid, preventing lactase-producing bacteria from being killed. Lactase activity varies among yogurt brands; Dannon yogurt has the highest lactase activity (Wytock & DiPalma, 1988). Most commercially available yogurt can be tolerated by lactose-intolerant clients, but unflavored yogurt generally has a higher lactase activity (Martini et al, 1987). Many commercially available frozen yogurts have been pasteurized to increase their shelf life. Since this process decreases lactase activity and kills lactose-producing bacteria, most frozen yogurts are not well tolerated by lactose-intolerant clients.

When is milk tolerated better; which type is tolerated best? How does yogurt help lactose intolerance?

Commercially available lactase in tablet or liquid form can be beneficial. Lactose tablets, taken with a lactase-containing food, are effective in the stomach's acidic environment for approximately 45 minutes. Liquid lactase is effective in a neutral pH. The enzyme, added to milk before it is consumed, hydrolyzes lactose before its ingestion. Specialized lactose-reduced products are also commercially available.

NURSING APPLICATIONS

Assessment

Physical—for frequent stomach cramping, diarrhea, and gas after ingestion of dairy products; ethnic origin; recent GI disease; type of lactose intolerance.
Dietary—for intake of dairy products; adequacy of intake of calcium and riboflavin.
Laboratory—for breath hydrogen or glucose levels following lactose tolerance test; reducing substances (sugars) in the stool, stool pH (acidic).

Interventions

1. Encourage use of lactose-reduced dairy products such as yogurt, aged cheese, and lactose-reduced milk to provide calcium, phosphorus, riboflavin, and vitamins.

Evaluation

* Client is able to plan a daily intake of 500 to 800 mg calcium using foods that minimize abdominal flatus, cramping, and diarrhea.

Client Education

- Lactose is used as an additive in some drugs and food products as a filler or carrier; clients should be taught to scrutinize labels.
- Teach clients approximate calcium composition of milk products tolerated (see Chapter 9, Table 9-2).
- Low lactose-containing milks, such as acidophilius or LactAid milk, are available.
- Unpasteurized yogurt, which is better tolerated by lactose-intolerant individuals, provides nutrients lacking from the omission of other milk products.
- Protein and fat absorption are not affected.

Gluten-Sensitive Enteropathy

GSE appears in familial clusters, implicating a hereditary factor. GSE is perceived as a malabsorption syndrome of childhood, but increasing numbers of adults are being diagnosed (Kelly et al, 1990). Infantile and adult forms are now thought to be the same.

Causes and Physical Consequences

GSE causes fewer villi, which are blunted or may disappear, so the mucosa becomes partially flattened (Fig. 23–2). These damaged cells produce fewer digestive enzymes. In many cases, this is due to an abnormal sensitivity to **gluten.** Symptoms include diarrhea or foul-smelling, frothy, bulky stools; bloating; anorexia; muscular wasting; and cramping abdominal pain. Even when large amounts of food are eaten, underweight is common since protein, fat, and carbohydrate are poorly absorbed. Other manifestations include iron deficiency anemia, chronic fatigue, and weakness.

Gluten is a protein found mainly in wheat, with less in rye, oat, and barley. Actually, only the gliadin (another protein) part of gluten causes mucosal damage in these clients.

Projectile vomiting, a bloated abdomen, and growth failure are frequently observed in children. Infants may exhibit no symptoms until cereals are introduced, at which time, in addition to the aforementioned symptoms, they refuse to eat and become irritable.

Name 5 symptoms of GSE.

Nutritional Care

When damage occurs to the lining of the small intestine, many nutrients cannot be digested and absorbed. The small intestine repairs itself when gluten-containing foods are totally removed from the diet. Gluten-containing foods can cause severe villi damage even in clients without symptoms. Thus, the keystone of treatment of primary GSE requires elimination of wheat and rye from the diet for life; however, if GSE is secondary to another condition, malabsorptive symptoms may not recur when the underlying condition has resolved. Following diagnosis, implementation of a gluten-free diet usually results in a rapid response or disappearance of GI symptoms within 1 to 2 weeks (Trier, 1991). This response confirms the diagnosis.

A primary concern of parents is possible adverse effects of celiac disease on future health (Anson et al, 1990). Parents or clients need to be knowledgeable of the overall role of celiac disease on health and long-term adverse effects and should be able to plan a nutritionally adequate diet without gluten-containing foods. Noncompliance with the diet during childhood or adolescence may result in stunted growth. Overall incidence of lymphoma is increased in clients with GSE (Trier, 1991).

When the condition has stabilized, some clients (especially adolescents) are able to consume small amounts (0.06-2 gm/day) of gluten occasionally without overt symptoms (Mayer et al, 1991).

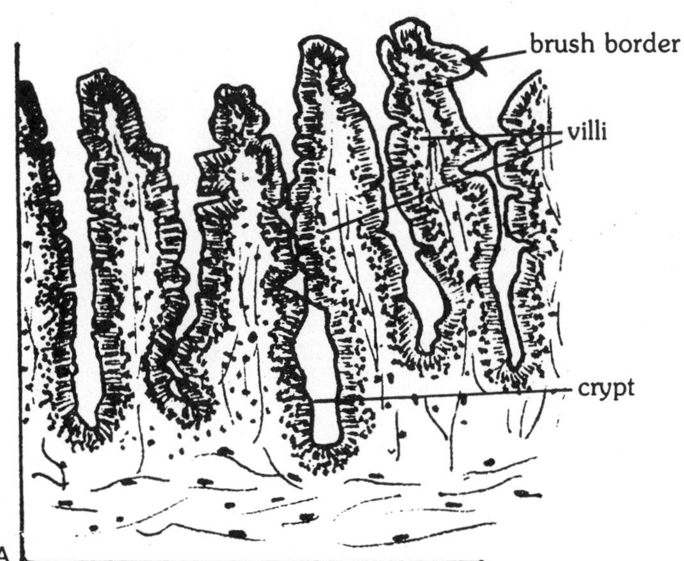

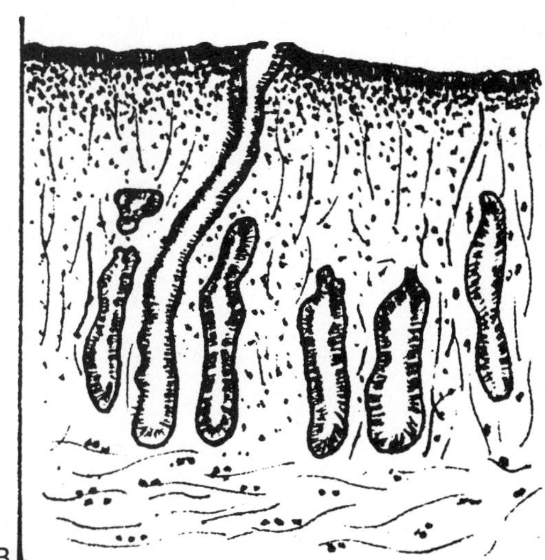

Figure 23–2 *A*, Normal small intestine. *B*, Intestine, untreated celiac. (From Hartsook E. Fact sheet on celiac sprue. Seattle, The Gluten Intolerance Group, 1982.)

The gluten-free diet is a real challenge because of the ubiquitous use of wheat products in processed foods, i.e., hot dogs and luncheon meats, or staple foods, such as vinegar (cider and wine are acceptable). Although 98% of gluten-sensitive clients report following a gluten-free diet, about 88% indicate that lapses in adherence occur accidentally about once a month (Campbell et al, 1991). Malt and malt flavoring derived from barley is unacceptable, but some malt is made from corn. Reading labels is a must to avoid these products. Other less readily recognized foods that may need to be excluded because of intolerance include creamed soups and vegetables, ice cream, spaghetti, macaroni and other pastas, mixed infant and junior dinners, malted milk, processed cheese, commercial salad dressings, Postum, and Ovaltine.

Becoming familiar with products and recipes using allowable foods improves dietary compliance and variety in the diet. Wheat flour can be replaced with corn flour or meal and potato and rice flour (see Table 23–7). Elimination of wheat, rye, oats, and barley means labels must be carefully read for cereal, starch, flour, thickening agents, emulsifiers, gluten, and stabilizers. (Wheat starch is acceptable because the gluten has been removed.) Hydrolyzed vegetable protein may be from soybeans, corn, wheat, or a mixture of these; vegetable protein may include soybeans, corn, wheat, rye, oats, and barley. The diet should initially be low in fiber since mucosal villi are flattened. Gradually fiber content can be increased. If steatorrhea is present, MCT oil is usually well tolerated.

Because of a long history of malabsorption before diagnosis, clients with celiac disease are at greater risk of developing nutrient deficiency–related disorders, such as osteoporosis. Calcium supplements may be needed to reverse bone demineralization. Since the major grain sources used in this diet are refined and unenriched, vitamin (especially the B vitamins) and mineral (iron, calcium, and trace elements) intake may be inadequate, and a multivitamin-mineral supplement is encouraged. Fat-soluble vitamins should be provided in a water-miscible form because of decreased fat absorption.

Name 6 foods to be avoided. What can wheat flour be replaced with in recipes? Why are vitamin/mineral supplements encouraged?

Villi are affected during exacerbations, causing temporary intolerance to lactose. Fat intake may increase steatorrhea during acute stages and may need to be decreased.

NURSING APPLICATIONS

Assessment

Physical—for frequency and consistency of bowel movements; muscle weakness and cramping; weight, height, IBW; for infants and children, percentile on growth charts; type of vomiting, bloating.

Dietary—for dietary intake of gluten-containing products; knowledge related to gluten-free diet and gluten-containing products.

Laboratory—for albumin; potassium, sodium, calcium; serum carotene and folate; CBC with differential; fecal fat, stool cultures.

Interventions

1. Refer to a dietitian to help with the diet and provide clients/parents with information about reading labels and food preparation.
2. Emphasize to client to check all labels for cereal, starch, flour, thickening agents, emulsifiers, gluten, stabilizers, hydrolyzed vegetable protein, and other additives.
3. If client does not improve within 6 to 8 weeks following implementation of the diet, investigate for inadvertent gluten intake.

Evaluation

* Client should comply with gluten-free diet and should verbalize foods allowed. Adults should gain weight, and children's height and weight should be maintained above the 25th percentile on growth charts.

Client Education

- Adherence to a strict, lifelong gluten-free diet is recommended until the relation of gluten ingestion to the development of malignant disease is clarified (Trier, 1991).
- When starch is listed as an ingredient on a product made in the US, it is cornstarch.
- Some instant coffees contain gluten, as do beer and ale.
- Inform clients of support groups, i.e., American Celiac Society and Gluten Intolerance group (see Appendix E-1).
- Inform clients of companies that provide gluten-free flours and breads (see Chapter 29, Table 29-6).

PHARMACOLOGICAL FOOD INTOLERANCES

Food intolerances due to biochemical reactions that result from food additives and natural ingredients in foods are called **pharmacological food reactions.** Several different substances with pharmacological properties are present in foods. Vasoactive amines, or histamine and monoamines (tyramine and phenylethylamine), and methylxanthines (caffeine, theobromine, and theophylline) have pharmacological potential. Symptoms appear following ingestion of large quantities of food containing these substances. Clients may have a lowered threshold because of a disease process occurring at the same time or a medication being taken. Degree of reaction varies, but the offending ingredient may affect anyone.

A pharmacological food reaction is an adverse reaction to a natural constituent of a food or chemical added to a food that produces a drug-like effect.

Histamine

Foods containing a large quantity of histamine may result in a reaction that is clinically indistinguishable from an IgE-mediated food allergy. Elevated histamine levels correlate with migraine attacks in susceptible clients (Mansfield, 1990). Foods with a high content of histamine include several cheeses (parmesan, blue, roquefort), Chianti and Burgundy wines, yeast extract, and several fishes (mackerel, tuna). Improper refrigeration of these products causes a dramatic rise in histamine content. Smaller amounts of histamine are present in chicken liver, sausage, sauerkraut, spinach, and tomatoes (Zeitz, 1991).

What foods have a high histamine content?

Monoamines

Vasoactive amines, principally tyramine and phenylethylamine, mainly affect the GI tract and CNS and have been associated with migraine headaches. Tyramine releases norepinephrine from tissue stores and causes a rise in blood pressure. Tyramine can also cause migraines and MAO inhibitor reactions (Monro, 1987). Currently MAO inhibitor medications are not widely used, but clients taking these medications for depression should avoid foods containing tyramine to prevent migraine headaches and hypertensive crises (see Chapter 20).

Tyramine is found in most aged cheese, brewer's yeast, concentrated yeast extracts, Chianti wine, pickled herring, and chicken liver.

Tyramine may be a contributing factor in chronic urticaria (Saifer & Saifer, 1987). This intolerance may be due to low levels of MAO (Zeitz, 1991).

High phenylethylamine intake may adversely affect individuals susceptible to dietary-related migraine headaches. It is found in the same products as tyramine

What foods are high in tyramine; phenylethylamine?

(principally cheese and red wine). However, phenylethylamine is also found in chocolate.

Salicylate

List foods high in salicylate.

Foods with a high content of natural salicylate include dried fruits, oranges, berries, apricots, pineapples, cucumbers, gherkins, endive, olives, grapes, almonds, licorice, peppermint, honey, tomato sauce, tea, wines, and liqueurs. Several herbs and spices contain salicylate, e.g., thyme, mint, paprika, rosemary, oregano, and curry. Salicylates have been accused of causing hyperactivity, although scientific studies have been unable to confirm this. Although 10 to 20% of asthmatics react negatively to aspirin, it is rarely necessary to restrict salicylate-containing foods.

Methylxanthines

Caffeine, theobromine, and theophylline are methylxanthines found in many medications and foods, especially tea, coffee, and chocolate (see Appendix A-3). When large quantities are consumed, CNS stimulation may cause hypertensive/hyperactivity symptoms. Caffeine stimulates gastric secretion and can cause esophageal reflux, nausea or vomiting, and diarrhea.

Methylxanthines also function as bronchodilators. They may be advantageous for clients who suffer from bronchospasms, or they may intensify the effects of theophylline medications, increasing risk of anorexia, insomnia, and cardiac arrhythmias.

INTOLERANCE TO FOOD ADDITIVES

Food additives can also cause adverse reactions. Despite extensive testing of food additives before their being allowed on the market, sensitive clients may experience adverse effects.

Sulfites

Sulfites are sulfur dioxide, sulfurous acid, and any salt of sulfurous acid. Sulfites are a very versatile additive with many functions.

Sulfites occur naturally in many foods, especially fermented foods, and are often added to products, such as salad greens, vegetables, and fruits, to maintain freshness. In 1986, the FDA banned use of sulfites in raw produce and fresh meats. Sulfites have an adverse effect on thiamin stability; they cannot be used in foods that are a good source of thiamin, i.e., enriched bread and flour. They are also present in some wines and beers and dried fruits.

Sulfite sensitivity affects only a rather small subgroup of asthmatics. Following ingestion of sulfites, anaphylactic-like reactions have been documented. Because of severe, life-threatening reactions in sensitive clients, use of sulfites has been curtailed or banned in many products. The search for an effective alternative continues; where possible, sulfites have been replaced. Packaged foods containing more than 10 ppm residual of sulfite equivalents must state the presence of sulfites on food labels. No evidence exists to suggest that foods having less than this amount are hazardous to sulfite-sensitive clients (Taylor et al, 1991).

A client's degree of sensitivity determines the amount of food that can be safely consumed. For example, a client with a 200-mg threshold for sulfites would be unlikely to have a severe reaction to most sulfite-containing foods because very few have this amount (except lettuce or greens from salad bars, dried fruit, guacamole, and hash-brown potatoes with the sulfite heavily added). Additionally, concentration of residual sulfite in the food and the form of sulfite present are influential factors in reactions.

What group of clients is most affected by sulfites? What foods are high in sulfite? What 3 factors influence reactions?

Monosodium Glutamate

Monosodium glutamate (MSG) is one of the most widely used food additives worldwide. The most commonly reported adverse reaction associated with MSG consumption is Chinese restaurant syndrome because MSG is frequently used as a flavor enhancer in Asian foods. Symptoms, which occur 15 to 30 minutes after a meal, include headache, chest tightness, nausea, and sweating. Severe attacks of asthma and dizziness have also been associated with ingestion of MSG. Bronchospasms as a reaction to MSG may appear 1 to 2 hours after ingestion or as long as 12 hours after ingestion. Younger children may experience shudder attacks, and older children and adults may experience migraine headaches (Allen, 1991).

What signs and symptoms may occur in MSG-sensitive clients?

Nitrates

Nitrates and nitrites are widely used as preservatives. They are popular because of the flavoring and coloring attributes they contribute to products. Nitrates are potentially involved in migraine headaches. Hot dogs, bacon, ham, luncheon meats, smoked fish, and some imported cheeses have high concentrations of nitrates.

What foods are high in nitrates?

Tartrazine (FD&C Yellow #5)

Tartrazine gives a lemon-yellow color to foods and some medicines. Since 1980, government regulations require identification of the dye on food and drug labels (package inserts). This has resulted in many manufacturers removing tartrazine from their products, but it is still present in hundreds of products. Tartrazine is added to vitamin supplements, pickles, cakes, gelatins, packaged soup, custard, instant puddings, colored candies, cheese dishes, soft drinks (orange and lime), jelly, ice cream, mustard, and yogurt. Adverse reactions to tartrazine include bronchospasms and urticaria. Individuals who are sensitive to aspirin are frequently sensitive to tartrazine.

What foods contain tartrazine?

NURSING APPLICATIONS

Assessment

Physical—for migraine; increased blood pressure and heart rate; bronchospasms, Chinese restaurant syndrome symptoms and duration; history of similar reactions.
Dietary—for foods eaten in the past 24 hours, offending pharmacological agent or food additives, adequacy of diet, diet history.
Laboratory—for histamine level.

Interventions

1. Help client identify offending food substances and avoid serving.
2. Refer to dietitian.
3. Provide support.

Continued

Evaluation

* Client should be able to identify foods to avoid and state why avoidance is necessary. Additionally, symptoms caused by offending foods should decrease or not occur.

Client Education

- Numerous naturally occurring chemicals or additives are possible precipitating factors for migraine (Walling, 1990). In addition, other lifestyle factors, such as fatigue, stress, or too much or too little exercise, may increase vulnerability to an acute attack, as shown in Table 23–13.
- Restriction of MSG is advised for clients with migraine headaches (Perkin, 1990).
- Fresh meats are more advisable than cured meats; hot dogs, bacon, ham, and salami have been demonstrated to cause vascular headache in some clients.
- Three well-balanced meals a day are recommended. Skipped meals, prolonged fasting, or excessive amounts of carbohydrates at any single meal are associated with headaches.

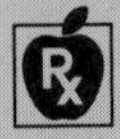
Cafergot, sometimes prescribed for migraine headaches, may cause nausea, vomiting, drowsiness, and edema.

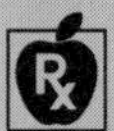
If sedatives, tranquilizers, antidepressants, or diuretics are used for migraine, alter diet accordingly (see Table 23–13), especially alcohol.

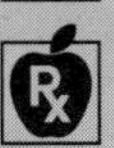
Isoniazid (INH) is a strong histaminase inhibitor; a large intake of histamine-containing foods concurrent with isoniazid therapy may result in headache and reddening of the eyes, face, and palms.

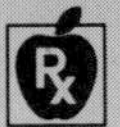
Sulfite sensitivity appears to occur more frequently in clients receiving corticosteroids (Bush et al, 1986).

TABLE 23–13

POSSIBLE DIETARY FACTORS PRECIPITATING MIGRAINE HEADACHES

Food Categories	Specific Foods
Beverages	Alcohol, particularly red wine, champagne, and beer
	Caffeine-containing beverages (large amounts), including colas, tea, and coffee
Dairy products	Aged and processed cheese, especially cheddar
	Sour cream
	Yogurt
Meats and other protein foods	Aged, cured, or processed meats containing nitrates or nitrites such as bacon, sausage, hot dogs, luncheon meats
	Peanuts and peanut butter
Grains	Homemade yeast bread
Miscellaneous	Chocolate
	Caffeine-containing medications
	Food additives, including meat tenderizers, monosodium glutamate, soy sauce, and yeast extracts
Eating habits	Missing or skipping meals

Data from Sutherland JE. Headaches. *Am Fam Phys* 1983; 27(2):137–142.

SUMMARY

A dietary history, including symptoms and environmental factors, is useful in diagnosing and treating food allergies; a food diary is an important part of this history. Despite several laboratory tests that can provide additional information, the most valuable and least expensive procedure for diagnosis is the elimination diet followed by food challenge testing. However, when food avoidance does not produce desired results, a rotation diet may allow some foods to be consumed with less severe allergic reactions.

Basic principles to prevent as well as treat adverse food reactions include the following:

1. Offer a varied diet; avoid excessive quantities of any one food.
2. Replace each food that is omitted from the diet with one of similar nutrient value.
3. Know what a client is actually eating. Identification and treatment of adverse food reactions is a complex problem and must involve active participation of client and nurse.

NURSING PROCESS IN ACTION

A client has migraine headaches and wants to know what foods to avoid or use in moderation. She has heard some conflicting data and does not want to give up her favorite foods unnecessarily.

 Nutritional Assessment

- IBW, height, weight, family history, auras.
- Knowledge of nutrition, migraines.
- Intake of food, food additives, and pharmacological agents.
- Intake in the last 24 hours.
- Histamine levels.

 Dietary Nursing Diagnosis

Knowledge deficit: Nutritional aspects of migraines RT inappropriate/insufficient information.

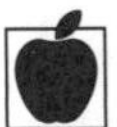 Nutritional Goals

Client will state foods to avoid, plan and consume nutritious meals, and have fewer migraine headaches.

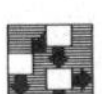 Nutritional Implementation 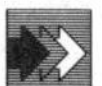

Intervention: Teach her to avoid aged cheeses, especially parmesan, blue, roquefort cheeses; Chianti and Burgundy wines; beer; yeast extract; and anchovy, sardines, tuna, pickled herring, and chicken livers.

Rationale: These foods are high in histamine and tyramine. Histamine can cause vasodilation and intensify migraine attacks. Tyramine releases norepinephrine from tissue stores and causes a rise in blood pressure, thereby compounding migraine pain.

Intervention: Encourage use of chocolate in moderation.
Rationale: This contains phenylethylamine, which may be offensive for clients susceptible to dietary-related migraines.

Intervention: Explain how to avoid nitrates in processed foods (hot dogs, bacon, ham, luncheon meats), smoked fish, and imported cheeses, and MSG.
Rationale: Nitrates can worsen or precipitate a migraine attack. MSG can precipitate attacks.

Evaluation

Client should be able to say, "I will try to stay away from processed foods, MSG, Chinese food, wines, and beers." She would also be able to plan 3 meals a day without the offending foods and still include a variety of foods from all food groups. Additionally, frequency of migraines would decrease. She would say, "I haven't had an attack in 1 month."

STUDENT READINESS

1. Plan meals for 1 day for a wheat-free diet.
2. Why is a food diary important?
3. A client asks what foods are high in histamine and sulfites. How would you respond?
4. How can an infant be protected from potential allergies?
5. Name 5 of the most common foods that cause allergic reactions in children and adults.

CASE STUDY

Susan P. is a college freshman who has had asthma since she was 4 years old. During her first semester, she lived in the dormitory and ate in the university's cafeteria. The second semester she moved into her own apartment. Since she dislikes cooking and wants to lose 5 lbs, she has been eating salads at a local restaurant frequently. She has noted a dramatic increase in asthmatic episodes this semester.

1. What changes in Susan's life have taken place in the past year?
2. Differentiate between food intolerance and food allergies.
3. List procedures that might be used to diagnose a food allergy.
4. What food allergies are the least likely to resolve with age?

5. List foods Susan should avoid.
6. What do you think caused an increase in her asthmatic attack?
7. Write one nursing diagnosis and goal for Susan.

CASE STUDY

On examination at the clinic, a woman tells the nurse she frequently experiences bloating, cramping, and diarrhea. She has lost 20 lbs. Milk is a preferred beverage rather than coffee, tea, or cola beverages. Several diagnostic studies are performed, and a diagnosis of lactose intolerance is made. She is placed on a restricted lactose-containing diet and referred for diet counseling.

1. What types of tests were performed to help diagnose lactose intolerance?
2. Why is a restricted diet ordered?
3. Name at least 1 nursing diagnosis and goal for this client.
4. What foods will she need to avoid?
5. What tips can you tell her that will help her consume adequate amounts of calcium; for ingestion of milk?
6. What products are available for her to use?
7. How can she increase kilocaloric intake to regain weight lost?
8. She wants to eat at restaurants; what foods would you advise her to avoid; to consume?
9. Would you recommend yogurt in her diet? Why or why not?
10. How would you evaluate nursing care of this client?

REFERENCES

Allen DH. Monosodium glutamate. *In* Metcalfe DD, et al, eds. *Food Allergy Adverse Reactions to Foods and Food Additives.* Boston, Blackwell Scientific Publications, 1991: 261–266.

American College of Physicians. Allergy testing. *Ann Intern Med* 1989 Feb 15; 110(4):317–320.

Anderson JA. The establishment of common language concerning adverse reactions to foods and food additives. *J Allergy Clin Immunol* 1986 July; 78(1):140–144.

Anson O, et al. Celiac disease: Parental knowledge and attitude of dietary compliance. *Pediatrics* 1990 Jan; 85(1):98–103.

Arshad SH, et al. Effect of allergen avoidance on development of allergic disorders in infancy. *Lancet* 1992 June 20; 339(8808): 1493–1497.

Bock SA. Perspective of appraisal of complaints of adverse food reactions to foods in children during the first three years of life. *Pediatrics* 1987 May; 79(5):683–688.

Bock SA, Atkins FM. Patterns of food hypersensitivity during sixteen years of double-blind, placebo-controlled food challenges. *J Pediatr* 1990 Oct; 117(4):561–567.

Bock SA, et al. Double-blind, placebo-controlled food challenge as an office procedure: A manual. *J Allergy Clin Immunol* 1988 Dec; 82(6):986–997.

Bush RK, et al. Prevalence of sensitivity to sulfiting agents in asthmatic patients. *Am J Med* 1986 Nov; 81(5):816–820.

Bush RK, et al. Soybean oil is not allergenic to soybean sensitive individuals. *J Allergy Clin Immunol* 1985 Aug; 76(2 pt 1):242–245.

Campbell JA, et al. Dietary aspects from national survey of persons with celiac disease and dermatitis herpetiformis. *J Can Diet Assoc* 1991 Fall; 52(3):161–165.

Chandra RK. Food allergy: Diagnosis and strategies for prevention. *Nutr & the MD* 1991 Apr; 17(4):1–3.

Chandra RK. Food allergy. *In* Shils ME, Young VR, eds. *Modern Nutrition in Health and Disease.* 7th ed. Philadelphia, Lea & Febiger, 1988: 1298–1305.

Council on Scientific Affairs. In vitro testing for allergy: Report II of the allergy panel. *JAMA* 1987 Sept 25; 258(12):1639–1643.

Devlin J, David TJ. Intolerance to oral and intravenous calcium supplements in atopic eczema. *J Roy Soc Med* 1990 Aug; 83(8):497–498.

Gern JE, et al. Allergic reactions to milk-contaminated "non-dairy" products. *N Engl J Med* 1991 April 4; 324(14):976–979.

Hunter JO. Provocation testing and food sensitivity (letter). *N Engl J Med* 1991 Oct 17; 325(16):1171–1174.

Jewett DL, et al. A double-blind study of symptom provocation to determine food sensitivity. *N Engl J Med* 1990 Aug 16; 323(7):429–433.

Kelly CP, et al. Diagnosis and treatment of gluten sensitive enteropathy. *Adv Intern Med* 1990; 35:341–363.

Mansfield LD. The role of antihistamine therapy in vascular headaches. *J Allergy Clin Immunol* 1990 Oct; 86(4 Pt 2):673–676.

Martini MC, et al. Lactose digestion from flavored and frozen yogurts, ice milk, and ice cream by lactase deficient persons. *Am J Clin Nutr* 1987 Oct; 46(4):636–640.

Mayer M, et al. Compliance of adolescents with coeliac disease with a gluten free diet. *Gut* 1991 Aug; 32(8):881–885.

Monro J. Food induced migraine. *In* Brostoff J, Challacombe SJ, eds. *Food Allergy and Intolerances.* Philadelphia, Bailliere Tindall, 1987: 633–665.

Perkin JE. *Food Allergies and Adverse Reactions.* Gaithersburg, MD, Aspen, 1990.

Saifer PL, Saifer M. Clinical detection of sensitivity to preservatives and chemicals. *In* Brostoff J, Challacombe SJ, eds. *Food Allergy and Intolerances.* Philadelphia, Bailliere Tindall, 1987: 416–430.

Sampson HA, et al. Fatal and near-fatal anaphylactic reactions to food in children and adolescents. *N Engl J Med* 1992 Aug 6; 327(6):380–384.

Sampson HA. Food allergy. *J Allergy Clin Immunol* 1989 Dec; 84(6 Pt 2):1062–1067.

Sampson HA. Food allergies and the infant at risk. *JAMA* 1988 Dec 16; 260(23):3507.

Sampson HA, et al. Food allergy. *JAMA* 1987 Nov 27; 258(20):2886–2890.

Sampson HA, Metcalfe DD. Food Allergies. *JAMA* 1992 Nov 25; 268(20):2840–2844.

Scrimshaw NS, Murray EB. Lactose tolerance and milk consumption. *Am J Clin Nutr* 1988; 48(suppl):1083–1159.

Taylor SL, et al. Sulfites. *In* Metcalfe DD, et al, eds. *Food Allergy Adverse Reactions to Foods and Food Additives.* Boston, Blackwell Scientific Publications, 1991:239–260.

Trier JS. Celiac sprue. *N Engl J Med* 1991 Dec 12; 325(24):1709–1719.

Van Arsdel PP Jr, Larson EB. Diagnostic tests for patients with suspected allergic disease. Utility and limitations. *Ann Intern Med* 1988 Feb 15; 110(4):317–320.

van Bavel JH. Immunological principles of allergies. Summary Report by Locniskar MF. *Nutr Today* 1988 Sept-Oct; 23(5):31–32.

Van Hooser B, Crawford LV. Allergy diets for infants and children. *Compr Ther* 1989 Oct; 15(10):38–47.

Van Metre TE Jr. Unproven procedures for diagnosis and treatment of food allergy. *New Engl Reg Allergy Proc* 1987 Jan 15; 8(1):17–21.

Walling AD. Drug prophylaxis for migraine headaches. *Am Fam Phys* 1990 Aug; 42(2):425–432.

Wytock DH, DiPalma JA. All yogurts are not created equal. *Am J Clin Nutr* 1988 March; 47(3):454–457.

Zeigler RS, et al. Effectiveness of dietary manipulation in the prevention of food allergy in infants. *J Allergy Clin Immunol* 1986 July; 78(1 pt 2):224–238.

Zeitz HJ. Pharmacologic properties of foods. *In* Metcalfe DD, et al, eds. *Food Allergy Adverse Reactions to Foods and Food Additives.* Boston, Blackwell Scientific Publications, 1991: 311–318.

SECTION

V

Diet Therapy

Many diseases or conditions affect the body's ability to handle various nutrients or types of food. These situations may require diet modification to avoid further problems. Working with these clients requires all your previous learned skills and nutritional knowledge because making dietary changes is very difficult, even if one recognizes the need and importance to health. After all, eating is supposed to be fun and enjoyable! This section will provide you with dietary knowledge and practical methods to keep eating as rewarding as possible and to maintain optimal nutrition.

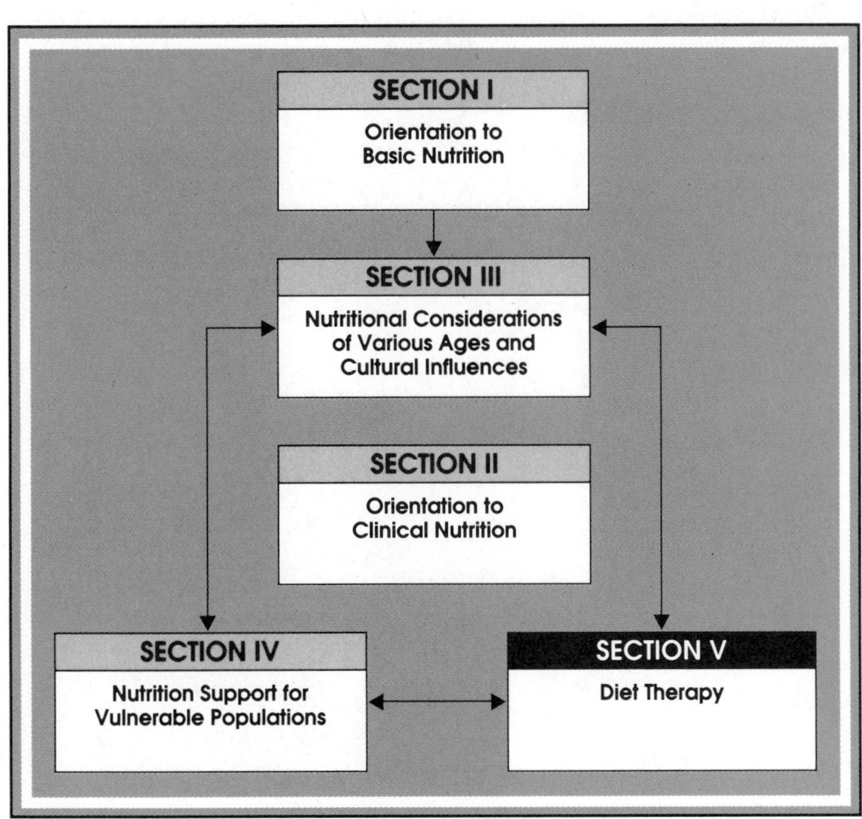

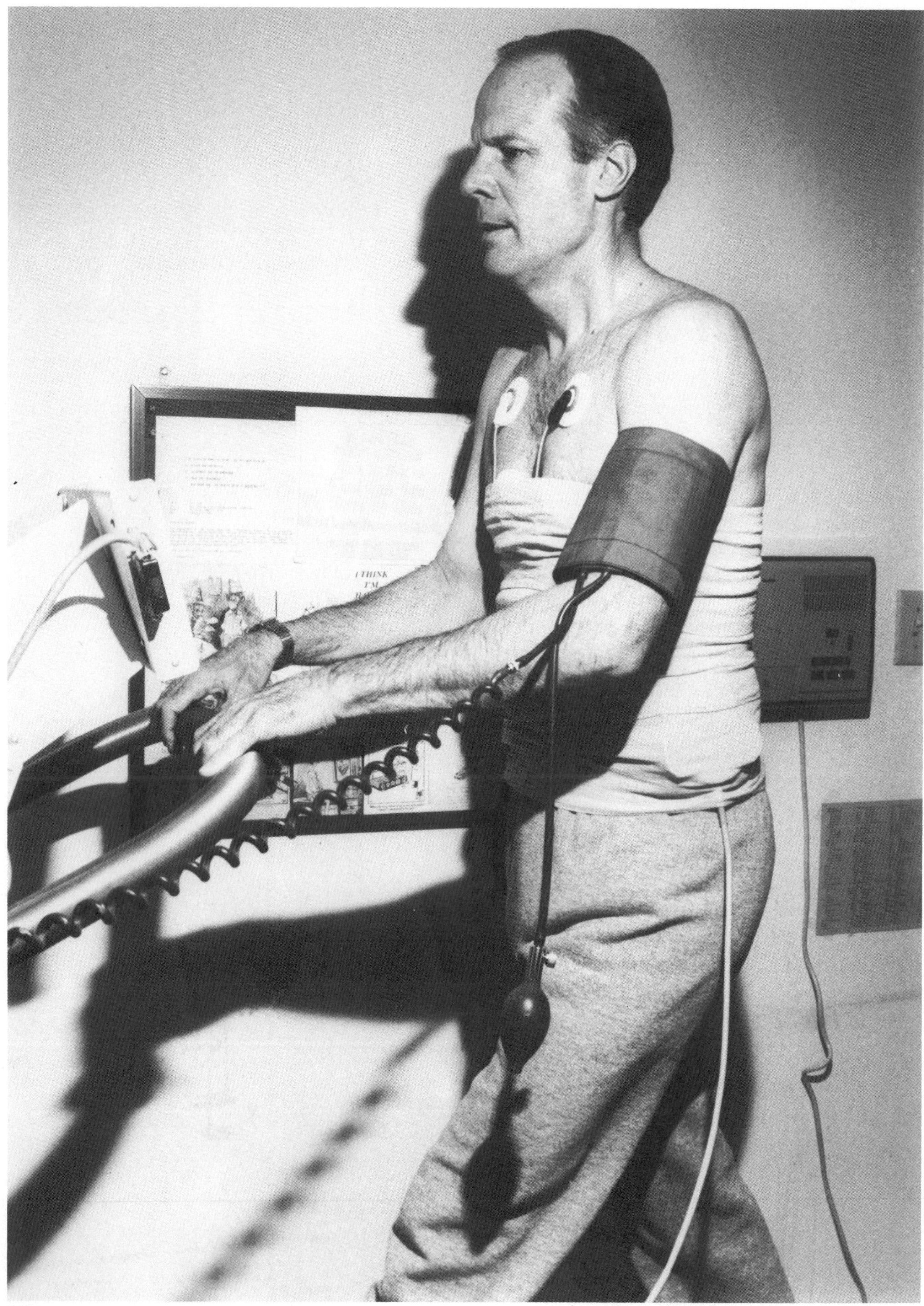

Dietary Management Of Cardiovascular Disease

CHAPTER 24

OUTLINE

I. CORONARY HEART DISEASE
II. HYPERTENSION
  A. Causes
  B. Nutritional Risk Factors Related to Hypertension
    1. Weight/Energy Overconsumption
    2. Sodium
    3. Potassium
    4. Calcium
    5. Alcohol
    6. Caffeine
    7. Dietary Fat
  C. Management
  D. Nutritional Care
    1. Weight Control
    2. Sodium
    3. Potassium
    4. Calcium
    5. Alcohol
    6. Fat
  Nursing Applications
III. HYPERLIPIDEMIA
  A. Risk Factors Related to Coronary Heart Disease and Hyperlipidemia
  B. Lipoproteins
  C. Laboratory Tests
  D. Hyperlipoproteinemia
  E. Nutritional Factors Affecting Serum Lipids
    1. Cholesterol
    2. Type and Quantity of Dietary Fat
    3. Kilocalorie Level
    4. Fiber
    5. Carbohydrates
    6. Dietary Antioxidants
    7. Alcohol
    8. Garlic
    9. Coffee
  F. Management
  G. Nutritional Care
  Nursing Applications

OBJECTIVES

THE STUDENT WILL BE ABLE TO:

- List dietary guidelines for managing hypertension.
- Discuss the dietary management for hyperlipidemia, congestive heart failure, acute myocardial infarction, and stroke.
- Plan a day's menus using the Step-1 diet.
- Identify methods of reducing serum cholesterol.
- Name factors that modify HDL-cholesterol and LDL-cholesterol levels.
- Discuss nursing applications for cardiovascular diseases.
- Identify client education principles for cardiovascular diseases.

TEST YOUR NQ (True/False)

1. Sodium should be severely restricted in hypertensive clients.
2. Hypertensive clients should consume 800 mg/day of calcium.
3. A high serum level of HDL is desirable.
4. Lowering cholesterol intake is the best way to lower serum cholesterol levels.
5. Soluble fiber found in apples, legumes, and oats can decrease cholesterol levels.
6. The Step-1 diet may be ordered for clients with hyperlipidemia.
7. Restricting sodium intake is beneficial for a client with CHF.
8. Limiting saturated fat intake to less than 30% of the kilocalories is recommended for clients following an MI.
9. One or 2 alcoholic beverages should be encouraged for clients with CHD to lower cholesterol levels.
10. CVA clients may forget they have food in their mouth.

Cardiovascular disease is still the leading cause of death in the US. Cardiovascular disorders include coronary heart disease (CHD) or coronary artery disease (CAD), hypertension, peripheral vascular disease, congestive heart failure (CHF), and congenital heart disease. Nearly one-fourth of all persons who die from cardiovascular disease are under age 65.

Annually approximately 1.25 million Americans may have a heart attack, and more than 500,000 die of CHD. Approximately $58 billion is spent on direct and indirect costs from CHD each year (NHLBI, 1991). Nutrition intervention can play a significant role in alleviating some of these problems.

Atherosclerosis is caused by an accumulation of fatty materials (such as cholesterol) within and on smooth inner walls of medium and larger arteries. As this plaque thickens, arteries become progressively narrow and rough, and blood flow, which carries oxygen and nutrients, may be disrupted.

CORONARY HEART DISEASE

The primary cause of CHD is **atherosclerosis,** which occurs particularly in coronary arteries (Fig. 24–1). Arteries afflicted with atherosclerosis may gradually lead to **arteriosclerosis.** An artery may become blocked from atherosclerosis or **thrombus; ischemia** results in damage to the part of the body supplied by the blocked artery. In the heart, a partially occluded artery may result in chest pain (angina pectoris); complete occlusion leads to myocardial infarction (MI) and sometimes death. If occlusion occurs in an artery supplying the brain, a cerebral vascular accident (CVA) or stroke results. Occlusion of a leg artery may cause claudication (leg pain on activity) and/or gangrene; occlusion of renal arteries may cause hypertension and poor renal function.

Arteriosclerosis is a poorly defined term for atherosclerotic arteries that have lost their elasticity, commonly known as hardening of the arteries.

Thrombus—a blood clot.

Ischemia—inadequate blood flow and lack of oxygen due to constriction or obstruction of arteries.

What are potential consequences of atherosclerosis?

HYPERTENSION

Hypertension is one of the high risk factors for CHD; it may also result in MI, CVA, and CHF. For every increment of blood pressure above normal levels, there is a commensurate increase in risk of cardiovascular complications. Uncon-

Hypertension is defined as a persistent elevation of systolic blood pressure above 140 mmHg in clients less than 45 years of age (greater than 150 mmHg in those over 45) and diastolic pressure above 90 mmHg. Mild hypertension refers to a diastolic blood pressure of 90 to 104 mmHg.

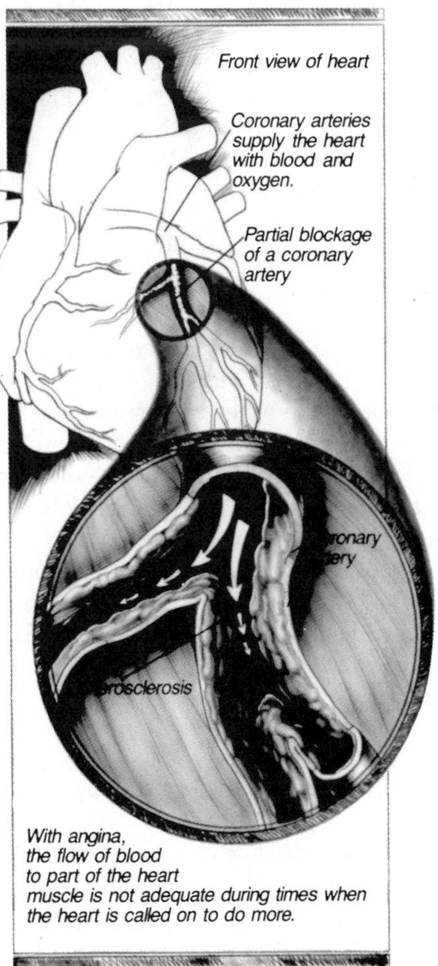
Front view of heart
Coronary arteries supply the heart with blood and oxygen.
Partial blockage of a coronary artery
With angina, the flow of blood to part of the heart muscle is not adequate during times when the heart is called on to do more.

Figure 24–1 Diagram of the natural history of atherosclerosis. (Reproduced with permission. *Fact Sheet on Heart Attack, Stroke, and Risk Factors.* 1991 Copyright. American Heart Association.)

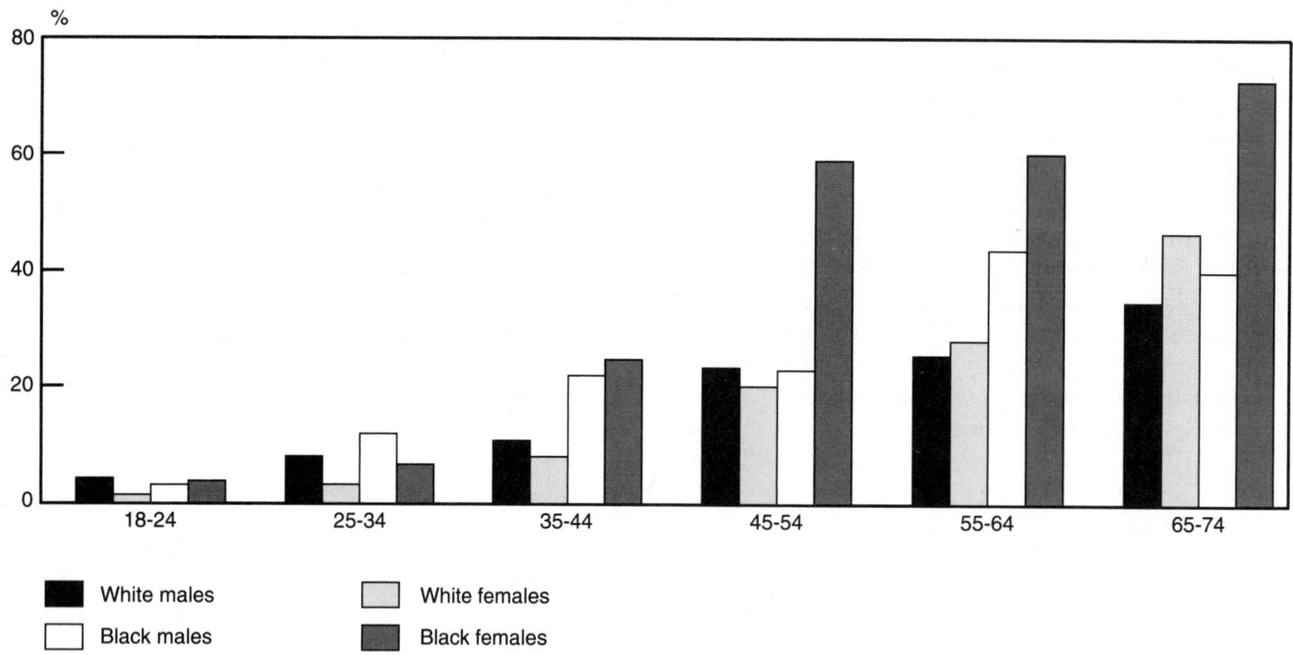

Figure 24–2 Prevalence of definite hypertension, US adult population, 1976 through 1980. (Data from National Health Survey Series 11, No. 234. US Department of Health and Human Services. DHHS Publication 86–168, July; 1986.)

trolled hypertension can affect blood vessels of the eyes, kidneys, and nervous system.

Hypertension has been called mankind's most common disease. Approximately 1 in 5 adult Americans has hypertension. Women develop hypertension more frequently than men but are less dramatically affected by a sustained elevation of blood pressure. Hypertension is about twice as common among blacks as whites; chances of developing the disease increase with age (Fig. 24–2).

Causes

Viscosity—thickness.

Vascular constriction is caused by increased sympathetic nervous system activity or increased levels of vasoconstrictors such as angiotensin and norepinephrine.

What determines blood pressure? How can salt and water retention elevate blood pressure?

Blood pressure is determined by cardiac output and peripheral resistance (elasticity) of blood vessels. An increase of either of these without commensurate decrease of the other causes an elevation in blood pressure. For instance, normally the heart pumps approximately 60 ml of blood with each beat about 70 times a minute. If arterial lumens become constricted, the heart pumps harder to force blood through these arteries. This leads to an increase in blood pressure, causing stress to both heart and blood vessels.

Resistance is determined by both **viscosity** of blood and width of blood vessels. Peripheral resistance may result from increased **vascular constriction** leading to narrowing of the arterial lumen. Blood pressure can also rise as a result of expansion of extracellular and plasma volume precipitated by increased salt and water retention.

Nutritional Risk Factors Related to Hypertension

Hypertension is nonexistent in primitive cultures. Therefore, almost all dietary factors that are significantly changed in industrialized societies have been studied for their effects on blood pressure: kilocaloric overconsumption (obesity), sodium, potassium, calcium, fiber, alcohol, caffeine, and dietary fat.

Weight/Energy Overconsumption

Throughout Western societies, obesity and hypertension are highly correlated. In addition to excessive weight being an accompanying symptom of hypertension, it is a reliable factor for predicting hypertension. Lean hypertensives are more likely to gain weight with increasing age than normotensives. Elevation of blood pressure is related to the degree of obesity. Body fat deposited in the trunk increases risk for developing essential hypertension independent of the overall level of obesity, whereas peripherally deposited fat does not (Selby et al, 1989).

Kilocaloric-restricted diets result in lower blood pressure before weight loss is significant; this has been correlated to suppression of sympathetic activity (Kushiro et al, 1991). Greatest reductions in blood pressure occur during the first half of weight loss (Schotte & Stunkard, 1990). Based on predictions from the Framingham studies, a 10% weight change (gain or loss) would result in a rise or fall in systolic blood pressure of 6.6 mmHg in men and 4.5 mmHg in women (Ashley & Kannel, 1974). It is estimated that about 50% of all hypertensive cases could be prevented entirely with weight control.

What type of body fat predisposes to hypertension? Predict the effect of a 20-lb weight loss for a 200-lb male client whose BP was 160/100 mmHg before the weight loss.

Sodium

Hypertension does not occur in societies where sodium intake is low. In contrast to no-salt cultures, blood pressures of all populations that use salt rise with age. Likewise, individuals originally from populations with low blood pressure who have become acculturated to Western civilization often develop higher blood pressure as they age.

Clients who consume comparable amounts of salt do not have the same probability of developing hypertension. Only about 50% of clients with essential hypertension are **salt sensitive.** The incidence of salt sensitivity is higher in blacks, and elderly and obese clients (Salt, 1993). Genetic factors may make some clients salt sensitive, but the physiological association is unclear. Unfortunately, there is no clear-cut method of identifying salt sensitivity.

Clients whose blood pressure responds to changes in salt intake are salt sensitive.

Despite the fact that sodium restriction does not always result in lower blood pressure, consensus from a survey of studies is that sodium reduction lowers mean blood pressure (Cutler et al, 1991). Sodium restriction improves blood pressure–lowering effects of diuretics and other pharmacological treatments.

Is decreased sodium intake always effective in lowering blood pressure? Why or why not?

Potassium

High potassium intake has a protective effect against hypertension. Potassium causes **natriuresis,** inhibits renin production by the kidney, and causes vasodilatation. Indeed, a low potassium intake, particularly when sodium consumption is high, may contribute to essential hypertension associated with decreased sodium excretion (Krishna & Kapoor, 1991). Customary high-sodium, low-potassium diets consumed when most foods are highly processed may be detrimental to normal blood pressure regulation. Potassium supplementation does not alleviate the need for pharmacological therapy even with a sodium-restricted diet (Grimm et al, 1990). However, increasing dietary potassium intake from natural foods may decrease the amount of medication needed (Siani et al, 1991).

Natriuresis—large amounts of urinary sodium excretion.

Why does high potassium intake protect against hypertension?

Calcium

An association linking higher incidence of hypertension in areas with **soft drinking water** resulted in numerous studies regarding the role of calcium intake in hypertension. Calcium plays an active role in regulating numerous physiological processes that influence blood pressure, but the mechanism is not well defined at this time. Higher intakes of calcium and potassium are associated with lower mean

Soft drinking water contains less calcium than hard water.

systolic blood pressure and lower risk of hypertension in the general population. Currently, evidence that calcium intake may affect blood pressure is provocative; further research is needed. By decreasing dairy products (all contain sodium) to lower sodium intake, a negative effect occurs because calcium intake is decreased. Hypertensive clients with low serum ionized calcium levels and low plasma renin activity are frequently salt sensitive and respond favorably to an increase in calcium intake (Moore, 1989).

Why may lowering dairy products cause a negative effect?

Alcohol

Moderate to heavy alcohol consumption (> 1 to 2 oz daily) is associated with hypertension; 10% of hypertension in the general population may be attributed to alcohol (Adlin, 1988). The mechanism for this hypertensive effect is not well defined. During alcohol withdrawal, blood pressure is elevated; however, abstinence results in a return to normal levels. Although heavy alcohol intake is associated with high blood pressure, no effect is noted for less than 2 or 3 oz per day of 40% alcohol (Einhorn & Landsberg, 1988).

How does alcohol affect blood pressure?

Caffeine

Even a single cup of regular caffeine-containing coffee can cause a significant transient rise in blood pressure. However, according to most studies, clients who regularly consume caffeine develop a tolerance to its hypertensive effects (MacDonald et al, 1991; van Dusseldorp et al, 1991). Therefore, it is believed that caffeine intake is not a significant factor in most cases of hypertension.

What is the effect of regular caffeine intake on blood pressure?

Dietary Fat

Consumption of the amount of and type of dietary fats has been studied for effects on blood pressure. Some short-term studies have shown a beneficial effect of increasing the **polyunsaturated/saturated fat ratio (P/S)** combined with an overall low fat intake (25% of the kcal) on blood pressure. PUFAs are precursors of prostaglandin biosynthesis and may reduce blood pressure by increasing production of prostaglandins that enhance renal sodium excretion and lower peripheral resistance. However, some studies have not shown a decrease in blood pressure with dietary adjustments of fat.

P/S ratio is the amount of PUFAs present as compared with the saturated fatty acid content.

Omega-3 fatty acids have been associated with a lower diastolic blood pressure in short-term studies (Radack et al, 1991; Kestin et al, 1990a; Bonaa et al, 1990). Dietary supplementation with fish oil did not affect blood pressure in clients who normally ate fish at least 3 times a week (Bonaa et al, 1990).

Management

In 1988, the National High Blood Pressure Education Program (Joint National Committee, 1988) reevaluated guidelines for managing hypertension. Because of the multifactorial diversity of hypertension, several modalities, including nonpharmacological therapies and drug treatments, are used. A step-care approach is advocated involving clients, emphasizing quality of life and cost of care. Mild hypertension in clients at relatively low risk of developing CHD is treated with nonpharmacological approaches—weight loss, exercise, sodium restriction, and other dietary factors (Applegate et al, 1992).

Behavioral stress and certain social factors are often considered to have a contributing effect on hypertension. Biofeedback and muscular relaxation have been noted to be helpful in mild hypertension, but long-term effectiveness needs further evaluation. Numerous studies have found that physically active individuals report less hypertension. Regular aerobic exercise is helpful in weight control and lowering blood pressure. Prolonged use of tobacco is not associated with hypertension, but nicotine smoking increases CHD risk. Cessation of smoking is strongly recommended.

If the aforementioned measures are ineffective, pharmacological treatment is initiated. When needed, medications recommended include thiazide diuretics, beta blockers, calcium antagonists, or angiotensin-converting enzyme (ACE) inhibitors. If the initial medication is ineffective, the dose may be increased, another medication may be added, or another drug may be substituted. Many medications used for hypertension have nutritional implications, either affecting nutritional status or recommended intake (Table 24–1). A daily intake of less than 2 gm (60 mEq) sodium enhances effectiveness of antihypertensive drugs. Diuretics increase excretion of sodium and water. Diuretics may be classified into 2 groups by their effect on potassium excretion: potassium-wasting agents or potassium-sparing agents. Thiazide and loop diuretics (potassium-wasting agents) cause potassium excretion, whereas potassium-sparing agents do not.

TABLE 24–1

COMMONLY USED MEDICATIONS FOR HYPERTENSION AND THE NUTRITIONAL IMPLICATIONS

Class/Generic (Trade/Brand Names)	Nutritional Implications
Diuretics	
Thiazide and other potassium-wasting diuretics	
Bendroflumethiazide (Naturetin) Benzthiazide (Exna) Chlorothiazide (Diuril) Chlorthalidone (Hygroton) Cyclothiazide (Anhydron) Hydrochlorothiazide (Esidrix, HydroDIURIL, Oretic) Hydroflumethiazide (Saluron) Indapamide (Lozol) Methyclothiazide (Enduron) Metolazone (Diulo, Zaroxolyn) Polythiazide (Renese) Quinethazone (Hydromox) Trichlormethiazide (Metahydrin, Nagua)	Moderate sodium restriction helps prevent hypokalemia. Replace potassium excreted with high potassium food supplements. Increased blood glucose and lipid levels (high total cholesterol, LDL, and triglyceride; high HDL) may warrant further dietary intervention. Increased calcium resorption may retard osteoporosis. May increase zinc requirement as urinary zinc excretion is increased. Hypomagnesemia; hyperuricemia. Alcohol may cause orthostatic hypotension. Natural licorice may cause hypokalemia
Loop diuretics	
Bumetanide (Bumex) Ethacrynic acid (Edecrin) Furosemide (Lasix)	Same as for thiazides
Potassium-sparing agents	
Amiloride (Midamor) Spironolactone (Aldactone) Triamterene (Dyrenium)	Moderate sodium restriction increases effectiveness of medication. Avoid excess potassium intake from food or salt supplements to prevent hyperkalemia. Take with food to avoid GI disturbances and increase bioavailability. May elevate blood glucose level, increase calcium excretion, and decrease folate utilization
Adrenergic Inhibitors	
Beta-adrenergic blockers	
Acebutolol (Sectral) Atenolol (Tenormin) Metoprolol (Lopressor) Nadolol (Corgard) Penbutolol sulfate (Levatol) Pindolol (Visken)* Propranolol (Inderal) Timolol (Blocadren)	Take with food to enhance absorption. Low-kilocalorie, low-sodium diet recommended. May cause hypoglycemia in diabetics on oral agents. May elevate serum triglycerides and reduce HDL. (*Pindolol absorption is not affected by food and does not elevate triglycerides)

Table continued on following page

TABLE 24–1

COMMONLY USED MEDICATIONS FOR HYPERTENSION AND THE NUTRITIONAL IMPLICATIONS
Continued

Class/Generic (Trade/Brand Names)	Nutritional Implications
Centrally acting alpha-blockers	
Clonidine (Catapres) Guanabenz (Wytensin) Guanfacine (Tenex) Methyldopa (Aldomet)	Low-kilocalorie, low-salt diet may be recommended. Reduces food intake due to dry mouth. Natural licorice may cause orthostatic hypotension. May cause weight gain due to edema. Methyldopa may cause malabsorption associated with folate and vitamin B_{12} losses
Peripheral-acting adrenergic antagonists	
Guanadrel (Hylorel) Guanethidine (Ismelin) Rauwolfia (Harmonyl, Moderil, Raudixin, Rauwiloid) Reserpine (Serpasil)	Take with food to prevent GI distress. Low-salt, low-kilocalorie diet may be recommended for weight loss and to prevent edema. Alcohol may cause orthostatic hypotension. Reserpine requires reduced levels of pressor amines (MAO inhibitors); tyramine-restricted diet recommended
Alpha-adrenergic blockers	
Prazosin (Minipress) Terazosin (Hytrin)	Low-kilocalorie; low-sodium diet recommended to prevent edema. Alcohol may cause orthostatic hypotension
Vasodilators	
Hydralazine (Apresoline)† Minoxidil (Loniten, Minoxidil)	Take with food to enhance absorption. Low-kilocalorie, low-sodium diet recommended. (†Pyridoxine supplementation may correct drug-induced peripheral neuropathy)
Angiotensin-Converting Enzyme	
Captopril (Capoten) Enalapril (Vasotec)‡ Lisinopril (Prinivil, Zestril)	Take on empty stomach to enhance drug absorption. (‡Enalapril may be taken with food.) Low-kilocalorie, low-sodium diet may be recommended. Avoid potassium-containing salt substitutes and potassium supplements to prevent hyperkalemia
Calcium antagonists	
Diltiazem (Cardizem) Nicardipine (Cardene) Nifedipine (Procardia) Verapamil (Calan)	Avoid calcium supplements, as effectiveness of the drug may be decreased. May cause hyperkalemia. High-fiber diet may be needed to promote regular bowel function. Strict sodium restriction may reduce effectiveness of the medication

Describe management of hypertension. Why is it beneficial to lower sodium intake even though a diuretic is prescribed?

Since both hypokalemia and hyperkalemia can be life-threatening, monitoring potassium levels while using diuretics is imperative. Renal, muscle, and cardiac function may be adversely affected by hypokalemia. Adverse side effects of diuretics and other antihypertensive medications include increased risk of CHD, as shown in Table 24–1.

Nutritional Care

Dietary modifications lower blood pressure for many clients with mild to moderate hypertension. Weight control and reduced sodium intake are not only useful initial therapies, but also they enhance antihypertensive effects of drugs (Treat-

TABLE 24–2

GUIDELINES FOR NONPHARMACOLOGICAL MANAGEMENT OF HYPERTENSION

1. Control weight
   a. Weight loss to within 15% of desirable weight for obese clients
   b. Weight loss to IBW for overweight clients
   c. Maintenance of IBW for clients with normal weight
2. Limit sodium intake to 2–3 gm daily
3. Maintain recommended calcium intake
4. Increase intake of fresh fruits and vegetables to increase dietary fiber and potassium
5. Lower total fat intake to 30% of total kcal with 10% from saturated fats
6. Consume fatty fish (for example, mackerel, herring, salmon) several times a week to provide omega-3 fatty acids and to help lower saturated fat intake
7. Consume a well-balanced diet using a variety of foods to ensure adequate intake of magnesium
8. Restrict alcohol intake to 1–2 drinks daily or less
9. Do not use potassium, calcium, or magnesium supplements unless recommended by the physician/dietitian
10. Avoid tobacco
11. Participate in some type of relaxation therapy
12. Participate in a regular aerobic exercise program. Initiate an exercise program gradually

ment, 1991; Naslund et al, 1990; Oberman et al, 1990). Other dietary considerations include adequacy of potassium, magnesium, and calcium intake; dietary fat intake; and limited use of alcohol (Table 24–2).

Weight Control

Weight loss is the most effective nonpharmacological intervention for reducing blood pressure in clients with mildly elevated diastolic blood pressure (Trials of Hypertension, 1992). Participation in weight control programs is more effective in attaining goals. A goal of being within 15% of IBW is realistic for these clients. Weight loss of >4.5 kg lowers blood pressure similar to pharmacological treatment and potentiates drug effects (Wassertheil-Smoller et al, 1992). In addition to a reduced kilocaloric intake, behavior modification and exercise should be an integral part of the program (see Chapter 11). Realistic kilocalorie levels should be identified for each client. Approximately 10 kcal/lb IBW is usually effective to promote weight loss; i.e., for a client whose IBW is 130 lbs, 1300 kcal/day would promote loss.

Sodium

A reduction in kilocalories usually results in a similar decrease in sodium intake. However, clients must be knowledgeable about natural sodium content of foods, the amount of sodium added to commercially prepared foods, and other sources of sodium.

The level of sodium restriction is determined by the physical condition and a client's ability to follow a diet (Table 24–3). A mild sodium restriction (2 to 3 gm/day) is effective in lowering blood pressure (Table 24–4). This is about one-third of the typical sodium intake. Reductions to 1 gm sodium or less are usually ineffective for further decreases in blood pressure. They may, however, be used on a short-term basis for clients with edema or severe CHF.

An order of "no extra salt" may be a significant decrease in sodium, especially for clients with excessive intakes. (The average American diet contains 6 to 15 gm sodium.) An intake of 4 gm (170 mEq) sodium per day can be achieved by avoiding salty foods and by not adding salt to food at the table; small amounts may be used in cooking. Suggestions for no-extra-salt diets are listed in Table 24–5.

Approximately 2 to 3 gm sodium (87 to 130 mEq) is allowed on a mild sodium restriction. Salt is not added at the table, but foods can be lightly salted in cooking. Foods high in salt are omitted: pickles, olives, bacon, ham, chips, canned soups, and salted nuts and crackers. Some prepared foods are limited or omitted.

In general, when sodium is restricted, all potential sources of sodium should be considered. Sodium is a natural constituent of most foods; animal foods such as meat, saltwater fish, eggs, dairy products, and some vegetables (beets, carrots, celery, spinach, and other dark-green leafy vegetables) contain appreciable amounts of sodium. They should be used in moderation. A generalized listing of the sodium content of foods is in Chapter 8, Table 8–3; for specific amounts of sodium content, see Appendix A–1.

Processed foods provide more than 77% of sodium intake (Mattes & Donnelly, 1991). Sodium bicarbonate and other sodium products are used as leavening agents. Sodium benzoate is a preservative in margarine and relishes; sodium citrate and monosodium glutamate are both flavor enhancers used in gelatin desserts, beverages, and meats. Thus, teaching clients to read labels is important for determining the amount of sodium added. Many low-sodium products are available. A product can be labeled low sodium if it contains less than 140 mg per serving and per 100 gm of food.

Some medications, such as antacids, add significant amounts of sodium, particularly when taken regularly and frequently (Table 24–6). Laxatives and cough medicines may also contain significant amounts of sodium. A pharmacist can help clients choose OTC products low in sodium.

Despite reduced-sodium diets being used so frequently, they are difficult to follow. The chief complaint is that they are bland and tasteless. Americans are accustomed to higher amounts of salt on foods and may be unaware of the myriad of spices other than salt (Table 24–7). If a high-salt intake has been established, sodium intake can gradually be decreased. The preferred salt level decreases after about 3 months of moderately lowered intake.

How much sodium is allowed on a mild sodium restriction? List foods that naturally have a high sodium content. What are some other sources of sodium listed on labels? What is the difference between no-extra-salt diet and a 2- to 3-gm sodium diet?

Urinary sodium output closely reflects sodium intake. A 24-hour urine specimen of a client on moderate salt restriction contains 90 to 120 mEq of sodium; with no sodium restriction, the specimen contains over 200 mEq. Reporting this sodium output to hypertensive clients is an effective motivational factor.

TABLE 24–3

LEVELS OF DIETARY SODIUM RESTRICTION

	Condition	Sodium Content mEq/day	Sodium Content mg/day
No added salt	Mild hypertension; mild fluid retention	174	4000
Mild restriction	Hypertension; cirrhosis with ascites	87	2000
Moderate restriction	Congestive heart failure	43	1000
Severe restriction	Congestive heart failure; cirrhosis with massive ascites	22	500

TABLE 24–4

COMPARISON OF THREE LEVELS OF LOW-SODIUM DIETS

Food Groups[1]	Serving Size	Average Natural Sodium Content per Serving (mg)	Number of Servings Allowed 500 mg*	1 gm (1000 mg)	2 gm (2000 mg)
Milk[2]	8 oz	120	2	2	2
Low-sodium milk	8 oz	7	Unlimited	Unlimited	Unlimited
Meats, fish, poultry, or low-sodium cheese[3]	1 oz	25	4	4	6
Egg	1	60	1	1	1
Regular breads and cereals[4a]	1 slice/¾ oz/ ½ cup	200	0	2	5
Low-sodium breads and cereals[4b]	1 slice/¾ oz/ ½ cup	5	7	7	4 or more
High-sodium vegetables[5a,b]	½ cup	50	0	1	Unlimited
Low-sodium vegetables[5c]	½ cup	9	2	2–4	Unlimited
Fruits[6]	Varies	2	Unlimited	Unlimited	Unlimited
Salted butter or margarine[7a]	1 tsp	50	0	2	6
Unsalted fats[7b]	1 tsp	5	5	Unlimited	Unlimited
Sweets[8]	Varies	2	Unlimited	Unlimited	Unlimited
Desserts[9]	Varies	20	0	1	Unlimited

* 500-mg diet is not recommended for longer than 2–3 days.

[1] No sodium is added to foods in cooking or at the table in the form of salt or sodium-containing flavor enhancers or additives.

[2] Exclude buttermilk, evaporated milk, condensed sweetened milk, malted milk, and milkshakes.

[3a] Include fresh or frozen meats (beef, lamb, pork, veal, game, poultry), unbreaded fish and shellfish, low-sodium canned tuna, salmon, or sardines, low-sodium cottage cheese and peanut butter, and dried beans and peas.

[3b] Exclude smoked, cured, salted, or canned meats, such as bacon, chipped beef, corned beef, luncheon meats or cold cuts, ham, hot dogs, sausage, sardines, anchovies, marinated herring, and pickled meats; eggs; regular hard or processed cheese; cheese spreads; regular peanut butter; canned tuna; and kosher meats, kidneys, brains.

[4a] Consists of regular whole-grain or enriched bread; regular biscuits, pancakes, cornbread, and waffles; graham crackers, unsalted crackers, and yeast doughnuts.

[4b] Consists of puffed rice, puffed wheat, shredded wheat, low-sodium cornflakes, unsalted popcorn, matzo; cooked cereals, rice, macaroni, noodles, and pastas cooked without salt; melba toast, low-sodium crackers.

[5a] Consists of artichoke, beets, carrots, celery, dark leafy greens (mustard, turnip, dandelion, kale, spinach), blackeyed peas, sweet potato.

[5b] Omit regular canned vegetables and vegetable juices, frozen peas, lima beans, mixed vegetables, and corn; frozen vegetables in sauce; sauerkraut, pickles, and other vegetables prepared in brine.

[5c] Consists of fresh, frozen, or canned without salt: asparagus, bean sprouts, broccoli, Brussels sprouts, cabbage, cauliflower, cucumbers, eggplant, green beans, green pepper, lettuce, mushrooms, okra, onions, potatoes, radishes, rhubarb, rutabaga, summer squash, tomatoes, zucchini, and low-sodium tomato and vegetable juices.

[6] Exclude dried fruit with sodium sulfite added, crystallized or glazed fruits, and maraschino cherries.

[7a] Includes cream cheese, salted butter, regular margarine, and mayonnaise-type salad dressing.

[7b] Includes vegetable oils, unsalted butter and margarine, nondairy coffee creamer, low-sodium mayonnaise, cream, and sour cream.

[8] Allow sugar, syrup, honey, jelly, marmalade, jam, hard candy and other sugar candies, molasses, marshmallows.

[9] Allow desserts made with plain gelatin and fruit juice or dietetic gelatin with no sodium added, unsalted bakery goods, ice cream, pudding and custard (made from milk and/or egg allowance), sherbet, water ice, flavored gelatin (limit to <1 cup/day).

Other tips:

Allowed beverages: Tea, coffee, lemonade, carbonated beverages (limit to 16 oz/day).

Many spices can be used. Exclude sauces and seasonings such as bouillon cubes; barbecue sauce; catsup; celery salt, seeds, or leaves; chili sauce; garlic salt; horseradish made with salt; meat extracts, sauces, and tenderizers; monosodium glutamate, prepared mustard; olives, onion salt; saccharin; soy sauce; Worcestershire sauce.

Potassium

Increasing intake of fresh fruits and vegetables is usually beneficial. These items are not only low in kilocalories and sodium, but also high in potassium and fiber. Increased potassium intake is advisable for most clients with hypertension

TABLE 24–5

GUIDELINES FOR NO EXTRA-SALT DIETS

The object of this restriction is to limit the amount of sodium intake to between 4–5 gm (170–220 mEq) daily by avoiding (1) foods that are concentrated sources of sodium and (2) adding salt to foods

1. Avoid adding salt to food at the table
2. Use small amounts of salt in food preparation: 1/4 tsp of salt/lb of meat; 1/8 tsp salt/serving of cooked cereal and vegetables
3. Avoid the following high-sodium processed foods:
   Meats: Smoked, cured, salted, or canned meats, fish, or poultry: bacon, chipped beef, corned beef, cold cuts, ham, frankfurters, and sausages; sardines, anchovies, marinated herring, pickled meats or eggs
   Dairy products: Processed cheese, roquefort, buttermilk
   Vegetables: Sauerkraut, pickled vegetables prepared in brine, commercially frozen vegetable mixes with sauces
   Breads and cereals: Breads, rolls, and crackers with salted tops
   Soups: Canned soups, dried soup mixes, broth, bouillon (except salt-free)
   Fats: Salad dressings containing bacon bits, salt pork, dips made with instant soup mixes, and processed cheese
   Beverages: Commercially softened water, cocoa mixes, club soda, Gatorade, tomato or vegetable juice
   Miscellaneous: Casserole and pasta mixes; salted chips, popcorn, and nuts; olives; commercial stuffing; gravy mixes; seasoning salts (garlic, celery, onion), lite salt, monosodium glutamate; meat tenderizer; catsup, prepared mustard, prepared horseradish, soy sauce

TABLE 24–6

CHECKING SODIUM IN MEDICATIONS

Over-the-Counter Drugs*

Some drugs contain large amounts of sodium. Make it a practice to read carefully the labels on all OTC drugs. Look at the ingredient list and warning statement to see if sodium is in the product. A statement of sodium content must appear on labels of antacids containing 5 mg sodium or more per dose unit (tablet, teaspoon). Some companies are now producing low-sodium OTC products. If in doubt after reading the label, ask a physician or pharmacist if the drug is appropriate

Prescription Drugs*

Consumers have no way of knowing whether a prescription drug contains sodium. Ask a physician or pharmacist about the sodium content of prescription drugs

Some Sodium Compounds Used in Drugs and Medicines†

Sodium Compound	***Product Type***
Sodium cloxacillin	Antibiotic
Sodium ampicillin	Antibiotic
Sodium pentobarbitol	Sedative (sleep aid)
Sodium sulfosuccinate	Laxative
Sodium sulfacetamide	Ophthalmic (eye) drug
Sodium bicarbonate	Antacid
Sodium salicylate	Analgesic (pain reliever)
Sodium citrate	Cough medicine
Sodium saccharin	Various medicines

* From *Salt, Sodium and Blood Pressure: Piecing Together the Puzzle.* Dallas, TX, American Heart Association, 1979.

† From *Straight Talk about Salt and Sodium in Your Diet.* Salt Institute, Alexandria, VA, 1989.

TABLE 24–7

SPICES TO COMPLEMENT FOODS

Food	Herb
Soups	Bay, French tarragon, marjoram, parsley, rosemary
Poultry	Garlic, oregano, rosemary, sage
Beef	Bay, chives, cloves, cumin, garlic, hot pepper, marjoram, rosemary
Lamb	Garlic, marjoram, oregano, rosemary, thyme (make little slits in lamb to be roasted and insert herbs)
Pork	Coriander, cumin, garlic, ginger, hot peper, pepper, sage, thyme
Cheese	Basil, chives, curry, dill, fennel, garlic, marjoram, oregano, parsley, sage, thyme
Fish	Dill, fennel, French tarragon, garlic, parsley, thyme
Fruit	Cinnamon, coriander, cloves, ginger, mint
Bread	Caraway, marjoram, oregano, poppy seed, rosemary, thyme
Vegetables	Basil, chives, dill, French tarragon, marjoram, mint, parsley, pepper, thyme
Salads	Basil, chives, French tarragon, garlic, parsley, rocket-salad, sorrel (these are best used fresh or added to salad dressing; otherwise, use herb vinegars for extra flavor)

Adapted from Shimizu HH. Do Yourself a Flavor. *FDA Consumer*. US Department of Health and Human Services. Pub No. 84–2192. 1984.

(Table 24–8); however, it should not be recommended to clients with abnormal renal function or taking drugs known to raise serum potassium levels, such as potassium-sparing diuretics and ACE inhibitors.

Potassium chloride may be partially substituted for sodium chloride in cooking and at the table. When clients use salt substitutes, this source of potassium can be significant and should be considered to prevent hyperkalemia. One teaspoon per day of a salt substitute supplies approximately 60 mEq of potassium. This is within the range of potassium supplementation usually prescribed. Other salt substitutes are available that may have more taste appeal (Table 24–9).

Which clients should be cautioned against increasing potassium intake?

Calcium

Adequate amounts of dairy products should be included in the diet. Even if cholesterol intake is restricted, avoidance of dairy products and possible dietary deficiency of calcium are undesirable. Calcium intake should be maintained at least at the RDA level of 800 mg/day (see Chapter 9, Table 9–2). If a client cannot tolerate dairy products, calcium supplements of 1 gm/day may reduce blood pressure.

Currently data are too limited to recommend supplementation of calcium, mag-

TABLE 24–8

GUIDELINES FOR INCREASING POTASSIUM INTAKE

1. Increase high-potassium fruits and vegetables: apricots, raisins, citrus fruits, bananas, tomatoes and tomato products, green leafy vegetables (broccoli, Brussels sprouts, parsley, spinach), carrots, potatoes (white and sweet), and corn
2. Use whole-grain products
3. Include adequate amounts of high-protein foods (2–3 cups of milk/milk products; 4–6 oz meat)
4. Use minimal amounts of water in cooking foods
5. Use all liquids from cooked fruits, vegetables, and meats in soups, gravies, or sauces
6. Use a potassium-containing salt substitute
7. Use an economical high-potassium, low-kilocalorie food supplement by combining vegetable scraps that are ordinarily discarded (e.g., carrot or potato peelings, celery stalks, outside pieces of lettuce, cabbage, and snipped ends from green beans). The use of parsley increases the potassium content. These are covered with water and simmered for about 1 hour before being strained and seasoned to taste. It can be served hot or cold or substituted for water in many recipes

TABLE 24–9

COMMERCIAL SALT SUBSTITUTES

Brand	Sodium (mg/tsp)	Potassium (mg/tsp)
Nu-Salt	0.17	528
NoSalt	< 10	2502
Seasoned NoSalt	< 5	1332
Morton Salt Substitute	trace	2790
Morton Lite Salt Mixture	1100	1466
Adolph's Salt Substitute	< 0.5	2580
Adolph's Seasoned Salt	trace	1750
Diamond Crystal	trace	2208
Co-Salt	trace	1964
Mrs. Dash, Original	4	38
Mrs. Dash, Extra Spicy	4	38
Mrs. Dash, Table Blend	4	30
Mrs. Dash, Lemon and Herb	4	49
Mrs. Dash, Garlic and Herb	4	128
Lite, Lite, Lite Papa Dash	360	trace
Salt Lover's Blend (Papa Dash)	960	trace

nesium, or any other electrolytes. A well-balanced diet using a variety of foods usually contains adequate amounts of these nutrients.

Alcohol

Alcohol consumption should be limited to 1 to 2 oz ethanol per day, if at all. This is equal to 1½ oz of 80-proof whiskey, 4 oz of table wine, or 12 oz of beer.

Fat

Because of the prevalence of CHD and obesity in clients with hypertension and undesirable effects of many prescribed medications, fat restriction is advisable, with emphasis on lowering total fat and saturated fat intake and increasing polyunsatu-

TABLE 24–10

OMEGA-3 FATTY ACID (EPA AND DHA) CONTENT OF FISH

Fish	Omega-3 Fatty Acid Content
Atlantic mackerel	2.5
King mackerel	2.2
Dogfish, spiny	1.9
Atlantic salmon	1.8
Chub mackerel	1.9
Pacific herring	1.7
Atlantic herring	1.6
Lake trout	1.6
Bluefin tuna	1.6
Atlantic sturgeon	1.5
Chinook salmon	1.4
Sablefish	1.4
Anchovy, European	1.4
Lake whitefish	1.3
Coho	1.2
Sockeye salmon	1.2
Atlantic bluefish	1.2
Sardines, canned	1.1
Chum salmon	1
Pink salmon	1

From Nettleton JA. w-3 fatty acids: Comparison of plant and seafood sources in human nutrition. *J Am Diet Assoc* 1991 March; 91(3):331–337.

rated fats. Currently the health benefits of fish oil have not been proven, but eating fish that is rich in omega-3 fatty acids may be encouraged (Table 24–10).

NURSING APPLICATIONS

Assessment

Physical—for height, weight, IBW, history of weight gain, waist-to-hip ratio; exercise; edema, BP and changes in BP with position changes; I&O, psychosocial (compliance) and environmental factors; use of OTC medications.

Dietary—for diet ordered, adequacy of intake, calcium and potassium intake, frequency of eating out; use of salt at the table, prepared foods, high-fat foods, alcohol; sodium content of water and fluid intake.

Laboratory—for sodium, potassium; cholesterol, triglyceride, calcium, magnesium, glucose, BUN; urinary calcium and sodium.

Interventions

1. Provide adequate amounts of sodium when requirements are increased. The normal sodium requirement for healthy adults is 200 to 250 mg sodium. With heavy perspiration and during lactation, requirement is increased. Even in these conditions, 2 gm sodium is sufficient to prevent hyponatremia.
2. Monitor elderly clients closely when antihypertensive medications or a low-sodium diet is initiated. Older clients are more sensitive to volume depletion and sympathetic inhibition secondary to impaired cardiovascular reflexes that make them more susceptible to orthostatic hypotension.
3. When a strict dietary restriction is imposed, monitor food intake because some clients, especially the elderly, have more difficulty adjusting to dietary changes. If food intake is severely curtailed as a result of the diet, other alternatives are preferable.
4. Encourage use of Weight Watchers, TOPS, support groups, and so forth.
5. Refer to dietitian if on sodium restriction.
6. Praise for dietary compliance and weight loss (if this is a goal).

Evaluation

* Of course, BP would decrease. Other desirable outcomes include the following: Client consumes recommended levels of potassium, sodium, calcium, and fat; maintains ideal body weight; verbalizes positive and negative feelings about diet; uses support groups.

Client Education

- Follow guidelines in Tables 24–2, 24–4, 24–5, 24–6, and 24–7.
- Teach rule of 6 S's to decrease salt intake: Avoid (1) soups (canned or freeze dried), (2) sauces, (3) snacks (processed), (4) smoked meats or fish, (5) sauerkraut, and (6) seasonings (horseradish, soy sauce, Worcestershire, lemon pepper) (Beare & Myers, 1990).
- Client experimentation with salt substitutes should be anticipated, and the life-threatening risks of hypokalemia or hyperkalemia should be discussed before a problem develops.
- Although a high-potassium diet probably inhibits the pressure-raising effect of sodium, a high-potassium intake poses a definite risk for those with compromised renal function.
- Sodium depletion does not usually result from dietary restriction alone but may occur in combination with excessive losses because of vomiting, diarrhea, surgery, or profuse perspiration from exercise or fever. Symptoms of hyponatremia include lethargy, muscle weakness and twitching, oliguria, mental confusion, anxiety, and hypotension, progressing to convulsions and altered levels of consciousness. Inform clients to notify physician if these symptoms occur.

Continued

- Hypertension cannot be cured, but it can be controlled.
- Refer to American Heart Association. Offer low-sodium cookbooks such as *Cooking Without Your Salt Shaker, Living With High Blood Pressure,* and *The Secrets of Salt-Free Cooking.*
- Diet therapy can be a worthwhile option when expenses or side effects of antihypertensive drug therapy become a serious problem.
- Although some studies have indicated that a small amount of alcohol may reduce risk of cardiovascular disease, hazards associated with alcohol consumption for the sole purpose of improving health definitely outweigh benefits.

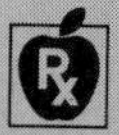
If a potassium-wasting diuretic is prescribed, encourage intake of high potassium-containing foods.

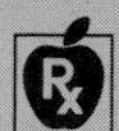
Clients taking diuretics for hypertension should be informed of beneficial effects of reducing sodium intake: (1) A modest but definite reduction of elevated blood pressure can be expected, (2) potassium supplements or relatively expensive potassium-sparing diuretics may not be necessary, and (3) antihypertensive effect of the diuretic is enhanced.

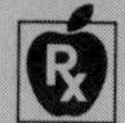
Clients receiving potassium-sparing diuretics and/or similar medications should be warned that they are likely to store potassium and not excrete it appropriately. Salt substitutes may cause hyperkalemia in these clients.

Refer to Table 24–1 for other information.

HYPERLIPIDEMIA

Hyperlipidemia is an elevation of major lipid components of lipoprotein particles as a result of one or more abnormalities of lipid metabolism or transport. In sporadic hyperlipidemia, there are no known genetic or secondary causes. In familial hyperlipidemia, the presence of this disorder in closely related family members indicates a genetic predisposition.

Primary **hyperlipidemia** (of unknown cause) is usually classified as **sporadic** or **familial.** Differentiation between primary and secondary hyperlipidemia is important because of differing treatment methods. Secondary causes of hyperlipidemia include weight gain in adults, pregnancy, high-carbohydrate/high-kilocalorie/high-saturated fat diets, alcohol excess, medications (steroids, thiazide, oral contraceptives), diabetes mellitus, hypothyroidism, nephrosis, chronic renal failure, obstructive jaundice, liver disease, or uremia. In contrast to primary hyperlipidemia, secondary hyperlipidemia may not require diet therapy; when possible, this condition is corrected by withdrawal of the drug or by treating the causative disease/condition.

Hyperlipidemia, or increased plasma levels of cholesterol and/or triglycerides, appears to be a major risk factor in CHD. Because of the prevalence of hyperlipidemia in the US and its role in CHD, a wide-scale cholesterol education program has been launched by the National Heart, Lung, and Blood Institute (NHLBI), National Institutes of Health (NIH), and the US Department of Health and Human Services (USDHHS). In 1989, the Report of the Expert Panel on Detection, Evaluation, and Treatment of High Blood Cholesterol in Adults was published, which established guidelines for detection and treatment (dietary and drug) of hyperlipidemia (USDHHS, 1989), as shown in Table 24–11.

Hypercholesterolemia—serum cholesterol levels over 200 mg/dl.

Based on many studies, including the Framingham Study (Dawber, 1980), **hypercholesterolemia** is a good predictor of the development of atherosclerosis. Results from a 10-year study called the Lipid Research Clinic's Coronary Primary Prevention Trial (LRC-CPPT) determined that CHD can be reduced in men at high risk for CHD by reducing serum cholesterol using diet and/or drugs. Therefore, the Consensus Development Panel (1985) concluded that (1) individuals with high-risk and moderate-risk blood cholesterol levels should be treated intensively by diet and/or drugs, and (2) all Americans should be advised to change dietary habits to lower blood cholesterol levels. This conclusion is in line with recommendations from the American Heart Association.

TABLE 24–11

TREATMENT RECOMMENDATIONS BASED ON TOTAL AND LOW-DENSITY LIPOPROTEIN CHOLESTEROL

	Cholesterol (mg/dl)		Recommendations		
Risk Category	*Total*	*Low-Density Lipoprotein*	*Diagnosis*	*Diet*	*Drugs*
Desirable	< 200	< 130	Remeasure in 5 years		
Borderline					
Without CHD or 2 other risk factors*	200–239	130–159	Recheck annually	Initiate Step-1 diet if LDL ≥ 130†	
With CHD or 2 other risk factors*				Initiate Step-1 diet if LDL > 130†	May initiate drug treatment
High					
Without CHD or 2 other risk factors*	≥ 240	≥ 160	Lipoprotein assay	Initiate Step-1 diet†	Initiate drug treatment if LDL ≥ 190
With CHD or 2 other risk factors*			Lipoprotein assay	Initiate Step-1 diet†	Initiate drug treatment if LDL ≥ 160

* Risk factors for increasing risk of developing coronary heart disease (CHD): (1) male sex, (2) family history of premature CHD (myocardial infarction or sudden death before age 55 of a parent or sibling), (3) cigarette smoking (> 10 cigarettes/day), (4) hypertension, (5) low HDL concentration (< 35 mg/dl), (6) diabetes mellitus, (7) history of cerebrovascular or occlusive peripheral vascular disease, and (8) severe obesity (> 30% overweight).

† The Step-1 diet is initiated first; blood lipid levels are measured and dietary compliance is assessed at 4 to 6 weeks and at 3 months. If the goals for blood lipids are met, no change is made. If the goals for the blood lipids have not been achieved, the client is referred to a registered dietitian for implementation of the Step-2 diet, which is followed by another reassessment after 4 to 6 weeks and 3 months.

Adapted from Report of the National Cholesterol Education Program Expert Panel on Detection, Evaluation and Treatment of High Blood Cholesterol in Adults. US Department of Health and Human Services, National Institutes of Health Pub No. 89–2925. Washington D.C., US Government Printing Office, 1989.

Risk Factors Related to Coronary Heart Disease and Hyperlipidemia

The principal risk factor associated with hyperlipidemia is elevated blood cholesterol and LDL levels. The Panel encouraged that everyone tested for blood cholesterol be assessed for other risk factors (see Table 24–11) with appropriate recommendations. Obvious risk factors include CHD, as defined by prior MI or ischemia such as angina pectoris. Heredity is a risk factor that cannot be controlled; however, individuals from families in which heart disease is common can follow a preventive diet. Diet can be manipulated to alter several of the risk factors: obesity, hyperlipidemia, and hypertension.

List risk factors for CHD.

Lipoproteins

Lipids are available to the body from the diet or can be synthesized by the liver and intestine. Lipids from dietary sources, breakdown of bile, or intestinal synthesis compose the exogenous lipid pathway; the endogenous pathway involves lipids synthesized by the liver.

Four different types of lipoproteins transport lipids in the blood; each contains triglycerides, **phospholipids,** and cholesterol bound to protein. The ratio of lipid to protein in serum lipoproteins varies widely, and these variations affect their density. As a rule, density increases as lipids decrease and the protein increases, i.e., HDLs,

Phospholipids—phosphorus combined with a lipid.

TABLE 24–12

CHARACTERISTICS OF LIPOPROTEINS

Types of Lipoprotein	Density	Protein	Cholesterol	Triglyceride	Source
Chylomicrons	Lowest density	Low	Low	Very high	Exogenous
Pre-beta-lipoproteins	Very low density	Low	Moderate	High	Principally endogenous
Beta-lipoproteins	Low density	Moderate	Very high	Low	Endogenous
Alpha-lipoproteins	High density	High	Moderate	Low	Endogenous

which are protective, contain larger amounts of protein and less lipid. Therefore, lipoproteins are classified according to their density and composition, as shown in Table 24–12. Phospholipids in lipoproteins are present in approximately the same proportions in all individuals.

Lipoproteins have different sources and functions even though they may be derived from one another in an interrelated process. Chylomicrons, formed in the intestine to transport recently absorbed dietary fat, carry some cholesterol to the liver and most of the triglycerides to peripheral tissues. **Hyperchylomicronemia** is a natural phenomenon dependent on the fat content of each meal. Normally hyperchylomicronemia peaks 3 to 4 hours after a fatty meal and is cleared within 12 to 14 hours.

Hyperchylomicronemia—high levels of chylomicrons in the blood.

VLDLs transport endogenously synthesized triglycerides for adipose tissue storage. VLDLs are primarily synthesized in the liver but can also be produced in the intestine. Lipoprotein lipase, an enzyme in peripheral tissues, releases fatty acids from chylomicrons or VLDL for muscle or adipose tissue to be used for energy or stored as fat.

Following triglyceride removal from VLDL and chylomicrons, a cholesterol-rich, intermediate-density lipoprotein (IDL) or VLDL remnant is left. IDL is a precursor of LDL and is believed to be **atherogenic.** The remaining cholesterol returns to the liver and is secreted into the intestine, mostly as bile acids, or it is changed into VLDL and recirculated.

Atherogenic—causing the formation or deposits of lipids within arteries.

LDL transports cholesterol chiefly to peripheral tissues, with some going to the liver. Approximately two-thirds of the LDL binds to LDL receptors in peripheral tissues or the liver, thus removing LDLs from circulation. The number of LDL receptors on cell membranes determines the amount of LDL degradation. In other words, the more receptors on cells, the more LDL is broken down. Anything that decreases the number or function of receptors, such as cholesterol, saturated fatty acid, or kilocaloric intake, increases the LDL level. Approximately 75% of total plasma cholesterol is in LDLs, which are believed to be atherogenic. Cholesterol transported by LDLs may infiltrate the arterial intima. Thus, a high serum LDL level is a positive risk factor for CHD.

Beta-adrenergic—specific sites on cells that respond to epinephrine.

Normally when the transport of LDL cholesterol to cells is elevated, the body regulates the cholesterol level by several mechanisms: Rate of endogenous cholesterol synthesis is reduced, cholesterol storage is increased, and manufacture of new LDL receptors is inhibited.

The most important but smallest group of lipoproteins is HDL. HDLs are available from hepatic and intestinal secretion and from breakdown of chylomicrons and VLDLs after triglyceride is removed. They contain moderate amounts of cholesterol. This cholesterol is being transported to the liver for catabolism and excretion and may have a protective effect against CHD.

Thus, elevated levels of HDL and low levels of LDL and serum cholesterol are believed to be the best preventive lipid profile for CHD (Table 24–13). HDL-cholesterol levels are not directly affected by diet. Major causes of low serum HDL-cholesterol levels are cigarette smoking, obesity, lack of exercise, medications (steroids and **beta-adrenergic** blocking agents), and genetic factors.

How is serum cholesterol regulated? Why is LDL the "bad cholesterol"? Differentiate between exogenous and endogenous pathways for lipid synthesis. What happens to lipoprotein density when the amount of lipids decreases and protein increases? What is the function of chylomicrons? What is the function of VLDL; LDL; HDL? How is IDL made? What are some causes of a low HDL? What will an increase in serum cholesterol cause; an increase in triglycerides?

Even though a high HDL level is generally considered beneficial, the protective effect of a high HDL in the face of high LDL is unknown. Generally increases in cholesterol are associated with an elevated LDL level and increases in triglyceride with a rise in VLDL.

Laboratory Tests

Total serum cholesterol is based on cholesterol in VLDL, LDL, and HDL. Lipoprotein analysis involves measuring fasting levels of total cholesterol, total triglyceride (TG), and HDL cholesterol. Cholesterol content of other lipoproteins is usually estimated by laboratories. Approximately 20% of the fasting triglyceride level (if less than 300 mg/dl) is VLDL. LDL cholesterol is estimated from the following equation:

$$\text{LDL cholesterol} = \text{total cholesterol} - \text{HDL cholesterol} - (\text{TG}/5)$$

Hepatic production of cholesterol, tissue LDL receptor activity, and sterol excretion require about a week to show changes. Thus, total cholesterol levels and HDL cholesterol are not affected by postprandial swings and do not require a fasting state.

Triglycerides are affected by fasting. Since the laboratory equation used to determine LDL cholesterol levels is based on triglyceride levels, a fasting state is required (Fraser, 1990). Cholesterol values fluctuate significantly even when fasting blood levels are used. Acute mental stress and orthostatic position elevate serum cholesterol concentrations, reflecting changes in fluid content of the blood (Muldoon et al, 1992). For an accurate assessment, several blood samples taken at the same time of day are checked. Levels considered to be high and low risk are shown in Table 24–13. Normal levels for triglycerides are 50 to 200 mg/dl.

Why is a fasting blood sample needed? What laboratory values indicate a high risk; a low risk?

Hyperlipoproteinemia

In 1967, Frederickson et al developed a system for classifying 5 types of **hyperlipoproteinemia** to distinguish individual causes and identify appropriate treatment (Table 24–14). In the past, dietary management of hyperlipoproteinemia has been based on this classification. The most prevalent hyperlipidemic profiles are type II or III. In recent years, nutritional treatment of all forms of hyperlipidemia has become more universal. Dietary recommendations are usually addressed by using the Step-1 or Step-2 diet (see section on nutritional care). Despite the cause of alteration, treatment is based on whether the cause is endogenous or exogenous and whether or not it is a primary factor or induced by secondary factors.

Hyperlipoproteinemia refers to specific high patterns of various plasma lipoproteins.

Nutritional Factors Affecting Serum Lipids

Numerous dietary factors are known to affect serum lipid levels. Thus, diet is believed to have direct effects on hyperlipidemia/hyperlipoproteinemia.

TABLE 24–13

DESIRABLE AND UNDESIRABLE LEVELS OF SERUM LIPIDS

Types of Serum Cholesterol	Low Risk (mg/dl)	High Risk (mg/dl)
Total cholesterol	< 200	≥ 240
High-density lipoprotein cholesterol	≥ 50	< 40
Low-density lipoprotein cholesterol	< 130	≥ 140

TABLE 24–14

HYPERLIPOPROTEINEMIA SUMMARY TABLE

Type and Prevalence	Cholesterol Level	Triglyceride Level	Signs and Symptoms	Coronary Heart Disease Risk	Therapeutic Diet
I—rare	++	++++	Abdominal pain Hepatosplenomegaly	Low	Low-fat diet (25–35 gm/day)
II—common	+++	+	Tendon xanthomas Accelerated atherosclerosis	Very high	Weight reduction Step-1 or Step-2 diet
III—fairly common	+++	+++	Accelerated atherosclerosis	Very high	Step-1 or Step-2 diet
IV—common	++	+++	Accelerated coronary atherosclerosis Abnormal glucose tolerance	High	Step-1 or Step-2 diet
V—uncommon	++	++++	Abdominal pain Hepatosplenomegaly Abnormal glucose tolerance	Low	Low-fat diet (25–35 gm/day) Limit Alcohol

Adapted from Frederickson DS, Levy RK. *Dietary Management of Hyperlipoproteinemia.* US Department of Health and Human Services No. (NIH) 75-110, Washington D.C., US Government Printing Office, 1974.

Cholesterol

Average cholesterol intake in the US is 450 mg/day. Approximately 60% of dietary cholesterol is absorbed. The body synthesizes approximately 2 to 4 times more cholesterol than it obtains from exogenous sources.

Unfortunately, the simple theory of lowering serum cholesterol by lowering dietary intake of cholesterol is not effective. Of all the dietary changes recommended, dietary cholesterol probably has the least effect on plasma cholesterol concentrations for most clients. This can be attributed to less endogenous cholesterol production in response to cholesterol absorption (Johnson & Greenland, 1990; Kestin et al, 1989; Miettenen & Kesaniemi, 1989).

Approximately 1 in 3 clients is sensitive to dietary cholesterol (McNamara et al, 1987). Reducing dietary cholesterol results in lower plasma cholesterol levels (VLDL and LDL) in these dietary cholesterol–sensitive individuals (Johnson & Greenland, 1990). This appears to be related to an inappropriate feedback mechanism to regulate endogenous cholesterol synthesis (increased cholesterol intake does not result in decreased synthesis).

Explain why lowering dietary cholesterol is not effective. What is the recommended intake of cholesterol?

The National Cholesterol Education Program has recommended a reduction of dietary cholesterol to less than 300 mg/day. For dietary cholesterol–sensitive clients, this reduction is associated with a 10 to 15% lower total plasma cholesterol concentration. In other words, a cholesterol level of 260 mg/dl is expected to decrease by 25 to 35 mg/dl. Clients who initially have a total plasma cholesterol level closer to normal levels are expected to have less effect from cholesterol restriction. Cholesterol levels of popular foods are listed in Table 24–15.

TABLE 24–15

FATTY ACID AND CHOLESTEROL CONTENT OF SELECTED FOOD

Food	Portion	Total Fat (gm)	Saturated Fatty Acids (gm)	Monounsaturated Fatty Acids (gm)	Polyunsaturated Fatty Acids (gm)	Cholesterol (mg)
Milk and Milk Products						
Cheddar cheese	1 oz	9.4	6	2.7	0.27	30
Monterey Jack cheese	1 oz	8.6	5.4	2.5	0.26	25
2% cottage cheese	½ cup	2.2	1.4	0.6	0.07	10
Cream cheese	1 oz	10	6.3	2.8	0.36	31
1% milk	1 cup	2.4	1.5	0.7	0.09	10
2% milk	1 cup	4.9	3	1.4	0.18	19
Whole milk	1 cup	8.1	5.1	2.4	0.30	33
Ice cream, 10% fat	1 cup	14.3	8.9	4.1	0.53	59
Meats, Fish, and Eggs						
Lean beef tenderloin	3 oz	8.6	3.2	3.2	0.32	71
Beef liver	3 oz	4.2	1.6	0.6	0.91	331
Skinless chicken breast	3 oz	3	0.9	1.1	0.65	72
Chicken breast (with skin)	3 oz	6.6	1.9	2.6	1.42	72
Skinless chicken thigh	3 oz	9.3	2.6	3.5	2.11	80
Lean pork chop	3 oz	13	4.5	5.8	1.59	81
Lean veal loin	3 oz	5.9	2.2	2.1	0.49	90
Canned salmon	3 oz	6.2	1.4	2.4	1.94	37
Cod fish	3 oz	0.7	0.1	0.1	0.25	47
Shrimp	3 oz	0.9	0.2	0.2	0.37	166
Whole egg	1	5.3	1.6	2.04	0.71	213
Egg white	1	0	0	0	0	0
Egg yolk	1	5.1	1.6	2	0.71	213
Fats and Oils						
Butter	1 tbsp	11.4	7.1	3.3	0.42	31
Half-and-half cream	¼ cup	7	4.3	2	0.26	22
Corn oil margarine, hard	1 tbsp	11.4	1.8	6.6	2.4	0
Corn oil margarine, soft	1 tbsp	11.4	2.1	4.5	4.5	0
Corn oil	1 tbsp	13.6	1.7	3.3	8	0
Vegetable shortening	1 tbsp	12.8	3.3	7.4	1.56	0
Mayonnaise-type salad dressing	1 tbsp	4.9	0.7	1.3	2.65	3.8

Nutrient data from Nutritionist III, version 7.0. N-Squared Computing, Salem, OR.

Type and Quantity of Dietary Fat

Currently the American diet contains approximately 40% of the total kilocalories as fat, with 17% of the fat from saturated fats (animal origin, palm oil, coconut oil, cocoa butter, hydrogenated margarine) and only 6% from PUFA. The remainder of ingested fat is derived from monounsaturated sources, such as olive, canola, and peanut oils, which may be significant in lowering cholesterol. Monounsaturated fats, previously believed to be neutral with respect to serum cholesterol levels, can effectively lower plasma LDL concentrations without reducing HDL-cholesterol levels (Ginsberg et al, 1990; Grundy, 1989; Mattson, 1989).

Most studies have found that reductions in total dietary fat lower serum cholesterol. Many of these studies have not controlled the type of fats used, and findings have not all been consistent. Because lower fat consumption generally coincides with decreased saturated fat intake, changes in blood lipids may be related more to type of fat consumed rather than total fat.

The general consensus of research indicates that fat quantity has less effect than quality or types of fatty acids on total cholesterol levels (Barr et al, 1992; Kris-Etherton et al, 1988). High saturated fat intake appears to suppress LDL receptor activity (Vega et al, 1991). A diet limited to 30% of the kilocalories from fat with a P/S ratio of 1 reduces total and LDL cholesterol concentrations in most hypercholesterolemic clients. Even small changes in the P/S ratio may have a general cholesterol-lowering effect. Long-term use of large quantities of PUFA is questionable. Therefore, saturated fatty acids are replaced partially with monounsaturated fatty acids and some PUFA, with an overall decrease in total fat (see Table 24–15). This results in LDL-cholesterol lowering without increasing plasma triglyceride concentrations and decreasing HDL concentrations (Grundy, 1990) and allows a more palatable diet that is better received by Americans.

PUFAs naturally occur in the "cis" configuration, i.e., the carbon chain bends so hydrogens stick out on the same side of the molecule. During processing, the groups rotate so they are on opposite sides of the bond, in the "trans" position.

During hydrogenation of oils to make shortening or "soft" margarines, the shape of the fatty acid is altered, resulting in **trans** fatty acids. Recently concerns have been raised about the effects of these trans fatty acids on CHD. Results of the Harvard Nurses' Health Study indicated that consumption of partially hydrogenated vegetable oils may increase the risk of CHD (Willett et al, 1993). However, further studies are needed to confirm these findings. Trans fatty acids are similar to oleic and stearic acids in their physical and chemical properties; neither oleic nor stearic acids appear to be hypercholesterolemic (Denke & Grundy, 1991).

One of the newer areas being intensively investigated is omega-3 fatty acids. Eicosapentaenoic acid (EPA) and docosahexaenoic acid (DHA) are omega-3 fatty acids that occur in fish lipid. Greenland Eskimos and British Columbian coastal Indians consume large amounts of fatty fish; low rates of CHD are observed in these populations. Although all deep-sea, cold-water species of fish and some that live in cold fresh water have some EPA, amounts vary with seasons and diet of the fish (see Table 24–10).

Like vegetable oils (corn, safflower, and sunflower) that contain omega-6 fatty acids, fish oils rich in omega-3 fatty acids significantly lower triglyceride levels (as much as 30%) when substituted for saturated fatty acids (Davidson et al, 1991; Green et al, 1990; Harris et al, 1990). Response of LDL is variable (Davidson et al, 1991; Kestin et al, 1990b). Habitual EPA intake more closely correlates with lower triglyceride and higher HDL levels than DHA (Bonaa et al, 1992). However, benefits may be principally due to the changes in plasma viscosity and effects on blood platelets and other blood-clotting mechanisms (Green et al, 1990). High dietary levels of omega-3 fatty acids prolong bleeding time as a result of altered prostaglandin synthesis (London et al, 1991).

Thus, 3 meals weekly containing fish and shellfish with high levels of EPA are recommended. Increasing fish intake may have other benefits by decreasing animal protein and saturated fatty acid intake.

Tropical oils or palm and coconut oils are known to increase plasma LDL concentrations. The recent movement to change the type of oil used in manufacturing processed foods is commendable. However, only about 2% of overall fat intake is from these oils. Its removal from the diet will have little impact on average plasma cholesterol concentration.

Explain the benefits of monounsaturated fats and omega-3 fatty acids.

Kilocalorie Level

Obesity, especially upper body obesity, is often associated with increased rates of cholesterol, elevated VLDL levels (as a result of overproduction and reduced catabolism of triglycerides), and low concentrations of plasma HDL, in addition to other risk factors for CHD (Thompson et al, 1991; Wing et al, 1991; Manson et al, 1990). There is a linear correlation between body weight and hepatic VLDL production, i.e., with overweight, hepatic VLDL production is high.

When a client loses weight, what happens to VLDLs?

Weight reduction is usually associated with an increase in plasma HDL concentration and improved lipoprotein profile. Although kilocaloric restriction to normalize body weight is an ideal goal, loss to IBW may not be necessary to correct hyperlipidemia.

Fiber

Some plant fibers, especially soluble carbohydrates (pectin, guar gum, carrageenan, or oat bran) found in apples, citrus fruit, legumes, oats, and barley, can have significant hypocholesterolemic effects, with a reduction in plasma LDL concentration and a rise or no change in plasma HDL (Ripsin et al, 1992; Whyte et al, 1992; McIntosh et al, 1991). Mechanisms involved are not clearly established. These substances may bind with bile acids, leading to a reduction in both plasma LDL and hepatic cholesterol availability.

Decreased serum cholesterol levels are more pronounced in hypercholesterolemic clients. Total plasma cholesterol levels have been lowered by 6 to 19% when 15 to 45 gm of soluble fiber was added (Kris-Etherton, 1988). Psyllium hydrophilic mucilloid, a soluble fiber added to cereal and used as a laxative (Metamucil), also reduces serum cholesterol (Anderson et al, 1992; Anderson et al, 1991).

In studies using insoluble fibers (alfalfa, wheat bran, or cellulose), no hypocholesterolemic effect is seen (Kashtan et al, 1992; Whyte et al, 1992). However, insoluble fiber may reduce constipation and should also be increased in the diet.

What are sources for soluble and insoluble fibers? Which fiber lowers cholesterol levels?

Carbohydrates

Triglyceride levels and CHD are consistently lower among populations who habitually consume a high percentage of kilocalories as carbohydrates. A transient rise in basal triglyceride levels is reported on high carbohydrate diets, but within 2 weeks, triglyceride levels (even in some clients with hypertriglyceridemia) spontaneously return to lower than basal levels. Thus, a higher percentage of total kilocalories from carbohydrate is probably desirable, even in clients with hypertriglyceridemia. Beneficial side effects of complex carbohydrates are increased levels of fiber and lower total fat intake.

List benefits of high-carbohydrate diets.

Dietary Antioxidants

Oxidation of LDL cholesterol within the arterial wall may be a contributing factor to the atherogenic effect. Diets high in monounsaturated fatty acids can cause LDL cholesterol to be less susceptible to oxidation than diets high in PUFA (Berry et al, 1991; Steinberg, 1990). The role of dietary antioxidants, selenium, beta-carotene, and vitamins E and C, is being studied. Vitamin E is carried in LDL and can retard LDL oxidation (Esterbauer et al, 1991; Gey et al, 1991). Ascorbic acid is able to protect lipids in plasma and LDL against oxidative damage and has been demonstrated as being more potent for preventing oxidation of LDL cholesterol than vitamin E and beta-carotene (Frei, 1991; Jialal et al, 1990). While studies continue to probe the role of food antioxidants in heart disease, the recommendation is to encourage intake of more fruits and vegetables (natural sources of antioxidants).

Alcohol

On the one hand, light to moderate alcohol consumption (2 drinks a day) is associated with an increase in HDL and may be protective against CHD (Suh et al, 1992; Jackson et al, 1991). On the other hand, high alcohol intake causes hypertriglyceridemia. A level of 1 to 2 drinks a day may have an important CHD risk-reduction effect, but the overall balance of harm and benefit does not favor a recommendation to drink alcohol to prevent CHD. If a client is trying to lose weight, alcohol contributes empty kilocalories to the diet, making weight loss harder to achieve.

Garlic

Many cultures have used garlic as a medicinal treatment for CHD. Evidence suggests that use of certain formulations of garlic is accompanied by favorable effects on coagulation, platelet aggregation, vasodilatation, and serum lipid concentrations (Mansell & Reckless, 1991). A controlled study performed in India resulted in decreased mortality rates and lower reinfarction rates and cholesterol levels in postinfarction clients (Garlic, 1991). Large doses of fresh garlic (7 to 28 cloves a day) had beneficial effects on cardiovascular risk factors, but the effects of commercial preparations were questionable (Kleijinen et al, 1989). This may be attributed to loss of active ingredients in processing. A major side effect of garlic is a detectable aroma caused by **allicin.** Although actual commercial preparations may be odorless, if allicin is released, there is substantial risk of a detectable odor. The role of garlic in hyperlipidemia warrants further investigation.

Allicin—the principal active agent of garlic.

Coffee

Analysis of data from research studying the effects of coffee on cholesterol are conflicting and controversial (Burke, 1991). Therefore, it may be wise to recommend a moderate coffee intake (fewer than 4 cups/day) until further research is more definitive.

Management

Approximately 60 million Americans are believed to need medical advice and intervention to treat hyperlipidemia (Sempos et al, 1989). Treatment is based on levels of cholesterol/LDL and the presence of identifiable risk factors. Dietary treatment is the initial therapy to lower LDL cholesterol (see section on Nutritional Care). Regular exercise (3 to 4 times/week) at intensities as low as 40 to 50% of maximal heart rate for 20 to 60 minutes is also encouraged to enhance improvement in plasma lipoprotein levels (Bankhead, 1991; Wood et al, 1991). If dietary changes are not effective in lowering serum cholesterol levels within 6 months or if LDL cholesterol levels are extremely high, drug treatment is recommended.

Bile acid sequestrants (cholestyramine and colestipol) have been used to lower LDL cholesterol levels. These bind with bile acids in the intestine, interrupting enterohepatic circulation of bile acids. Thus, hepatic synthesis of bile acids from cholesterol is increased. Bile acid sequestrants tend to increase triglyceride levels.

Nicotinic acid (a form of niacin) lowers total and LDL cholesterol and triglycerides and raises HDL cholesterol levels. Nicotinic acid is the preferred medication for clients with triglycerides >250 mg/dl.

Lovastatin inhibits biosynthesis of cholesterol and has shown a 25 to 45% reduction in LDL. Long-term effects on CHD have not been determined.

Gemfibrozil is used to lower triglyceride levels to reduce risk of pancreatitis and is not routinely used to reduce the risk of CHD. Probucol may function as an antioxidant to inhibit the oxidation of LDL and also reduce LDL. However, HDL may also be reduced. Nutritional implications for medications are shown in Table 24–16.

What are some drugs used to treat hyperlipidemia? What is the effect of each type?

Nutritional Care

Ideally dietary changes effect lower levels of LDL. The National Cholesterol Education Program has recommended a 2-step approach to diet therapy to reduce intake of saturated fatty acids and cholesterol gradually and promote weight loss in clients who are overweight (Table 24–17). These diets are nutritionally adequate and use readily available foods. They are based on healthy eating patterns, and the goal is to achieve a permanent change in eating behavior.

TABLE 24–16

COMMONLY USED DRUGS TO TREAT HYPERLIPIDEMIA

Drugs	Nutritional Implications
Bile acid sequestrants	
Cholestyramine (Questran) Colestipol (Colestid)	Take with water or milk. Low-fat, low-cholesterol diet recommended. Increase fluid and fiber to promote normal bowel function. Long-term intake may cause folate depletion and depletion of fat-soluble vitamins due to malabsorption. Take with food and cold liquids
Nicotinic acid	Low-fat, low-cholesterol diet recommended. May cause hyperglycemia and hyperuricemia, edema, and GI disturbances (nausea and vomiting, flatulence)
HMG-CoA reductase Lovastatin (Mevacor) Pravastatin (Pravachol) Simvastatin (Zocor)	To enhance effect, take with evening meal. Low-fat, low-cholesterol diet recommended. May cause GI disturbances (flatulence, abdominal pain, diarrhea)
Gemfibrozil (Lopid)	Take 30 minutes before meals. Low-fat, low-cholesterol diet is important. May cause GI disturbances (diarrhea, abdominal pain, dyspepsia, nausea and vomiting)
Clofibrate (Atromid-S)	Fatty foods promote drug absorption but may cause nausea, vomiting, and abdominal gas. Increases anti–vitamin K effect of warfarin. May cause weight gain. May have unpleasant taste sensation. Decreases absorption of glucose, iron, electrolytes, and vitamin B_{12}.
Probucol (Lorelco)	Take with food to enhance absorption. Low-fat, low-cholesterol, low-kilocalorie diet recommended. May cause GI upset (nausea, vomiting, bloating)

Data from Roe DA. *Drug and Nutrient Interactions: A Problem-Oriented Reference Guide.* 4th ed. Chicago, The American Dietetic Association, 1989; Allen AM. *Food Medication Interactions.* 7th ed. Pottstown, PA, Ann Moore Allen, 1991.

The Step-1 diet is normally prescribed by physicians and/or their staff (Table 24–18). Major obvious sources of saturated fats and cholesterol are reduced and can be achieved without a radical alteration in dietary habits. Serum cholesterol level is remeasured at 4 to 6 weeks and at 3 months after initiating this diet.

If the Step-1 diet is not effective in lowering serum cholesterol, the client is referred to a registered dietitian for adoption of the Step-2 diet. On this diet, an evaluation of overall eating patterns is necessary to reduce intake of saturated fatty acids and cholesterol to minimal levels (see Table 24–18) while maintaining adequate nutrients (Retzlaff et al, 1991). Even if drug therapy is initiated, diet therapy should be continued to enhance effectiveness of the medication.

What is the current recommendation regarding treatment of hyperlipidemia?

TABLE 24–17

DIETARY THERAPY OF HIGH BLOOD CHOLESTEROL

Nutrient	Recommended Intake		
	Step-1		***Step-2***
Total fat	30% of kcal		< 30% of kcal
Saturated fat	< 10% of kcal		< 7% of kcal
Polyunsaturated fatty acids		Up to 10% of total kcal	
Monounsaturated fatty acids		10–15% of total kcal	
Cholesterol	< 300 mg		< 200 mg
Carbohydrates		50 to 60% of total kcal	
Protein		10 to 20% of total kcal	
Total kilocalories		To achieve and maintain desirable weight	

From National Cholesterol Education Program Expert Panel on Detection, Evaluation, and Treatment of High Blood Cholesterol in Adults. US Department of Health and Human Services, Public Health Service, NIH Publication. Pub No. 89-2925. Washington, D.C., US Government Printing Office, 1989.

TABLE 24–18

RECOMMENDED DIET MODIFICATIONS TO LOWER BLOOD CHOLESTEROL: GUIDELINES FOR STEP-1 AND STEP-2 DIETS

Food Group and Servings per Day/Week	Choose	Decrease
Meat, Poultry, Fish, and Shellfish Step-1—6 oz/day Step-2—6 oz/day	***Lean cuts*** of meat with fat trimmed: beef—round, sirloin, chuck, loin; lamb—leg, arm, loin, rib; pork—tenderloin, leg, shoulder (arm or picnic); veal—all trimmed cuts except ground Poultry without skin Fish, shellfish	"Prime" grade ***Fatty cuts*** of meat: beef—corned beef, brisket, regular ground, short ribs; pork—spareribs, blade roll Goose, domestic duck Organ meats: liver, kidney, sweetbread, brain Sausage, bacon Regular luncheon meats Frankfurters Caviar, roe
Eggs Step-1—3 yolks/week Step-2—1 yolk/week	Egg whites Cholesterol-free egg substitutes	Egg yolks
Breads, Cereals, Pasta, Rice, Dried Peas, and Beans Step-1—4–7 servings/day* Step-2—5–8 servings/day*	Breads: whole wheat, pumpernickel, rye, and white breads; pita; bagels; English muffins; sandwich buns; dinner rolls; rice cakes	Croissants, butter rolls, sweet rolls, Danish pastry, doughnuts
	Low-fat crackers: matzo, bread sticks, rye krisp, saltines, zwieback	Most snack crackers: cheese crackers, butter crackers, those made with saturated fats
	Hot cereals; most cold dry cereals	Granola-type cereals made with saturated fats
	Pasta: plain noodles, spaghetti, macaroni Any grain rice Dried peas and beans: split peas, blackeyed peas, chick peas, kidney beans, navy beans, lentils, soybeans, soybean curd (tofu)	Pasta and rice prepared with cream, butter, or cheese sauces; egg noodles
Dairy Products Step-1—3 servings/day Step-2—2 servings/day	Skim milk, 1% milk, cultured buttermilk, evaporated skim or nonfat milk Low-fat yogurt and low-fat frozen yogurt Low-fat soft cheeses: cottage, farmer, pot cheeses labeled no more than 2 to 6 gm fat/oz	Whole milk: regular, evaporated, condensed Cream, half-and-half, most nondairy creamers and products, real or nondairy whipped cream Cream cheese Ice cream Sour cream Custard-style yogurt Whole-milk ricotta High-fat cheeses: Neufchatel, Brie, Swiss, American mozzarella, feta, cheddar, muenster
Fruits and Vegetables Step-1—3 fruit/4 vegetable servings/day Step-2—3 fruit/4 vegetable servings/day	Fresh, frozen, canned, or dried fruits and vegetables	Vegetables prepared in butter, cream, or sauce
Sweets and Snacks Step-1—2 servings/day Step-2—2 servings/day	Low-fat frozen desserts: sherbet, sorbet, Italian ice, frozen yogurt, Popsicles Low-fat cakes: angel food cake Low-fat cookies: fig bars, gingersnaps	High-fat frozen desserts: ice cream, frozen tofu High-fat cakes: most store-bought, pound, and frosted cakes Store-bought pies Most store-bought cookies

TABLE 24–18

RECOMMENDED DIET MODIFICATIONS TO LOWER BLOOD CHOLESTEROL: GUIDELINES FOR STEP-1 AND STEP-2 DIETS *Continued*

Food Group and Servings per Day/Week	Choose	Decrease
	Low-fat candy: jelly beans, hard candy Low-fat snacks: plain popcorn, pretzels Nonfat beverages: carbonated drinks, juices, tea, coffee	Most candy, like chocolate bars Potato and corn chips prepared with saturated fat Buttered popcorn High-fat beverages, like frappes, milkshakes, floats, and eggnogs
Fats and Oils Step-1—4–6 servings/day* Step-2—5–7 servings/day*	Unsaturated vegetable oils: corn, olive, peanut, rapeseed (canola oil), safflower, sesame, soybean Margarine or shortening made with unsaturated fats: liquid, tub, stick, diet Mayonnaise, salad dressings made with unsaturated fats Low-fat dressings	Saturated oils and fat: butter, coconut oil, palm kernel oil, palm oil, lard, bacon fat Margarine or shortening made with saturated fats Dressings made with egg yolk

* Variations in quantity reflect different kilocaloric intake—1600 or 2000 kcal/day.

Adapted from National Cholesterol Education Program. *Step to the Beat of a Healthy Heart: Lower Your High Blood Cholesterol.* US Department of Health and Human Services, National Heart, Lung, and Blood Institute. Serving sizes taken from *Dietary Treatment of Hypercholesterolemia: A Handbook for Counselors,* published by the American Heart Association in cooperation with the National Heart, Lung, and Blood Institute, 1988.

Other factors discussed earlier under the dietary factors have not been addressed, as it is premature to implement all of them at this time because of lack of scientific evidence.

NURSING APPLICATIONS

Assessment

Physical—for height, weight, IBW, waist-to-hip ratio; BP, presence of xanthomas, smoking habits, occupation.

Dietary—for dietary pattern, intake of saturated fat, PUFA, cholesterol, kilocalories, fiber, garlic, alcohol.

Laboratory—for cholesterol, fasting triglyceride, HDL/LDL; uric acid, BUN, sodium, potassium, magnesium, calcium.

Interventions

1. Encourage a diet of 30% fat, 55% carbohydrates, and 15% protein.
2. Involve the person who will be purchasing and cooking meals in diet modification care and education. Use specific examples and food models to demonstrate portion sizes.
3. Monitor intake of fat-soluble vitamins, calcium, and iron. Intake may be severely curtailed on a low-fat, low-cholesterol diet unless appropriate substitutes are made.
4. If serum lipids do not decrease after dietary counseling, monitor compliance.
5. Allow for gradual, progressive changes in diet, i.e., client can mix low-fat and whole milk in increasing proportions so that eventually only low-fat milk is being drunk. This practice can also be used with other foods (Burke, 1991).
6. Encourage spouse participation in nutritional care.
7. Refer to dietitian if the Step-2 diet is needed.
8. Provide support and praise, as these diets need to be life-long habits.

Continued

9. Problem solve possible situations that may provoke a relapse in diet, i.e., eating out, eating when stressed, lack of support from significant others, making wise menu selections, snacking, food preparation (Hadley & Saarmann, 1991).

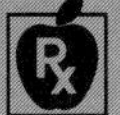

Anabolic steroids are atherogenic because of their effect on lipoproteins; LDL levels are elevated and HDL levels are depressed (Glazer, 1991).

Evaluation

* Desired outcomes include triglyceride and cholesterol levels below 200 mg/dl, IBW is maintained, appropriate diet is consumed, and exercise is performed 3 times a week.

Client Education

- Do not completely eliminate meat (including beef) from the diet. Eat 6 oz meat, poultry, and fish a day. Using food models, show clients this portion size (Burke, 1991).
- Cholesterol is found only in foods from animal sources.
- To help clients remember the difference between HDLs and LDLs, explain HDL means *h*ealthy and LDL means *l*ousy. Keep cholesterol level below 200 mg/dl.
- Family members with all types of hereditary hyperlipidemia should be screened for premature CHD and encouraged to adopt preventive treatment early in life.
- Low-fat diets may seem dry and unpalatable to clients accustomed to high-fat intakes. Discuss new ideas for moistening foods without adding fat, i.e., the use of jellies, low-fat yogurt, fat-free gravy, and so forth.
- Discuss food sources of saturated fats, PUFAs, and cholesterol. Assist client in making suitable substitutions.
- Explain how to read labels so client can decrease saturated and total fat and increase PUFA in the diet (see Chapter 1, Fig. 1–5).
- To increase PUFA content of the diet, safflower-containing oils and margarines are necessary (Smith-Schneider et al, 1992).
- Discuss kilocalorie-controlled diets, if indicated, and how to change eating habits.
- Discuss types of lipoproteins and their meaning to CHD.
- Explain how to prepare foods (use stir fry, broiling, steaming, baking) and make wise food choices at restaurants (consider method of preparation, fruit, vegetable plate, sherbet, and so forth) (Hadley & Saarmann, 1991).
- During pregnancy, serum lipids are increased markedly. Serum cholesterol levels should be monitored and prophylactic measures enacted to maintain the level close to 220 mg/dl. Careful food choices can ensure nutrient needs.

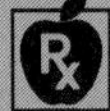

If taking Questran or Colestid, give 1 hour before other drugs or 2 to 4 hours after meal ingestion. If client is hypertriglyceridemic, consult with physician to discontinue these drugs.

CONGESTIVE HEART FAILURE

Causes and Physical Consequences

In CHF, the reduced pumping capacity of the heart is unable to maintain adequate blood circulation to supply the body's oxygen needs.

Congestive heart failure (CHF) can be caused by CHD, lung disease, severe anemia, hypothyroidism, or diseases that affect the myocardium or other cardiac structures. Decreased cardiac output results in less blood flow through the kidney. Tubular resorption of sodium is increased, and more water is retained.

Symptoms associated with CHF, such as anorexia, nausea, a feeling of fullness, shortness of breath and fatigue from eating, and abdominal pain, cause a decrease in food intake. Unpalatability of a sodium-restricted diet may also detrimentally affect intake (Belmin, 1992). Clients often lose lean body mass and are undernourished. Loss of lean tissue may be detrimental, but this is somewhat protective as a result of reduced oxygen requirement and circulating fluid volume (Heymsfield & Casper, 1989). Weight loss is also related to impaired delivery of oxygen and nutrients to body tissues and possibly to increased energy expenditure (Heymsfield & Casper, 1989).

Severe malnutrition or **cardiac cachexia** is frequently observed in advanced CHF. It is not clear why this condition occurs, but it may be related to poor intake that is due to factors already discussed and elevated BMR that is due to increased cardiac and pulmonary functions. Other factors that need to be considered are depression, weakness, pain, sedation, and side effects of medications. For instance, diuretics contribute to zinc excretion, which may cause **hypogeusia** and **hyposmia.**

Cardiac cachexia is a life-threatening condition with severe muscle and fat loss related to cardiac disorders.

Hypogeusia—diminished sensitivity to taste.
Hyposmia—diminished sensitivity to odors.

How does CHF affect nutrition?

Management

The primary objective in treatment of CHF is to reduce the work load of the heart and promote diuresis. An important therapeutic component is diet management. Additionally, important advances in therapy include the use of combined diuretic therapy, digitalis, and ACE inhibitors. ACE inhibitors can relieve symptoms and prolong life (Arai & Greenberg, 1990).

Nutritional Care

Restricting sodium intake reduces the cardiac work load by decreasing extracellular fluids. A low-salt diet, generally with a limitation of 1.5 to 3 gm sodium/day, may be prescribed. In severe conditions in a hospital setting, the sodium restriction may be 500 to 1000 mg. As the edema is controlled, sodium restriction may be raised to improve meal acceptance.

Generally moderate sodium restriction (1 gm sodium) is achieved by removing most high-sodium foods and not adding salt at the table or in cooking (see Table 24–4). This diet is more difficult for many persons to follow because many canned or processed foods (vegetables and meats) containing added salt are omitted. Four servings of regular bread are allowed (salt-free bread is not limited). Vegetables and other foods containing naturally high amounts of sodium are restricted; meat and milk products are used in moderation. Although this diet is more difficult for an individual to follow at home, compliance is better than for a severely restricted diet.

Severe restriction, or about 500 mg (33 mEq) of sodium, may be impractical for clients to achieve. In addition to items that must be omitted, milk is limited to 2 cups/day, meat to a total of 5 or 6 oz, and no more than 1 egg. Salt-free margarine is used, and high-sodium vegetables are omitted (see Table 24–4).

Because water may account for up to 10% of a client's daily sodium consumption, sodium content of drinking water is especially important for clients on severe sodium restriction. Approximately 42% of the nation's water supplies contain sodium in excess of the optimal level. A maximum of 20 mg of sodium per liter or quart of water is advisable for clients who require a low-sodium diet because of heart or kidney diseases. Consumption of 2 L of fluid (water or water-based liquids such as coffee or tea) containing 270 mg/L of sodium provides 540 mg sodium from this basic fluid. This is more than half of a 1-gm sodium diet. If assessment indicates a fluid intake in this range of high sodium-containing water, bottled water may be required.

Several small meals are provided to avoid excessive stress and exertion by the heart. Caffeine and alcohol intake is controversial. They may provoke cardiac arrhythmia, a common hazard under these conditions. The amount of kilocalories furnished must be individualized. For overweight clients, weight loss is essential.

Increasing kilocalorie intake may be indicated for malnourished clients. Enteral feedings may be used to promote anabolism and improve lean muscle mass in clients with cardiac cachexia (Heymsfield & Casper, 1989). Enteral feedings should be started as soon as it is recognized that clients are unable to consume adequate nutrients from oral intake. In the presence of malnutrition, feedings are initiated slowly to prevent pulmonary edema. Fluid and sodium restrictions require an enteral formula that is kilocalorie dense (1.5 to 2 kcal/ml) and low in sodium. Excess extracellular fluid diuresis may result in weight loss when feedings are begun, but clients soon establish a state of anabolism if adequate kilocalories are provided (1.1 to 1.8 BEE) (Heymsfield & Casper, 1989). Excessive kilocalories are avoided to prevent any additional stress on the heart and decrease oxygen requirements.

What guidelines should be followed on a 1-gm sodium diet? What foods must be limited on a 500-mg diet?

NURSING APPLICATIONS

Assessment

Physical—for height, weight, IBW, weight loss; edema, BP, I&O, elevated temperature, cardiac assessment.

Dietary—for acceptance of low-sodium diet, anorexia, potassium intake.

Laboratory—for BUN, creatinine, albumin, prealbumin; lipoprotein profile; glucose, PT; sodium, potassium, chloride; Hgb, Hct; nitrogen balance, GFR.

Interventions

1. Provide adequate potassium to replace potassium losses.
2. Provide 5 or 6 small feedings a day to avoid stomach distention and subsequent diaphragm depression and increased cardiac work load.
3. Limit fluid intake, as ordered.
4. If ordered, restrict caffeine intake.
5. Encourage a soft-type diet to lessen heartburn, distention, and flatulence and to reduce the amount of chewing.

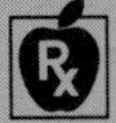
Salt substitutes may contain potassium. Avoid them if potassium-sparing diuretics or ACE inhibitors are prescribed.

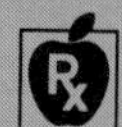
If digoxin is prescribed, give 1 hour before or 2 hours after meals, and provide high-potassium foods to prevent hypokalemia, which predisposes clients to digitalis toxicity. Absorption of digoxin is slowed by high-fiber foods, so avoid providing this medication when high-fiber food, i.e., bran cereal, is eaten.

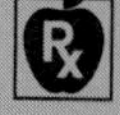
Digoxin may increase risk of weight loss when the diet is hypokilocaloric or low in potassium. Digitalis toxicity may cause anorexia and nausea, which may interfere with food intake and cause weight loss.

Evaluation

* Client should faithfully consume the sodium-restricted diet as ordered.

Client Education

- Explain the low-sodium diet and its importance (see Table 24–4). (Sodium retains water, making the heart pump harder.)
- If client experiences a sudden weight gain of 1 to 2 lbs in 1 day or gains 5 lbs within a week, the physician should be notified (Nagelhout, 1991).
- Spices rather than salt can improve palatability of the diet (see Table 24–7).
- Refer to American Heart Association and low-sodium cookbooks previously mentioned.

ACUTE MYOCARDIAL INFARCTION

Approximately 1.5 million Americans suffer a **myocardial infarction (MI)** each year, resulting in approximately 300,000 coronary bypass surgeries annually (AHA, 1990). Medical costs for 5 years following an acute MI are over $50,000 (Task Force, 1990). Reductions in death rates from acute MIs are attributable to efforts in primary prevention (smoking cessation, reduction in serum cholesterol, treatment of hypertension, and so forth) and improved therapies (Manson et al, 1992).

MI, commonly called a heart attack, is the occlusion of a coronary artery in the heart muscle. Oxygen deprivation results in necrosis (death) in the area affected.

Management

Initially following an MI, clients are placed on bed rest to reduce the work load of the heart. Measures are taken to prevent arrhythmias and heart stimulation and avoid constipation and flatulence. Aspirin affects the tendency of platelet aggregation and may be used to prevent **restenosis.** Aspirin is a gastric irritant and may cause occult bleeding.

Restenosis—recurrent narrowing of blood through blood vessels.

Anticoagulant medications, such as coumadin or heparin, may be given to prevent blood clots. Additionally, clients may be on antihypertensive, antiarrhythmic, and hypocholesterolemic medications, as needed.

Nutritional Care

Initially a liquid diet may be used to lessen the risk of aspiration or vomiting that may occur. Caffeine-containing foods should be reduced/omitted, as ordered by the physician, to prevent potential arrhythmias. As treatment progresses, soft, easily digested foods are provided. Small frequent feedings reduce cardiac work load but should provide a minimum of 1000 to 1200 kcal daily (Bagatell & Heymsfield, 1984). Gas-forming foods are omitted to prevent flatulence and distention. Foods that are low in saturated fats and cholesterol are provided.

Sodium restriction may be used, but restriction is based on the individual client's profile. Sodium restriction reduces circulating blood volume and may cause excessive sodium loss. Sodium restriction is more important if clients show signs of CHF or pulmonary edema.

Before discharge, clients should be instructed about appropriate long-term diet. Following an acute MI, aggressive management of high serum levels of cholesterol (and other risk factors) and pharmacologic treatments can lead to a 10% reduction in cholesterol and can reduce the rate of nonfatal reinfarction by 19% and of fatal infarction by 12% (Rossouw et al, 1990). The Step-1 or Step-2 diet may be advisable, especially if weight maintenance is a goal. Decreased intake of saturated fats and limiting total fat intake to 30% of the kilocalories are recommended. Additionally, soluble fiber intake should be increased to help lower serum lipid levels.

If weight loss is desirable, kilocaloric restriction may be necessary. A knowledge of healthy alternatives for weight loss is important for clients. A weight loss of more than 2 lbs a week is undesirable because of elevation of plasma free fatty acids and fluid and electrolyte alterations that accompany rapid weight loss.

What are some possible nutritional interventions for a client who has had an MI?

NURSING APPLICATIONS

Assessment

Physical—for height, weight, IBW, heart rhythm, chest pain; BP; stress level, psychosocial factors.

Dietary—for intake of salt, saturated fat, cholesterol, potassium, sodium, magnesium, caffeine, alcohol, and fiber.

Laboratory—for LDH, cholesterol, triglycerides, lipid profile; sodium, potassium; BUN; cardiac isoenzymes; ABGs; PT, PTT.

Interventions

1. Position client and arrange utensils; cut up foods to avoid or lessen fatigue and oxygen demand.
2. Encourage relaxation at mealtimes.
3. Prevent constipation with dietary measures to decrease the necessity of the Valsalva maneuver.
4. Temperatures of food and beverages should not be extremely hot or cold immediately following an MI (Kirchhoff et al, 1990), so avoid offering these types of food and beverages.
5. Severe sodium restriction may precipitate or aggravate shock by compounding extensive sodium loss occurring as a result of profuse diaphoresis immediately following an MI. Monitor sodium intake and blood pressure.
6. Initiate nutrition education to these clients as soon as possible; the fear produced by a coronary event is a strong motivation for changes.

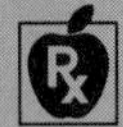

Administer aspirin with foods. Monitor clients taking aspirin regularly for prolonged bleeding time, gastric distress, and anemia.

Evaluation

* Client's laboratory tests should return to normal, and client does not reinfarct and ingests 70 to 100% of ordered diet.
* Other desirable outcomes include client can state rationale for diet ordered and types of food allowed.

Client Education

- Discuss the type of diet prescribed, and explain roles of dietary fats, cholesterol, sodium, potassium, calcium, magnesium, caffeine, and fiber.
- Refer to cardiac rehabilitation groups, American Heart Association, and self-help groups.

CEREBROVASCULAR ACCIDENT

Physical Consequences

Approximately 25 to 45% of all stroke clients initially have difficulty swallowing (Gresham, 1990). Prognosis for full return of the swallowing mechanism is good—76% of clients who present with swallowing disorders are discharged receiving adequate nutriment from various types of oral diets (Gresham, 1990).

Apraxia—inability to perform familiar purposeful movements caused by loss of sensory or motor impairment.

Dysphagia can occur with either left or right hemisphere CVA. Strong correlations have been observed between dysphagia and speech impairment (comprehension and expression) and with facial weakness (Barer, 1989). Generally, left-side CVA is characterized by difficulty following simple instructions and initiating coordinated motor activity, impaired oral stage swallowing function, and **apraxia.** Damage on the right side is more likely to result in laryngeal pooling, **penetration,** and aspiration (Smith & Dodd, 1990). Clients with brain stem CVA have difficulties handling their own secretions (saliva, mucus) and are more likely to require alternate means of feeding (Schultz, 1992).

Aspiration is the passage of food/fluid past the true vocal cords into the trachea. Penetration is when the bolus coats an area below the epiglottis but does not go below the vocal cords; this places the client at risk of aspiration because the material could be aspirated if not coughed up.

Management

Immediate life-saving measures consist of maintaining fluid-electrolyte balance. Evaluation of sensory and motor system deficits and cognitive status is paramount in recovery. One of the primary initial concerns is prevention of aspiration. Because of the danger of aspiration, early referral to a speech-language pathologist (SLP) or occupational therapist (OT) is essential. Medications frequently used for CVA include antihypertensives, anticoagulants, anticonvulsants, and stool softeners.

Nutritional Care

The general procedure has been to begin with a clear liquid diet within 24 to 48 hours, but this practice has been challenged because of the high prevalence of swallowing disorders and difficulties in safely handling thin liquids. Clinically undetected aspiration of swallowed fluids is common (Groher & Bukatman, 1986). Therefore, thickened liquids are advocated initially with gradual progressions to pureed and soft foods, as recommended by the SLP/OT. Easy to chew foods are used to minimize chewing and to increase a client's ability to control a bolus.

If dysphagia is a problem or if the client is comatose, tube feedings may be needed. Management of dysphagia is discussed in Chapter 25; dysphagia diets are discussed in Chapter 12.

Other problems increase risks of feeding. Cognitive deficits may result in poor attention to task; i.e., clients may place food in their mouths and promptly forget about the food. Short-term memory loss may lead to a client insisting that he or she has just eaten when it is time for the next meal. Impulsiveness results in putting too much food in the mouth or eating too fast. With visual field problems, clients may not be able to see food on the tray. Apraxia or judgment problems may cause clients not to know how much food to take or what to do with food in the mouth. Communication about what foods are preferred or disliked is frustrating for both the aphasic client and the nurse. Coordination problems may cause an inability to self-feed. Thus, clients with CVA are dealt with on the basis of their individual needs.

Based on the diagnoses and laboratory profile, saturated fats, cholesterol, and sodium may be restricted. Intake is checked frequently to ensure adequate provision of kilocalories and protein. In general, 35 to 45 kcal/kg and 1.2 to 1.5 gm protein/kg are recommended. Adequate fluids (6 to 8 cups) and fiber are needed to promote normal bowel function.

What are some possible problems affecting the client's nutritional status that may be encountered following a CVA?

If the client is subject to migraine headaches, foods that are frequently associated with headaches may be avoided (see Chapter 23). As the client progresses, long-term problems such as weight loss are addressed, as appropriate.

NURSING APPLICATIONS

Assessment

Physical—for height, weight, IBW; area of infarct; hand to mouth coordination, ability to handle saliva, chewing and swallowing ability, food pocketing; frequency of bowel movements, BP, I&O.
Dietary—for adequacy of intake; food preferences, fluid intake.
Laboratory—for cholesterol, triglycerides, lipid profile; albumin, protein; sodium, potassium, magnesium; urine specific gravity, PT, PTT.

Continued

Interventions

1. Do not offer thin liquids until an objective examination has been completed by the SLP/OT for diagnosis and treatment of the swallow reflex.
2. Have suction available.
3. Assist client with the tray; arrange and prepare foods in a ready to eat form. Assist to sitting position. Keep client upright (> 45-degree angle) for 30 minutes after eating.
4. Consult with PT and OT for adaptive devices and positioning for eating.
5. If client must be fed, place food on unaffected side and toward back of the tongue.
6. Provide oral hygiene frequently.
7. Encourage small bites and slow, thorough chewing.
8. If constipation is a problem, monitor fluid intake and check for any constipating medications; offer prune juice.

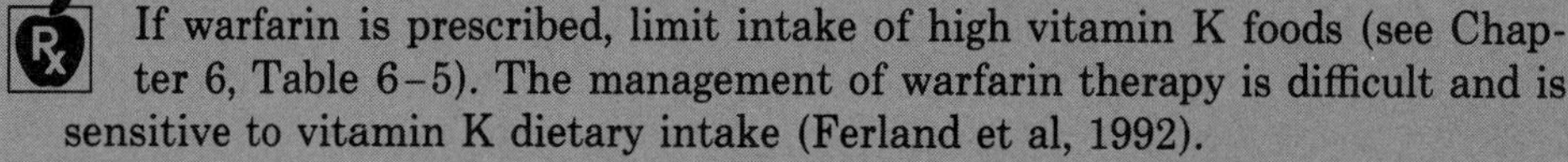

If warfarin is prescribed, limit intake of high vitamin K foods (see Chapter 6, Table 6–5). The management of warfarin therapy is difficult and is sensitive to vitamin K dietary intake (Ferland et al, 1992).

Evaluation

* Client should maintain weight and not aspirate.

Client Education

- Explain the type of diet prescribed and rationale.
- Refer to SLP/OT to help with improving the swallowing reflex.
- Teach client/family to check client's mouth after eating to avoid "pocketing" food.

NUTRITION UPDATE 24–1: LIPID LEVELS IN CHILDREN AND ADOLESCENTS

Controversy has existed concerning screening procedures for serum cholesterol and LDL levels of children and adolescents and how these factors may predispose young clients to CHD in adulthood (Newman et al, 1992; Clarke & Lauer, 1992). Several studies have reported high risk factors in childhood and adolescence that correlate highly with development of CHD later in life: (1) obesity, (2) increased diastolic blood pressure, and (3) elevated total cholesterol levels. A weight of 15% above IBW or greater than the 75th percentile on weight charts, a diastolic blood pressure of 90 mmHg or above, and an elevated total cholesterol level are indicative for later onset of CHD (Table 24–19). Even though lowering serum cholesterol levels during younger years has not been proven to reduce risk of CHD during later years, conclusive evidence drawn from adult studies supports this phenomenon. Therefore, to help detect, prevent, and treat abnormal serum cholesterol levels, the National Cholesterol Education Program (NCEP, 1991) has devised some guidelines for screening procedures and dietary modifications. In general, the American Academy of Pediatrics (1992) has endorsed these guidelines.

Not all children and adolescents need to be screened for increased serum cholesterol levels. Universal screening is not advocated by NCEP for several reasons: (1) High cholesterol levels in children may not develop into high levels in adulthood, (2) anxiety levels may be increased unnecessarily, (3) children may be placed on cholesterol-lowering drugs needlessly, and (4) therapy has proved effective when initiated in young adulthood. Testing is recommended for offspring whose parents/

TABLE 24–19

CUTPOINTS OF TOTAL AND LDL CHOLESTEROL FOR DIETARY INTERVENTION IN CHILDREN AND ADOLESCENTS WITH A FAMILY HISTORY OF HYPERCHOLESTEROLEMIA OR PREMATURE CARDIOVASCULAR DISEASE

Category	Total Cholesterol (mg/dl)	Low-Density Lipoprotein Cholesterol (mg/dl)	Dietary Intervention
Acceptable	< 170	< 110	Recommended population eating pattern
Borderline	170–199	110–129	Step-1 diet prescribed, other risk factor intervention
High	≥ 200	≥ 130	Step-1 diet prescribed, then Step-2 diet if necessary

From the National Cholesterol Education Program. Report of the Expert Panel on Blood Cholesterol Levels in Children and Adolescents. US Department of Health and Human Services, National Institutes of Health. 1991. NIH Publication No 91-2732.

grandparents have or have had the following conditions before the age of 55: coronary atherosclerosis, MI, angina, or serum cholesterol level of 240 mg/dl or above. Wilson and Lewis (1992) determined the most reliable parameters for predicting serum cholesterol levels in children were weight for height measurement and saturated fat intake.

As established from adult studies, diet and serum cholesterol levels are correlated. Generally school-age children eat a typical American diet, i.e., a high intake of sodium, animal protein, and fat and a low intake of potassium, calcium, and complex carbohydrates. Approximately 36% of total kilocalories comes from fat intake. Cholesterol intake exceeds 100 mg/1000 kcal.

Diets for children and adolescents must provide essential nutrients and kilocalories to promote normal growth and development. Diet therapy is the first line of treatment for elevated serum cholesterol levels, but concerns have been expressed about deleterious effects a low-fat diet may have in total kilocalories and essential nutrients (Nicklas et al, 1992). As recommended for adults, dietary treatment consists of a 2-step diet. Step-1 diet in children over 2 years old involves following a prudent diet: limit total fat intake to 30% of kilocalories, no restrictions on kilocalories or protein, less than 300 mg cholesterol intake. Additionally, if the serum cholesterol level is greater than 200 mg/dl or LDL greater than 130, the Step-1 diet is prescribed and monitored by a physician or dietitian. In the Bogalusa Heart Study, children consuming a low-fat diet obtained less vitamin B_6, B_{12}, thiamin, riboflavin, and niacin than those consuming a high-fat diet. Additionally, sugar intake was higher in the low-fat group (Nicklas et al, 1992). Therefore, close supervision is recommended anytime a low-fat diet is prescribed to ensure normal growth and development (Table 24–20).

If the Step-1 diet does not produce a lower cholesterol or LDL level (less than 200 mg/dl and less than 130 mg/dl, respectively) within 3 months, the Step-2 diet is prescribed (see Table 24–20). Saturated fat is limited to less than 7% of kilocalories and dietary cholesterol to less than 200 mg/day. Initiation of drug therapy to lower serum cholesterol is not advised unless serum levels of LDL are not lowered (less than 190 mg/dl) after being on the Step-2 diet for 6 months to 1 year. This applies to children over 10 years of age. Although one might question the validity of the same recommendations as for adults, if you will remember, dietary cholesterol is the least effective dietary measure for changing serum cholesterol levels.

For infants, NCEP values the importance of breast milk. After age 2 or following weaning, these children should partake of the family diet, which, it is hoped, observes guidelines in the Step-1 diet.

In light of these recommendations, nurses must become familiar with screening procedures and dietary measures to lower serum cholesterol and LDL levels. This knowledge will help dispel mistaken information and decrease undue anxiety in

TABLE 24–20

STEP-1 AND STEP-2 DIETS: HOW NUTRIENT RECOMMENDATIONS CAN BE TRANSLATED INTO SERVINGS PER DAY FOR DIFFERENT AGE GROUPS

Step-1 Diet

	Age (years)						
	CHILD 2–3	**CHILD 4–6**	**CHILD 7–10**	**MALE 11–14**	**FEMALE 11–14**	**MALE 15–18**	**FEMALE 15–18**
Food group							
Meat, poultry, and fish (oz)	2	5	6	6	6	6	6
Eggs (per week)*	3	3	3	3	3	3	3
Dairy products (servings)	3	3	4	4	4	4	4
Fats and oils (servings)	4	5	5	7	5	10	5
Breads and cereals (servings)†	5	6	7	9	8	12	8
Vegetables (servings)	3	3	3	4	3	4	3
Fruits (servings)	2	3	3	3	3	5	3
Sweets and modified fat desserts (servings)	1	2	2	4	3	4	3
Nutrients							
Recommended Dietary Allowance (RDA) for energy (kcal)	1300	1800	2000	2500	2200	3000	2200
Actual energy (kcal)	1317	1786	2025	2522	2221	3011	2221
Fat (gm)	46	62	70	86	73	103	73
(% kcal)	(30)	(31)	(31)	(30)	(29)	(30)	(29)
Carbohydrate (gm)	177	230	255	338	294	418	294
(% kcal)	(52)	(50)	(49)	(52)	(52)	(54)	(52)
Protein (gm)	59	87	104	114	109	125	109
(% kcal)	(18)	(19)	(20)	(18)	(19)	(16)	(19)
Fatty acids‡ and cholesterol							
Saturated fatty acids (gm)	15	20	23	26	24	29	24
(% kcal)	(10)	(10)	(10)	(9)	(9)	(9)	(9)
Monounsaturated fatty acids (gm)	16	23	25	31	26	37	26
(% kcal)	(11)	(11)	(11)	(11)	(11)	(11)	(11)
Polyunsaturated fatty acids (gm)	10	14	14	20	16	26	16
(% kcal)	(7)	(7)	(6)	(7)	(6)	(8)	(6)
Cholesterol (mg)	183	256	294	295	295	296	295
(mg chol/1000 kcal)	(139)	(143)	(145)	(117)	(133)	(98)	(133)
Fat-soluble vitamins							
Vitamin A (IU)	10,945	11,451	11,891	15,163	12,066	16,282	12,066
(% RDA)	(> 100)	(> 100)	(> 100)	(> 100)	(> 100)	(> 100)	(> 100)
Water-soluble vitamins							
Vitamin C (mg)	122	148	153	184	158	233	158
(% RDA)	(306)	(329)	(339)	(367)	(316)	(387)	(316)
Thiamin (mg)	1.3	1.7	2.0	2.4	2.1	2.9	2.1
(% RDA)	(188)	(190)	(196)	(184)	(195)	(196)	(195)
Riboflavin (mg)	1.7	2.1	2.5	2.8	2.6	3.2	2.6
(% RDA)	(213)	(188)	(206)	(186)	(200)	(175)	(200)
Niacin (mg)	13.4	20.9	24.2	28.1	25.9	32.9	25.9
(% RDA)	(149)	(174)	(186)	(165)	(173)	(165)	(173)
Vitamin B_6 (mg)	1.6	2.2	2.5	2.8	2.6	3.4	2.6
(% RDA)	(160)	(198)	(175)	(165)	(184)	(172)	(184)

TABLE 24–20

STEP-1 AND STEP-2 DIETS: HOW NUTRIENT RECOMMENDATIONS CAN BE TRANSLATED INTO SERVINGS PER DAY FOR DIFFERENT AGE GROUPS
Continued

Step-1 Diet

	Age (years)						
	CHILD 2–3	**CHILD 4–6**	**CHILD 7–10**	**MALE 11–14**	**FEMALE 11–14**	**MALE 15–18**	**FEMALE 15–18**
Folacin (mcg)	267	316	351	431	379	537	379
(% RDA)	(535)	(422)	(351)	(287)	(252)	(269)	(252)
Vitamin B_{12} (mcg)	3.4	4.7	5.8	6.1	6.0	6.6	6.0
(% RDA)	(492)	(472)	(415)	(307)	(299)	(330)	(299)
Minerals							
Calcium (mg)	889	948	1190	1287	1226	1380	1226
(% RDA)	(111)	(119)	(149)	(107)	(102)	(115)	(102)
Phosphorus (mg)	1100	1365	1651	1852	1738	2073	1738
(% RDA)	(138)	(171)	(206)	(154)	(145)	(173)	(145)
Magnesium (mg)	265	327	377	449	406	547	406
(% RDA)	(332)	(272)	(222)	(166)	(145)	(137)	(145)
Iron (mg)	10.8	14.5	16.5	20.3	18.1	24.7	18.1
(% RDA)	(108)	(145)	(165)	(169)	(121)	(206)	(121)
Zinc (mg)	7.8	11.6	13.8	15.2	14.4	16.9	14.4
(% RDA)	(78)	(116)	(138)	(101)	(120)	(112)	(120)
Sodium§	2093	2780	3234	3859	3479	4485	3479

Step-2 Diet

	Age (years)						
	CHILD 2–3	**CHILD 4–6**	**CHILD 7–10**	**MALE 11–14**	**FEMALE 11–14**	**MALE 15–18**	**FEMALE 15–18**
Food group							
Meat, poultry, and fish (oz)	2	5	6	6	6	6	6
Eggs (per week)*	2	2	1	1	1	1	1
Dairy products (servings)	3	3	4	4	4	4	4
Fats and oils (servings)	5	7	7	9	7	13	7
Breads and cereals (servings)†	5	6	7	9	8	12	8
Vegetables (servings)	3	3	3	4	3	4	3
Fruits (servings)	2	3	4	3	3	5	3
Sweets and modified fat desserts (servings)	1	2	2	4	3	4	3
Nutrients							
(RDA) for energy (kcal)	1300	1800	2000	2500	2200	3000	2200
Actual energy (kcal)	1275	1775	2037	2475	2178	2999	2178
Fat (gm)	41	61	66	81	69	102	69
(% kcal)	(28)	(30)	(29)	(29)	(28)	(30)	(28)
Carbohydrate (gm)	176	228	268	337	293	417	293
(% kcal)	(54)	(50)	(51)	(53)	(53)	(54)	(53)
Protein (gm)	59	88	106	115	110	125	110
(% kcal)	(18)	(20)	(20)	(18)	(19)	(16)	(19)
Fatty acids‡ and cholesterol							
Saturated fatty acids (gm)	10	15	17	19	17	22	17
(% kcal)	(7)	(7)	(7)	(7)	(7)	(7)	(7)
Monounsaturated fatty acids (gm)	16	24	26	32	27	40	27
(% kcal)	(11)	(12)	(11)	(12)	(11)	(12)	(11)

Table continued on following page

TABLE 24–20

STEP-1 AND STEP-2 DIETS: HOW NUTRIENT RECOMMENDATIONS CAN BE TRANSLATED INTO SERVINGS PER DAY FOR DIFFERENT AGE GROUPS
Continued

Step-1 Diet

	Age (years)						
	CHILD 2–3	**CHILD 4–6**	**CHILD 7–10**	**MALE 11–14**	**FEMALE 11–14**	**MALE 15–18**	**FEMALE 15–18**
Polyunsaturated fatty acids (gm)	11	16	17	23	18	30	18
(% kcal)	(8)	(8)	(7)	(8)	(8)	(9)	(8)
Cholesterol (mg)	138	211	214	215	214	216	214
(mg chol/1000 kcal)	(108)	(118)	(105)	(87)	(98)	(72)	(98)
Fat-soluble vitamins							
Vitamin A (IU)	10,930	11,561	12,154	15,230	12,067	16,539	12,067
(% RDA)	(> 100)	(> 100)	(> 100)	(> 100)	(> 100)	(> 100)	(> 100)
Water-soluble vitamins							
Vitamin C (mg)	123	148	172	184	158	233	158
(% RDA)	(307)	(329)	(383)	(367)	(316)	(388)	(316)
Thiamin (mg)	1.3	1.7	2.0	2.4	2.2	2.9	2.2
(% RDA)	(188)	(191)	(202)	(185)	(196)	(196)	(196)
Riboflavin (mg)	1.6	1.9	2.3	2.6	2.4	3.0	2.4
(% RDA)	(197)	(177)	(194)	(173)	(186)	(164)	(186)
Niacin (mg)	13.5	21.0	24.7	28.3	26.1	33.1	26.1
(% RDA)	(150)	(175)	(190)	(166)	(174)	(166)	(174)
Vitamin B_6 (mg)	1.6	2.2	2.6	2.8	2.6	3.4	2.6
(% RDA)	(158)	(199)	(186)	(165)	(184)	(172)	(184)
Folacin (mcg)	271	320	368	434	381	540	381
(% RDA)	(542)	(426)	(368)	(289)	(254)	(270)	(254)
Vitamin B_{12} (mcg)	3.5	4.9	6.0	6.3	6.2	6.8	6.2
(% RDA)	(496)	(492)	(428)	(316)	(308)	(339)	(308)
Minerals							
Calcium (mg)	891	951	1203	1289	1227	1383	1227
(% RDA)	(111)	(119)	(150)	(107)	(102)	(115)	(102)
Phosphorus (mg)	1217	1500	1830	2019	1904	2241	1904
(% RDA)	(152)	(187)	(229)	(168)	(159)	(187)	(159)
Magnesium (mg)	261	323	383	445	402	542	402
(% RDA)	(326)	(270)	(226)	(165)	(143)	(136)	(143)
Iron (mg)	10.9	14.7	16.9	20.6	18.4	24.9	18.4
(% RDA)	(109)	(147)	(169)	(171)	(122)	(208)	(122)
Zinc (mg)	8.1	12.1	14.5	15.9	15.1	17.5	15.1
(% RDA)	(81)	(121)	(145)	(106)	(126)	(117)	(126)
Sodium (mg)§	2441	3162	3697	4344	3941	5032	3941

* Nutrient analysis is for 3 eggs per week; with 4 eggs per week, the average dietary cholesterol increases by 30 mg/day.
† The breads and cereals food group includes bread, cereal, pasta, rice, starchy vegetables, and dry beans and peas.
‡ The values for total fat are greater than the sum of saturated, monounsaturated, and polyunsaturated fatty acids since total fat includes fatty acids plus other fatty substances and glycerol.
§ Values include a standard amount of salt added to foods in the meat, poultry, and fish group; vegetables group; and breads and cereals group. Value does not include salt added at the table or sodium present in the water supply.
From the National Cholesterol Education Program. Report of the Expert Panel on Blood Cholesterol Levels in Children and Adolescents. NIH Publication No. 91-2732, Sept. 1991.

clients. Assessment of children and adolescents for risk factors and a positive family history may assist in identifying high-risk children to initiate earlier treatments. Further research is needed to provide proven, effective treatment measures. For those who have identified high-risk factors or require the Step-2 diet, referral to a dietitian is vital so individualized preventive or maintenance measures may be instituted promptly.

Besides individualization of diets, educational programs beginning with school-age children are necessary. Educating the whole US population on methods for implementing and adhering to a prudent diet is needed. Additionally, not only is nutrition education important, but also equally important is education about risk factors, fast food choices, exercise, life-long behavioral skills, and self-esteem factors. All these areas need to be addressed to provide a comprehensive, holistic approach to childhood cholesterol nutrition.

SUMMARY

Inadequate nutrient intake as well as excesses can contribute to hypertension. In general, energy and sodium intake is excessive. However, frequently calcium and potassium intake may be below RDA levels. Weight control and sodium restriction are important dietary factors for treating hypertension with or without pharmaceutical therapies.

Relaxation therapy and a calm lifestyle can reduce hypertension. An exercise program is highly recommended for any type of cardiovascular problem, not only to reduce tension, but also for weight control.

Dietary control of hyperlipidemia is one of the most promising ways to treat CHD and to help prevent it in those genetically at risk. The 3 basic goals of any preventive program for cardiovascular disease include (1) limiting total dietary fat to not more than 30% and to divide it equally among polyunsaturated (especially linoleic acid as well as omega-3), saturated, and monounsaturated fatty acids; (2) restricting cholesterol to 300 mg/day or less; and (3) increasing intake of complex carbohydrates. Excessive weight increases chances for hyperlipidemia; weight loss is recommended for these clients. If these measures are followed, it is hoped that the incidence of hypertension, MIs, and CVAs will continue to decrease.

Nurses are vital to a successful cardiovascular disease program. Since sodium and fat restriction are so widespread (even if only moderately restricted), there are not enough dietitians available for the desired consultation and monitoring. In addition to teaching the client about the diet and reinforcing information taught by the dietitian, an informed nurse can honestly compliment clients on even a modest reduction in weight or sodium intake. This feedback can be most encouraging and a motivating factor to clients. Nurses are in a prime position to help clients and families adjust successfully to dietary modifications, address practical behavioral changes, possible stressors, nutrient–drug interactions, and physical activity levels.

NURSING PROCESS IN ACTION

A CVA client in rehabilitation is having some difficulties swallowing. He is oriented and can follow commands. He is paralyzed on his left side and is right-handed. Weight (150 lbs) is appropriate (within IBW). The speech-language pathologist has recommended thickened liquids and a dysphagia diet that consists of ground foods.

 Nutritional Assessment

- Blood pressure.
- Hand to mouth coordination.
- Which hand eats with—right.

- Ability to swallow and chew.
- Emotional adjustment, such as depression, denial, anger.
- Food preference, fluid/nutrient intake, kilocalories needed.
- Cholesterol, triglyceride, lipid levels, sodium, and potassium.

Dietary Nursing Diagnosis

Altered nutrition: High risk for less nutrients than body requirements RT impaired swallowing and muscle paralysis.

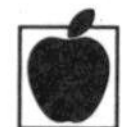

Nutritional Goals

Client will maintain weight of 150 lbs, consume thickened liquids and ground food without aspiration, and enjoy eating.

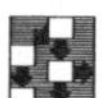

Nutritional Implementation 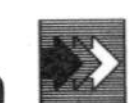

Intervention: Elevate head of bed during and for 30 minutes after feedings.
Rationale: This minimizes possible aspiration by the use of gravity.

Intervention: Monitor diet for appropriateness of food texture, per SLP recommendation. Be sure foods are moistened with gravy or sauces.
Rationale: Clients handle these types of food better than liquids and are at less risk of aspiration.

Intervention: Monitor for adequate intake of kilocalories and protein.
Rationale: In general, 35 to 45 kcal/kg and 1.2 to 1.5 gm protein/kg are recommended.

Intervention: Offer 6 to 8 cups of preferred juice, thickened.
Rationale: Thickened fluids are less likely to be aspirated, but fluid requirements remain the same. Adequate fluid intake allows water to be drawn into stool, making it soft. The client should not have to strain during defecation because this may increase intracranial pressure.

Intervention: Refer to dietitian, OT, PT, SLP.
Rationale: This is a chronic disease, and support is needed for dietary management to maintain ideal body weight. Dietitian can help with consulting and monitoring intake for nutrient adequacy; OT for fitting and use of assistive devices for eating; PT for positioning; and speech therapist for swallowing problems.

Intervention: Have suction available.
Rationale: If aspiration/choking occurs, effects may be minimized with suction.

Intervention: Follow guidelines provided by SLP/OT for feeding. Frequently the following are recommended: (1) Place food on right side of mouth toward the back of the tongue, (2) provide oral hygiene, (3) check for pocketing, (4) tilt head forward as client swallows.
Rationale: His unaffected side (good side) is the right side since he is paralyzed on the left. Oral hygiene stimulates saliva and heightens taste sensation. CVA clients may pocket food on affected side (left) and not know it. Tilting the head forward facilitates swallowing by closing the epiglottis.

Intervention: Crush medications and mix with applesauce/low-fat pudding, or provide in liquid form (thickened, if needed).
Rationale: Client is likely to aspirate on water or large pills.

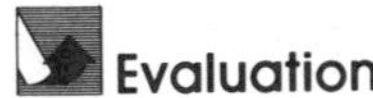

Evaluation

Client weighs 150 lbs, consumes food and medication without complications (aspiration), and verbalizes positive feelings about eating.

STUDENT READINESS

1. How can cholesterol levels be reduced in the body?
2. List the sodium levels for various restricted diets.
3. Define high-density lipoproteins and discuss factors that influence their levels.
4. When are low-sodium diets ordered?
5. What are the 2 steps of diets for hyperlipidemia?

CASE STUDY:

Mr. A. C. is a 43-year-old bank vice-president who has been experiencing chest pain for the past 5 years. His family history is positive for CHD; his father died at age 58 of an MI, and his brother, who is in his early 40s, has had 2 MIs. He is approximately 22 kg overweight and smokes 2 packs of cigarettes per day.

At his yearly physical examination, the physician noted a blood pressure of 168/100 mmHg. All laboratory findings were within normal limits except for the serum cholesterol (305 mg/dl) and serum triglycerides (176 mg/dl).

1. What risk factors for CHD does Mr. A. C. have?
2. Is it important that the type of hyperlipoproteinemia be identified before diet counseling?
3. What would be the impact of weight loss on Mr. A. C.'s serum cholesterol and triglycerides; blood pressure?
4. What is the range of cholesterol intake allowed for the client with hyperlipidemia?
5. What P/S ratio is desirable for this client?

CASE STUDY

On physical examination, Mr. H. G., a 63-year-old postal worker, was found to have a blood pressure of 192/114 mmHg. There were no other significant findings except for his being 25 lbs overweight. After an unsuccessful trial of hygienic measures (weight reduction, increased exercise, and decreased salt intake), the physician prescribed a thiazide diuretic, continuation of the hygienic measures, and increased intake of foods high in potassium.

1. Why were weight reduction and increased activity initially prescribed for Mr. H. G.?
2. Why is the increased potassium intake necessary?
3. Prepare a list of at least 10 foods that are high in potassium.
4. What prepared snacks are particularly high in sodium and should be avoided?

5. What prepared snacks are lower in sodium and should be suggested to Mr. H. G.?
6. What flavoring agents should be recommended to replace salt?

REFERENCES

Adlin EV. Edema and hypertension. *In* Kinney JM et al, eds. *Nutrition and Metabolism in Patient Care.* Philadelphia, WB Saunders, 1988: 445–464.

American Academy of Pediatrics Committee on Nutrition. Statement on Cholesterol. *Pediatrics* 1992 Sept; 90(9):469–473.

American Heart Association (AHA). *1990 Heart and Stroke Facts.* Dallas, TX, American Heart Association, 1990.

Anderson JW, et al. Cholesterol-lowering effects of psyllium-enriched cereal as an adjunct to a prudent diet in the treatment of mild to moderate hypercholesterolemia. *Am J Clin Nutr* 1992 *July;* 56(1):93–98.

Anderson JW, et al. Hypocholesterolemic effects of different bulk-forming hydrophilic fibers as adjuncts to dietary therapy in mild to moderate hypercholesterolemia. *Arch Intern Med* 1991 Aug; 151(8):1597–1602.

Applegate WB, et al. Non-pharmacologic intervention to reduce blood pressure in older patients with mild hypertension. *Arch Intern Med* 1992 June; 152(6):1162–1166.

Arai AE, Greenberg BH. Medical management of congestive heart failure. *West J Med* 1990 Oct; 153(4):406–414.

Ashley FW Jr, Kannel WB. Relation of weight change to changes in atherogenic traits: The Framingham study. *J Chron Dis* 1974 March; 27(3):103–114.

Bagatell CJ, Heymsfield SB. Effect of meal size on myocardial oxygen requirements. Implications for postmyocardial infarction diet. *Am J Clin Nutr* 1984 March; 39(3):421–426.

Bankhead CD. Intensity of exercise. *Med World News* 1991 Sept; 32(9):22–23.

Barer DH. The natural history and functional consequences of dysphagia after hemispheric stroke. *J Neurol Neurosurg Psychiatry* 1989 Feb; 52(2):236–241.

Barr SL, et al. Reducing total dietary fat without reducing saturated fatty acids does not significantly lower total plasma cholesterol concentrations in normal males. *Am J Clin Nutr* 1992 March; 55(3):675–681.

Beare P, Myers J. *Principles and Practice of Adult Health Nursing.* St. Louis, CV Mosby, 1990.

Belmin J. Low-sodium diet and congestive heart failure. *J Am Geriatr Soc* 1992 March; 40(3): 298–299.

Berry EM, et al. Effects of diets rich in monounsaturated fatty acids on plasma lipoproteins—the Jerusalem Nutrition Study: High MUFAs vs high PUFAs. *Am J Clin Nutr* 1991 Apr; 53(4):899–907.

Bonaa KH, et al. Habitual fish consumption, plasma phospholipid fatty acids, and serum lipids: The Tromso study. *Am J Clin Nutr* 1992 June; 55(6):1126–1134.

Bonaa KH, et al. Effect of eicosapentaenoic and docosahexaenoic acids on blood pressure in hypertension. A population-based intervention trial from the Tromso study. *N Engl J Med* 1990 March 22; 322(12):795–801.

Burke LE. Dietary management of hyperlipidemia. *J Cardiovas Nurs* 1991 Jan; 5(2):23–33.

Clarke WR, Lauer RM. The predictive value of childhood cholesterol screening. A response. *JAMA* 1992 Jan 7; 267(1):101–102.

Consensus Development Panel. Lowering blood cholesterol to prevent heart disease. *JAMA* 1985 Apr 12; 253(14):2080–2086.

Cutler JA, et al. An overview of randomized trials of sodium reduction and blood pressure. *Hypertension* 1991 Jan; 17(1 suppl):I27–I33.

Davidson MH, et al. Marine oil capsule therapy for the treatment of hyperlipidemia. *Arch Intern Med* 1991 Sept; 151(9):1732–1740.

Dawber TR. *The Framingham Study: The Epidemiology of Atherosclerotic Disease.* Cambridge, MA, Harvard University Press, 1980.

Denke MA, Grundy SM. Effects of fats high in stearic acid on lipid and lipoprotein concentrations in men. *Am J Clin Nutr* 1991 Dec; 54(6):1036–1040.

Einhorn D, Landsberg L. Nutrition and diet in hypertension. *In* Shils ME, Young VR, eds. *Modern Nutrition in Health and Disease.* 7th ed. Philadelphia, Lea & Febiger, 1988: 1269–1282.

Esterbauer H, et al. Role of vitamin E in preventing the oxidation of low-density lipoprotein. *Am J Clin Nutr* 1991 Jan; 53(suppl 1):314S-321S.

Ferland G, et al. Development of a diet low in vitamin K-1 (phylloquinone). *J Am Diet Assoc* 1992 May; 92(5):593–597.

Fraser GE. Cholesterol values and the fasting state. *JAMA* 1990 Dec 19; 264(23):3063–3067.

Frederickson DS, et al. Fat transport in lipoproteins—an integrated approach to mechanisms and disorders. *N Engl J Med* 1967 Jan 5; 276(1):34–42.

Frei B. Ascorbic acid protects lipids in human plasma and low-density lipoprotein against oxidative damage. *Am J Clin Nutr* 1991 Dec; 54(suppl):1113S–1118S.

Garlic—the next wonder drug? *Nutr & the MD* 1991 May; 17(5):4.

Gey KF, et al. Inverse correlation between plasma vitamin E and mortality from ischemic heart disease in cross-cultural epidemiology. *Am J Clin Nutr* 1991 Jan; 53 (suppl 1): 326S–334S.

Ginsberg HN, et al. Reduction of plasma cholesterol levels in normal men on an American Heart Association step 1 diet or a step 2 diet with added monounsaturated fat. *N Engl J Med* 1990 March 1; 322(9):574–579.

Glazer G. Atherogenic effects of anabolic steroids on serum lipid levels. A literature review. *Arch Intern Med* 1991 Oct; 151(10):1925–1933.

Green P, et al. Effects of fish oil ingestion on cardiovascular risk factors in hyperlipidemic subjects in Israel: A randomized double-blind crossover study. *Am J Clin Nutr* 1990 Dec; 52(6):1118–1124.

Gresham SL. Clinical assessment and management of swallowing difficulties after stroke. *Med J Aust* 1990 Oct 1; 153(7):397–399.

Grimm RH Jr, et al. The influence of oral potassium chloride on blood pressure in hypertensive men on a low-sodium diet. *N Engl J Med* 1990 March 1; 322(9):569–574.

Groher M, Bukatman R. The prevalence of swallowing disorders in two hospitals. *Dysphagia* 1986; 1(1):3–6.

Grundy SM. Cholesterol and coronary heart disease. Future directions. *JAMA* 1990 Dec 19; 264(23):3053–3059.

Grundy SM. Monounsaturated fatty acids and cholesterol metabolism: Implications for dietary recommendations. *J Nutr* 1989 Apr; 119(4): 529–533.

Hadley SA, Saarmann, L. Lipid physiology and nutritional considerations in coronary heart disease. *Crit Care Nurse* 1991 Oct; 11(10):28–37.

Harris WS, et al. Fish oils in hypertriglyceridemia: A dose-response study. *Am J Clin Nutr* 1990 March; 51(3):399–406.

Heymsfield SB, Casper K. Congestive heart failure: Clinical management by use of continuous nasoenteric feeding. *Am J Clin Nutr* 1989 Sept; 50(3):539–544.

Jackson R, et al. Alcohol consumption and risk of coronary heart disease. *Br Med J* 1991 July 27; 309(6796):211–216.

Jialal I, et al. Physiologic levels of ascorbate inhibit the oxidative modification of low-density lipoprotein. *Atherosclerosis* 1990 June; 82(3): 185–191.

Johnson C, Greenland P. Effects of exercise, dietary cholesterol, and dietary fat on blood lipids. *Arch Intern Med* 1990 Jan; 150(1):137–141.

Joint National Committee. The 1988 Report of the Joint National Committee on detection, evaluation, and treatment of high blood pressure. *Arch Intern Med* 1988 May; 148(5):1023–1038.

Kashtan H, et al. Wheat-bran and oat-bran supplements' effect on blood lipids and lipoproteins. *Am J Clin Nutr* 1992 May; 55(5):976–980.

Kestin M, et al. n-3 fatty acids of marine origin lower systolic blood pressure and triglycerides but raise LDL cholesterol compared to n-3 and n-6 fatty acids from plants. *Am J Clin Nutr* 1990a June; 51(6):1028–1034.

Kestin M, et al. Comparative effects of three cereal brans on plasma lipids, blood pressure, and glucose metabolism in mildly hypercholesterolemic men. *Am J Clin Nutr* 1990b Oct; 52(4): 661–666.

Kestin M, et al. Effect of dietary cholesterol in normolipidemic subjects is not modified by nature and amount of dietary fat. *Am J Clin Nutr* 1989 Sept; 50(3):528–532.

Kirchhoff KT, et al. Electrocardiographic response to ice water ingestion. *Heart Lung* 1990 Jan; 19(1):41–48.

Kleijinen J, et al. Garlic, onions, and cardiovascular risk factors. A review of the evidence from human experiments with emphasis on commercially available preparations. *Br J Clin Pharmacol* 1989 Nov; 28(5):535–544.

Kris-Etherton PM, et al. The effect of diet on plasma lipids, lipoproteins, and coronary heart disease. *J Am Diet Assoc* 1988 Nov; 88(11): 1373–1396.

Krishna GG, Kapoor SC. Potassium depletion exacerbates essential hypertension. *Ann Intern Med* 1991 July 15; 115(2):77–83.

Kushiro T, et al. Role of sympathetic activity in blood pressure reduction with low calorie regimen. *Hypertension* 1991 June; 17 (6 Pt 2):965–968.

London SJ, et al. Comparison of three species of dietary fish: Effects on serum concentrations of low-density lipoprotein cholesterol and apolipoprotein in normotriglyceridemic subjects. *Am J Clin Nutr* 1991 Aug; 54(2):334–339.

MacDonald TM, et al. Caffeine restriction: Effect on mild hypertension. *Br Med J* 1991 Nov 16; 303(6812):1235–1238.

Mansell P, Reckless JPD. Garlic (editorial). *Br Med J* 1991 Aug 17; 303(6799):379–380.

Manson JE, et al. The primary prevention of myocardial infarction. *N Engl J Med* 1992 May 21; 326(21):1406–1414.

Manson JE, et al. A prospective study of obesity and risk of coronary heart disease in women. *N Engl J Med* 1990 March 29; 322(12):882–889.

Mattes RD, Donnelly D. Relative contributions of dietary sodium sources. *J Am College Nutr* 1991 Aug; 10(4):383–392.

Mattson FH. A changing role for dietary monounsaturated fatty acids. *J Am Diet Assoc* 1989 March; 89(3):387–391.

McIntosh GH, et al. Barley and wheat foods: Influence on plasma cholesterol concentrations in hypercholesterolemic men. *Am J Clin Nutr* 1991 May; 53(5):1205–1209.

McNamara DJ, et al. Heterogeneity of cholesterol homeostasis in man: Response to changes in dietary fat and cholesterol quantity. *J Clin Invest* 1987 June; 79(6):1729–1739.

Miettenen TA, Kesaniemi Y. Cholesterol absorption regulation of cholesterol synthesis and elimination and within-population variations of serum cholesterol levels. *Am J Clin Nutr* 1989 Apr; 49 (4):629–635.

Moore TJ. The role of dietary electrolytes in hypertension. *J Am College Nutr* 1989; 8(suppl): 68S–80S.

Muldoon MF, et al. Acute cholesterol responses to mental stress and change in posture. *Arch Intern Med* 1992 Apr; 152(4):775–780.

Nagelhout JJ. Pharmacologic treatment of heart failure. *Nurs Clin North Am* 1991 June; 26(2):401–415.

Naslund T, et al. Low sodium intake corrects abnormality in beta-receptor-mediated arterial vasodilation in patients with hypertension: Correlation with beta-receptor function in vitro. *Clin Pharmacol Ther* 1990 July; 48(1):87–95.

National Cholesterol Education Program (NCEP). *Report of the Expert Panel on Blood Cholesterol Levels in Children and Adolescents.* Bethesda, MD, National Heart, Lung, and Blood Institute, 1991.

National Heart, Lung, and Blood Institute (NHLBI), National Institutes of Health, US Department of Health and Human Services. National cholesterol education program. Report of the expert panel on population strategies for blood cholesterol reduction: Executive summary. *Arch Intern Med* 1991 June; 83(6):1071–1084.

Newman TB, et al. Childhood cholesterol screening: Contraindicated. *JAMA* 1992 Jan 1; 267(1):100–101.

Nicklas TA, et al. Nutrient adequacy of low fat intakes for children: The Bogalusa Heart Study. *Pediatrics* 1992 Feb; 89(2):221–228.

Oberman A, et al. Pharmacologic and nutritional treatment of mild hypertension: Changes in cardiovascular risk status. *Ann Intern Med* 1990 Jan 15; 112(2):89–95.

Radack K, et al. The effects of low doses of n-3 fatty acid supplementation on blood pressure in hypertensive subjects. A randomized controlled trial. *Arch Intern Med* 1991 June; 151(6):1173–1180.

Retzlaff BM, et al. Changes in vitamin and mineral intakes and serum concentrations among free-living men on cholesterol-lowering diets: The dietary alternatives study. *Am J Clin Nutr* 1991 Apr; 53(4):890–898.

Ripsin CM, et al. Oat products and lipid lowering. A meta-analysis. *JAMA* 1992 June 24; 267(24): 3317–3325.

Rossouw JE, et al. The value of lowering cholesterol after myocardial infarction. *N Engl J Med* 1990 Oct 18; 323(16):1112–1119.

Salt sensitivity and essential hypertension. *Nutr & MD* 1993 Jan; 19(1):1.

Schotte DE, Stunkard AJ. The effects of weight reduction on blood pressure in 301 obese patients. *Arch Intern Med* 1990 Aug; 150(8):1701–1704.

Schultz AF. Identifying dysphagia and working to resolve it. ASPEN 16th Clinical Congress, Jan 19–22, 1992.

Selby JV, et al. Precursors of essential hypertension: The role of body fat distribution pattern. *Am J Epidemiol* 1989 Jan; 129(1):43–53.

Sempos C, et al. The prevalence of high blood cholesterol levels among adults in the United States. *JAMA* 1989 July 7; 262(1):45–52.

Siani A, et al. Increasing the dietary potassium intake reduces the need for antihypertensive medication. *Ann Intern Med* 1991 Nov 15; 115(10):753–759.

Smith DS, Dodd BA. Swallowing disorders in stroke. *Med J Aust* 1990 Oct 1; 153(7):372–373.

Smith-Schneider LM, et al. Dietary fat reduction strategies. *J Am Diet Assoc* 1992 Jan; 92(1):34–38.

Steinberg D. Lipoproteins and atherogenesis. Current concepts. *JAMA* 1990 Dec 19; 264(23): 3047–3052.

Suh H, et al. Alcohol use and mortality from coronary heart disease: The role of high-density lipoprotein cholesterol. *Ann Intern Med* 1992 June 1; 116(11):881–887.

Task Force on Cholesterol Issues, American Heart Association. The cholesterol facts. A summary of the evidence relating dietary fats, serum cholesterol, and coronary heart disease. A joint statement by the American Heart Association and the National Heart, Lung, and Blood Institute. *Circulation* 1990 May; 81(5): 1721–1731.

Thompson CJ, et al. Central adipose distribution is related to coronary atherosclerosis. *Arterioscler Thromb* 1991 March-Apr; 11(2):327–333.

Treatment of Mild Hypertension Research Group. The treatment of mild hypertension study: A randomized, placebo-controlled trial of a nutritional hygienic regimen along with various drug monotherapies. *Arch Intern Med* 1991 July; 151(7):1413–1423.

Trials of Hypertension Prevention Collaborative Research Group. The effects of nonpharmacologic interventions on blood pressure of persons with high normal levels. *JAMA* 1992 March 4; 267(9):1213–1220.

US Department of Health and Human Services (USDHHS). Expert Panel on Detection Evaluation and Treatment of High Blood Cholesterol in Adults. Washington, D.C., Government Printing Office, 1989.

van Dusseldorp M, et al. Boiled coffee and blood pressure. A 14-week controlled trial. *Hypertension* 1991 Nov; 18(5):607–613.

Vega GL, et al. Metabolic basis of primary hypercholesterolemia. *Circulation* 1991 July; 84(7): 118–128.

Wassertheil-Smoller S, et al. The trial of antihypertensive interventions and management (AIM) study. *Arch Intern Med* 1992 Jan; 152(1):131–136.

Whyte JL, et al. Oat bran lowers plasma cholesterol levels in mildly hypercholesterolemic men. *J Am Diet Assoc* 1992 Apr; 92(4):446–449.

Willett WC, et al. Intake of *trans* fatty acids and risk of coronary heart disease among women. *Lancet* 1993 March 6; 341(8845):581–585.

Wilson DKW, Lewis NM. Weight-for-height measurement and saturated fatty acid intake are predictors of serum cholesterol level in children. *J Am Diet Assoc* 1992 Feb; 92(2):192–196.

Wing RR, et al. Waist to hip ratio in middle-aged women. Associations with behavioral and psychosocial factors and with changes in cardiovascular risk factors. *Arterioscler Thromb* 1991 Sept-Oct; 11(5):1250–1257.

Wood PD, et al. The effects on plasma lipoproteins of a prudent weight-reducing diet, with or without exercise in overweight men and women. *N Engl J Med* 1991 Aug 15; 325(7):461–466.

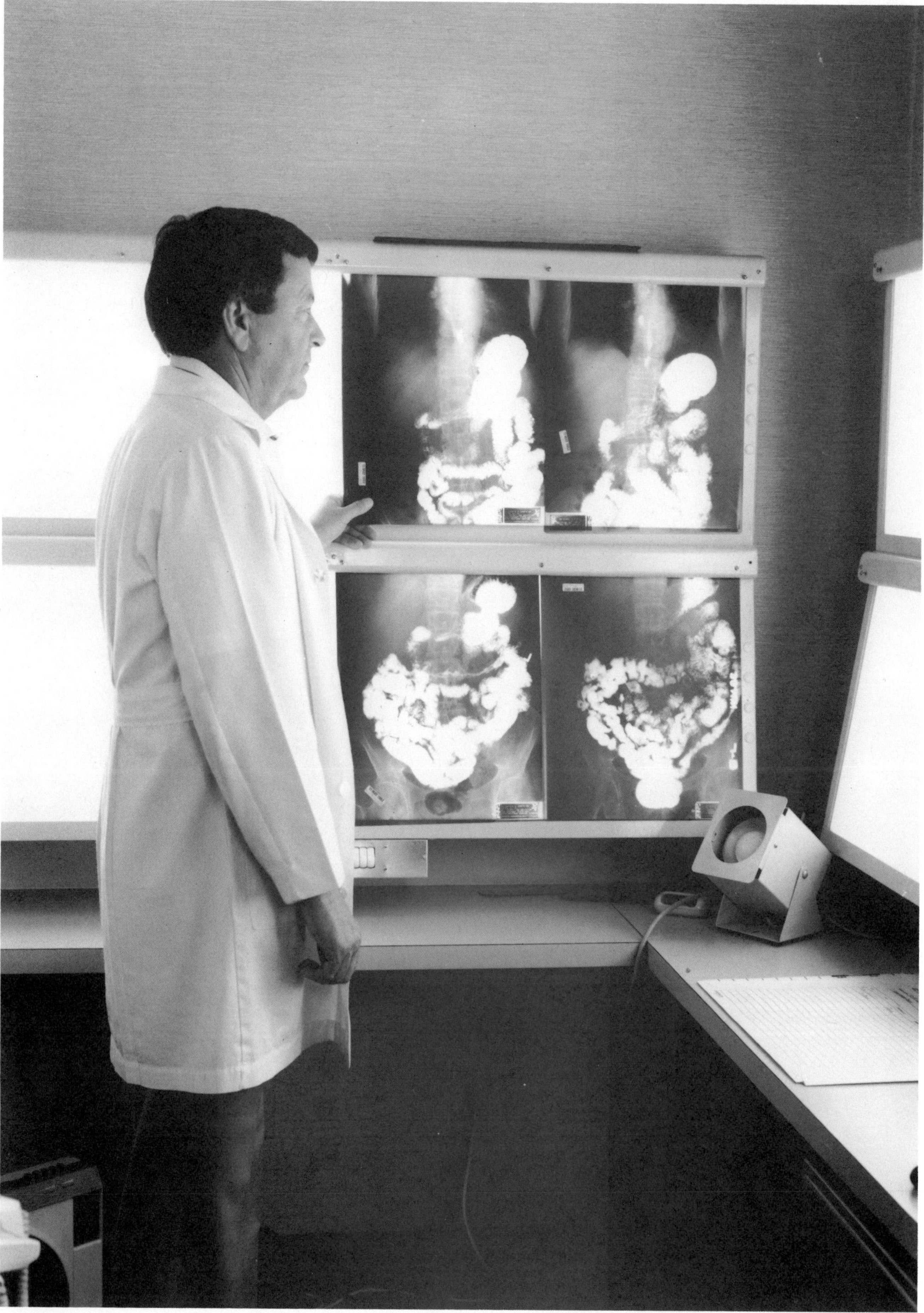

Dietary Management of Oral and Gastrointestinal Disorders

CHAPTER 25

OUTLINE

2. Chronic Diarrhea
3. Osmotic Diarrhea

B. Treatment

C. Nutritional Care

1. Acute Diarrhea
2. Chronic Diarrhea
3. Osmotic Diarrhea

Nursing Applications

VII. CROHN'S DISEASE (REGIONAL ENTERITIS)

A. Physical Consequences

B. Treatment

C. Nutritional Care

1. Goals
2. Nutritional Deficiencies
3. Nutritional Modalities
4. Fat
5. Vitamins and Minerals

Nursing Applications

VIII. ULCERATIVE COLITIS

A. Physical Consequences

B. Treatment

C. Nutritional Care

Nursing Applications

IX. IRRITABLE BOWEL SYNDROME

A. Causes

B. Treatment

C. Nutritional Care

Nursing Applications

X. DIVERTICULAR DISEASE

A. Causes

B. Treatment

C. Nutritional Care

1. Diverticulitis
2. Diverticulosis

Nursing Applications

XI. HEMORRHOIDS

A. Causes

B. Nutritional Care

Nursing Applications

XII. SURGICAL INTERVENTION

XIII. ORAL AND ESOPHAGEAL SURGICAL INTERVENTION

A. Nutritional Care

Nursing Applications

XIV. TONSILLECTOMY

A. Nutritional Care

Nursing Applications

XV. GASTRIC SURGERY

A. Complications

1. Dumping Syndrome
2. Malabsorption
3. Anemia
4. Osteoporosis

B. Nutritional Care

1. Postoperative Progression
2. Dumping Syndrome Diet

Nursing Applications

XVI. INTESTINAL SURGERY WITH CREATION OF AN OSTOMY

A. Nutritional Care

1. Progression
2. Effluent Consistency
3. Obstructions

OBJECTIVES

THE STUDENT WILL BE ABLE TO:

- Discuss general methods of dealing with dysphagia.
- Discuss the treatment of hiatal hernia.
- Explain the role of diet for ulcer disease.
- List foods included on high-fiber diets and discuss low fiber dietary regimens.
- Define and discuss diverticulosis/diverticulitis.
- Explain the steps and precautions for nutritional care of a client with an ostomy.
- Apply nursing application principles to clients experiencing GI disorders/surgeries.
- Identify client teaching tips for clients with GI disorders/surgeries.

TEST YOUR NQ (True/False)

1. Tilt the head backwards to facilitate swallowing.
2. Digestive enzyme tablets decrease heartburn.
3. A bland diet is the most common treatment for peptic ulcers.
4. Eating ice in a foreign country may cause diarrhea.
5. Dried fruits are good food choices for clients with constipation.
6. Chewing gum can cause flatus.
7. Malnutrition rarely occurs in clients with Crohn's disease.
8. A high-fiber diet is recommended for clients with diverticulitis.
9. Dumping syndrome is emesis.
10. Tapioca, creamy peanut butter, and cheese are foods ostomy clients can eat.

GI disorders can be particularly devastating because the GI tract is the only natural way of providing nutriment to the body. When GI functions are altered, digestion and/or absorption may be compromised. One out of 9 Americans is affected by some type of digestive disorder, which is the leading cause of hospitalization.

DYSPHAGIA

Stages of Swallowing

Dysphagia is a symptom of an underlying condition that affects deglutition, or chewing/swallowing in the oral cavity, pharynx, or esophagus.

Bolus—masticated (chewed) food mass.

Peristalsis—wave-like contractions in the GI tract that propel digested food.

Normally a swallow is a rapid, dynamic, and complex process, involving oral, pharyngeal, and esophageal phases (Fig. 25–1). The oral phase is voluntary. During this phase, the tongue propels a **bolus** of food posteriorly until a swallow reflex is triggered.

This reflexive swallow carries the bolus through the pharynx, thereby initiating the involuntary pharyngeal phase. Respiration ceases momentarily as the bolus passes the trachea, while coordinated muscle movements of the tongue, epiglottis, pharynx, and larynx react so the epiglottis protects the trachea to prevent aspiration. Gravity and **peristalsis** aid in moving the bolus down the esophagus. In the

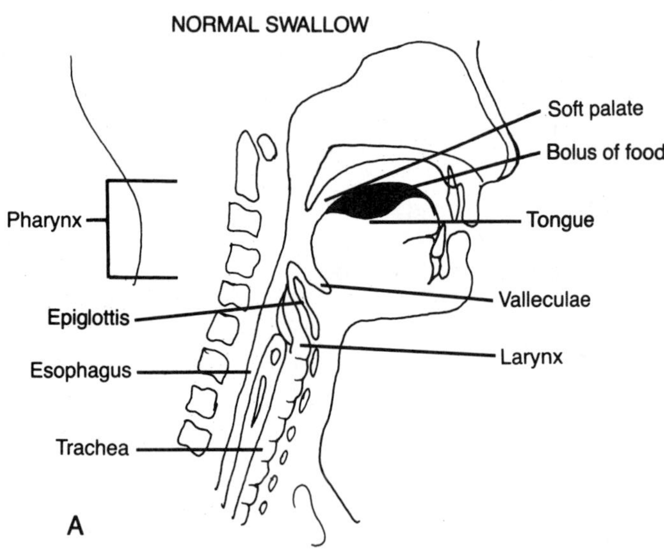

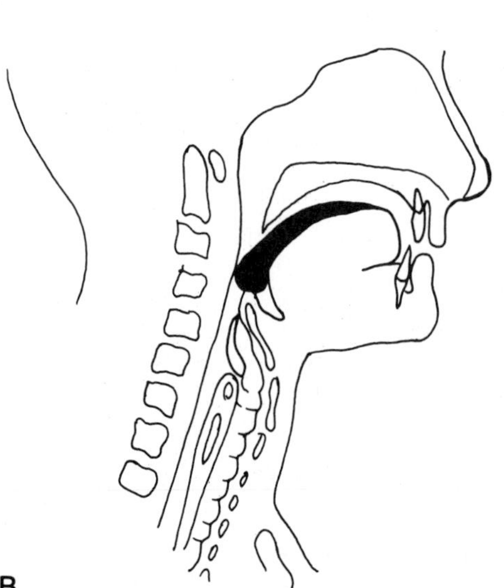

PICTURES OF A DYSFUNCTIONAL SWALLOW AS VIEWED ON VIDEOFLUOROSCOPY

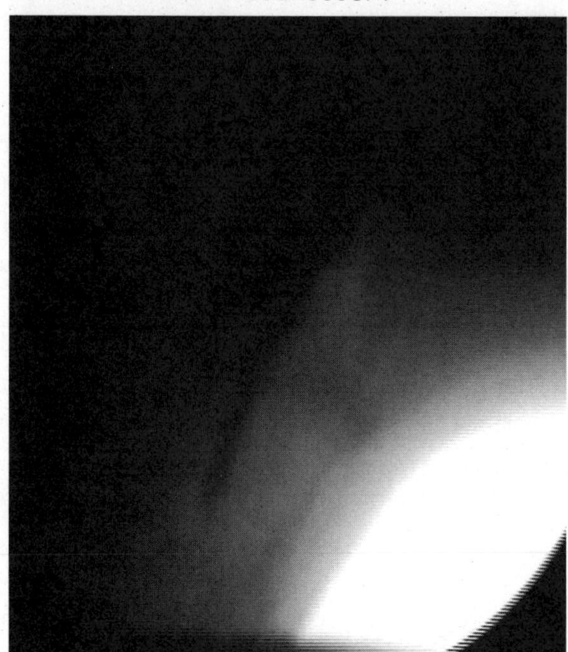

Figure 25–1 Lateral view of the intricate pharyngeal area and videofluoroscopy of dysphasic swallow. *A*, Oral phase of swallow in which food is chewed and manipulated until a bolus is formed. The anterior tongue elevates and squeezes the bolus against the hard palate, pushing the bolus backward toward the pharynx. This phase may be observed on videofluoroscopy but also may be assessed at the bedside by the SLP/physician. *B*, The back of the tongue moves down, the soft palate moves up, and the pharynx opens to receive the bolus. C, The esophagus is beginning to open as the bolus penetrates below the vocal cords with subsequent aspiration.

esophageal phase, peristalsis pushes the bolus down the esophagus toward the stomach; gastroesophageal sphincter muscles relax, allowing the bolus to enter the stomach.

Describe 3 phases of swallowing.

Causes

Achalasia is excessive sphincter tone at the junction of the esophagus and stomach (LES) preventing a normal flow of food into the stomach.

Approximately 12 to 13% of hospitalized clients have dysphagia (Martin, 1991) as a result of numerous structural or neuromotor abnormalities. Structural problems include an esophageal tumor, **achalasia,** or surgery associated with cancer of the

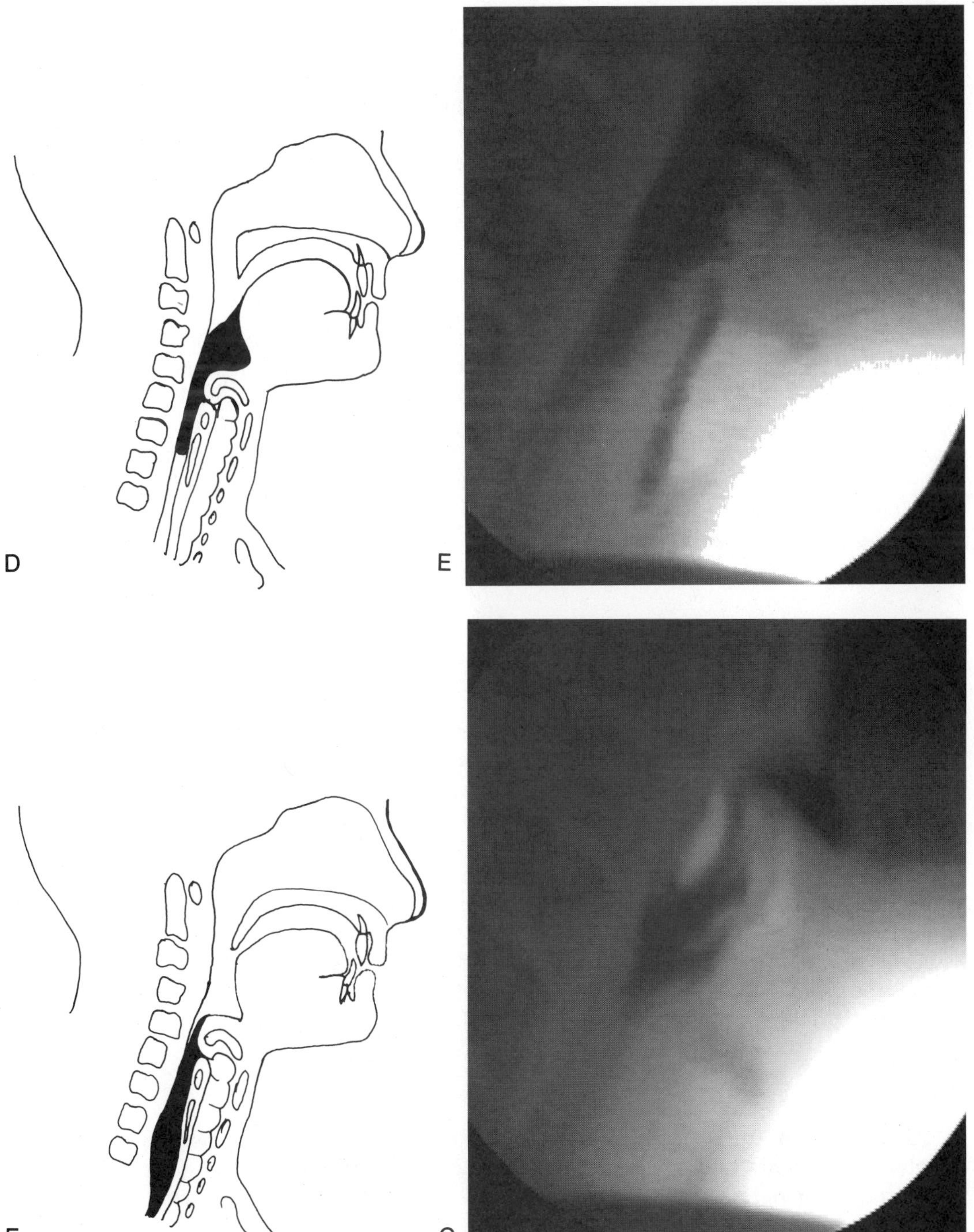

Figure 25–1 *Continued* (D–G) *D*, As the food reaches the opening of the pharynx, the swallow reflex is triggered as the bolus is moved toward the esophagus, initiating a series of coordinated movements of the tongue, epiglottis, and vocal cords and elevation of the larynx, which normally protects the airway. *E*, On videofluoroscopy, the esophagus is opening to receive the bolus with significant aspiration. *F*, During the esophageal phase, peristalsis (originated in the pharynx) moves through the esophagus, and the LES sphincter opens to allow the bolus to enter the stomach. *G*, Residue in the pharyngeal area and in the airway (aspirated material).

Name 3 structural and 3 neuromuscular causes of dysphagia.

tongue or another organ involved in swallowing. Neuromuscular disorders include cerebral vascular accident, head trauma, Parkinson's disease, multiple sclerosis, salivary gland dysfunction, cerebral palsy, amyotrophic lateral sclerosis, cerebellar degeneration, and myotonic dystrophy. Dysphagia should be suspected if a client has facial muscle weakness (drooping mouth); if a client has weak oral, neck, or tongue muscles; or if a client coughs or chokes frequently when taking foods or fluids. Neurologically impaired clients may deny having swallowing problems.

Complications

Silent aspiration is when there is no reflexive cough when foods or liquids enter the trachea.

Problems associated with dysphagia range from malnutrition related to inadequate intake to death secondary to aspiration. Any number of problems can trigger aspiration. For example, poor tongue movement can allow food to fall into the pharynx and enter the trachea before a reflexive swallow is initiated. Aspiration can also occur in clients receiving enteral feedings by the following mechanisms: (1) incorrectly inserted tube, (2) dislodged tube, or (3) gastric reflux (Meehan, 1992). Coughing is an unreliable index of aspiration because clients may be **silent aspirators.**

Nutritional Assessment

A small amount of liquid barium, barium paste, and a cookie coated with barium are ingested by the client, and the swallowing mechanism is recorded on videotape for review in slow motion.

Assessment of clients with suspected dysphagia includes taking a client history, taking a diet history, performing physical and neurological examinations, and videotaping a barium swallow. A speech language pathologist (SLP) typically participates in assessment and treatment of dysphagia. (Or in some areas, the occupational therapist (OT) performs this function). The **modified barium swallow** or **videofluoroscopy** allows assessment for physiological and anatomical abnormalities. The main concerns during videofluoroscopy are the latter part of the oral phase and the pharyngeal stage (see Fig. 25–1).

Nutritional Care

Individualizing Care Through Teamwork

An individualized treatment protocol is based on diagnosis (oropharyngeal or esophageal dysphagia). Usually various exercises are used to strengthen weakened oral-pharyngeal muscles. A SLP/OT uses appropriate techniques to teach clients to swallow in a safe way, such as thermal stimulation, body and head positioning, food placement in the mouth, and modifying food textures.

Interdisciplinary communications and teamwork are essential. A SLP may coordinate team efforts. Nurses may be responsible for implementing guidelines established by the SLP/OT for feedings at mealtime (Table 25–1), providing nourishment and liquids between meals, administering oral medications, and evaluating effectiveness of therapy. A dietitian is responsible for ensuring adequate nutriment using appropriate texture recommended by a SLP.

Preventing Aspiration

If more than 10% of a particular food texture is aspirated, this texture is restricted until clients can safely swallow. Placing clients on NPO status while being fed enterally or parenterally may be indicated. This allows time for clients to receive oral-pharyngeal muscle therapy to relearn how to swallow.

TABLE 25–1

GUIDELINES FOR FEEDING A DYSPHAGIC CLIENT

If a client needs to be fed:

1. Apply slight downward pressure on the tongue when removing a spoon from the mouth
2. Watch the thyroid cartilage (Adam's apple) to determine if client has swallowed before giving another bite or drink
3. Allow client to indicate readiness for the next mouthful
4. Converse with client only as needed. Communication may be distracting for clients who are relearning the swallowing process, but verbal direction for eating may be necessary

When oral feedings are initiated, if the client experiences difficulty with foods or liquids or coughs and chokes, discontinue the feeding. Suction equipment should be within reach. Proper positioning or having the client in an upright sitting position with 90 degrees flexion at the hips during eating is important to prevent aspiration. A semi-upright position (45-degree angle) is maintained for at least a half hour following feedings.

Sufficient time for eating must be allowed. However, after eating for about 30 minutes, clients may tire, which would increase risks of a dysfunctional swallow. Thus, small, frequent (4 to 6) feedings promote adequate nutrition without tiring clients.

If one side of the face is weak or paralyzed, head rotation toward the weaker side improves swallowing. Neck flexion during swallowing facilitates glottis closure by the epiglottis and enhances the pharyngeal phase of swallowing.

If too much food is put into the mouth too rapidly, place a single food item in front of the client and provide a spoon with a small bowl to limit bite size. Washing food down with liquids increases aspiration risk. If allowed by treatment protocol, use flexible straws. Checking a client's mouth after meals and removing any **pocketed** food with a toothette decreases chance of a client unknowingly retaining and inadvertently aspirating food.

In neurologically affected clients, sensation may be decreased; food remaining in the mouth, especially between gums and cheeks, is called pocketing.

Papain—commercially available enzyme from papaya.

Describe 3 ways to prevent aspiration.

If excessive drooling or salivation occurs, or excessive thick phlegm is produced, avoid uncooked milk products (milk and ice cream). Cream soups and puddings are acceptable. Some juices, such as cranberry, pineapple, and grapefruit (thicken if needed), or **papain** may help cut mucous (Wood, 1989; Groher, 1984).

Modifying Textures, Aromas, and Temperatures

Modifying food consistency may be recommended for dysphagic clients. If food is tolerated, a diet order specifies a texture or consistency of foods and beverages. Normal diet texture progression is from thick pureed foods (semi-solid consistency), to foods requiring little chewing (ground), to chewable foods in bite-sized pieces (sugar cube size). Unless recommended by a SLP/OT, pureed foods are avoided because their lack of texture fails to stimulate a swallow reflex, thereby increasing aspiration risk.

Slippery foods are easier to swallow but may be difficult to control in the mouth for mastication. Thus, toast is tolerated better than bread; a boiled potato is more easily controlled than mashed potatoes. Moistened foods allow clients to form a bolus easier; using gravies, sauces, mayonnaise, or ketchup to moisten foods may be desirable. Foods that fall apart easily, such as corn kernels or peas, plain ground meat, rice, and dry cottage cheese, can be easily aspirated. Sticky foods such as peanut butter or soft bread with a hard crust should be avoided. Foods with a combination of textures, such as soups, are difficult for clients to control orally until a swallow is initiated.

Mildly sweetened and salted foods are generally favored because flavor initiates a better swallow by increasing saliva production. Temperature guidelines provided by the SLP/OT are important since food temperatures (hot or cold) may be necessary to stimulate the swallow reflex. When nerve function is impaired, cold temperatures stimulate swallowing.

Thin beverages are the most difficult to manipulate. Beverages may be thickened to nectar, honey, or pudding consistency. Thickened beverages are easier for the tongue to manipulate and help initiate the oral phase of swallowing. Beverages and some foods may need to be thickened using a modified food starch, such as Thick-it (Milani) or Thick and Easy (American Institutional Products). Hydration status is frequently overlooked. Because thickened beverages are not well accepted, clients may consume limited amounts of allowed fluids.

What are some foods to provide; to avoid? Describe beverage considerations for these clients.

NURSING APPLICATIONS

Assessment

Physical—for difficulty swallowing, drooling, frequent pneumonia, choking or coughing associated with food/fluid intake; poor initiation of swallowing, food pocketing; gurgling voice or breathing; hydration status (I&O, skin turgor, mucous membranes), level of consciousness.

Dietary—for various food textures that appear to present problems, type of diet ordered, SLP's recommendations.

Interventions

1. Do not allow client to self-feed unless the client will be safe and alert throughout the meal. Client safety is paramount.
2. Monitor client for deterioration of nutritional status, as client may inadvertently reduce food intake because of decreased palatability, apathy, poor endurance, or depression; note and report intake and weight loss to a dietitian/physician.
3. Make sure client is well rested before feeding, and remove distractions during feeding to allow concentration on chewing and swallowing.
4. If the client must be fed, begin by offering a quarter teaspoonful of food. Never give more than ½ a heaping teaspoon (Meehan, 1992).
5. Use adaptive equipment per SLP's recommendation.
6. Note any particular types of foods or textures that cause problems for a client (such as coughing) and report to physician, SLP/OT, or dietitian.
7. If client complains of "food sticking in the throat," alternate thickened liquids and solids. Liquids may assist solids through the pharynx, promoting more food intake (Rubin-Terrado & Linkenheld, 1991).
8. For clients who can close lips but have a weak or delayed swallow reflex, offer fluids in a glass that is ¾ full to prevent tilting the head too far back to take a drink. Use nosey cutout glass if recommended by the SLP/OT (see Chapter 16, Fig. 16–7). For clients who have difficulty propelling liquids back into the mouth but have a functional swallow reflex, offer fluids in a glass that is ⅓ or less full to promote tilting the head back so fluid flows further back into the throat (Rubin-Terrado & Linkenheld, 1991).

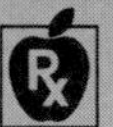

If on anticholinergic drugs, monitor swallowing. Anticholinergic medications decrease saliva and make swallowing more difficult.

Evaluation

* Aspiration should not occur, and texture-modified, nutritionally balanced meals are consumed by clients in sufficient quantity and variety to meet nutritional requirements.

Client Education

- Plain or flavored gelatin, thick sauces, creamed soups, and pureed fruits and vegetables in an appropriate consistency can be used to increase fluid intake.
- Nutritional supplements (thickened or puddings) can provide complete nutrition in a concentrated form when appetite is poor.
- Place food on stronger side of mouth if client has had a stroke affecting one side of the body.

LOWER ESOPHAGEAL SPHINCTER INCOMPETENCE: GASTROESOPHAGEAL REFLUX, HIATAL HERNIA, AND ESOPHAGITIS

One of the most common problems encountered in clinical practice is **gastroesophageal reflux (GER)** (heartburn). Because many clients assume heartburn is normal, they do not report it to their physician.

GER is a return of gastric contents into the esophagus, causing severe burning sensations under the sternum.

Acidity from the stomach, alkalinity, pepsin, or bile may be damaging to the esophageal mucosa. This reflux occurs most frequently about 30 minutes to 1 hour following a meal. The LES usually keeps caustic stomach juices from refluxing into the esophagus. If esophageal pressure is less than stomach pressure, juices reflux into the esophagus and cause pain. If this condition is not treated, **esophagitis** may result.

Esophagitis is inflammation of the lower esophagus.

When does this reflux occur most often?

Causes

Increased levels of serum progesterone are correlated with increased GER. Sphincter pressures are progressively decreased during pregnancy, in women taking birth control pills containing progesterone, and even in late stages of normal menstrual cycles. Vigorous exercise can induce GER in normal clients with greater amounts of reflux related to postprandial exercise (Clark et al, 1989). GER is also associated with achalasia. A **hiatal hernia** affects LES pressure and may cause GER (Fig. 25–2). Various medications may also lower LES pressure and cause GER (Table 25–2).

A partial stomach protrusion (herniation) through the esophageal opening into the chest cavity is called a hiatal hernia.

GER is an important cause of chronic bronchitis and asthma (Sontag et al, 1990; Mansfield, 1989). Recognition and treatment of GER can lead to improvement of these pulmonary problems.

Name 5 causes of GER.

Treatment

A few lifestyle changes are recommended in addition to antacid use. These include elevation of the head of the bed, avoidance of tight-fitting clothes (belts, undergarments) and some medications (Table 25–2), remaining upright for 1 to 3 hours after eating, and restriction of alcohol intake and smoking. Weight loss may be encouraged if needed; other dietary changes include abstaining from eating foods that aggravate the condition and for at least 2 to 4 hours before bedtime. Nurses

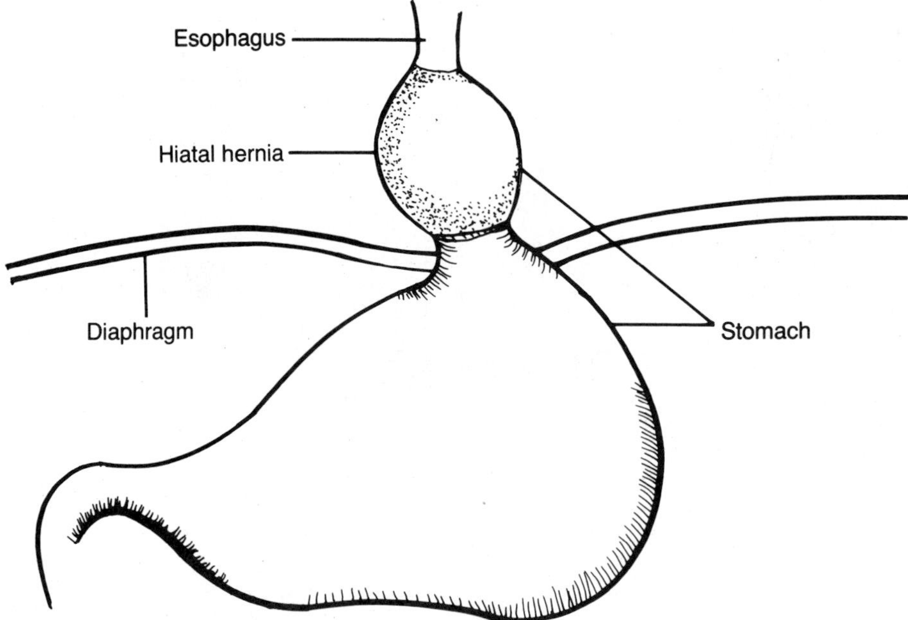

Figure 25–2 Hiatal hernia.

are in a prime position to advise clients of benefits of these changes and to educate clients on how best to implement these changes based on a client's lifestyle (Mitchell & Parry-Billings, 1992).

Antacids help alleviate pain by neutralizing stomach acidity but do not deter reflux. They are more effective if food is present in the stomach. Antacids differ not only in duration and strength, but also in their side effects (e.g., inducing constipation or acting as a laxative) on nutritional status (Table 25–3).

Other medications, i.e., histamine (H_2) receptor antagonists are effective in reducing acid production; long-term effects on acid production can cause malabsorption of vitamins B_{12} and folate. The use of these medications has resulted in less emphasis on the simplistic traditional modes of therapy already mentioned, but these simple lifestyle modifications are based on sound physiological principles (Kitchin & Castell, 1991).

TABLE 25–2

ALTERATION OF LOWER ESOPHAGEAL SPHINCTER PRESSURE BY DRUGS AND FOODS

Increase	Decrease
Drugs	
Cholinergics (Reglan, Urecholine)	Theophylline
	Alcohol
	Anticholinergics (atropine, Bentyl, Librax)
	Beta-blockers
	Calcium channel blockers (Isoptin)
	Prednisone
	Valium (Diazepam)
	Oral contraceptives
	Tobacco smoking
Foods	
High-protein foods (meats, eggs, fish)	Fatty foods
	Chocolate
	Carminatives (spearmint, peppermint)
	Caffeine
	Garlic

TABLE 25–3

ADVANTAGES AND DISADVANTAGES OF ANTACIDS

Components	Advantages	Disadvantages	Trade Name
Aluminum hydroxide	Hypophosphatemia with renal insufficiency Floats on gastric contents Reduces tendency to reflux Combines with bile salts	Lowers serum phosphorus with continuous use Constipation Hypercalciurea, resorption of bone calcium and phosphate Chalky taste Inactivates thiamin	AlternaGel, Amphojel, Basaljel
Magnesium hydroxide	Can be used as a laxative	Hypermagnesemia, especially in renal failure Diarrhea Decreases vitamin A absorption Hypophosphatemia Resorption of bone calcium and phosphate	Milk of Magnesia
Calcium carbonate	Source of calcium	Constipation Milk-alkali syndrome Rebound hyperacidity Hypercalcemia Decreases iron absorption	Tums, Titralac
Sodium bicarbonate	Can alkalinize urine to enhance excretion in drug overdoses	High in sodium Possible milk-alkali syndrome Hypercalcemia Reduces folate and iron absorption	Baking soda, Citrocarbonate
Hydroxymagnesium aluminate		High in aluminum and magnesium Hypermagnesemia, especially in renal failure Decreased vitamin A absorption May inhibit gastric emptying May cause hypophosphatemia	Riopan
Magnesium carbonate		May cause rebound hyperacidity Inhibits gastric emptying	Gaviscon (Extra Strength, Liquid)
Magnesium/aluminum hydroxide	Low sodium	Decreased vitamin A absorption Inactivates thiamin Decreased calcium absorption and may lower serum phosphorus with long-term use Chalky taste	Maalox, Mylanta, Gelusil

TABLE 25–4

FREQUENTLY CONSUMED FATTY FOODS
Fried foods
Gravies
Pastries
Fatty meats (bacon, sausage, choice grade meats, frankfurters, luncheon meats)
Cheese (aged cheese and cream cheese)
Nuts
High-fat snacks (potato chips, some crackers, dips)
Salad dressing, mayonnaise, sour cream

Nutritional Care

Dietary factors may decrease LES pressure, stimulate acid production, and irritate the esophageal mucosa. Thus, goals of nutrition therapy are to increase LES pressure and decrease reflux and esophageal irritation.

Lower Esophageal Sphincter Pressure

Carminatives, such as spearmint, peppermint, or garlic, are oil extracts of plants used as food seasonings or flavorings.

Fatty foods, chocolate, and **carminatives** decrease LES pressure and worsen GER (see Table 25–2). Alcohol also lowers LES pressure. Conversely, a high-protein diet is advocated since protein increases sphincter pressure.

What foods increase or decrease LES pressure?

What foods should be avoided to decrease acid secretions or decrease esophageal irritation?

Esophageal Irritants

Caffeine, cola, coffee (regular and decaffeinated), alcohol, beer, and milk stimulate acid secretion, which irritates the esophageal mucosa. Onions promote esophageal reflux. Coffee, red peppers, citrus juices, and tomato products are directly irritating to the esophagus (Kitchin & Castell, 1991; Allen et al, 1990).

Intragastric Pressure

Decreasing intragastric pressure may lessen GER symptoms; gastric retention or dilation increases intragastric pressure. Therefore, small, frequent (4 or more) feedings are better tolerated. Fluids can be taken between meals with small amounts at mealtimes to decrease volume of a meal. Weight loss, if appropriate, is recommended. Chewing gum and using straws are also discouraged because this increases flatus and intragastric pressure.

Foods high in fats (Table 25–4) decrease LES pressure and delay gastric emptying; thus, gastric reflux may occur for up to 3 hours after eating (Kitchin & Castell, 1991). Since fatty foods remain in the stomach longer than proteins and carbohydrates, a low-fat diet (<45 gm/day) may be used for treating GER; it may also be effective in promoting weight loss.

Name 3 ways to decrease intragastric pressure.

NURSING APPLICATIONS

Assessment

Physical—for amount and type of medications used, smoking habits; heartburn; height, weight, IBW.

Dietary—for adequacy of intake; caffeine, fat, alcohol, protein intake; knowledge of foods that increase/decrease LES and intragastric pressure.

Interventions

1. Implement measures using gravity to facilitate movement of food from mouth to stomach (decreasing intragastric pressure and esophageal exposure to gastric acid). Clients should (1) sit in an upright position while eating and (2) avoid waterbeds.
2. If weight loss is needed, refer to a dietitian or weight loss program such as Weight Watchers or TOPS for counseling and a nutritionally sound reduction program.
3. Give H_2 antagonists and antacids at least 1 hour apart. Antacids inhibit cimetidine (Tagamet) absorption.
4. Monitor for possible interactions of drug therapy. Cimetidine and ranitidine (Zantac) increase risk of warfarin-induced bleeding. Cimetidine may increase risk of intoxication related to elevated blood alcohol levels (DiPadova et al, 1992).

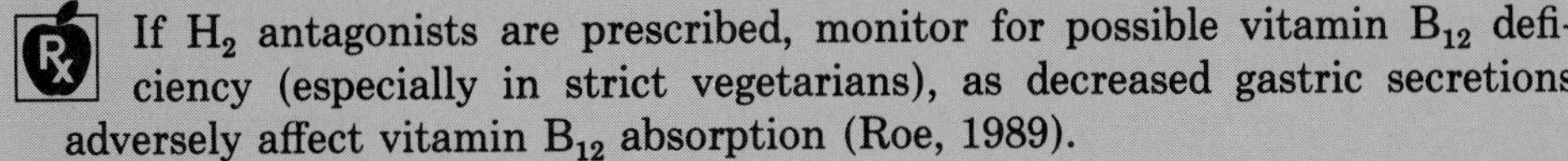
If H_2 antagonists are prescribed, monitor for possible vitamin B_{12} deficiency (especially in strict vegetarians), as decreased gastric secretions adversely affect vitamin B_{12} absorption (Roe, 1989).

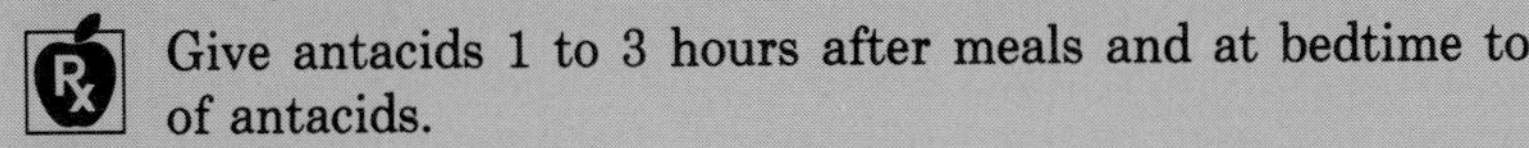
Give antacids 1 to 3 hours after meals and at bedtime to prolong effects of antacids.

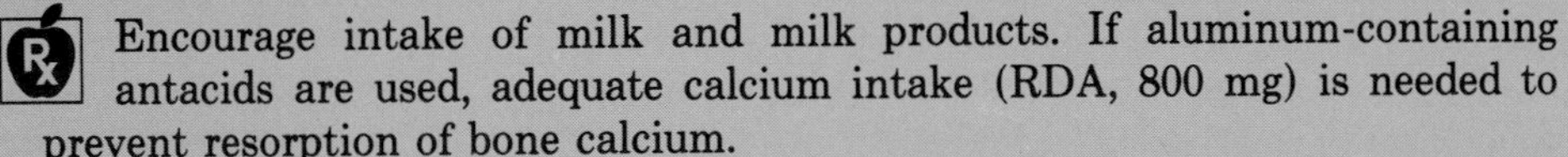
Encourage intake of milk and milk products. If aluminum-containing antacids are used, adequate calcium intake (RDA, 800 mg) is needed to prevent resorption of bone calcium.

Evaluation

* Client should plan a meal that will not adversely affect LES pressure and describe foods allowed and those foods that decrease LES pressure and irritate the esophagus.

Client Education

- Avoid foods listed in Tables 25–2 and 25–3 that decrease LES pressure.
- Drink fluids between meals.
- Since citrus fruits and tomato products are avoided, other sources of vitamin C intake include cantaloupe, potatoes, and strawberries.
- GER is a frequent occurrence in pregnancy, but is temporary.
- Heartburn is not caused by inadequate digestion; therefore, digestive enzyme tablets are not appropriate.
- GER may be accompanied by a feeling of fullness or regurgitation, but it can masquerade as chest pain or pulmonary disorder.

PEPTIC ULCER

A peptic **ulcer** may occur in any part of the GI tract exposed to pepsin and gastric acid. A stomach erosion is called a gastric ulcer, whereas a peptic ulcer in the duodenum is termed a duodenal ulcer. Stress ulcers are common from trauma (burns, major illness, or injuries). Maintaining a gastric pH above 4.0 appears to reduce morbidity and mortality associated with such stress-induced ulcers (Rogers, 1990).

An ulcer is tissue erosion of skin or mucous membrane.

Causes and Physical Consequences

The fundamental cause of peptic ulcer is unclear. In some instances, secretion of HCl with or between meals is excessive; mucosal lining of the stomach is not sufficiently protected; or peristalsis of the digestive tract is reduced, allowing acid to remain in the GI tract longer than usual. When mucosal erosion allows submucosal exposure to gastric juices, an ulcer may develop. Excessive production of acid and pepsin may be the main cause of duodenal ulcer, whereas decreased tissue resistance may be more important in gastric ulcers. Gastric ulcers have also been associated with gastritis from the *Helicobacter pylori* organism, which impairs mucosal defense.

Melena—tarry stools.

Ordinarily burning epigastric pain similar to heartburn occurs, but some ulcers are discovered by hemorrhage or **melena.** Other symptoms, including aching, burning, gnawing, and boring sensations, occur before meals. Pain from duodenal ulcers occurs 1 to 4 hours after a meal or in the middle of the night when the stomach is empty; in gastric ulcers, pain occurs on eating, and pain is not relieved by food intake.

What may cause an ulcer? What is the main problem in a client with a duodenal or gastric ulcer?

Treatment

GI peristalsis and secretions are directly affected by tension and strain. A basic component of treatment involves modifying lifestyle toward a more relaxed and slower pace with less strain and pressure. Nicotine from tobacco products increases acid secretion and should be limited, or better yet, eliminated.

Antacids are frequently used to neutralize acidity. In addition to having different effects on nutritional status (see Table 25–3), each has a different acid-neutralizing capacity. Antacids are most effective in sustaining acid neutralization if taken 1 hour after eating.

Nurses must remember to watch for sodium overload if antacids are given over a long-term period. This sodium overload could contribute significantly in clients with renal disease or congestive heart failure (Esberger, 1991).

H_2 antagonists inhibit gastric secretions, accelerate healing, and reduce pain. Use of these medications usually reduces the need for antacids, and antacids may interfere with their absorption. However, many of these medications affect nutritional status (Table 25–5). Since intrinsic factor secretion may be decreased, clients on long-term therapy with these drugs should be monitored for vitamin B_{12} deficiency. Sucralfate (Carafate) enhances prostaglandin synthesis, binds with bile salts and pepsin, and coats the ulcer (Szabo & Hollander, 1989; Friedman, 1988). Treatment for *Helicobacter pylori* usually includes colloidal bismuth (Pepto-Bismol) and emeprazole (Prilosec).

Surgery is sometimes necessary, especially when hemorrhage or perforation occurs. Fortunately, use of H_2 medications has decreased the need for surgical procedures (discussed in the section on surgical interventions). Because of the availability of H_2 inhibitors and sucralfate, clients with peptic ulcers are no longer placed on severely restrictive diets, and surgical procedures are necessary less frequently.

Nutritional Care

In the past, the principal treatment for ulcers was frequent feedings of milk and cream to coat the stomach lining. Currently milk is not used as a therapy since large amounts of calcium and protein are potent stimulants of gastric acid secretion. Milk has a transient buffering effect, so it does not need to be eliminated, but frequent milk intake is not advised.

Why is milk not used as therapy?

Bland Diet

There is much disagreement about which foods to include or exclude. Research shows that a bland diet does not decrease gastric acid secretion or increase healing rate.

TABLE 25–5

ADVANTAGES AND DISADVANTAGES OF ANTIULCER MEDICATIONS

Generic (Trade) Name	Advantages	Disadvantages
Cimetidine (Tagamet)	May be given with meals	Reduced effectiveness with caffeine, cigarette smoking, and alcohol Can cause confusion in the elderly May cause diarrhea Decreased gastric secretion results in less iron, folate, vitamin B_{12} absorption Hyperglycemia Decreased absorption if given with antacids or Reglan Increases risk of bleeding associated with warfarin-induced vitamin K deficiency
Ranitidine (Zantac)	Associated with fewer side effects and interactions than cimetidine	Abdominal discomfort May cause constipation or diarrhea Elevated liver enzymes (SGOT (AST), SGPT (ALT), gamma glutamyl transferase) Increases risk of bleeding associated with warfarin-induced vitamin K deficiency Decreased vitamin B_{12} absorption with long-term use
Sucralfate (Carafate)	Protects ulcer from acid, bile, and pepsin	Interferes with absorption of fat-soluble vitamins; deficiencies associated with long-term use May cause GI discomfort, constipation, diarrhea; dry mouth Decreases bioavailability of tetracycline and cimetidine if taken with sucralfate

Data from Allen AM. *Powers & Moore's Food Medication Interactions.* 7th ed. Tempe, AZ, Ann Moore Allen, 1991; and Roe DA. *Handbook on Drug and Nutrient Interactions.* 4th ed. Chicago, American Dietetic Association, 1989.

A bland diet is now considered a transitional diet used during severe inflammation and to determine food intolerances. It is designed to avoid chemical, thermal, and mechanical irritations of the GI tract and decrease peristalsis. Fried and raw foods are usually excluded. Small, frequent feedings buffer gastric acidity and reduce symptoms during acute stages (Pemberton et al, 1988). When pain disappears, intervals between feedings may be lengthened and larger amounts of food eaten. Although a bland diet is safe, it does not hasten the healing process nor prevent recurrences.

Dietary Modifications

Symptoms of food intolerance are related more to individual response than to intake of specific foods or presence of disease. A client is the best person to decide which foods are eliminated, if any. Most condiments do not cause gastric irritation, with the exception of black pepper and chili powder, and should be allowed, as tolerated by clients. A person with an ulcer may continue a normal diet or a diet as tolerated. However, an individual should maintain a regular eating schedule and eat moderate amounts to avoid gastric distention. A relaxed atmosphere is important to allow clients to eat slowly and chew food thoroughly to decrease workload on the stomach.

Small, frequent feedings have not been shown to be more effective than 3 meals a day and may be contraindicated because of increased acid secretion.

Coffee and decaffeinated coffee stimulate acid secretion (Elta et al, 1990). If the client insists, caffeine-containing beverages may be taken with or near mealtime even though this may increase gastric acid production. Other foods present buffer effects of caffeine and may minimize stress in an already stressed client. Some clients experience discomfort from citric acid juices. Alcohol is a potent gastric acid stimulator and should be avoided.

What foods can cause gastric irritations?

Fiber

Increased dietary fiber has been studied in ulcer management. Insoluble fibers (whole-grain products) increase GI motility. Soluble fiber (from fruits, vegetables, and oatmeal) affects acid, pepsin, and bile and may delay gastric emptying. Adequate chewing is important for any ulcer client; fiber-rich diets, which have an added benefit of satiety, require more oral processing. Clinical studies to date do not support fiber for ulcer healing or prevention. However, a low-fiber diet may result in constipation, a frequent problem when antacids are a principal form of therapy (Rydning et al, 1986).

NURSING APPLICATIONS

Assessment

Physical—for smoking, time of pain in relation to meals, medications taken.
Dietary—for intake of caffeine, fiber, alcohol; eating patterns (frequency, speed, environmental factors); knowledge of gastric irritants.
Laboratory—for Hgb, Hct, sodium.

Interventions

1. Encourage client to eat slowly and chew foods well. Teeth are designed to prepare food for digestion, not the stomach.
2. Allow client to decide which foods to eliminate since responses to specific foods are unique to an individual.
3. Give antacid 1 hour after meals and at bedtime (see Table 25–3) and schedule so it is not given with any H_2 antagonists prescribed.

Rx Ranitidine (Zantac) may be more effective if given 2 hours before meals rather than with food; greater acid inhibition is achieved (Cole et al, 1992).

Rx Increase intake of high fiber foods to prevent constipation if sucralfate is prescribed (Roe, 1989).

Rx Sucralfate may be given prophylactically for trauma clients (burns, major illness, or injuries); monitor these clients closely for hypophosphatemia because sucralfate binds with phosphate in the GI tract (Millet & Simpson, 1991).

Evaluation

* Desirable outcomes of care are that a client eats in a relaxed manner and plans a menu that decreases gastric discomfort.

Client Education

- Skim milk is quite acceptable as part of a dietary regimen.
- Decrease or avoid alcohol, coffee (caffeinated and decaffeinated), cocoa, and spicy foods since these increase acid production.
- Avoid smoking.
- Use acetaminophen or buffered aspirin rather than aspirin or nonsteroidal anti-inflammatory agents (e.g. ibuprofen) for pain.

INTESTINAL GAS AND FLATULENCE

Causes

Excess **flatus** can be produced by **aerophagia** from eating with the mouth open, digestion of certain foods, or intestinal bacteria. Chronic air swallowing accounts for 60 to 80% of intestinal gas. This can be related to anxiety, nervousness, or breathing problems in addition to practices associated with foods and types of foods. Gulping food or fluids or carbonated beverages, using a straw, and frequent sucking of hard candy or chewing gum or food with the mouth open encourage air swallowing.

Flatus—gas in the GI tract. Aerophagia—air swallowing.

Most gases in the large intestine are formed as a result of bacterial action. Some foods serve as a suitable medium for gas-forming bacteria, but other foods are irritating to the large intestine, resulting in expulsion of gas before they are absorbed.

Name 3 ways flatus can be produced.

Nutritional Care

Gas-forming foods (e.g., beans, peas, cabbage, broccoli, Brussels sprouts) contain nonabsorbable **oligosaccharides,** which remain in the bowel, increasing bacterial action and forming gas. These foods can be eliminated or taken in moderation depending on the client's preferences and tolerances. Other vegetables reported to be gas-forming include cauliflower, onions, turnips, corn, and cucumbers. Since fats produce carbon dioxide (a gas), their intake may be reduced.

Oligosaccharide—a carbohydrate that contains several (3–10) simple sugars.

Describe nutritional care for flatulence.

NURSING APPLICATIONS

Assessment

Physical—for flatus.

Dietary—for speed of intake, drinking and snacking habits, intake of gas-forming foods.

Interventions

1. If habits associated with air swallowing are practiced, discuss with the client so behavior can be modified.
2. Monitor for possible lactose intolerance, which also causes increased flatus.

Evaluation

* Relief of discomfort and flatulence are the desired outcomes as well as minimizing dietary habits that increase air swallowing.

Client Education

- If gas-forming foods appear to be associated with increased flatus, curtail their use. However, intestinal response to these foods is variable between clients.
- Ambulation may help relieve gas pains.
- Remain erect after eating meals for at least 30 minutes.

CONSTIPATION

Causes

Constipation is prolonged retention of feces in the colon resulting in small volume and difficult evacuation of hard, dry stools.

Decreased peristalsis results in prolonged transit time in the GI tract, allowing more fluid absorption. Possible causes include (1) inadequate fiber intake, (2) inadequate fluid intake, (3) lack of exercise, (4) habitually not responding to defecation urges, or (5) habitual use of laxatives or enemas. In addition to the aforementioned reasons, hospitalized clients are frequently constipated as a result of poor intake, inactivity, depression, and/or medications or anesthetics.

TABLE 25–6

DRUGS USED FOR CONSTIPATION

Type of Agent and Generic Name	Trade Name	Nutritional Implications
Bulk-forming agents (increases bulk)		
Psyllium	Metamucil	Least likely to cause nutrient malabsorption
Methylcellulose	Fiberall	Increase fluid intake (8–10 glasses/day)
Polycarbophil	Perdiem	Can reduce appetite
	Citrucel	Can reduce riboflavin absorption
	Konsyl	Long-term use can alter transport of electrolytes and lower plasma cholesterol
	FiberCon	
		Creates a feeling of fullness
Stimulants (increases peristalsis)		
Bisacodyl	Correctol	Decreases absorption of vitamins D and C
Senna	Ex-Lax	With prolonged use or abuse, may cause potassium depletion and malabsorption with weight loss
Phenolphthalein	Feen-A-Mint	
	Dulcolax	
	Senokot	Encourage increased fluid intake unless contraindicated
		Do not give bisacodyl with milk or antacids, as this dissolves enteric coating, releasing irritating content
		Long-term use of phenolphthalein can adversely affect vitamin D, potassium, protein, and calcium absorption
Saline cathartics (draws water into the GI tract)		
Magnesium hydroxide/sulfate	Milk of Magnesia	Can cause severe dehydration and hypermagnesemia
	Epsom salts	
		Encourage increased fluid intake unless contraindicated
Emollient (lubricant) laxative (reduces surface tension by coating stool and intestines)		
Mineral oil	Agoral plain	Decreased absorption of vitamin D and fat
	Kondremul	May decrease absorption of vitamins A, E, K
		Impairs calcium and phosphorus absorption
		Take 2 hours after food intake
		Do not take at bedtime; possibility of oil aspiration
Surfactants (increases bulk, softens stool)		
Docusate calcium/potassium/sodium	Surfak	Encourage fluid intake unless contraindicated
	Dialose	Alters electrolyte absorption
	Colace	Docusate calcium and potassium useful with low-sodium diet
	Modane	

Numerous medications cause constipation, including aluminum and calcium antacids, anticholinergics, iron supplements, anticonvulsants, diuretics, antidepressants, and some narcotics. Certain conditions predispose to constipation: stroke, multiple sclerosis, Parkinson's disease, spinal cord injuries, hypothyroidism, and colon cancer.

Atonic constipation results from ignoring the urge to defecate or overuse of laxatives. Intermittent constipation can result from obstructions such as **impaction, adhesions,** or tumors. This type of constipation may allow small, ribbonlike stools to be passed.

Impaction—hardened feces that may block the intestinal tract. Adhesions—fibrous bands connecting 2 surfaces that are normally separate.

Name 5 causes of constipation.

Treatment

The most important factor regulating colonic function is diet (Taylor, 1990). Different types of laxatives are relied on frequently because of their ease of use and client compliance (Table 25–6). More than $200 million are spent for OTC laxatives annually (Donatelle, 1990). Bulk-forming agents such as methylcellulose (Citrucel) are the safest and most effective agents used for constipation. Surfactants function as stool softeners and are particularly useful in immobile clients to soften hard stools. Saline laxatives draw water into the bowel and promote easier passage of stools; long-term use results in loss of body salts. Stimulant laxatives (such as bisacodyl, senna, and phenolphthalein) should be used infrequently since they may damage GI nerves and muscles. Mineral oil should not be taken for extended periods because it interferes with absorption of fat-soluble vitamins.

Nutritional Care

Dietary recommendations include (unless contraindicated by other conditions) providing sufficient fluids (at least 8 to 10 glasses daily) and foods with fiber such as raw fruits and vegetables and whole-grain breads and cereals. Fluids allow water to be drawn into the stool, making feces soft and easier to pass.

Fiber provides bulk, which stimulates peristalsis. Many secondary effects of fiber (flatulence, bloating) decrease with time, probably as a result of alterations in colonic microflora. These effects can be minimized by increasing fiber intake gradually (Taylor, 1990). Bran may be added to a wide variety of foods. One of the most important effects of dietary fiber is reducing laxative use by clients.

What are dietary recommendations for constipation?

NURSING APPLICATIONS

Assessment

Physical—for I&O; irregular bowel habits; use of laxatives, drug intake, conditions that may cause hard, dry stools.

Dietary—for fiber and fluid intake, knowledge of fiber content of foods.

Interventions

1. Offer clients a hot beverage on arising, such as coffee, tea, or lemon water, to enhance peristalsis.
2. If possible, assist client to the toilet, as squatting is the natural position for defecation.
3. Caution clients about the hazards of laxative abuse.
4. Encourage increasing fiber and fluid intake, especially if stool softeners, saline laxatives, or bulk laxatives are prescribed.

Rx Administer medications as ordered (see Table 25–6) and monitor for side effects. These agents alter nutrition in varying ways while alleviating constipation.

(Continued)

Evaluation

* Client should lessen or eliminate laxative use, plan/consume a high-fiber diet, and pass soft stools.

Client Education

- Infrequency of bowel movements does not mean constipation. A normal elimination pattern may be only 2 to 3 times per week; everyone is different in their elimination patterns.
- Increasing fiber and fluids can relieve constipation, but does not cure it; therefore, these dietary changes should be life-long.
- Fiber intake must be increased gradually to prevent diarrhea and flatus.
- Dried fruits (especially prunes) stimulate peristalsis by acting as natural laxatives.
- Fiber tablets cannot be considered an adequate substitute for dietary fiber.
- Exercise/activity may decrease incidence of constipation by stimulating peristalsis.

DIARRHEA

Causes and Physical Consequences

Diarrhea may be defined as excess liquidity of stools that causes increased frequency of stools.

Diarrhea may have a number of causes, including the presence or lack of microorganisms, dietary substances, organic changes, or malabsorption syndromes. Intestinal contents are rapidly propelled through the small intestine with excessive loss of fluids, electrolytes (especially sodium and potassium), and nutrients by diminishing absorption time.

Acute Diarrhea

Pathogenic—disease producing.

Acute diarrhea is usually of short duration and caused by **pathogenic** organisms. Food-borne pathogenic microorganisms are responsible for tens of millions of cases of diarrheal illness in the US each year, costing an estimated $1 billion to $10 billion (Hecht, 1991). A summary of more prevalent food-borne–related pathogenic organisms is provided in Table 25–7. Antibiotics reduce microflora, and chemotherapeutic agents affect intestinal villa, reducing absorption. These medications may cause transient acute diarrhea.

Travelers' diarrhea, frequently called "turista," "Montezuma's revenge," or "green-apple two-step," affects 20 to 50% of Americans traveling abroad (Cohn, 1991). Poor sanitation may result in foods being contaminated with a variety of infectious agents; *Escherichia coli* is the most common. This untimely illness is usually not severe; high fever, vomiting, or bloody stools occur in only a minority of cases.

Name 5 foods associated with travelers' diarrhea.

Clients should be aware of measures to prevent travelers' diarrhea; foods and beverages likely to produce diarrhea should be avoided. Improperly handled, cooked or uncooked foods may be implicated. Raw vegetables, meat, and seafood are especially risky foods. Other items associated with increased risk of travelers' diarrhea include tap water, ice, unpasteurized milk and dairy products, and unpeeled fruits. Only canned or bottled carbonated beverages using water that has been boiled or chemically treated are safe.

TABLE 25–7

SUMMARY OF COMMON FOOD-BORNE ORGANISMS

Illness or Organism	Incubation Period	Duration	Symptoms	Foods Implicated	Prevention	Treatment
Salmonella	6–36 hours (usually 12 hours)	1–3 days	Diarrhea, nausea, abdominal cramps, prostration, chills, fever, and vomiting. Severe cases resemble typhoid	Raw meat and poultry; cracked eggs and egg products; salads; milk and milk products; gravies, sauces, and warmed-over food	Wash hands; adequately cook foods; immediate and adequate refrigeration of foods; clean work surfaces	Rehydration
Clostridium perfringens	8–24 hours	12–24 hours	Abdominal cramps, intestinal gas, and diarrhea; rarely, fever or vomiting	Meats inadequately cooked and allowed to cook slowly or stand at room temperature	Serve meats directly after cooking or refrigerate rapidly between cooking and serving	Self-limited disease
Clostridium botulinum	8–72 hours	Weeks; death may occur in 4–8 days	Early signs include fatigue, weakness, vertigo, and dry mouth followed by blurred vision and progressive difficulty in speaking and swallowing; bilateral sixth nerve dysfunction with or without ptosis or pupillary abnormalities	Home-canned vegetables improperly processed—especially string beans, asparagus, spinach, and smoked fish	Pressure cooking of home canned foods, especially vegetables	Maintain adequate ventilation; trivalent antitoxin
Staphylococcus	2–4 hours	Less than 24 hours	Abrupt and violent onset of nausea, vomiting, explosive diarrhea, prostration. No fever	Cooked ham or other meats, cream-filled or custard pastries, and other dairy products; chicken, fish, meat, or potato salads; gravies, sauces, and dressings	Handle food as little as possible with bare hands. Thoroughly cook foods; refrigerate foods immediately after cooking; frequent hand washing. Persons with infected lesions or nasal discharges should not be permitted to handle food	Rehydration; antiemetics
Trichinosis	24–72 hours (acute)	Year or more	Vomiting, cramps, and diarrhea for 2–3 days; followed by muscle pain and tenderness, fever, periorbital edema, which subsides about 1 month after onset	Inadequately cooked pork and pork products; whale, bear, walrus, and seal meats	Adequate cooking of pork and pork products	Adrenocorticotropic hormone or corticosteroids

Chronic Diarrhea

Chronic diarrhea is usually of long duration (3 to 6 months) and is frequently caused by intestinal lesions or irritations associated with GI diseases such as irritable bowel syndrome, colon cancer, inflammatory bowel disease, and AIDS. Magnesium-containing antacids and vitamin/mineral supplements may precipitate chronic diarrhea. Nutritional deficiencies are common secondary to impaired absorption. Malabsorption results in loss of electrolytes, vitamins, minerals, protein, and fats.

Osmotic Diarrhea

Cations—electrolytes that have positive charges in a solution. Divalent cations include calcium and magnesium, which have 2 positive charges.

Osmotic diarrhea is the result of fluid drawn into the GI tract to dilute osmotically active substances.

Carbohydrate intolerance, **divalent cations,** or saline laxatives result in **osmotic diarrhea.** Lactose or gluten intolerance results in osmotic diarrhea. In children, carbohydrate malabsorption following the ingestion of common fruit juices may cause a nonspecific osmotic diarrhea (Hyams et al, 1988). Because of low albumin levels, osmotic diarrhea is associated with PEM when refeeding is initiated. Osmotic diarrhea can be caused by medications, especially when enteral feedings are provided.

Treatment

Second to fluid and electrolyte replacement, which is of utmost concern in all types of diarrhea, is the importance of a correct diagnosis to prescribe appropriate medications that will not worsen diarrhea. In addition to a diet history to determine where clients have been and eaten, other medical conditions that may reveal organic causes, types of foods consumed recently, medications taken, a thorough physical examination, and a stool culture are important to determine presence of pathogenic organisms. Nonspecific antidiarrheal agents, used to slow peristalsis or thicken stools, may be harmful to a client infected with pathogenic organisms, which may require antibiotics specific for the type of organism. A decreased transit rate may allow bacterial overgrowth.

Adsorbents (bismuth preparations, kaolin, and pectin) and bulk-forming agents (methylcellulose) have no major nutritional side effects. The use of aluminum hydroxide on a long-term basis lowers phosphate levels. Anticholinergics used to relieve cramping associated with diarrhea should be given 30 minutes to 1 hour before meals. Opioid preparations (Lomotil, loperamide, paregoric, and opium tincture) suppress peristalsis to allow absorption of water and electrolytes and are used especially to decrease propulsive diarrhea reactions. They may precipitate nausea and constipation (Table 25–8).

Little can be done to relieve symptoms or shorten the course of travelers' diarrhea, but suggestions for diarrhea in general may be followed. Drugs can be used to reduce severity of diarrhea; prophylactic antimicrobial drugs are not recommended.

In antibiotic-induced diarrhea, microorganisms can be replaced using *Lactobacillus acidophilus,* yogurt, or buttermilk. Osmotic diarrhea can sometimes be corrected by removing the offending substance or diluting hyperosmolar solutions/medications provided. Hypoalbuminemia-induced diarrhea is corrected as a client's nutritional status is improved. Use of cholestyramine (Questran) to control chronic diarrhea is discussed with small bowel resection. TPN may be the only way to provide nourishment for clients with intractable diarrhea.

Nutritional Care

Goals of therapy for all types of diarrhea are to replace fluid plus electrolytes and decrease the number and frequency of stools. Without fluid replacement, dehydration and acidosis may result. Thus, IV replacement may be necessary.

TABLE 25–8

ADVANTAGES AND DISADVANTAGES OF ANTIDIARRHEALS

Generic (Trade Name)	Advantages	Disadvantages
Diphenoxylate (Lomotil)	May be taken with food	Nausea, vomiting, bloating, anorexia, dry mouth, swollen gums
Pectin/kaolin (Kaopectate)	Occurs naturally in some foods Has a local effect, not systemic	Constipation, dry mouth, altered taste perception
Loperamide (Imodium)		Abdominal pain, constipation, bloating, dry mouth, vomiting, nausea
Paregoric (camphorated tincture of opium)	Can give with food May help decrease pain	Nausea, vomiting, constipation, sedation, dry mouth, anorexia Extreme CNS toxicity leading to decreased breathing, disorientation, and seizures if given with cimetidine Can be habit-forming
Difenoxin (Motofen)	Can give with food to negate GI side effects	Can be habit-forming Nausea, vomiting, dry mouth, epigastric distress

Acute Diarrhea

Because acute diarrhea of bacterial origin is self-limiting, nutrition therapy is not a major concern for most healthy clients. Adults can usually maintain electrolyte and hydration status with additional intake. This consideration is more serious in infants and elderly clients because of their limited capacity to maintain fluid balance and in clients who are already ill or whose immune systems are suppressed.

In severe cases, NPO status may serve to relieve the digestive tract; but as a rule, it is unnecessary to withhold all feedings. Fluids that help replace sodium and potassium losses are advocated. Diarrheal dehydration can be prevented with the use of oral rehydration therapy (ORT). **Oral rehydration solutions** are initiated at the onset of diarrhea to prevent and treat dehydration. These solutions are much safer than the commonly used soft drinks, fruit juices, or sports beverages (Avery & Snyder, 1990). Additionally, plain water, juice, carbonated beverages, flavored gelatin, and other clear liquids may aggravate diarrhea, especially in children and infants, and lead to further electrolyte imbalances (Leung, 1989).

Oral rehydration solutions are a mixture of sugar or cereals, salts, and water in proportions similar to body fluids. The American Academy of Pediatrics has recommended a solution for rehydration with more sodium than the one used for maintenance. Because of cost and ease of distribution, the use of 2 different solutions has not proved practical.

Numerous studies have found that early refeeding did not adversely affect the course of diarrhea in infants and children (Lifschitz & Shulman, 1990; Margolis et al, 1990). Early refeeding using lactose-free formulas is generally recommended since it appears to minimize weight loss and adverse nutritional effects of prolonged fasting (Brown et al, 1988).

Frequently diarrhea may precipitate temporary lactose intolerance. Milk or lactose-containing products are withheld for at least 6 hours after the last episode of diarrhea to prevent osmotic diarrhea.

Eliminating raw fruits (except bananas) and vegetables, colas, coffee, tea, and alcoholic beverages may be beneficial. Extremely hot or cold foods, foods high in insoluble fiber, caffeine, and alcohol may increase peristalsis and should be avoided.

As acute diarrhea subsides, increase bananas, rice, applesauce, and tapioca (BRAT) intake. The BRAT diet may decrease transit time and bind liquids. (Bananas provide potassium and pectin; applesauce supplies pectin, which binds free water and improves consistency of stools).

Foods containing fat should be used in moderation. As a result of increased peristalsis, fats cannot be digested and may lead to **steatorrhea.**

Steatorrhea—abnormal amounts of fat in feces.

What do oral rehydration solutions treat? What foods should be withheld for at least 6 hours after the last episode of diarrhea and why? What foods are on the BRAT diet?

Chronic Diarrhea

What type of diet is recommended to prevent nutritional deficiency in chronic diarrhea?

Hyponatremia (lethargy, mental confusion) and hypokalemia (muscle weakness) may occur because of significant losses of sodium and potassium. To prevent nutritional deficiency in chronic diarrhea, high-protein, high-kilocalorie diets and nutrition supplements are recommended. Other nutritional factors such as fat, fiber, or lactose are dependent on specific disease processes.

Osmotic Diarrhea

Fluid loss may be significant in osmotic diarrhea. For information on osmotic diarrhea related to enteral feedings see Chapter 17; lactose or gluten intolerance is discussed in Chapter 23.

NURSING APPLICATIONS

Assessment

Physical—for hydration status (I&O, skin turgor, and mucous membranes); weight changes; recent travel and location, medications used.
Dietary—for caffeine, fiber, carbohydrate, and fluid intake.
Laboratory—for sodium, potassium; albumin; stool culture.

Interventions

1. Maintain accurate records concerning frequency, amount, and consistency of stool to determine client's response to treatment.
2. Administer antidiarrheal drugs as ordered.
3. For intractable diarrhea, suggest TPN to physician/dietitian to replace fluid and nutrients lost.
4. Explain that carbonated beverages may further aggravate diarrhea because of their high osmolality.

Evaluation

* Desired outcomes include soft formed stools and normal hydration levels as evidenced by good skin turgor and moist mucous membranes.

Client Education

- Fluid and electrolyte intake is critical; solids may be added when preferred if diarrhea is of short duration.
- Apple juice is not beneficial since it contains little sodium and has been associated with osmotic diarrhea.
- Foods containing soluble fiber (oatmeal, bananas, apple) are helpful in binding fluid and decreasing fluidity of stools, whereas insoluble fiber (bran, whole-grain products) increases peristalsis and may worsen diarrhea.
- Until the problem is resolved, avoid fatty foods (see Table 25–4).
- During bouts of diarrhea, avoid caffeine, which increases peristalsis.
- When traveling, eat only hot well-cooked meals, self-peeled fruits, and packaged foods. Be sure milk products are pasteurized (Cohn, 1991).

CROHN'S DISEASE (REGIONAL ENTERITIS)

Physical Consequences

One of the 2 types of inflammatory bowel disease (IBD) is Crohn's disease. This inflammatory process involves ulcerations through all layers of the intestinal wall, with a characteristic cobblestone appearance, primarily affecting the ileum and the proximal colon (although it can affect any part of the GI tract). Because affected areas are scattered among normal sections, some absorption is maintained. Crohn's disease affects mainly children and young adults. Scarring, thickening, and narrowing of the intestinal wall restrict nutrient absorption and cause a narrowed lumen with increased risk/frequency of intestinal obstructions. Thus, diarrhea, abdominal pain, and fever result; steatorrhea may also occur. Peristalsis precipitated by food intake is associated with cramping pain.

This condition is intimately tied to nutritional status. Inadequate nutrient intake, even for short periods, produces morphological and functional changes that may further increase malabsorption and depress a body's ability to heal.

What is the characteristic appearance of Crohn's disease and what part of the intestine does it primarily affect?

Treatment

Currently there is no medical treatment totally effective in curing Crohn's disease. During critical periods of Crohn's disease, corticosteroids, such as prednisone and sulfasalazine (Azulfidine) are used, but neither is effective in maintaining remission. Many clients with Crohn's disease who require surgery to remove the diseased area ultimately experience a postoperative recurrence at the **anastomotic** site (Sachar, 1990). Metronidazole (Flagyl) may also be prescribed to reduce anaerobic bacteria. Azathioprine (Imuran), an immunosuppressive drug, is commonly used. If diarrhea is severe, antidiarrheal agents such as loperamide (Imodium) are given (Perucca, 1992).

Anastomotic—connection between 2 normally distinct structures joined in a surgical procedure.

Nutritional Care

Goals

Goals of nutritional care include (1) removal of irritating and poorly absorbed foods and (2) reversal of nutritional deficiencies and growth failure in children.

Nutritional Deficiencies

Nutritional deficiencies are related to the extent, severity, and location of ulcerations. Problems related to nutritional deficiencies include anemia, hypoalbuminemia, poor wound healing, and suppressed immune response. As shown in Table 25–9, clients are frequently malnourished because of inadequate intake, anorexia, malabsorption, intolerance to many different food components (fat, lactose, and fiber), and nutrient–drug interactions (Perucca, 1992).

Adequate nutrition support to correct or prevent nutritional deficiencies is a challenge. A team approach in the treatment of this condition is vital. Because of effects of food, i.e., abdominal discomfort and diarrhea, clients are finicky and ap-

TABLE 25–9

NUTRITIONAL PROBLEMS RELATED TO INFLAMMATORY BOWEL DISEASE

Inhibiting food intake	Anorexia, nausea, pain, malaise, fever, food intolerances, restrictive diet
Increasing nutritional requirements	Inflammation, fever, infection, cell proliferation
Increasing nutrient losses	Morphological and functional changes secondary to inadequate nutrients, malabsorption due to scarred, thickened, and narrowed mucosa surface area; bacterial overgrowth; increased peristalsis and diarrhea; steatorrhea related to poor bile salt absorption; drugs; bleeding; protein-losing enteropathy
Affecting nutrient utilization	Corticosteroids, sulfasalazine

prehensive about eating. Spontaneous food intake does not usually maintain or increase weight in clients.

Nutritional Modalities

Different nutritional modalities are used, depending on disease severity (Table 25–10). Clients with acute Crohn's disease may require TPN or elemental diets to rest the bowel and improve healing and closure. This curtails drainage and induces remission. It is generally believed that TPN has no significant advantage over oral feedings except in clients with severe obstruction and severe malnutrition (Cravo et al, 1991), and its widespread use is discouraged. Numerous studies have documented favorable responses on elemental and polymeric formulas (Rigaud et al, 1991; Giaffer et al, 1990; O'Keefe et al, 1989). However, because of varied results of other studies, the only conclusion is that nutrition, whether provided by TPN, elemental diets, or oral diet, can reverse nutritional deficiencies caused by Crohn's disease and can aid in the healing process in conjunction with standard medical treatment (Culpepper-Morgan & Flock, 1991; Singleton, 1991).

With improvement, foods are gradually added, progressing to a semi-regular diet and eliminating foods that cause problems for clients. A diet high in kilocalories (40 to 50 kcal/kg IBW), protein (>1.5 gm/kg IBW), vitamins, and minerals is needed to replenish depleted stores secondary to the inflammatory process, fever, and catabolic effects of corticosteroid therapy. Small, frequent meals are better tolerated to increase adequacy of intake. Even though clients can tolerate some foods, supplementation with polymeric formulas may be necessary to augment nutrient intake.

Fat

In clients with Crohn's disease of the distal ileum or an ileal resection, a low-fat diet (40 gm/day) is required to control diarrhea. Rapid transit rate (increased peristalsis) decreases fat absorption, resulting in decreased bile salt reabsorption, which further reduces fat absorption and may cause steatorrhea. Therefore, a low-fat diet using principally emulsified fats, such as in homogenized milk and nutrition supplements, or MCT oils that do not require bile for absorption, are better toler-

TABLE 25–10

NUTRITION MODALITIES IN INFLAMMATORY BOWEL DISEASE

Severity of Disease	Goal of Treatment	Helpful Hints
Mild stage	Restrict foods that are irritating and/or poorly absorbed	Decrease fiber intake, especially popcorn, seeds (sesame, pepper, tomato), nuts, fruit peels, broccoli, dried beans Restrict lactose-containing foods (milk and milk products) Restrict fatty foods. Foods with short-chain or medium-chain fats are better tolerated; use to increase kilocalories
Mild to moderate stage	Increase kilocalorie intake and correct nutritional deficiencies	Counsel client or parents regarding nutritional needs and a well-balanced diet. Increase kilocalories >300–500 kcal/day; protein requirement, 1.5–3 gm/kg/day Supplement with a multivitamin containing 100–150% of the RDA
Moderate to severe stage	Induce clinical remission by providing bowel rest	Use enteral elemental nutrition orally or via tube feedings Use TPN when obstruction is almost total or when fistula cannot be bypassed by feeding tube

ated. A low-fat diet is also important to decrease **oxalate** absorption and potential renal stone formation.

Oxalates, formed from oxalic acid that is present in dark green leafy vegetables, rhubarb, chocolate and cocoa, and nuts, normally bind with calcium and are excreted. If steatorrhea is present, calcium is bound and excreted with fats, and more oxalate is absorbed.

Vitamins and Minerals

Anemia may result from inadequate intake of iron, folate, and vitamin B_{12}. Because of malabsorption, clients may need more than the RDAs for water-soluble vitamins and minerals, especially vitamins C, B_6, and B_{12}; iron; zinc; copper; calcium; potassium; folate; and magnesium, to prevent or correct subclinical deficiencies. Supplements of fat-soluble vitamins should be given every other day. Intramuscular injections of vitamin B_{12} may be needed. If sepsis occurs and the client is receiving corticosteroid therapy, hyperglycemia may result. Insulin may be required to decrease serum glucose levels to normal.

Name 2 goals for Crohn's disease. What can cause malnutrition in Crohn's disease? What type of diet is needed to replenish depleted stores?

NURSING APPLICATIONS

Assessment

Physical—for age, height, weight, weight changes, growth rate for children (use growth charts); diarrhea, steatorrhea, abdominal cramping/pain; fever.

Dietary—for appetite; food, caffeine, alcohol intake; self-imposed dietary restrictions.

Laboratory—for Hgb, Hct, RBCs, MCV; potassium, calcium, magnesium; albumin, nitrogen balance, transferrin, glucose.

Interventions

1. Refer clients to the dietitian for nutrition counseling.
2. Encourage client to eat by discussing/alleviating fears associated with feedings. Provide medications as prescribed to lessen pain.
3. Discuss rationale for fiber, nutritional supplements, and fluids.
4. Monitor for lactose intolerance as milk products are not well tolerated. Discuss other sources of calcium for bone mineralization (see Chapter 23, Table 23–12).
5. Monitor for gluten intolerance. Damage to the villa may produce a temporary intolerance to wheat products (see Chapter 23).
6. If nutrition supplements are needed, maintain a container of client's favorite type and flavor in the room in an iced container.
7. Provide empathy and support because this disease may cause lost time from school/work, financial concerns, disrupted relationships, numerous hospitalizations, an uncertain future, and emotional upheavals (depression, irritability, fear, anxiety, and so forth).

Rx Corticosteroid use has numerous nutritional implications. If corticosteroids are prescribed, implement the following measures: (1) If edema develops, restrict sodium intake; (2) for hypokalemia, encourage intake of high-potassium foods; (3) for hyperglycemia, encourage omission of concentrated sweets; (4) if client appears to be in negative nitrogen balance (weight loss, muscle wasting), encourage nutritional supplements; (5) for osteoporosis, encourage appropriate sources of calcium, phosphorus, and vitamin D; (6) if blood lipid levels are elevated, encourage low-cholesterol, low-fat foods. Be aware that corticosteroids may be administered rectally through a retention enema to cause direct contact with GI mucosa and reduce side effects (Percucca, 1992).

Rx Encourage an intake of 8 to 10 cups of fluid if client is on Azulfidine. Azulfidine may precipitate sulfa crystals in the urine and is irritating to gastric mucosa.

(Continued)

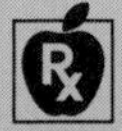 Absorption of iron and folate is decreased by Azulfidine; increase foods rich in iron and folate, and monitor Hgb, Hct, and MCV levels.

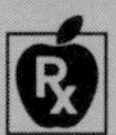 If antibiotics are used, microflora may be diminished; monitor PT (blood clotting test) and encourage intake of foods that contain vitamin K.

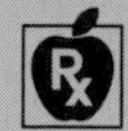 A metallic taste coupled with dry mouth may decrease intake in clients taking Flagyl. Offer clients mouth care and sugarless lozenges.

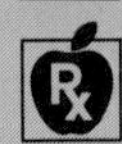 Administer Flagyl with food to decrease epigastric distress.

Evaluation

* Client should consume 60 to 75% of required diet and increase weight.

Client Education

- Resources available to these clients are "Reach Out for Youth with IBD" and the newsletter *The Community* for clients with Crohn's disease and ulcerative colitis, and Crohn's & Colitis Foundation of America (see Appendix E-1).
- Remissions may last a few weeks to many years (Perucca, 1992).
- If steatorrhea is present, use MCT oils to increase kilocalorie intake, as they do not require bile for absorption.
- When diarrhea is present, be sure a well-balanced diet is consumed with increased intake of potassium, magnesium, and zinc, which are lost in large amounts.
- Most multivitamin supplements omit folate, so clients need to look for folate on the nutrient label.
- High-calcium, low-oxalate intake helps decrease incidence of oxalate renal stones.
- Clients with extensive involvement or resection of the ileum from Crohn's disease require vitamin B_{12} IM every month.
- For clients taking Flagyl, it is normal for urine to turn dark.
- Abstain from alcohol while taking Flagyl; the concurrent intake causes a disulfiram-like reaction.

ULCERATIVE COLITIS

Physical Consequences

The second type of inflammatory bowel disease, ulcerative colitis, is colon inflammation, sometimes extending into the rectum and less frequently involving the terminal ileum. Ulcerative colitis and Crohn's disease are so similar that they are often hard to distinguish. However, in ulcerative colitis, the mucosa becomes very fragile and bleeds easily. It is usually continuous along the GI tract, whereas Crohn's disease affects only segments.

Diarrhea, occurring when scar tissue fills in ulcerations of the mucosa and destroys absorptive areas of the colon, is the most critical factor. Diarrhea and malabsorption, caused by bacterial overgrowth within the bowel lumen, create deficiencies of nutrients and trace elements (see Table 25–9). Fever may occur with the disease itself or from secondary infections. Exacerbations often follow emotional upsets, illness, or dietary indiscretions involving milk and fried or fatty food.

How are Crohn's disease and ulcerative colitis different?

Growth failure in children is probably multifactorial. In addition to problems already discussed, endocrinologic problems may contribute to growth failure (Michener & Wyllie, 1990).

Treatment

As with Crohn's disease, corticosteroids are used during critical periods. Sulfasalazine is the principal drug used during mild to moderate phases and sometimes during remission.

Nutrition support is an integral part of therapy to promote healing and prevent further deterioration of nutritional status while allowing bowel rest. Elemental formulas have become a key therapy for clients with acute inflammatory bowel disease; TPN is used when fistulas, obstruction, or abscesses are present. Such treatment can result in remission without surgical intervention.

Nutritional Care

Counseling is extremely important to help clients understand reasons for dietary intervention. Abdominal discomfort with expectations of GI discomfort and diarrhea causes clients to become reluctant to eat. Clients are encouraged to eat whatever foods they desire; restrictions are unnecessary.

Irritating foods are excluded (see Table 25–10). Extremely hot and cold foods and high-fiber foods are avoided because they increase peristalsis. Milk and milk products that contain large amounts of lactose are discouraged. Lactase deficiency may precipitate worsening of symptoms. If the terminal ileum is involved, fat intake should be decreased to 40 gm/day, as described in Crohn's disease.

During bouts of diarrhea, a well-balanced diet is advocated to replace potassium, magnesium, and zinc losses. **Toxic megacolon** may be precipitated by hypokalemia. Not only is potassium lost during severe diarrhea, but also magnesium may be lost, sometimes resulting in hypomagnesemia. When diarrhea is bloody, anemia may develop. Insufficient intake of iron, folate, and vitamin B_{12} may also contribute to anemia. Vitamin and mineral concerns are the same as in Crohn's disease.

Toxic megacolon—a complication of ulcerative colitis that causes colonic dilatation.

Teamwork is needed to help stimulate the client's appetite. Nutrition supplements may be necessary, especially in children. When symptoms are under control, a low-residue diet (Table 25–11), high in protein and kilocalories (40 to 50 kcal/kg IBW), is initiated. A low-residue diet is easier to digest and places less strain on intestines; high protein (>1.5 gm/kg IBW) intake provides amino acids for healing.

As a client progresses, fiber is introduced, gradually increasing to a high-fiber diet. Soluble fibers, or guar and pectin, are especially helpful because of their water-retaining capacity. Exercise is an important adjunct.

When symptoms are under control, what diet is recommended and why? What foods are avoided?

NURSING APPLICATIONS

Assessment

Physical—for findings in Table 25–9; IBW, weight/height percentile on growth charts (for children), weight loss, bloody diarrhea.

Dietary—for appetite, adequacy of intake, intake of protein, kilocalories, residue, magnesium, zinc, potassium.

Laboratory—for Hgb, Hct, MCV; sodium, potassium; glucose, lipids.

Interventions

See the section on Crohn's disease.

Evaluation

* Client should gain or maintain weight. Additionally, symptoms should be controlled or alleviated.

Client Education

See the section on Crohn's disease.

TABLE 25–11

LOW-FIBER/LOW-RESIDUE FOODS

Milk/milk products	Limited to 2 cups/day
Fruits*	Fruit juices without pulp (excluding prune) Canned fruit Ripe bananas
Vegetables*	Vegetable juices without pulp Lettuce Cooked tender vegetables: asparagus, beets, green beans, tomato sauce/puree; spinach, eggplant, acorn squash, white potatoes (without skin)
Bread/cereals	White or refined breads and cereals (cream of wheat, cornflakes, puffed rice)
Meats	Lean tender meats without grease: ground or well-cooked beef, lamb, ham, veal, pork, poultry, fish, organ meats, eggs, cheese

* To reduce residue further, eliminate all fruits and vegetables except strained fruits and vegetable juices and white potatoes without skin.

IRRITABLE BOWEL SYNDROME

Causes

IBS is defined as recurrent or chronic abdominal pain, accompanied by alternating periods of constipation and diarrhea and bloating, or feelings of abdominal distention without diagnosable organic cause.

Irritable bowel syndrome (IBS) is as "common as the common cold" and the most frequent problem seen by physicians. Functional abnormalities may occur in the small bowel. GI symptoms are worse following a meal, especially a large meal; attacks are frequently associated with emotional stress.

Many clients attribute their abdominal pain to specific foods, but there is little evidence that specific food sensitivities are involved. Numerous studies have tested for a connection between food allergy and IBS, but an immunological response is not present in many clients. Conversely, many clients have a strong history of atopy and improve on an elimination diet (Mullin, 1991). Other causative factors include laxative and caffeine abuse, previous GI illness, lack of fluid intake, and irregular bowel movements.

Treatment

Because of the diversity of symptoms, a combination of medications are used. Anticholinergic medications relieve abdominal pain that is due to GI spasms. When diarrhea is present, antidiarrheal agents are used to slow intestinal motility, and bulking agents for constipation result in softer stools with increased volume.

Nutritional Care

In acute stages of IBS, the goal is to minimize residue and feces (if a client has diarrhea); therefore, a low-fiber, low-residue diet may be ordered (see Table 25–11). Elemental formulas may be used, especially for lactose-intolerant clients; elemental formulas are completely absorbed, resulting in no fecal residue.

As the condition improves, soft, nonirritating foods are added along with a high fluid intake. Gradually fiber is introduced. Increased dietary fiber has become the cornerstone of therapy. However, results of various studies with fiber have produced conflicting results (Dietary, 1990).

A low-fat diet that also eliminates gas-forming foods may improve postprandial discomfort by decreasing gas formation. Wheat bran is more effective for clients with abdominal pain and predominant constipation. Bulking agents such as psyllium (Metamucil) may be more effective than unprocessed bran in decreasing constipation (Shaw et al, 1989). Other foods reported to provoke symptoms include cereals, dairy products, caffeine, alcohol, citrus fruits, onions, and potatoes (Shaw et al, 1989). Allowing a client to identify specific food intolerances with elimination of that item may be the most effective treatment (Dietary, 1990).

What types of food are used in acute stages of IBS; as the condition improves?

NURSING APPLICATIONS

Assessment

Physical—for cigarette use; weight loss, IBW, stress level.
Dietary—for rich food, caffeine, gas-producing foods, and alcohol intake.

Interventions

1. If client is lactose intolerant, discuss ways of maintaining adequate calcium intake (see Chapter 23, Table 23–12).
2. Discuss ways of handling stress.
3. Assist client in maintaining a food diary to help identify food sensitivities.

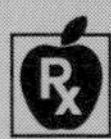 Provide anticholinergic and antidiarrheal medications 30 minutes to 1 hour before meals.

Evaluation

* Client consumes a diet that relieves symptoms and provides nutrients and kilocalories to regain/maintain normal body weight.

Client Education

* Regular mealtimes and nourishing meals may help decrease symptoms.
* Increase fiber gradually to 20 to 30 gm to prevent discomfort from flatus. If flatus occurs, reduce fiber and gradually increase again. Increased fiber is encouraged for constipation rather than laxatives, which may precipitate diarrhea (Drossman et al, 1992).
* Abstain from gas-forming foods (beans, cabbage, Brussels sprouts, and so forth) if not tolerated.
* Diarrhea may be associated with excessive sorbitol intake from candies, gums, and other dietetic foods and drinks (Drossman et al, 1992).
* Avoid foods listed in Table 25–4.
* Exercise regularly.

DIVERTICULAR DISEASE

Causes

More than half of the population in the US will have diverticular disease by age 60 (Weck, 1987). A protrusion of intestinal mucosa through the muscular coat is called a colon **diverticulum** (Fig. 25–3). Greater pressure exerted to remove hard, dry stools may cause the diverticula; diverticulosis is thought to be precipitated by chronic constipation.

Diverticulosis is the term for protruding colon pouches; diverticulitis refers to inflammation in these pouches that occurs because of inadequate drainage or impacted feces.

Treatment

In diverticulitis, treatment depends on the nature and degree of inflammation. Severe cases may require bed rest. In addition to dietary changes, antibiotics (usually ampicillin or tetracycline) and analgesics may be indicated. Surgery may be re-

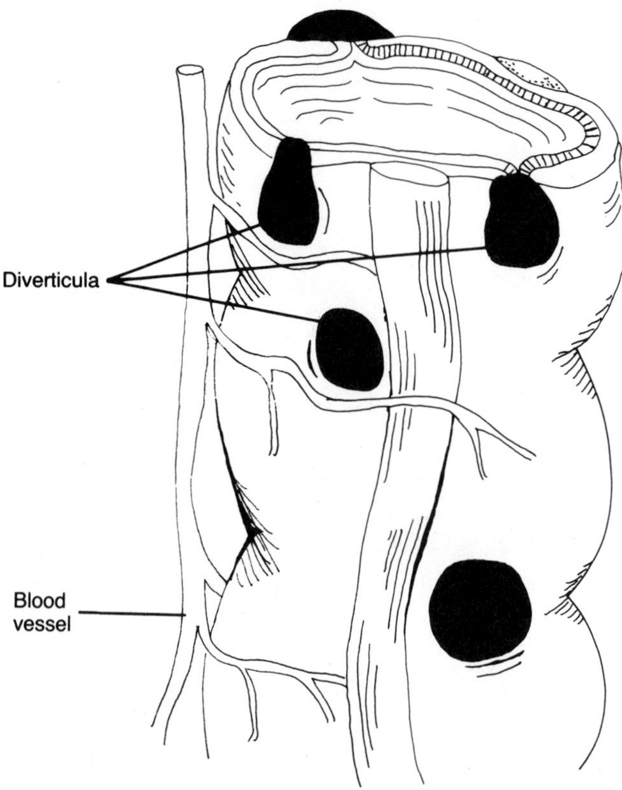

Figure 25–3 Diverticula in the large intestine. Protrusion of the intestinal mucosa through the muscular wall.

quired for complications such as abscesses, peritonitis, fistulas, hemorrhage, or obstruction.

Nutritional Care

Diverticulitis

What diet is recommended during diverticulitis; if inflammation is severe, how do clients receive nutriment?

If inflammation is severe, clients may be NPO with nasogastric tube and IV therapy, as this allows bowel rest and decreases inflammation by placing no food or fluid in the GI tract. More frequently, clients can tolerate a clear liquid diet and progress to a low-fiber diet (12 gm) to prevent fiber from accumulating in pouches (see Table 25–11). Low-fiber foods help to lessen pain and stresses of defecation by decreasing stool weight and bulk and delaying intestinal transit time. Legumes, whole-grain bread and cereal products, nuts, fibrous vegetables, and fruits with seeds and skins are avoided. As inflammation subsides, fiber is gradually increased to reduce strain during defecation.

Diverticulosis

Both insoluble and soluble fiber should be increased. Insoluble fibers (whole-grain products) increase volume and weight of fecal residue to maintain normal colonic size and increase GI motility. Soluble fibers (in oatmeal, bananas, and apples) bind free water, thus softening stools. At first, bran intake may result in flatulence, but this subsides. Initially 1 tsp bran is added daily, progressing to 2 tsp 3 times daily (10 gm of dietary fiber), with modifications made according to individual needs. Although fiber is not a cure, it may prevent diverticula formation and also offer relief from pain and bowel dysfunction in uncomplicated diverticular disease.

Importance of fluid intake should be emphasized. Bulk-forming laxatives and fiber necessitate large amounts of fluid intake to keep the stool and body hydrated. Fiber is preferred over laxative use because harsh laxatives may further damage the colon.

Nuts, seeds, and celery are avoided, as they may become trapped in pouches and cause inflammation. If client is overweight, weight loss may decrease symptoms by decreasing intraabdominal pressure.

NURSING APPLICATIONS

Assessment

Physical—for bowel habits, inflammation (fever, chills, nausea/vomiting).

Dietary—for dietary patterns and fiber intake, recent ingestion of indigestible roughage and seeds.

Interventions

1. Administer antibiotics as ordered to decrease inflammation. Monitor for diarrhea since antibiotics may decrease microflora.
2. Explain that the human digestive tract is unable to digest insoluble dietary fiber. This contributes to increased stool volume and decreased intracolonic pressure, which promote normal bowel movements.

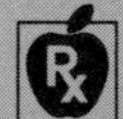
Do not give tetracycline with meals that contain milk or milk products because calcium decreases absorption of the medication and calcium.

Evaluation

* Client consumes a high-fiber diet unless symptoms of diverticulitis occur. Thus, client should be able to identify signs and symptoms of diverticulitis and how to change diet if these symptoms occur.

Client Education

- Increase intake of whole-grain products, including bran, and fruits and vegetables, especially legumes (see Chapter 4, Table 4–6).
- A high-fiber diet requires at least 8 glasses of water daily.
- Avoid nuts and seeds (such as in tomatoes, strawberries, raspberries, and blackberries), fibrous vegetables such as celery, and hulls (popcorn) that may become trapped in the diverticula.
- Chew food slowly and thoroughly.
- Eliminate fiber if fever or left lower quadrant abdominal pain develops.

HEMORRHOIDS

Enlarged veins in the anal canal or the anal orifice are called internal **hemorrhoids**; external hemorrhoids lie distal to the anal sphincter. This disorder becomes more serious as degenerations occur after many years.

Hemorrhoids are enlarged veins in the mucous membrane inside or outside the rectum.

Causes

Pregnancy, straining to defecate, infiltrating carcinoma, or portal hypertension may cause hemorrhoids. The position while sitting on the toilet impairs blood flow and puts added pressure on anal vessels; time spent in this position should be minimal.

Nutritional Care

The same fiber modifications as listed for diverticulosis also apply to hemorrhoids. Fiber increases stool bulk, exercising the digestive tract muscles by increasing colon radius and preventing intestinal muscles from being chronically contracted. Highly seasoned foods or relishes may not be well tolerated.

NURSING APPLICATIONS

Assessment

Physical—for elimination patterns and habits, use of the Valsalva maneuver.
Dietary—for dietary fiber intake.
Laboratory—for iron, Hgb, Hct; PT; stool for occult blood.

Interventions

1. Explain the benefits of a high-fiber diet.
2. If client must strain while having a bowel movement, tell client to open mouth while straining as this will diminish the effect of the Valsalva maneuver.
3. Implement measures to prevent straining on defecation, i.e., increasing fluid and fiber intake, offering prune juice, suggesting exercise.

Evaluation

* Complications from hemorrhoids are avoided as a result of proper eating habits (high fiber).

Client Education

- A high-fiber diet helps decrease discomfort of hemorrhoids, but fiber may need to be decreased during a flare-up.
- Drink at least 8 cups of fluid daily.
- Routine exercise is important.
- If persistent or recurrent bleeding occurs, contact a physician.

SURGICAL INTERVENTION

Clients undergoing GI surgery are at nutritional risk because of protracted periods of abstinence from food both preoperatively and postoperatively. Decreased serum albumin levels and total lymphocyte counts have been associated with an increased incidence of postoperative morbidity and mortality. Nutritional status should be assessed before surgery (see Chapter 11). If a client will be NPO for more than 5 to 7 days, nutrition support (enteral feedings or TPN) should be implemented.

When surgery involves the GI tract, a low-residue diet may be used preoperatively for 2 to 3 days to minimize intestinal residue. An elemental formula or TPN can provide adequate nutrients without residue.

ORAL AND ESOPHAGEAL SURGICAL INTERVENTION

Surgical procedures in the oral cavity, pharynx, and esophagus may be necessitated by injury, neoplasms, or obstructions.

Nutritional Care

After surgery involving the mouth, throat, or neck, clients may not be able to chew or swallow. If eating is not anticipated for more than several days, it is essential that adequate nutrients be provided. Enteral feedings are a viable alternative since the remainder of the GI tract is intact; adequate nutrients are provided.

When the ability to chew food is interrupted because of pain or physical immobility for more than 1 week, clients should receive nutritional counseling to avoid nutritional deterioration and optimize wound healing. Frequently hospitalization is brief; this group may easily be overlooked by dietitians unless a nurse specifically requests a consultation visit.

When a client's condition improves, attention should be given to reestablishing oral feedings. Initially milk is avoided, as it tends to coat the mucous lining of the mouth and increase phlegm production. Clients are usually apprehensive about taking foods orally. Therefore, foods are provided that are moist and nonirritating, using gravies and sauces (unless contraindicated); hard foods such as toast or cookies can be softened by dunking in a beverage.

Gradual advances from nonirritating liquids to ground or blenderized foods are followed by soft foods. This promotes better appetite and increases variety.

Adequate fluid intake is important. Liquids of thick consistency are better tolerated than thin fluids.

What types of foods can be served to decrease a client's apprehension about eating?

NURSING APPLICATIONS

Assessment

Physical—for type of surgery, pain, difficulty swallowing; weight, recent weight loss.
Dietary—for diet order; adequacy of intake.
Laboratory—for albumin, TLC.

Interventions

1. Offer small, frequent feedings to augment intake.
2. Monitor intake and weight to determine adequacy of diet. If intake is poor, confer with dietitian or physician for nutrition supplements or enteral feedings.

Evaluation

* Desirable outcomes are adequate nutrition, no weight loss, and resumption of a regular diet.

Client Education

• For clients on enteral feedings or nutrition supplements, assure them that this nutritionally complete formula will hasten the healing process.

TONSILLECTOMY

Nutritional Care

Following a tonsillectomy, a tonsillectomy and adenoidectomy (T&A) diet may be ordered. The purpose of this diet is to protect the sensitive throat from foods that are chemically, mechanically, and thermally irritating. Although the diet is not nutritionally adequate, the convalescent period is relatively short and poses no serious nutritional problems.

Foods allowed are generally the same as for a full-liquid diet, omitting citrus juices and hot foods (soups, hot chocolate, or coffee). Citrus juices may be irritating to a sensitive throat area, and hot foods may increase bleeding from vasodilation. Milk, fruit nectars, punches, popsicles, and plain gelatin desserts are given during the first 24 hours. Some physicians prefer that milk be omitted for the first 12 to 24 hours to avoid excessive mucus production.

What is the general progression of the T&A diet?

As tolerated, very soft textured foods (strained soups and cereals, soft-cooked eggs, and mashed potatoes) are added. Clients gradually return to a normal diet within 1 week.

NURSING APPLICATIONS

Assessment

Physical—for mouth/throat bleeding, difficulty swallowing.
Dietary—for diet order, preferences for nonirritating foods.

Interventions

1. Before surgery, encourage adequate intake to promote optimal glycogen stores.
2. Offer preferred cold foods that are nonirritating.

Evaluation

* Client consumes a T&A diet, progressing to a normal diet within 1 week without complications (bleeding).

Client Education

- Large swallows are more comfortable than small sips.
- Use of a straw may increase bleeding.
- Within 2 to 3 days, soft protein foods, such as soft-cooked eggs and puddings, can be tolerated. These are needed to promote healing.
- Avoid raw vegetables, hot spicy foods, and hard items, such as toast, chips, and crackers, until full recovery to prevent throat irritation.

GASTRIC SURGERY

Perforated ulcers and neoplasms may necessitate gastric surgery. Many clients may be underweight and malnourished before surgery as a result of adverse effects related to eating, or their nutritional status may deteriorate following surgery. Insufficient intake or malabsorption leads to inadequate nutrients available for anabolism. However, several types of GI surgeries are used to promote weight loss in extremely obese clients. The type of gastric surgery and client's presurgical nutritional status and response to the insult all affect nutritional outcomes. Nutritional effects of these physiological changes are summarized in Table 25–12.

Complications

Dumping Syndrome

Chyme—viscous, semifluid contents produced by gastric digestion of food.

One of the main functions of the stomach is to act as a reservoir, releasing small amounts of **chyme** into the intestine at appropriate intervals (controlled by the pyloric sphincter). Following gastric resection, this function of the stomach is

TABLE 25–12

EFFECTS OF GASTRIC SURGERY ON DIGESTIVE FUNCTIONS WITH NUTRITIONAL IMPLICATIONS

Type Gastric Surgery	Digestive Alterations	Nutritional Implication
Vagotomy Billroth I Billroth II Total gastrectomy	Decreased amount of gastric juices	Protein digestion occurs in the small intestine. Intrinsic factor reduced or missing. Iron not converted to its absorbable form
Total gastrectomy Billroth II	No "holding" area; food is dumped into the jejunum instead of being gradually released	Dumping syndrome; individuals are not able to eat adequate amounts of food
All types of gastric surgery	Less mixing of foods	Fats not well mixed with digestive juices Anemia caused by decreased availability of absorbable iron
Vagotomy	Stomach becomes atonic	Food may ferment and cause flatus and diarrhea
Billroth II	Pancreatic and bile insufficiency	Malabsorption of fats and proteins

impaired leading to **dumping syndrome.** As clients begin to eat foods in larger quantities and variety, large amounts of partially digested food are propelled rapidly into the jejunum.

Dumping syndrome is a physiological response to rapid emptying of the stomach contents into the jejunum that may occur when more than two-thirds of the stomach is removed.

Ten to 15 minutes following a meal, abdominal cramping and fullness, nausea, sweating, tachycardia, dizziness, and diarrhea are frequent complaints. This syndrome occurs when nutrients in the jejunum are hydrolyzed, producing a hypertonic solution. Fluid is drawn into the intestine, decreasing vascular fluids and causing hypotension and dizziness. This hyperosmolar solution, caused principally by carbohydrate intake, may precipitate diarrhea.

Late dumping syndrome occurs about 1 to 2 hours later, when the concentrated carbohydrate solution is rapidly absorbed. Blood glucose rises, stimulating an overproduction of insulin, which results in hypoglycemia and symptoms of weakness, perspiration, hunger, nausea, and tremors.

Describe symptoms of early and late dumping syndrome.

Malabsorption

In addition to dumping syndrome, which increases risk of hyperosmolar diarrhea, malabsorption or steatorrhea may develop, particularly when a gastrojejunostomy is performed. When the duodenum is bypassed, diminished pancreatic secretions lead to incomplete digestion, especially of fats. Bile acid malabsorption may also precipitate diarrhea because excess bile acids prevent absorption of water and electrolytes in the colon.

Malabsorption may also result from secondary lactase intolerance. Consequently, consumption of lactose-containing products results in flatus and diarrhea.

Anemia

After surgery, anemia is frequently observed, especially in menstruating women. Iron absorption may be decreased as a result of rapid stomach emptying and less mixing of chyme in the stomach. Ferric iron must be mixed with HCl to change it to the absorbable form, ferrous. If the duodenum is bypassed, where most of the iron is absorbed, iron must be given parenterally. If adequate amounts of intrinsic factor are not available, vitamin B_{12} absorption is affected, and pernicious anemia can develop. Diminished amounts of HCl may lead to bacterial overgrowth, which also interferes with vitamin B_{12} absorption. Malabsorption may also implicate inadequate folate absorption.

Osteoporosis

Approximately one-third of these clients develop latent osteoporosis. This may be secondary to malabsorption that decreases calcium absorption and the fat-soluble vitamins, especially vitamin D. Inadequate intake of these nutrients, especially in lactose-intolerant clients, may possibly contribute to this problem.

Nutritional Care

What is the nutritional goal for clients undergoing gastric surgery?

Dietary modification can reduce signs and symptoms and prevent excess weight loss if the functioning GI tract is provided with easily digested, low-bulk foods in small amounts that lessen discomfort. The goal is not to restrict but restore nutritional status by minimizing complications.

Postoperative Progression

Immediately following surgery, clients are NPO for 24 to 48 hours, with IV feedings given until peristalsis returns. Edema and swelling must also have subsided enough for fluids to pass the surgical area. When clear water is tolerated, small amounts (30 to 60 ml) of liquids are given hourly, gradually progressing to soft foods and a regular diet with frequent feedings. Progressions may take as much as 2 weeks following surgery but are determined by a client's progress and tolerance. If a diet order is written "as tolerated," progression is determined by the nurse and client.

What is the typical progression for gastric surgery?

Since the stomach size has been decreased, early satiety or a feeling of "fullness" after a few bites decreases intake. Thus, 5 or 6 small feedings are recommended daily. Portion size depends on client's tolerance. However, as tissue heals and becomes stronger, the stomach gradually expands. Within a year, some clients are able to eat 3 regular meals. Total gastrectomy clients may need to eat several small meals a day for the rest of their lives.

Dumping Syndrome Diet

This syndrome is treated with a diet referred to as the "dumping syndrome diet." A high-protein (1.5 to 2 gm/kg of IBW), moderate-fat, high-kilocalorie (35 to 45 kcal/kg of IBW) diet is recommended. Protein and some fats are better tolerated and delay gastric emptying time; this decreases dumping, maintains weight, and rebuilds tissue. If steatorrhea is present, MCT oil and short-chain fatty acids are better tolerated and can provide necessary kilocalories, if needed.

Simple carbohydrates (candy, desserts, and sweetened beverages) are used sparingly. Hypertonic liquids such as many fruit juices and carbonated beverages are likely to precipitate dumping symptoms. Complex carbohydrates (bread, rice, and vegetables) are better tolerated because they are digested slowly. Pectin, a dietary fiber in fruits and vegetables, may help delay gastric emptying and increase tolerance to foods not previously tolerated by decreasing dumping symptoms (Harju, 1990). However, clients who have had gastric surgery (Billroth I and II, vagotomy, pyloroplasty, or Roux-en-Y) have less gastric acid secretion or decreased GI motility and may encounter impaction or **bezoar** formation if dietary fiber is increased.

Bezoar—compacted mass of ingested material, usually fruit and vegetable fibers, in the intestine.

Describe recommendations for protein, fat, and carbohydrates and why these are needed.

The amount of liquids provided at mealtime is limited; by providing liquids ½ to 1 hour after a meal, gastric emptying is delayed. Environmental (eating habits) and emotional (stress) factors and extreme food/fluid temperatures may alter peristalsis and worsen malabsorption.

NURSING APPLICATIONS

Assessment

Physical—for previous weight, weight changes following surgery, type of surgery, findings summarized in Table 25–12, dumping syndrome; diarrhea, constipation/bezoar formation; lactase deficiency.
Dietary—for knowledge of diet ordered, understanding of causes/symptoms of dumping syndrome; intake of sodium, calcium, vitamin B_{12}, folate, iron, kilocalories, carbohydrate, protein, fat.
Laboratory—for albumin, TLC; glucose; sodium, potassium, calcium; RBCs, MCV, Hgb, Hct, iron.

Interventions

1. Frequently check with client regarding responses to foods and portions. Report intolerances to the dietitian.
2. Explain the role of the diet in preventing dumping syndrome.
3. Introduce milk-containing items, such as puddings or custards, slowly into the diet and observe for signs of intolerance. If lactose intolerance is present, discuss other ways of maintaining adequate calcium intake (see Chapter 23, Table 23–12).

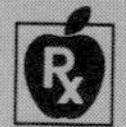
Provide antidiarrheal medications before meals.

Evaluation

* Dumping syndrome should be reduced or eliminated, and client should be eating adequate amounts; mineral and vitamin complications as well as diarrhea and lactose intolerance are reduced or prevented.

Client Education

- Oat products, apples, and citrus fruits may reduce dumping symptoms by delaying gastric emptying.
- Simple carbohydrates are not tolerated well by clients because rapid digestion of sugars triggers a "dumping" into the intestines quicker than proteins or fat. Food exchange lists (listed in Appendix D–1) can be used to identify carbohydrate-containing foods.
- To minimize malabsorption, advise clients to (1) eat meals slowly in a relaxed atmosphere, (2) lie down for 30 minutes to 1 hour after eating, and (3) avoid extremely hot or cold foods.
- Iron absorption can be improved by delaying gastric emptying time (such as lying down after eating and increasing foods containing pectin).
- Discuss foods that are rich sources of iron, vitamin B_{12}, and folate, especially if supplements are not ordered.
- Use salt in moderation (about 3 gm) because salt draws fluid into the GI tract.

INTESTINAL SURGERY WITH CREATION OF AN OSTOMY

An ileostomy or colostomy may be performed to treat Crohn's disease, colonic cancer, intestinal lesions or obstruction, or severe ulcerative colitis or bowel trauma. The affected intestinal section is removed with the remaining end attached through an opening in the abdominal wall for defecation (Fig. 25–4).

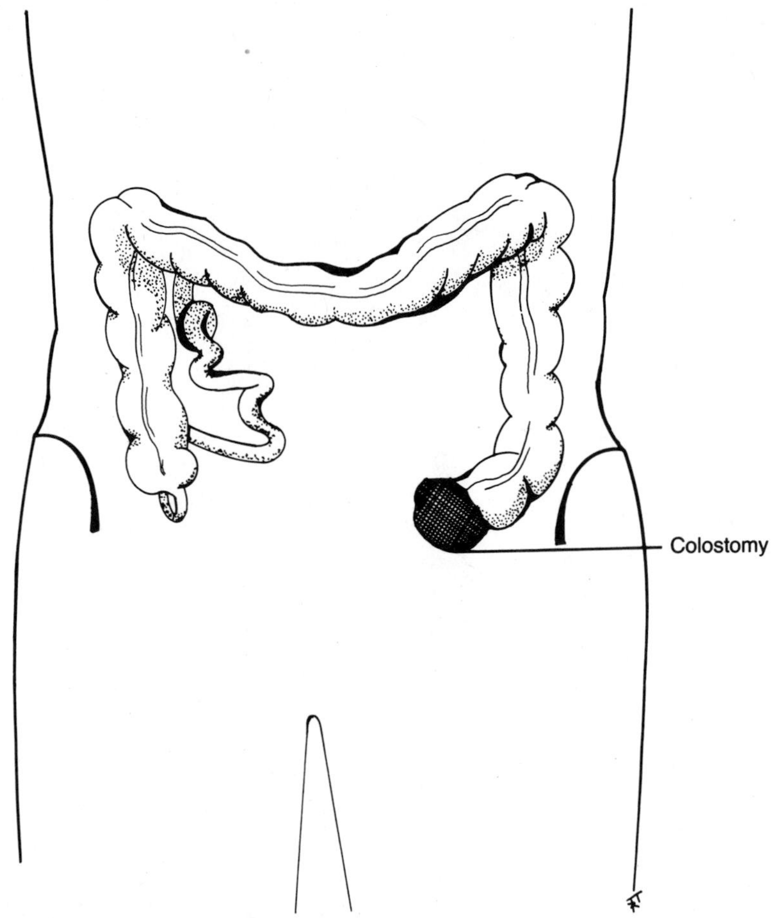

Figure 25–4 Colostomy. A part of the colon is brought through an artificial outlet on the abdomen for defecation.

Effluent — excrement.

For an ileostomy, the ileum is brought through an artificial outlet in the abdomen. **Effluent** from an ileostomy is fluid and irritating to skin. An ileostomy may drain almost continuously. Because of the large amount of intestinal resection, nutrient losses are great. Fluid, sodium, potassium, and vitamin B_{12} absorption are reduced or absent.

Describe differences between an ileostomy and colostomy.

For a colostomy, part of a colon section is brought through the abdominal wall. Because some water is reabsorbed from the chyme, fecal material is mushy to fairly well formed. Bowel regularity can be established by some clients. A greater percentage of electrolytes are reabsorbed.

Nutritional Care

Progression

Diet is a primary concern of ostomy clients. Consistency of stool and presence of flatus depend on the types of foods eaten. Following postoperative IV feedings and a clear-liquid period, a low-residue diet is usually prescribed, progressing to a high-protein (1 to 1.5 gm/kg), high-carbohydrate diet within 2 to 3 weeks. Kilocalories are increased principally using carbohydrates to regain weight lost and maintain a desirable weight. Small, frequent feedings are recommended.

Foods may be added individually to determine their effect. Milk may not be tolerated by these clients; foods or environmental factors that increase peristalsis may need to be avoided. Clients must observe their own tolerances regarding food and bowel movements and then eat accordingly. When a problem is observed, the food should be eliminated for a while and then tried again. Preferred foods that cause problems can be eaten infrequently or in small amounts.

Describe progression of an ostomy diet. How are food intolerances treated?

Effluent Consistency

Because less fluid in the GI tract is reabsorbed, liberal fluid intake is needed (8 to 10 cups daily), especially for ileostomy clients. Usually the principal concern is to thicken the effluent if needed; foods that affect fluidity of the stool are listed in Table 25–13. Diphenoxylate (Lomotil) may be permitted to decrease GI motility and thicken effluent.

TABLE 25–13

FOODS THAT AFFECT EFFLUENT OF OSTOMY CLIENTS

Affect Thickness of Effluent	
Increase (control diarrhea)	*Loosen output* (cause diarrhea)
Ripe bananas	Beans
Rice	Beef
Creamy peanut butter	Caffeinated beverages
Cheese	Leafy vegetables
Potatoes	Apple juice
Applesauce	Prune juice
Tapioca	Raw fruits (except bananas)
	Raw vegetables
	Spicy or highly seasoned foods
	Cabbage
	Broccoli
Affect Odor	
Increase	*Decrease*
Beans	Chlorophyll in green leafy vegetables and parsley
Fish	Buttermilk
Eggs	Yogurt
Asparagus	
Coffee	
Onions	
Beer	
Possible Obstruction	
Popcorn	
Chinese vegetables (bean sprouts, bamboo shoots)	
Raw apples	
Pineapple	
Whole kernel corn	
Celery	
Tomatoes	
Nuts	
Coconut	
Fruits with seeds	
Increase Flatus	
Beef	
Carbonated beverages	
Dried beans and peas	
Milk and milk products	
Onions	
Vegetables in cabbage family (broccoli, Brussels sprouts)	
Radishes	
Cucumbers	
Chamomile tea	
Turnips	
Corn	
Spicy foods	

Name 5 foods that can increase thickness of effluent.

Emotional upsets affect bowel function and may cause changes in the effluent. It is important for clients to eat in a relaxed, pleasant atmosphere.

Obstructions

Name 3 foods that may cause obstructions in ostomy clients.

In addition to the possibility of constipation causing obstructions, fibrous foods and foods with seeds and kernels that may cause obstructions should be eliminated (see Table 25–13). Foods should be chewed thoroughly.

Odors

Odors are usually caused by steatorrhea or bacterial action on foods. Foods that are more frequently associated with malodorous odors are listed in Table 25–13. Again, this is an individual matter, and clients are encouraged to determine effects for themselves. Antibiotics and vitamin/mineral supplements also increase odor. In addition to foods that are natural intestinal deodorizers, commercial deodorants may be placed in an ostomy bag. Bismuth subgallate used for this purpose may be constipating.

Name foods that decrease/increase odor.

Flatus

Loss of sphincter means that clients have no control over expulsion of flatus and no sensations to indicate when flatus will occur. Excessive gas may cause accidental dislodgment of the pouch. In addition to foods listed in Table 25–13, certain behaviors increase flatus. Chewing gum and drinking straws are discouraged because they increase flatus by encouraging air swallowing. Clients should eat in a sitting position and chew with the mouth closed. Simethicone and activated charcoal can be used to decrease flatus.

Name 5 foods that can increase flatus formation.

Vitamins and Minerals

Loss of absorptive surface may reduce absorption of nutrients, especially vitamins and minerals. If the terminal ileum has been removed, parenteral vitamin B_{12} is needed. A multivitamin-mineral supplement may be needed.

NURSING APPLICATIONS

Assessment

Physical—for hydration status (skin turgor, I&O, mucous membranes), location of stoma.
Dietary—for dietary habits and nutrient intake; knowledge of foods that cause odor, flatus and obstruction.
Laboratory—for albumin, TLC; sodium, potassium.

Interventions

1. Refer to enterostomal therapy (ET) nurse, if available.
2. Maintain a nonjudgmental approach while caring for an ostomy; your reaction can either hinder or help clients.
3. If many fruits and vegetables are eliminated, discuss foods that can be used to provide adequate amounts of vitamin C.

Evaluation

* Desirable outcomes are client looks at and cares for ostomy and adheres to diet that decreases flatus, odor, and obstruction.

Client Education

- Inform of United Ostomy Association (see Appendix E–1).
- Despite some limitations of foods tolerated, a nutritionally balanced diet is possible.
- Reduction of fluid intake does not decrease effluent volume but results in dehydration or constipation. Maintain adequate intake of 8 to 10 cups of fluid daily.
- As a result of watery stools, sodium and potassium losses are increased. Both sodium and potassium intake should be increased.

SMALL BOWEL RESECTION

Small bowel resection may be necessary secondary to many conditions, such as Crohn's disease, neoplasm, and fistula. Normally most nutrients are absorbed in the first 150 cm of the small intestine. Nutritional status can be seriously affected by this surgery, especially if more than 50% of the small bowel is removed. An understanding of nutrient absorption in the GI tract (see Chapter 2, Fig. 2–5) and knowledge of how much of the small intestine is removed (less than 50% is best), what section is removed (resection of jejunum is better tolerated than the ileum), and condition of the remaining bowel are necessary to provide nutrition support. Prognosis is better if the ileocecal valve remains. If principally the jejunum is removed, the ileum becomes stronger with increasing absorptive capabilities. However, there is no compensatory action if the ileum is resected.

Complications

Short bowel syndrome, resulting when large amounts of the small intestine are surgically resected, is characterized by significant malabsorption, diarrhea, severe malnutrition, and weight loss (Table 25–14). Large amounts of bacteria in the GI tract (of unknown cause) increase risk of viral **gastroenteritis.** In addition to malabsorption problems, there are several other potential complications. GI motility and peristalsis are increased, decreasing the length of time chyme is present for absorption. Fat malabsorption may lead to steatorrhea. Indirectly this may lead to **cholelithiasis** and **nephrolithiasis.** Osteoporosis may occur as a result of chronic

Gastroenteritis—inflammation of the stomach and intestines.

Cholelithiasis—the presence or formation of gallstones. Nephrolithiasis—renal calculi.

TABLE 25–14

PHYSIOLOGICAL CONSEQUENCES OF SHORT BOWEL SYNDROME

Alteration	Consequences
Gastric	Hyperacidity Delayed gastric emptying Dumping syndrome
Small bowel	Diarrhea Excessive loss of fluid and electrolytes
Specific nutrients	Fat malabsorption Vitamin and mineral malabsorption Lactose intolerance Oxalate kidney stones

Adapted from Edes TE. Clinical management of short bowel syndrome: Enhancing the patient's quality of life. *Postgrad Med* 1990 Sept 15; 88(4):91–95.

calcium and vitamin D malabsorption. If the ileum is lost, absorption of vitamin B_{12} is nonexistent.

Treatment

Cimetidine (Tagamet) is usually given to decrease hyperacidity. Most clients receive drugs such as propantheline bromide (Pro-Banthine), Lomotil, and others, as necessary, to decrease intestinal transit time. When less than 100 cm of the ileum is resected, cholestyramine (Questran) is effective in decreasing diarrhea associated with bile salt wastage. Pancreatic enzymes may be provided to improve fat and protein absorption, especially if part of the jejunum is resected. Antibiotics (usually tetracycline) reduce bacterial content of the intestinal tract. Subcutaneous injections of vitamin K may be necessary to prevent bleeding problems.

In some clients, home enteral feedings may be needed for extended periods of time; extensive resection (less than 100 cm remaining) necessitates TPN for life.

Nutritional Care

Progressions

Nutritional management of these clients is complicated, involving a combination of individually tailored oral and parenteral feedings for a period of 2 years or more. Because of poor absorption, large amounts of all nutrients are required to maintain weight. Team work is essential for individualizing diets for these clients.

What are the goals for short bowel syndrome clients initially? Describe the 3 phases of nutrition support.

Initially or during the first month, goals are to control fluid and electrolyte abnormalities and infections. Nutrition support is through TPN solely during the first phase, which lasts approximately 7 to 10 days. Phase 2, lasting from 1 to 3 months, involves the use of enteral and parenteral feedings. Phase 3 begins 3 to 12 months after surgery; gradual increases in enteral/oral feedings should occur with tapering of TPN (Hennessy, 1989).

Oral Intake

Oral intake of food stimulates the release of GI hormones, which subsequently induces the remaining small intestine to expand its absorptive surface area. Therefore, as soon as possible, oral intake is encouraged to reestablish gut function and provide nutrients. Initially, simple hypotonic fluids are provided. Elemental diets may be used, but they should be diluted so they are not hypertonic. In addition to their rather unpalatable taste, studies indicate that simple amino acids do not stimulate intestinal adaptations. Lactose-free polymeric formulas are more popular; when tolerance permits, nutrient-dense formulas (1.5 to 2 kcal/gm) may be used.

Describe why oral intake is initiated as soon as possible.

When liquids are tolerated, foods are introduced gradually until adequate oral intake is reached. Small, frequent (4 to 6) meals are tolerated best. Clients need to be aware of their tolerance for various foods; a food diary helps.

Nutrient Requirements

A high-kilocalorie (up to 5000 kcal), high-protein (175 gm protein) diet is advocated. Nutrition supplements may be needed to help increase intake.

What are requirements for kilocalories and protein? Why may fat need to be limited?

Fats increase kilocalorie intake but may need to be restricted to 40 to 60 gm. If the distal part of the ileum is removed, bile salts cannot be reabsorbed. Since bile salts are recirculated several times a day, when they are lost in the stool, the liver is unable to compensate. Adequate amounts of bile salts are not available for fat absorption. Fats in the form of MCT oil, homogenized milk, and margarine are better tolerated by clients. Fat intake should be as high as possible to increase kilocalorie intake but prevent steatorrhea.

Vitamins and Minerals

Absorption of vitamin B_{12} occurs only in the ileum; removal of the ileum necessitates parenteral injections for life. Decreased absorption of fat-soluble vitamins (as well as calcium and magnesium) results from fat malabsorption. Daily vitamin supplements (especially fat-soluble ones) twice the RDA may be necessary.

Unabsorbed bile salts precipitate watery diarrhea with loss of fluid and minerals. Daily supplements of minerals (especially calcium and magnesium) may be necessary.

Decreased calcium absorption leads to increased absorption of oxalates, which can precipitate gallstones and renal stones. Thus, dark green leafy vegetables, chocolate, cola, nuts, and plums are avoided (Hennessy, 1989). Hypercalciuria and oxaluria can be treated with the addition of unprocessed wheat bran (Gleeson et al, 1990).

What foods should be avoided to minimize stone formation?

NURSING APPLICATIONS

Assessment

Physical—for hydration status, weight, weight loss, IBW; extent and location of intestinal removal and whether ileocecal valve remains; dehydration, diarrhea/steatorrhea.
Dietary—for diet order, intake of nutrients/kilocalories.
Laboratory—for albumin, prealbumin, TLC; sodium, potassium, magnesium, phosphorus; RBC, MCV, Hgb, Hct, PT.

Interventions

1. Assist with food diary to determine food intolerances.
2. Provide elemental or polymeric formulas well chilled or on ice to improve acceptance. If elemental formulas are prescribed, dilute so they are initially isotonic. Flavor packets (available from manufacturers) can be added to elemental formulas to increase palatability.

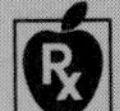
Closely monitor clients taking Questran for malabsorption that may lead to vitamin A, D, and K deficiencies.

Evaluation

* Client should gain weight.

Client Education

- Avoid use of laxatives, unless approved by the physician.
- Generally gut functioning improves.
- Very hot or cold items, alcohol, and caffeine are discouraged because they stimulate GI activity.

RECTAL SURGERY

Nutritional Care

A clear liquid or nonresidue diet may be indicated following rectal surgery, such as hemorrhoidectomy, to permit healing and decrease risk of wound infection. A minimal-residue diet or monomeric formula may be used. Foods allowed on a minimal-residue diet are almost completely digested and absorbed in the intestine, resulting in nominal feces. A normal diet is resumed when tolerated, after which clients should consume a high-fiber diet to increase bulk and stimulate peristalsis.

List diets used for rectal surgery clients.

NURSING APPLICATIONS

Assessment

Physical— for fluid deficit (poor skin turgor, dry mucous membranes), type of surgery.

Dietary—for diet order, fiber and fluid intake.

Interventions

1. Give stool softener as prescribed to prevent anal irritations.
2. Discuss the role of fiber and fluid in promoting normal bowel movements.

Evaluation

* Expected outcomes include a soft formed stool passed with minimal discomfort because of appropriate food choices (minimal residue, progressing to high fiber).

Client Education

• Drink at least 8 cups of fluids daily.

SUMMARY

Generalized therapy necessary for the healing process in gastric disorders includes small, frequent feedings to minimize irritation while maintaining nutritional status. Treatment of GI disorders necessitates a team approach for a desirable outcome. Factors such as reduction of stress, anxiety, and frustration may be as important as providing adequate nutrition. In some cases, medical and surgical procedures are necessary. All clients with GI problems need personal attention and an individualized plan of care to correct and maintain their nutritional status.

NURSING PROCESS IN ACTION

While in the recovery phase following ostomy surgery, your client expresses concerns about flatus and odor leakage as well as possible ostomy obstruction. He wants to know what foods he should eat.

Nutritional Assessment

- Dietary habits and nutrient intake.
- Motivation to learn.
- Food preferences.

Dietary Nursing Diagnosis

High risk for altered health maintenance RT inadequate knowledge of dietary adjustments for altered bowel elimination.

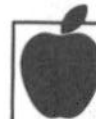

Nutritional Goals

Client plans a nutritionally balanced diet that will minimize nutrient losses, flatus, and odor.

Nutritional Implementation 

Intervention: Suggest adding foods one at a time and maintaining a food diary.

Rationale: This determines client's tolerance to foods.

Intervention: Suggest (1) avoiding popcorn, Chinese vegetables, raw apples, whole kernel corn, celery, nuts, coconut, fruits with seeds, tomatoes, pineapple and (2) chewing foods adequately.
Rationale: Certain foods should be avoided to prevent obstructions. Chewing foods well lessens chances of obstruction.

Intervention: Suggest using in moderation: beef, carbonated drinks, dried beans and peas, milk and milk products, onions, vegetables in the cabbage family, turnips, cucumber, radishes, corn, and spicy foods. Avoid chewing gum and use of a straw.
Rationale: Loss of sphincter means that client will not have control of passage of flatus. These foods and behaviors increase flatus.

Intervention: Explain that seafood, asparagus, onions, and beer should be avoided.
Rationale: These foods increase odor.

Intervention: Encourage deodorizing agents (Pals, Chloresium) and chlorophyll-containing foods such as parsley, dark green leafy vegetables, buttermilk, and yogurt.
Rationale: These are intestinal deodorizers.

Intervention: Administer bismuth subgallate if ordered.
Rationale: Bismuth subgallate has a deodorizing effect. However, it may be constipating.

Intervention: If permitted by the physician, give Lomotil.
Rationale: Lomotil decreases motility and thickens excrement.

Intervention: Encourage bananas, rice, applesauce, tapioca, peanut butter (creamy), cheese, potatoes.
Rationale: These foods increase thickness of effluent.

Intervention: Avoid beans, beef, caffeinated beverages, leafy vegetables, apple juice, prune juice, raw fruits and vegetables, spicy foods, cabbage, and broccoli.
Rationale: These foods loosen effluent, particularly with sigmoid colostomy.

Intervention: Emphasize drinking 8 to 10 cups of fluid daily.
Rationale: Because less fluid in the GI tract is reabsorbed, liberal fluid intake is needed to prevent dehydration. Reducing fluid intake does not decrease effluent volume.

Intervention: Refer to enterostomal therapy (ET) nurse or United Ostomy Association.
Rationale: These are knowledgeable resources for clients and can provide support and empathy.

Intervention: Offer foods high in potassium and sodium.
Rationale: These nutrients are lost in feces and need to be replaced.

Evaluation

Client plans/consumes a nutritionally balanced diet that minimizes flatus (moderate use of carbonated drinks, dried beans and peas, onions, and vegetables in the cabbage family), odor (avoids seafood and asparagus, but includes parsley, buttermilk, and yogurt in diet), and compensates for nutrient losses (drinks 8 to 10 cups of fluid/day, increases sodium and potassium intake).

STUDENT READINESS

1. Discuss ways to treat heartburn.
2. What are some special nursing interventions for a peptic ulcer client?
3. List conditions requiring a low-fiber diet and state reasons for its use; list conditions requiring a high-fiber diet and state reasons for its use.
4. Why are clients undergoing gastric or intestinal surgery at a greater nutritional risk than other surgical clients?

CASE STUDY

Mrs. A. B. is a 60-year-old personnel director who has complained of increasing indigestion following meals, particularly after her evening meal. Her usual schedule is to work until 7 PM, then eat a heavy meal and retire by 10 PM. The heartburn following her evening meals is so severe, she cannot lie down at night and sleeps propped up on pillows in a sitting position. Following a physical evaluation, her physician diagnoses hiatal hernia. Six small feedings are ordered, plus elevating the head of the bed on 4- to 6-inch blocks.

1. What is the effect of caffeine and nicotine on the lower esophageal sphincter?
2. What foods have the same effect?
3. What nursing diagnoses could you develop from the data? Develop goal(s) for each.
4. As you plan Mrs. A. B.'s nursing interventions, what would you teach her regarding lying down after meals, tight belts and foundation garments, and meal spacing?
5. If antacids are added to the therapeutic regimen, when is the best time for them to be administered?
6. Why did the physician order head of bed elevated on 4- to 6-inch blocks?

CASE STUDY

Ms. S. J. is a 26-year-old secretary who is the sole support of her 4-year-old son. She has been diagnosed with ulcerative colitis for the past 3 years. During the latest flare-up of her disease, she lost 10 lbs. She now weighs 97 lbs, and her height is 64 inches. After discharge from the hospital, she is referred to a nutritionist for diet counseling. Her physician orders a 2500-kcal, low-residue diet with vitamin and mineral supplements.

1. What dietary restrictions are imposed during the acute phase of this disease?
2. Why are foods with lactose often restricted?
3. Why may long-chain triglycerides cause steatorrhea in ulcerative colitis clients? What substitutions are possible?
4. Plan a low-fiber diet for 1 day.
5. In counseling this client about her diet, what activities will help avoid episodes of diarrhea?

REFERENCES

Allen ML, et al. The effect of raw onions on acid reflux and reflux symptoms. *Am J Gastroenterol* 1990 Apr; 85(4):377–380.

Avery ME, Snyder JD. Oral therapy for acute diarrhea. *N Engl J Med* 1990 Sept 27; 323(13):891–893.

Brown KH, et al. Effect of continued oral feeding on clinical and nutritional outcomes of acute diarrhea in children. *J Pediatr* 1988 Feb; 112(2):191–200.

Clark CS, et al. Gastroesophageal reflux induced by exercise in healthy volunteers. *JAMA* 1989 June 23–30; 261(24):3599–3601.

Cohn JP. Preventing "turista" and other traveler's ailments. *FDA Consumer* 1991 March; 25(2):24–27.

Cole AT, et al. Ranitidine, aspirin, food, and the stomach. *Br Med J* 1992 Feb 29; 304:544–545.

Cravo M, et al. Nutritional support in Crohn's

disease: Which route? *Am J Gastroenterol* 1991 March; 86(3):317–321.

Culpepper-Morgan JA, Flock MH. Bowel rest or bowel starvation: Defining the role of nutritional support in the treatment of inflammatory bowel disease (editorial). *Am J Gastroenterol* 1991 March; 86(3):269–271.

Dietary fiber, food intolerance and irritable bowel syndrome. *Nutr Rev* 1990 Sept; 48(9):343–344.

DiPadova C, et al. Effects of ranitidine on blood alcohol levels after ethanol ingestion. *JAMA* 1992 Jan 1; 267(1):83–86.

Donatelle EP. Constipation: Pathophysiology and treatment. *Am Fam Phys* 1990 Nov; 42(5):1335–1342.

Drossman DA, et al. Approaching IBS with confidence. *Patient Care* 1992 Aug 15; 26(13):175–178, 183, 201–203.

Elta GH, et al. Comparison of coffee intake and coffee-induced symptoms in patients with duodenal ulcer, non-ulcer dyspepsia, and normal controls. *Am J Gastroenterol* 1990 Oct; 85(10):1339–1342.

Esberger KK. Guide to gastrointestinal problems of elders. *Geriatric Nurs* 1991 March-Apr; 12(2):74–75.

Friedman G. Peptic ulcer disease. *Clin Symp* 1988; 40(5):1–32.

Giaffer NH, et al. Controlled trial of polymeric versus elemental diet in treatment of active Crohn's disease. *Lancet* 1990 Apr 7; 335(8693):816–819.

Gleeson MJ, et al. Effect of unprocessed wheat bran on calciuria and oxaluria in patients with urolithiasis. *Urology* 1990 March; 35(3):231–234.

Groher ME. *Dysphagia. Diagnosis and Management.* Stoneham, MA, Butterworth Publishers, 1984.

Harju E. Metabolic problems after gastric surgery. *Int Surg* 1990 Jan-March; 75(1):27–35.

Hecht A. The unwelcome dinner guest—preventing food-borne illness. *FDA Consumer* 1991 Jan-Feb; 25(1):19–25.

Hennessy K. Nutritional support and gastrointestinal disease. *Nurs Clin North Am* 1989 June; 24(2):373–382.

Hyams JS, et al. Carbohydrate malabsorption following fruit juice ingestion in young children. *Pediatrics* 1988 July; 82(1):64–67.

Kitchin LI, Castell DO. Rationale and efficacy of conservative therapy for gastroesophageal reflux disease. *Arch Intern Med* 1991 March; 151(3):448–454.

Leung AKC. Acute diarrhea in children: What to do and what not to do. *Postgrad Med* 1989 Dec; 86(8):161–174.

Lifschitz CH, Shulman RJ. Nutritional therapy for infants with diarrhea. *Nutr Rev* 1990 Sept; 48(9):329–336.

Mansfield LE. Gastroesophageal reflux and respiratory disorders: A review. *Ann Allergy* 1989 March; 62(3):158–163.

Margolis PA, et al. Effect of unrestricted diet on mild infantile diarrhea. *Am J Dis Child* 1990 Feb; 144(2):162–164.

Martin A. Dietary management of swallowing disorders. *Dysphagia* 1991; 6(3):129–134.

Meehan M. Nursing diagnosis: Potential for aspiration. *RN* 1992 Jan; 92(1):30–34.

Michener WM, Wyllie R. Management of children and adolescents with inflammatory bowel disease. *Med Clin North Am* 1990 Jan; 74(1):103–115.

Millet SH, Simpson J. Medication-nutrient interactions: Hypophosphatemia associated with sucralfate in the intensive care unit. *Nutr Clin Pract* 1991 Oct; 6(5):199–201.

Mitchell C, Parry-Billings K. Gastroesophageal reflux disease. *Nurs Standard* 1992 March 4; 6(24):25–28.

Mullin GE. Food allergy and irritable bowel syndrome. *JAMA* 1991 Apr 3; 265(13):1736.

O'Keefe SJD, et al. Steroids and bowel rest versus elemental diet in the treatment of patients with Crohn's disease: The effects on protein metabolism and immune function. *JPEN* 1989 Sept-Oct; 13(5):455–460.

Pemberton CM, et al. *Mayo Clinic Diet Manual.* 6th ed. Philadelphia, BC Decker, 1988.

Perucca R. Understanding Crohn's disease. *J IV Nurs* 1992 May-June; 15(3):164–169.

Rigaud D, et al. Controlled trial comparing two types of enteral nutrition in treatment of active Crohn's disease: Elemental versus polymeric diet. *Gut* 1991 Dec; 32(12):1492–1497.

Roe DA. *Drug and Nutrient Interactions: A Problem-Oriented Reference Guide.* Chicago, The American Dietetic Association, 1989.

Rogers AI. Medical treatment and prevention of peptic ulcer disease. *Postgrad Med* 1990 Oct; 88(5):57–60.

Rubin-Terrado, M, Linkenheld I. Don't choke on this: A swallowing assessment. *Geriatr Nurs* 1991 Nov-Dec; 12(6):288–291.

Rydning A, et al. Healing of benign gastric ulcer with low-dose antacids and fiber diet. *Gastroenterology* 1986 July; 91(1):56–61.

Sachar DB. The problem of postoperative recurrence of Crohn's disease. *Med Clin North Am* 1990 Jan; 74(1):183–188.

Shaw J, et al. Advances in the understanding and management of the irritable bowel syndrome. *Med J Aust* 1989 July 17; 151:92–99.

Singleton JW. Enteral feeding versus drug therapy in Crohn's disease: A continuing story. *Gastroenterology* 1991 Oct; 101(4):1127–1128.

Sontag SJ, et al. Effect of positions, eating and bronchodilators on gastroesophageal reflux in asthmatics. *Dig Dis Sci* 1990 July; 35(7):849–856.

Szabo S; Hollander D. Pathways of gastrointestinal protection and repair: Mechanisms of action of sucralfate. *Am J Med* 1989 June 9; 86(6A):23–31.

Taylor R. Management of constipation. 1. High fibre diets work. *Br Med J* 1990 Apr 21; 300(6731):1063–1064.

Weck E. New hope for those with diverticular disease. *FDA Consumer* 1987 July-Aug; 20(6):24–27.

Wood P. Differential diagnosis and prescriptive team management of dysphagia. *J Am Diet Assoc* 1989 Sept; 89(suppl 9):A142.

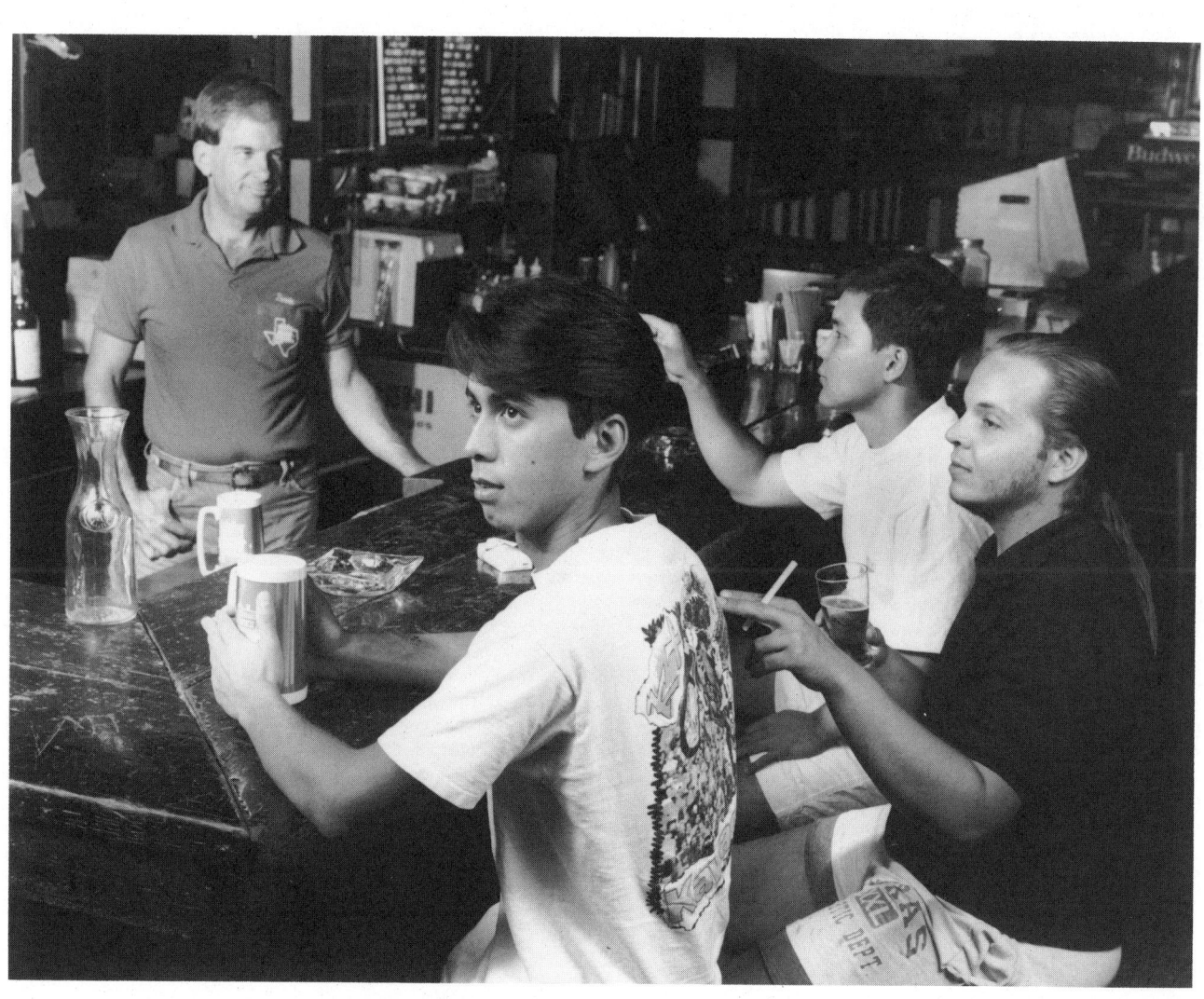

Dietary Management of Disorders of Accessory Gastrointestinal Organs

CHAPTER 26

OUTLINE

OBJECTIVES

THE STUDENT WILL BE ABLE TO:

- Relate the diseased conditions of the liver and pancreas to nutritional status.
- Identify the role of protein in liver disease.
- State the role of fat in gallbladder disease.
- Explain dietary management of pancreatitis.
- Assist clients in planning adequate diets for cystic fibrosis.
- Modify a normal diet to meet the requirements for a client with each of these conditions: hepatitis, cirrhosis, hepatic encephalopathy, gallbladder disease, pancreatitis, and cystic fibrosis.
- Discuss nursing applications for the above conditions.
- Identify client teaching tips for each disorder.

TEST YOUR NQ (True/False)

1. Lipid deficiency is the most common nutritional cause of steatosis.
2. Hepatitis clients need a high intake of protein.
3. Dairy products and eggs should not be served to clients with hepatitis.
4. Laennec's cirrhosis is a result of malnutrition and biliary disease.
5. The portal vein carries nutrients from the liver to the GI tract.
6. Dietary cholesterol plays an important role in the cause of gallstones.
7. In acute gallbladder attacks, a low-fat diet is used.
8. Pancreatitis can result in hypercalcemia.
9. A high-protein, high-carbohydrate, low-fat diet is used for chronic pancreatitis.
10. Cystic fibrosis clients need a high-protein diet.

Because digestion of all foodstuffs is accomplished by the actions of enzymes, bile salts, and other substances secreted into the GI tract, an alteration in their availability affects digestion and, ultimately, absorption of nutrients. The liver and pancreas produce important digestive substances to facilitate absorption; the gallbladder stores, concentrates, and releases bile on stimulation. Additionally, the liver has many other physiological functions that affect health and well-being; it can be adversely affected by ingested substances.

THE LIVER AND LIVER DISORDERS

As discussed in Chapter 2, the liver is the chemical governor of the body, storing and regulating the release of most of the body's nutrients. All digested substances, except long-chain fatty acids, are transported directly to the liver. From there, they may be altered before distribution to the rest of the body. Not only are nutrients handled in this manner, but also ingested poisons, medications, antigens, and possibly some bacteria are detoxified or destroyed for excretion. Thus, the liver changes nutrients into a usable form for the body and stores some nutrients until they are needed (Fig. 26–1). Liver function not only affects normal metabolism of many nutrients, but also its structure and functions are affected by nutritional

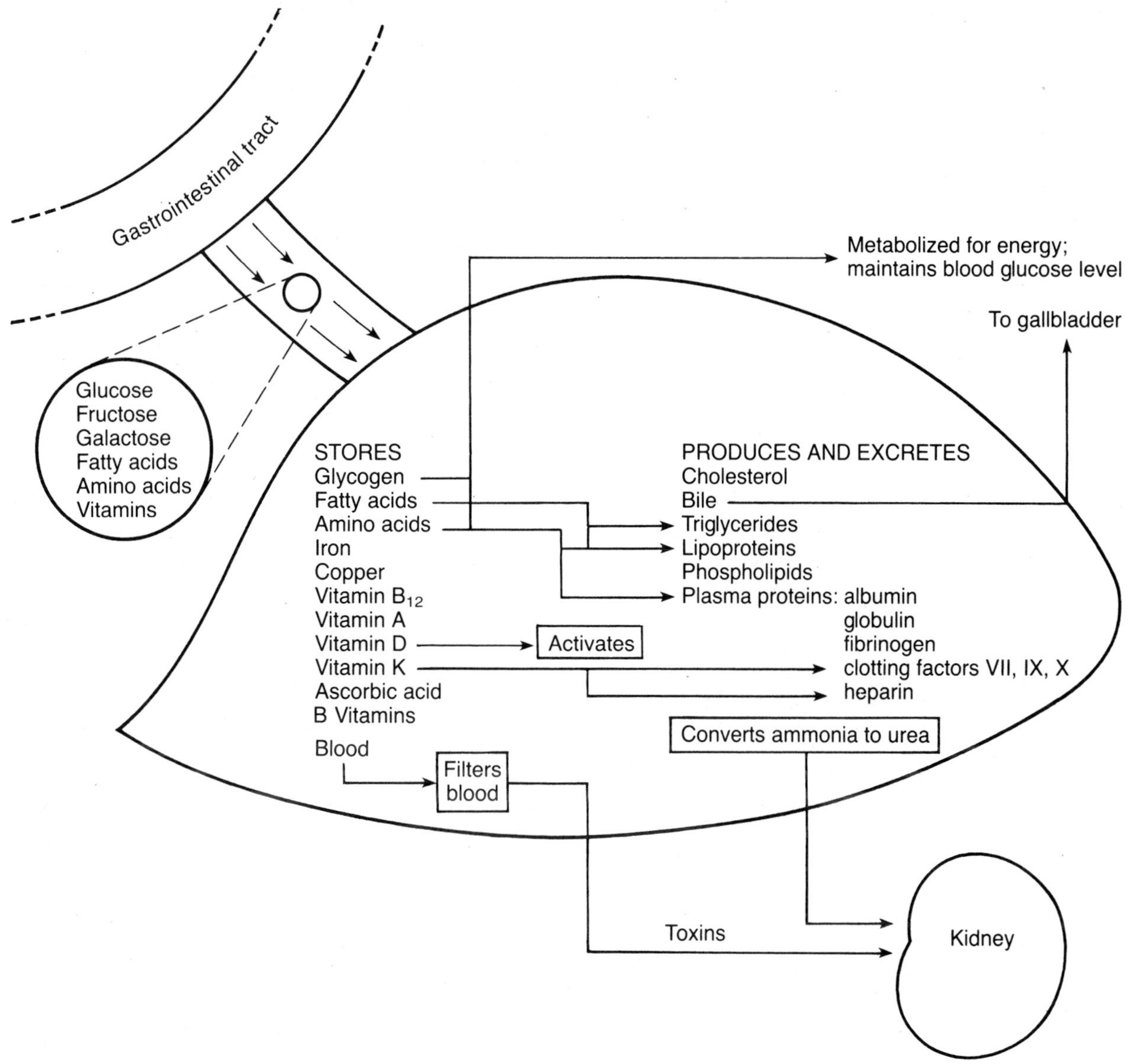

Figure 26–1 **Functions of the liver affecting nutritional status. The liver is the chemical governor of the body; any damage to the liver may affect nutritional status.**

TABLE 26–1

IMPLICATIONS OF COMMON LIVER FUNCTION TESTS

Diagnostic Test	Alteration due to Liver Damage	Significance
Serum/urine bilirubin	Elevated	Bile formation and excretion
Albumin, globulin, total protein	Decreased	Inability to synthesize protein or decreased protein intake
Prothrombin time	Decreased	Prothrombin and fibrinogen production reduced
Urea	Decreased	Liver cannot produce urea to remove ammonia, or too much ammonia is entering the blood stream from action of colonic bacteria
Ammonia	Elevated	
Urine N, total		Measures the amount of nitrogen required (from the diet)
Cholesterol (total or ester)	Elevated	Cholesterol not being converted to bile acids
Bromsulphalein	Elevated	Liver is unable to filter at normal rate
SGOT or AST	Elevated	Reflects enzyme production
SGPT or ALT	Elevated	Reflects enzyme production
Alkaline phosphatase	Elevated	Increase indicates deterioration
Transferrin	Decreased	Failure of liver to synthesize

TABLE 26–2

COMPARISON OF DIETARY GUIDELINES FOR LIVER DISEASE

Nutrients	Hepatitis	Cirrhosis	Encephalopathy
Kilocalories	3000 or more	2000–3000 kcal	1800 kcal minimum
Carbohydrate	300–400 gm	300–400 gm	450 gm
Protein	High: 1.5–2 gm/kg (100–150 gm)	Moderate: 1–1.5 gm/kg (70 gm)	Low: 0.5 gm/kg (20–30 gm)
Fat	35% of kcal	Moderate: 25 to 30% of kcal as tolerated	Initially none Increase as tolerated up to 20 to 25% of kcal
Other	Vitamin supplement including folic acid	Vitamin supplement, especially thiamin, folic acid, vitamin B_6 and B_{12} Possible sodium and fluid restrictions	Vitamin supplement

status. Various liver function tests (LFTs) are invaluable and reflect the functions and changes as they occur during therapy (Table 26–1).

Dietary treatment for liver disorders is aimed at relieving disease symptoms; in most instances, a modified diet does not cure the underlying disease. A diet for a liver condition should be as pleasant and tolerable as possible. Nutritional care should maintain or improve nutritional status by providing adequate kilocalories, protein, fluids, and other nutrients and allow the liver to "rest" as much as possible. Depending on the extent of liver damage, various nutrients are tolerated in different amounts, as compared in Table 26–2.

Describe the general nutritional care for liver problems.

STEATOSIS

Steatosis is the accumulation of fat globules (triglycerides) in the liver.

The liver can be injured from infections, parasites, nutritional deficiencies, metabolic disorders, obstructions, alcohol, toxins, and malignancy. Protein deficiency is the most common nutritional cause, but deficiencies of lipids, carbohydrates, vitamins, or minerals can lead to liver abnormalities. Medications such as steroids and tetracycline can cause liver damage. Degenerative processes can lead to steatosis, necrosis, and fibrosis.

A fatty liver is a symptom of an underlying problem. Treatment of the causative factor (for example, abstinence from alcohol, correction of nutritional deficiency) corrects the liver problem. Steatosis is often accompanied by anorexia, nausea, vomiting, and food intolerance. A well-balanced diet is an important factor in reversing steatosis.

NURSING APPLICATIONS

Assessment

Physical—for malaise, anorexia, nausea, vomiting, weakness, liver tenderness.

Dietary—for actual intake and food intolerances.

Laboratory—for increased bromsulphalein (BSP) retention, elevated globulin and transaminase, depressed albumin; triglycerides.

Interventions

1. Encourage bed rest.
2. Encourage abstinence from alcohol.
3. Provide a nutritious diet.

Evaluation

* LFTs and triglyceride levels return to normal.

Client Education

- Discuss the food pyramid or US Dietary Guidelines.
- Adequate nutrients are important for the liver to heal.
- If the problem is not corrected, it may progress to a more serious liver problem and, if unattended, even death.

HEPATITIS

Causes and Physical Consequences

Hepatitis is an inflammation of the liver, which can result in destruction of liver cells.

In healthy, well-nourished clients, the liver can regenerate destroyed cells, but when excessive amounts of liver tissue are wasted, normal liver functions are inhibited.

Infectious hepatitis is usually caused by a viral microorganism. Type A is transmitted through drinking water, food, or sewage (via the fecal-oral route). Hepatitis B can be transmitted through blood transfusions, improperly sterilized medical instruments, and body fluids such as tears, saliva, and semen. Hepatitis C (formerly called non-A, non-B) is predominately associated with blood transfusions.

Hepatitis can also be caused by chemical toxins such as chloroform, carbon tetrachloride, or alcohol. In most cases, hepatitis is completely reversible. However, these clients are usually anorexic and malnourished. Sometimes the condition deteriorates with increased fatty infiltration and impending hepatic coma. This condition requires a lower quantity of protein and is discussed in the section on hepatic encephalopathy.

What are the different types of hepatitis? What can cause hepatitis?

Nutritional Care

All types of hepatitis are treated in the same manner. Currently no medication is available to cure hepatitis; the major components of therapy are bed rest and dietary management to prevent further injury to the liver and to allow or hasten healing and regeneration of damaged cells.

During the initial stage of anorexia and vomiting, IV solutions of dextrose may provide hydration and prevent hypoglycemia in severe hepatitis since the liver's ability to store glycogen is compromised (Cerrato, 1992). If prolonged parenteral feedings are indicated, protein should be added to the IV feeding. Enteral formulas can also be given via tube feeding or orally, as the condition permits.

As soon as the client is able to tolerate food orally, persistent and persuasive efforts are implemented to ensure the client's intake of a nutritionally adequate diet. Even though the client may feel hungry, nausea may be experienced after eating only a few bites.

Energy intake should be 3000 to 4000 kcal, with at least 40% being furnished from carbohydrates (300 to 400 gm) to promote glycogen synthesis and spare protein (see Table 26–2). Protein intake should be relatively high (1.5 to 2 gm/kg or 100 to 150 gm) to maintain positive nitrogen balance, as LFTs permit. This should be comprised of adequate amounts (>60%) of high-quality protein. When protein is supplied from both animal and vegetable sources (meats, fish, eggs, dairy products, legumes, and cereals), adequate amounts of lipotropic agents (e.g., choline, inositol, and methionine) accompany these foods to prevent further development of fatty liver. Additionally, fluid intake should be high (2500 to 3000 ml/day).

Food and Meal/Snack	Portion Size for Cirrhosis	Portion Size for Hepatitis
Breakfast		
banana	1/2	1/2
bran flakes	1 cup	1 cup
low-fat fruit-flavored yogurt	1 cup	1 cup
whole milk	1 cup	1 cup
coffee with non-dairy creamer and	1 cup/1 tsp	1 cup/1 tsp
sugar	1 tsp	1 tsp
Mid-morning Snack		
pineapple juice	6 oz	8 oz
whole wheat toast	1	1
margarine	1 tsp	1 tsp
jelly	1 packet	1 packet
Lunch		
lean broiled pork chop	3 oz	3 oz
mashed potatoes	1/2 cup	
salt-free scalloped potatoes		1/2 cup
cooked carrots	1/2 cup	1/2 cup
whole wheat bread	1	1/2 slice
margarine	2 tsp	2 tsp
baked apple	1	1
tea	Not limited	Not limited
Mid-afternoon snack		
canned pear halves	2	2
cheddar cheese	1/4 cup	2 oz
saltines		4
low-sodium crackers	4	
Dinner		
beef cubes in salt-free broth	3 oz	
beef stroganoff		1/2 cup
cooked noodles	1/2 cup	1/2 cup
cooked broccoli	1/2 cup	1/2 cup
cheese sauce		1/4 cup
whole wheat bread	1 slice	1/2 slice
margarine	1 tsp	
cream pie		1 slice
baked custard with	1/2 cup	
blueberry sauce	1/4 cup	1/4 cup
tea	Not limited	Not limited
Evening snack		
ice cream	1 cup	
1/2 sandwich: whole wheat bread,		1 slice
sliced turkey,		1 oz
mayonnaise		1 tbsp

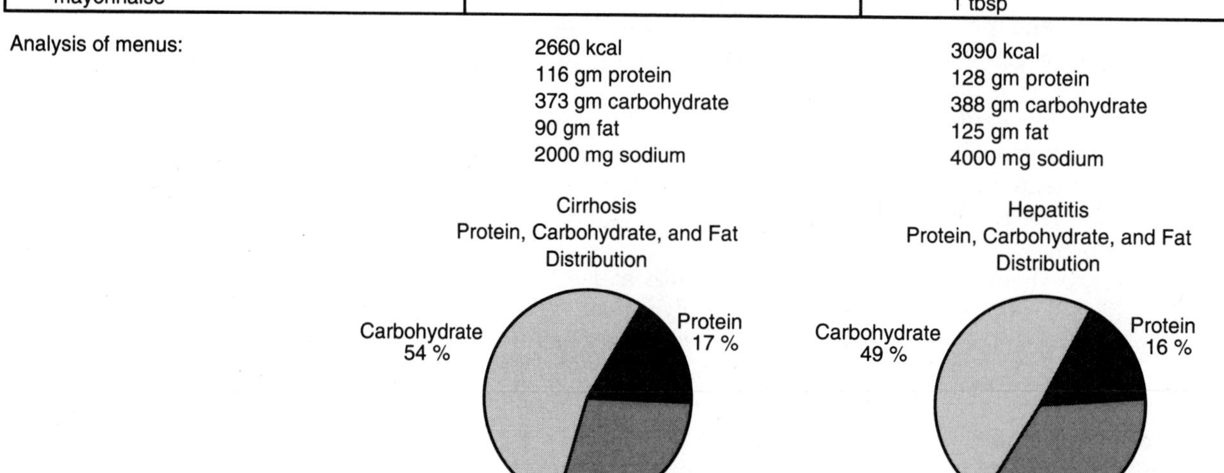

Figure 26–2 Sample menus for hepatitis and cirrhosis. (Nutrient data from Nutritionist III, version 7.0 software. N-Squared Computing, Salem, OR.)

Fat restriction below the normal level of 30 to 35% of total energy intake is unnecessary unless fats are not well tolerated. Fat increases the diet's palatability and also decreases the enormous volume of food necessary to provide 3000 kcal. However, a high-fat diet is not well tolerated. Fats in dairy products and eggs are usually better tolerated than fried foods and fatty meats (Fig. 26–2).

On the one hand, the reduced plasma prothrombin level usually does not respond to vitamin K therapy since it is a result of impaired liver function. On the other hand, if intrahepatic biliary obstruction occurs, parenteral or oral, water-miscible vitamin K improves prothrombin levels. Usually intake before onset has been poor. As a result of this poor intake coupled with poor appetite and poor utilization of nutrients, a daily multivitamin that includes folic acid is recommended.

What are the requirements for energy, protein, and fat in hepatitis?

NURSING APPLICATIONS

Assessment

Physical—for fatigue, weakness, anorexia, fever, hepatomegaly, nausea and vomiting, abdominal discomfort, diarrhea, jaundice, pressure sores, weight/weight loss, dark urine, yellow sclera.

Dietary—for alcohol consumption, appetite and dietary intake, especially kilocalories, carbohydrate, protein, and fat.

Laboratory—elevated transaminase, glutamate dehydrogenase, AST (SGOT), ALT (SGPT), LDH, alkaline phosphatase, bilirubin, increased prothrombin time; total protein, albumin, cholesterol; sodium, potassium, hypoglycemia.

Interventions

1. For a malnourished client, provide a high-kilocalorie, high-protein diet.
2. For a client in good nutritional status, provide a well-balanced diet.
3. For a client with anorexia or nausea, offer small, frequent meals with nutrition supplements.
4. For severe hepatitis, IV glucose may be necessary to avoid fasting hypoglycemia.
5. Take proper precautions to prevent further spread of the infectious form of the disease: (a) Disposable dishes should be used and disposed of in the client's room. (b) Inform visitors/family that they should not eat foods from the client's tray.
6. Adequate fluid intake is necessary to replace losses and prevent dehydration: At least 2500 to 3000 ml/day is needed.
7. Serve small, frequent feedings consisting of simple foods for better tolerance and acceptance.
8. Serve foods attractively to stimulate appetite.
9. Monitor I&O, especially the color of urine and stool.
10. Provide a pleasant eating environment since hepatitis clients are sensitive to odors.

Evaluation

* Evaluation parameters include the following: The client's appetite will increase, weight will be maintained or gained, nausea and vomiting will diminish, laboratory results will be normal, and complications associated with hepatitis will not develop.

Client Education

- For the liver to repair itself, dietary intake must furnish adequate nutrients.
- Include foods from all the food groups.
- Choose high-kilocalorie fluids (fruit juices, milkshakes).

Continued

- Increase high-protein foods.
- If nauseated, eat small, frequent meals during the day and choose nutrient-dense foods.
- Inflammation of the liver may cause the liver to be more vulnerable to any hepatotoxic agents, including alcohol. Therefore, alcohol should be avoided, especially during the acute phase and for 4 to 6 months after recovery.
- Even after recovery from viral hepatitis, the liver is more susceptible to the toxic effects of alcohol; moderation (<20 gm/day) is advisable. Moderation is considered 2 beers, 1–2 3½ oz glasses of wine, and 2 jiggers of hard liquors.
- Clients with alcoholic hepatitis should be clearly advised in a firm manner to abstain from alcohol and referred to Alcoholics Anonymous (AA) or other alcohol/drug abuse programs.

CIRRHOSIS

Causes and Physical Consequences

Cirrhosis is characterized by prolonged fatty degeneration with fibrous connective tissue replacing destroyed liver cells.

Hemochromatosis is a metabolic disorder with large deposits of iron in the liver.

Laennec's cirrhosis is a result of alcoholism and malnutrition.

Nutrients from the GI tract are carried via the portal vein to the liver.

Portal hypertension is a result of increased blood pressure in the liver because of the resistance to blood flow in the scarred liver tissue. Increased portal pressure causes enlargement and dilatation of the collateral circulatory blood vessels in the esophagus, stomach, and rectum. When this occurs in the lower esophagus, it is called esophageal varices; in the rectum, hemorrhoids may occur.

Ascites is the accumulation of large quantities of fluid in the abdomen.

What can cause cirrhosis; ascites?

Cirrhosis is a further degenerative stage of severe chronic liver disease than hepatitis. Cirrhosis may be caused by improperly treated hepatitis or toxic or viral hepatitis, chronic autoimmune disease, metabolic disorders such as Wilson's disease or **hemochromatosis,** obstruction of biliary drainage or biliary disorders, or chronic use of hepatotoxic drugs (acetaminophen). It is most frequently associated with chronic alcohol abuse or **Laennec's cirrhosis.**

Since blood cannot flow easily through the fibrous liver tissue, it backs up into the **portal vein,** causing further deterioration in hepatic function. **Portal hypertension** and **esophageal varices** are usually observed. Low-sodium antacids or anticholinergics may be prescribed.

Increased intrahepatic pressure results in another complication of cirrhosis, **ascites.** It may be caused by obstruction of the damaged liver, decreased osmotic pressure from hypoalbuminemia, sodium retention, or impaired water excretion.

Branched-Chain Amino Acids

BCAAs include leucine, isoleucine, and valine; aromatic amino acids include phenylalanine, tyrosine, and tryptophan.

Explain why serum levels of BCAA may be low, whereas aromatic amino acids are increased. Give examples of BCAA and aromatic amino acids.

In hepatic diseases, catabolism and increased gluconeogenesis occur. Skeletal muscle breakdown releases a variety of amino acids. **BCAA** are decreased, and **aromatic amino acids** and methionine are increased. Since BCAA can be metabolized by muscles, they are used for energy. Aromatic amino acids depend primarily on the liver for their catabolism. These aromatic amino acids may bypass the liver or cannot be catabolized by the diseased liver; increased levels in the blood also affects the CNS. These amino acids are precursors of neurotransmitters (norepinephrine). High levels of aromatic amines function as "false neurotransmitters," which are involved in the pathogenesis of hepatic coma and other neurological and cardiovascular problems.

Methods of Therapy

Primary treatments are removal of the causative agent (for example, alcohol, drug), bed rest, and nutrition support. Effective management of nutrition problems depends on nutritional status, as determined by physical assessment and laboratory results of LFTs.

Drug therapy is limited because of a reduced ability of the liver to metabolize drugs. Antibiotics, such as neomycin or ampicillin, are instituted to decrease colonic bacteria, which produce ammonia from protein, thereby decreasing the amount of nitrogenous wastes in the blood. These drugs, however, cause malabsorption. The medication lactulose (Cephulac, Chronulac) is a synthetic nonabsorbable disaccharide that reduces the absorption of ammonia and increases peristalsis.

What are methods of treatment for cirrhosis?

Nutritional Care

Nutritional care is more complex than mere nutritional replenishment, which may be corrected while the individual is in the hospital. A typical alcoholic exhibits many self-abusive behaviors, including disinterest in food. This is commonly associated with excessive coffee consumption, heavy smoking, and heavy use of prescription and OTC drugs. Counseling is used to overcome personal and situational factors that contribute to these problems and to deal with anxiety and depression with a motivational approach.

The goal of diet therapy in the cirrhotic client is to (1) provide adequate kilocalories and other nutrients, (2) correct nutritional deficiencies, (3) enhance tissue repair, (4) prevent or correct protein intolerances, and (5) manage other life-threatening complications. Recovery is enhanced by a high-kilocalorie, normal to high-protein, normal-fat, and vitamin-enriched diet (see Table 26–2 and Fig. 26–2). Because of poor nutritional status and appetite, enteral feedings supplying adequate nutrients have been advocated with improved clinical outcome (Kearns et al, 1992; Cabre et al, 1990).

The metabolic rate is elevated (Green et al, 1991). Thus, the energy requirement is approximately 2000 to 3000 kcal/day or 40 to 50 kcal/kg of **dry body weight.** Protein intake must be adequate to prevent nitrogen wasting. However, too much protein can result in further degeneration of the liver. Protein intake may be 1 to 1.5 gm/kg dry weight, depending on the client's ability to tolerate protein. When the diet is adequate in protein, supplementation with choline and methionine is not necessary.

Dry body weight is an estimate of actual weight without the weight of the ascites fluid. A recent premorbid weight might be used.

Alcohol dependency may be accompanied by pancreatic insufficiency and alterations in bile salt metabolism; fat must be used judiciously to prevent steatorrhea. Dietary fat should be as high as possible for greater palatability of food given to the anorectic client but low enough so as not to precipitate steatorrhea. If fat malabsorption is present, dietary fat may need to be lowered to constitute 25% of the energy level (about 50 gm fat) (Fig. 26–3). Emulsified fats (homogenized milk and eggs) decrease the demand for bile. Also, MCT oils can be used safely to supply necessary kilocalories without further liver damage.

Thiamin deficiency in alcoholics is common because of inadequate consumption and malabsorption. Severe deficiency (contributing to amnesia and personality changes) is known as the Wernicke-Korsakoff syndrome. Vitamin deficiencies are seldom limited to a single vitamin. Water-soluble vitamins are usually supplemented 2 to 3 times the RDAs (without known harmful effects) for the first week or 2 of therapy or until the client is able to eat adequately. Precursor blood cells in the bone marrow can be damaged by alcohol, which increases the requirements for vitamins used in the maturation of red and white blood cells. This includes folacin and vitamins B_6 and B_{12}. Initially vitamin supplements are used to correct deficiencies and for repletion but are not necessary once the client is eating well.

Although the diet ordered and the diet planned by the dietitian may be important, it is the food eaten by the client that affects the condition. The provision of 6 small daily feedings generally results in an increased total intake. Therefore, nursing's role is to encourage and support the client, especially if alcohol withdrawal is part of the treatment.

Decreased motility and increased intra-abdominal pressure secondary to ascites

Food and Meal/Snack	Portion Size for 50 gm fat	Portion Size for 30 gm fat
Breakfast		
pineapple juice	6 oz	6 oz
banana	1/2	1/2
bran flakes	1 cup	1 cup
low-fat fruit-flavored yogurt	1 cup	1 cup
whole wheat toast	1 slice	1 slice
margarine	1 tsp	0
jelly	1 packet	1 packet
1% low fat milk	1 cup	0
skim milk, protein fortified	0	1 cup
coffee with nondairy creamer and	1 cup/1 tsp	1 cup/1 tsp
sugar	1 tsp	0
Lunch		
baked cod fish	3 oz	3 oz
scalloped potatoes	1/2 cup	1/2 cup
cooked carrots	1/2 cup	1/2 cup
whole wheat roll	1	1
margarine	1	0
jelly	0	1 packet
cranberry juice	6 oz	6 oz
baked apple	1	1
1% low fat milk	1 cup	0
skim, protein fortified milk	0	1 cup
tea	Not limited	Not limited
Dinner		
beef cubes in salt-free broth	2.5 oz	2.5 oz
cooked noodles	1/2 cup	1/2 cup
cooked summer squash	1/2 cup	1/2 cup
relishes: cherry tomatoes, celery sticks	Not limited	Not limited
whole wheat bread	1 slice	1 slice
jelly	1 packet	1 packet
low fat custard with	1/2 cup	0
blueberry sauce	1/4 cup	0
tea	Not limited	Not limited
Evening snack		
sherbet	1/2 cup	1/2 cup

Analysis of menus:	2240 kcal 100 gm protein 373 gm carbohydrate 48 gm fat	2169 kcal 103 gm protein 395 gm carbohydrate 28 gm fat

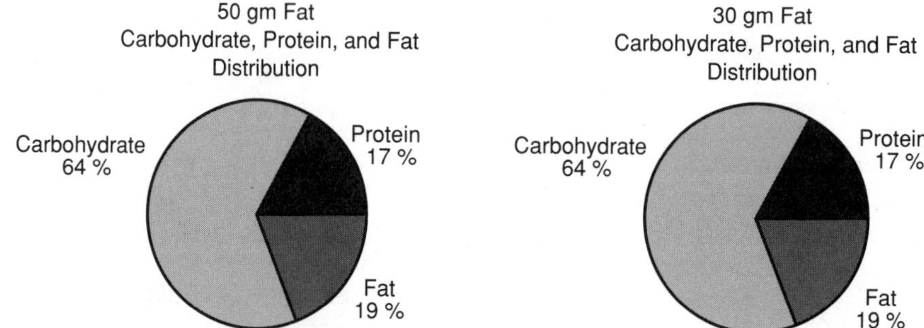

Figure 26–3 Sample menus for 50-gm and 30-gm low-fat diets. (Nutrient data from Nutritionist III, version 7.0 software. N-Squared Computing, Salem, OR.)

contribute to poor appetite. Therefore, ingenuity is needed to serve food attractively. Efforts to furnish clients with foods they feel they can eat can be frustrating; clients may become nauseated after eating only a few bites of their favorite dish. These attempts may, however, entice the client to try to eat. They also offer an opportunity to stress the importance of diet. As the client's condition improves, appetite also improves.

The level of sodium restriction for ascites depends on whether the physician simultaneously orders a diuretic and the client's ability to eliminate sodium and fluids. Spironolactone is the preferred diuretic for liver disease because potassium depletion and excessive diuresis are avoided (Bruckstein, 1987). Sodium may need to be severely restricted because diuretics may be contraindicated in some cirrhotic clients. Diuretics that are not potassium sparing may precipitate hypokalemic alkalosis with further deterioration of status (more ammonia is produced). A severe sodium restriction (0.5 gm) is not well received by clients and is recommended for only a brief period (3 to 4 days). Compliance on a 1 gm sodium level is difficult at home and is not recommended unless absolutely essential.

When the sodium content of the diet is severely restricted, protein foods must necessarily be limited (see Chapter 24, Table 24–4). Low-sodium milk, such as Lonalac, and low-sodium breads can be used. Because the client already has a depressed appetite, these substitutions may not be well received. Sodium intake is gradually liberalized as the rate of diuresis increases. A low-sodium diet is not easy to follow but can be made reasonably palatable. Most clients accept this restriction as preferable to the discomfort of severe ascites.

Sodium restriction is not without risks; unless fluid intake is restricted, severe symptomatic hyponatremia may occur. Fluid intake may be restricted to 1000 to 2000 ml/24 hours. (Helpful hints for easing the client's discomfort are listed in Chapter 8, Table 8–1). This limitation may be followed by oliguria, which may not be noticed for several days without accurate recording of I&O.

NURSING APPLICATIONS

Assessment

Physical—for malaise, lethargy, dyspepsia, bloating, breath odor (musty), nausea, vomiting (especially of blood), anorexia, ascites (abdominal girth), edema, diarrhea, oliguria, weight/weight changes, SF thickness, MAMC, dry scaly skin, jaundice.

Dietary—for adequacy of kilocalorie, protein, and sodium intake.

Laboratory—for depressed Hgb, Hct, and WBC; increased ALT (SGPT), AST (SGOT), LDH, BSP retention, globulin, bilirubin, ammonia, transaminase, alkaline phosphatase (normal to markedly increased), prolonged PT, PTT; decreased electrolytes (sodium, potassium); serum transferrin, albumin, BUN; occult blood.

Interventions

1. Chart daily dietary intake.
2. Weigh and measure abdominal girth daily in clients with ascites to assess changes in fluid balance.
3. Maintain I&O.
4. If the client does not have an order for a multivitamin (including folacin, vitamins B_6, B_{12}, C, K, and the mineral magnesium), notify the physician/dietitian.
5. Provide a large breakfast when the appetite is best and less nausea is present.
6. Restrict dietary fat or use MCT oils if malabsorption or jaundice occurs.

Continued

7. When prothrombin levels are prolonged, emphasize the importance of including foods high in vitamin K (green leafy vegetables).
8. When esophageal varices are present, avoid GI irritants, such as caffeine and spices, and provide foods that are smooth in texture to prevent the danger of rupture.
9. Provide a diabetic type diet (see Chapter 27) if glucose intolerance develops.
10. Encourage the client to enroll in some type of psychotherapy program for behavior therapy. The program should focus on long-term rehabilitation of the alcoholic and incorporate nutrition education into therapy sessions.
11. For ascites, follow a low-sodium diet because decreased sodium retards fluid retention.
12. Avoid salt substitutes that contain ammonia chloride because they amplify the high ammonia levels caused by the liver disease.
13. Provide salt substitutes that contain potassium chloride (if the potassium level is low or normal).
14. For clients with Wilson's disease, eliminate copper from the diet (grains, shellfish, organ meats).
15. For hemochromatosis, limit dietary iron (meats and iron-fortified foods).

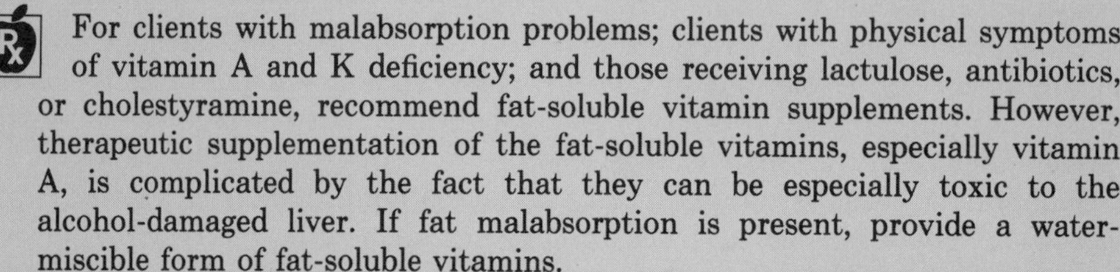
For clients with malabsorption problems; clients with physical symptoms of vitamin A and K deficiency; and those receiving lactulose, antibiotics, or cholestyramine, recommend fat-soluble vitamin supplements. However, therapeutic supplementation of the fat-soluble vitamins, especially vitamin A, is complicated by the fact that they can be especially toxic to the alcohol-damaged liver. If fat malabsorption is present, provide a water-miscible form of fat-soluble vitamins.

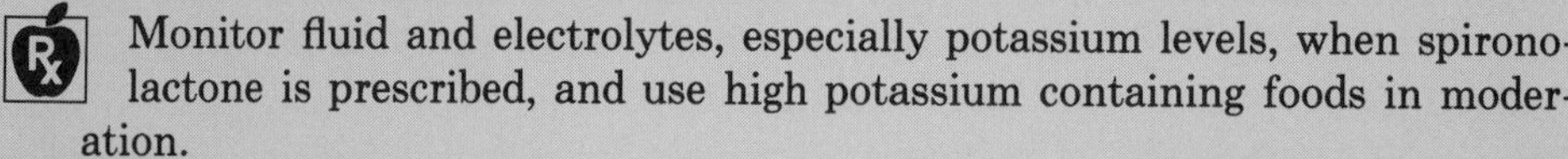
Monitor fluid and electrolytes, especially potassium levels, when spironolactone is prescribed, and use high potassium containing foods in moderation.

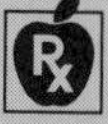
Monitor magnesium, potassium, and zinc levels of clients receiving diuretics.

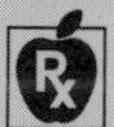
Monitor for zinc deficiency when client is receiving lactulose or neomycin.

Evaluation

* For evaluation of goals, have client state 3 high-protein foods, 3 foods low in salt, and why these restrictions are necessary.
* The client should also gain dry body weight and decrease ascites.

Client Education

- Clients with ascites may try to "diet away" the added weight by not eating all the foods on the tray. Explain that the additional pounds are due to water retention or the ascites; the weight will be lost by diuresis or removal of ascitic fluid.
- Development of alcoholic liver disease (fatty liver, hepatitis, or cirrhosis) cannot be prevented by supplements of a nutrient or a combination of nutrients. However, if alcohol intake is terminated, liver functions return toward normal if promoted by nutrition support.
- Supplements of methionine, choline, and liver extract do not have any special benefits and may sometimes be dangerous because of the additional nitrogen load.
- Hypervitaminosis may occur if too many vitamin supplements are taken by alcoholics to help prevent damage to the liver.
- Hyperabsorption of iron in genetically predisposed alcoholics causes hemochromatosis. Caution clients to abstain from iron-fortified foods and to consume iron-rich foods in moderation.

HEPATIC ENCEPHALOPATHY

Further liver disease may lead to **hepatic encephalopathy.** As portal blood circulation decreases and collateral circulation develops, increasing amounts of blood bypass the liver. Toxic substances are not eliminated, and amino acids are not metabolized normally. Excess ammonia and nitrogenous waste products and a deficiency of BCAA all appear to play a role in the development of hepatic encephalopathy. Although the exact cause has yet to be determined, it is known that although protein is needed for recovery, clients cannot tolerate it.

Advanced liver disease or hepatic encephalopathy is reflected in a disturbance of consciousness that can readily progress into deep coma (hepatic coma).

What are some possible causes of hepatic encephalopathy?

Ammonia

Intestinal flora break down dietary protein and blood (from GI bleeding) into ammonia, which is absorbed. It is important to arrest GI bleeding. Ammonia not converted to urea by the damaged or bypassed liver accumulates in amounts that are toxic to the CNS.

Ammonia levels can be lowered in several ways. Neomycin, an antibiotic, is used to interfere with the bacterial conversion of urea to ammonia. By reducing the numbers of colonic bacteria, more dietary protein can be given. Lactulose produces an acidic diarrhea, reduces GI flora, and may depress absorption of aromatic amino acids. The use of these drugs has decreased the need for special low-protein diets.

Describe methods to decrease ammonia.

Nutritional Care

Although metabolism of all nutrients in hepatic failure is abnormal, intolerance to protein makes nutrition support treacherous. The basic objectives of diet therapy in hepatic coma are to (1) remove the sources of excess ammonia (dietary and pharmacological), (2) furnish adequate amounts of energy to prevent hypoglycemia and excessive tissue catabolism, (3) promote regeneration of liver tissue, and (4) balance fluids and electrolytes.

Initial therapy for encephalopathy is focused on decreasing absorption of toxic materials (especially ammonia) from the GI tract by using poorly absorbed antibiotics. Purgatives may be used to remove any protein present in the GI tract (from blood or dietary source). Protein may be completely withheld for about 3 days.

For numerous reasons, elemental or parenteral feedings are frequently necessary. The combination of dietary restrictions—protein, sodium, fluid, and food consistency—contributes to an unpalatable diet. Large quantities of kilocalories are needed for the anabolic process. Additionally, eating is hindered by anorexia and cognitive status. If the GI tract is functional, enteral feedings are preferred over parenteral feedings. Enteral nutrition improves hepatic perfusion and enhances GI immunity. GI bleeding and hypoactive bowel sounds contraindicate enteral feedings.

The amount of protein allowed is regulated according to the client's level of consciousness or tolerance. A very low-protein diet (20 to 30 gm) composed of high-quality protein is associated with improvement in the encephalopathic client's mental condition. The narrow range of protein tolerance requires that increases are closely monitored. With an excess of protein, coma may occur; without enough, the illness is prolonged. The diet may progress from 20 gm of protein and is increased in 10-gm increments every few days, to a total of 50 gm, as tolerated and as the client's condition improves. Therefore, the objective is to provide adequate amounts of high-quality protein to prevent negative nitrogen balance. Protein intake can be increased to 70 to 100 gm daily with the use of neomycin or lactulose (Cephulac, Chronulac) (Lee, 1988).

For rough calculations of protein levels, the amounts of protein from the food exchange lists can be used (see Appendix D–1). Thirty grams of protein can be

TABLE 26–3

USING DIABETIC FOOD EXCHANGES TO CALCULATE 30 GRAMS PROTEIN

Food Item	Protein (gm)
2 oz of meat	14
8 oz of whole milk	8
2 servings of bread/cereal	6
2 servings of vegetables	2
Total	30

provided, as shown in Table 26–3. Maximum amounts of high-quality protein are given in small amounts throughout the day. Complex carbohydrate foods also provide some protein that cannot be ignored. (They are necessary to increase energy content of the diet and for their protein-sparing role). Kilocaloric requirement is high, approximately 35 to 45 kcal/kg of dry body weight. Excess carbohydrate may cause a fatty liver, so dietary fat is important to provide the kilocalories necessary for protein sparing. Also, many clients have carbohydrate intolerance; high-carbohydrate diets may further aggravate hyperglycemia.

By modifying amino acid mixtures and providing increased amounts of protein, liver protein synthesis is stimulated. Although natural foods cannot be manipulated to increase the amounts of BCAA, several preparations are available for enteral feeding (oral or supplements)—Travasorb Hepatic (Clintec) and Hepatic Aid (Kendall McGaw)—or for parenteral use—Hepatamine (Kendall McGaw). (Hepatic Aid does not contain vitamins and electrolytes, necessitating supplementation). Approximately 50% of the total amino acids are provided by BCAA-fortified formulas, whereas foods usually contain about 22% BCAA. Clients with hepatic encephalopathy in poor nutritional status and who are intolerant to regular protein are candidates for BCAA supplementation to reestablish positive nitrogen balance (Fischer, 1990; Skeie et al, 1990). BCAA have been used successfully in chronic hepatic encephalopathy and for comatose clients (Marchesini et al, 1990). Additionally, casein-based formulas are well tolerated in clients with encephalopathy (ADA, 1988).

What are the goals of diet therapy in hepatic coma?

Comatose clients are given IV glucose solutions only without any protein until some response is seen. As soon as signs of recovery are observed (or the level of consciousness increases), protein can be instituted in 10-gm increments, progressing as previously discussed. Although 0.5 gm/kg/day promotes nitrogen balance in clients with advanced liver disease, the ultimate goal is 1 gm/kg/day to provide protein for anabolism.

Describe how protein intake is regulated in hepatic clients.

As protein is being increased and is better tolerated, up to 40 to 50 gm of fat can be gradually added (20 to 25% of the kilocalories). MCT oils may be used if malabsorption is present. Increases in fat should be closely monitored because alcoholic clients are at risk for pancreatitis. At least 1800 kcal are necessary to prevent catabolism.

What are the requirements for protein, fat, carbohydrate, and kilocalories?

NURSING APPLICATIONS

Assessment

Physical—for sweet putrid odor of the breath, loss of concentration, apathy, personality changes, intellectual and speech deterioration, weight, muscle spasms, ascites, edema, GI bleeding, stupor, confusion, disorientation, xerosis, night blindness, stomatitis, neuromuscular irritability.

Dietary—for actual kilocalorie, protein, carbohydrate, fat, and sodium intake.

Laboratory—(in addition to those listed for cirrhosis) for elevation of ammonia and CSF glutamine levels.

Interventions

1. Monitor clients carefully for adherence to the prescribed diet and for any GI bleeding.
2. Since serum levels of aromatic amino acids are elevated in clients with liver disease, avoid the use of the sweetener aspartame (an aromatic amino acid). Besides, clients need the additional kilocalories provided by sugar.
3. Weigh the client daily to assess hydration status.
4. Monitor for muscle wasting since a prolonged low-protein diet can result in PEM.

Evaluation

* Clients should receive the appropriate amounts of kilocalories, protein, fat, and carbohydrate based on the severity of their condition.

Client Education

- Do no actual teaching while client is in a coma but converse with the client while providing care.
- Vegetable and dairy proteins contain fewer aromatic amino acids and are better tolerated than meat proteins.

LIVER TRANSPLANTATION

There is no curative medical treatment for severe hepatic failure; thus, liver transplantation may be appropriate in selected clients. Clients scheduled for a liver transplant are in poor nutritional status because of protein, fluid, and salt restrictions and poor appetite.

Nutritional Care

A nutritional assessment is the first step of developing a nutrition care plan for these clients. Before and following the transplant, a low-bacteria diet (see Chapter 22) is needed because of immunosuppressive medications. Following the transplant, TPN is recommended until the client has a functioning GI tract. TPN with either standard or BCAA-enriched amino acids is well tolerated immediately after a successful liver transplant (Reilly et al, 1990). This is especially important in clients with a compromised nutritional status. Anabolism and nitrogen balance can be achieved with a high-kilocalorie (1.5 kcal × BEE) and high-protein (1.5 gm/kg) intake (Hasse, 1990). High levels of glucocorticoids accelerate protein losses and cause sodium and fluid retention. Initially fat intake may be relatively high unless triglycerides are elevated.

When bowel sounds are present with no gastric bleeding, tube feedings may be provided until the client can eat 75% of estimated nutritional requirements. A 1 kcal/ml formula may be used unless fluid restriction is needed for edema or ascites (Hasse, 1991). When clients are able to consume 50% of their needs orally, tube feeding may be provided nocturnally to promote appetite at meals. Kilocalorie counts are needed to assess actual kilocaloric and protein intake. The diet should be high kilocalorie, high protein. Serum magnesium and phosphorus levels are monitored; supplements are provided when serum levels are low.

In the long-term post-transplant client, kilocaloric and protein requirements are decreased to amounts recommended for healthy clients (1.2 × BEE and 0.8 to 1 gm/kg, respectively). Fats should be decreased to 30% of the kilocalorie requirement. Many clients develop hypertension, obesity, hyperlipidemia, hyperkalemia,

Describe nutritional care for transplant clients.

edema, and hyperglycemia. Immunosuppressive medications are believed to contribute to these conditions.

NURSING APPLICATIONS

Assessment

Physical—for weight loss/gain, hydration status, edema, bowel sounds, NG drainage, high blood pressure, type of drugs taken, mental status (physical and psychological), urine output.
Dietary—for any restrictions, especially protein, fluid, salt; appetite; diet intake records.
Laboratory—for cholesterol, triglycerides; glucose; electrolytes, especially magnesium, phosphorus; LFTs.

Interventions

1. Monitor liver function and mental status to ensure the client is adequately metabolizing protein.
2. If the glucose level is above 200 mg/dl, eliminate concentrated sweets.
3. When edema and ascites are present, restrict sodium and fluids, as ordered.
4. Monitor clients for complications such as sepsis, renal failure, and rejection of the transplant.

Evaluation

* A high kilocalorie, high protein diet is consumed and gradually replaced by a diet containing 1.2 × BEE and 0.8 to 1 gm/kg protein.

Client Education

- During periods of rejection, increased amounts of immunosuppressive drugs are needed. Encourage the client to make dietary modifications, as indicated in Chapter 22, in the section on transplants.
- Long-term sodium restriction (3 to 4 gm) is appropriate for clients with hypertension.
- The transplanted liver must be monitored for the rest of the client's life; routine laboratory tests are monitored for signs of rejection.

GALLBLADDER

Causes and Physical Consequences

Stones, composed of cholesterol, calcium, bilirubin, and inorganic salts, form in the gallbladder, causing a condition called cholelithiasis. An inflammation of the gallbladder is called cholecystitis. Choledocholithiasis is an obstruction of the common bile duct.

Common diseases of the gallbladder are **cholelithiasis, cholecystitis,** and **choledocholithiasis,** which occur more frequently in obese women over 40 years of age, particularly those with previous multiple pregnancies. Several conditions are associated with an increased incidence of gallstones, including hemolytic disorders, obesity, diabetes, familial hypercholesterolemia, cardiovascular disease, multiple pregnancies, and use of oral contraceptives. In all of the conditions, pain occurs when the gallbladder contracts.

Most gallstones are about 85% crystallized cholesterol, but cholesterol intake plays only a small role in the cause of gallstones (Maclure et al, 1990). Hypomotility appears to be a more important factor in stone formation. During fasting and TPN, the risk of stone formation is increased secondary to lack of gallbladder stimulation. Cholecystokinin may be provided during TPN to decrease this risk. Elevated progesterone levels inhibit smooth muscle contractions, resulting in increased bile in the gallbladder (Paumgartner & Sauerbruch, 1991). A high-fiber diet has been associated with decreased incidence of gallstones. Studies have shown various insoluble fibers change the proportion of bile acids and reduce the formation of calculi (MacDonald, 1988).

Methods of Therapy

In the past, the only treatment was to surgically remove stones or the gallbladder. However, 2 bile acids, chenodeoxycholic acid (CDCA) and ursodeoxycholic acid (UDCA), can be used to dissolve small stones. This is a slow process, and the medication must be taken daily for at least 6 months. Their use is contraindicated in clients with liver disease or obstructed bile ducts. CDCA is more effective when taken at bedtime (single dose) and while following a low-cholesterol diet (Maudgal & Northfield, 1991). Because of the distinctly different chemical properties of the 2 bile acids, a combination of them may prove to be more effective than monotherapy (Sauerbruch & Paumgartner, 1991). Extracorporeal shock wave lithotripsy (ESWL) is the newest therapy, which breaks the stones into smaller fragments. Either of the 2 bile acids already discussed may be given to help dissolution rate. Laser surgery is another option for treatment of gallstones.

Name 3 methods to treat gallstones.

Nutritional Care

The goal for nutritional care in gallbladder conditions is to minimize discomfort. Clients usually quickly learn which foods cause distress. Although a low-fat diet for gallbladder has been a traditional therapy, research indicates that the action of the gallbladder is independent of a meal's fat content.

In acute gallbladder attacks, a low-fat, clear liquid diet is used with IV fluids and electrolytes to replace losses and rest the gallbladder. As soon as possible, the client can progress to soft foods, very restricted in fats (20 to 30 gm) (see Fig. 26–3).

If inflammation is present or the client is obese, the physician may postpone surgery, and nutritional therapy is implemented during this period. Clients awaiting gallbladder surgery as well as those with chronic gallbladder problems should eliminate foods that cause discomfort. Fats may be reduced to alleviate pain. By reducing fat intake, weight loss can usually be accomplished since fat is the most concentrated source of energy. Fried foods, fatty meats, and rich desserts are avoided. Spicy foods (chili or curry) may also cause discomfort. Many strongly flavored or gas-forming vegetables (onions, sauerkraut, cabbage, radishes, turnips, or cucumbers) may be poorly tolerated. These need not be restricted unless they cause problems.

Following a cholecystectomy, clear liquids are initiated within 24 to 48 hours. The client gradually progresses toward resumption of a regular diet. Postoperatively bile enters the small intestine continually rather than being secreted in response to food intake. Some clients have less distress on a low-fat diet for the first several weeks after surgery (see Chapter 1, Table 1–6, and Chapter 24, Step-1 Diet). Whether or not fat is controlled in this progressive diet depends on the client's tolerance and the physician's preferences. There is little reason to restrict the diet beyond 1 month following surgery.

Diarrhea after a cholecystectomy indicates a dietary intolerance. Spicy foods, such as Mexican food, may cause diarrhea. Six small feedings are better tolerated and may increase nutrient intake.

Who is the main decision maker in regard to the amount of fat allowed in the diet?

NURSING APPLICATIONS

Assessment

Physical—for weight gain; number of pregnancies; use of birth control pills; pain, especially in the right shoulder; nausea and vomiting; flatulence.
Dietary—for foods that cause distress.
Laboratory—for triglycerides, cholesterol; vitamin K, PT; bilirubin.

Interventions

1. Preoperatively, give vitamin K if ordered to prevent bleeding problems resultant of poor absorption of this vitamin.
2. Postoperatively, allow the client to make food choices, as he or she is the best judge of which foods cause discomfort.
3. Refer to the dietitian.

Evaluation

* Possible parameters to evaluate care include the following: The client verbalizes and consumes a diet that helps avoid further attacks or complications; pain is absent after eating; and weight is lost, if indicated.

Client Education

- If client is at risk for gallbladder disease, encourage a high-fiber diet.
- When bile acids are given to dissolve gallstones, provide information about a high-fiber diet, which helps bind cholesterol and reduce weight.
- Clients may gain considerable weight after a cholecystectomy, enjoying many fatty foods previously not tolerated.
- Encourage clients to consume a well-balanced diet and eliminate only foods that cause discomfort.
- Cholesterol restriction is unnecessary unless indicated from blood cholesterol levels and lipid profile.

PANCREATITIS

Pancreatitis is an inflammatory state of the pancreas resulting in decreased amounts of pancreatic enzymes secreted.

Pancreatitis can be caused by gallbladder diseases, mumps, tumors, or bacterial infections, but it is usually related to excessive use of alcohol. Pancreatitis can be acute or chronic (long-term pancreatic insufficiency). Acute pancreatitis may or may not progress to chronic pancreatitis.

Blocked pancreatic enzymes somehow become activated and begin to digest pancreatic cells. This enzyme autodigestion may be limited to a small area or may be generalized throughout the gland.

Pancreatic enzymes are essential for the digestion of all nutrient constituents of foods. Their secretion is stimulated by foodstuffs in the duodenum. In addition to the nonfunctional GI tract to absorb needed nutrients, the body is hypermetabolic (Sax, 1987).

Pancreatitis can result in the following problems:

1. Fluid and electrolyte imbalances, particularly hypocalcemia and dehydration.
2. Impaired acid–base balance, particularly hypochloremic (decreased chloride) alkalosis.
3. Malabsorption of nutrients, especially fats and fat-soluble vitamins and vitamin B_{12}. Digestion is impaired depending on the availability of pancreatic secretions. Steatorrhea increases calcium excretion.
4. Impaired utilization of nutrients.
5. Impaired growth, healing, and resistance.

Describe the causes of pancreatitis. What regulates the secretion of pancreatic enzymes? Name 3 problems resulting from pancreatitis.

Insulin-dependent diabetes mellitus is also present when the islets of Langerhans are destroyed.

Methods of Therapy

Primary objectives of care are to rest the pancreas by minimizing pancreatic secretions, yet provide "optimal" nutritional support and fluid–electrolyte balance. Pancreatic enzymes are secreted in response to any oral intake, even water. To rest the organ, alimentary feedings may be withheld for a time or the types of foods modified, depending on the severity of the condition.

In addition to antacids and anticholinergic medications used, enzyme replacements (Pancreatin, Pancrease) provide symptomatic and nutritional benefits to clients with chronic pancreatitis. These enzymes are contained in the core of enteric-coated tablets or in the form of acid-resistant granules so they will not be hydrolyzed by the gastric acid. They should be swallowed whole; the protective coating is destroyed if the medication is crushed or given with hot foods or liquids.

What are some methods used to rest the pancreas?

Nutritional Care

Proper nutrition support is essential and often difficult. During acute pancreatitis, IV feedings are given to rest the GI tract and provide some form of nutrition support. Rehydration should be closely monitored as well as repletion of sodium, potassium, and calcium lost from vomiting and steatorrhea. This period usually lasts for 2 or 3 days and may also include the use of NG suction and anticholinergics. In severe protracted pancreatitis or pancreatic abscess, nutrition support in the form of TPN may be implemented to prevent nutritional depletion. TPN is recommended within 1 week of onset of the attack if an oral diet is not considered imminent (McMahon, 1988). The implementation of TPN within 72 hours of onset of severe acute pancreatitis results in fewer complications and deaths (Kalfarentzos et al, 1991; Robin et al, 1990).

Oral feedings may be instituted when the client is able to do so without pain or discomfort. Anytime the GI tract is used, the pancreas is stimulated to some degree (McMahon, 1988). A gradual transition beginning with fat-free clear liquids is implemented to determine tolerance. This is followed with full liquids then low-fat solid foods.

Elemental formulas can be used. The use of hydrolyzed or "predigested" nutrients causes less stimulation of secretions than regular or full liquid diets (Koruda & Feurer, 1989). The principal value of elemental feedings is to enhance absorption of nutrients while pancreatic enzyme secretion is low. Elemental formulas are especially advantageous when nutritional status is poor.

Because of limited pancreatic secretions, digestion of fat may be impaired. For chronic pancreatic insufficiency, limited amounts of dietary fat (40 to 50 gm) are usually sufficient to prevent symptoms of steatorrhea. MCT oils are recommended to increase the kilocaloric level, relieve steatorrhea, and help restore weight. The level of fat is gradually increased to promote weight gain and absorption of fat-soluble vitamins until the client's limit is reached, as indicated by steatorrhea.

A high-fiber diet may be contraindicated in clients with pancreatic insufficiency on pancreatic enzyme therapy. Steatorrhea may be caused by a reduction in the enzyme activity by the dietary fiber.

Most clients with acute pancreatitis exhibit an impaired glucose tolerance. This is controlled with a carbohydrate-restricted diet similar to diabetic management (see Chapter 27).

Sample Menu

Breakfast
1 banana
1 cup bran flakes
1 cup low-fat fruit-flavored yogurt
1 cup skim, protein-fortified milk
coffee with non-dairy creamer and sugar

Mid-morning snack
6 oz pineapple juice
1 slice whole wheat toast
1 tsp margarine
1 packet jelly

Lunch
3 oz baked codfish
1/2 cup mashed potatoes
1/2 cup cooked carrots
1 slice whole wheat bread
1 tsp margarine
1 baked apple
1 cup protein-fortified skim milk
tea

Mid-afternoon snack
2 pear halves
1/4 cup grated low-fat cheese
4 low-sodium crackers

Dinner
3 oz beef cubes
1/2 cup cooked noodles
1/2 cooked summer squash
1 slice whole wheat bread
1 tsp margarine
1/2 cup baked custard with 1/4 cup blueberry sauce
tea

Evening snack
1 cup sherbet
4 oz grape juice

Nutrient	RDA: Male–25 to 50 years	Actual	% RDA
Kcal		2628 kcal	91
Protein		121 gm	192
Carbohydrate		445 gm	123
Fat		52 gm	54
Fiber–dietary		46 gm	157
Vitamin A		3075 RE	308
Thiamin		1.9 mg	124
Riboflavin		3.3 mg	195
Niacin		22 mg	115
Vitamin B_6		3.4 mg	169
Folate		415 mcg	208
Vitamin B_{12}		8.7 mcg	437
Pantothenic acid		6.4 mg	116
Vitamin C		84 mg	139
Vitamin D		9.7 mcg	195
Vitamin K		110 mcg	138
Sodium		2288 mg	95
Potassium		4942 mg	247
Calcium		1566 mg	196
Phosphorus		2018 mg	252
Magnesium		510 mg	146
Iron		36 mg	361
Zinc		20 mg	130
Copper		2.2 mg	96
Manganese		6.4 mg	183
Selenium		0.2 mg	220
	^0 ^50 ^100 ^150 ^200		

Carbohydrate, Protein, and Fat Distribution

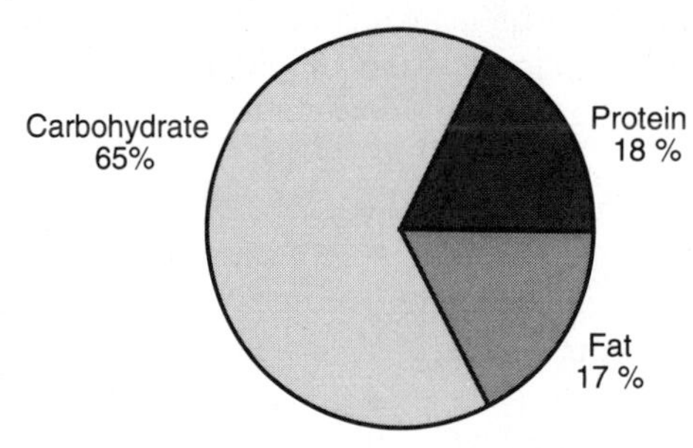

Figure 26–4 High-carbohydrate, high-protein, low-fat diet. (Nutrient data from Nutritionist III, version 7.0 software. N-Squared Computing, Salem, OR.)

As the client improves, a bland, low-fat diet with 6 feedings a day is instituted. A high-protein (120 gm), high-carbohydrate (450 gm), low-fat (50 gm) diet is used for chronic pancreatitis (Fig. 26–4). Clients are usually anorectic and nauseous; efforts should be made to provide foods that the client prefers and can tolerate.

NURSING APPLICATIONS

Assessment

Physical—for nausea, vomiting, diarrhea, steatorrhea, dehydration, abdominal pain (left upper quadrant) exacerbated by food intake, fever, edema, weight loss.

Dietary—for alcohol and fat consumption, adequacy of nutrient intake, frequency of meals/feedings.

Laboratory—for increased serum and urine amylase, serum lipase; Hgb and Hct, WBC, vitamin B_{12} levels; glucose; decreased serum calcium, magnesium, sodium, chloride, potassium; ABGs; BUN; hyperlipidemia, elevated alkaline phosphatase and LDH; hyperglycemia; depressed albumin, transferrin; PT.

Interventions

1. Monitor for deficiencies of fat-soluble vitamins and vitamin B_{12}, calcium, magnesium, zinc, and trace elements.
2. Monitor I&O.
3. For clients receiving TPN, monitor physical and laboratory values closely to identify renal or hepatic complications promptly or fluid or electrolyte imbalances that may occur.
4. After oral feedings are initiated, observe the client's response. If nausea, vomiting, or abdominal distention occurs, notify the physician.
5. Refer to the dietitian.
6. If steatorrhea is present, provide water-miscible form of fat-soluble vitamins.

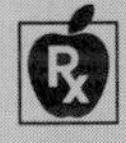
Provide pancreatic enzymes immediately before or just after the start of a meal.

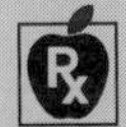
Provide antacids ½ hour before meals to reduce gastric acid secretion (gastric acid inactivates enzymes) and decrease pancreatic stimulation.

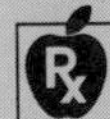
Provide anticholinergics as ordered before meals to reduce pancreatic secretions. These enhance the effects of antacids by allowing them to remain in the stomach longer.

Evaluation

* Desired outcomes include the client can explain dietary restrictions and choose appropriate food from the menu, weight appropriate for height, diminished or no steatorrhea, and attendance at AA meetings.

Client Education

- Completely eliminate alcohol intake.
- Enzyme replacements are the primary treatment for steatorrhea; a low-fat diet may bring additional benefits. Fiber intake should be moderate.
- Teach clients what a well-balanced diet consists of (appropriate number of servings from the food groups) to ensure adequate amounts of vitamins, minerals, and trace elements.
- Discuss foods that are high in carbohydrate and fat.
- The client must understand the diet and its importance to comply with it at home and to prevent future attacks.
- Large meals are to be avoided; small feedings low in fat are needed.
- Gastric stimulants, including coffee, tea, spices, and condiments, should be avoided.
- Although the cause is not known, vitamin B_{12} is not absorbed in clients with pancreatitis and must be given parenterally.
- Refer to AA or other alcohol/drug abuse programs, if appropriate.

CYSTIC FIBROSIS

Causes and Physical Consequences

CF affects the exocrine glands, interfering with normal pulmonary and pancreatic function.

Cystic fibrosis (CF) is the most common fatal autosomal recessive disease in the white population, affecting approximately 1 in 2000 white infants (Bines & Israel, 1991). The average life span for a CF client is approximately 24 years (Naccarato & Kresevic, 1989).

Viscous pancreatic secretions may obstruct the pancreatic and bile ducts. The condition is characterized by recurrent respiratory infections, excessive losses of sodium and chloride in the sweat, and usually (but not always) pancreatic insufficiency and GI malabsorption. Treatment involves controlling respiratory symptoms and infections (asthma-like attacks, recurrent pneumonia, and sinusitis) and maintaining nutritional status. Most adults with CF develop pancreatic insufficiency secondary to obstruction of the islets of Langerhans by pancreatic fibrosis. Clients with end stage CF may be candidates for lung transplantation.

What organs are affected in CF?

Nutritional Care

Malnutrition occurs frequently during infancy and childhood when nutritional demands are great because of increased growth rates. Deficits of body fat and muscle mass implicate chronic catabolic stress. The degree of malabsorption affects the nutritional requirement and severity of nutritional deficiencies. Good nutritional status enables clients to combat pulmonary infection better. Additionally, when clients are infection free, they have a better appetite and are able to consume increased amounts to compensate for malabsorption. However, there is no evidence of improved pulmonary function by nutritional care.

Almost all nutrients are affected by CF, including the energy requirement; protein; fat (and essential fatty acids); fat-soluble vitamins; and sodium, calcium, iron, zinc, and selenium. The use of pancreatic enzyme supplements with each meal (see the section on pancreatitis) enhances the intestinal absorption of fat and protein. These enzyme supplements have permitted the liberalization of dietary recommendations.

Routine monitoring of nutritional status and the amount of energy absorbed is recommended. Total energy requirement for CF may be more than the RDAs for the age group and sex because (1) malabsorption results in energy nutrients not being absorbed, (2) labored breathing requires extra energy, and (3) frequent infections and fever increase basal metabolic rate (Dodge, 1988; Goodchild, 1987). Intake is compromised because of fatigue from breathing, chest physical therapy, and chronic coughing, which leads to anorexia and vomiting.

Protein requirement is high; 15 to 20% of the total daily energy intake should be furnished by protein. Protein deficiencies in CF are frequently seen during the first year of life and early childhood, as reflected by a stunted growth rate. Hypoalbuminemia is observed more commonly in breast-fed than in formula-fed infants. Breast-fed infants who do not grow at an appropriate rate may need supplements to increase kilocalories provided, but this is not essential for all CF infants (Holliday et al, 1991). Infants with failure to thrive usually do well on casein hydrolysates (predigested peptides and amino acids). Stunted growth can be corrected by treatment with oral pancreatic enzyme supplements, multiple vitamin supplements, and additional vitamin E (Sokol et al, 1989). For many growing children, the use of powdered or liquid nutrition supplements is important for continued growth and nutritional status.

Simple sugars (monosaccharides and disaccharides) are better tolerated than complex starches, which may cause flatulence. When insulin is used to control glucose levels, the intake of simple sugars needs to be regulated.

Because of the importance of fat in improving the palatability of the diet and providing kilocalories and essential fatty acids, the fat content should be as high as the client can tolerate without discomfort from abdominal cramps. As much as 40 to 50% of the total kilocalories may be provided by fats. MCTs are better absorbed and can be used to decrease the characteristic steatorrhea. They are most appropriately used as a dietary additive or partial replacement of long-chain fatty acids. Even with use of pancreatic enzymes, many clients continue to have steatorrhea. Taurine, a conditionally essential amino acid that is involved in fat digestion, has been used in CF clients to lessen steatorrhea (Smith et al, 1991). To prevent fatty acid deficiency, an absorbable form of linoleic acid should be supplied.

Fat-soluble vitamins are of concern because of fat malabsorption. Water-miscible forms of these vitamins are better absorbed. Vitamin A deficiencies have been observed, and 2000 IU of a water-soluble preparation is recommended. Bone demineralization is seen frequently, but no additional supplementation of vitamin D over the 400 IU present in a multivitamin supplement is recommended. Water-soluble vitamin E supplements should contain 50 IU/day for infants or 200 IU/day for adults. Although vitamin K deficiency is not a common problem, a daily dose of 50 to 100 mcg or 2.5 to 5 mg/week is recommended.

Calcium intake is especially important; because many clients with CF are lactase-deficient, calcium supplements are necessary. Lactose-free polymeric formulas containing MCT oil or lactose-free milk products can be used for supplementation or during an acute phase of the disease.

The sodium content of sweat is abnormally high; salt depletion is a risk. Although clients with CF need 2 to 4 times the amount of sodium required normally, sodium supplements are unnecessary unless environmental conditions precipitate profuse sweating (exercise or fever) for extended periods. In this case, salt tablets are recommended rather than overly salted foods because they can be better monitored, are more acceptable for the client, and are less influenced by daily fluctuations in food choices.

Aggressive nutrition support using other feeding methods may be necessary for CF clients with low body weight and impaired growth. Polymeric formulas may be effective in improving nutritional status if pancreatic enzymes are given. Elemental formulas may improve nutritional status, but palatability affects acceptance. These have been provided enterally at night, allowing the client to eat regularly during the daytime. The nocturnal use of elemental formulas has resulted in dramatic weight gains (Huang et al, 1988).

In general, the diet should be high in protein and energy, with the fat content as high as tolerated to improve growth rate and prognosis. Supplementation of all vitamins is needed; a daily multivitamin supplement is advised.

Foods high in fat or containing concentrated carbohydrates and heavily spiced foods may cause distress. Clients should be encouraged to eat slowly. Small, frequent feedings are better tolerated.

Why is nutritional status affected in CF clients? What are the requirements for energy, protein, carbohydrate, fats, vitamin, calcium, and sodium in CF clients?

NURSING APPLICATIONS

Assessment

Physical—for weight, serial weights (plot on growth chart), poor weight gain (in infants and children), TSF, MAMC, frequent, bulky, foul-smelling greasy bowel movements, repeated vomiting, frequent infections, psychological state, especially rebellion.

Continued

Dietary—for actual intake of kilocalories, carbohydrate, protein, and fat using a 3- to 5-day dietary record.
Laboratory—for fecal fat; decreased serum albumin; sodium, potassium, chloride, magnesium, carotene; triglycerides, cholesterol; iron, Hgb, CBC with differential, sweat test, 3-day fat balance study.

Interventions

1. Refer to a dietitian with special interest and training in the care of clients with CF.
2. Provide adequate kilocalories based on degree of pulmonary involvement and GI complications.
3. Provide pancreatic enzymes to infants mixed in applesauce or banana before feedings.
4. Introduce new foods gradually; observe the client for any distress.
5. Omit any food that causes distress.
6. Include dietary counseling in one of the initial teaching sessions (Huang et al, 1988).
7. If client's weight to height ratio falls between 85 and 90% of ideal or rate of weight gain declines, refer to the dietitian (Ramsey et al, 1992).

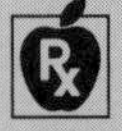 Provide riboflavin supplements when CF clients are given chloramphenicol to prevent cheilosis (Huang et al, 1988).

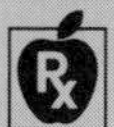 During antibiotic therapy, be sure clients are receiving vitamin B complex and vitamin C and K supplements.

Evaluation

* A high kilocalorie, high protein diet is consumed.

Client Education

- Required nutrient intake for children with CF is frequently more than that for normal children, depending on activity level.
- Although appetites are perceived as voracious, assessments show that actual intake is only 80 to 90% of the RDA (Luder, 1991).
- Explain the rationale for and administration of pancreatic enzymes. Explain that enzymes should be taken anytime food is consumed, not just at mealtime. Enzymes are needed with all types of milk products, including predigested formulas and breast milk.
- Supplementation of the diet with pancreatic enzyme preparation partly corrects the deficiency. Generic enzymes are frequently not biologically equivalent to brand name products (Hendeles et al, 1990).
- Advise clients to use corn or soy oil in their diets daily to prevent EFA deficiency.
- Cholesterol levels in these clients are normally low; clients are encouraged to eat eggs for their protein content.
- The nutritional status of clients with CF can be improved (as evidenced by increased body fat) by nutrition counseling at frequent intervals (not just at the time of diagnosis) (Luder & Gilbride, 1989).
- It is extremely important that all CF clients adhere to recommended levels of intake all of their life.
- Assist the parent in planning a specific schedule regarding meals and snacks and the kinds of foods and beverages to include. (Anticipatory guidance is important for an awareness of potential trouble areas) (Huang et al, 1988).
- Discuss the detrimental effects of allowing high sugar containing beverages such as carbonated beverages in place of nutrient-dense liquids such as whole milk, milkshakes, or nutritional supplements.

- Instruct parents to add ¼ to 1 tsp salt to infant formula or foods since the salt content of baby foods has been reduced; breast-fed infants also require additional amounts of salt, especially during summer months (Ramsey et al, 1992).
- For children and young people, additional salt (1 to 2 gm) is needed to offset losses through perspiration during summer months.
- Dietary restrictions make the child feel different; keep dietary manipulations to a minimum by using enzyme preparations.
- Adequate nutrition support should be provided during and after each episode of pulmonary disease, which adversely affects protein-energy balance.
- Encourage liberal fluid intake to prevent dehydration and help liquefy secretions.
- Refer to cystic fibrosis resources and social workers.

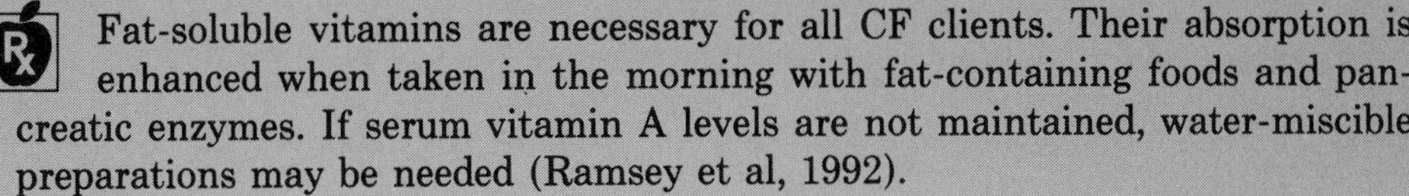

Fat-soluble vitamins are necessary for all CF clients. Their absorption is enhanced when taken in the morning with fat-containing foods and pancreatic enzymes. If serum vitamin A levels are not maintained, water-miscible preparations may be needed (Ramsey et al, 1992).

SUMMARY

The accessory GI organs—the liver, gallbladder, and pancreas—all have special functions affecting digestion and absorption of foods. When they are unable to function properly, malabsorption results, negatively affecting nutritional status. In most cases, nutritional care is imperative to restore health; it is not a cure for the disease.

When the liver is diseased, protein is crucial for its healing. However, since protein can frequently worsen a severe condition, the amount of protein allowed depends on the amount of damage to the liver (as measured by various laboratory tests).

Nutritional care for clients with gallbladder disease may involve control of total dietary fat to minimize discomfort. Diseases affecting the pancreas, including pancreatitis and cystic fibrosis, affect the digestion and absorption of all nutrients because of pancreatic insufficiency. The use of pancreatic enzyme replacements may be encouraged to improve absorption and increase intake. Large amounts of all nutrients are required.

NURSING PROCESS IN ACTION

A client is admitted to the hospital with a diagnosis of Laennec's cirrhosis. Ascites and steatorrhea are present. He drinks 15 cups of coffee and smokes 2 packs of cigarettes a day. He admits he does not eat well but states he does not feel hungry. A 1-gm sodium diet is ordered with a multivitamin supplement.

Nutritional Assessment

- Dyspepsia, delirium tremens, nausea, vomiting, abdominal girth, weight, height, portal hypertension.
- Kilocaloric need, diet ordered, supplements used, food and fluid intake.
- Alcohol, caffeine, sodium, and nicotine consumption, time of last alcohol consumption.

- Use/abuse of prescription or street drugs.
- Psychological status.
- ALT (SGPT), AST (SGOT), LDH, protein, albumin, ammonia level.

Dietary Nursing Diagnosis

Altered nutrition: Less than body requirements RT anorexia, intake of alcohol rather than nutrients and impaired absorption of vitamins.

Nutritional Goals

Client will consume a high-energy, normal to high protein, normal fat, and vitamin-enriched diet.

Client will gain dry body weight appropriate for height.

Client will state foods he is allowed to consume.

Nutritional Implementation 

Intervention: Provide 2000 to 3000 kcal daily.

Rationale: This provides the needed energy for the elevated metabolic rate.

Intervention: Calculate the amount of protein needed (provide 1 to 1.5 gm/kg daily).

Rationale: Protein intake must be adequate to prevent nitrogen wasting and help liver cells regenerate but not too much since further degeneration of the liver is possible.

Intervention: (1) Encourage low-fat diet (about 50 gm). (2) Offer eggs and some milk. (3) Provide MCT oil as ordered.

Rationale: (1) Since client has steatorrhea, fat must be restricted. (2) Because alcoholism causes an alteration in bile salt metabolism, foods that decrease the demand for bile (eggs, milk) are better tolerated. (3) These supply necessary kilocalories without further liver damage.

Intervention: Provide 6 small feedings daily with the largest meal at breakfast.

Rationale: This increases total intake by applying less pressure to an already pressured (ascites) area. Appetite is usually best with less nausea in the morning.

Intervention: (1) Offer Lonalac, low-sodium breads; avoid foods with high sodium content. (2) Make sure fluids are less than 2000 ml/day.

Rationale: (1) This follows the 1-gm sodium order and helps reduce ascites by retarding fluid retention since water follows sodium. (2) Unless fluid intake is restricted, severe symptomatic hyponatremia may occur.

Intervention: Allow client to rest before meals.

Rationale: Fatigue can enhance the anorexia experienced.

Intervention: Monitor abdominal girth and weight.

Rationale: An increase in abdominal girth reflects worsening of ascites. Conversely, a decrease in abdominal girth means the ascites is lessening. Weight provides an indication of fluid balance: An increase means ascites is worsening; a decrease means ascites is lessening. Client should lose 0.5 to 1 kg/day until ascites is no longer present.

Intervention: Monitor I&O.

Rationale: Sodium and fluid restriction may precede oliguria, which may not be noticed unless I&O is performed.

Intervention: (1) Monitor for Wernicke-Korsakoff syndrome. (2) Offer legumes, beans, oranges, lean pork, and enriched grain products.
Rationale: (1) Thiamin deficiency in alcoholics is common because of inadequate consumption and malabsorption. (2) These foods are high in thiamin.

Intervention: Monitor for bleeding.
Rationale: Increased portal pressure causes enlargement and dilatation of the collateral circulatory blood vessels called esophageal varices. These are prone to rupture and bleed.

Intervention: Monitor for impending coma.
Rationale: Further dietary restrictions are warranted if this condition occurs.

Intervention: Discourage the use of coffee and cigarettes but do not remove completely.
Rationale: This is how the client copes. Since 1 method of coping has been removed (alcohol), it would be unrealistic to remove all coping mechanisms.

Intervention: Teach to avoid salt substitutes that contain ammonia chloride.
Rationale: These amplify the high ammonia levels caused by the liver disease.

Intervention: Teach about hazards of nutrition-related problems, i.e., dieting, supplements.
Rationale: The additional pounds are due to the ascites; when the ascites improves, weight will decrease. Supplements of methionine, choline, and liver extract do not have any special benefits and may be dangerous because of the additional nitrogen load. Hypervitaminosis may occur if too many vitamin supplements are taken.

Intervention: Refer to dietitian, AA, and social worker.
Rationale: Expert knowledge is needed to handle this chronic disease. This also treats the client holistically.

Evaluation

If client consumed 75 to 100% of ordered diet, gained dry body weight, and verbalized appropriate low-sodium foods allowed on his diet, goals were achieved. Additionally, if he avoids salt substitutes with ammonia, states he will not buy OTC nutritional preparations (especially proteins and vitamins), does not experience hepatic coma or Wernicke-Korsakoff syndrome, and attends AA meetings, nursing care was excellent.

STUDENT READINESS

1. Why is protein important in liver disease? Discuss the different amounts of protein recommended for initial treatment of hepatitis, cirrhosis, and encephalopathy. Discuss the reasons for the different levels.
2. A client with liver disease wants to know why branched-chain amino acids are beneficial. What would you say?
3. When is sodium restriction necessary for liver disease?
4. Why might a client with gallbladder disease choose to eliminate potato chips, mayonnaise, and pecan pie from his diet?
5. Why would an elemental diet be better tolerated than a bland diet by a client with pancreatitis?
6. Plan a menu for a 7-year-old school child with cystic fibrosis who carries her lunch to school. She weighs 18.1 kg and should have at least 3000 kcal, 50 gm of protein, and 50 gm of fat.

Case Study

Three weeks following ingestion of contaminated oysters, Mr. C. M., a 26-year-old accountant, showed signs of hepatitis A. At the physician's office, he complains of weight loss, right upper abdominal quadrant tenderness, anorexia, nausea, and a loss of taste for cigarettes. His skin and sclerae are slightly jaundiced. After his admission, he is placed on a high-kilocalorie, high-protein diet with vitamin supplements.

1. Why is a high-kilocalorie, high-protein diet indicated for this client?
2. What precautions must be observed in caring for this client, particularly concerning food left on his tray?
3. What alterations should be made in meal times and the quantity of food served at each meal?
4. Is a soft diet indicated for this client?
5. List a nursing diagnosis and goal for this client.

Case Study

Dr. B. D. has consumed an increasing amount of alcohol over the past 5 years. Staff members have noted his decreasing ability to function in the office. Over the past 2 months, they have also noted discoloration of the skin and sclerae, increasing size of his abdomen, and ankle edema. On his admission to the hospital, tests reveal serum albumin, 2.5 gm/dl; prothrombin time, 25 seconds; and elevated serum ammonia. He is confused, irritable, and uncoordinated. He is placed on a soft diet of 20 gm of protein and 1000 mg of sodium.

1. Why is the protein restriction deemed necessary at this time?
2. What is the physiological basis for the sodium restriction?
3. In planning Dr. B. D.'s care, prepare a meal plan for the protein and sodium restrictions.
4. Are vitamin supplements indicated for this client?
5. Why is magnesium an important electrolyte for the client with alcoholic cirrhosis?
6. Why is a soft diet often indicated for this type of client?
7. What should the nurse teach this client?

REFERENCES

American Dietetic Association (ADA). *Manual of Clinical Dietetics.* Chicago, American Dietetic Association, 1988.

Bines, JE, Israel EJ. Hypoproteinemia, anemia, and failure to thrive in an infant. *Gastroenterology* 1991 Sept; 101(3):848–856.

Bruckstein AH. Management of the patient with ascites. *Postgrad Med* 1987 Oct; 82(5):277–283;286.

Cabre E, et al. Effect of total enteral nutrition on the short-term outcome of severely malnourished cirrhotics. *Gastroenterology* 1990 March; 98(3):715–720.

Cerrato P. When your patient has liver disease. *RN* 1992 March; 55(3):77–80.

Dodge J. Nutritional requirements in cystic fibrosis. A review. *J Pediatr Gastroenterol Nutr* 1988; 7(suppl 1):S8–S11.

Fischer JE. Branched-chain-enriched amino acid solutions in patients with liver failure: An early example of nutritional pharmacology. *JPEN* 1990 Sept-Oct; 14(5 suppl):249S-256S.

Goodchild M. Nutritional management of cystic fibrosis. *Digestion* 1987; 37(suppl 1):61–67.

Green JH, et al. Are patients with primary biliary cirrhosis hypermetabolic? A comparison between patients before and after liver transplantation and controls. *Hepatology* 1991 Sept; 14(3):464–472.

Hasse J. Role of the dietitian in the nutrition management of adults after liver transplantation. *J Am Diet Assoc* 1991 Apr; 91(4):473–476.

Hasse JM. Nutritional implications of liver transplantation. *Henry Ford Hosp Med J* 1990; 38(4):235–240.

Hendeles L, et al. Treatment failure after substitution of generic pancrelipase capsules. *JAMA* 1990 May 9; 263(18):2459–2461.

Holliday KE, et al. Growth of human milk-fed and formula-fed infants with cystic fibrosis. *J Pediatr* 1991 Jan; 118(1):77–79.

Huang NN, et al. Cystic fibrosis. *In* Kinney J, et al, eds. *Nutrition and Metabolism in Patient Care.* Philadelphia, WB Saunders, 1988: 405–428.

Kalfarentzos FE, et al. Total parenteral nutrition in severe acute pancreatitis. *J Am Coll Nutr* 1991 Apr; 10(2):156–162.

Kearns PJ, et al. Accelerated improvement of alcoholic liver disease with enteral nutrition. *Gastroenterology* 1992 Jan; 102(1):200–205.

Koruda MJ, Feurer ID. Pancreatic fistulas. *In* Blackburn GL, et al, eds. *Nutritional Medicine: A Case Management Approach.* Philadelphia, WB Saunders, 1989: 39–43.

Lee SP. Diseases of the liver and biliary tract. *In* Kinney JM, et al, eds. *Nutrition and Metabolism in Patient Care.* Philadelphia, WB Saunders, 1988: 313–341.

Luder E. Nutrition care of patients with cystic fibrosis. *Topics Clin Nutr* 1991 March; 6(3):39–50.

Luder E, Gilbride JA. Teaching self-management skills to cystic fibrosis patients and its effect on their caloric intake. *J Am Diet Assoc* 1989 March; 89(3):259–264.

Maclure KM, et al. Dietary predictory of symptom-associated gallstones in middle-aged women. *Am J Clin Nutr* 1990 Nov; 52(5):916–922.

MacDonald I. Carbohydrates: General. *In* Shils ME, Young VR, eds. *Modern Nutrition in Health and Disease.* 7th ed. Philadelphia, Lea & Febiger, 1988: 38–51.

Marchesini G, et al. Long-term oral branched-chain amino acid treatment in chronic hepatic encephalopathy: A randomized double-blind casein-controlled trial. *J Hepatol* 1990 July; 11(1):92–101.

Maudgal DP, Northfield TC. A practical guide to the non-surgical treatment of gallstones. *Drugs* 1991 Feb; 41(2):185–192.

McMahon MJ. Diseases of the exocrine pancreas. *In* Kinney JM, et al, eds. *Nutrition and Metabolism in Patient Care.* Philadelphia, WB Saunders, 1988: 386–404.

Naccarato M, Kresevic D. Caring for adults who have cystic fibrosis. *Am J Nurs* 1989 Nov; 89(11):1462–1465.

Paumgartner G, Sauerbruch T. Gallstones: Pathogenesis. *Lancet* 1991 Nov 2; 338(8775):1117–1121.

Ramsey BW, et al. Nutritional assessment and management in cystic fibrosis: A consensus report. *Am J Clin Nutr* 1992 Jan; 55(1):108–116.

Reilly J, et al. Nutritional support after liver transplantation: A randomized prospective study. *JPEN* 1990 July-Aug; 14(4):386–391.

Robin AP, et al. Total parenteral nutrition during acute pancreatitis: Clinical experience with 156 patients. *World J Surg* 1990 Sept-Oct; 14(5):572–579.

Sauerbruch T, Paumgartner G. Gallbladder stones: Management. *Lancet* 1991 Nov 2; 338(8775):1121–1124.

Sax HC. Pancreatitis. *In* Lang CE, ed. *Nutrition Support in Critical Care.* Rockville, MD, Aspen, 1987:15–72.

Silk DB, et al. Nutritional support in liver disease. *Gut* 1991 Sept; Suppl:S29–S33.

Skeie B, et al. Branch-chain amino acids: Their metabolism and clinical utility. *Crit Care Med* 1990 May; 18(5):549–571.

Smith SJ, et al. Taurine decreases fecal fatty acid and sterol excretion in cystic fibrosis. A randomized double blind trial. *Am J Dis Child* 1991 Dec; 145(12):1401–1404.

Sokol RJ, et al. Fat soluble vitamin status during the first year of life in infants with cystic fibrosis identified by screening of newborns. *Am J Clin Nutr* 1989 Nov; 50(5):1064–1071.

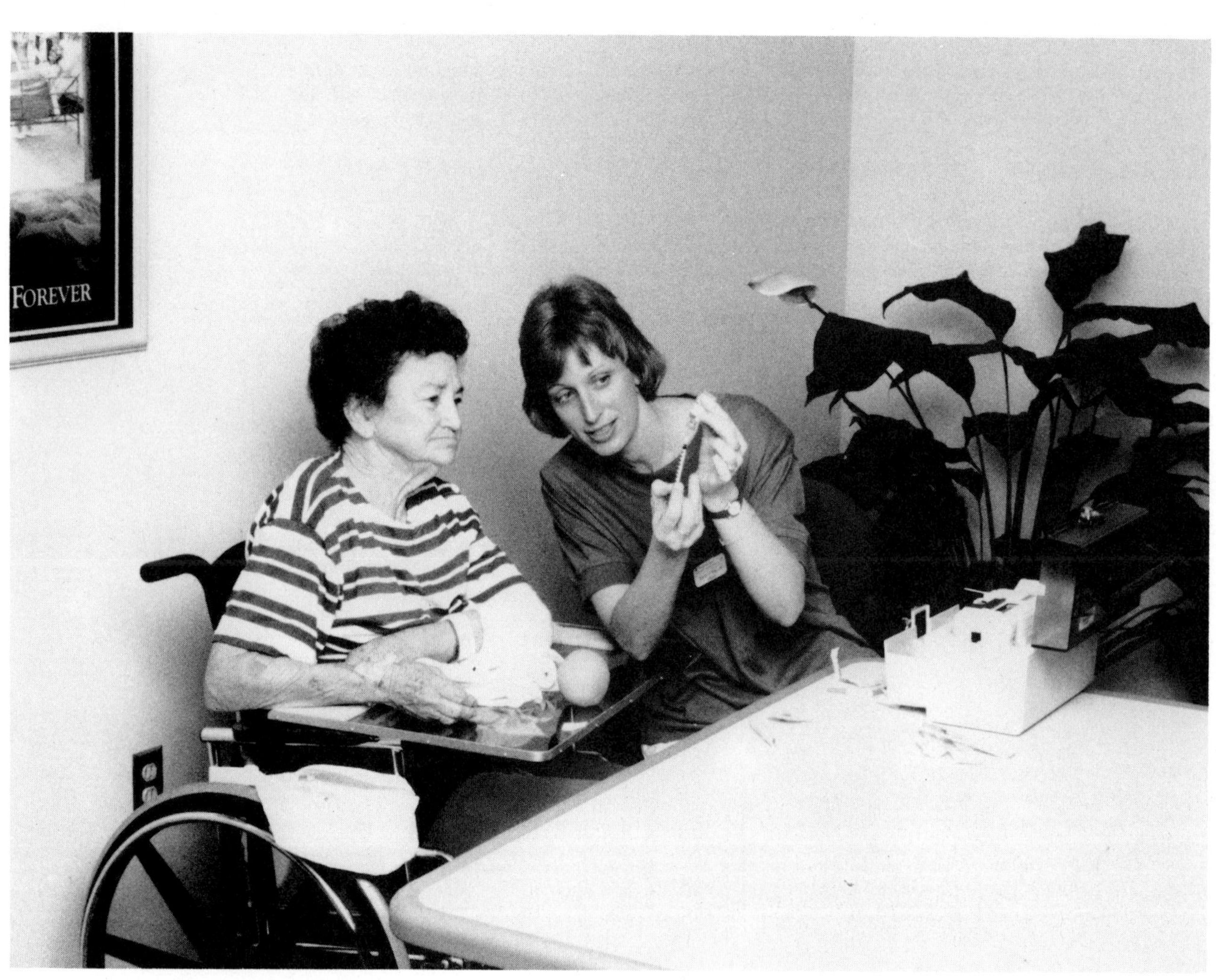
FOREVER

CHAPTER 27

Dietary Management of Diabetes Mellitus

OUTLINE

VIII. SPECIAL CONSIDERATIONS IN INSULIN-DEPENDENT DIABETES MELLITUS
   A. Insulin
   B. Exercise
   C. Nutritional Care
   Nursing Applications
IX. SPECIAL CONSIDERATIONS OF NONINSULIN-DEPENDENT DIABETES MELLITUS
   A. Oral Hypoglycemic Agents
   B. Exercise
   C. Nutritional Care
      1. Very-Low-Calorie Diet
   Nursing Applications
X. SPECIAL CONSIDERATIONS FOR ILLNESS OR SURGERY
   Nursing Applications
XI. SPECIAL CONSIDERATIONS FOR NUTRITION SUPPORT
   Nursing Applications
XII. SPECIAL CONSIDERATIONS FOR PREGNANCY
   A. Treatment
   B. Nutritional Care
   Nursing Applications
XIII. COUNSELING FOR SELF-MANAGEMENT
   Nursing Applications

OBJECTIVES

THE STUDENT WILL BE ABLE TO:

- Plan food intake for 1 day using the exchange lists.
- Discuss the role of diet in the treatment for diabetes mellitus.
- Explain basic dietary principles of managing diabetes.
- List recommendations of the American Diabetic Association for the amount of dietary carbohydrate, protein, and fat.
- Explain the role of insulin and how the meal plan varies according to the type of insulin prescribed.
- Discuss the role of oral hypoglycemic agents and their effect on diet.
- State the causes, symptoms, and treatment for hyperglycemia and hypoglycemia.
- Discuss effects of exercise on insulin and dietary requirements.
- Plan dietary management for a diabetic who is ill, undergoing surgery, receiving nutrition support, or pregnant.
- Apply nursing application principles to all types of diabetic clients.
- Discuss client teaching tips for diabetics.

TEST YOUR NQ (True/False)

1. Insulin is a hormone that decreases blood glucose.
2. Overeating can cause hyperglycemia in diabetic clients.
3. If a diabetic client is experiencing hypoglycemia, give insulin.
4. Glycosylated hemoglobin reflects an average of blood glucose levels for 2 to 3 months.
5. Legumes and whole-grain cereals delay glucose emptying from the stomach.
6. Lower levels of protein intake are beneficial for clients with diabetic nephropathy.
7. A diabetic client needs to purchase dietetic foods.

8. IDDM clients can use oral hypoglycemics and diet for control of their condition.
9. A nutritional goal for NIDDM clients is to achieve and maintain IBW.
10. A pregnant diabetic client should consume at least 200 gm carbohydrate.

Diabetes mellitus (DM) is a heterogeneous group of endocrine diseases in which carbohydrates are ineffectively metabolized, leading to disturbances in lipid and protein metabolism. Progress toward identifying the cause of the disease with its many complications has greatly increased our understanding of body metabolism. Although much progress has been made, it is a complex condition about which there is much more to learn.

This condition is specifically related to hormonal pancreatic secretions but also involves the entire endocrine system. The main manifestation of diabetes mellitus is **hyperglycemia.** However, glucose homeostasis involves a complex network of many **hormones,** as shown in Table 27-1.

Hyperglycemia—elevated blood glucose.

Hormones are "messengers" produced by a group of cells that stimulate or retard the functions of other cells. Hormones principally control different metabolic functions that affect growth and secretions.

DM is presently one of the most common diseases. Incidence of DM is increasing worldwide, affecting 7% of US households in 1990 (Surveys, 1991). Estimates indicate that fewer than half of the cases are diagnosed. Lower-income groups have the highest incidence of DM (Surveys, 1991). In addition to metabolic complications secondary to DM, life expectancy is about 70 to 80% that of the general population (Harris & Hamman, 1985).

PHYSICAL CONSEQUENCES

Glucagon, insulin, and somatostatin are hormones produced by different types of pancreatic cells. Beta cells in the islets of Langerhans produce insulin, which transports glucose into cells and aids in converting glucose to glycogen or fat tissue. The overall effect is to decrease serum glucose. Insulin inhibits **lipolysis** and **glycolysis.**

Lipolysis is breakdown of body fat; glycolysis is breakdown of glucose.

Pancreatic alpha cells secrete another hormone, glucagon, which works in opposition to insulin. Other hormones also function to counterbalance the effects of insulin by raising blood glucose levels: epinephrine, cortisol, and growth hormone (Table 27-1). Blood glucose level increases as a result of **glucogenesis.** As such, it increases **glycemic** level. It also causes adipose tissue to release free fatty acids and glycerol that can be used for energy.

Glucogenesis—glycogen is broken down to glucose.

Glycemic level is the amount of glucose in the blood.

Normally hormonal secretions are controlled by the glycemic level. When the blood glucose level is high, insulin is secreted, which lowers blood glucose level. Insulin binds to receptors on cell membranes; glucose is transported through cell membranes at these sites. In DM, insulin is absent, deficient, or ineffective; gluca-

TABLE 27-1

ACTIONS OF HORMONES AFFECTING BLOOD GLUCOSE LEVELS

Decreases Blood Glucose	Increases Blood Glucose
Insulin	Cortisol
↑ peripheral glucose utilization	↑ gluconeogenesis (mobilizes amino acids)
↑ amino acid transport into cells	Glucagon
↑ fatty acid storage	↑ glycogenesis (mobilizes glycogen)
↓ gluconeogenesis	Growth hormone
Somatostatin	↑ gluconeogenesis (mobilizes fatty acids)
↓ glucagon secretion	Thyroxine
↓ release of growth hormone	↑ insulin degradation
↓ gastric emptying and intestinal absorption	Somatostatin
	↓ insulin secretion

Renal threshold is the concentration of a substance (i.e., glucose) in plasma at which it is excreted in the urine. Normal renal threshold for sugar is about 180 mg/dl but varies between individuals.

Glycosuria is glucose spilled in the urine; this occurs when the glucose level exceeds the kidney's ability to reabsorb glucose (renal threshold).

gon is present in excessive amounts. These problems then precipitate clinical manifestations.

Insulin deficiency results in hyperglycemia. Because glucose cannot be transported into the cell or converted into glycogen, blood glucose level rises, increasing osmotic pressure within the blood vessels and pulling fluid out of cells. This results in cellular dehydration. When blood glucose exceeds the **renal threshold,** glucose is excreted in the urine (Fig. 27–1).

Thus, hyperglycemia results in **glycosuria.** Glycosuria increases osmotic pressure of urine, which prevents water reabsorption, thereby causing **polyuria.** Along with excretion of large amounts of water, sodium (from extracellular fluid) and po-

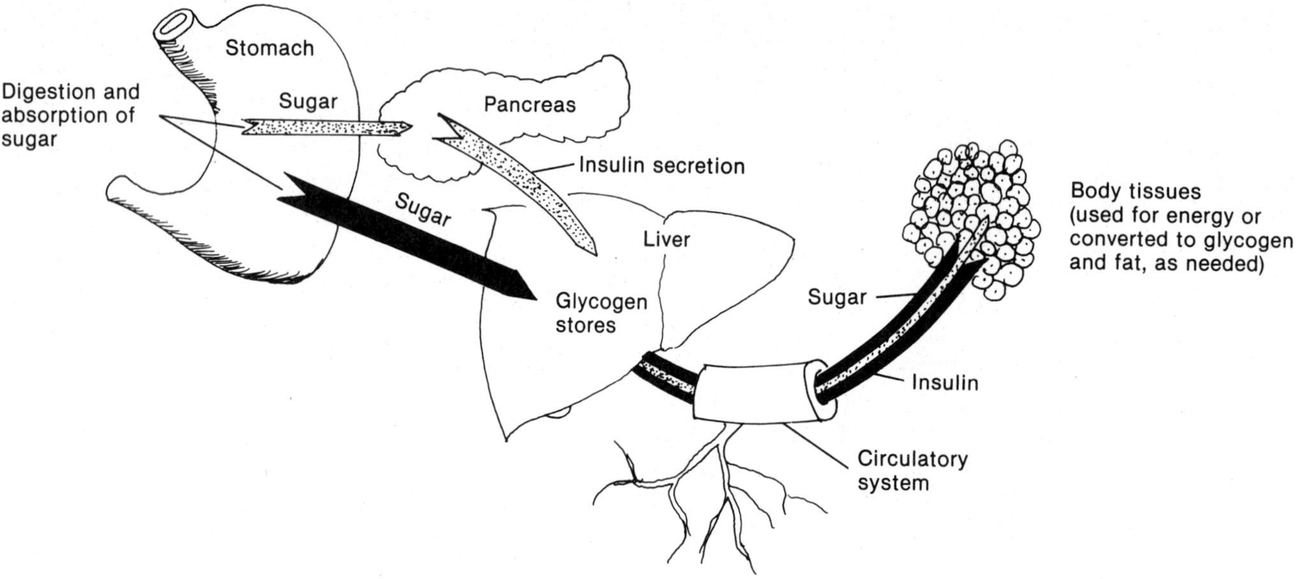

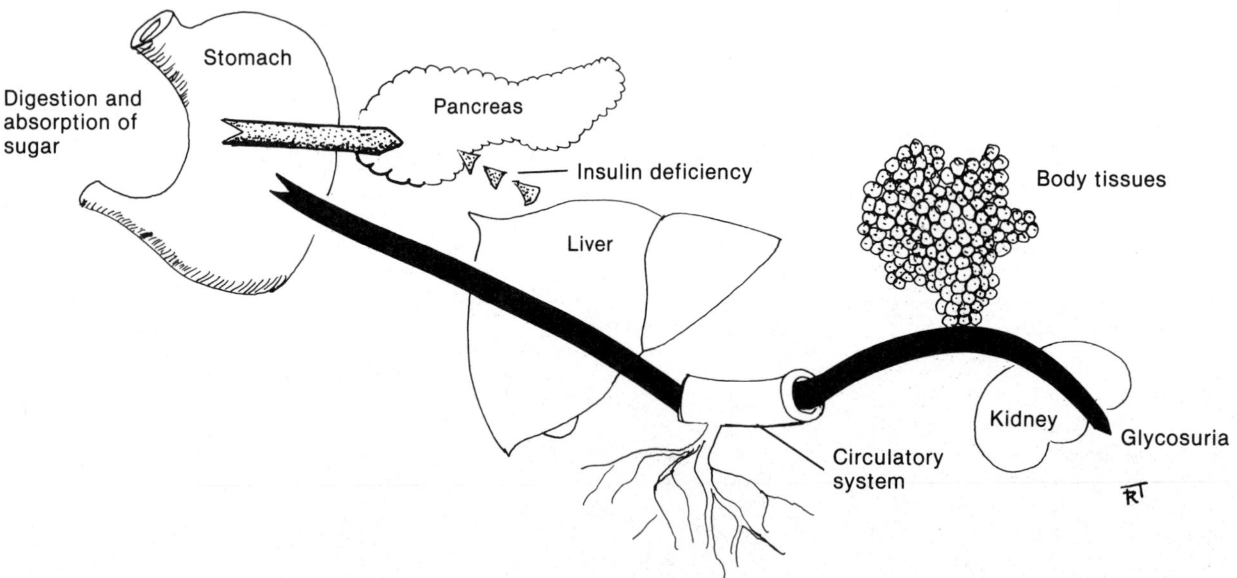

Figure 27–1 Comparison of carbohydrate utilization of the nondiabetic and diabetic client. (Adapted from What is Diabetes? Indianapolis, Eli Lilly & Co, 1975.)

tassium (from intracellular fluid) are also excreted. Polyuria results in **polydipsia,** which is symptomatic of fluid depletion.

Insulin deficiency results in **polyphagia** and **asthenia.** Because cells are unable to use available glucose, they have no energy supply. Muscle protein and adipose tissue are catabolized to supply energy needs. Muscle catabolism results in weight loss and negative nitrogen balance.

Catabolism of large amounts of fatty tissue results in **ketosis.** When excessive amounts of fatty acids are being broken down, muscles cannot use them fast enough, so they are changed into ketone bodies by the liver. The body tries to rid itself of ketones, so **ketonuria** develops. Ketonuria is accompanied by excretion of sodium and potassium. With continued accumulation of ketone bodies, **ketoacidosis** may occur. Physiological adjustments are made in an attempt to compensate for ketoacidosis: (1) Respiration rate increases to eliminate carbon dioxide, and (2) kidneys excrete excess acid. If this continues, compensatory mechanisms are overwhelmed with loss of sodium, potassium, and bicarbonate (base) ions. Consequently, the body is depleted of its reserves to neutralize acids, and blood pH decreases further, causing severe ketoacidosis. Failure to correct ketoacidosis results in **hypovolemia,** which can lead to diabetic coma and death.

Therefore, diabetes is not only an abnormality of carbohydrate metabolism, but also involves metabolism of protein, fat, and fluid and electrolyte balance.

Polyuria is excessive amounts of water excreted in the urine.

Polydipsia is increased thirst.

The "starved" state results in an increased appetite, or polyphagia. Asthenia —a lack of energy.

Ketosis is accumulation of ketone bodies. Ketone bodies or ketones are acidic substances.

Ketonuria—urinary excretion of ketone bodies.

Since ketones are acids, they disrupt acid–base balance, lowering blood pH. Thus, ketoacidosis is caused by excess accumulation of ketones in body tissues and fluids.

Hypovolemia—decreased circulating plasma.

Which cells produce insulin; glucagon? What is the principal function of insulin; glucagon? What happens in the body when insulin secretion is inadequate?

CLASSIFICATIONS

There are 2 prevalent types of DM. They are characterized by different basic metabolic defects and can appear to be very different conditions (Table 27–2).

TABLE 27–2

COMPARISON OF TYPE I AND TYPE II DIABETES

	Type II (NIDDM)	**Type I (IDDM)**
Age of onset	Frequently over 35	Most frequently during childhood or puberty
Type of onset	Usually gradual	Sudden
Family history of diabetes	Usually positive	Frequently positive
Nutritional status at time of onset	Usually obese	Frequently undernourished
Symptoms	Frequently none	Polydipsia, polyphagia, polyuria
Hepatomegaly	Uncommon	Rather common
Stability	Blood glucose fluctuations are less marked	Blood glucose fluctuates widely in response to changes in insulin, dose, exercise, and infection
Control of diabetes	Easy, especially if a diet is followed	Difficult
Ketosis	Uncommon except in the presence of unusual stress or moderate to severe sepsis	Frequent
Plasma insulin	Plasma insulin may be low, but not absent, or high	Negligible to zero
Vascular complications and degenerative changes	Frequent	Occurs after diabetes has been present for about 5 years
Diet	Diet therapy may eliminate the need for hypoglycemic agents	Required
Insulin	Used for a few clients	Necessary for all clients
Oral agents	Effective	Not suitable

Adapted from Waife SO, ed. *Diabetes Mellitus,* 8th ed. Indianapolis, Eli Lilly & Co, 1980.

TABLE 27-3

SORTING OUT THE OLD AND THE NEW

Clinical Categories *New Names*	*Old Names*	*Clinical Characteristics*
Type I: IDDM	Juvenile diabetes Juvenile-onset diabetes Ketosis-prone diabetes Brittle diabetes	Clients have little or no endogenous insulin and need injections to preserve life. New clients may be of any age but are usually young; they often have islet-cell antibodies. Scientists believe causes may be genetic, environmental, or acquired, probably involving abnormal immune responses
Type II: NIDDM	Adult-onset diabetes Maturity-onset diabetes Ketosis-resistant diabetes Stable diabetes Maturity-onset diabetes of youth	Except during infection or other stress, clients rarely develop ketosis. They vary in amount of endogenous insulin and may need injections to avoid hyperglycemia. New clients may be of any age but are usually over 40. Most are obese. NIDDM is thought to be caused by genetic susceptibility plus environmental factors
Diabetes mellitus associated with other conditions or syndromes	Secondary diabetes	This type of diabetes is accompanied by conditions known or suspected to cause the disease, including pancreatic or hormonal disease, drug or chemical toxicity, abnormal insulin receptors, or certain genetic syndromes
Impaired glucose tolerance Type a: nonobese Type b: obese	Asymptomatic diabetes Chemical diabetes Subclinical diabetes Borderline diabetes Latent diabetes	Glucose levels are between those of normal people and those of diabetics. Clients have above-normal susceptibility to atherosclerotic disease. Renal and retinal complications generally do not become clinically significant
Gestational diabetes mellitus	Gestational diabetes	This classification is retained for women whose diabetes begins or is recognized during pregnancy. They have an above-normal risk of perinatal complications. Their glucose intolerance may be transitory, but it frequently recurs

From Nemchik R. Diabetes today: A startling new body of knowledge. *RN* 1982; 45(10):31. Published in *RN*, the full-service nursing journal. Copyright© 1982, Medical Economics Company, Inc, Oradell, NJ.

Glucose intolerance and the clinical characteristics of diabetes are listed in Table 27-3.

Insulin-Dependent Diabetes Mellitus

Insulin-dependent diabetes mellitus (IDDM) is distinguished by little or no endogenous insulin production. This condition most commonly manifests itself in young people but can occur at any age. Onset is sudden with all the clinical symptoms associated with this condition. Clients are ketosis prone and must receive exogenous insulin for life.

Tight control—maintaining blood glucose levels between 70 and 180 mg/dl.

How much insulin is produced in IDDM?

About 5 to 10% of DM cases in the US are IDDM (Fig. 27-2). **"Tight control"** has been proposed as the best method of preventing or alleviating chronic complications that may develop.

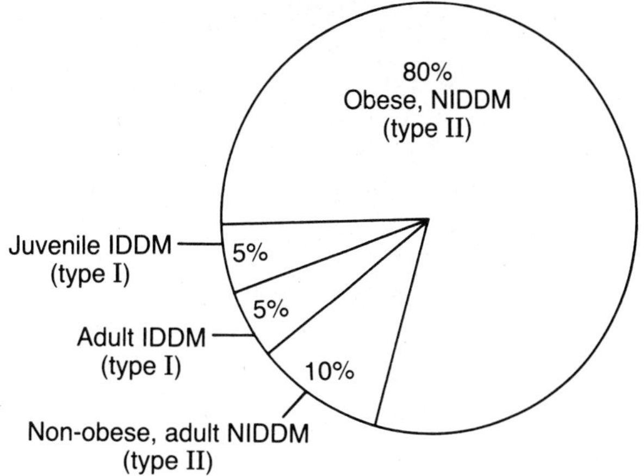

Figure 27–2 The incidence of various types of diabetes mellitus. (Data from Basic Facts About Diabetes. Indianapolis, Eli Lilly & Co, 1985.)

Noninsulin-Dependent Diabetes Mellitus

About 90% of cases of DM in the US are noninsulin-dependent diabetes mellitus (NIDDM) (see Fig. 27–2), affecting about 10 million Americans. It is diagnosed most frequently in overweight individuals over 40 years of age; only about 10% are not obese. This type of diabetes develops more slowly; clinical symptoms are mild. In most cases, clients with NIDDM are **insulin resistant.** Numbers of available cell receptors are inversely correlated with basal insulin levels. Hepatic cells do not decrease glucose production in response to hyperglycemia.

Insulin is secreted in adequate or higher than normal amounts in NIDDM; decreased numbers of cell receptors, leading to decreased uptake of glucose by all body cells (except for the brain), is called insulin resistance.

Obesity and weight gain are associated with insulin resistance. Obese individuals with upper body obesity, particularly women, are at greater risk of developing NIDDM and CHD than clients with lower body fat distribution.

Which fat distribution makes clients more susceptible to NIDDM? In general practice, will you be working with more IDDM or NIDDM clients?

NIDDM also includes diabetes that is secondary to other conditions or syndromes (pancreatitis, pancreatic resection, use of glucocorticoid medications, liver disease, and others).

ETIOLOGICAL FACTORS

Although heredity and DM are related, genetic mechanisms are poorly understood. It has been proposed that the human leukocyte antigen may transmit a predisposition for IDDM. Karjalainen et al (1992) reported that proteins in cow milk could be the key trigger of the autoimmune response that affects pancreatic beta cells in genetically susceptible clients, thus precipitating DM. Since some clients develop IDDM without exposure to cow milk, further studies are needed (Maclaren & Atkinson, 1992). Onset of IDDM is associated with viral infections and autoimmune reactions, which may result in damage to or destruction of pancreatic beta cells.

Studies have demonstrated a relationship between magnesium deficiency and insulin resistance. Hypomagnesemia has been demonstrated in both IDDM and NIDDM. Increased urinary losses secondary to urinary glycosuria may result in magnesium deficiency in DM. An American Diabetes Association Consensus Panel (1992) has concluded that magnesium deficiency may play a role in insulin resistance and carbohydrate intolerance. Assessment for hypomagnesemia is recommended, but levels should be repleted only if hypomagnesemia is demonstrated (ADA, 1992).

In NIDDM, diet may play an indirect role. Prevalence of diabetes in adults is closely related to adiposity throughout several populations. Precisely how diet contributes to diabetes other than overconsumption of energy-containing nutrients, which produces obesity, is unknown. Several conclusions have been made. High starch consumption is negatively correlated with diabetes incidence. (This does not mean that starch prevents diabetes, but that eating a diet high in complex carbohydrates does not contribute to incidence of DM.) Although sugar consumption has been suspected, epidemiological evidence has found no relationship between sugar consumption and prevalence of diabetes. Colditz et al (1992) determined BMI (>29) was a positive risk factor for diabetes, but energy, protein, sucrose, carbohydrate, or fiber intake was not associated with risk of diabetes.

Hemochromatosis is a disorder of iron metabolism with excessive deposits of iron in the liver and pancreas.

Hemochromatosis is associated with a high incidence of NIDDM. Zinc deficiency is associated with decreased glucose tolerance in rats but has not been documented as a causative factor or a consequence of diabetes in humans. Chromium supplementation improves glucose tolerance and circulating insulin and glucagon levels of hyperglycemic individuals with low chromium intake (Anderson et al, 1991). Chromium deficiency is not indicated in IDDM; clients with NIDDM should have a dietary assessment for chromium intake before arbitrarily using chromium supplements.

What are some possible causes for IDDM? Explain how diet may affect NIDDM.

NURSING APPLICATIONS

Assessment

Physical—for age, weight, height, IBW, fat distribution; polyuria, polyphagia, polydipsia, asthenia, weight changes, BP, dehydration (skin turgor, mucous membranes), stress, infections, trauma, weakness, fatigue, irritability.

Dietary—for intake of complex carbohydrate, protein, sugar, fat, iron and chromium.

Laboratory—for increased glucose, sodium, potassium; urine ketones, ABGs.

Interventions

1. Monitor I&O and blood glucose levels.
2. Monitor for blurred vision, tingling or numbness in extremities, drowsiness, slow healing time, and frequent skin infections, as these may signal NIDDM.
3. Consult with the physician if you suspect a client has DM to obtain appropriate diagnosis and treatment.
4. Monitor clients at high risk of hypomagnesemia (excessive urinary losses, decreased GI absorption or decreased dietary intake) for magnesium deficiencies.

Evaluation

* Client's predisposition to DM is identified and presented to physicians so treatment can be initiated. If diagnosed, clients should also be able to describe the type of DM they have.

Client Education

- DM causes interruptions in carbohydrate, fat, and protein metabolism.
- Explain the reasons for all the physical changes that occur.
- Insulin makes glucose available to cells; it does not metabolize glucose.
- Using Table 27–2, explain the different types of DM.
- DM is a life-long disease.
- Food and stress elevate the blood glucose, whereas insulin and activity lower glucose levels. All these aspects must be kept in balance to stabilize blood glucose.

DIABETIC COMPLICATIONS

Complications are numerous as a result of metabolic and endocrine derangements caused by diabetes. Hyperglycemia and hypoglycemia are acute complications. Hyperglycemia leading to ketoacidosis, as described earlier, occurs in undiagnosed/uncontrolled IDDM; hyperglycemia resulting in hyperosmolar nonketotic coma typically presents in NIDDM clients. Recognition of symptoms of hyperglycemia or hypoglycemia facilitates diagnosis and treatment of these life-threatening situations.

Other complications are chronic, developing slowly over long periods of time as body tissues are adversely exposed to acute complications of hyperglycemia and hypoglycemia.

Acute Complications

Hyperglycemia/Ketoacidosis

A high blood glucose level causes various signs and symptoms, as described in Table 27–4. Hyperglycemia in elderly diabetic clients is associated with cognitive impairment, which may lead to poor compliance (Morley & Perry, 1991). If hyperglycemia is untreated, ketosis, ketoacidosis, and then diabetic coma can occur (Table 27–5).

Diabetic ketoacidosis (DKA) can result in death; prevention is of key importance. DKA usually develops rapidly in juvenile diabetics, but onset is slower in adults. DKA occurs more frequently in IDDM than in NIDDM; 5 to 8% of all diabetic-related deaths are due to ketoacidosis (Fishbein, 1985).

DKA is caused by metabolic derangements (insulin deficiency relative to counterregulatory hormones) because of failure to take insulin or because of an excess of the counterregulatory hormones that occur with stress.

This type of hyperglycemia is precipitated when insulin levels are inadequate relative to glucose level. Glucose levels may be elevated from dietary intake, noncompliance, or stressful conditions (infectious diseases, trauma) in which catecholamine secretions cause an impaired glucose insulin homeostasis. Amino acids and free fatty acids are presented to the liver for gluconeogenesis and lipid metabolism. Increased hepatic glucose output results in progressive hyperglycemia that is due to the tissue's inability to use glucose. This results in glycosuria, dehydration, ketosis, and acidosis.

Describe signs and symptoms of hyperglycemia. What occurs in DKA?

Hyperglycemia/Hyperosmolar Nonketosis

The syndrome, hyperosmolar hyperglycemic nonketosis (HHNK) is more prevalent in NIDDM clients over age 60 who have CHD or renal disease. Hyperglycemia develops without ketoacidosis because clients have enough insulin present to inhibit

TABLE 27–4

HYPERGLYCEMIA: WARNING SIGNS, CAUSES, AND TREATMENT

Warning Signs	Causes	Treatment
Gradual onset	Inadequate insulin	Administer usual or increased dose of insulin
Drowsiness, weak	Overeating	Rest
Flushed, hot, dry skin	Omission of routine exercise	Keep warm
Extreme thirst	Nausea or vomiting	Force fluids
Frequent urination with large amounts of glucose	Infection	Call physician
Ketonuria	Illness	
Blurred vision	Surgery	
Irritability	Stress	
Frequent infections		
Slow-healing cuts or sores		

TABLE 27-5

DIABETIC KETOACIDOSIS: WARNING SIGNS, CAUSES, AND TREATMENT

Warning Signs	Causes
Excessive thirst	Undiagnosed IDDM
Frequent urination	Mismanagement of sick days
Sudden weight loss	Decrease/omission of insulin dose or error in the type of insulin
Nausea and vomiting	Overeating
Stomach pains	Sudden withdrawal of insulin when initiating hypoglycemic agents
Fruity odor breath (ketotic breath)	Exercise when blood glucose is >240 mg/dl
Fatigue, weakness, listlessness	Infections
Kussmaul respiration (deep labored breathing) and coma in 12-23 hours	Trauma
	Stress
	Medications (steroids, thiazide diuretics, birth control pills, antihypertensives)

Treatment

1. For confused or comatose clients, do not give food
   a. Administer insulin plus IV fluids and electrolytes
   b. Monitor blood and urine profiles every 1-2 hours
   c. Hypotension and shock secondary to dehydration may be treated with artificial plasma expanders or plasma transfusion. IV dextrose is added when blood glucose levels fall to 250 mg/dl
2. Resume oral feedings when the client is mentally alert
   a. Provide small amounts of fluids to assess nausea and vomiting.
   b. Progress to a liquid diet with milk, fruit juices, and broth to provide some glucose, potassium, and phosphate
   c. Progress slowly to a regular diabetic diet as tolerated

excessive fat mobilization and development of ketosis but not enough to prevent hyperglycemia. Dehydration develops rapidly because glucose levels may exceed 900 mg/dl. HHNK frequently may be precipitated by severe stress—pancreatitis, burns, severe infections. Other causes include large carbohydrate intake; total parenteral nutrition; decreased fluid intake; and use of steroids, diuretics, or beta blockers (Peterson & Drass, 1991; Huzar, 1989).

What causes HHNK? How is it treated?

HHNK must be treated promptly. Treatment consists of insulin to lower the blood glucose level and administration of fluids and electrolytes to correct fluid/electrolyte imbalance. Blood glucose must be lowered gradually. When glucosuria and hyperglycemia begin to drop, glucose may be added in the form of IV dextrose to prevent too rapid a drop in glycemic levels.

Dawn Phenomenon

Dawn phenomenon is early morning hyperglycemia related to diminished sensitivity to insulin.

Another complication of blood glucose control is the **dawn phenomenon.** This early AM hyperglycemia may be due to a surge of growth hormone or cortisol released during sleep, which may be confirmed by measuring a 3 AM blood glucose level.

NURSING APPLICATIONS

Assessment

Physical—for lung and heart sounds, skin turgor; see Tables 27-4 and 27-5.
Dietary—see Tables 27-4 and 27-5.
Laboratory—for serum glucose, urine ketones, potassium, phosphate, urine specific gravity.

Interventions

1. Monitor glucose every hour for the first 12 to 24 hours to determine client's physical response to treatment.
2. Provide mouth care. Client's mouth is usually dry secondary to dehydration.
3. Administer IV fluid (usually 0.9 or 0.45% saline) as ordered to replace fluid lost from polyuria and to prevent hypovolemia.
4. If potassium level is 4 mEq or below, consult the physician to add potassium to IV fluid. Low potassium levels, caused by polyuria, may lead to cardiac problems.
5. Monitor 3 AM blood glucose if dawn phenomenon is suspected. If it is high, consult the physician to adjust insulin dosage or timing of insulin injection.
6. Refer to Tables 27–4 and 27–5.

Evaluation

* These hyperglycemic complications should not occur, but if they do, correct treatment should be initiated to minimize adverse effects. Additionally, insulin should be given at the appropriate time, in the appropriate amount.

Client Education

- Infection is the main cause of DKA.
- The diabetic treatment plan is important and should be followed closely.
- Teach how to recognize signs of hyperglycemia and how to check blood glucose and urine ketones.
- Test for ketones when blood glucose is above 250 mg/dl. Call the physician if ketones are positive.

Hypoglycemia

A hypoglycemic reaction in diabetes is frequently called an insulin reaction (Table 27–6), although it may be caused by other factors such as inadequate intake. Hypoglycemia can appear at any time—even on a simple outing or while sleeping. Hypoglycemic symptoms may develop suddenly. Unfortunately, IDDM clients may adapt to hypoglycemic reactions and not recognize them to initiate corrective action (Kerr et al, 1991).

Subnormal blood glucose levels are physically and emotionally upsetting and can cause CNS damage because brain cells are glucose dependent. Even mild hypoglycemia may have significant implications for school-age children, with deficits in learning, attention, and concentration (Puczynski et al, 1992). Over an 8-year period, incidence of hypoglycemic coma in children with IDDM increased from 4.4/100 persons/year over the first 4 years to 7.4/100 persons/year during the latter 4 years. It is believed this may be precipitated by tighter glycemic control to prevent chronic diabetic complications (Egger et al, 1991).

Immediate treatment is essential; a readily available source of glucose, such as dextrose tablets, sugar, or fruit juice, is given. The needed boost in blood glucose can be supplied by any readily available source of sugar. Foods containing complex carbohydrates or protein, such as crackers or milk, respectively, are used to maintain the blood glucose level until the next meal.

Why is hypoglycemia detrimental? What is the treatment for hypoglycemia?

Somogyi Effect

Rebound hyperglycemia or Somogyi effect is a rapid swing from hypoglycemia to hyperglycemia (within 1 to 2 hours) to correct hypoglycemia caused by overinsulinization.

In **rebound hyperglycemia** or **Somogyi effect,** the body's normal defense mechanisms overreact to hypoglycemia caused by overinsulinization and secrete large amounts of counterregulatory hormones (cortisol, growth hormone, glucagon, and catecholamines). This causes a skyrocketing blood glucose level. Subclinical hypoglycemia is followed by spontaneous hyperglycemia and ketonuria. Insulin doses

TABLE 27–6

HYPOGLYCEMIA: WARNING SIGNS, CAUSES, AND TREATMENT

Warning Signs	Causes
Sudden onset	Too much insulin or oral hypoglycemic agents
Mild shakiness or lightheadedness	Failure to eat the prescribed diet (omission of evening/afternoon snack)
Nervous	Meal delayed following insulin injection
Irritable	Vomiting
Confused, disorientation, loss of coordination	Diarrhea
Sudden hunger	Increased heavy exercise/activity
Pale color	Alcohol intake
Faster heartbeat	Error in insulin dosage
Rapid, shallow breathing	Weight loss without decreasing insulin dosage
Sweating	Renal insufficiency with decreased renal clearance of insulin
Headache	
Blurred vision	
Nausea	
Anger, bad temper, combative	
Seizures	
Unconsciousness	
Coma	

Treatment

1. Treatment should be administered promptly
2. For mild reactions, administer a readily absorbable source of carbohydrate by mouth. Each of the following can be used to elevate the blood glucose level

Food/Glucose Source	*Amount**
Regular gelatin (prepared)	½ cup
Life Savers	6
Honey/corn syrup	1 tbsp
Fruit juice	1 exchange
Regular carbonated beverages	½ cup
Raisins	2 tbsp
Granulated sugar	4 tsp
Sugar cubes	6
Sugar-sweetened frozen ice	½ twin
Thirst quencher (Gatorade)	1 cup
Candy bar	½
Milk†	1 cup
Glucose tablets (5 gm)	3 tablets
Glutose	½ 80-gm bottle
Insta Glucose	½ 31-gm tube
Insulin Reaction Gel	1 ½ 25-gm packet

3. When the reaction is from too much insulin, additional carbohydrates may be needed for several hours because of the duration of the insulin. For this type of reaction, some complex carbohydrates or additional protein may be given along with a simple sugar, such as milk, bread and jelly, or crackers and cheese
4. For more severe reactions, administer glucagon injection along with oral glucose sources
5. If client cannot safely swallow, use glucagon injection to prevent aspiration
6. For clients who are unconscious or experiencing seizures, provide IV glucose, or use glucagon if IV glucose is not available

* Do not subtract this food from the daily carbohydrate intake.
† Preferred treatment if available because of its long-lasting effects due to its protein content.

may be increased to alleviate hyperglycemia, but glycemic levels increase. By increasing insulin, the problem is compounded. Correction of this problem is to decrease insulin to the point at which it no longer triggers a rebound effect.

What causes rebound hyperglycemia; how does the nurse test for this; why does increasing the insulin not work?

Rebound hyperglycemia occurs principally in clients receiving high insulin doses (>1 units/kg/day for children and >1.5 units/kg day for adolescents and adults). Rebound hyperglycemia can be investigated by testing blood glucose levels during the night; negative urine ketones and hypoglycemia at 3 AM with hyperglycemia and ketonuria at 7 AM usually indicate Somogyi effect. This effect may be precipitated by stressful situations, such as pregnancy or surgery. Occasionally the Somogyi effect is diagnosed when the problem is related to dietary deviations.

NURSING APPLICATIONS

Assessment

Physical—for signs and symptoms described in Table 27–6.
Dietary—for noncompliance (see Table 27–6).
Laboratory—for decreased plasma glucose; urine ketones.

Interventions

1. Refer to Table 27–6.
2. If client is NPO for surgery or tests, check with the physician before giving insulin or oral hypoglycemics, as they may result in hypoglycemia.
3. Suspect rebound hyperglycemia if wide fluctuations occur in serum glucose levels over several hours or if nocturnal hypoglycemia is occurring. If rebound hyperglycemia is suspected, consult physician to perform an early AM blood glucose test.

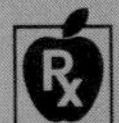
Monitor for use of aspirin, sulfa drugs, and marijuana, as these increase hypoglycemic risk.

Evaluation

* Hypoglycemia should not occur, but if it does, treatment is rendered to correct hypoglycemia and prevent adverse effects. Additionally, blood glucose remains or is maintained near normal levels.

Client Education

- Insulin shock, insulin reaction, and hypoglycemia all mean the same thing.
- Teach signs and symptoms of hypoglycemia.
- Always carry some form of glucose.
- To prevent hypoglycemia, the following must be stressed: meal and snack regularity, correct dosage of insulin or oral hypoglycemics, and regular exercise and daily activity.
- Before changing the evening insulin dose, the 3 to 4 AM blood glucose level should be checked for rebound hyperglycemia.

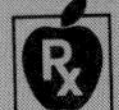
Hypoglycemia may provoke marked hypertensive reactions, particularly in clients taking beta blocker antihypertensive medications.

Long-Term Complications

Because of metabolic alterations secondary to DM, treatment should be implemented as soon as possible after diagnosis to prevent retinal, renal, neurological, and cardiovascular problems. Most diabetic authorities believe that early control of diabetes can postpone and minimize many of these severe complications.

Accelerated **macrovascular** disease is the major chronic complication. This multifactorial process is not well defined, but vascular changes are thought to result from hyperlipidemia, hypertension, hyperinsulinemia, and hyperglycemia (Ronnemaa et al, 1991; Iwai et al, 1990). High or moderate-high total cholesterol levels are observed in 70% of adults under treatment for IDDM and 77% of all untreated cases (Harris, 1991). After 20 years of DM, 45% of clients have **arteriosclerosis obliterans.** Diabetic clients, especially those with NIDDM, have problems with slow wound healing, frequent abscesses, skin irritations, pruritus, numbness and tingling of the extremities, and visual problems. These are generally associated with vascular problems.

Macrovascular—refers to larger blood vessels.

Arteriosclerosis obliterans is proliferation of the intima (inside lining) causing complete blockage of an artery.

Microangiopathy can be identified as a thickening of the capillary basement membrane.

Microangiopathy is unique to DM. These changes result in renal complications (leading to renal failure), obstruction of circulation in the extremities (leading to gangrene), and progressive blood vessel damage in the retina of the eye (leading to blindness).

Both renal function and structure can be affected by DM. Approximately 30 to 50% of IDDM clients develop diabetic nephropathy (Shyh et al, 1985). Hyperglycemia is a significant risk factor for development of proteinuria and subsequent renal failure (Klein et al, 1991); high protein intake may be a contributing factor. The earliest manifestation of this process is proteinuria.

Diabetic clients are often hypertensive. To prevent devastating end-organ damage associated with hypertension, adequate control of both blood pressure and glycemic levels is advocated. Weight reduction, sodium restriction, and exercise are beneficial in treating hypertensive diabetic clients by lowering blood pressure, improving glycemic control, and modifying other cardiovascular risk factors (Tjoa & Kaplan, 1991).

Neuropathy, or deterioration of nervous tissue, is also frequently seen in DM. Impaired sensations attributable to diabetic neuropathy are a contributing factor in gangrene. Neuropathy in the autonomic nervous system involves viscera nerves and is particularly disabling and occasionally fatal. Abnormalities in the GI tract interfere with food intake and absorption. Such GI disturbances include dysphagia, diarrhea, constipation, and pancreatic enzyme insufficiency. Diabetic gastroparesis causes delayed gastric emptying, resulting in a mismatch between the therapeutic action of insulin and food absorption. Clients exhibit nausea, early satiety, and frequent vomiting.

What causes macrovascular problems in DM? List examples of microangiopathy.

NURSING APPLICATIONS

Assessment

Physical—for obesity, activity level, tobacco use, stress, hypertension, visual problems, dysphagia, diarrhea, constipation, nausea, vomiting, anorexia.
Dietary—for saturated fat, cholesterol, and sodium intake; alcohol use.
Laboratory—for lipid levels (total, LDL, HDL, triglycerides), glucose, proteinuria, BUN, creatinine.

Interventions

1. Explain long-term complications of DM and treatments to clients.
2. If gastroparesis is a problem, consult physician for initiation of Reglan and erythromycin (Peeters et al, 1992).
3. Praise clients when they adhere to the prescribed diet or choose appropriate foods.
4. Normalize blood pressure, reduce dietary protein intake to 0.8 gm/kg IBW, and control hyperglycemia to retard progression of diabetic nephropathy (Narins, 1991).

Evaluation

* Long-term complications are delayed or minimized in clients. BP should be below 140/90 mmHg; IBW should be maintained or achieved; cholesterol and triglyceride levels should be below 200 mg/dl.

Client Education

- To help clients remember how to prevent long-term complications, remember the word CHANGE (Colwell & Jewler, 1990):

Cholesterol and lipid control—keep cholesterol and triglyceride levels below 200 mg/dl.

*H*ypertension control—keep BP below 140/90 mmHg.
*A*ppropriate weight management—maintain IBW.
*N*o smoking—quit or do not start smoking.
*G*lycemic control.
*E*xercise.

LABORATORY TESTS

DM is diagnosed and monitored using laboratory tests. Classification of DM affects how the condition is treated (Table 27–7). A diagnosis is based on any of the following criteria (Lebovitz, 1988):

1. Marked elevation of plasma glucose (>200 mg/dl) accompanied by symptoms of polydipsia, polyuria, polyphagia, and weight loss.
2. Elevated fasting plasma glucose (>140 mg/dl) on more than one occasion.
3. Elevated plasma glucose of >200 mg/dl 2 hours after an oral glucose tolerance test with previous documentation of a blood glucose >200 mg/dl.

The classic symptoms listed in the first criterion are enough to diagnose DM, but less than half of all diabetic clients present with these symptoms.

Fasting Blood Glucose

Normally **fasting blood glucose** level is 70 to 110 mg/dl for clients under 50 years of age. Fasting blood glucose levels are elevated (over 120 mg/dl) in DM; normal fasting blood glucose levels increase approximately 1% per year after age 50. Mental, emotional, or physical stress elevates cortisol secretion, which increases blood glucose levels.

Fasting blood glucose levels are determined from plasma after a client has fasted for 8 hours.

TABLE 27–7

CRITERIA FOR DIAGNOSIS OF DIABETES MELLITUS AND IMPAIRED GLUCOSE TOLERANCE

	Plasma	
	Venous* *mg/dl (mmol/L)	***Capillary* *mg/dl (mmol/L)***
*Diabetes Mellitus**		
Fasting glucose	≥ 140 (7.8)	≥ 140 (7.8)
2-hour postglucose+	≥ 200 (11.1)	≥ 220 (12.2)
*Impaired Glucose Tolerance**		
Fasting glucose	< 140 (7.8)	< 140 (7.8)
2-hour post glucose+	140–200 (7.8–11.1)	160–220 (8.9–12.2)
Gestational Diabetes		
1. WHO criteria are the same as those given for diabetes mellitus		
2. American Diabetes Association‡ criteria: 2 or more of the following values must be met or exceeded:		
Venous Plasma Glucose		
Fasting—105 (5.8)		
1 hour—190 (10.6)		
2 hour—165 (9.2)		
3 hour—145 (8.1)		

* Data from Shuman Cr. Diabetes mellitus. *In* Kinney JM et al (eds): *Nutrition and Metabolism in Patient Care.* Philadelphia, WB Saunders, 1988: 360–385.

+ Oral glucose challenge is 75 gm for adults and 1.75 gm/kg to 75 gm for children. Diagnostic criteria for children are same as those for adults.

‡ Data from American Diabetes Association (ADA). Gestational diabetes mellitus. *Diab Care* 1992 Apr; 15(suppl 2):5–6.

TABLE 27–8

INTERPRETATION OF GLYCOSYLATED HEMOGLOBIN LEVELS IN DIABETES MELLITUS

HbA_{1c} Level	5.4–7.4	7.5–8.5	8.6–10.5	10.6–13	> 13
Average Blood Glucose (mg/dl)	70–105	120–150	150–200	200–300	> 300
Control	Normal	Excellent	Good	Fair	Poor

OGTT measures blood glucose levels at 1-hour intervals for 2 hours following a carbohydrate challenge of 75 gm glucose. The diet should contain 150 gm or more of carbohydrates daily for at least 3 days before the test followed by a 12-hour fast.

Postprandial blood glucose test—blood drawn 2, 3, and 4 hours after a regular meal to determine blood glucose levels.

HbA_{1C}, the glycosylated form of hemoglobin, is produced when glucose molecules attach to normal hemoglobin in a high-glucose environment.

Oral Glucose Tolerance Test

Oral glucose tolerance test (OGTT) may be ordered to confirm a diabetic diagnosis. This test can be affected by illness and medications that affect glucose tolerance (hormones, hypoglycemic agents, diuretics, and salicylates). A gradual deterioration of glucose tolerance is observed after the age of 50.

Normally 2-hour values are 120 to 140 mg/dl. A diabetic response results in a higher glycemic level that returns to normal more slowly than in a nondiabetic. A **postprandial blood glucose test** is being used more frequently.

Glycosylated Hemoglobin (HbA_{1C})

Another diagnostic test for determining long-term glucose levels is **hemoglobin A_{1C} (HbA_{1C})** (Table 27–8). The reaction is nearly irreversible, so levels remain high until cells die and are replaced by new cells. Therefore, it reflects an average of blood glucose levels for 2 to 3 months (RBCs have a life span of 120 days). Regular measurements of HbA_{1C} can be used to change diabetic treatments, improve metabolic control, and motivate compliance (Larsen et al, 1990).

Self-Monitoring Blood Glucose

With the advent of affordable accurate blood glucose meters (more frequently referred to as glucometers), self-monitoring blood glucose levels is encouraged for all diabetics to maintain better control of blood glucose levels. By monitoring blood glucose levels on a regular basis, acute and chronic problems associated with hyperglycemia and hypoglycemia can be averted. Records of blood glucose levels allow clients to make appropriate changes in diet, exercise, or medication levels and are useful for physicians to evaluate effectiveness of treatments.

Other Tests

Urine specimens are tested to determine total urine volume (for a 24-hour period), specific gravity, and ketone bodies. Ketonuria indicates that excessive amounts of fats are being metabolized; this requires an immediate adjustment of diet and insulin. Measurement of glucose in the urine has been replaced with blood glucose measurements because of unreliable results of urine testing.

Choose 1 laboratory test, describe how it is performed, and what the results would be if a client has DM.

Other laboratory tests are performed to assess risk of diabetic-associated complications. These include a fasting lipid profile (including triglycerides and total, LDL, and HDL cholesterol). BUN, creatinine, and 24-hour urine protein are measured to assess renal function.

DIABETIC MEAL PLANS

Numerous types of meal planning systems have been devised to achieve comparable diabetic control. Some options are basic food groups; healthy food choices; US dietary guidelines; food exchange lists; high-carbohydrate, high-fiber diet (HCF);

kilocalorie counting; **total available glucose (TAG); point system;** and ***Month of Meals.*** The structured diets (food exchange lists, HCF diet, kilocalorie counting, and point system) are best for those who require structure and consistency in a diet. The TAG system is appropriate for those who want maximum glucose control, but because of extensive planning required, it is generally reserved for the most compliant clients. Planned menus are appropriate for clients who prefer specified food choices and appropriate amounts or for clients who do not understand the concept of other meal planning options. The food exchange list system is the most widely used.

Total available glucose is a system to regulate insulin requirements to food intake. An individualized glucose to insulin ratio is determined, and generalized categories of foods are defined in TAG units. A point system is used to control kilocalorie intake using a simple to use, easy to count method. Foods are assigned a point value (1 point = 75 kcal). (A client on a 1200 kcal diet would have 16 points for the day, and intake is limited to 16 points.) *Month of Meals* and *Month of Meals 2*, published by the American Diabetes Association, are 28-day planned menus designed to provide 1500 kcal/day.

Individualizing the Diet

Ideally a client's personal needs, learning abilities, nutritional requirements, and lifestyle are assessed before determining an appropriate meal plan. Since proper diet is definitely a matter of self-management, input from a client regarding the type of meal plan preferred may result in better compliance. A meal plan should not be regarded as a diet but rather a guide to good eating and for making healthy food choices (Pastors, 1992).

An important consideration of a diabetic meal plan is that it should be flexible in allowing wide choices of foods and adaptable to specific needs and individual preferences. Increased flexibility and minimal disruptions in a client's lifestyle are associated with improved compliance. Special foods are not necessary; foods can be the same as those purchased for the rest of the family. Differences in schedules and activity levels over the weekend versus weekdays should be considered and discussed with clients.

Goals of a diabetic diet include the following: (1) improve overall health of a client by attaining and maintaining optimum nutrition; (2) attain and/or maintain an ideal body weight; (3) provide for normal physical growth in a diabetic child; (4) provide adequate nutrition for the pregnant woman, her fetus, and lactation needs, if she chooses to breast-feed her infant; (5) maintain plasma glucose as near the normal physiological range as possible; and (6) prevent and/or delay development or progression of cardiovascular, renal, retinal, neurological, and other complications associated with diabetes, insofar as these are related to metabolic control.

Name 3 goals of a DM diet.

Food Exchange Lists

The American Diabetes Association, the American Dietetic Association, and the US Public Health Service compiled the "Exchange System" more than 30 years ago. Changes have been made as needed to reflect increased knowledge. Exchange lists are frequently referred to as the ADA diet. These exchange lists were developed primarily to provide optimum nutrition for DM while counting carbohydrate intake.

Food exchange lists allow flexibility of the diet in addition to achieving a reasonable constancy of carbohydrate, protein, fat, and energy intake. These exchange lists divide food into 6 groups; within each group, all food items are approximately equal in kilocalories and in amount of carbohydrate, protein, and fat content. Serving sizes vary, so foods in each list are kilocalorically equivalent. Therefore, foods within any group can be traded, or exchanged, with other foods in the same group. Table 27–9 shows the major exchange lists, kilocalorie content, and distribution of energy nutrients (carbohydrate, protein, and fat) for each exchange. Additionally, a free food list includes foods or beverages that contain less than 20 kcal per serving. Some items contain no kilocalories; others could be considered low kilocalorie and should be limited to 2 or 3 servings per day.

Foods are categorized somewhat differently than in the basic food groups. Instead of classifying all milk products together, food exchange lists categorize cheese

TABLE 27–9

MAJOR EXCHANGE LISTS

List	Exchange Group	Carbohydrate (gm)	Protein (gm)	Fat (gm)	Kilocalories
1	Starch/bread	15	3	0.9*	80
2	Meat				
	Lean	—	7	3	55
	Medium-fat	—	7	5	75
	High-fat	—	7	8	100
3	Vegetable	5	2	—	28
4	Fruit	15	—	—	60
5	Milk				
	Skim	12	8	1	90
	Low-fat	12	8	5	120
	Whole	12	8	8	150
6	Fat	—	—	5	4

* This is typically not calculated.

From *Exchange Lists for Meal Planning,* which is the basis of a meal planning system designed by a committee of the American Diabetes Association and the American Dietetic Association, Copyrighted © 1989 by the American Diabetes and the American Diabetes Association.

with meats because of its low-carbohydrate, high-protein content. Vegetables with higher carbohydrate content are in the bread/starch exchange; only nonstarchy vegetables are in the vegetable exchange. Fruits are in a separate list. Foods within each exchange and serving sizes are provided in Appendix D–1.

Although foods within an exchange list are interchangeable, it is not permissible to exchange foods from 1 list for another because each group contains different amounts of carbohydrate, protein, and fat. Any interchange between groups could disrupt diet balance. Foods cannot be saved from a meal and eaten at another meal, but with the physician's permission, a food from 1 list can be "saved" for a later snack. However, if snacking is a regular habit, it should be calculated as such into a meal plan.

What is the purpose of food exchange lists? What are the 6 categories of foods in the exchange lists? Give examples of foods in each. How is it different from the basic food groups? Can foods from different groups be interchanged? Why or why not?

Lactovegetarian and ovolactovegetarian diets can be used by diabetic clients since they are nutritionally adequate. Both milk and egg products are recommended. Peas, lentils, and legumes are substituted for lean meats; eggs and nonfat or low-fat cheese make up the meat exchange list; nuts and nut butters are also used to provide protein.

ADA Diet Order

The physician's diet order should indicate kilocaloric level, kilocaloric distribution, and number of feedings daily. If this specific breakdown is not ordered by the physician, the standard ADA recommendation is followed with 3 meals and a bedtime snack.

Total food allotment is divided into the number of exchanges from each group allowed for the day. Then they are divided among the number of feedings so the food (especially the carbohydrate) is distributed equally throughout the day or to coincide with insulin activity.

NURSING APPLICATIONS

Assessment

Physical—for personality, lifestyle, sex, age.

Dietary—for preferred foods; fad diets; vegetarian type (if applicable).

Interventions

1. Provide exchange list for fast foods, especially for adolescents, to allow "fitting in" with peers while still following their diet (Appendix D–2).

2. For clients who dislike milk, add an extra fruit and 1 lean meat exchange; discuss other sources of calcium (cheese, cottage cheese, calcium-fortified orange juice) to ensure adequate calcium intake.
3. Monitor a client's attitude and motivation, as these affect compliance.
4. Monitor family involvement and understanding since these also affect adherence to diet.
5. Involve client/family in nutritional care.

Evaluation

* Client should adhere to and consume the meal pattern decided on and explain rationale for its use.

Client Education

* It is extremely important to teach both the client and the person who prepares meals how to use the exchange lists.
* Clients frequently become overly concerned about understanding food "exchanges." Discuss food groups rather than exchange lists.
* A nutritionally balanced diet is important; fad diets should be avoided.
* Dietary requirements and recommendations for diabetic clients are based on sound principles of nutrition.
* A diabetic diet is a healthful way to eat; this fact should be stressed to new diabetic clients and family food providers. It helps them recognize that the whole family benefits by eating in a similar manner.
* Because of the liberal amount of carbohydrate allowed, diabetic diets are no more expensive than a regular diet.
* Several special products may be used, such as fruits canned without sugar.
* Fruits canned in their own juice may be more economical than those labeled "dietetic" and packed with artificial sweeteners.
* "Dietetic" or "sugar-free" may not be synonymous with "nonkilocaloric."
* Clients need to be able to distinguish between "dietetic" and "diabetic" (neither are required). Some dietetic products are intended for salt restrictions or other types of diets. Labels must be read carefully.

GENERAL PRINCIPLES FOR NUTRITIONAL CARE

Diabetes mellitus is a chronic, lifelong disease. Consensus supports diet therapy as the cornerstone for preventing hyperglycemia and hypoglycemia as well as decreasing complications. No single dietary plan can be appropriate for all people with different personalities and lifestyles. The objective of the diet is to enable clients to maintain good control of their diabetes or to promote near normal blood glucose and lipid levels.

Because of different philosophies regarding diabetic control, physicians differ in their approach to diet therapy. Clients may be allowed to eat anything so long as they do not have any clinical symptoms (no ketosis or hypoglycemia) and maintain or gain weight as appropriate. Glycosuria and hyperglycemia are permitted. Insulin dosages are adjusted frequently. This approach is known as clinical control. A more popular practice is chemical control. A measured diet and a certain or predetermined amount of insulin is used to maintain blood glucose between 80 and 200 mg/dl.

TABLE 27-10

CALCULATING KILOCALORIE LEVEL FOR DIABETIC CLIENTS

Determine Kilocalorie Requirements

A. For *children**
  1. For the first year of life, 1000 kcal
  2. For children over age 1, 1000 kcal plus 100 kcal for each year of age up to 2000 kcal at age 11
     Example: 7-yr-old—1000 kcal + 700 (kcal/yr) = 1700 kcal/day
  3. From age 12 to 15, 100 kcal/year for girls and 200 kcal per year for boys
     Example: 14-yr-old boy—200 kcal × 14 (age) = 2800 kcal/day

B. For *adults*†
  1. For obese or inactive clients: 10 × IBW (lbs)
  2. For clients over age 55 or sedentary clients: 13 X IBW (lbs)
  Example: 35-yr-old secretary, weight 130 lbs within her IBW, no regular exercise: 13 (kcal/lb) × 130 (lbs) = 1690 kcal/day
  3. For desirable weight or moderately active clients: 15 × IBW (lbs)
  4. For thin or very active clients: 20 × IBW (lbs)

Adjust Kilocalories for Weight Loss

Since 3500 kcal are in each stored pound of fat, 500 kcal less should be consumed per day to lose 1 lb a week.
Example: 180-lb male (5′8″), moderately active, who needs to lose about 25 lbs:
155 (lbs IBW) × 15 (kcal/lb for moderate activity level) = 2325 kcal/day
2325 (kcal/day) − 500 kcal/day for weight loss = 1825 kcal/day

* From Pricilla White, MD, Joslin Clinic.
† Adapted from *Calculation of a Diabetic Diet Prescription.* Minneapolis, MN, International Diabetes Center.

Energy

Sufficient kilocalories are necessary to achieve full growth potential in children and achieve or maintain IBW (Table 27-10). (Usually the minimum level of average range of weight for height is advisable.) When kilocalorie content is controlled, all foods containing carbohydrate, protein, fat, and alcohol are restricted to some degree. All these sources of energy are potential sources of glucose (carbohydrate, 100%; protein, 58%; fat, 10%).

Recommendations for distribution of kilocalories represented by carbohydrate, protein, and fat are shown in Table 27-11. The total amount of energy needed is based on IBW (kg) and activity. Steps for calculating a diabetic meal pattern using the exchange lists are described in Table 27-12.

TABLE 27-11

DISTRIBUTION OF MAJOR NUTRIENTS IN NORMAL AND IN DIABETIC DIETS (AS PERCENTAGES OF TOTAL KILOCALORIES)

	Starch and Other Polysaccharides* (%)	Sugars† and Dextrins (%)	Fat (%)	Protein (%)	Alcohol (%)
Typical American diet	25-35	20-30	35-45 P/S ratio 1:3	12-19	0-10
Traditional diabetic diets	25-30	10-15‡	40-45	16-21	0
Newer diabetic diets	35-45§	5-15‡	< 30§ P/S ratio 1:1	12-20	0-6

* Almost all of these kilocalories are starch, but complex carbohydrates also include cellulose, hemicellulose, pentosans, and pectin.
† Monosaccharides and disaccharides, mainly sucrose, but also includes fructose, glucose, lactose, and maltose.
‡ Almost exclusively natural sugars, mainly in fruit and milk (lactose).
§ The ideal diet is probably even higher in starch and lower in saturated fat, but in typical affluent Western societies, it is usually not feasible to achieve higher ratios of starch to fat than shown on the bottom line of this table.
Adapted from West KM. Diabetes mellitus. *In* Schneider HA, et al, eds. *Nutritional Support of Medical Practice,* 2nd ed. Philadelphia, Harper & Row, 1983.

TABLE 27–12

STEPS IN PLANNING DIET PRESCRIPTIONS USING EXCHANGE LISTS

STEP 1. Assess desirable weight

Use height/weight tables or the rule of "5's and 6's" as described in Chapter 9

Example: NIDDM female; medium frame, height 68 inches; current weight, 160 lbs

For 5′ = 100 lbs
For 8″ (8 × 5) = 40 lbs
Total 140 lbs

Client is approximately 20 lbs above desirable body weight

STEP 2. Calculate total daily kilocalorie requirement

Using desirable weight, use Table 22–10 to determine kilocaloric requirements

Example: Activity level sedentary; weight loss is desirable

140 lb (IBW) × 13 = 1820 kcal/day

1820 kcal/day − 500 (kcal for wt loss) = 1320 kcal

Figures are normally rounded off; 1300 kcal/day for weight loss

STEP 3. Determine distribution of the energy nutrient in grams

(This may be stipulated by the physician's order). Using a distribution of 50% carbohydrate, 20% protein, and 30% fat, divide the total kilocalories of each nutrient by the amounts of kilocalories the nutrient provides

Example

Carbohydrate: 1300 kcal × 0.50 = 650 kcal ÷ 4 kcal/gm = 162.5 gm
Protein: 1300 kcal × 0.20 = 260 kcal ÷ 4 kcal/gm = 65 gm
Fat: 1300 kcal × 0.30 = 390 kcal ÷ 9 kcal/gm = 43 gm

So 163 gm carbohydrate, 65 gm protein, and 43 gm fat is needed.

STEP 4. Determine distribution of servings from each exchange group

This calculation is based on the amount of carbohydrate, protein, and fat contributed by each exchange list and the client's preferences regarding each list

A.

Decide from the client's diet history the desirable number of servings from the milk, vegetable, and fruit lists

Example	SERVINGS	CARBOHYDRATE	PROTEIN	FAT
List 5—Milk, skim	1	12	8	1
List 3—Vegetables	3	15	6	
List 4—Fruits	4	60		
Subtotal A		87	14	1

B.

To determine the number of servings from the starch/bread list, subtract the total grams of carbohydrate (87) from milk, vegetables, and fruit lists from the total grams of carbohydrate (163). This amount is divided by 15 (gm carbohydrate/serving) to determine the number of servings from the starch/bread list

Example	SERVINGS	CARBOHYDRATE	PROTEIN	FAT
Subtotal A		87	14	1
List 1—Starch/bread	5	75	15	3
Subtotal B		162	29	4

C.

To determine the number of servings from the meat list, subtract the total protein (29) from the milk, vegetable, and starch/bread lists from the total desired amount (65) and divide by 7 (gm protein/serving)

Example	SERVINGS	CARBOHYDRATE	PROTEIN	FAT
Subtotal B		162	29	4
List 2—Meat/lean	5		35	15
Subtotal C		162	64	19

Table continued on following page

TABLE 27–12

STEPS IN PLANNING DIET PRESCRIPTIONS USING EXCHANGE LISTS *Continued*

D.

To determine the number of servings from the fat list, subtract the total fat from the sum of the milk, starch/bread, and meat lists (19) from the total grams of fat (43) and divide by 5 (gm fat/serving)

Example	**SERVINGS**	**CARBOHYDRATE**	**PROTEIN**	**FAT**
Subtotal C		162	64	19
List 6—Fat	5			25
Final total		162	64	44

Thus, the daily distribution of the exchange list is as follows:

LIST	**FOOD GROUP**	**SERVINGS**	**CARBOHYDRATE**	**PROTEIN**	**FAT**
1	Starch/bread	5	75	15	3
2	Meat (lean)	5		35	15
3	Vegetable	3	15	6	
4	Fruit	4	60		
5	Milk (skim)	1	12	8	1
6	Fat	5			25

STEP 5. Divide the number of servings from each group into 3 meals and the number of snacks ordered

The distribution is based on the client's eating habits, work schedule and peak action of insulin. Clients on oral hypoglycemic agents normally receive only 3 meals

Example

Breakfast	
2 Fruit Exchanges	1 banana
1 Bread Exchange	¾ cup dry cereal
1 Milk Exchange	1 cup skim milk
Lunch	
2 Meat (lean) Exchanges	1½ oz 95% fat-free luncheon meat
	1 oz diet cheese
2 Bread Exchanges	2 slices rye bread
Free Exchange	Lettuce slices, mustard, Kosher pickle
2 Fat Exchanges	2 tsp mayonnaise
1 Vegetable Exchange	Tomato juice
1 Fruit Exchange	1 kiwi
Supper	
3 Meat (lean) Exchanges	3 oz charcoal broiled loin pork chop
2 Vegetable Exchanges	½ cup spinach
	½ cup yellow squash
2 Bread Exchanges	¼ cup baked beans
	1 dinner roll
Free Exchange	Tossed salad
3 Fat Exchanges	2 tsp margarine
	2 tbsp reduced-kilocalorie salad dressing
1 Fruit Exchange	1 cup cantaloupe cubes

Carbohydrate

Diets that are high in complex carbohydrates are well tolerated by most diabetics. The American Diabetes Association has endorsed a high-carbohydrate diet (55 to 60% of total kilocalories) using principally complex carbohydrates, in the absence of carbohydrate-induced hypertriglyceridemia (ADA, 1992a). As shown in Table 27–11, recommended carbohydrate content is similar to the typical American diet. Unrefined carbohydrates are preferable because they supply required nutrients, including fiber.

A high-carbohydrate diet actually increases the sensitivity of peripheral tissues to both endogenous and exogenous insulin. This improves glucose tolerance, especially if dietary fiber is also increased (Vinik & Jenkins, 1988). Another plus for a high-carbohydrate diet is that substitution of complex carbohydrates for saturated fats results in lower LDL cholesterol levels (Howard et al, 1991). Some clients with NIDDM exhibit sustained carbohydrate-induced hypertriglyceridemia. In such cases, reduction of dietary carbohydrate may be needed.

What are the advantages of a high-carbohydrate diet?

Simple Sugars

Use of simple sugars is generally limited because of their lack of nutritive value and kilocaloric density. Simple saccharides offer less satiety, and hunger develops sooner than with polysaccharide-rich foods. Typically 10 to 15% of the carbohydrate kilocalories are derived from sugars, principally natural sugars.

In the past, it was believed that simple sugars would cause a rapid rise in blood glucose levels. If consumed as a part of a meal, the blood glucose level may not differ greatly from other complex carbohydrate intake. A controlled study of IDDM children providing 10% of total kilocalories from sucrose versus a sugar-free diet resulted in similar glycemic responses (Loghmani et al, 1991). Although diabetic clients are advised to limit simple or refined sugars, modest amounts are acceptable contingent on metabolic control and body weight (ADA, 1992a). Simple sugars are used as a replacement for complex carbohydrates, not additive carbohydrates.

Fiber

The ADA (1992a) recommends a maximum of 40 gm/day or 25 gm/1000 kcal. To achieve this, most clients should increase their fiber intake gradually to minimize abdominal cramping, discomfort, diarrhea, and flatulence. Adequate amounts of fluid are necessary with a higher fiber intake. Diabetic clients are at risk of **phytobezoar** formation when increasing fiber intake because of the prevalence of neuropathy and gastric **hypotony.**

Phytobezoar—an impaction composed of vegetable fibers that does not pass through the intestine. Hypotony refers to decreased tone or strength in the GI tract that deters transit time.

Considerable debate surrounds the guidelines to increase carbohydrate because of elevated triglyceride levels and increased insulin requirements in some individuals in response to a high-carbohydrate diet. These adverse effects are neutralized when fiber and carbohydrate are increased simultaneously (Riccardi & Rivellese, 1991).

Soluble fiber delays gastric emptying and glucose absorption. Thus, advantages of increasing soluble fiber are improved carbohydrate metabolism and reduced dosage of oral hypoglycemic agents or insulin, lower blood lipids, and enhanced satiety for NIDDM clients on weight reduction diets (Anderson & Akanji, 1991). Soluble fibers found in legumes, whole-grain cereals, green leafy vegetables, and fruits tend to lower plasma glucose concentrations and total cholesterol (especially LDL cholesterol).

How does soluble fiber help glucose levels? List examples of soluble fibers.

Glycemic Index

Glycemic index is a method of dividing foods according to physiological effect on blood glucose. The blood glucose curve for 50 gm of carbohydrate from a food is evaluated and expressed as a percentage of the effect induced by white bread. A higher glycemic index results in greater elevations of the blood glucose level.

Until recently, complex carbohydrate foods were considered to have similar effects on blood glucose concentrations, whereas simple sugars were assumed to elicit a higher response. As shown in Chapter 4, Table 4–4, blood glucose responses to various carbohydrates overlap so simple and complex carbohydrates cannot be distinguished as separate groups having different glycemic responses. Research studies have determined a **glycemic index** for specific effects of carbohydrate foods. Glycemic response may not be as dramatic when various carbohydrates are given as part of a mixed meal instead of by themselves.

At this time, use of glycemic indexes is not widely practiced because of many unanswered questions. Although definite recommendations cannot be made based on current information, several facts have been established: (1) Starchy foods do not all have the same effect, and (2) minimally processed and leguminous carbohydrates generally have lower glycemic effects (the blood glucose level does not rise as rapidly).

Self-monitoring blood glucose allows a diabetic client to test individual responses to specific foods or food combinations. The glycemic index can be used to interpret unexpected blood glucose variations and thereby fine-tune the diet by emphasizing foods that have lower glycemic responses for that particular client.

What 2 facts have been established based on glycemic index findings?

Protein

Protein required by diabetic clients is the same as for individuals with normal hepatic and renal status, 0.8 gm/kg body weight for adults. This is generally 12 to 20% of total kilocaloric intake.

As is true for any other client, stress, strain, or an illness increases protein requirements (1 to 1.5 gm/kg body weight). Protein requirements are modestly increased during gestation (60 gm/day), lactation (65 to 62 gm/day), and periods of rapid growth (1 to 2.2 gm/kg).

Although diabetic recommendations have emphasized protein in the past, it is now believed that protein intake should be reduced in individuals who are identified at risk or who have clinical evidence of nephropathy. Lower levels of protein intake (0.6 to 0.8 gm/kg IBW) can preserve renal function and decrease albuminuria (Brouhard & LaGrone, 1990; Yue et al, 1988).

What is the basic protein recommendation for a healthy diabetic client; for clients who are ill; for client with nephropathy?

Fat

Atherosclerosis appears to be accelerated as a result of serum lipid derangements. Low HDL and elevated LDL levels are associated with poorly controlled DM. Thus, prudent dietary measures are implemented to improve lipid profile. Current recommendations include daily fat intake limited to 30% of total kilocalories, with polyunsaturated, saturated, and monounsaturated fats each contributing 10% of the kilocalories. Cholesterol is limited by selection of unsaturated fat sources; recommended intake is less than 300 mg/day (ADA, 1992a). In NIDDM clients with elevated triglycerides and HDL cholesterol, complex carbohydrates may be replaced with monounsaturated fats to improve glycemic control and hypertriglyceridemia (Bonanome et al, 1991; Garg et al, 1988).

Inclusion of omega-3 fatty acids may reduce incidence of CHD (Bagdade et al, 1990; Wahlqvist et al, 1989). Providing capsules of EPA or 8 oz fatty fish weekly has been shown to have a protective effect in both IDDM (Mori, 1991) and NIDDM (Hendra et al, 1990). Although omega-3 fatty acids may decrease plasma triglyceride concentrations, deleterious effects on glucose control and clotting factors require close monitoring (Hendra et al, 1990).

What is the recommended fat intake?

Alcohol

Alcohol intake has several disadvantages in DM, but an occasional alcoholic beverage is allowed if there are no medical restrictions. Alcohol is primarily metabolized by the liver and does not require insulin (Table 27–13). Alcohol is high in energy (7 kcal/gm). If it is taken with a mixed meal, blood glucose control is not compromised.

Large quantities of alcohol have been associated with hyperglycemia, especially in malnourished diabetics. Conversely, diabetics are actually more vulnerable to hypoglycemic effects from alcohol. Hypoglycemia may develop up to several hours

TABLE 27–13

EXCHANGE EQUIVALENTS FOR ALCOHOLIC BEVERAGES

Beverage	Serving (oz)	Alcohol (gm)	Carbohydrate (gm)	Kilo-calories	Exchanges for Type II Diabetes
Beer					
Regular beer	12	13	13.7	151	1 starch/bread, 2 fat
Light beer	12	10.1	6	90	2 fat
Extra-light beer	12	8.1	3.3	70	1½ fat
Near beer	12	1.5	12.3	60	1 starch/bread
Nonalcoholic beer	11	0.3	9.7	50	1 starch/bread
Distilled spirits					
86 proof (gin, rum, vodka, whiskey, scotch)	1½	15.3	Trace	107	2 fat
Dry Brandy or Cognac	1	10.7	Trace	75	1½ fat
Table wines					
Red or rosé	4	11.6	1	85	2 fat
Dry white	4	11.3	0.4	80	2 fat
Sweet wine	4	11.8	4.9	102	⅓ starch/bread, 2 fat
Light wine	4	6.4	1.3	48–58	1 fat
Wine coolers	12	15	22	192	1½ fruit, 3 fat
Sparkling Wines					
Champagne	4	11.9	3.6	98	2 fat
Sweet kosher wine	4	11.9	12	132	1 starch/bread, 2 fat
Appetizer/Dessert wines:					
Sherry	2	9.4	1.5	73	1½ fat
Sweet sherry, port, muscatel	2	9.4	7	94	½ starch/bread, 1½ fat
Vermouths					
Dry	3	12.6	4.2	105	2 fat
Sweet	3	12.2	13.9	141	1 starch/bread, 2 fat

From Franz MJ. *Exchanges For All Occasions.* Minneapolis, International Diabetes Center, © 1987.

after alcohol ingestion because of reduced gluconeogenesis in the liver. This problem is especially significant when ingestion follows a fasting period (15 to 36 hours) because glycogen reserves are depleted or if alcohol is taken with readily absorbed carbohydrates.

Since many NIDDM clients are concerned with maintaining or losing body weight, these superfluous kilocalories become even more undesirable, interfering with the discipline required to stay on their prescribed diet.

What are possible consequences of drinking alcohol? When is hypoglycemia most likely to occur when drinking alcohol?

Vitamins and Electrolytes

Supplemental vitamins and minerals are not ordinarily required for diabetic clients. However, clients with poorly controlled DM, infection, malabsorption, or other complications may require supplements. Additionally, IDDM clients with recent weight loss may initially benefit from vitamin supplements since growth and development might have been compromised before diagnosis.

A moderate salt restriction (3 to 4 gm daily) is advisable for well-controlled DM. DM clients are prone to hypertension, renal disease, and CHF. However, if DM is poorly controlled, the resulting diuresis may produce deficits of water, sodium, potassium, and chloride; thus, sodium is not restricted in this circumstance.

When is vitamin supplementation necessary?

Alternative Sweeteners

Alternative sweeteners have been developed because of inborn desires for sweetness. As much as possible, diabetic clients should be encouraged to eat foods without added sweeteners. However, their use may improve dietary compliance. Alternative sweeteners, both nonkilocaloric (e.g., aspartame and saccharin) and kilocaloric varieties (e.g., fructose and sorbitol), are not encouraged but acceptable in moderation (see Chapter 4, Table 4–8).

Fructose, sorbitol, and mannitol are kilocaloric sweeteners that have been recommended for use in diabetic diets or incorporated into "sugar-free" products. Use of kilocaloric sweeteners (glucose, lactose, fructose, and sorbitol) could perhaps undermine efforts to lose or maintain weight if not substituted for carbohydrate.

Fructose is better tolerated (lower hyperglycemia and insulin response) for most diabetic clients than sucrose or glucose (Thorburn et al, 1990; Grigoresco et al, 1988). However, in some NIDDM clients with hypertriglyceridemia, insulin and triglyceride levels may rise dramatically (Henry et al, 1991). Use of fructose should be limited so intake can still be nutritively adequate. The American Diabetes Association has warned that fructose should be used with caution in a diabetic diet (ADA, 1987).

Regular ingestion of sorbitol has been linked to "idiopathic" diarrhea in DM. Diabetics appear to be especially sensitive to sorbitol and are frequently unaware of its presence in foods and medications (Badiga et al, 1990).

NURSING APPLICATIONS

Assessment

Physical—for weight, height, IBW, weight changes, age, activity level, special medical problems, impaction, bowel sounds, diarrhea, malabsorption, client's lifestyle, stress, infection, illness, BP, poorly controlled DM, infection.

Dietary—for dietary preferences, usual eating patterns, intake of fiber, simple and complex carbohydrates, protein, fat, alcohol, fish preferences, vitamin supplements, alternative sweetener.

Laboratory—for glucose, insulin, cholesterol, triglycerides, LDL/HDL, proteinuria, BUN, creatinine, PT, PTT; sodium, potassium, chloride.

Interventions

Regarding carbohydrate:

1. If a client is on a high carbohydrate diet, monitor triglycerides. If triglycerides are elevated, consult the physician or dietitian to lower the carbohydrate diet.
2. Encourage legumes, beans, and whole-grain rice to improve control of blood glucose concentration without compromising overall nutrition and health (Jenkins et al, 1988).
3. In clients increasing their fiber intake, monitor for hypoglycemic reactions, as these may occur more often.
4. Individualize diet by working with client and dietitian.

Regarding protein:

1. Offer high-quality proteins including milk, egg whites, and meats to provide adequate amounts of protein and delay progression of renal disease (Zeller et al, 1991).
2. Provide specific information about correct portion sizes for meat (use food models, pictures, demonstrate on a scale).

Regarding alcohol:

1. Incorporate alcohol into the diet as 2 to 3 saturated fat exchanges or a combination of bread and fat exchanges, as shown in Table 27–13.

Regarding vitamins and electrolytes:

1. For clients with fluid retention, restrict dietary sodium (1000 mg/1000 kcal) to decrease adverse effects of diuretics on DM management.

Regarding alternative sweeteners:

1. If undetermined diarrhea occurs, collaborate with clients to see if ingestion of sorbitol is occurring.
2. Monitor blood glucose levels after ingestion of kilocaloric sweeteners.

Evaluation

* Client should achieve control of blood glucose by maintaining desired nutritional intake. Client/family should be able to plan a diabetic menu and choose/consume a well-balanced diet following their meal pattern.

Client Education

Regarding energy:

- It is recommended that kilocalories be distributed as follows: less than 20% from protein, less than 30% from fat, and the rest from carbohydrates.
- Three well-balanced meals are needed; do not skip meals or consume all the food at 1 meal.

Regarding carbohydrate:

- Unrefined complex carbohydrates (whole grains, legumes, brown rice, fruits, vegetables) are more desirable than simple carbohydrates.
- High glycemic index foods include cereals, bread, and root vegetables (carrots, parsnips, potatoes). Fruit juices have a higher postprandial glycemic effect than fresh fruits (Sullivan & Scott, 1991).
- At least 80 gm of carbohydrate must be consumed daily to prevent ketosis in adult diabetic clients.
- Increase fiber intake slowly; undesirable GI symptoms associated with increased fiber intake may require up to 3 to 4 months to subside (Hockaday, 1990).
- Fiber supplements are not recommended; they appear to be beneficial only if at least 50% of the kilocalories are from carbohydrates (ADA, 1992a). Raw fruits and vegetables are encouraged.

Regarding protein:

- Use of egg substitutes can add variety to diet.
- Fresh fruits or starches are recommended as snacks to maintain moderate protein intake.

Regarding fat:

- Some dietetic products can actually be hazardous; sugar-free products may contain more kilocalories in the form of fat than the original product.

Regarding alcohol:

- Excessive alcohol consumption without some food intake may cause hypoglycemia.
- Limit alcohol intake to 1 or 2 drinks in the course of an evening no more than once or twice a week.
- Hypoglycemic symptoms may be obscured by the cerebral effects of alcohol.
- Clients with peripheral neuropathy should limit alcohol intake to a single drink daily since excessive amounts may aggravate this condition.

Continued

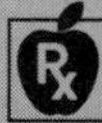 Hypoglycemia or antabuse-like reactions may occur in clients taking first-generation sulfonylurea drugs and drinking alcohol concurrently.

Regarding vitamins and electrolytes:

- Vitamin supplements, including thiamin and vitamin B_{12}, have been given to prevent diabetic neuropathy but have not been proven effective.
- Any diet restriction containing less than 1200 kcal requires vitamin supplementation.

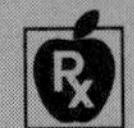 Diabetic clients are at greater risk for hyperkalemia with the use of potassium supplements or beta blockers.

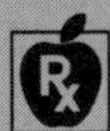 Diuretics combined with a beta blocker for hypertension may worsen diabetic control (blood glucose levels).

Regarding alternative sweeteners:

- Special foods are not required except perhaps sweeteners.
- Nonkilocalorie sweeteners, i.e., aspartame and saccharin, may be used in moderation. A variety of non-nutritive sweeteners is recommended to minimize potential risk from excessive consumption of any single type.
- The use of cinnamon, vanilla, spearmint, and anise exhibit properties related to sweetness and may be helpful in decreasing sugar content or the need for artificial sweeteners (Blank & Mattes, 1990).

SPECIAL CONSIDERATIONS IN INSULIN-DEPENDENT DIABETES MELLITUS

Maintaining HbA_{1C} levels less than 8% is associated with growth acceleration; inhibition of growth occurs when HbA_{1C} is greater than 16% (Wise et al, 1992). Early stages of puberty are most vulnerable to growth suppression. Glycemic equilibrium is basically managed by diet and insulin control. Other factors, such as variation in physical activity and emotional stresses, are more difficult to control. Lifestyle and physical activity must be considered when establishing the type and amount of insulin and distribution of nutrients for these clients.

A timetable for eating becomes tiresome and tedious but, if ignored, can cause unpleasant hypoglycemic consequences. For most people, unavoidable problems, such as airport delays and traffic jams, are annoying; for diabetic clients on insulin without access to food, such problems become frightening and even dangerous. Although most people never consider it, diabetic clients must always think about going from fed to fasted states because insulin secretions are not automatic. To adhere to a lifelong commitment of the diabetic regimen takes a great deal of discipline, and occasional dietary deviations should be put into a perspective of overall control rather than trying to elicit guilt. The psychological implications of a child never having a birthday cake may be worse than the effects of sugar in the cake. Other foods can be consumed simultaneously to moderate the effects of sugar.

Treatment of IDDM demands a multidisciplinary approach. Clients and their families are taught about the disorder and usual complications and receive guidance about daily management along with some insight into problems they may face. Additionally, teachers and school nurses must be aware of the situation. Although degenerative changes usually seen in diabetes should not be ignored, a positive approach is helpful.

Nurses who work with children and adolescents should understand behaviors and stages of growth and development. They should also have an acute awareness of everyday challenges to parents as well as to the child or adolescent. Preschool children must eat meals on time, take injections, and be protected against hypoglycemia. Later, the child must cope with school activities and lunches and hypoglycemia at school or parties and during other usual activities of childhood. For adolescents, being different is not the "in" thing; efforts should be made to normalize their diet as much as possible. There may be increased requirements for insulin, instability of the DM, accidents, and the usual stresses as an adolescent searches for independence.

Insulin

Endogenous insulin may be present when diabetes is first diagnosed, but it becomes nonexistent within a few years. Since the body does not produce insulin, daily lifelong injections are required. As a child grows or during illnesses, insulin dosages increase. This should be explained to parents so they do not interpret it as a deteriorating condition. During stable periods, the amount of insulin may be adjusted downward.

Approximately 76% of clients receiving insulin have NIDDM, which is not well controlled with oral hypoglycemic agents (Galloway, 1990). Insulin therapy may sometimes be required in NIDDM clients who are controlled with oral hypoglycemics, especially during illness or following surgery.

Timing and constancy of food intake for clients on insulin are the most important considerations (Table 27–14), but both diet and insulin intake must be tailored for a client's lifestyle. For instance, if an individual becomes nauseated when forced to eat breakfast, insulin and meal patterns should take this into consideration. In other words, familiarity with routine eating patterns influences insulin prescription.

Originally insulin was derived from beef and pork pancreas glands. Humulin insulin is identical to human insulin; because it is a synthetic product, it contains no impurities and is associated with fewer immunologically mediated allergic reac-

TABLE 27–14

DIETARY STRATEGIES FOR THE TWO MAIN TYPES OF DIABETES

Dietary Strategy	Type II (NIDDM)	Type I (IDDM)
Decrease kilocalories	Yes	No
Protect or improve beta cell function	Very urgent priority	Seldom important because beta cells are usually extinct
Increase frequency and number of feedings	Usually no*	Yes
Day to day consistency of intake of kilocalories, carbohydrates, protein, and fat	Not crucial if average kilocaloric intake remains in low range	Very important
Day to day consistency of the ratios of carbohydrate, protein, and fat for each of the feedings†	Not crucial	Desirable
Consistency of timing of meals	Not crucial	Very important
Extra food for unusual exercise	Not usually appropriate	Usually appropriate
Use of food to treat, abort, or prevent hypoglycemia	Not necessary	Important

* There are some theoretical advantages in dividing the diet into 4 or 5 feedings even in mild diabetes *if* this can be done without increasing kilocaloric consumption. However, because limitation of kilocalories has highest priority in obese diabetics, there are some potential disadvantages in providing extra feedings. Giving overweight people an opportunity to eat at bedtime is particularly "risky" if weight reduction is the prime goal.

† The total daily insulin requirement is apparently not much affected when dietary constituents are changed *under isocaloric conditions*. But insulin requirement *immediately* after a high-carbohydrate meal is higher than immediately after a low-carbohydrate meal, even if the meal is isocaloric.

From West KM. Diet therapy of diabetes: An analysis of failure. *Ann Intern Med* 1973; 79(3):425.

TABLE 27–15

TYPES OF INSULIN

Insulin	Onset (hr)*	Peak (hr)*	Duration (hr)*
Short Acting			
Regular	½	2–4	4–6
Semilente	½–2	3–10	8–10
Intermediate Acting			
NPH	1–2	6–12	10–14
Lente	1–3	6–12	12–18
Long-Acting			
Ultalente	4–6	Minimal	18–36
NPH and Regular Premixed			
(30% R/70% N)	½+	2–4/8±	8+18–24

* These times are averages and vary between clients, as the insulins are dependent on the dosage given and injection site.

Adapted from Ignatavicius DD, Bayne MV. *Medical-Surgical Nursing.* Philadelphia, WB Saunders, 1991.

tions. Clients need to be aware of which insulin source has been prescribed; absorption rate and duration of action are different.

Several types of insulin are available; their action is different with regard to onset, peak, and duration of activity (Table 27–15). The type, dosage, and frequency of insulin are individually tailored for clients, depending on the stage of growth, physical status, and activity level. Coordination between peak action of insulin and timing of meals/snacks is important. This provides available glucose when insulin level is high. If glucose is insufficient relative to the amount of insulin present or if a meal is omitted, hypoglycemia may occur.

Regular insulin is used for immediate effects such as for surgery or ketoacidosis. Regular insulin may be used in IDDM to give a more balanced level of blood glucose. Because of the number of injections needed daily, it is seldom used on a regular basis by itself except with an insulin pump.

Continuous subcutaneous insulin infusion, or **insulin pumps,** can dramatically improve a diabetic's ability to maintain a stable and satisfying life (Fig. 27–3). Insulin delivery can be preprogrammed for continuous infusion of small amounts of insulin or larger amounts administered before meals or when blood glucose levels are elevated. Regular insulin is used to simulate normal physiological response to dietary intake or elevated glucose levels. Clients have a great advantage for controlling timing and amount of insulin in relation to the time and size of a meal. Self-monitoring blood glucose is used to adjust insulin injections appropriately.

A continuous subcutaneous insulin infusion or insulin pump is a small lightweight pump worn 24 hours a day that provides insulin through tubing via a needle inserted subcutaneously.

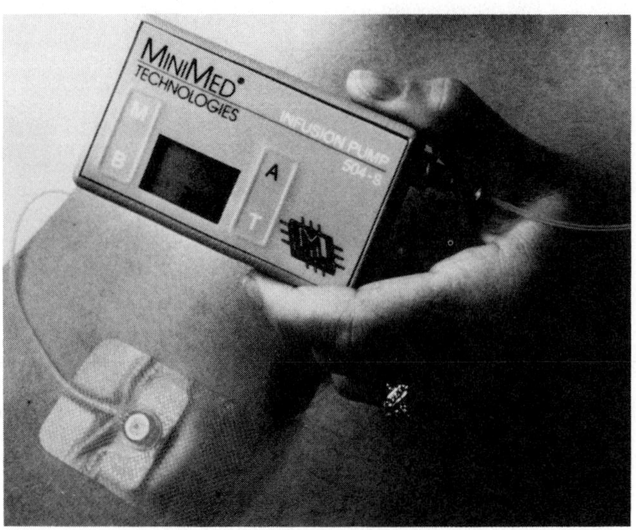

Figure 27–3 Subcutaneous insulin pumps allow more normal insulin infusion when food is consumed and insulin is needed to metabolize glucose. (Courtesy of MiniMed Technologies, Sylmar, CA.)

Intermediate-acting insulins are presently the most popular because their action is more intermediate in duration and intensity; they are injected once or twice daily alone or in conjunction with regular insulin. An afternoon and bedtime snack is usually given. The breakdown of food exchanges and a sample menu are provided in Figure 27–4 for an IDDM client using an intermediate-acting insulin.

Diet Prescription: 2000 kcal (275 gm carbohydrate, 70 gm protein, 65 gm fat)

Mealtime Division:

20% Breakfast
30% Lunch
10% Midafternoon snack
30% Dinner
10% Bedtime snack

% Energy Nutrient Distribution:

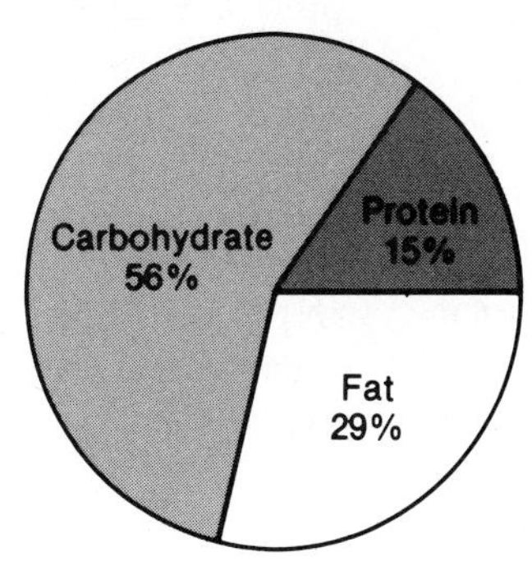

Total Daily Division of Food into Exchanges:

Exchange List	No. of Exchanges
Starch/bread	8
Meat, lean	4
Vegetables	3
Fruit	8
Milk, nonfat	2
Fats	9

Sample Meal Plan	No. of Exchanges	Sample Menu
Breakfast		
Fruit	1	1/2 banana
Starch/bread	2	3/4 cup bran flakes
		1 slice whole-wheat toast
Fat	2	2 tsp safflower margarine
Milk	1	1 cup skim milk
Free		2 tsp sugar-free jam
Lunch		
Meat, lean	2	2 oz lean broiled pork chop
Starch/bread	2	1/2 cup scalloped potatoes
		1 whole-wheat roll
Vegetable	1	1/2 cup cooked carrots
Free		1/2 cup cabbage slaw
Fats	3	1 tbsp reduced-kilocalorie mayonnaise (in slaw)
		2 tsp safflower margarine (in scalloped potatoes and for roll)
Fruit	3	1/3 cup pineapple chunks (in slaw)
		1 baked apple
Snack		
Fruit	1	2 pear halves canned in juice
Starch/bread	1	6 crackers
Dinner		
Meat, lean	2	2 oz beef cubes
Starch/bread	3	1/2 cup noodles
		2 slices whole-wheat bread
Vegetable	2	1/2 cup broccoli
		1/2 cup steamed summer squash
Free		Relishes: cherry tomato, celery sticks, radishes, cucumber slices
Fat	2	2 tsp safflower margarine
Fruit	2	1 1/2 cup fresh blueberries
Bedtime Snack		
Milk, nonfat	1	1 cup plain yogurt
Fruit	1	2 tbsp raisins (in yogurt)
Fat	2	2 tbsp chopped nuts (in yogurt)

Coffee, tea, and artificially sweetened beverages are allowed as desired.

Figure 27–4 Meal planning for an insulin-dependent diabetic using a combination of regular and intermediate-acting insulin.

Long-lasting insulin is not widely used because of its prolonged action (approximately 24 hours). When this type is used, a bedtime feeding is essential. Carbohydrate distribution may be divided into 3 meals and a snack, as follows: 20% at breakfast, 25% at lunch; 35% at dinner, and 20% at bedtime.

Types of insulin can be mixed to approximate glycemic equilibrium and to fit into a client's lifestyle. Usually the insulin regimen consists of multiple injections using a combination of regular plus intermediate-acting insulins; various regimens are based on a client's status and physician's preference. Intermediate-acting insulin may be given alone twice a day—before breakfast and before supper. Or regular and intermediate-acting insulin may be given together before breakfast and supper. A multidose insulin (MDI) therapy involves 3 or 4 injections of regular insulin before meals coupled with intermediate-acting or long-acting insulin, i.e., premeal regular insulin plus long-acting insulin once or twice a day, or regular insulin before meals with an injection of intermediate-acting insulin at bedtime. For instance, a farmer who enjoys a large breakfast might be given a combination of regular and NPH insulin in the morning and evening. Carbohydrate distribution would then be divided to provide a larger breakfast (30%), smaller lunch (30%) and dinner (20%), with mid-afternoon and bedtime snacks each consisting of 10% of the total kilocalories.

How long must the IDDM client take insulin? When do NIDDM clients need insulin? Why is timing of meals and insulin important?

Exercise

Diabetic clients experience the same benefits from exercise as nondiabetics. In addition, muscular exercise improves the body's ability to use glucose, increases effectiveness of insulin, and improves risk factors related to heart disease (increases HDL cholesterol and lowers serum triglycerides). If exercise is performed routinely, insulin requirements may be decreased (does not replace insulin).

Diabetic children should be encouraged to participate in active sports, e.g., soccer or basketball. They should also understand the effects of exercise on insulin usage. Consistent, regular exercise 3 times a week is more advantageous than sporadic and taxing workouts. Physical activity is erratic in most people, but it has profound effects on insulin needs.

Exercise should be done when the blood glucose level is between 100 and 200 mg/dl (30 to 60 minutes after a meal) rather than when insulin is at its peak. If the blood glucose level is over 250 mg/dl, glucose uptake by the cell is decreased, and glucose production by the liver is increased. Thus, exercise at this time worsens hyperglycemia, leading to ketosis.

Short exercise periods of modest intensity do not require additional feedings. When a diabetic client anticipates an extensive special exercise, additional carbohydrate is needed. A typical allowance might include 10 to 15 gm/hour for moderate exercise, such as playing golf, or 20 to 30 gm/hour for a vigorous exercise, such as playing soccer or digging (Table 27–16).

Diabetic clients active in sports or vigorous activities can increase their food intake earlier in the day or in days preceding the event along with an increase in short-acting insulin (Greenhalgh, 1990). Diabetic athletes are at greater risk of delayed absorption of carbohydrate, gastric stasis, and vomiting. A large meal just before vigorous activity is discouraged, and clients might be better advised to eat a complex carbohydrate snack to maintain glycemic level until the next regular meal.

How is exercise beneficial to IDDM clients? At what blood glucose level should exercise not be initiated?

Nutritional Care

Nutritional care for IDDM clients is to provide adequate kilocalories for growth and weight gain and to help avoid wide fluctuations in glycemic levels. Several factors should be considered when planning a diet for these individuals: (1) meal tim-

TABLE 27–16

MAKING FOOD ADJUSTMENTS FOR EXERCISE: GENERAL GUIDELINES

Type of Exercise and Examples	If Blood Glucose Is:	Increased Food Intake By:	Suggestions of Food to Use
Exercise of short duration and of low to moderate intensity (walking a half mile or leisurely bicycling for less than 30 minutes)	Less than 100 mg/dl	10 to 15 gm carbohydrate per hour	1 fruit or 1 starch/bread exchange
	100 mg/dl or above	Not necessary to increase food	
Exercise of moderate intensity (one hour of tennis, swimming, jogging, leisurely bicycling, golfing, etc)	Less than 100 mg/dl	25 to 50 gm carbohydrate before exercise, then 10 to 15 gm/hour of exercise	½ meat sandwich with a milk or fruit exchange
	100 to 180 mg/dl	10 to 15 gm carbohydrate	1 fruit or 1 starch/bread exchange
	180 to 300 mg/dl	Not necessary to increase food	
	300 mg/dl or above	Don't begin exercise until blood glucose is under better control	
Strenuous activity or exercise (about one to two hours of football, hockey, racquetball, or basketball games; strenuous bicycling or swimming; shoveling heavy snow)	Less than 100 mg/dl	50 gm carbohydrate, monitor blood glucose carefully	1 meat sandwich (2 slices of bread) with a milk and fruit exchange
	100 to 180 mg/dl	25 to 50 gm carbohydrate, depending on intensity and duration	½ meat sandwich with a milk or fruit exchange
	180 to 300 mg/dl	10 to 15 gm carbohydrate	1 fruit or 1 bread exchange
	300 mg/dl or above	Don't begin exercise until blood glucose is under better control	

Reprinted, with permission, from *Diabetes Actively Staying Healthy (DASH): Your Game Plan for Diabetes and Exercise,* by Marion J. Franz, MS, RD and Jane Norstrom, MA. Minneapolis: International Diabetes Center, 1990.

ing, (2) diet composition, (3) energy content, (4) amount of physical activity, and (5) insulin regimen.

Diet composition should be in the percentages recommended earlier. Protein allowances for juvenile diabetics should be on the generous side because of requirements for growth and development. After severe infections or episodes of ketoacidosis, protein needs are increased to replenish protein catabolized during the stressful situation.

Energy needs for these clients are the same as for nondiabetics. Growth spurts and hormonal changes influence energy requirements. Since many are thin when first diagnosed, energy allowances should be adequate for normal growth and development to attain a desirable body weight. Variations in exercise patterns may require adjustments in food intake.

Food intake should be spaced so it takes into account the type of insulin (and the period of peak action). Consistency of meal timing is essential.

IDDM clients are more effectively treated when several snacks are allowed to avoid hypoglycemia. However, these snacks should be planned to suit the circumstances under which a client is supposed to consume them. Snacks that fit into a client's regular schedule become a pleasant habit and a dependable element of their therapeutic program. Clients who use an insulin pump can enjoy a more flexible meal schedule.

NURSING APPLICATIONS

Assessment

Physical—for height, weight, patterns of growth; BP; type of insulin, physical activity level.

Dietary—for dietary compliance; frequency of intake; intake of fast foods, fiber, alcohol.

Laboratory—for blood glucose levels, HgA_{1C}, lipoprotein profile, albuminuria, urine ketones.

Interventions

1. Problem solve different situations that may interfere with adhering to meal plans (activities, eating out, dates, weekend schedules). Anticipatory guidance can enhance compliance.
2. Offer support and empathy for clients and family. Focus on the positive. Tell parents they did nothing wrong to cause this disease and that they are not at fault (McEvilly, 1991).
3. Provide information on less obvious sources of fat. IDDM adolescents routinely consume increased amounts of energy, principally from fat sources (Schmidt et al, 1992).
4. Monitor a client's tray after each meal to be certain he or she is eating well. If an IDDM client does not eat everything, substitutions should be made to prevent hypoglycemia. In addition to the replacement of actual carbohydrate, potential glucose available from protein (58%) and fat (10%) should be replaced.
5. Refer clients to a dietitian or physician for suggestions dealing with irregular schedules, for instance, being a guest in another's home or traveling that results in jet lag.
6. Administer insulin injections 45 minutes before meals to prevent hypoglycemia and obtain the most acceptable pattern of glucose concentrations.
7. Introduce client/family to other families who have a child with DM.

Evaluation

* Client should maintain weight for height, comply/consume ordered diet, recognize the importance of meal timing and insulin administration (verbalize how to adjust diet and insulin), exercise regularly, maintain blood glucose near normal, and avoid hypoglycemic reactions.

Client Education

- Physical activity should be considered in relation to meal scheduling and insulin dosage to avoid hypoglycemia and ketosis.
- For many children, peak insulin activity is in the afternoon, at which time hypoglycemia is most likely to occur if participating in after-school sports activities. A planned or extra snack may be used to compensate for this extra exercise, or glucose tablets or other quick-acting carbohydrate should be available.
- Regularity of food intake and exercise are of paramount importance.
- Exercise should be avoided if blood glucose levels are greater than 250 to 300 mg/dl and ketones are present.
- Hypoglycemia may occur during exercise and for up to 24 hours after strenuous exercise.

- To avoid unexpected hypoglycemia, inject insulin into areas that will not be used when exercising. Insulin will be used faster in the exercised area, i.e., if client is going to jog, do not inject insulin into thigh.
- A snack consisting of 15 gm carbohydrate (fruit or bread exchange or equivalent) may be consumed 1 hour before exercise (see Table 27–16). This does not need to be counted as part of the daily allowance.
- Since insulin injections are given at a specific time, meals and snacks should be eaten at consistent times.
- Glucose should be carried at all times, and a medical identification bracelet is a sensible precaution.

SPECIAL CONSIDERATIONS OF NONINSULIN-DEPENDENT DIABETES MELLITUS

Most cases of NIDDM are secondary to excessive kilocaloric intake and resultant obesity; in some cases, weight loss alone (to within about 15% IBW) is often all that is necessary to produce lower and sometimes acceptable blood glucose levels. There is no relationship between amount of weight lost and improvement of insulin response. Every pound counts. Wing et al (1990) found that improvement of glycemic control with weight loss was more profound in clients with higher initial glucose levels.

A fat cell response to insulin is inversely proportional to its size; the larger the cell, the less responsive it is to insulin. Abnormal glucose tolerance is found even though plasma insulin level is high, indicating insulin resistance or inadequate cell receptors. Primary treatment modalities for NIDDM are nutrition, exercise, and, if necessary, medication.

NIDDM clients are normally not prone to ketosis, but it may occur during stress or infection. Vascular complications and degenerative changes are common.

Explain how fat cell size or obesity affects insulin.

Oral Hypoglycemic Agents

Oral hypoglycemic agents may be necessary to control glycemic levels in some NIDDM clients. Others are able to obtain good control with diet and exercise. Sulfonylureas (Orinase, DiaBeta) lower blood glucose concentrations primarily by stimulating insulin secretion (Groop, 1992). These drugs are effective only if the pancreas is able to produce insulin. Oral hypoglycemic medications are listed in Table 27–17. Second-generation compounds, glipizide and glyburide, are more po-

TABLE 27–17

PHARMACOKINETICS OF ORAL HYPOGLYCEMICS

Drug	Duration of Activity
First-generation sulfonylureas	
Acetohexamide (Dymelor)	12–18+ hours
Chlorpropamide (Diabinese)	24–72 hours
Tolazamide (Tolinase)	10–16+ hours
Tolbutamide (Orinase)	6–12 hours
Second-generation sulfonylureas	
Glyburide (DiaBeta, Micronase)	24 hours
Glipizide (Glucotrol)	16–24 hours

Adapted from Shimizu HH. Do Yourself a Flavor. *FDA Consumer*. US Department of Health and Human Services. Pub No. 84–2192. 1984.

tent in insulin-releasing capacity and have fewer side effects. They may elicit insulin secretion only when hyperglycemia is present. These drugs are popular with clients because the necessity for dieting is often not emphasized.

Insulin is not recommended for obese clients because of the large amounts that must be given to normalize their blood glucose. In these large doses, appetite may be increased along with decreased insulin utilization. This results in increased food intake, weight gain, and the need for even more insulin. Additionally, insulin, an anabolic hormone, may increase fat deposits and fluid retention. Therefore, insulin should be given only as a last resort or for specific conditions such as ketoacidosis or pregnancy.

Why is insulin not routinely given to NIDDM?

Exercise

In addition to benefits of exercise by normal clients, NIDDM clients may benefit with lower blood pressure (and chronic problems attributed to hypertension) and weight loss. Exercise can lower blood glucose levels and reverse insulin resistance, resulting in decreased dependency on hypoglycemic agents. Regular activities combined with a weight loss diet often control NIDDM.

Exercise does not automatically cause weight loss. Increased use of muscle causes some increase in lean body mass and therefore a small weight increase.

What are the benefits of exercise for NIDDM?

Nutritional Care

Clients can frequently be managed successfully with diet alone or with a combination of diet and oral hypoglycemics. A blood glucose level less than 180 to 200 mg/dl responds better to dietary intervention. Basic objectives of diet therapy in NIDDM are to provide adequate nutrition at regular intervals; maintain IBW; and prevent secondary complications of retinopathy, neuropathy, nephropathy, and macrovascular disease. An individualized meal plan, considering age, physical activity, daily routine, and medications, is important to promote client compliance.

Clients who are within their IBW are encouraged to maintain their body weight and modify food composition and eating patterns to minimize glucose fluctuations. The goal for overweight clients is to achieve IBW or to be on the low side of IBW range for their height. Weight reduction can be accomplished by reducing total energy intake to levels below energy expenditure and increasing activities.

The diet should provide adequate nutrients with appropriate kilocaloric intake to cause weight loss. Because weight loss is not an easy task, a diet program requires incentive, vigor, and skill on the part of all involved. A client should have an appreciation of the benefits of weight reduction on the disease course. Rate of weight loss is slow; a single eating binge may undo several weeks of successful dieting efforts. It is believed that by restricting energy, glucose tolerance is improved via several mechanisms: (1) Fat cell size is decreased, (2) available insulin increases the rate of glucose metabolism, and (3) more fatty acids are synthesized from glucose. Weight loss is also successful in lowering cholesterol and triglycerides.

Meals should be regular, and the relationship of meals to physical activity is important. However, this requirement is less important than decreased energy intake. Meals are normally distributed equally, with one-third of the carbohydrate being given at each meal. They are evenly spaced throughout the waking hours (every 4 to 5 hours). Snacks are usually discouraged to allow the blood glucose to return to normal and prevent further weight gain. There may be metabolic advantages in allowing more frequent feedings, but the possibility of overconsumption and its adverse effects on weight must be considered (Jenkins et al, 1992).

A typical diet prescription provides 10 to 30% of the energy in breakfast, 25 to 35% in lunch and dinner, and sometimes 0 to 25% for between-meal snacks. This

Diet Prescription: 1200 kcal (125 gm carbohydrate, 70 gm protein, 45 gm fat)

Mealtime Division:

Equally divided into 3 meals

% Energy Nutrient Distribution:

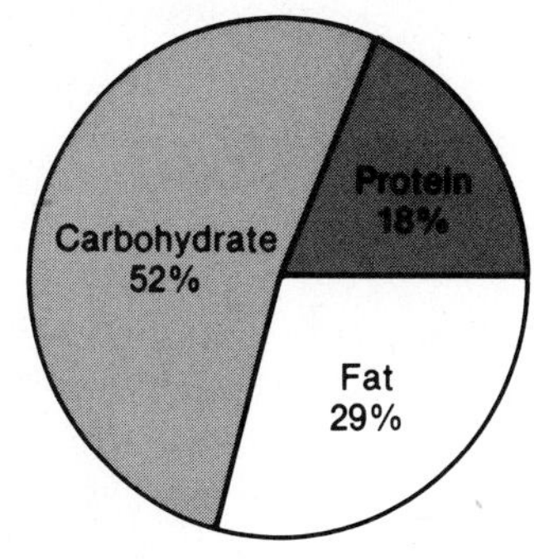

Total Daily Division of Food into Exchanges:

Exchange List	No. of Exchanges
Starch/bread	5
Meat, lean	4
Vegetables	2
Fruit	4
Milk, nonfat	1
Fat	4

Sample Meal Plan	No. of Exchanges	Sample Menu
Breakfast		
Fruit	1	1/2 banana
Starch/bread	2	3/4 cup bran flakes 1 slice whole-wheat toast
Fat	1	1 tsp safflower margarine
Milk, nonfat	1/2	1/2 cup skim milk
Free		2 tsp sugar-free jam
Lunch		
Meat, lean	2	2 oz lean broiled pork chop
Starch/bread	1	1/2 cup scalloped potatoes
Vegetable	1	1/2 cup cooked carrots
Free		1/2 cup cabbage slaw
Fats	2	1 tbsp reduced-kilocalorie mayonnaise (in slaw) 1 tsp safflower margarine (in scalloped potatoes and for roll)
Fruit	2	1 baked apple

Sample Meal Plan	No. of Exchanges	Sample Menu
Dinner		
Meat, lean	2	2 oz beef cubes
Starch, bread	2	1/2 cup noodles 1 slice whole-wheat bread
Vegetable	2	1/2 cup broccoli
Free		Relishes: cherry tomato, celery sticks, radishes, cucumber slices
Fat	1	1 tsp safflower margarine
Milk, nonfat	1/2	1/2 cup skim milk
Fruit	1	1 3/4 cup fresh blueberries

Coffee, tea, and artificially sweetened beverages are allowed as desired.

Supplement with multivitamin supplement and calcium.

Figure 27–5 Meal planning for a noninsulin-dependent diabetic client.

distribution must take into account a client's preferences and lifestyle. A sample menu for NIDDM is shown in Figure 27–5.

What are the goals for NIDDM diet therapy?

Very-Low-Calorie Diets

As a result of frustrating efforts and the difficulty of achieving weight loss using regular 1000 to 1200 kilocalorie diets, 600 to 800 kcal liquid diets have been employed in NIDDM to provide a structured weight loss program. With careful monitoring, very-low-calorie diets (VLCD) can be safe and effective in obese NIDDM. Glucose control and associated coronary risk factors have shown short-term improvement (Henry & Gumbiner, 1991; Uusitupa et al, 1990). Weight loss is rapid. However, in long-term follow-up studies, clients treated with VLCD gained more weight during the year following this dietary regimen than the control group. Even with this weight gain, fasting insulin levels and OGTT continued to be improved (Wing et al, 1991).

NURSING APPLICATIONS

Assessment

Physical—for weight, type of oral hypoglycemic medication or insulin, activity level, BP.
Dietary—for food preferences, dietary compliance, frequency of intake, use of fad diets, previous weight loss attempts.
Laboratory—for glucose, lipoprotein profile.

Interventions

1. Involve client and family in nutritional care, especially weight loss measures to enhance compliance.
2. Praise the client for appropriate food choices and weight loss since praised behavior is repeated.

Evaluation

* Client should consume a high-carbohydrate, low-fat, moderate-protein diet; maintain IBW; exercise; and verbalize a desire to adhere to the DM management plan.

Client Education

- Oral hypoglycemics should be used in conjunction with reduction diets and exercise.
- Oral hypoglycemics are not advisable for clients with other diseases, such as liver or kidney disorders, or during pregnancy.
- About a week is necessary for metabolic processes to stabilize when oral hypoglycemics are given; doses should not be changed too quickly.
- NIDDM clients who take insulin are insulin requiring, not insulin dependent. Because NIDDM clients produce some insulin, they are not ketosis prone and do not require insulin for survival. Inappropriately high levels of insulin cause polyphagia, leading to increased weight.
- NIDDM clients who are over 30 years of age or have had diabetes for 10 years or more should consult their physician before beginning an exercise program.
- Weight loss for obese clients with NIDDM results in lower glucose levels.
- Exercise is recommended for all NIDDM clients to help decrease insulin resistance. No additional food is needed if insulin or oral agents are not prescribed.

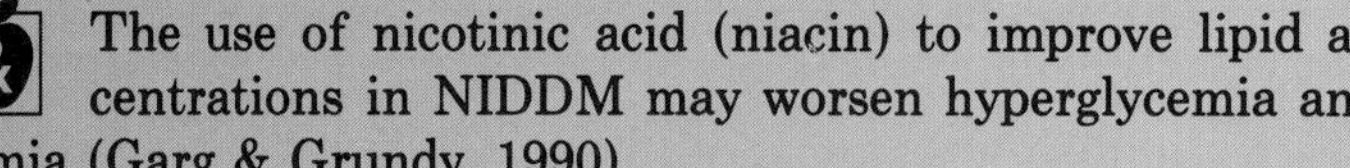

The use of nicotinic acid (niacin) to improve lipid and lipoprotein concentrations in NIDDM may worsen hyperglycemia and cause hyperuricemia (Garg & Grundy, 1990).

SPECIAL CONSIDERATIONS FOR ILLNESS OR SURGERY

Special measures are required for diabetic clients when illness decreases the appetite or interferes with eating habits. Even though the client is ill, insulin is necessary and may actually need to be increased during febrile illnesses. Increased levels of counterregulatory hormones increase glycemic levels, and cellular insulin utilization is decreased. Insulin prevents lipolysis, which leads to ketoacidosis. NIDDM clients may require insulin temporarily during illness or infections.

Vomiting or diarrhea that may be minor for most persons may become complicated in a diabetic client. Because of rapid fluid and electrolyte losses, the physician should be notified if either condition occurs.

Hourly or frequent liquid intake helps replace fluid losses. Carbohydrate is necessary to prevent hypoglycemia and provide a source of glucose to curb ketone production. When sickness impairs appetite and digestion, simple sugars in the form of juices, custards, ice cream, and sweetened beverages are used to replace the normal carbohydrate value of solid foods (see Table 27–6). These foods may be used on an emergency basis for a 3-day period. If used longer, the physician should be consulted. To replace sodium, potassium, and water lost from vomiting and diarrhea, salty foods such as crackers and broth should be included. Small, frequent, high-carbohydrate feedings can be used. Protein and fat allowances may be ignored in attempts to provide adequate carbohydrate-containing foods.

If the illness is not gastrointestinal, semi-liquid foods such as dairy foods and soft-cooked eggs or custards are desirable. Table 27–18 shows an example of a replacement meal. It can be taken in small, frequent amounts, rather than as a meal. Dietary carbohydrate portion can be met on a clear-liquid diet; the entire carbohydrate, protein, and fat requirements can be met on a full-liquid diet.

Following uncomplicated surgery that does not interfere with GI function, a client is usually able to resume oral feedings within 2 to 3 days. Normally the traditional progression from clear liquids to full liquids, followed by regular consistency is followed. Advances should be made as quickly as possible to meet nutrient needs.

If intake is inadequate, the diet can be boosted using supplemental formulas or adding modular protein, fat, and carbohydrate components to soups, milk, or other foods tolerated. A nutritional supplement should be composed of 50% carbohydrate, 20% protein, and 30% fat. Supplements can be calculated as a part of the diet plan.

Why do diabetic clients who are ill need insulin? Describe nutritional measures to follow when a client is ill.

NURSING APPLICATIONS

Assessment

Physical—for type of illness, surgery, fever, vomiting, diarrhea, dehydration.
Dietary—for type of foods/fluid ingested, time of last intake.
Laboratory—for glucose, urine ketones.

Interventions

1. Monitor blood glucose levels and urinary ketones every 3 to 4 hours to determine effectiveness of care and physical status of client.
2. Emphasize the need for providing obligatory glucose during illness or infections so clients do not become overly concerned when a clear liquid tray is served.
3. Offer at least 50 gm of carbohydrate every 3 to 4 hours unless blood glucose is higher than 240 mg/dl to prevent ketosis.
4. Offer kilocalorie-free drinks (broth, bouillon, tea, water, sugar-free soda) to replace fluids lost from fever and diaphoresis if client is eating well at meals.

Evaluation

* Client should verbalize correct fluid/meal replacement regimen illness.

Client Education

- During illness, insulin or an oral hypoglycemic agent is needed to prevent ketoacidosis or hyperglycemia. Monitor blood glucose and urine ketones every 3 to 4 hours.
- Explain how illness increases blood glucose.
- Call the physician when urine ketones are positive or blood glucose level remains high (>200 mg/dl).

TABLE 27–18

REPLACEMENT CARBOHYDRATE FOR ILLNESS

Usual Meal Pattern	Carbohydrate	Replacement Carbohydrates	Carbohydrate
3 meat exchanges	0	2 cups broth	0
2 bread exchanges	30	1 cup ginger ale	20
2 fat exchanges	0	½ cup regular fruit-flavored gelatin	20
1 fruit exchange	15	⅓ cup grape juice	15
1 milk exchange	12	Hot tea (no sugar)	0
Total	57	Total	55

SPECIAL CONSIDERATIONS FOR NUTRITION SUPPORT

Enteral feedings are appropriate for diabetic clients with inadequate oral intake and a functioning GI tract. Risks are the same as for any normal client receiving an enteral feeding. Diabetic clients with frequent hypoglycemic episodes may exhibit slow gastric emptying; risk of aspiration may be exaggerated. Contributing factors relating to gastroparesis include secretory abnormalities, peptic ulcer disease, gastric mucosal alterations, and increased antibody production. Hyperosmolar formulas may contribute to the problem. Hyperglycemia may also inhibit HCl secretion.

Intermittent feedings improve metabolic control in diabetic clients; simulation of a normal meal pattern may result in increased nutrient absorption and glucose utilization (Phillips, 1987; Jones et al, 1980). However, bolus feedings may increase aspiration risk. In many critically ill clients, continuous feedings are necessary, promoting gradual absorption of carbohydrate and other nutrients, and insulin may be provided with continuous peripheral IV infusion or sliding scale coverage. Blood glucose should be maintained below 200 mg/dl. Use of an IV insulin drip is rather treacherous if the enteral feeding stops but the insulin drip continues to run; this practice is not advisable unless constant monitoring is available.

Carbohydrate content of the formula has a significant effect on glycemic response (Peters & Davidson, 1992). A commercial formula, Glucerna (Ross), is specially designed for diabetic clients. Carbohydrates (as glucose polymers and fructose) are restricted (33%), and soluble fiber is added. Fat content is high (50%); a large portion of the fat is monounsaturated, which promotes normal levels of lipoproteins (Brackenridge & Campbell, 1990). One study associated the use of Glucerna with more stable blood glucose levels (Peters et al, 1989). Because of the formula's high cost and variability among individual client responses, it may be advantageous to initiate a diabetic client (especially if NIDDM) on a regular formula with a normal distribution of energy nutrients. Blood glucose levels are closely monitored, especially initially. If blood glucose level is exceptionally high, the formula is changed.

Many elemental formulas contain greater than 60% carbohydrate and minimal amounts of fat, and most have a high osmolality. If an elemental formula is needed, it is best to use one of the newer products in which the energy nutrient distribution is similar to recommended levels, and osmolality is lower.

What is the goal of maintaining serum glucose levels when on continuous tube feedings? If an elemental formula is used, what considerations should be followed? Why is TPN more desirable than PPN?

PPN can be safely used in DM for supplemental or short-term nutrition support. PPN solutions for DM should contain fat emulsions in addition to the traditionally used amino acids and dextrose solutions. TPN is favored because of decreased amounts of glucose infusions as a result of lipid infusions, which are well utilized. PN infusions are initiated slowly with close monitoring of blood glucose levels; insulin is added to the infusion. A client is weaned from TPN gradually to avoid hypoglycemia.

NURSING APPLICATIONS

Assessment

Physical—for reason for nutrition support, type of nutrition support; baseline weight, serial weights (2 to 3 times/week).
Dietary—for type of formula used.
Laboratory—for glucose, triglyceride levels.

Interventions

1. Keep head of bed elevated at all times with tube feedings to prevent aspiration.
2. Monitor gastric residual at least every 4 to 8 hours or before each bolus feeding to prevent overfilling of the stomach, possibly leading to aspiration and to determine that volume of feeding is appropriate for client.
3. Throughout TPN, monitor blood glucose every 4 hours to ensure proper insulin coverage.
4. Keep accurate I&O records to detect polyuria or possible impending dehydration.
5. Monitor urine ketones every 6 hours to ensure that excessive lipolysis is not occurring.

Evaluation

* Client's blood glucose should remain below 200 mg/dl while receiving nutrition support.

Client Education

- Explain why nutrition support is needed.
- Discuss why the client's blood glucose may be high at this time. Assure the NIDDM client that when the blood glucose is above 200 mg/dl, medicines are used to control the blood glucose, but this is probably temporary.

SPECIAL CONSIDERATIONS FOR PREGNANCY

Good diabetic or near-normal glycemic control in early pregnancy reduces the frequency of congenital abnormalities (Gregory & Tattersall, 1992; Kitzmiller et al, 1991). If DM is controlled, fertility of diabetic women is normal, maternal mortality is almost negligible, and fetal survival rate approaches that of nondiabetics. Without strict control of DM, major congenital anomalies affect 4 to 12% of infants of diabetic mothers (Jovanovic-Peterson et al, 1991).

Most fetal malformations occur during the first trimester of pregnancy as a result of any of the metabolic disorders associated with DM affecting glucose, insulin, or ketone levels (Miodovnik, et al, 1988). A woman may not even be aware of the pregnancy; therefore, a great concern is for prepregnancy counseling with control of the diabetic condition before conception. Hyperglycemia is a potential risk for both mother and infant. Maternal obesity or poor glycemic control increases risk of infant **macrosomia** (Jovanovic-Peterson et al, 1991; Thompson et al, 1990).

Macrosomia—larger body size.

Numerous changes during pregnancy affect DM control and insulin utilization, when euglycemia is most important but harder to achieve. Hormones and enzymes produced by the placenta are antagonistic to insulin or increase its degradation. Elevated levels of estrogen (especially in the first trimester) and progesterone indirectly affect carbohydrate metabolism by their effects on insulin. Maternal insulin does not cross the placenta, but glucose does. When the fetal blood glucose level is too high, the fetus's pancreas increases insulin production. Insulin is the "growth" hormone for the developing fetus, causing macrosomia. These high insulin levels are also implicated in infant hypoglycemia that frequently occurs shortly after birth. Another problem caused by increased insulin levels is hypokalemia, which leads to flaccid muscles and can cause fatal arrhythmias in an infant. Newborn infants may present other problems such as respiratory difficulties, hypocalcemia, and/or jaundice.

Ketones are passed to the developing fetus; currently it is controversial whether they cause lasting damage to the infant. Avoidance of exposing the fetus to ketones seems prudent. Ketones should be monitored because during pregnancy, blood glucose may be normal even though the gravida may be approaching a state of ketoacidosis. Therefore, weight loss is not advisable for obese diabetic women.

As a consequence of metabolic changes, insulin requirements vary during pregnancy. Insulin dosage must be reduced early in pregnancy when the mother tends to become hypoglycemic, but the dose may be doubled or tripled later with a leveling off by about the eighth month.

Gestational diabetes is the occurrence of hyperglycemia that develops during pregnancy.

Gestational diabetes occurs in about 2 to 3% of all pregnancies, probably caused by the potentially diabetogenic hormones present to support a pregnancy. If endogenous insulin secretions are inadequate, hyperglycemia occurs. During standard obstetric care, blood glucose levels are screened initially and again at 24 to 26 weeks of pregnancy. Women at risk for gestational diabetes include obese clients or those with a family history of DM or a personal history of large babies, spontaneous abortion, **hydramnios,** or glycosuria. Gestational diabetes usually disappears after delivery unless the DM is actually a preexisting mild condition first discovered during pregnancy. Periodic checkups following the pregnancy are suggested since there is an increased risk for developing DM later in life.

Hydramnios—excessive amniotic fluid.

Why is glucose control difficult during pregnancy?

Treatment

Team management during pregnancy to minimize possible congenital abnormalities may include an internist (diabetologist), obstetrician (perinatologist), pediatrician (neonatologist), nurse-educator, dietitian, and social worker. Perinatal complications can be reduced by intense efforts to control DM by means of hospitalization, bed rest, and close supervision by specialized team members.

Adequate nutrients for a normal pregnancy plus avoidance of hyperglycemia and hypoglycemia are the goals for a pregnant diabetic. Maintaining maternal fasting blood glucose levels between 60 and 80 mg/dl and postprandial blood glucose levels between 100 and 140 mg/dl in both pregestational and gestational diabetic clients is believed to maintain normal fetal weight and reduce perinatal mortality (Kitzmiller et al, 1991). Exercise is advocated to help control blood glucose and prevent excessive weight gain and hypertension. If diet and exercise are not effective in controlling blood glucose, insulin injections are implemented, which will be necessary for the remainder of the pregnancy. Self-monitoring blood glucose is required if insulin is necessary (ADA, 1992b).

Nutritional Care

Desired weight gains and nutrient requirements are the same as for nondiabetics (see Chapter 14)—32 kcal/kg IBW for the first trimester and 38 kcal/kg IBW thereafter. Lowered energy intake is not usually recommended even for an obese client since weight reduction may induce ketosis or nutritional inadequacy. Utilization of insulin may be favored over kilocaloric reduction to improve glucose regulation. However, recent studies indicate that a modest kilocaloric reduction (1200 to 1800 kcal) has resulted in healthy infants with normal birth weights (Hollingsworth & Ney, 1992; Dornhorst et al, 1991; Knopp et al, 1991). Further studies are needed. To ensure adequate amounts of protein, approximately 18 to 20% of total daily kilocalories are from protein sources.

Glycemic response of gestational diabetes is highly correlated with the percentage of dietary carbohydrate. The recommendation that only 40% of kilocalories should be from carbohydrates is lower than the normal ADA recommendation (Jovanovic-Peterson, 1992); carbohydrate intake should not be less than 200 gm. (The fetus requires about 50 gm glucose daily; inadequate carbohydrate intake may induce maternal ketosis). Fiber intake of 30 to 40 gm daily is important to improve glucose tolerance and reduce insulin requirements.

No more than 25% of the kilocalories are taken at breakfast. An evening snack is always included, but 6 feedings daily may provide better control. A high ketone level in the morning may indicate a feeding is necessary during the middle of the night. No meal, especially breakfast, should be omitted.

Gestational diabetes is usually controlled by diet alone. By merely restricting the amount of simple carbohydrates and providing 6 small meals a day, incidence of infant macrosomia and hypoglycemia is decreased. In addition to elimination of all concentrated sweets, artificial sweeteners, caffeine, and alcohol are avoided.

Describe nutritional care for the pregnant client with DM.

NURSING APPLICATIONS

Assessment

Physical—for weight, height, preconceptual weight and weight gain/loss patterns.

Dietary—for intake of simple and complex carbohydrate, fats, protein, artificial sweeteners, caffeine, alcohol, diet patterns, especially breakfast intake.

Laboratory—for glucose, urine ketones, urine protein.

Interventions

1. Offer small, frequent meals to provide a steady source of glucose and prevent the body from using fat stores.
2. Praise client for adherence to the diet.
3. Monitor for hypertension and eclampsia, as these are more common in diabetic clients.

Evaluation

* Client should adhere to individualized diabetic diet and gain appropriate amount of weight based on her prepregnant status. Additionally, hyperglycemia and hypoglycemia are prevented. Blood glucose range should be 60 to 140 mg/dl.

Client Education

- Oral hypoglycemic agents should be discontinued even before conception, if possible, because they tend to produce fetal deformities.
- Reassure diabetic mothers that an increased need for insulin in the second trimester is not harmful; this normal response of a healthy developing pregnancy is due to antagonistic effects of placental hormones on insulin.
- Hospitalization during the last 4 weeks is not uncommon for a diabetic with edema.
- A diabetic newborn may remain in the hospital to be monitored for blood glucose levels and particularly to determine respiratory adequacy.
- Teach client self-monitoring blood glucose.
- Eat a bedtime snack every day.

COUNSELING FOR SELF-MANAGEMENT

When a client is diagnosed as having DM, many adjustments must be made that affect emotional well-being and lifestyle. It is a matter of adjusting to a condition that must be given constant attention every day. Initially clients are overwhelmed and anxious; basic information is introduced to help them to cope. Clients are responsible for learning many new things about DM. This education process takes time; clients cannot be expected to learn everything in a single session. A minimum of 3 counseling sessions is needed to cover basic nutritional concerns.

A team approach is necessary for teaching clients about the many facets of self-care for which they are responsible. They must be taught about the disease, diet, and type of medication (insulin or oral hypoglycemics). Dunn et al (1990) found that knowledge about diabetes does not predict better glycemic control, but as clients become participants in their own care, diabetic control is improved. They must believe that benefits of compliance exceed disadvantages.

Clients must be taught to self-monitor their daily status (glucose and ketone testing) as well as how to avoid hypoglycemia and hyperglycemia and what to do when they do occur. Benefits and effects of exercise must be explained.

Although individual counseling is important, group instruction classes are more effective for clients as well as more economical for the hospital. These are taught by several specialists—nurses, dietitians, physical therapists, and physicians. Many visual teaching aids are available that can help explain all facets of this disease.

Cognitively alert hospitalized clients should be started on an educational program regarding diabetes as soon as possible, not at the time of discharge. Although all aspects of the condition are important, many clients express that diet and diet-related issues are the most difficult problems. Recognizing these problems, the Task Force for the American Diabetes Association (1987) developed a simplified meal planning tool (entitled "Healthy Food Choices") for initial education of diabetic clients. Its simplified approach has planned stages for further teaching as appropriate. Initially clients are counseled on how they can use less salt, sugar, and fat and increase dietary fiber. In the second stage, foods are divided into 6 groups by approximate portion sizes and kilocalories. Dietitians can offer specific suggestions for implementation of and living with these dietary changes.

An appropriate family member must also understand and be able to implement the daily meal plan, if necessary. Every effort should be made to work with family members so the meal plan neither creates conflicts nor disrupts usual household activities.

In addition to explaining how food exchange lists work and which foods are in each exchange, both the person who prepares the food and the client must be taught the importance of careful measurements. If 1 tbsp margarine is mistakenly used for 1 tsp, for example, the number of kilocalories is tripled. Many people are not familiar with cooking measurements; measuring devices such as scales are useful teaching tools. Food models may also be used as a reference.

Diabetic clients should eventually learn to calculate and plan their diets. They also need to know what may happen when they do not adhere to the diet. Changing eating patterns may be difficult; sticking to a set regimen can be even more upsetting for some people. Diabetic clients should understand the important distinctions between short-term effects of occasional overconsumption and more harmful effects of persistent dietary noncompliance. For a successful continuing education program, children receive nutritional counseling at least every 3 to 6 months; adults may need to be seen only once or twice a year.

There is so much for clients to learn that it is virtually impossible for them to comprehend it all while in the hospital. They should know whom to call when they have problems putting it all into action. Many hospitals have regular meetings for diabetic clients. The American Diabetes Association has local chapters in most communities that can function as a support group and furnish reading and reference materials.

NURSING APPLICATIONS

Assessment

Physical—for emotional state, motivation, lifestyle, personality, coping patterns, education level.

Dietary—for dietary compliance, knowledge of dietary regimen.

Interventions

1. Refer to diabetic educator, social services, diabetes support groups, suppliers of diabetes products, and American Diabetes Association on admission; do not wait until discharge.
2. Involve family and client in nutritional care to enhance compliance.
3. Provide support and empathy to both client and family. Since DM affects all areas of life, anger, denial, fear, and grief are all common responses.

Evaluation

* Clients should verbalize feelings and concerns, maintain prior activities (as much as possible), and make decisions concerning diabetes management.

Client Education

- Wear a Medic Alert bracelet.
- Encourage subscription to *Diabetes Forecast, Diabetes Self-Management, Diabetes,* and *Diabetes Talk.* The ADA cookbook can also be helpful in meal planning.
- Teach client how to monitor blood glucose.
- Avoid buying OTC drugs, as they may contain sugar, i.e., cough syrups, cold remedies, throat lozenges.
- See the registered dietitian every 6 months or at least annually.

SUMMARY

DM is a complex disorder that requires a regimen of insulin (for IDDM and some NIDDM), diet, and exercise. The most important objective of the diet is control of total kilocalorie intake to attain ideal body weight. Obesity is diabetogenic. Meals must be eaten on a regular schedule. A flexible approach that takes into consideration a client's lifestyle, socioeconomic and ethnic factors, food preferences, and eating habits results in better compliance.

The exchange lists are designed to help all populations, whether diabetic, obese, cardiovascular, or even normal populations, to improve their quality of life by making wise food choices based on kilocaloric content and/or energy nutrients. Basically the diet involves (1) increasing complex carbohydrates (50 to 60%) for higher fiber intake, (2) reducing total fat to 25 to 30%, and (3) limiting cholesterol to less than 300 mg/day. Diets planned by the exchange lists actually could be considered as plans for optimum wellness rather than menus for specific diseases.

Regular preplanned meals based on the exchange lists, exercise regimens, adequate rest, and systematic monitoring of glucose levels, lipids, and body weight are significant factors that contribute to vitality, energy, and good health.

NURSING PROCESS IN ACTION

A newly diagnosed 16-year-old IDDM client is concerned about what to do if he becomes ill at home with a cold, flu, or vomiting. He is on insulin, 38 units NPH and 6 units regular insulin.

Nutritional Assessment

- Knowledge of pathophysiology of illness, IDDM, diet, community resources.
- Motivation to learn, support system.
- Home environment: who cooks, what type of cooking facilities are available, amount of money available for food, frequency of eating out, and use of fast foods.
- Food preferences, carbohydrates, fat, protein, alcohol, drug intake, current meal plan.
- Amount of insulin used, technique.
- Kilocalories needed.
- Anthropometric measures: skinfold, height, weight, IBW.
- Education and economic level.

Dietary Nursing Diagnosis

Knowledge deficit: Sick-day care RT no previous exposure to this event and lack of information.

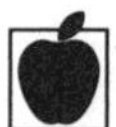

Nutritional Goals

Client will state how to care for self when he is sick at home, state 3 foods to ingest when sick, and verbalize when to call the physician.

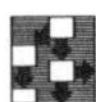

Nutritional Implementation 

Intervention: Refer to dietitian or diabetes educator.
Rationale: This is a lifelong disease that requires day to day decisions; follow-up care is essential.

Intervention: Involve client/family member in care.
Rationale: IDDM clients are usually young and still live with someone. For better compliance, all people affected need to be involved.

Intervention: Stress the need to continue insulin.
Rationale: Illness (stress) increases blood glucose by stimulating the sympathetic nervous system, which enhances the release of hormones (glucagon, epinephrine, cortisol), causing a rise in blood glucose. Without insulin, ketoacidosis may occur.

Intervention: Encourage him to follow a meal plan as closely as possible. If he can follow meal plan, he should drink extra broth, bouillon, tea, sugar-free carbonated beverages or water (sips are better). If food intake is not tolerated, he should consume the following every hour: ½ cup ice cream, ½ cup pudding, ½ cup custard, 1 piece toast, ½ cup fruited yogurt, ½ cup regular carbonated beverages, or 6 crackers (anything high in carbohydrate).
Rationale: These measures will provide the needed carbohydrates to prevent ketosis.

Intervention: Emphasize checking blood glucose every 4 hours; if blood glucose is above 250 mg/dl, check for urine ketones.

Rationale: Blood glucose levels help determine glycemic control, and ketones determine if fats are being used for energy rather than carbohydrate leading to possible DKA.

Intervention: Teach client to call the physician for the following: (1) vomiting or diarrhea lasting more than 6 hours; (2) urine ketone results are moderate to large; (3) blood glucose levels remain above 250 mg/dl; (4) mouth is dry, lips are cracked, eyes are sunken, or skin is dry and red; (5) breath has fruity smell; and (6) temperature is above 101°F.
Rationale: These all indicate home treatment is ineffective, and more intervention is needed to prevent DKA.

Intervention: Instruct the client/family regarding the most important aspects of care using short words and short clear sentences, using concrete specific statements. Review information, and provide written instructions.
Rationale: When client is sick, concentration of client/family may be impaired. If information is written down, compliance is enhanced.

Intervention: Make sure client/family has the following phone numbers: physician, ambulance, pharmacy, hospital, diabetic educator.
Rationale: Client safety is of utmost importance during emergencies. Preparation is necessary to avoid complications.

Evaluation

Nursing care was effective if client stated he will test his blood glucose, urine for ketones when glucose is greater than 250 mg/dl; consumes some form of nourishment when sick; calls the physician when blood glucose or urine ketones are elevated or nausea and vomiting continue longer than 6 hours. Additionally, DKA does not develop, and hospitalization is avoided.

STUDENT READINESS

1. How are the basic food groups different from the exchange lists? Cite 3 differences in classification other than those mentioned in the text.
2. Tally all the foods you eat in a day, then calculate the number of food exchanges. Can you see any changes in food choices that would be beneficial to you and why?
3. Why are complex carbohydrates especially important for the client using the exchange lists?
4. Plan 3 meals for a day to meet a diet prescription of 2500 kcal with 70 gm protein, 364 gm carbohydrate, and 85 gm fat.
5. A client asks, "Why are some vegetables in the vegetable exchange and others in the bread exchange, instead of all being in the vegetable exchange?" How would you respond?
6. Why do current dietary recommendations for DM emphasize increased carbohydrate and fiber and low fat intake?
7. Your client is on a 2000-kcal diabetic diet with NPH insulin. What important facts should you stress to him about the diet? Discuss the total management of the client's medication, exercise, and diet.
8. What advice should you give your diabetic client to avoid having a hypoglycemic reaction? What precautionary measures are recommended?
9. Why is it important for the obese NIDDM client to reduce weight?
10. What are the effects of pregnancy on the diabetic condition? What changes would clients expect with regard to diet and insulin?

CASE STUDY

Mrs. S. M. is a 42-year-old woman who has had IDDM for 19 years. She has a family history of DM (mother and maternal grandfather). She has been admitted to the hospital twice in the past 2 years for ketoacidosis.

On examination, her height is 165 cm and her weight is 77.8 kg; she has a medium frame. Mrs. S. M. also demonstrates diabetic retinopathy. Laboratory studies reveal a fasting serum glucose of 310 mg/dl, 4+ urine protein, negative urine acetone, and a serum creatinine of 2.3 mg/dl. Her blood pressure is 158/92.

She has been receiving NPH insulin U-100 42 units and regular insulin U-100 8 units each morning. With further questioning, Mrs. S. M. admits to frequently deviating from her 1500-kcal diet. She is again referred to the center for diabetic education classes and individual dietary counseling.

1. What additional dietary information is needed before a plan of care can be developed?
2. Identify 2 nursing diagnoses (include relevant supporting data) and appropriate goals for each.
3. What is Mrs. S. M.'s ideal weight?
4. What is the desirable range for her blood glucose?
5. Outline a meal plan for a 1500-kcal diet (220 gm carbohydrate, 60 gm protein, 40 gm fat).
6. What insulin adjustments would be made if Mrs. S. M. were to increase her level of physical activity? If she were to develop a systemic infection?

CASE STUDY

Mr. M. P. is a 63-year-old postal worker currently undergoing his annual physical examination. The physician notes hypertension; a weight gain of 15 lbs since the last examination (current weight 194 lbs); and elevated serum glucose, cholesterol, and triglycerides. Following a glucose tolerance test, the diagnosis of NIDDM is made. He is started on glyburide (DiaBeta) and referred to the nutritionist for dietary counseling.

Since his son and daughter-in-law have moved out of his house into a home of their own 8 months ago, Mr. M. P. has been eating frequently at restaurants. When he eats at home, he uses prepackaged food.

1. What additional assessment data do you need?
2. List at least 2 nursing diagnoses that can be derived from the history.
3. List a goal for each diagnosis.
4. Why is it important to reduce his serum glucose?
5. Calculate Mr. M. P.'s kilocaloric requirements with the proportions of carbohydrate, protein, and fat.
6. What lifestyle factors should be considered when planning his diet plan?
7. As you are evaluating the effectiveness of the diet counseling, Mr. M. P. states, "Well, if I can't eat the proper foods every day, can't I just take an extra pill?" What should you say?

CASE STUDY

Sarah is 29 years old, single, and works every day with little time for exercise programs. Since graduating from college, she has gained 22 lbs and realizes that her energy level is lower and that her appearance is not as attractive with this additional weight.

1. Plan meals and snacks (including brown-bag lunches) for Sarah for 3 days using the exchange lists to provide a weight loss of 2 lbs a week by reducing dietary intake.

REFERENCES

American Diabetes Association (ADA). Position Statement. Nutritional recommendations and principles for individuals with diabetes mellitus. *Diab Care* 1992a Apr; 15(suppl 2):21–28

American Diabetes Association (ADA). Gestational diabetes mellitus. *Diab Care* 1992b Apr; 15(suppl 2):5–6.

American Diabetes Association (ADA) Consensus Statement. Magnesium supplementation in the treatment of diabetes. *Diabetes Care* 1992 Aug; 15(8):1065–1066.

American Diabetes Association (ADA). Statement on sweeteners. *Diab Care* 1987 July-Aug; 10(4):526.

Anderson JW, Akanji AO. Dietary fiber—an overview. *Diab Care* 1991 Dec; 14(12):1126–1131.

Anderson RA, et al. Supplemental-chromium effects on glucose, insulin, glucagon, and urinary chromium losses in subjects consuming controlled low-chromium diets. *Am J Clin Nutr* 1991 Nov; 54(5):909–916.

Badiga MS, et al. Diarrhea in diabetics: The role of sorbitol. *J Am Coll Nutr* 1990 Dec; 9(6):578–582.

Bagdade JD, et al. Effect of ω-3 fish oils on plasma lipids, lipoprotein composition, and post heparin lipoprotein lipase in women with IDDM. *Diabetes* 1990 Apr; 39(4):426–431.

Blank DM, Mattes RD. Sugar and spice: Similarities and sensory attributes. *Nurs Res* 1990 Sept-Oct; 39(5):290–292.

Bonanome A, et al. Carbohydrate and lipid metabolism in patients with non-insulin-dependent diabetes mellitus: Effects of a low-fat, high carbohydrate diet vs a diet high in monounsaturated fatty acids. *Am J Clin Nutr* 1991 Sept; 54(3):586–590.

Brackenridge BP, Campbell RK. Enteral nutritional support and supplementation in diabetes. *Diab Ed* 1990 Nov-Dec; 16(6):463–465.

Brouhard BH, LaGrone L. Effect of dietary protein restriction on functional renal reserve in diabetic nephropathy. *Am J Med* 1990 Oct; 89(4):427–431.

Colditz GA, et al. Diet and risk of clinical diabetes in women. *Am J Clin Nutr* 1992 May; 55(5):1018–1023.

Colwell J, Jewler D. Lowering the risk. *Diab Forecast* 1990 Feb; 43(2):57–62.

Dornhorst A, et al. Calorie restriction for treatment of gestational diabetes. *Diabetes* 1991 Dec; 40(suppl 2):161–164.

Dunn SM, et al. Knowledge and attitude change as predictors of metabolic improvement in diabetes education. *Soc Sci Med* 1990; 31 (10):1135–1141.

Egger M, et al. Increasing incidence of hypoglycemic coma in children with IDDM. *Diab Care* 1991 Nov; 14(11):1001–1005.

Fishbein HA. Diabetic ketoacidosis, hyperosmolar nonketotic coma, lactic acidosis, and hypoglycemia. *In* Harris MI, Hamman RF, eds. *Diabetes in America.* NIH Publication No. 85–1468, Washington, D.C., Government Printing Office, 1985.

Galloway JA. Treatment of NIDDM with insulin antagonists or substitutes. *Diab Care* 1990 Dec; 13(12):1209–1239.

Garg A, Grundy SM. Nicotinic acid as therapy for dyslipidemia in non-insulin-dependent diabetes mellitus. *JAMA* 1990 Aug 8; 264(6):723–726.

Garg A, et al. Comparison of a high-carbohydrate diet with a monounsaturated-fat diet in patients with non-insulin-dependent diabetes mellitus. *N Engl J Med* 1988 Sept 29; 318(13):829–834.

Greenhalgh PM. Competitive sport and the insulin-dependent diabetic patient. *Postgrad Med J* 1990 Oct; 66(780):803–806.

Gregory R, Tattersall RB. Are diabetic pre-pregnancy clinics worthwhile? *Lancet* 1992 Sept 12; 340(8820):656–657.

Grigoresco C, et al. Lack of detectable deleterious effects on metabolic control of daily fructose ingestion for 2 months in NIDDM patients. *Diab Care* 1988 July-Aug; 11(7):546–550.

Groop LC. Sulfonylureas in NIDDM. *Diab Care* 1992 June; 15(6):737–754.

Harris MI. Hypercholesterolemia in diabetes and glucose intolerance in the U.S. population. *Diab Care* 1991 May; 14(5):366–374.

Harris M, Hamman R, eds. *Diabetes in America.* NIH Publication No. 85–1468, Washington, D.C., Government Printing Office, 1985.

Hendra T, et al. Effects of fish oil supplements in NIDDM subjects. Controlled study. *Diab Care* 1990 Aug; 13(8):821–829.

Henry RR, Gumbiner B. Benefits and limitations of very-low-calorie diet therapy in obese NIDDM. *Diab Care* 1991 Sept; 14(9):802–823.

Henry RR, et al. Current issues in fructose metabolism. *Annu Rev Nutr* 1991; 11:21–39.

Hockaday TD. Fibre in the management of diabetes. 1. Natural fibre useful as part of total dietary prescription. *Br Med J* 1990 May 19; 300(6735):1224–1226.

Hollingsworth DR, Ney DM. Caloric restriction in pregnant diabetic women: A review of maternal obesity, glucose and insulin relationships as investigated at the University of California, San Diego. *J Am Coll Nutr* 1992 June; 11(3):251–258.

Howard BV, et al. Evaluation of metabolic effects of substitution of complex carbohydrates for saturated fat in individuals with obesity and NIDDM. *Diab Care* 1991 Sept; 14(9):786–795.

Huzar JG. Diabetes now: Preventing acute complications. *RN* 1989 Aug; 52(8):34–39.

Iwai M, et al. Abnormal lipoprotein composition in normolipidemic diabetic patients. *Diab Care* 1990 July; 13(7):792–796.

Jenkins DJ, et al. Metabolic advantages of spreading the nutrient load: Effects of increased meal frequency in non-insulin-dependent diabetes. *Am J Clin Nutr* 1992 Feb; 55(2):461–467.

Jenkins DJ, et al. Low glycemic-index starchy

foods in the diabetic diet. *Am J Clin Nutr* 1988 Aug; 48(2):248-254.

Jones BJM, et al. Indications for pump-assisted enteral feeding. *Lancet* 1980 May 17; 1(8177):1057-1058.

Jovanovic-Peterson L. Guest editorial: Nutritional management of the obese gestational diabetic pregnant woman. *J Am Coll Nutr* 1992 June; 11(3):246-250.

Jovanovic-Peterson L, et al. Maternal postprandial glucose levels and infant birth weight: The Diabetes in Early Pregnancy Study. The National Institute of Child Health and Human Development—Diabetes in Early Pregnancy Study. *Am J Obstet Gynecol* 1991 Jan; 164(1 Pt 1):103-111.

Karjalainen J, et al. A bovine albumin peptide as a possible trigger of insulin-dependent diabetes mellitus. *N Engl J Med* 1992 July 30; 327(5):302-307.

Kerr D, et al. Importance of insulin in subjective, cognitive, and hormonal responses to hypoglycemia in patients with IDDM. *Diabetes* 1991 Aug; 40(8):1057-1062.

Kitzmiller JL, et al. Preconception care of diabetes. Glycemic control prevents congenital anomalies. *JAMA* 1991 Feb 13; 265(6):731-736.

Klein R, et al. The incidence of gross proteinuria in people with insulin-dependent diabetes mellitus. *Arch Intern Med* 1991 July; 151(7):1344-1349.

Knopp RH, et al. Metabolic effects of hypocaloric diets in management of gestational diabetes. *Diabetes* 1991 Dec; 40(suppl 2):165-171.

Larsen ML, et al. Effect of long-term monitoring of glycosylated hemoglobin levels in insulin-dependent diabetes mellitus. *N Engl J Med* 1990 Oct 11; 323(15):1021-1025.

Lebovitz HE, ed. *The Physician's Guide to Type II Diabetes (NIDDM): Diagnosis and Treatment.* 2nd ed. Alexandria, VA, American Diabetes Association, 1988.

Loghmani E, et al. Glycemic response to sucrose-containing mixed meals in diets of children with insulin-dependent diabetes mellitus. *J Pediatr* 1991 Oct; 119(10):531-537.

Maclaren N, Atkinson M. Is insulin-dependent diabetes mellitus enviromentally induced? *N Engl J Med* 1992 July 30; 327(5):348-349.

McEvilly A. Taloring a lifestyle for a diabetic child. *Midwife Health Visitor and Community Nurse* 1991 Feb; 27(2):39-41.

Miodovnik M, et al. Major malformations in infants of IDDM women. Vasculopathy and early first-trimester poor glycemic control. *Diab Care* 1988 Oct; 11(9):713-718.

Mori TA. Comparison of diets supplemented with fish oil or olive oil on plasma lipoproteins in insulin-dependent diabetics. *Metabolism* 1991 March; 40(3):241-246.

Morley JE, Perry HM 3d. The management of diabetes mellitus in older individuals. *Drugs* 1991 Apr; 41(4):548-565.

Narins RG. Diabetic nephropathy: Can the natural history be modified? *Am J Med* 1991 Feb 21; 90(2A):70S-75S.

Pastors JG. Alternatives to the exchange system for teaching meal planning to persons with diabetes. *Diab Educ* 1992 Jan-Feb; 18(1):57-62.

Peeters TL, et al. Effect of motilin on gastric emptying in patients with diabetic gastroparesis. *Gastroenterology* 1992 Jan; 102(1):97-101.

Peters AL, Davidson MB. Effects of various enteral feeding products on postprandial blood glucose response in patients with Type I diabetes. *JPEN* 1992 Jan-Feb; 16(1):69-74.

Peters AL, et al. Lack of glucose elevation after simulated tube feedings with low carbohydrate high fat enteral formula in patients with Type I diabetes. *Am J Med* 1989 Aug; 87(8):178-182.

Peterson A, Drass J. Managing acute complications of diabetes. *Nursing 91* 1991 Feb; 21(2):34-39.

Phillips M. Enteral nutrition support in diabetes mellitus. *Nutr Clin Pract* 1987 July-Aug; 2(4):152-154.

Puczynski S, et al. Hypoglycemia in children with insulin-dependent diabetes mellitus. *Diab Educ* 1992 March-Apr; 18(2):151-153.

Riccardi G, Rivellese AA. Effects of dietary fiber and carbohydrate on glucose and lipoprotein metabolism in diabetic patients. *Diab Care* 1991 Dec; 14(12):1115-1125.

Ronnemaa I, et al. High fasting plasma insulin is an indicator of coronary heart disease in non-insulin-dependent diabetic patients and nondiabetic subjects. *Arterioscler Thromb* 1991 Jan-Feb; 11(1):80-90.

Schmidt LE, et al. Compliance with dietary prescriptions in children and adolescents with insulin-dependent diabetes mellitus. *J Am Diet Assoc* 1992 May; 92(5):567-570.

Shyh E-D, et al. Treatment of the uremic diabetic. *Nephron* 1985 June; 40(2):129-138.

Sullivan MJ, Scott RL. Postprandial glycemic response to orange juice and nondiet cola: Is there a difference? *Diab Ed* 1991 July-Aug; 17(4):274-278.

Surveys show socioeconomic trends in diabetes. *Hospitals* 1991 Feb 20; 65(4):14.

Task Force for the American Diabetes Assocation. Nutritional recommendations and principles for individuals with diabetes mellitus: 1986. *Diab Care* 1987 Jan-Feb; 10(1):126-132.

Thompson DJ, et al. Prophylactic insulin the management of gestational diabetes. *Obstet Gynecol* 1990 June; 75(6):960-964.

Thorburn AW, et al. Long-term effects of dietary fructose on carbohydrate metabolism in non-insulin-dependent diabetes mellitus. *Metabolism* 1990 Jan; 39(1):58-63.

Tjoa HI, Kaplan NM. Nonpharmacological treatment of hypertension in diabetes mellitus. *Diab Care* 1991 June; 14(6):449-460.

Uusitupa MI, et al. 5-year incidence of atherosclerotic vascular disease in relation to general risk factors, insulin level, and abnormalities in lipoprotein composition in non-insulin-dependent diabetic and nondiabetic subjects. *Circulation* 1990 July; 82(1):27-36.

Vinik AJ, Jenkins DA. Dietary fiber in management of diabetes. *Diab Care* 1988 Feb; 11(2):160-173.

Wahlqvist ML, et al. Fish intake and arterial wall

characteristics in healthy people and diabetic patients. *Lancet* 1989 Oct 21; 2(8669):944–946.

Wing RR, et al. Effects of a very-low-calorie diet on long-term glycemic control in obese type 2 diabetic subjects. *Arch Intern Med* 1991 July; 151(7):1334–1340.

Wing RR, et al. Variables associated with weight loss and improvements in glycemic control in type II diabetic patients in behavioral weight control programs. *Int J Obes* 1990; 14(6):495–503.

Wise JE, et al. Effect of glycemic control on growth velocity in children with IDDM. *Diab Care* 1992 July; 15(7):826–830.

Yue DD, et al. Proteinuria and renal function in diabetic patients fed a diet moderately restricted in protein. *Am J Clin Nutr* 1988 Aug; 48(2):230–234.

Zeller K, et al. Effect of restricting dietary protein on the pregression of renal failure in patients with insulin-dependent diabetes mellitus. *N Engl J Med* 1991 Jan 10; 324(2):78–84.

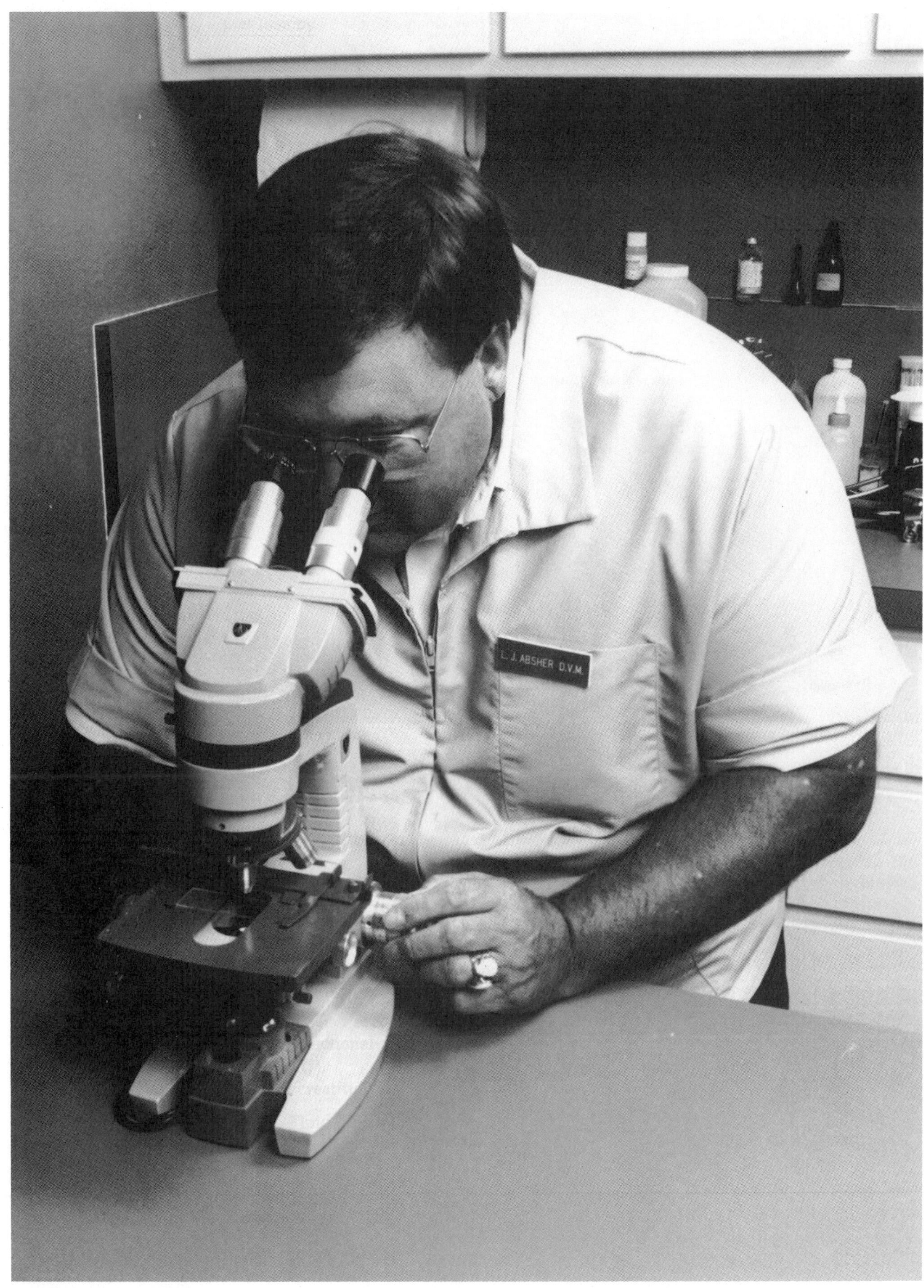
L. J. ABSHER D.V.M.

Dietary Management of Endocrine and Genetic Disorders

CHAPTER 28

OUTLINE

OBJECTIVES

THE STUDENT WILL BE ABLE TO:

- Identify nutritional care for endocrine disorders.
- Discuss the prevention and treatment of phenylketonuria.
- Name some foods high in purines.
- Discuss nutritional concerns of sickle cell anemia and thalassemia.
- Apply the nursing process to endocrine, genetic, and metabolic disorders.
- Discuss client teaching tips for endocrine, genetic, and metabolic disorders.

TEST YOUR NQ (True/False)

1. For hypoglycemia, a low-carbohydrate, high-protein diet is recommended.
2. A low-protein, moderate-carbohydrate diet is given to clients with Addison's disease.
3. Vitamin C supplementation is advocated for Cushing's syndrome.
4. Clients with Graves' disease need a low-kilocalorie diet.
5. Iodized salt intake is beneficial for clients with hypothyroidism.
6. Clients with tetany need low calcium intake.
7. A diet limited in phenylalanine is necessary for infants born with PKU.
8. In pregnant women with PKU, dietary manipulations keep plasma phenylalanine levels around 8 mg/dl.
9. An acid ash diet may be prescribed for clients with hypercalcemia.
10. Clients with gout should eat organ meats.

Metabolism includes all the chemical processes required to build and maintain a body. When the activity of a hormone, enzyme, or cofactor is abnormal (i.e., excessive, absent, or reduced), metabolism of that compound and the entire body is detrimentally affected.

Hormones secreted by pancreas, adrenal cortex, thyroid, and parathyroid glands are very potent; imbalances (too much or too little) of these hormonal secretions have a direct effect on how the body handles nutrients. With modern technology, the most effective treatment is hormonal replacement. Treatment of some of these metabolic problems involves nutritional care, especially during the acute phase to restore homeostasis.

A genetic disorder, also called an inborn error of metabolism, is a physiological problem caused by a defective gene in which a metabolic block is produced by an enzymatic abnormality (excess or deficiency). Pathological consequences may be manifest soon after birth or later in life. Nutritional care for these problems usually involves preventing accumulation of the nonmetabolized substrate, which becomes toxic in excessive amounts, and/or replacing the deficient product.

Although early detection and diagnosis of metabolic disorders by a physician are important, effective treatment involves active participation of a nurse and dietitian to plan and implement effective nutritional care and help a client and family understand the disorder and follow the frequently rigid guidelines.

PANCREATIC DYSFUNCTION

As discussed in Chapter 27, glycemic levels are normally maintained at a fairly stable level by a complex, but well-coordinated hormonal system (see Chapter 27, Table 27–1). Following food intake, blood glucose rises, causing insulin to be released. Insulin secretion lowers glucose by promoting glucose storage (glycogenesis) and cellular uptake. Then when no more glucose is entering the blood stream, insulin secretion decreases, and counterregulatory hormones (glucagon, epinephrine, cortisol, growth hormone) take over and maintain a normal blood glucose level (70 to 110 mg/dl) from glycogen stores, followed by protein and fat stores. Diabetes mellitus is a metabolic disorder involving insulin utilization that is discussed in Chapter 27; pancreatic disorders affecting GI secretions (cystic fibrosis, pancreatitis) are discussed in Chapter 26.

Describe how blood glucose is maintained at a stable level.

Hypoglycemia

Hypoglycemia is not a distinct disease but a symptom of problems involving insulin secretion and carbohydrate metabolism. This type of hypoglycemia is not caused by administration of hypoglycemic drugs. Symptoms may occur within 2 to 4 hours of food intake or more than 5 hours after eating.

Reactive hypoglycemia is postprandial (following food intake) appearance of hypoglycemic symptoms with concomitant blood glucose levels <50 mg/dl.

Reactive Hypoglycemia

Symptoms (weakness, anxiety, sweating, shakiness) occurring soon after the meal are due to secretion of epinephrine to restore normal glucose levels. Symptoms may coincide with oversecretion of insulin following rapid carbohydrate absorption. This is known as **reactive hypoglycemia.**

Depending on results of the oral glucose tolerance test (OGTT), reactive hypoglycemia is classified as functional, **alimentary,** or prediabetic hypoglycemia. Clients with functional hypoglycemia may have normal blood glucose concentrations at the time of their symptoms. Responses to OGTT in these clients may not

Alimentary hypoglycemia, more frequently referred to as dumping syndrome, is precipitated by rapid emptying of a hyperosmolar solution into the small intestine, which is absorbed rapidly, resulting in oversecretion of insulin. It is usually precipitated by gastric surgery such as gastrectomy or gastrojejunostomy.

Leucine sensitivity results in oversecretion of insulin and hypoglycemia when infants consume high-protein feedings such as milk.

Describe the differences between functional, alimentary, and prediabetic hypoglycemia.

be reliable; some health care professionals prefer to use self-monitoring of blood glucose levels when symptoms occur. Blood glucose should be measured during the spontaneous occurrence of symptoms or after ingestion of a typical meal that precipitates symptoms (Snorgaard et al, 1991; Palardy et al, 1989; Service, 1989). Functional hypoglycemia is indicated if glucose levels are low when a client is symptomatic, or it is strongly suspected if symptoms are relieved with carbohydrate ingestion and blood glucose levels are low. Prediabetic stages have a delayed secretion of insulin (180 minutes compared with the normal 35 to 60) (Cerrato, 1989), allowing longer periods of hyperglycemia, followed by hypoglycemia.

Reactive hypoglycemia may also be associated with certain inherited metabolic disorders such as **leucine sensitivity** and hereditary fructose intolerance.

Organic or Fasting Hypoglycemia

Insulinoma—benign tumor of the beta cells of the islet of Langerhans.

What are the signs and symptoms of organic hypoglycemia, and when do they occur? What are some causes of fasting hypoglycemia?

Postabsorptive or fasting hypoglycemia, caused by a slowly decreasing blood glucose level, may occur more than 5 hours following food intake. Fasting hypoglycemia is more serious than postprandial hypoglycemia. This type of hypoglycemia principally affects the brain (approximately two-thirds of glucose use occurs in the CNS). Common symptoms include headache, blurred vision, diplopia, abnormal behavior, unconsciousness, and amnesia. Symptoms may occur in healthy clients following exercise or fasting or may be precipitated when meals are delayed or if 1 or 2 meals are missed. Fasting hypoglycemia may develop within 6 to 36 hours of moderate amounts of alcohol intake by chronically malnourished clients.

Postabsorptive hypoglycemia may be the result of **insulinoma,** chronic liver disease, tumor-related hypoglycemia, or endocrine deficiencies (Marks, 1989). It is also associated with systemic lupus erythematosus, rheumatoid arthritis, and Graves' disease (Polonsky, 1992). Insulinoma may be diagnosed by inappropriately elevated levels of insulin for the amount of glucose present.

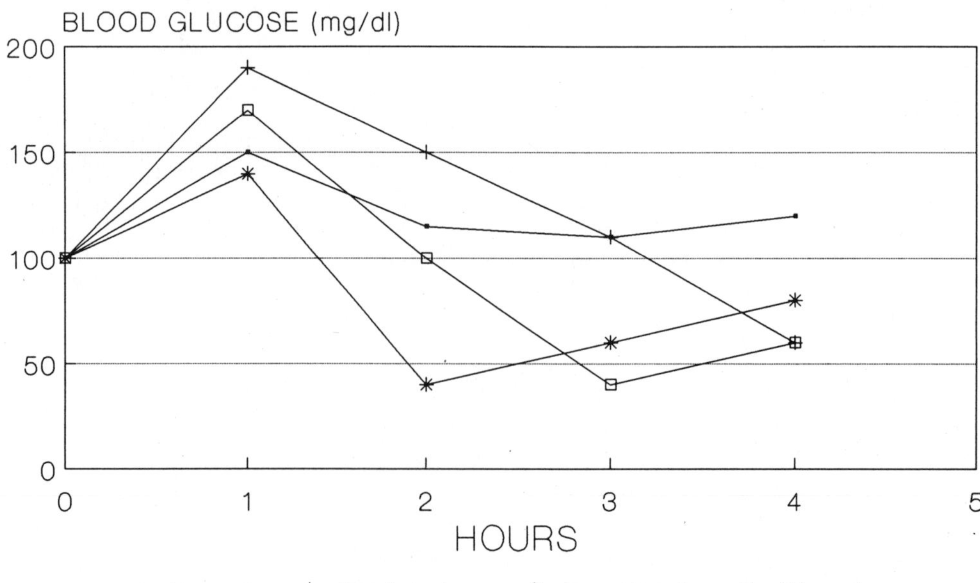

Figure 28–1 Oral glucose tolerance curves in hypoglycemia syndromes. (Adapted from Bacchus H. *Rational Management of Diabetes.* University Park Press, Baltimore, MD, 1977.)

Diagnosis

Because of the complexity of underlying causes of hypoglycemia, numerous diagnostic tests are used to document hypoglycemia and determine its cause. Correct diagnosis is important for appropriate treatment.

A low blood glucose level is normally diagnosed with a 4- to 5-hour OGTT that demonstrates a circulating glucose level of less than 50 mg/dl. Tests are extended beyond the normal 2 hours used for diabetes to aid in hypoglycemic diagnosis (Fig. 28–1). Of course, if the blood glucose level drops to a dangerously low level (<50 mg/dl), the physician is contacted, and the test is discontinued. As shown in Figures 28–2 and 28–3, other tests used to determine causes include fasting blood glucose, IV glucose tolerance tests (for dumping syndrome), prolonged fast (48 to 72 hours for organic hypoglycemia), **intravenous tolbutamide response** (to help differentiate fasting hypoglycemia), fructose loading (for hereditary fructose intolerance), and serum insulin levels (for insulinoma).

In a tolbutamide response test, tolbutamide is given intravenously, followed by measurements of glucose levels. This test avoids the prolonged fast.

What are some tests used for hypoglycemia?

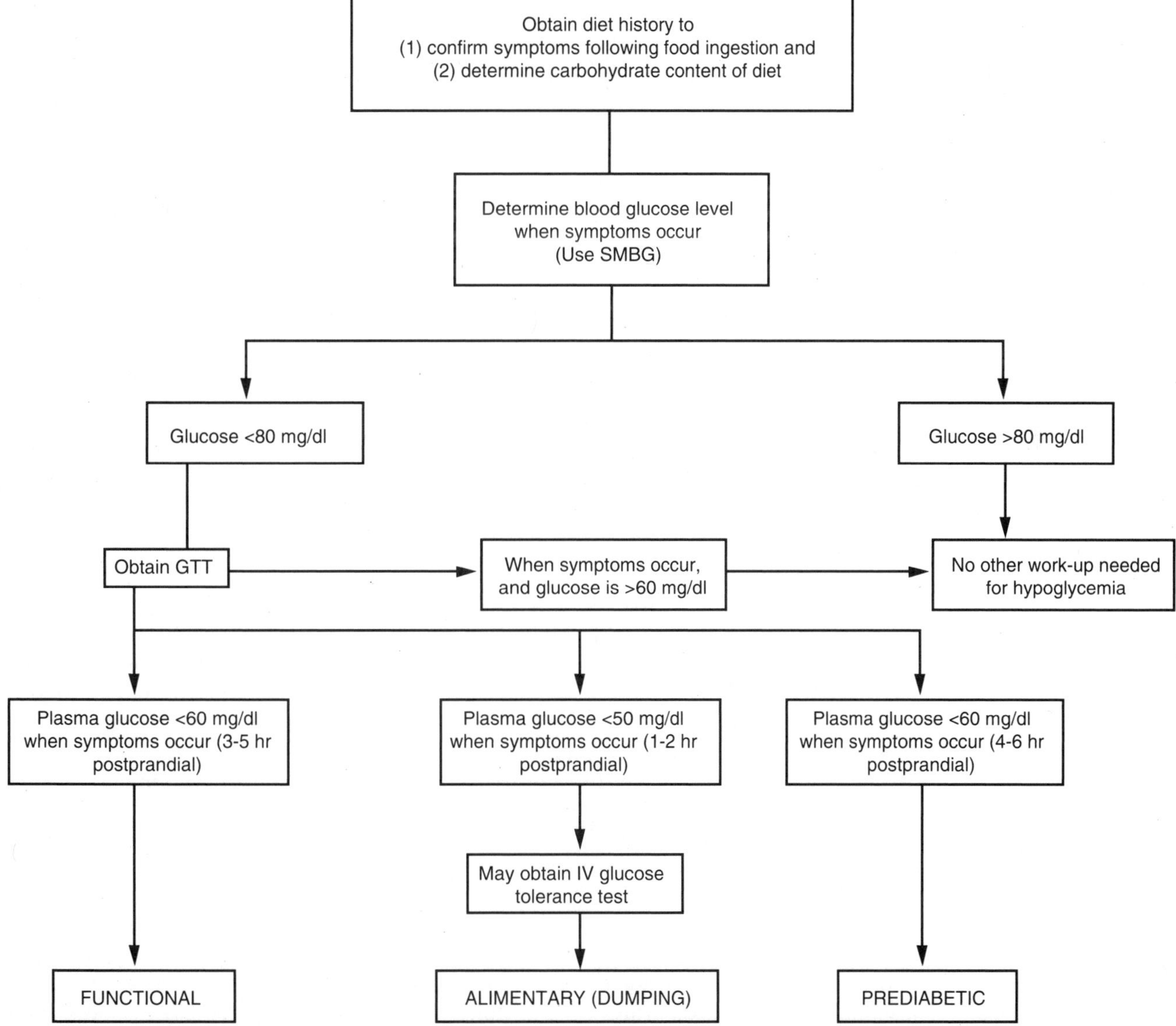

Figure 28–2 Testing for reactive hypoglycemia. (Adapted from Georgopoulos A, Margolis S. Hypoglycemia. *In* Harvey AM, et al, eds. *The Principles and Practice of Medicine.* 22nd ed. Norwalk, CT, Appleton-Lange, 1988:968–975.)

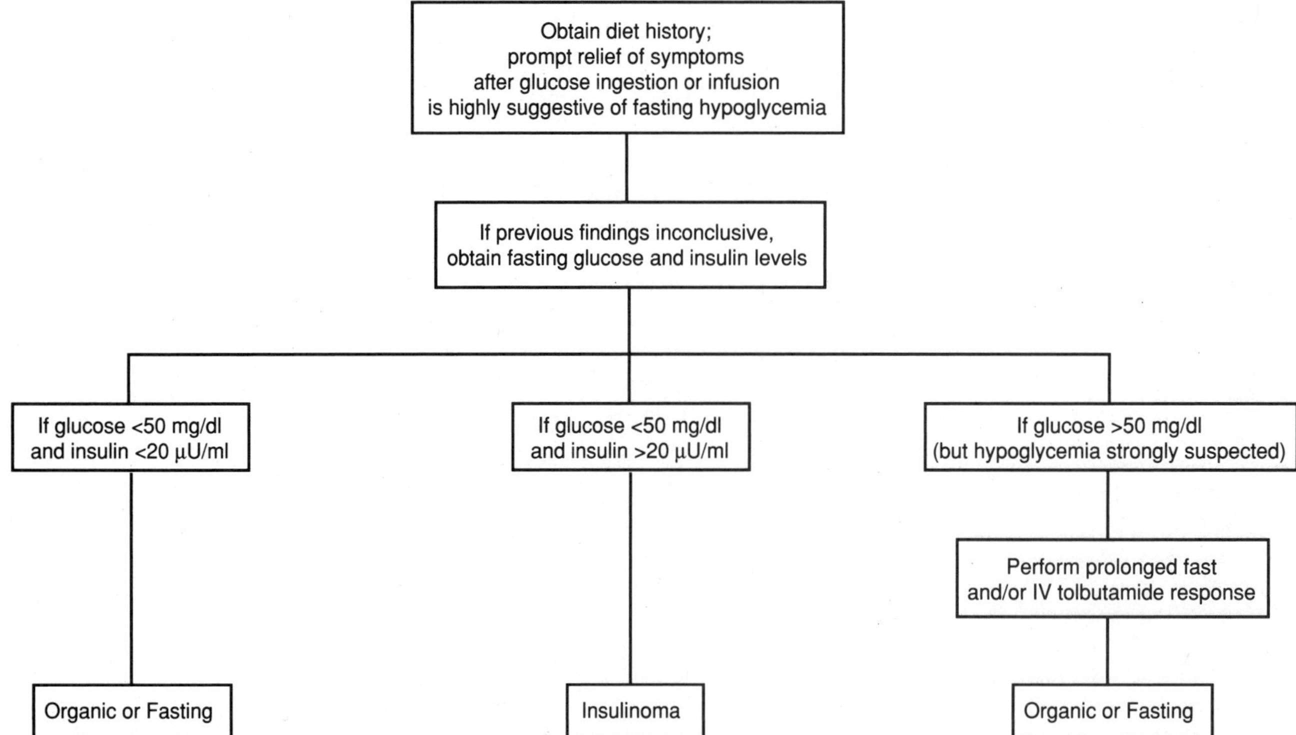

Figure 28–3 Testing for fasting/organic hypoglycemia. (Adapted from Georgopoulos A, Margolis S. Hypoglycemia. *In* Harvey AM, et al, eds. *The Principles and Practice of Medicine.* 22nd ed. Norwalk, CT, Appleton-Lange, 1988:968–975.)

Treatment

A careful diagnosis, using endocrine and metabolic testing procedures, may determine a correctable cause of hypoglycemia. The principal treatment of organic hypoglycemia is correction of the underlying cause. Dietary measures may reduce symptoms; however, as stated by Danowski et al (1975), "It is a disservice to clients to limit treatment to diet manipulations without seeking the origins of the hypoglycemia."

Nutritional Care

The purpose of nutrition support for hypoglycemia is to provide a more even release of glucose; carbohydrate causes hypoglycemia in those with reactive hypoglycemia. The most common diet recommended is low carbohydrate (80 to 120 gm), high protein (120 to 140 gm) with frequent feedings. Five to 6 feedings help to maintain euglycemia. Three high-protein snacks are provided in addition to 3 meals daily, as shown in Figure 28–4. Nutritional care for clients with dumping syndrome is covered in Chapter 25.

For fasting hypoglycemia, total energy intake should meet a client's requirements to maintain IBW, as described in Chapter 27, Table 27–10. Carbohydrate restriction is widely practiced, although it is neither necessary nor practical; approximately 45% of the total kilocaloric intake should be provided by carbohydrate (Anderson & Herman, 1975). Carbohydrate content is generally 80 to 100 gm to prevent ketosis. All forms of sugar-sweetened desserts and concentrated sweets are avoided. Use of fresh fruits or vegetables is preferred over fruit juices or beverages with high sugar content, which are absorbed more rapidly. Carbohydrates are distributed equally in feedings throughout the day. Food exchange lists (see Appendix

Breakfast

1/2 cup tomato juice
1/2 slice toast
1 tsp margarine
6 oz low-fat plain yogurt with 2 tsp sugar-free jam
Decaffeinated coffee

Mid-morning snack

1 1/2 oz sunflower seeds
12 oz sugar-free, caffeine-free carbonated beverage

Lunch

3.5 oz broiled pork chop
1/2 cup cooked carrots with 1 tsp margarine
Cole slaw with 2 tbsp mayonnaise
Small baked apple
Decaffeinated tea

Mid-afternoon snack

1 oz cheddar cheese
4 crackers

Dinner

4 oz beef cubes
1/4 cup cooked noodles
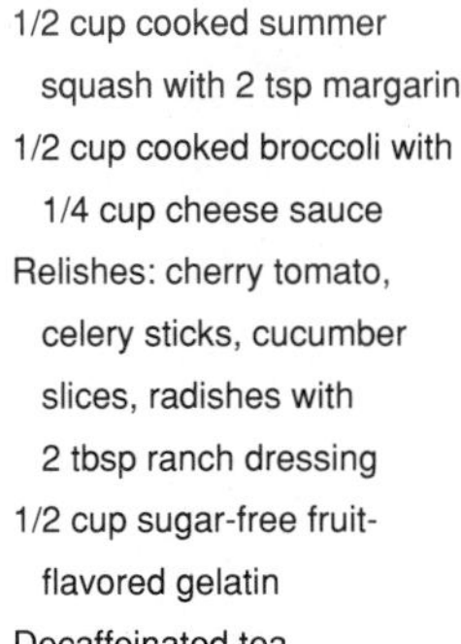
1/2 cup cooked summer squash with 2 tsp margarine
1/2 cup cooked broccoli with 1/4 cup cheese sauce
Relishes: cherry tomato, celery sticks, cucumber slices, radishes with 2 tbsp ranch dressing
1/2 cup sugar-free fruit-flavored gelatin
Decaffeinated tea

Evening snack

1 cup whole milk
2 tbsp peanut butter
1 multigrain rice cake

Nutrient	RDA: FEMALE–25 TO 50 years	Actual	% RDA
Kilocalories		2155 kcal	98
Protein		102 gm	204
Carbohydrate		120 gm	44
Fat		147 gm	200
Cholesterol		260 mg	87
Fiber–dietary		21.5 gm	98
Vitamin A		2694 RE	337
Thiamin		5.3 mg	480
Riboflavin		2.2 mg	171
Niacin		19.7 mg	131
Vitamin B_6		2.1 mg	132
Folate		373 mcg	207
Vitamin B_{12}		5.1 mcg	257
Pantothenic Acid		8.0 mg	145
Vitamin C		104 mcg	173
Vitamin D		5.0 mg	99
Vitamin K		352 mcg	541
Sodium		3021 mg	126
Potassium		3657 mg	183
Calcium		1185 mg	148
Phosphorus		2042 mg	255
Magnesium		380 mg	136
Iron		11.6 mg	77
Zinc		16.8 mg	140
Copper		2.1 mg	91
Manganese		4.5 mg	127
Selenium		0.11 mg	192
	^0 ^50 ^100 ^150 ^200		

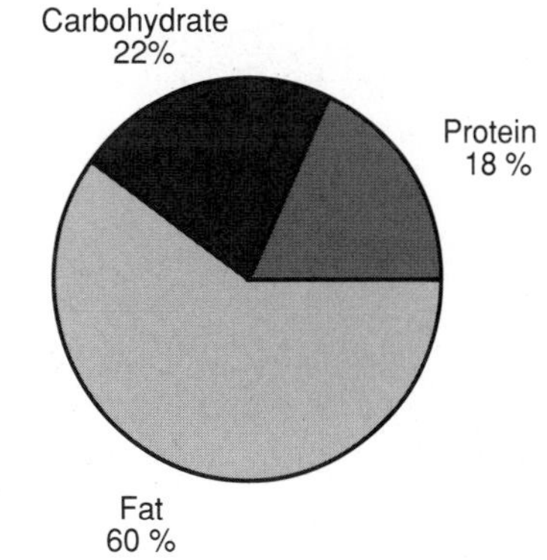

Figure 28–4 Sample menu for hypoglycemia. (Nutrient data from Nutritionist III software, version 7.0. N-Squared Computing, Salem, OR.)

D-1) are used to calculate the diet and help clients limit their consumption of carbohydrates.

Since proteins and fats are digested and absorbed more slowly and stimulate less insulin secretion than simple sugars, thereby providing a delayed source of glucose, they are better tolerated. Protein is usually 20% of the kilocalories (110 to 130 gm) and should also be distributed equally.

The remainder of the kilocalories is provided by fat. Alcohol can potentiate hypoglycemia by decreasing gluconeogenesis. Caffeine causes hypoglycemia by stimulating epinephrine.

NURSING APPLICATIONS

Assessment

Physical—for height, weight, IBW; medications; I&O; sweating, shakiness, anxiety, palpitations, weakness, headache, blurred vision, diplopia, unconsciousness, amnesia.
Dietary—for frequency of eating, nutritional adequacy of diet, time of last food intake, timing of symptoms in relation to meals, alcohol or caffeine intake.
Laboratory—for glucose, ketones, OGTT, serum insulin.

Interventions

1. Many of these clients have not been regularly eating well-balanced meals; review the food guide pyramid or dietary guidelines to be sure they are knowledgeable of basic nutrition principles. Suggest appropriate foods they can "eat on the run" (i.e., bagel, peanut butter and crackers, carrots).
2. Monitor diet for calcium and riboflavin adequacy; milk intake may be low because of its carbohydrate content. Supplementation may be necessary.
3. Consult the physician for chromium supplements. These have been effective for some reactive hypoglycemic clients (Cerrato, 1989).

Evaluation

* Client should verbalize foods to include and avoid; consumes complex carbohydrates at every meal/snack; does not experience hypoglycemia or, if it does occur, can tell how to correct this; and has normal glucose levels. Additionally, alcohol and caffeine intake are avoided or decreased.

Client Education

- Eat fiber-rich, whole-grain breads/cereal, fresh vegetables, and legumes to delay carbohydrate absorption, causing a slower, more even release of glucose into the blood stream.
- Avoid or limit alcohol and caffeine, which can lower blood glucose levels.
- Follow a specific schedule with regard to eating; eat small meals/snacks 5 to 6 times a day.
- Because of limited intake of fruits and vegetables, foods that are excellent sources of vitamin C should be routinely selected (see Chapter 7, Table 7–2).
- Some high-protein snacks are cheese, nuts, or cottage cheese.

ADRENAL DYSFUNCTION

Mineralocorticoids, principally aldosterone, affect extracellular fluid electrolytes, principally sodium and potassium. Glucocorticoids, mainly cortisol, have important effects on blood glucose concentration and protein and fat metabolism, with lesser influence on extracellular electrolyte concentration.

The adrenal cortex secretes 2 major types of adrenocortical hormones, the **glucocorticoids** and **mineralocorticoids,** that have significant effects on metabolic balance (Table 28–1).

Adrenocortical Insufficiency

Idiopathic adrenocortical insufficiency is called Addison's disease.

Insufficient production of one or more hormones by the adrenal cortex results in **Addison's disease,** a long-term and rare metabolic disorder. It may be caused by autoimmune disease, tumors, tuberculosis, histoplasmosis, or other infectious diseases.

TABLE 28–1

FUNCTIONS OF CORTISOL AND ALDOSTERONE

Cortisol*	Aldosterone+
Stimulates gluconeogenesis Increases breakdown of protein, thereby elevating serum protein levels Increases mobilization and utilization of fatty acids Stimulates anti-inflammatory processes	Increases sodium retention in kidneys with passive absorption of water Increases renal excretion of potassium

* ACTH is needed to stimulate release of cortisol from the adrenal glands.
\+ Aldosterone secretion is stimulated by the renin-angiotensin process.

Physical Consequences

In Addison's disease, cells in the cortex may be damaged, interfering with hormonal production of aldosterone and glucocorticoids. When insufficient amounts of aldosterone are secreted, renal absorption of sodium is decreased, precipitating excessive sodium and fluid excretion. Therefore, extracellular volume is decreased, acidosis develops, serum potassium levels are increased, and cardiac output decreases. If untreated, blood volume falls, precipitating an addisonian crisis (Fig. 28–5).

Glucocorticoid deficiencies cause decreased conversion of fats and proteins to glucose, resulting in weakness and weight loss. Symptoms of Addison's disease are similar to those of anorexia nervosa: weight loss, vomiting, poor food intake, hypotension, hypoglycemia, and abnormal (dark) skin pigmentation (Fig. 28–5).

Describe the physical consequences of Addison's disease.

Treatment

Lifelong replacement of deficient adrenal cortex hormones is necessary to lower serum potassium and decrease salt and water excretion. If medication is taken regularly, clients can lead a normal life. The use of a modified diet in conjunction with drug therapy may decrease drug dosage.

Nutritional Care

Depending on hormones administered, additional salt (4 to 6 gm/day) is often advised. Several salt tablets may be given along with high-salt foods. (Increase fluid intake to prevent dehydration). If aldosterone is replaced, salt intake is not increased.

A high-protein (1 gm/kg IBW/day), moderate-carbohydrate (120 to 150 gm/day) diet is used to prevent hypoglycemia (as described earlier). Six feedings are given with a substantial bedtime feeding to prevent nocturnal hypoglycemia. Between-meal snacks should be principally protein and complex carbohydrates; simple sugars are avoided. Because of an increased metabolism associated with disease management, vitamin B complex and C supplements may be needed. Depending on laboratory data results, clients are advised to avoid or increase potassium-containing foods.

NURSING APPLICATIONS

Assessment

Physical—for weight/weight loss, IBW, TSF; see Figure 28–5; vomiting, nausea, headache.
Dietary—for adequacy of food intake, sodium and potassium intake.
Laboratory—for sodium, potassium, magnesium level; glucose; BUN, protein; nitrogen balance, ACTH levels; cortisol.

Continued

Interventions

1. Monitor for hypokalemia or hyperkalemia.
2. Monitor I&O; fluid intake is important to detect dehydration.

Evaluation

* Client should not experience Addisonian crisis, and laboratory values should remain WNL.
* Client should salt food and eat cheese, milk, and meat.

Client Education

- Drink large amounts of fluids (3 L/day) to prevent dehydration.
- Meals should not be skipped; fasting is not well tolerated.
- Always carry a high-protein snack and wear a Medic Alert band.
- In times of emotional or physical stress, more cortisol may be needed.

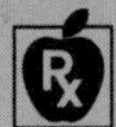
Corticosteroids should be taken with milk or antacids to minimize gastric irritation.

Cushing's Syndrome and Corticosteroid Therapy

Physical Consequences

Cushing's syndrome is a group of specific symptoms: fat deposits in the interscapular area (buffalo hump), facial area (moon face), and abdomen; impotence, amenorrhea, hypertension, general weakness, and loss of muscle mass due to elevated plasma cortisol levels.

Describe the appearance of a Cushing's syndrome client. What are the effects of increased glucocorticoids?

Pharmacological use of corticosteroids and endogenous secretion of excess cortisol, as seen in **Cushing's syndrome,** result in a state of hypercortisolism. Both conditions can be considered together. Cushing's syndrome caused by hypothalamic pituitary or adrenal tumors may be treated with surgical removal or radiation.

Increased amounts of glucocorticoids affect carbohydrate, protein, and lipid metabolism. Since glucocorticoids increase protein catabolism, clients may exhibit signs of muscle wasting, thin skin and subcutaneous tissues, poor wound healing, capillary fragility, and dissolution of vertebral bone matrix. Subcutaneous fat is lost in the arms and legs with excessive fatty deposits in the trunk and neck areas (Fig. 28–6). Growth retardation is a common finding among children.

Excess cortisol can have mineralocorticoid-like effects. Fluid and sodium retention is characterized by "moon face." Potassium depletion is associated with hypertension, weakness, and abnormal glucose tolerance.

Treatment

Death can ensue within 5 years of diagnosis if treatment is not followed. Surgery is the preferred treatment followed by radiation and pharmacological modalities. A combination of any of these 3 may be initiated. Adrenal enzyme inhibitors and/or ACTH inhibitors may be prescribed.

Nutritional Care

Nutrition support for Cushing's syndrome or clients on corticosteroid therapy should include an adequate amount of kilocalories, high levels of protein (100 gm), and moderate amounts of carbohydrate. Concentrated sugars are normally restricted to help maintain euglycemic levels. Fluid retention can be lessened by limiting sodium intake. Ascorbic acid supplementation is advised because ACTH depletes adrenal tissue of vitamin C, which is needed for collagen formation. High potassium intake is needed to prevent problems associated with hypokalemia.

Osteopenia—decreased bone mass.

Corticosteroids or Cushing's syndrome can cause **osteopenia** as a result of depressed bone formation with normal bone resorption (Prummel et al, 1991). When corticosteroids are given for a prolonged period, vitamin D (50,000 IU, 3 times a week) plus calcium (500 to 1000 mg/day) should be given to prevent osteopenia. Physical activity is also encouraged to enhance bone mineralization. In some cases of glucocorticoid therapy, oral zinc supplements have been used because of zinc depletion, and this may improve wound healing.

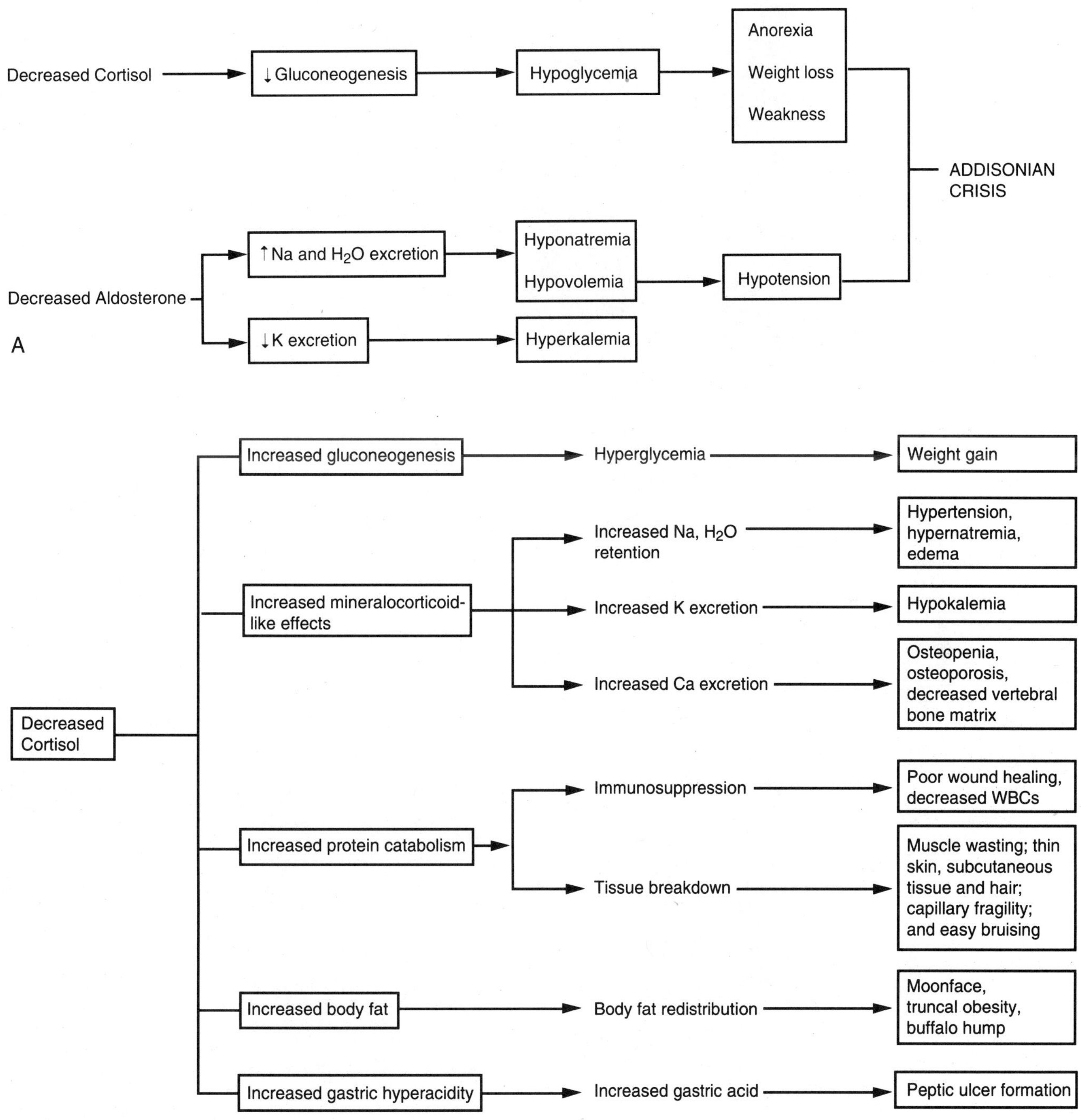

Figure 28–5 Comparison of Addison's and Cushing's diseases. *A*, Addison's (remember: this disease involves a lack of hormones that requires "added" (like *Add*ison's) cortisol and aldosterone). *B*, Cushing's and corticosteroid therapy (aldosterone is not affected). (Adapted from Beare PG, Myers JL. *Principles and Practices of Adult Health Nursing.* St. Louis, CV Mosby, 1990.)

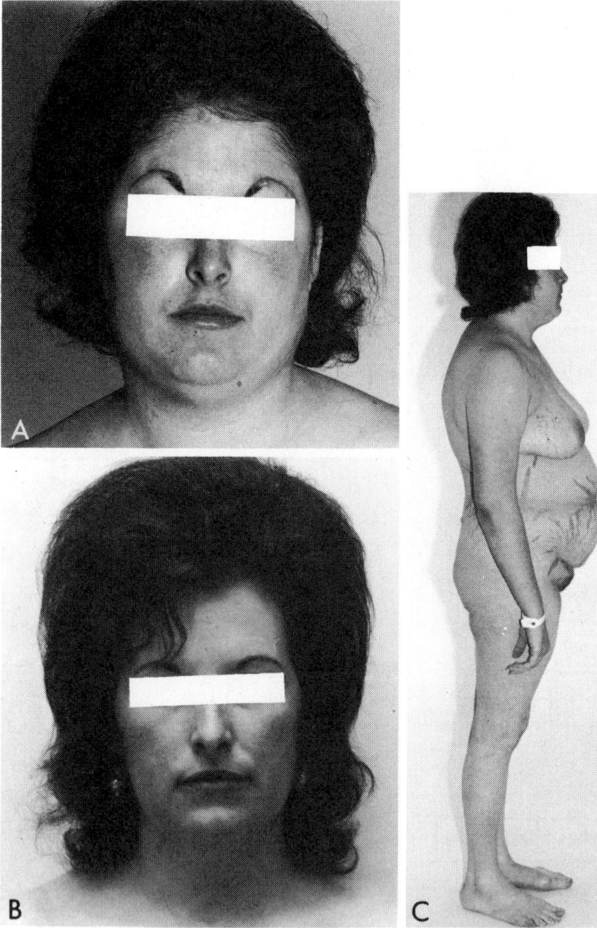

Figure 28–6 *A* and *C*, A client with Cushing's syndrome before and after treatment. *B*, One year after treatment (removal of an adrenal adenoma). (From Tyrrell JB, Baxter JD. Endocrine and reproductive diseases. *In* Wyngaarden JB, Smith LH Jr, eds. *Cecil Textbook of Medicine.* 18th ed. Philadelphia, WB Saunders, 1992.)

NURSING APPLICATIONS

Assessment

Physical—for weight; weight gain, height, IBW, MAMC, TSF, other symptoms shown in Figure 28–5.

Dietary—for increased appetite; concentrated sugar, sodium, potassium, calcium, vitamin C and D intake.

Laboratory—for glucose, abnormal GTT; potassium, calcium; cortisol; decreased WBC, TLC; ACTH.

Interventions

1. Offer empathy to deal with altered body image.
2. Refer to a dietitian.
3. Monitor for undesirable weight gain associated with hyperphagia and/or fluid retention.

Evaluation

* Desired outcomes include edema is reduced; laboratory values return to near-normal levels; and a diet adequate in kilocalories, high protein (with moderate amounts of carbohydrate), and adequate amounts of vitamins C and D, calcium, and potassium is consumed.

Client Education

- Eat foods high in potassium.
- Be sure to include vitamins C, D, and B_6 and calcium-rich foods in daily food choices.

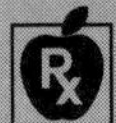 Prolonged usage of glucocorticoids is associated with osteoporosis, especially when calcium intake is low (<500 mg/day).

THYROID DYSFUNCTION

Thyroid hormones are secreted when stimulated by thyrotropin (TSH); they affect many metabolic processes; thyroid diseases are more prevalent than other endocrine diseases other than diabetes (Schimke, 1992). Dietary sources of iodine are an important constituent of these hormones. Thyroid hormones, thyroxine (T_4) and triiodothyronine (T_3), control the rate of biochemical processes. They increase oxidation of active cells (increasing kilocalorigenic activity), stimulate quantity and rate of enzymatic activity, increase glucose absorption and utilization, and regulate vitamin requirements because of vitamin functions in enzymes. These hormones are needed for normal growth and mental acuity. Since they increase anabolism and catabolism, an overabundance or deficiency affects metabolism of all energy nutrients—carbohydrate, protein, and fat. Thyroid gland enlargement is termed goiter and may be associated with either hypothyroidism or hyperthyroidism (see Chapter 9, Fig. 9–3).

The most sensitive marker for thyroid dysfunction is TSH (Stuck & McFarland, 1991). TSH is decreased in hyperthyroidism and increased in hypothyroidism.

List the effects of T3 and T4.

Hypothyroidism

Causes and Physical Consequences

Hypothyroidism may be related to (1) inadequate consumption of iodine, (2) an inborn error of metabolism, (3) high intake of **goitrogens,** (4) treatment of hyperthyroidism (surgical excision, irradiation, antithyroid drugs), (5) thyroid gland disorder, or (6) deficient secretion of thyrotropin (TSH) by the pituitary gland. Goitrogenic substances naturally present in broccoli, kale, kohlrabi, cabbage, rutabagas, turnips, cauliflower, Brussels sprouts, horseradish, and soybeans can precipitate hypothyroidism.

Thyroxine activity is decreased in hypothyroidism; BMR is decreased as much as 15 to 30%.

Goitrogens are chemicals that cause hypothyroidism by inhibiting thyroid iodine uptake.

Although goiter caused by iodine deficiency has been practically eliminated in the US with the use of iodized salt, some groups of people in Kentucky have a high prevalence of goiter despite sufficient iodine intake. These goiters occur mainly in children 12 to 13 years old. Apparently environmental and immunological factors play a role in this endemic goiter.

Cretinism develops as a result of hypothyroidism during childhood. In addition to mental retardation, lethargy and an increased susceptibility to respiratory infections are also observed.

Cretinism, caused by congenital lack of thyroid gland secretion, affects brain development, growth rate, and bone maturation.

Myxedema or **hypothyroidism** develops frequently after treatment for hyperthyroidism (Fig. 28–7). Hypothyroidism may be a result of an autoimmunity against the thyroid gland, which eventually destroys this gland but initially causes hyperthyroid secretion. Following **thyroiditis,** which causes gland deterioration that ultimately affects secretion of thyroid hormone, hypothyroidism may develop.

Advanced hypothyroidism or deficiency of thyroxine in adults is known as myxedema.

Thyroiditis—thyroid inflammation.

Recent studies have cited an increased incidence of hypothyroidism in elderly Americans (Bagchi et al, 1990; Griffin, 1990; Simons et al, 1990). In these clients,

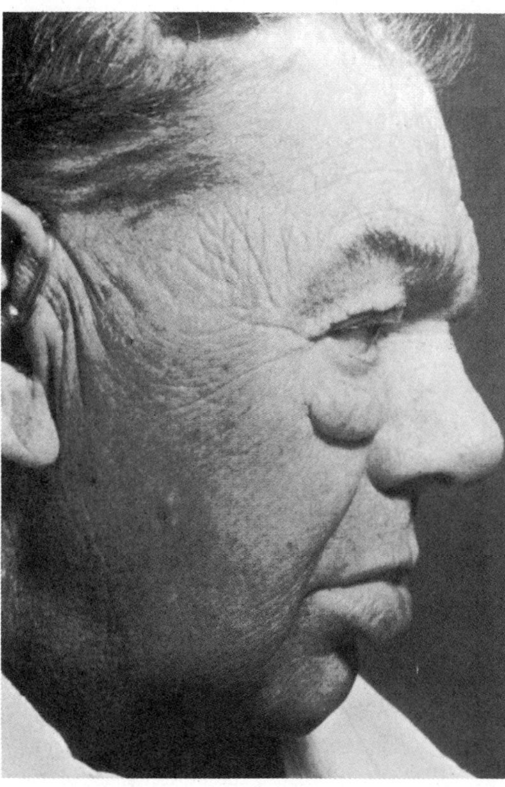

Figure 28–7 Myxedema. Note thick lips, baggy eyes, loss of hair, and dry skin. (From Jacob SW, Francone CA. *Elements of Anatomy and Physiology.* 2nd ed. Philadelphia, WB Saunders, 1989.)

nonspecific clinical findings mimicking the normal aging process may result in an oversight of hypothyroidism with serious consequences (Sawin, 1992).

What are causes of hypothyroidism? Why does weight gain occur? What else may occur in the body? What is hypothyroidism called in children? In adults?

Clients may gain weight despite a decreased appetite, exhibit an intolerance to cold, and have a decreased basal body temperature. Weight gain is due to increased fluid retention and excess adipose tissue along with decreased BMR (Katzeff & Rivlin, 1988). Lipid catabolism is decreased, resulting in increased serum triglycerides, cholesterol, and LDL. Decreased cellular uptake of glucose despite high levels of insulin leads to hyperglycemia. Macrocytic and pernicious anemia is common, which may be a result of vitamin B_{12} and folate metabolic abnormalities.

Treatment

Detection and treatment of subclinical hypothyroidism is important to prevent further decline in thyroid functioning (Drinka & Nolten, 1990). Overt hypothyroidism (elevated TSH and low T_4) requires lifelong hormonal replacement, or levothyroxine (Synthroid). Normal levels of thyroid activity can be maintained with daily oral doses of hormone(s). Nutritional measures may be needed to prevent weight gain and edema.

Nutritional Care

Kilocalories should be limited for overweight clients. Energy allotment is determined by the degree of overweight and metabolic rate. Fluids are encouraged to prevent constipation. High-fiber foods, such as bran and natural laxatives (prunes), help stimulate peristalsis. Iodized salt is important. A daily intake of 100 to 150 mcg of iodine can be obtained from approximately 1 tsp of iodized salt daily. This is feasible even if sodium intake is curtailed to 3 to 4 gm sodium to help decrease fluid retention.

NURSING APPLICATIONS

Assessment

Physical—for height, weight/weight gain, IBW; see Table 28–2.
Dietary—for adequacy of kilocalorie intake, iodine and goitrogenic foods, fluid intake, appetite.
Laboratory—for hyperlipidemia; sodium, potassium; vitamin B_{12}; glucose; decreased T_3, T_4; protein-bound iodine (PBI), TSH.

Interventions

1. Weigh daily; notify physician if weight increases by 10%.
2. Offer small portions to help offset impaired digestion from lack of HCl.
3. If hypothyroidism is induced by goitrogenic foods, encourage thorough cooking to inactivate goitrogens in foods.

Evaluation

* Desired outcomes include myxedema coma is prevented, weight gain does not occur; consumption of high-protein, low kilocalorie, high-fiber foods is maintained; and constipation and edema are alleviated.

Client Education

- Encourage use of iodized salt, as permitted.
- Encourage a low-fat, low-cholesterol diet and regular exercise to help control serum cholesterol levels.
- Eat fruits with skin, vegetables, and whole-grain breads and cereal to help maintain normal bowel function.
- Avoid cigarette smoking, as this increases vasoconstriction, enhancing cold sensitivity in arms and legs (Carpenito, 1991).

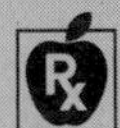 Thyroid hormones may elevate serum glucose and decrease cholesterol.

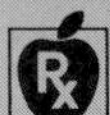 Thyroglobulin (Proloid) or levothyroxine (thyroid replacement hormones) should be given on an empty stomach to increase absorption; intake of goitrogens should be limited.

Hyperthyroidism or Graves' Disease

Causes

Hyperthyroidism may be caused by a tumor in the thyroid tissue that increases thyroid hormone secretion, but it is more frequently caused by **Graves' disease. Exophthalmos** is indicative of hyperthyroidism (Fig. 28–8). In addition to increased requirements for all nutrients because of an elevated metabolism, bone demineralization can be a complication if left untreated.

Hyperthyroidism is caused by excess secretion of thyroid hormones, resulting in an increased BMR and weight loss despite increased food intake.

In Graves' disease, antibodies to thyroid-stimulating hormone receptors stimulate thyroid hormone secretion.

Exophthalmos—protruding eyeballs.

Treatment

Several modes of treatment are used to decrease the amount of hormonal secretion: (1) antithyroid drugs, (2) surgery, or (3) radioiodine therapy. Iodine may be used as adjunctive therapy for hyperthyroidism; its major action is to inhibit hormonal release (Woeber, 1991). Antithyroid drugs inhibit biosynthesis of thyroxine.

What causes Graves' disease?

What are treatments for hyperthyroidism?

TABLE 28–2

COMPARISON OF HYPOTHYROIDISM AND HYPER-THYROIDISM

	Hypothyroidism	**Hyperthyroidism**
Basal metabolic rate	Weight gain	Weight loss
Body features	Thickened nose; periorbital edema; decreased sweating; thick, brittle fingernails	Exophthalmos (protruding eyes), increased sweating
Behaviors	Mental sluggishness, sleepy, fatigue, tired, "run down," cold intolerance	Restlessness, irritability, anxiety, mood swings, heat intolerance
Cholesterol level	Hypercholesterolemia (decreased lipid catabolism)	Hypocholesterolemia (increased lipid catabolism by the liver)
Gastrointestinal	Constipation, fecal impactions, decreased gastric and pancreatic* secretions, poor appetite	Diarrhea (rapid transit time), increased gastric secretions, hyperphagia
Proteins	Infections	Muscle proteins catabolized for energy
Blood glucose	Hypoglycemia	Hyperglycemia (decreased cellular glucose uptake)
Vitamins	Metabolic abnormalities of vitamin B_{12} and folate	Increased requirements due to increased BMR, causing accelerated use of vitamins in enzyme functions
Complications	Myxedema, coma	Thyroid crisis (storm)

* Gullo L, et al. Influence of the thyroid in exocrine pancreatic function. *Gastroenterology* 1991 May; 100(5, pt 1):1392–1396.

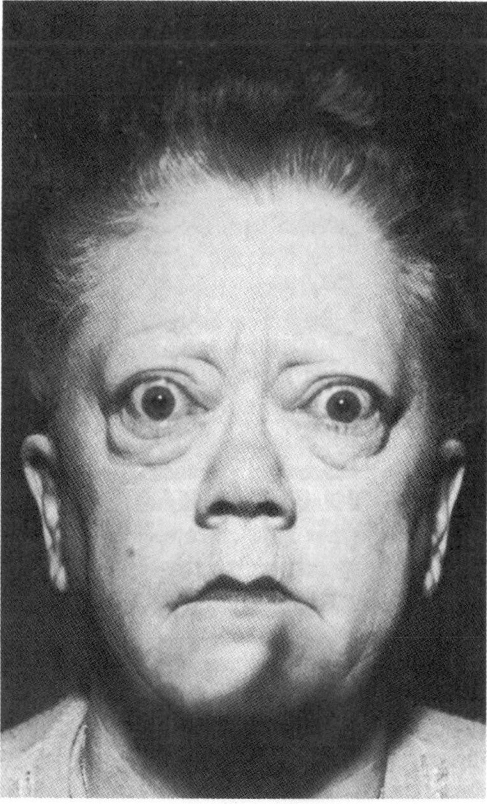

Figure 28–8 Exophthalmos. Note startled appearance and loss of eyebrows. (From Jacob SW, Francone CA. *Elements of Anatomy and Physiology.* 2nd ed. Philadelphia, WB Saunders, 1989.)

Nutritional Care

Until treatment results in a euthyroid state, a very high kilocalorie diet is indicated to prevent weight loss and body tissue destruction. There is no limitation on energy needs, but the diet should contain at least 3000 kcal; actual energy requirements are determined by the severity of the case. Liberal amounts of protein (1 to 2 gm/kg) are needed to offset negative nitrogen balance. Usually 100 gm protein is an adequate daily intake. Liberal use of carbohydrates and fats can increase kilocalorie intake. Snacks are usually beneficial in increasing total food consumption. Readily accessible foods should be available for clients in the hospital; "constant nibbling" is acceptable. Large amounts of fluid (3 to 4 L/day) are encouraged to offset excessive losses from sweating and heavy breathing.

GI transit time is significantly faster in untreated Graves' disease. Thus, high-fiber foods may need to be limited. Rapid transit time also may account for lactose malabsorption frequently observed (Szilagyi et al, 1991). Lactose-intolerant clients should increase intake of yogurt, buttermilk, and aged cheeses to provide needed calcium. If a client is not lactose intolerant, milk consumption (4 cups/day) is encouraged to compensate for calcium losses. Enhanced cellular metabolism increases requirements for riboflavin, ascorbic acid, pyridoxine, vitamin A and possibly B_{12}, and folate (Katzeff & Rivlin, 1988). Multivitamin supplements are usually advisable.

NURSING APPLICATIONS

Assessment

Physical—for height, weight/weight changes, IBW; other symptoms in Table 28-2.
Dietary—for appetite, adequacy of intake, calcium and lactose intake.
Laboratory—for glucose, calcium, potassium, sodium; T_3, T_4, PBI, TSH; cholesterol, triglyceride.

Interventions

1. Monitor for thyroid storm, which is caused by a sudden increase in thyroid hormone secretion (disorientation, fever, hypotension and tachycardia). Notify physician immediately.
2. Keep mealtimes calm and unhurried.

Evaluation

* Desired outcomes include client consuming a high kilocalorie, high protein, nutrient-dense diet, maintaining stable weight, and avoiding a thyroid storm.

Client Education

- To prevent further CNS stimulation, avoid or limit use of stimulants: caffeinated beverages and tobacco.
- Alcohol is excluded to prevent low blood glucose.
- After hyperthyroidism is controlled, appetite may not automatically decrease. Clients should be advised about the possibility of obesity if food intake is not altered.

PARATHYROID DYSFUNCTION

The parathyroid hormone (PTH) functions to maintain a constant serum calcium level, which is necessary for blood coagulation, cardiac and skeletal muscle contraction, and nerve function. Normally PTH secretion is inversely proportional

TABLE 28–3

NUTRITIONAL AND METABOLIC ACTIONS OF PARATHYROID HORMONE*

Increases renal calcium retention
Increases renal phosphate excretion
Stimulates intestinal calcium absorption
Stimulates bone resorption
Stimulates bone anabolism
Stimulates kidney production of the active form of vitamin D

* A low serum calcium level stimulates release of parathyroid hormone.

Adapted from Katzeff HL, Rivlin RS. Endocrine diseases. *In* Kinney JM, et al, eds. *Nutrition and Metabolism in Patient Care.* Philadelphia, WB Saunders, 1988: 342–359.

to serum calcium level. Thus, when serum calcium is low, PTH is increased, and when calcium is high, PTH is decreased. Intestinal absorption of calcium, bone homeostasis, and renal excretion of calcium and phosphate are controlled by the parathyroids, as shown in Table 28–3. When phosphate is high, calcium is excreted and vice versa.

Hypoparathyroidism

Physical Consequences

Tetany is characterized by hyperirritability of the nervous system, caused by an imbalance of calcium (low) and phosphorus (high), and is evidenced by carpopedal spasms, muscle twitching or abdominal cramps, convulsions, and occasionally laryngospasms.

A deficiency of PTH impairs conversion of precursor forms of vitamin D to its active form. Hypocalcemia results from lack of PTH and 1,25 dihydroxy-vitamin D_3 (active form of vitamin D). Hypocalcemia also occurs because a low PTH decreases calcium in 3 areas: bone reabsorption, renal reabsorption, and intestinal absorption. This decrease in PTH also causes phosphorus to increase.

Hypocalcemic **tetany** is the result of parathyroid hypofunction associated with rickets, osteomalacia, pregnancy, hypermagnesemia, steatorrhea, thyroid surgery, and renal insufficiency (Fig. 28–9). Alkalotic tetany may be caused by hyperventilation, vomiting, or injection of alkaline salts. Total plasma calcium may be as low as 4 mg/dl (normally 8.5 to 10.5 mg/dl).

Treatment

Treatment varies according to the cause. Administration of vitamin D, calcium, and PTH is used successfully to treat hypocalcemia and/or tetany from hypoparathyroidism. Tetany resulting from alkalosis is treated with large doses of an acid-producing salt, frequently ammonium chloride.

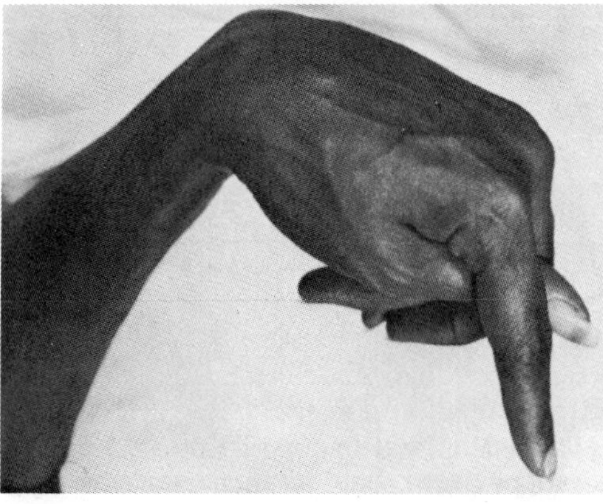

Figure 28–9 Hypocalcemic tetany in the hand, called "carpopedal spasm." (Courtesy of Dr. Herbert Langford; from Guyton AC. *Textbook of Medical Physiology.* 8th ed. Philadelphia, WB Saunders, 1991.)

Nutritional Care

Usual treatment is to increase calcium levels with a high-calcium diet. At least 1 to 1½ qt of milk daily are advisable. (Milk contains the most bioavailable form of calcium.) Calcium supplements (1.5 gm) are usually necessary since diet alone cannot adequately increase calcium levels. Vitamin D supplementation (25,000 to 200,000 IU/day) enhances calcium absorption. However, clients must be monitored for hypervitaminosis D. Calcium–vitamin D supplements may be needed for clients who dislike milk and milk products. Phosphorus intake may be restricted depending on laboratory results.

NURSING APPLICATIONS

Assessment

Physical—for symptoms, see Table 28–4.
Dietary—for calcium and phosphorus intake.
Laboratory—for calcium; low PTH, elevated phosphate.

Interventions

1. Offer high-calcium foods. For clients who are lactose intolerant, give calcium–vitamin D supplements, as ordered.

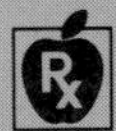
When phosphate levels are high, administer aluminum antacids (Amphojel, Basojel) to decrease absorption of dietary phosphorus.

Evaluation

* Client should have a normal calcium level, maintain an adequate intake of calcium, and have no seizures.

Client Education

- A prescription for quinine sulfate tablets (Quinamm) alleviates only the muscle cramping, not the condition (hypoparathyroidism).
- Use meats, poultry, fish, eggs, cheese, and cereal in moderation since they are high in phosphorus.

TABLE 28–4

COMPARISON OF HYPOPARATHYROIDISM AND HYPERPARATHYROIDISM

System	Hypoparathyroidism	Hyperparathyroidism
Musculoskeletal	Numbness, tingling in lips and fingertips, weak muscles, seizures, tetany; positive Chvostek's (tapping a client's jaw causes a facial spasm) and Trousseau's (spasms in the hand when BP cuff is inflated) signs, laryngeal spasms	Weight loss, muscle weakness, fatigue, diffuse bone pain, osteopenia, osteoporosis
Gastrointestinal	Abdominal cramping, diarrhea, possible steatorrhea	Anorexia, nausea, vomiting, constipation; hyperacidity and peptic ulcer disease, thirst
Cardiovascular	Conduction through the heart is slowed, leading to bradycardia, possible heart block, heart failure, or decreased cardiac output	Bounding pulse, calcification of arteries produces high BP and heart disease and arrhythmias; increased heart contractability
Renal		Kidney stones, renal pain, frequent UTIs, polyuria

Hyperparathyroidism

Causes and Physical Consequences

Hyperparathyroidism results in hypersecretion of PTH, leading to alterations in calcium, phosphorus, and bone metabolism, thus causing calcium resorption from skeletal tissue and decreasing bone integrity. An elevated calcium level is the classic sign of hyperparathyroidism. Physical findings are usually a result of the imbalance between calcium and phosphorus (see Table 28-4). However, nurses must remember that elevated calcium levels can also occur for other reasons; they may occur as a result of immobility (accompanied by hypophosphatemia) and other disorders including hyperthyroidism and bone disorders. Hypercalcemia is the most common life-threatening metabolic disorder associated with malignancy. Hypercalcemia is observed in vitamin A and D intoxication and **milk-alkali** syndrome.

Milk-alkali syndrome denotes excessive ingestion of milk and absorbable antacids, resulting in kidney damage and elevated blood calcium levels.

What can cause hypercalcemia?

Usually hyperparathyroidism is discovered incidentally in laboratory testing, but clients may present with vague symptoms. Since calcium is present in blood in a protein-bound and a free ionized form, it is important to ascertain that a client is truly hypercalcemic (see Chapter 9).

Treatment

Treatment for hyperparathyroidism is surgical removal of the gland. After surgery, low calcium levels are expected because calcium regulation is altered (removed PTH), and a client's demineralized bone reabsorbs available serum calcium.

Initial treatment for hypercalcemia is rehydration with IV normal saline (1000 ml/4 to 6 hr). Hemodilution decreases serum calcium concentration, and sodium increases urinary calcium excretion. Various medications differ in mechanisms for lowering calcium levels: Diuretics, such as furosemide (Lasix) (except for thiazide diuretics that worsen hypercalcemia), increase urinary calcium excretion; prednisone decreases calcium absorption; phosphate compounds (Phos-Tabs) promote deposition of calcium into skeletal tissue. Mithramycin (Mithracin) may be used for metastatic malignancies.

Nutritional Care

Since hypercalcemia is only a symptom, the underlying disorder is usually treated. However, several nutritional factors can be implemented until effective medical treatment is established. A high level of fluid intake is needed to prevent formation of kidney stones and constipation. As discussed in Chapter 2, an acid-ash diet may be prescribed to produce an acidic urine and prevent calcium stone formation (see Appendix D-4). Low calcium and vitamin D intake along with an increased vitamin K intake may be recommended (Gribbin, 1990).

NURSING APPLICATIONS

Assessment

Physical—for immobility, cancer, renal disease; bowel sounds, coma; see Table 28-4.

Dietary—for intake of vitamin A and D, use of megadose vitamins, appetite, anorexia.

Laboratory—for calcium, phosphate, BUN.

Interventions

1. Refer to OT and PT to increase muscular strength and endurance, especially for specialized eating utensils and for energy-conservation tips to prepare meals.

2. Encourage 2 to 3 L/day of fluid unless contraindicated as in renal or cardiac problems.
3. Monitor I&O for overhydration since client may be receiving numerous IV infusions (Gribbin, 1990).
4. If permitted, offer foods high in sodium, as this may enhance urinary calcium excretion.

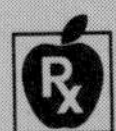 If on diuretics, monitor potassium and vitamin C intake.

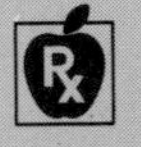 Monitor clients on phosphate solutions for signs of metastatic calcification and acute renal failure, as oral phosphates may cause GI symptoms and may increase absorption of oxalates.

Evaluation

* Client's calcium level should return to normal, intake of fluid should be high, and urinary tract should be free of stones.

Client Education

* Elevated calcium levels are dangerous but are not caused by calcium intake alone.
* Large doses of vitamin D supplements or increased intake of milk along with sodium bicarbonate may precipitate hypercalcemia.
* Remind clients of hypercalcemic symptoms with the catchy phrase, "stones, bones, abdominal groans, and emotional overtones." If these symptoms occur, notify the physician.

INBORN ERRORS OF METABOLISM

The discovery of many inborn errors of metabolism has increased dramatically, even though their occurrence is relatively rare. Successful therapeutic nutritional interventions have been developed. Success is varied with the type of disease and the ease with which dietary modifications can be achieved. Although this text discusses only one inborn error of metabolism (phenylketonuria), other less prevalent conditions also respond only to diet therapy, e.g., **maple syrup urine disease (MSUD), tyrosinemia,** and **galactosemia.** Because of the specialized diagnostics and treatments required for controlling these conditions, only large medical facilities are equipped to handle them.

MSUD, tyrosinemia, and galactosemia are genetic disorders characterized by an enzyme deficiency needed to metabolize branched-chain amino acids, tyrosine (an amino acid), and galactose (a monosaccharide), respectively.

In **aminoacidopathy,** restriction of the offending amino acid is essential to avoid accumulation of excessive amounts of the amino acid or its derivatives. However, adequate amounts must be provided for growth. Careful monitoring must continue to maintain such delicate balances.

Aminoacidopathy is an inborn error of metabolism in which a particular step in the utilization of an amino acid is blocked.

Phenylketonuria

Physical Consequences

In **phenylketonuria (PKU),** phenylalanine (an EAA) is not converted to tyrosine in a normal manner (Fig. 28–10), and phenylalanine accumulates, whereas tyrosine is inadequate. Thus, tyrosine becomes an EAA for these clients. High levels of circulating phenylalanine affect brain development. Infants in whom the condition is detected early and treatment initiated before 6 weeks of age are not mentally retarded. Approximately 1 in every 70 persons in the US is a carrier of PKU, an autosomal recessive disorder.

PKU is an inborn error of metabolism in which the enzyme, phenylalanine hydroxylase, is either absent or present in trace amounts.

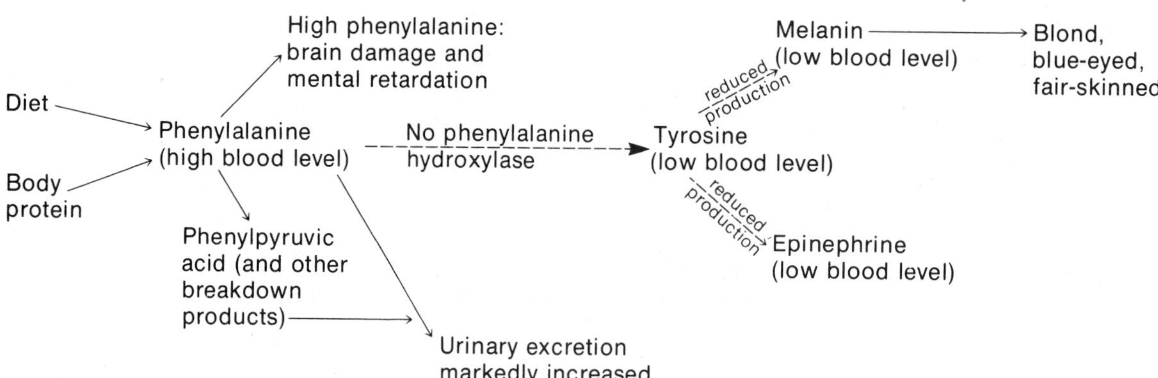

Figure 28–10 Absence of the enzyme phenylalanine hydroxylase prevents conversion of phenylalanine to tyrosine. Blood samples reveal high phenylalanine and low tyrosine. Urine samples show excessive phenylalanine and its breakdown products. Production of melanin and epinephrine is decreased. Mental retardation develops as a result of the toxic character of high levels of phenylalanine in the brain. (From Sorensen KC, Luckmann J. *Basic Nursing: A Psychophysiologic Approach.* 2nd ed. Philadelphia, WB Saunders, 1986.)

If an infant is not identified by testing, the first conspicuous sign of PKU is an inability of the child to sit unassisted at the normal age. Untreated PKU infants may not walk until early childhood or may never learn to walk. Motor development is slow, and electroencephalographic abnormalities are common in these blond, blue-eyed children. When compared with siblings, PKU clients usually have a slightly lower IQ with difficulty in math and conceptual thinking (Rylance, 1989).

What happens in PKU?

Screening Tests

Screening newborns for PKU has been mandatory in most states since 1961. This is normally performed before an infant is released from the hospital. At birth, serum phenylalanine levels are less than 2 mg/dl. Intake of phenylalanine, present in breast milk or formula, induces immediate increases in serum phenylalanine levels. A phenylalanine level measuring 4 to 8 mg/dl within 1 week of birth warrants further investigation, which may be conducted in a physician's office at 4 to 6 weeks of age.

What are normal levels of phenylalanine? What results require immediate implementation of dietary measures?

A phenylalanine level of 20 mg/dl or higher with normal tyrosine concentrations warrants immediate implementation of dietary measures. A small percentage of children develop an ability to convert phenylalanine to tyrosine during the first year of life; thus, the special diet should be challenged with milk about 3 months after initiating therapy. If dietary restrictions are lifted, laboratory tests are used to verify that phenylalanine restriction is not needed (results < 8 mg/dl).

Treatment

The only effective method of treating PKU is dietary control of phenylalanine intake. Enough must be provided to allow for growth, but accumulation of excessive amounts of phenylalanine must be prevented. Natural protein-containing foods can be added to provide the minimum requirement of phenylalanine and additional protein when plasma phenylalanine levels fall to 6 mg/dl.

Excessive vigorous dietary restrictions have resulted in profound malnutrition and even deaths during the first year. As a preventive measure, serum phenylalanine levels are measured once or twice a week during the first year. Serum protein and hemoglobin levels as well as height and weight are measured to determine adequacy of protein and energy intake.

A collaborative study in the US provided data indicating that blood phenylalanine levels should be maintained between 2 and 10 mg/dl at least through adolescence (Link, 1989). Liberalizing the diet too early is thought to be responsible for behavior patterns that interfere with normal mental functioning. Short attention span, poor short-term memory, impaired visual-motor perception, defective motor coordination, seizures, and musty odor may result when serum phenylalanine levels are allowed to increase (Azen et al, 1991; Smith et al, 1991; Thompson et al, 1990; Yannicelli et al, 1990). Therefore, lifelong dietary management may be beneficial.

A PKU child must be treated as normally as possible, even though rigid dietary regulations are required, and should not be pampered in his or her attitude or behavior. Because of social interactions, it becomes increasingly difficult to maintain a restricted diet after age 2. Positive attitudes regarding this diet must be initiated and cultivated during the toddler period and continued through early childhood and adolescence. Parents often discover that these dietary restrictions are more difficult for them than for their PKU child. An experienced multidisciplinary health care team can offer support and guidance on diagnosis and during difficult periods.

Parents must have a sincere commitment and considerable patience to keep a child on this special diet; struggles involved may place a serious emotional/financial burden on families. Expense of the PKU diet is considerable. Annual costs for PKU infants as compared with regular formula-fed infants were $1200 versus $600; for toddlers, $1920 versus $480; for grade school girls, $2400 versus $300; and for adolescents, $3480 versus $720. Costs for PKU boys were proportionately higher because of their increased requirements (McMurry et al, 1986).

As a child grows and matures, he or she must increasingly take responsibility for self-management of the diet. By 7 or 8 years of age, a child is taught to prepare the formula. By 12 years of age, a child should be calculating phenylalanine content of food. A major goal of the health care team is to encourage a child's independence.

Nutritional Care

Initially in infancy, all protein requirements can be met from a minimal phenylalanine formula such as Lofenalac (Mead Johnson), PKU-I (Milupa), and XPAnalog (Scientific Hospital Supplies) (Table 28–5). Adequate protein while limiting phenylalanine cannot be provided without using these products. Parents must be instructed how to calculate amounts of protein, phenylalanine, and fluid provided by these feedings as the infant grows and intake increases. Phenylalanine intake should be calculated daily.

Phenylalanine is present in all foods at a remarkably constant and relatively large amount—about 5% of the protein content of foods is phenylalanine. The diet can be modified by using **protein hydrolysates** in which phenylalanine is limited and tyrosine is added.

Protein hydrolysates are a mixture of amino acids prepared by splitting proteins.

As shown in Table 28–6, recommended intakes of phenylalanine gradually decrease (based on body weight) throughout infancy and childhood to 3 to 4 mg/kg/day by adulthood. This diet requires frequent adjustments. Because of the time-consuming task for manual calculations, a microcomputer program has been developed to aid in figuring the diet prescription.

Despite numerous restrictions, a well-balanced diet is needed. Low phenylalanine diets of PKU children are frequently below recommended levels of vitamins and minerals, especially selenium (Reilly et al, 1990; Link, 1989). Therefore, a multivitamin/mineral supplement may be recommended. Consistent with the diet during infancy, foods must provide nutrients necessary for growth, development, and general well-being, while preventing excess phenylalanine accumulation.

For older children with PKU, an appropriate diet consists of a low-phenylalanine or phenylalanine-free protein substitute, some phenylalanine-containing foods, and many low-protein products (Fig. 28–11). Low-protein products produced com-

TABLE 28-5

COMMERCIAL FORMULAS FOR PHENYLKETONURIA AND THEIR INTENDED USE

Target User Group	Product and Manufacturer	Comments
Infant	XP Analog (Scientific Hospital Supplies)	Complete formula
	Lofenalac* (Mead Johnson)	Complete formula
	PKU 1 (Milupa)	Requires additional carbohydrate and fat
	PKU-Aid* (Dietary Specialties)	Requires vitamin A, D, E, K, and C supplements
Child, age 2-8 years	XP Maxamaid (Scientific Hospital Supplies)	Requires additional fat, carbohydrates, and vitamin K
	Phenyl-Free (Mead Johnson)	Complete formula
	PKU-2 (Milupa)	Requires additional carbohydrate and fat
Child 8 years to adolescence	XP Maxamum (Scientific Hospital Supplies)	Requires additional fat and/or carbohydrate; plain or orange flavored
	Phenyl-Free (Mead Johnson)	Complete formula
	PKU-2 (Milupa)	Requires additional fat and carbohydrate
Adolescent	XP Maxamum (Scientific Hospital Supplies)	Requires additional fat and/or carbohydrate and vitamin K
	PKU-3 (Milupa)	Requires additional fat and carbohydrate
Pregnancy	XP Maxamum (Scientific Hospital Supplies)	Vitamin and mineral supplements may be necessary
	PKU-3 (Milupa)	Vitamin and mineral supplements may be necessary

* These products contain phenylalanine. For phenylalanine-free products, low-protein foods (fruits, vegetables, starchy foods, and low-protein starchy foods) are used to provide required phenylalanine.

mercially and low-protein recipes are used to incorporate variety (see Chapter 29, Table 29-5). Fruits, vegetables, and small amounts of other foods provide adequate amounts of phenylalanine and energy. The phenylalanine, protein, and kilocaloric content of vegetables, fruits, breads, and cereals used in a phenylalanine-restricted diet is important.

TABLE 28-6

APPROXIMATE DAILY RECOMMENDED INTAKE OF FLUID, KILOCALORIES, PROTEIN, PHENYLALANINE, AND TYROSINE FOR CHILDREN WITH PHENYLKETONURIA

Age	Fluid (ml/kg)	Kilocalories kcal/kg	Kilocalories kcal/day	Protein gm/kg	Protein gm/day	Phenylalanine mg/kg	Tyrosine* mg/kg
0-6 months	120-115	145-195		2.5		70-20	80-60
6-12 months	100	135-180		2.2		50-15	60-40
1-4 years	95		900-1800		25	40-15	60-30
4-7 years	90		1300-2300		30	35-15	50-25
7-11 years	75		1650-3300		35	30-15	40-20
11-15 years	50		1500-3700		45-50	30-15	30-15
15-19 years	50		1200-3900		45-55	30-10	30-10

* Data from Elsas LJ, Acosta PB. Nutrition support of inherited metabolic diseases. *In* Shils ME, Young VR, eds. *Modern Nutrition in Health and Disease.* 7th ed. Philadelphia, Lea & Febiger. 1988, 1337-1379.
Data from Martin SB, Acosta PB. Nutrition support of phenylketonuria and maple syrup urine disease. *Topics Clin Nutr* 1987; 2:3.

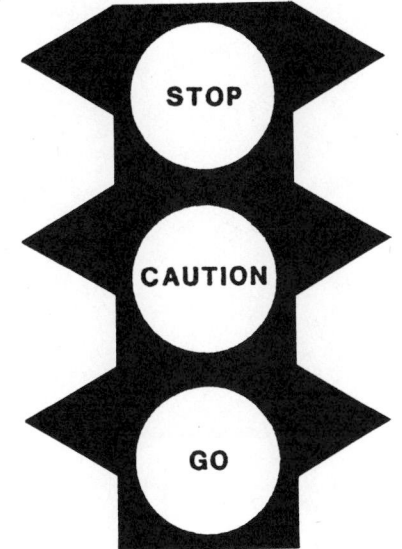

NOT ALLOWED—meat, fish, chicken, turkey, milk, cheese, ice cream, yogurt, eggs, beans, nuts, peanut butter, Nutra Sweet*

ALLOWED BUT CONTROLLED—fruits, fruit juices, vegetables, vegetable juices, breads, cereals, crackers, potato chips, pop corn, special low protein foods**

FREE FOODS*—soda, Kool-Aid, lemonade, popsicles, jelly, gum drops, suckers, hard candy

Figure 28–11 Examples of foods allowed and restricted in phenylketonuria.
*Products containing NutraSweet, Equal, or aspartame shoud be avoided by clients with phenylketonuria. **Some food manufacturers use special ingredients to make low-protein foods, such as pastas and baked goods, for the phenylketonuria diet. (From Kaufman M, Nardella M. *A Teacher's Guide to PKU.* Phoenix, AZ, Arizona Department of Health Services, 1985.)

NURSING APPLICATIONS

Assessment

Physical—for birth weight and growth record, length, developmental stages, marked irritability, rebellion, musty odor, eczema; severe vomiting, lethargy, anorexia, fever, seizures.

Dietary—for economic resources, intake of phenylalanine, tyrosine, and artificial sweetener, special diet consumed.

Laboratory—for phenylalanine, tyrosine, protein, Hgb.

Interventions

1. Refer to a dietitian.
2. Support and encourage parents in meal planning.
3. Encourage age-appropriate responsibilities for the diet.
4. Involve an adolescent in food choices and planning.
5. Suggest family counseling.

Evaluation

* Client should consume a low phenylalanine diet, have a relatively normal IQ, and grow/mature according to growth charts. Additionally, parents should be able to discuss joys, successes, fears, and concerns while providing the special diet.

Client Education

- Tell parents, "Do not let your child know you find the formula objectionable."
- Include the child in all special occasions, even when food is provided, to prevent feelings of being left out. Dietary restrictions should be enforced, but some of the foods served should be permitted.
- Serve formula cold in a glass. Formula can be partially frozen or combined with ice and blended to milkshake or slushy consistency.

Continued

- Add artificial flavors, pureed fruits, or juices (Tang, chocolate or strawberry flavoring, lemon or peppermint extract, fruit-flavored soft drink mix, banana) to alter formula flavor.
- Provide fruits and vegetables, sugars, and fats to furnish adequate kilocalories.
- Involving children in management of their own diet helps to develop a healthy attitude toward food.
- Inform a child's teacher about the diet. Encourage participation in school activities even though special arrangements may be necessary.
- Adolescents may prefer to refer to their diet as vegetarian.
- Do not completely omit phenylalanine from the diet, as the body cannot make it and phenylalanine is essential for growth.
- Refer to resources for low-protein foods: Dietary Specialties, Ener-G Foods, Inc., and Med-Diet, Inc. (see Chapter 29, Table 29–5).

Maternal Phenyketonuria

Increasingly healthy PKU women with normal IQs are reaching childbearing age and presenting new challenges for health care professionals. While these mothers may bear healthy, normal infants, the risks of pregnancy and alternatives must be explained to all women with PKU considering marriage and a family.

A fetus exposed to elevated levels of phenylalanine, which crosses the placenta, is likely to develop congenital anomalies, profound mental retardation, low birth weight, and congenital heart disease (Waisbren et al, 1988; Drogari et al, 1987). Untreated pregnant women with blood phenylalanine concentrations of 20 mg/dl or higher have a 95% chance of having at least one mentally retarded child, which is not due to PKU.

Microcephaly—smaller than normal-size head.

Dietary treatment should begin before conception (Davidson, 1989). Within a few weeks of conception, fetal damage has already occurred, resulting in reduced brain growth, **microcephaly,** and cardiac malformations. However, good dietary control of phenylalanine levels throughout pregnancy can foster normal fetal development and result in a healthy infant (Waisbren et al, 1988).

The diet, begun before conception, is manipulated to keep plasma phenylalanine around 8 mg/dl. Special products have been formulated to help provide nutritional requirements for pregnant PKU women (see Table 28–5). These formulas are used in conjunction with fruits and vegetables and low-protein starchy products to allow some variety in the diet.

NURSING APPLICATIONS

Assessment

Physical—for weight gain pattern.
Dietary—for economic resources, artificial sweetener use, special diet consumed, compliance.
Laboratory—for plasma phenylalanine, tyrosine.

Interventions

1. Monitor adherence to low phenylalanine diet, especially before conception.
2. Explain to women with PKU the importance of close monitoring by a physician from the onset of pregnancy.
3. Praise for dietary adherence.
4. Refer to a dietitian for dietary information.
5. Locate sources for commercial formulas (see Table 28–5) and economic resources if needed.

Evaluation

* Desired outcomes are infant and mother are healthy, mother consumes special diet, and blood phenylalanine levels stabilize around 8 mg/dl.

Client Education

- Low-protein products such as pastas and bread can be used to add variety and kilocalories (see Chapter 29, Table 29–5).
- Aspartame, a high-intensity sweetener, contains phenylalanine and another amino acid. Any product that contains aspartame is contraindicated for PKU clients and pregnant PKU carriers.

GOUT

Nearly 2 million (8 out of 1000) people in the US have **gout,** most of whom are men. Women rarely develop this painful form of arthritis until after menopause.

Gout is a metabolic disease in which increased levels of uric acid in the blood may be deposited in joints and tissues.

Physical Consequences

Uric acid is the end product of **purine** metabolism, which is normally excreted via the kidneys. In primary gout, **hyperuricemia** results in urate crystals deposited throughout the body. These needle-like crystals irritate joint lining and can cause severe inflammation, or acute attacks. In turn, crystal deposits form a **tophus** (Fig. 28–12). The joint in the big toe is affected in 3 out of 4 people, but any joint may be involved. Hyperuricemia may lead to uric acid kidney stones.

Purine—a nucleic acid or nucleoprotein.

Hyperuricemia is excessive accumulation of uric acid in the plasma.

Tophus—a nodular deposit.

What causes the pain and formation of tophus in gout? Why does this occur?

Treatment

Objectives of treatment include prevention of acute attacks, delaying of progressive disability from erosion of bone and joint cartilage, and slowing of progres-

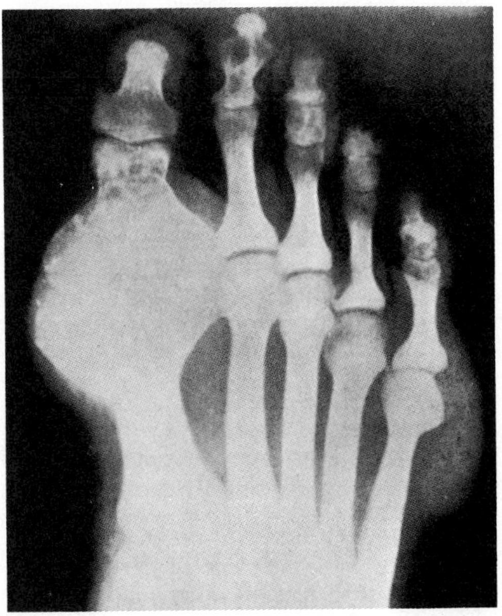

Figure 28–12 Deposit of sodium urate crystals from tophi in the big toe. Gouty involvement of the bones of the first metatarsophalangeal joint simulating a bone tumor. (From Bondy PK, Rosenberg LE. *Metabolic Control and Disease.* 8th ed. Philadelphia, WB Saunders, 1980.)

sive renal dysfunction. In clients with chronic gout, progressive renal dysfunction is the greatest threat to life.

Drug therapy is the main treatment for gout. Nonsteroidal anti-inflammatory drugs are effective during an acute attack. Uricosuric agents (allopurinol, probenecid, or sulfinpyrazone) lower uric acid levels and prevent further attacks. Colchicine is recommended mainly during acute attacks. Bicarbonate or citrate may be prescribed to alkalinize urine and increase uric acid solubility in urine. Acute medical or surgical illnesses may necessitate involuntary fasting for gout clients. Under these conditions, a high-carbohydrate intake is important as well as adequate fluids, even if parenteral fluids are administered. Diuretics (especially thiazides) cause increased tubular reabsorption of urate and may be a predisposing factor for gout, so these are not used (Hopkinson & Doherty, 1991).

Nucleoproteins—conjugated proteins consisting of nucleic acids and simple proteins.

What are objectives of treatment? Why does diet alone not cure gout?

Dietary intake decreases only exogenous sources of **nucleoproteins,** which account for less than half the uric acid found in blood. Uric acid is endogenously produced from available compounds such as carbon dioxide, ammonia, and glycine. Therefore, diet is used as an adjunctive therapy.

Nutritional Care

The single, most important dietary recommendation for a client with gout is to drink large volumes of fluids (3 L/day) to enhance uric acid secretion and decrease renal calculi formation.

A purine-restricted diet may be prescribed. Foods highest in purines include organ meats, anchovies, sardines, meat extracts, gravy, broth, and bouillon. Severe limitations on protein and purine content are necessary only during acute stages. A moderate protein diet results in a slightly increased rate of endogenous purine production and uric acid synthesis. Serum uric acid levels generally decrease as much as 0.5 to 1.5 mg/dl in clients on diets permitting up to 1 gm protein/kg IBW. Thus, protein intake should be moderate during interim stages to reduce gout medication.

Urate excretion is decreased by high fat intake; additionally, most clients have elevated triglyceride levels. A minimum of 100 gm carbohydrate should be consumed daily to prevent tissue catabolism or ketosis. Large amounts of fructose precipitate hyperuricemia (Henry et al, 1991).

Fasting may cause ketosis, which may precipitate an acute attack. Hyperuricemia is correlated to alcohol abuse in men. Large quantities of alcohol result in accumulation of lactic acid, which inhibits renal secretion of urates, and may precipitate acute attacks. When fasting is added to an increased alcoholic intake, effects are multiplied. Complete abstinence is not required; alcohol diluted with water and taken in moderation (not more than 100 gm/day) with food is acceptable (Table 28–7).

What foods are high in purine?

TABLE 28–7

DIETARY GUIDELINES FOR TREATMENT OF GOUT

1. The diet should be low in fat; a high-fat diet increases the frequency of acute attacks
2. Obese clients should follow a nutritionally balanced weight reduction program. The course of their gout may be favorably influenced by a slow steady weight loss. Fasting is recognized as a precipitating factor of acute attacks and should be avoided since it produces a metabolic situation comparable to that of a high-fat diet
3. A high intake of liquids lessens the incidence of kidney stones and prevents the dehydration associated with antigout medications. A minimum of 2 qt/day of water and fruit juices is advised
4. Purine and protein intakes are not rigidly restricted, but a high-protein diet does accelerate gout. Limiting protein to 50–75 gm/day with most of it in the form of plant and dairy products is often recommended

Nursing Applications

Assessment

Physical—for height, weight, IBW.
Dietary—for use of alcoholic beverages, intake of protein and purine-containing foods; compliance with purine-restricted diet.
Laboratory—for elevated uric acid; triglycerides; sodium, urine pH.

Interventions

1. See Table 28–7.
2. Identify clients who could benefit from dietary measures by evaluating a 3-day food diary for kilocalorie, protein, purine, and oxalate intake.
3. Offer a high-carbohydrate, moderate-protein, low-fat diet.
4. Demonstrate to clients how to measure urine pH with test tape. Urine should be alkaline to increase solubility of uric acid.

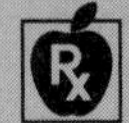 If client is on colchicine, encourage foods rich in vitamin B_{12} as colchicine impairs vitamin B_{12} absorption.

Evaluation

* Client should ingest a well-balanced meal, maintain IBW, restrict foods high in purine, and drink 3 L of fluid a day.
* Alcohol consumption should decrease or stop.

Client Education

- Organ meats should be eliminated.
- Do not exceed 3 to 4 oz meat at each meal.
- By lowering fat intake, acute attacks may be avoided, triglycerides lowered, and excess weight lost.
- Slow weight loss (1 to 2 lb/week) is desirable for overweight clients. (Provide 500 kcal below maintenance needs.)
- Optimal body weight for clients with gout is 10 to 15% below normal ranges.
- Liberal fruit and vegetable intake is recommended to maintain a slightly alkaline urine.
- Foods that are low in nucleoproteins include milk/milk products, eggs, and vegetables.

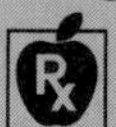 Clients taking uricosuric agents should consume 10 to 12 glasses of fluids daily to produce 2 L urine within a 24-hour period.

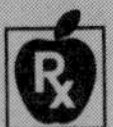 Maintenance of an alkaline urine is important for the effectiveness of uricosuric drugs. Vitamin C supplements should not be taken.

SICKLE CELL ANEMIA

Most cases of sickle cell anemia occur among blacks and Hispanics of Caribbean ancestry; however, persons from the Mediterranean area or southern Asian ancestry may also inherit this condition. About 1 in every 400 to 600 blacks and 1 in every 1000 to 1500 Hispanics have sickle cell disease. One in 10 black Americans carries this gene.

Physical Consequences

In sickle cell anemia, the oxygen-carrying RBC changes into a crescent or sickle shape instead of the usual round shape (Fig. 28–13). These sickle cells may become stuck in tiny blood vessels and rupture easily. This causes bouts of pain and

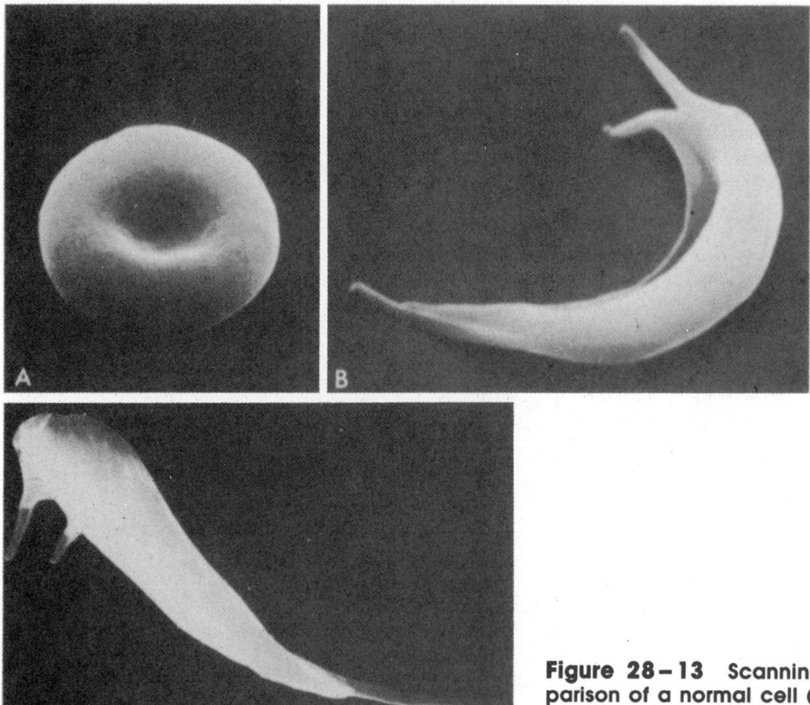

Figure 28–13 Scanning electron micrograph of erythrocytes. Comparison of a normal cell (*A*) and deoxygenated sickled cells (*B* and *C*). (Courtesy of Dr. James White; from Bunn HG, et al. *Human Hemoglobins.* Philadelphia, WB Saunders, 1977.)

What happens when RBCs sickle?

damage to vital organs, such as the brain, lungs, and kidneys, leading to disability or even death. Clients tire easily and may often be short of breath and prone to infections. Hematuria and urinary tract infections are more frequent in those with the sickle cell trait.

Treatment

A diagnosis of iron deficiency in sickle cell disease is difficult because usual iron values for blacks differ from the norms (Yip et al, 1984), yet a correct diagnosis is imperative before treatment is initiated. Iron deficiency may or may not occur with sickle cell anemia. If iron deficiency is not present, iron supplementation is contraindicated. If supplemental iron is required, it must be monitored closely because of the possibility of excess iron storage or reduced zinc absorption and utilization.

Nutritional Care

Growth retardation may be apparent as early as 6 months after birth. Impaired nutrient absorption and increased RBC hemolysis may contribute to deficiencies of zinc, iron, folate, and vitamins C and E. Iron intake should be relatively low. Caffeine and alcohol intake should also be low since both products can cause vasoconstriction and dehydration (from diuresis). This could aggravate sickle cell anemia (Rivers & Williamson, 1990).

Zinc, present in erythrocytes, is lost as the cells are lysed. Without adequate intake, zinc deficiency results. Zinc supplementation results in reduced numbers of sickled cells and increases oxygen affinity of RBCs (Muskiet et al, 1991). Zinc supplementation in adolescent boys significantly increases weight, growth of pubic hair, serum testosterone level, and zinc levels.

Rapid folate turnover (from destruction of RBCs) increases risk of megaloblastic anemia. Even though mild folate deficiency is routinely observed in children with sickle cell disease, folate supplementation should be reviewed on an individual basis (Sinow et al, 1987). Normally 400 to 600 mcg of folate per day is recommended.

NURSING APPLICATIONS

Assessment

Physical—for height, weight, weight history, TSF; bowel sounds, race.

Dietary—for appetite, food intake, vitamin/mineral supplements, caffeine and alcohol intake.

Laboratory—for serum iron, MCV, ferritin, Hgb, Hct, folacin, percentage transferrin saturation, RBC; nitrogen balance.

Interventions

1. Tubular concentrating ability may be reduced; even slight dehydration causes increased plasma viscosity and aggravation of sickling. Provide roughly 80 ml/kg of fluid in 24 hours (Evans, 1989).
2. Monitor I&O.
3. Weigh client daily.
4. Offer warm or tepid drinks rather than iced, cold drinks since cold beverages promote vasoconstriction (Rivers & Williamson, 1990).
5. Encourage high-kilocalorie, high-protein diet.

Evaluation

* Client should consume 80 ml/kg/day of fluid, a diet high in zinc, folate, and vitamins E and C.
* Laboratory values should return to normal.

Client Education

- Discuss foods that are good sources of high-quality protein; zinc; folate; riboflavin; and vitamins E and C.
- Following transfusions, do not consume large amounts of iron-rich foods (liver and iron-fortified cereals).
- Refer client/family to the National Association for Sickle Cell Disease (Appendix E-1) and genetic counseling.

OTHER ANEMIC CONDITIONS

Thalassemia

One of the most common inherited blood diseases in the US is thalassemia; some 2500 people are hospitalized every year for treatment. Usually, they are of Mediterranean, southern Asian, or African ancestry. The RBCs take on abnormal shapes, are fragile, and rupture easily. Blood transfusions lessen the effects of thalassemia, but a major problem is iron accumulation in the heart and other organs. Nutrient supplementation is of no benefit to these clients. It is important for these clients to consume a well-balanced diet with adequate amounts of water-soluble vitamins, especially folate. If transfusions are used frequently, iron-rich foods are avoided.

NURSING APPLICATIONS

Assessment

Physical—for race, weight gain/loss pattern; fatigue.
Dietary—for appetite, iron and folate intake.
Laboratory—for RBC, Hgb, Hct, iron, transferrin, TIBC, MCV, folate.

Interventions

If folate therapy is not initiated, consult physician, as these clients need folate for proper RBC production and maturation.

Evaluation

* Client should consume a well-balanced diet while avoiding iron-rich foods.

Client Education

- Avoid organ meats and iron-fortified cereals.
- Refer to genetic counseling.

SUMMARY

Dietary management in endocrine disorders can help alleviate symptoms. Nutritional care may be used in conjunction with drugs for an extended period of time or temporarily until other therapies can correct the endocrine dysfunction.

Inborn errors of metabolism, such as PKU, need prompt diagnosis and proper attention to prescribe exact dietary intakes and to avoid problems such as mental retardation and abnormal motor function.

Another metabolic disorder, gout, affects the musculoskeletal system. Although there is no nutritional "cure" for gout, proper nutritional interventions can minimize disabling symptoms.

Genetic disorders of RBCs can cause disabling symptoms; they may also be fatal. Well-balanced diets are necessary for clients with sickle cell anemia and thalassemia. However, special emphasis is on hydration for sickle cell clients and avoidance of iron-rich foods in thalassemia.

NURSING PROCESS IN ACTION

A client with hyperthyroidism is admitted to the hospital. She is not experiencing a thyroid storm but has been under a lot of stress lately. She mentions she has an insatiable appetite despite recent weight loss. Current medications include propranolol (Inderal) (to block the effects of hyperthyroidism on sympathetic nervous system), Propylthiouracil (PTU), and multivitamins.

Nutritional Assessment

- Duration of the disease.
- Definition/description of stressors.
- Favorite food and drink.
- Appetite, height, usual and current weight, bowel sounds, diarrhea.
- Tremors, insomnia, anxiety.
- Vital signs.
- Serum levels T_3, T_4, TSH.

Dietary Nursing Diagnosis

Altered nutrition: Less than body requirements RT an intake below metabolic needs secondary to hypermetabolic state.

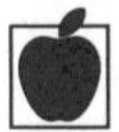

Nutritional Goals

Client will not lose weight, can verbalize type of diet needed, and consumes high-kilocalorie diet.

Nutritional Implementation 

Intervention: Provide a high-kilocalorie, high-protein, nutrient dense diet. Have client select appropriate foods from menu.

Rationale: Hyperthyroidism elevates metabolism, thereby increasing nutrient requirements. Kilocalories provide needed energy, protein offsets negative nitrogen balance, and carbohydrates increase kilocalorie content and prevent ketosis.

Intervention: Offer between-meal snacks and small, frequent meals. Allow access to kitchen.

Rationale: Snacks increase intake to help offset increased BMR. Small, frequent meals may seem less overwhelming. Access to kitchen allows increased intake because of availability and ease.

Intervention: Weigh daily. Report significant loses (>10%) to the physician.

Rationale: This determines if nutritional care is appropriate. A loss signifies current treatment is ineffective and needs to be modified.

Intervention: Offer favorite foods.

Rationale: Larger amounts of favorite foods usually result in increased nutrient intake.

Intervention: Offer favorite beverage hourly.

Rationale: This helps replace fluid losses from diaphoresis and tachypnea.

Intervention: Give multivitamins as ordered. Give Inderal with meals. Give antidiarrheals if needed. Give PTU as ordered.

Rationale: Accelerated utilization of vitamins increases vitamin requirements. Inderal can cause GI disturbances if taken on an empty stomach, and food can increase absorption of Inderal. Antidiarrheals decrease GI transit rate, allowing increased nutrient absorption. If diarrhea is present, nutrients cannot be absorbed. PTU helps decrease hyperthyroidism by inhibiting thyroxine synthesis.

Intervention: Explain why she should avoid high-fiber and gas-producing foods.

Rationale: Bowel transit time is significantly faster. Avoidance of high-fiber foods helps minimize increased peristalsis.

Intervention: Keep mealtimes stress free.

Rationale: When stressed, client stimulates the sympathetic nervous system, thus compounding an already hypermetabolic state.

Intervention: Offer foods high in calcium, i.e., milk, yogurt, cheese.

Rationale: Bone demineralization can be a complication if left untreated.

Intervention: Teach client to avoid/limit caffeine.

Rationale: Hyperthyroidism induces an elevated BMR. To prevent further stimulation, avoid or limit use of stimulants: caffeinated beverages and tobacco.

Intervention: Explain that appetite may not decrease even when the condition is stabilized.

Rationale: Obesity may be a possibility if food intake is not altered. Knowledge increases compliance.

Evaluation

If client maintained her IBW, stated she needed to increase food (nutrient) intake, and actually ingested more nutrients, nursing care was effective. Also, client should not experience thyroid storm.

STUDENT READINESS

1. Explain how and why the hypoglycemic diet differs from the diabetic diet.
2. What type of diet might be ordered for hypothyroidism, and why?
3. What is tetany, and what foods should be encouraged for a client with tetany?
4. How is PKU identified, and what dietary measures are taken to provide for normal growth? What are the consequences if the diet is not controlled?
5. What dietary recommendations would you offer a client who has gout?

CASE STUDY

Following a normal pregnancy, Mrs. A. J. delivers a 7-lb, 6-oz full-term infant. In compliance with state requirements, the baby is screened for PKU. After initial tests, more definitive studies are ordered. These also are positive. Mr. and Mrs. A. J. are angry and confused as they begin counseling for their daughter's dietary management.

1. What is the physiological basis of PKU?
2. What signs will the daughter demonstrate in the first 6 months without dietary modification?
3. What are the complications if this condition is left untreated?
4. Outline a diet plan for the first year.
5. What are the names of commercially available milk substitutes?
6. Mrs. A. J. asks, "Won't she ever be able to eat normally?" How would you counsel her?
7. What are some of the foods allowed as desired?
8. As the child grows, should she use the artificial sweetener aspartame?

REFERENCES

Anderson JW, Herman RH. Effects of carbohydrate restriction on glucose tolerance of normal men and reactive hypoglycemic patients. *Am J Clin Nutr* 1975 July; 28(7):748–755.

Azen CG, et al. Intellectual development in 12-year-old children treated for phenylketonuria. *Am J Dis Child* 1991 Jan; 145(1):35–39.

Bagchi N, et al. Thyroid dysfunction in adults over age 55 years. A study in an urban US community. *Arch Intern Med* 1990 Apr; 150(4):785–787.

Carpenito LJ. *Nursing Care Plans and Documentation: Nursing Diagnoses and Collaborative Problems.* Philadelphia, JB Lippincott, 1991.

Cerrato P. Hypoglycemia: Separating facts from fads. *RN* 1989 Apr; 89(4):81–83.

Danowski TS, et al. Hypoglycemia. *World Rev Nutr Diet* 1975; 22:288.

Davidson DC. Maternal phenylketonuria. *Postgrad Med J* 1989; 65(suppl 2):S10–S20.

Drinka PJ, Nolten WE. Prevalence of previously undiagnosed hypothyroidism in residents of a midwestern nursing home. *South Med J* 1990 Nov; 83(11):1259–1261, 1265.

Drogari E, et al. Timing of strict diet in relation to fetal damage in maternal phenylketonuria. *Lancet* 1987 Oct 24; 2(8565):927–930.

Evans JP. Practical management of sickle cell

disease. *Arch Dis Child* 1989 Dec; 64(12):1748–1751.

Gribbin ME. Could you detect these oncologic crises? *RN* 1990 June; 53(6):36–41.

Griffin JE. Hypothyroidism in the elderly. *Am J Med Sci* 1990 May; 299(5):334–345.

Henry RR, et al. Current issues in fructose metabolism. *Annu Rev Nutr* 1991; 11:21–39.

Hopkinson N, Doherty M. In patients with chronic cardiac failure who have diuretic induced gout, are certain diuretics less prone at causing problems? *Br J Rheumatol* 1991 June; 30(3):225.

Katzeff HL, Rivlin RS. Endocrine diseases. *In* Kinney JM, et al, eds. *Nutrition and Metabolism in Patient Care.* Philadelphia, WB Saunders, 1988: 342–359.

Link R. Phenylketonuria diet in adolescents—energy and nutrient intake—is it adequate? *Postgrad Med J* 1989; 65(suppl 2):S21–S24.

Marks V. Diagnosis and differential diagnosis of hypoglycemia (editorial). *Mayo Clin Proc* 1989 Dec; 64(12):1558–1561.

McMurry MP, et al. What does it cost to treat PKU? Analysis of the food expenses for children at different ages. Presented at the American Dietetic Association 69th Annual Meeting, Las Vegas, 1986.

Muskiet FA, et al. Supplementation of patients with homozygous sickle cell disease with zinc, alpha-tocopherol, vitamin C, soybean oil, and fish oil. *Am J Clin Nutr* 1991 Oct; 54(4):736–744.

Palardy J, et al. Blood glucose measurements during symptomatic episodes in patients with suspected postprandial hypoglycemia. *N Engl J Med* 1989 Nov 23; 321(21):1421–1425.

Polonsky KS. A practical approach to fasting hypoglycemia. *N Engl J Med* 1992 Apr 9; 326(15):1020–1021.

Prummel MF, et al. The course of biochemical parameters of bone turnover during treatment with corticosteroids. *J Clin Endocrinol Metab* 1991 Feb; 72(2):382–386.

Reilly C, et al. Trace element nutrition status and dietary intake of children with phenylketonuria. *Am J Clin Nutr* 1990 July; 52(1):159–165.

Rivers R, Williamson N. Sickle cell anemia: Complex disease, nursing challenge. *RN* 1990 June; 53(6):24–28.

Rylance G. Outcome of early detected and early treated phenylketonuria patients. *Postgrad Med J* 1989; 65(suppl 2):S7–S9.

Sawin CT. Thyroid dysfunction in older persons. *Adv Intern Med* 1992; 37:223–248.

Schimke RN. Hyperthyroidism: The clinical spectrum. *Postgrad Med* 1992 Apr; 91(5):229–236.

Service FJ. Hypoglycemia and the postprandial syndrome. *N Engl J Med* 1989 Nov 23; 321(21):1472–1474.

Simons RJ, et al. Thyroid dysfunction in elderly hospitalized patients. Effect of age and severity of illness. *Arch Intern Med* 1990 June; 150(6):1249–1253.

Sinow RM, et al. Unsuspected pernicious anemia in a patient with sickle cell disease receiving routine folate supplementation. *Arch Intern Med* 1987 Oct; 147(10):1828–1829.

Smith I, et al. Effect on intelligence of relaxing the low phenylalanine diet in phenylketonuria. *Arch Dis Child* 1991 March; 66(3):311–316.

Snorgaard O, et al. Glycaemic thresholds for hypoglycaemic symptoms, impairment of cognitive function and release of counterregulatory hormones in subjects with functional hypoglycaemia. *J Intern Med* 1991 Apr; 229(4):343–350.

Stuck LM, McFarland KF. Hypothyroidism in the elderly. When symptoms are not a 'normal' part of aging. *Postgrad Med* 1991 Dec; 90(8):141–143, 146.

Szilagyi A, et al. Reversible lactose malabsorption and intolerance in Graves' disease. *Clin Invest Med* 1991 June; 14(3):188–197.

Thompson AJ, et al. Neurological deterioration in young adults with phenylketonuria. *Lancet* 1990 Sept 8; 336(8715):602–605.

Waisbren SE, et al. The New England Maternal PKU Project. Identification of at-risk women. *Am J Pub Health* 1988 July; 78(7):789–792.

Woeber KA. Iodine and thyroid disease. *Med Clin North Am* 1991 Jan; 75(1):169–178.

Yannicelli S, et al. Nutrition support for the late-treated adult with phenylketonuria. *Metabolic Currents* 1990; 3(1):1–4 (Ross Laboratories).

Yip R, et al. Age-related changes in laboratory values used in the diagnosis of anemia and iron-deficiency. *Am J Clin Nutr* 1984 March; 39(3):427–436.

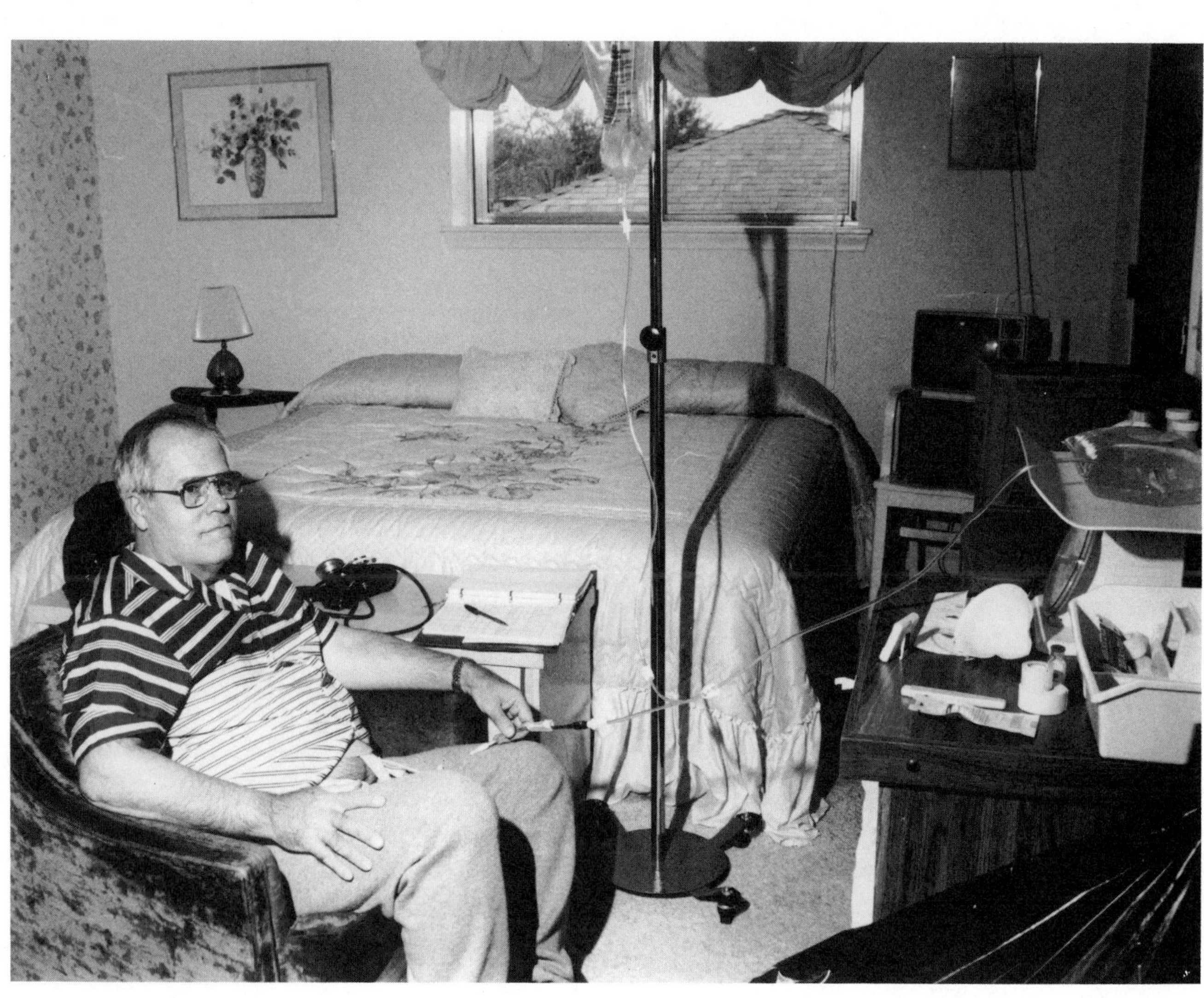

Dietary Management of Renal and Urinary Tract Disorders

CHAPTER 29

OUTLINE

2. Energy
3. Fluid and Electrolyte Balance
4. Nutritional Requirements

Nursing Applications

VI. CHRONIC RENAL FAILURE
A. Treatment
B. Nutritional Care
1. Effect of Nutrition on Progression of Renal Failure
2. Protein
3. Energy Intake
4. Fluid and Electrolyte Balance
5. Acid–Base Balance
6. Calcium and Phosphorus
7. Trace Elements
8. Vitamins
9. Cholesterol and Fats

Nursing Applications

VII. PLANNING THE RENAL DIET

Nursing Applications

VIII. SPECIAL CONSIDERATIONS FOR DIALYSIS
A. Dietary Compliance
B. Hemodialysis
1. Nutritional Care

Nursing Applications

C. Peritoneal Dialysis
1. Nutritional Care

Nursing Applications

IX. SPECIAL CONSIDERATIONS FOR TRANSPLANTATION

Nursing Applications

X. SPECIAL CONSIDERATIONS FOR CHILDREN WITH RENAL DISEASE

Nursing Applications

XI. NEPHROLITHIASIS AND UROLITHIASIS
A. Physical Consequences
B. Causes
C. Treatment
1. Calcium Oxalate Stones
2. Struvite or Triple Phosphate
3. Uric Acid

Nursing Applications

OBJECTIVES

THE STUDENT WILL BE ABLE TO:

- Discuss the complications of renal dysfunction.
- Explain reasons for the modifications of protein, sodium, and potassium in renal disease.
- Discuss nutrient supplements that are usually required with renal disorders.
- List the types of kidney stones, their causes, and the recommended dietary interventions.
- Discuss nursing application as it relates to renal and urinary tract disorders.
- Identify client education principles for UTI, renal diseases, and renal stones.

TEST YOUR NQ (True/False)

1. Cranberry juice should not be given to clients with urinary tract infections.
2. In acute glomerulonephritis, 35 kcal/kg is recommended.
3. Clients with nephrotic syndrome need additional protein intake.

4. The Step-1 diet is suggested for nephrotic clients with high serum lipid levels.
5. Low protein breads are not considered beneficial for clients with acute renal failure.
6. Diet modification is effective in preventing acidosis in renal failure.
7. Phosphorus should be increased in chronic renal failure clients with a blood creatinine level of 3 mg/dl.
8. Cola beverages are avoided when phosphate levels are elevated.
9. Intake of high calcium-containing foods is beneficial in transplant clients.
10. In clients with calcium oxalate stones, spinach and other green leafy vegetables are recommended.

RENAL DISORDERS

Renal disease affects approximately 8 million people in the US. The kidney is the primary organ that eliminates significant amounts of waste products; it also has metabolic and endocrine functions that are affected when disease is present (Table 29–1). Interferences with normal kidney functions may result from infections, inflammation, or blockages such as those from cysts, renal calculi, injuries, or tumors. Renal disease can affect the entire nephron or different parts of the urinary system: (1) Glomerulus, tubules, or interstitial renal tissue are affected in nephritis; (2) the glomeruli are damaged in glomerulonephritis; (3) very permeable renal tubules result in nephrosis; and (4) severe loss of renal function is a result of glomerular and/or tubular insufficiency. Since the problem is an accumulation of "waste products" because of the kidney's inability to remove them, the best solution is to lower the intake of foods that produce or contain too much "waste." Therefore, therapy for each condition varies since different parts of the kidney have distinct functions.

Metabolic nitrogenous wastes from protein catabolism, specifically urea, creatinine, and other nitrogenous products, are not removed from the blood; therefore, the BUN rises. Azotemia refers to elevation of nitrogenous products in the blood; uremia is a clinical syndrome that includes azotemia plus other clinical signs and symptoms that can affect all body systems.

Complications

Excessive retention of by-products from protein metabolism in the blood produces a toxic condition called **azotemia** or **uremia.** Initially, decreased renal reserves may not be symptomatic. As more nephrons are affected, renal insufficiency

TABLE 29–1

FUNCTIONS OF THE KIDNEY

Filtration, reabsorption of nutrients (amino acids, glucose, sodium, vitamins), and excretion of waste products (urea, creatinine, nitrogen, ammonia salts, uric acid, electrolytes, drugs, and toxins)
Maintenance of acid–base (bicarbonate reabsorption and hydrogen ion excretion) and electrolyte and fluid balance
Secretion of hormones, e.g., erythropoietin for RBC production, prostaglandin, and vitamin D_3 for calcium/phosphorus homeostasis
Secretion of renin for regulation of blood pressure
Production of carnitine (affects muscle strength, lipoprotein status, and heart function)
Catabolism of amino acids and hormones (insulin, glucagon, parathyroid hormone)

Polyuria—excessive urination. Nocturia—frequent excessive urination at night.

Oliguria—reduced urine secretion. Anuria—no urine secretion.

results in an inability to concentrate urine, which causes **polyuria** and **nocturia.** Further loss of nephron function results in azotemia and imbalances in electrolyte and acid-base balance. Hypertension with edema, particularly of the face, may develop. In the final phase, a client is uremic, with symptoms of **oliguria** or **anuria** and involvement of many organ systems (Table 29-2). Of course, not all clients with renal disease progress to these final stages, and these signs and symptoms may not appear in this order, but this is a generalized overview of what might be expected.

Protein Loss

Hypovolemia—abnormally low circulating plasma volume that could lead to hypotension.

How does hypoalbuminemia aggravate the edematous state? What conditionally EAA becomes essential in renal clients?

In renal diseases that cause massive protein losses, serum protein levels drop and may be as low as 1 gm/dl. Hypoalbuminemia leads to a concurrent decrease of colloid osmotic pressure with passage of circulatory fluids into interstitial areas (edema). This results in **hypovolemia;** less blood passes through the kidneys, and sodium and water are retained secondary to increased ADH secretion. This further aggravates the edematous state.

Synthesis of histidine is impaired in uremia; thus, for these clients, this amino acid is an EAA. Histidine supplements are effective in increasing hemoglobin levels and promoting positive nitrogen balance.

Fluid and Electrolyte Balance

GFR reflects the ability of the kidney to filter and reabsorb fluids. It is an important indicator of renal function. (The normal glomerular filtration rate is about 125 ml/min or 180 L/day.)

Water intoxication—fluid retention with sodium depletion, associated with lethargy, nausea, vomiting, and mental changes.

Disturbances in fluid and electrolyte balance accompany oliguria and tubular adaptations to reduce **glomerular filtration rate (GFR).** In uremic clients, excess fluid intake may result in **water intoxication,** or sodium retention with FVE. Hypertension may occur with water intoxication or FVE and water retention. Overhydration is a danger when the GFR falls below 2 to 5 ml/min.

Although sodium retention occurs in the majority of uremic clients, the amount of sodium reabsorbed decreases as renal insufficiency progresses. As kidney function deteriorates, excessive sodium and water loss on a normal sodium intake may occur. These clients are at risk of extracellular dehydration and hypotension. Sodium depletion may develop unless sodium intake is increased.

Fluid overload or dehydration must be controlled by balancing intake against output. Nurses frequently monitor blood pressure, which is indicative of fluid and electrolyte balance.

How is sodium affected by renal disease? How is potassium affected in renal disease?

Hyperkalemia is another possible consequence of reduced renal function, especially in clients with marked oliguria. Hyperkalemia usually does not occur as long as urine output is more than 1000 ml/day. The kidney is the major route for potassium excretion; hyperkalemia occurs predominately in acute renal failure and the latter stages of renal failure and is usually associated with (1) excessive potassium intake, (2) acidosis, (3) oliguria, (4) hypoaldosteronism, or (5) catabolic stress.

Acidosis

How does renal acidosis affect the body?

As renal failure advances (GFR <25 ml/min), acidosis increases. This phenomenon demineralizes bone; retards growth in children; exacerbates fatigue, nausea, and vomiting of uremia; and, if severe, can cause cardiovascular collapse. Despite physiological compensatory mechanisms to restore balance (increased depth and rate of respiration), mild acidosis remains. Acidosis is usually treated when serum bicarbonate falls below 18 mEq/L.

Calcium and Phosphorus Imbalances

Abnormalities in calcium and phosphorus metabolism are universally present, as evidenced by hyperphosphatemia, hypocalcemia, and increased levels of parathyroid hormone (PTH). Since the kidney has an important role in the conversion of

TABLE 29–2

EFFECTS OF UREMIA ON BODY SYSTEMS

Body System	Effects
Cardiovascular	Fluid overload; water intoxication; high blood pressure activates renin-angiotensin mechanism; CHF, CHD; arrhythmias; edema, peripheral and/or systemic cardiovascular collapse
Hematopoietic	Anemia; bleeding problems; decreased platelets
Immune	Decreased WBCs; susceptibility to infections (from protein, zinc deficiency)
Respiratory	Pulmonary edema; pneumonia; uremic pneumonitis; dyspnea (from CHF); Kussmaul's respirations (from metabolic acidosis)
Gastrointestinal	Anorexia, nausea, vomiting; metallic taste, hypogeusia (from zinc deficiency), stomatitis, gum ulceration and bleeding, uremic halitosis (ammonia-smelling breath); gastritis, GI bleeding; diarrhea or constipation; duodenal ulcers, pancreatitis
Integumentary	Pallor, yellowish bronze, dry, scaly skin; itching, uremic frost; purpura, ecchymosis (from clotting problems)
Neuromuscular	Drowsiness, confusion, irritability, coma; pain, burning and itching of legs and feet; altered perceptions, muscle wasting; tremors, twitching, convulsions, paresthesia
Endocrine	Stunted growth patterns in children; hyperlipidemia; infertility and decreased sex drive (in both sexes); amenorrhea in women, impotence and decreased sperm production in men; impaired vitamin D metabolism; glucose intolerance (from impaired carbohydrate metabolism)
Skeletal	Hypocalcemia, hyperphosphatemia, parathyroid hormone imbalance; muscle and bone pain; demineralization of bones; calcifications in brain, eyes, gums, joints, myocardium, and blood vessels; osteodystrophy (osteomalacia, osteoporosis, osteosclerosis)
Renal	Initially hyponatremia, causing hypotension, dry mouth, poor skin turgor, listlessness, fatigue, nausea, and confusion; later after nephrons are destroyed, hypernatremia and hyperkalemia; carnitine deficiency, metabolic acidosis, oliguria

Data compiled from Baer CL. Acute renal failure: Recognizing and reversing its deadly course. *Nursing* 1990 June; 20(6):34–39; and Weaver SH. Renal and urological care. *In* Shaw M, et al, eds. *Illustrated Manual of Nursing Practice.* Springhouse, PA, Springhouse, 1991: 603–680.

vitamin D into its active hormonal form, vitamin D metabolism is disturbed as renal function becomes impaired.

Serum phosphorus levels increase as less phosphorus is excreted by the faltering kidney. When the product of serum calcium and phosphate (Ca × P) is greater than 75 mg/dl, calcium phosphate salts are deposited in bone and soft tissues. Both phosphorus and calcium levels are lowered by calcium phosphate deposits. Other metabolic abnormalities may also contribute to hypocalcemia: (1) hypoalbuminemia, (2) low levels of vitamin D, and (3) decreased calcium intestinal absorption (Strauss et al, 1987). Hypocalcemia stimulates PTH secretion. Elevated PTH levels block phosphorus reabsorption and raise serum calcium levels by resorption of bone. Thus, normal plasma concentration of calcium and phosphorus is restored, but the PTH level remains elevated. As more damage occurs to nephrons, phosphorus is retained. These metabolic derangements lead to **renal osteodystrophy.**

Renal osteodystrophy describes various changes in bones associated with renal failure, i.e., classic hyperparathyroidism, osteomalacia, osteoporosis, and sometimes osteosclerosis.

How are calcium and phosphorus affected in renal disease?

Lipid Alterations

Cholesterol levels are frequently over 400 gm/dl, and triglycerides are over 250 gm/dl. Hyperlipidemia often correlates with the degree of hypoalbuminemia. This may be caused by decreased oncotic pressure, but it appears that as the liver compensates by increasing protein synthesis, lipid production (especially LDL) is also higher than normal (Joven et al, 1990).

What happens to cholesterol and lipoproteins in renal disease?

In uremia, enzymatic changes affect lipoprotein metabolism. Triglyceride turnover and catabolism of VLDL and IDL are decreased. Within the lipoprotein fractions, levels of cholesterol and triglycerides are increased. CHD is a common cause of mortality in chronic renal failure and post–renal transplant clients.

CRF is irreversible loss of kidney function that occurs over an extended period of time. In addition to involvement of excretory functions, endocrine and metabolic functions are also affected.

The role of carnitine deficiency in elevating lipid levels in clients with **chronic renal failure (CRF)** has been investigated. Carnitine, synthesized by the kidneys, plays a critical role in oxidation of long-chain fatty acids. Carnitine deficiency appears to be related to the high incidence of lipid abnormalities and cardiovascular problems observed in CRF (Hoppel & Ricanati, 1991).

Anemia

Why is anemia frequently observed in renal clients?

Anemia may be attributed to decreased production of RBCs in the bone marrow that is due to inhibited kidney production of erythropoietin, the hormone that stimulates RBC formation. GI bleeding, dietary deficiency of folate or vitamin B_{12}, and drug-induced hemolysis may also contribute to anemia. The severity of anemia is roughly related to the degree of azotemia. Each increment of 10 mg/dl of serum urea nitrogen (SUN) correlates to a hemoglobin decrease of 1 gm/dl. This relationship is useful in determining when anemia is disproportionately severe for the degree of renal failure.

Mineral and Vitamin Alterations

Hypogeusia–abnormally diminished taste sensitivity.

As a result of abnormal zinc metabolism, uremic clients may be zinc deficient. Zinc deficiency may be a major cause of impaired cellular immunity, **hypogeusia,** and poor appetite. Decreased taste perception in uremic clients usually affects appetite.

Frequently water-soluble vitamins are deficient in uremia because of poor intake of nutrient-dense food sources, dietary restrictions, and altered metabolism due to drugs and/or uremia. Pyridoxine, folate, and ascorbic acid are major concerns because of the body's low capacity for storing these vitamins.

Weight Loss

What causes negative nitrogen balance and muscle wasting in clients with renal disease?

Negative nitrogen balance and muscle wasting are frequently observed in clients with advanced renal failure because of altered amino acid metabolism. Body weight, adipose tissue, and muscle mass are decreased. Hormonal derangements, including insulin and parathyroid hormone, may also contribute to weight loss. Growth retardation in children may be related to a combination of problems. Food intake may be poor secondary to anorexia caused by uremic symptoms and unpalatable dietary restrictions.

Nutritional Assessment

Because of a high incidence of malnutrition in clients with renal disease, a thorough assessment is needed to evaluate multiple parameters: biochemical and hematological measures, anthropometries, medical and dietary history, metabolic status, and physical examination. A client's changing status necessitates frequent reassessments to evaluate appropriateness of therapy.

Dry weight is a client's normal body weight, without extraneous fluid, when serum sodium and blood pressure are WNL.

Fluid disturbances affect weights; therefore, estimated **dry weight** of a client is used as a measure of actual body weight.

In addition to assessing traditional serum proteins (albumin, transferrin) for nutritional status and TLC for immune function, products of protein catabolism must be monitored (Table 29–3). In renal disease, albumin, transferrin, and protein waste products are indicative of intake, but they also reflect renal function. Elevated serum nitrogen levels are a result of the breakdown of endogenous proteins.

BUN or SUN indicates the extent of renal failure. BUN levels are elevated with dehydration, catabolism, and GI bleeding, but if these factors are stable, BUN is closely correlated with protein intake.

TABLE 29–3

ASSESSMENT OF LABORATORY VALUES FOR RENAL DISEASE

Laboratory Value	Normal Range	Approximate Range in Renal Disease	Considerations for High Levels	Considerations for Low Levels
Albumin	3.5–5 gm/dl	Same	Fluid volume deficit; fluctuates rapidly	Fluid volume excess; inadequate protein intake (long-term or high-quality protein deficit), usually corresponds to low MAMC; possibly additional stresses (surgery or infection)
Serum ferritin	150 mcg/l (M) 68 mcg/l (F)	Same	Frequent transfusions; excessive supplementation	Decreased erythropoiesis; inadequate iron intake; possibly need supplement
Calcium	8.5–10.5 mg/dl	Same	Check serum phosphorus, intake of vitamin D–fortified milk; use of calcium supplements, thiazide diuretics; prolonged bed rest	Check serum phosphorus (high); if albumin is low (common in nephrotic syndrome), calcium will be low. Check calcium intake, type of supplement. Inquire about diarrhea; possibly need calcium supplement
Phosphorus	2.5–4.2 mg/dl	2.5–5 mg/dl	Check for low serum calcium; dialysis may not be sufficient; check prescription for binders and compliance	Check for use of binders—may be excessive; alcohol intake; check serum calcium; anorexia, dietary adequacy
Potassium	3.5–5 mEq/L	3.5–6 mEq/L	Check for acidosis (draws K^+ out of cell); check for intake of high-quality protein (too much), intake of salt substitutes, orange juice and other high K^+ fruits and vegetables, supplements, catabolism of tissue (muscle wasting, weight loss)	Check dietary intake (poor), especially intake of fruits and vegetables, anorexia; intake of low-quality protein; vomiting, diarrhea, excessive urine secretion; use of cardiac glycosides, corticosteroids (cause Na^+ retention, K^+ excretion); stress
BUN:SUN	5–20 mg/dl: 6–20 mg/dl	80–100 mg/dl (for both BUN and SUN)	Check for signs of uremia (vomiting, diarrhea); GI bleeding, catabolism; check K^+ and phosphorus levels, and intake to determine if dietary protein is too high; check for compliance with dialysis treatments; possible decreasing residual renal function, dehydration	Check for other signs of malnutrition (weight loss, MAMC); adequacy of protein intake, anorexia; fluid volume excess, excessive alcohol intake
Creatinine	0.7–1.5 mg/dl	10–20 mg/dl	Changes in dialysis; check for elevated BUN and K^+ that denote further renal decline	Changes very slowly with protein malnutrition—check long-term inadequate protein intake, MAMC, depressed BUN and albumin levels

MAMC, Mid-arm muscle circumference; SUN, serum urea nitrogen.

Creatinine, another nitrogenous waste of muscle metabolism, is affected less by diet and is not influenced by hydration status. Since meats contain creatinine, high meat intake slightly increases creatinine levels. Protein catabolism can be assessed by 3-methyl histidine level excreted in urine; higher levels reflect muscle catabolism.

Iron status of uremic clients is evaluated from serum ferritin levels. Besides measuring calcium levels, calcium homeostasis in bone can be determined by alkaline phosphatase levels. When calcium is released from bone, alkaline phosphatase rises.

A detailed dietary assessment must include data that affect fluid, sodium, potassium, and other electrolyte balance. Monitoring food intake or analyzing food diaries is essential. Other information to be determined includes use of low-protein products, salt substitutes, phosphate binders, compliance and difficulties with diet, and attitudes about diet. Determination of all medications used, including OTC, is important, as these significantly affect the dietary prescription.

Renal Health Care Team

Initially, ideal parameters are established for a client's treatment modality: height, weight, coexisting medical conditions that may have impact on nutrient parameter decisions, nutritional status, laboratory values, physician's orders or philosophy, and client's preferences. An energetic and enthusiastic health care team is vital for monitoring and promoting a nutritional program. In no other illness is the expertise of a registered dietitian to implement an individualized diet plan as important as in renal disease. The diet prescription is based on frequent laboratory tests, anthropometric measurements, and feedback from clients. Time spent planning the diet may be useless if a client is noncompliant or is wasting away because of anorexia. Data from assessment parameters (especially anthropometric and laboratory tests) can be used by nurses to encourage clients to continue the diet.

URINARY TRACT INFECTIONS

Causes and Physical Consequences

The simplest and most common kidney abnormality is urinary tract infection (UTI). It is caused by bacteria that may be secondary to an injury or obstruction, such as kidney stones. If untreated, chronic **pyelonephritis** and renal failure may develop.

Pyelonephritis—kidney inflammation.

Treatment

Currently antimicrobial agents are dependable, provide quick results, and effectively treat these infections. Short-term therapy is usually effective treatment, but long-term use of nitrofurantoin (Furadantin) is associated with decreased folate absorption and megaloblastic anemia. Nitrofurantoin should be taken with food or milk to increase its bioavailability. Methenamine mandelate (Mandelamine) for UTI is ineffective, unless the urine pH is 5.5 or less.

Nutritional Care

Increased fluid intake is the main dietary goal. Previously an acidic urine using an acid-ash diet or vitamin C was frequently prescribed. Although metabolism of most fruits yields alkaline residues, cranberries, prunes, and plums increase urinary acidity. The insignificant amount of cranberry juice in commercially prepared cranberry cocktail is ineffective in changing urinary pH. Nevertheless, cranberry juice and vitamin C supplements are commonly used for preventing and treating UTI and calculi. Beneficial results from the use of cranberry juice may be due to its ability to inhibit *Escherichia coli* from adhering to the mucosal cells of the bladder (Ofek et al, 1991). Fructose may also have this effect.

What is the main dietary goal in UTI?

NURSING APPLICATIONS

Assessment

Physical—for voiding patterns, urinary frequency/urgency, pain on urination, nocturia, fever.
Dietary—for excessive intake of concentrated sweets (may increase UTIs), cranberry, acid-ash food intake.
Laboratory—for urinalysis, urine culture, CBC with differential.

Interventions

1. Offer eggs, cheese, meats, and nuts to acidify urine.

Evaluation

* Pain and frequency of UTIs should decrease, and consumption of foods causing an acid-ash diet should increase.

Client Education

- Cranberry juice may be beneficial in preventing and recovering from UTIs.
- Use carbonated beverages, coffee, and tea in moderation because they are irritating to the bladder.
- Drink 2 to 3 L of fluid daily.

GLOMERULONEPHRITIS (ACUTE AND CHRONIC)

Causes and Physical Consequences

One to 2 weeks after an infection, particularly a streptococcal infection, acute **glomerulonephritis** may develop. In most cases, glomerulonephritis may be the result of an immune reaction to a bacterial or viral infection, a protein, or an autoimmune disease. Inflammation may lead to scarring and loss of filtering surface within the glomeruli. The accompanying **hematuria** and proteinuria contribute to symptoms of edema, shortness of breath, tachycardia, and mild hypertension. Anorexia contributes to poor nutritional status and deters efforts to increase food intake.

Inflammation or injury of glomeruli is called glomerulonephritis.

Hematuria—blood in the urine.

Each recurrence of glomerulonephritis destroys renal tissue and decreases renal function. Most children recover completely, but many adults may develop chronic glomerulonephritis, which can be inactive for long periods of time. Most clients with chronic glomerulonephritis may not have had acute glomerulonephritis. Since this disease may be asymptomatic indefinitely and is of unknown cause, clinical testing may be the only way of detection. Proteinuria and hematuria reflect glomeruli damage. As glomerulonephritis progresses, serum proteins decrease, hypertension and edema develop, and vascular changes occur. Chronic glomerulonephritis may progress to subacute glomerulonephritis (with destruction of nephrons) and renal failure several months later or to acute renal failure.

What are symptoms of chronic glomerulonephritis?

Treatment

Treatment of glomerulonephritis is aimed at improving renal functioning, preventing further renal damage and systemic complications, and maintaining adequate

TABLE 29–4 **GUIDELINES FOR RENAL FAILURE DIETS**

Disease State	Protein gm/kg IBW	Potassium mg/day	Phosphorus mg/day	Sodium mg/day	Fluid ml/day	Kilocalories kg/IBW/day	Comments
Acute/chronic glomerulonephritis	If BUN normal, no restriction For azotemia: 0.5–0.6 (60–70% HBV)	Monitor for oliguria; restrict if K^+ levels are elevated	Monitor for elevated phosphorus levels	Restrict to 500–1000 if edema, hypertension present	For oliguria: 500–700 + urine output	30–40	
Nephrotic syndrome	0.8 to 1; 60–70% HBV	High K^+ if thiazide diuretics are ordered	1200–1500	2000–3000 to control edema and hypertension	Variable; usually 500 ml + urine output	40–60; encourage PUFA or monounsaturated fatty acids	
Acute renal failure	0.55–0.60; 60–70% HBV (EAA supplements may be used) Increase as tolerated to 0.8 gm/kg	Oliguric phase: 1000–1500 Diuretic phase: replace losses, based on urine volume, serum urinary K^+ levels, drug therapy	Variable (300–1000); monitor closely	Oliguric phase: 500–1000 Diuretic phase: replace losses based on urinary and serum sodium level and edema	Oliguric phase: 500–600 ml + urine output Diuretic phase: encourage fluids to replace losses	30–35; 35–50 if catabolic	Monitor glucose levels due to insulin resistance and decreased insulin breakdown
Chronic renal failure	0.5–1 or higher based on stress or metabolic needs	Same as in Acute	Individualized; 800–1000	Individualized; 2000–3000	500–1000 + urine output	30–45	Vitamin supplement; folate, B-complex, C; minerals as needed
End-stage renal disease	0.6–0.8 (60–70% HBV); higher for protein losses	Individualized	Individualized	Individualized	500–800 ml + urine output	For weight maintenance: 35 For weight loss: 25–30 For weight gain or repletion: 40–45	

Hemodialysis (maintenance)*	1–1.2; individualized based on amino acid losses during treatment	2000–3000	800–1200 or 15 mg/gm of protein prescribed	2000–3000	Individualized based on urinary losses (500–1000 ml + urine output)	For weight maintenance: 35 For weight loss: 25–30 For weight gain or repletion: 40–45	
Peritoneal dialysis*	1.2–1.5 (50% HBV)	CAPD: restriction unnecessary unless serum K+ is high. CCPD/IPD: 2000–3000	800 to 1200	CAPD/CCPD: 2000–3000 IPD: 2000–3000	CAPD/CCPD: not restricted (monitor BP and weight) IPD: output plus 2–3 cups	For weight maintenance: 35 For weight loss: 20–25 For weight gain or repletion: 40–45	CAPD/CCPD: Monitor for hypertriglyceridemia and weight gain due to dextrose in hydrolysate
Renal transplant*	1–1.5	Individualized, approximately 3000, depending on drug therapy	Individualized; usually not restricted	2000–4000 to control hypertension	Unrestricted	For weight maintenance: 30–35 For weight loss: 20–25 For weight gain or repletion: 40–45	Dietary modification to minimize effects of immunosuppressive medication

General Information:
1. When <40 gm protein is provided, 75% HBV is needed. If >40 gm protein is provided, 60–75% HBV is given.
2. Phosphorus: Use of phosphate binders may be more acceptable than dietary phosphorus restriction.
3. Sodium: Monitor for adequate sodium intake.
4. Fluids: Normally insensible fluid losses are equal to the fluid content of foods.
5. Vitamin/mineral supplements are frequently indicated, especially water-soluble vitamins, B-complex, folate, and vitamin C; iron, calcium, and vitamin metabolites.

HBV, High biological value.

* Based on data from Wilkens KG, Schiro KB, ed. *Suggested Guidelines for Nutritional Care of Renal Patients,* 2nd ed. Chicago, American Dietetic Association, 1992.

CAPD, continuous ambulatory peritoneal dialysis; CCPD, continuous cyclic peritoneal dialysis; IPD, intermittent peritoneal dialysis.

nutrition support during recovery. Bed rest is important and is essential if anorexia is present. Antimicrobials are provided to control infectious organisms. If hypersensitivity is suspected, glucocorticoids may be used. Diuretics used to reduce edema may lead to hypokalemia and contribute to elevated BUN. Hypertension may be treated with antihypertensive medications. Dietary modifications are based on the progression of the disease. In chronic glomerulonephritis, dialysis and transplantation may be necessary. Both treatments are discussed later in this chapter.

Nutritional Care

Serum values that indicate accumulation of metabolic wastes (see Table 29–3) and clinical symptoms dictate appropriate dietary therapy. Dietary changes are made to restore or maintain optimum nutritional status (Table 29–4).

Protein

Protein must be supplied to replace losses, but at the same time, waste products of protein metabolism should be minimized to prevent azotemia. If the kidney is able to eliminate protein metabolic waste products, no protein restriction is necessary. Less protein intake does not alter the course of the disease, but moderate restriction may be recommended to ensure a client against developing renal failure. Initially, 0.5 to 0.6 gm protein/kg IBW or 40 gm/day is provided using principally high-quality proteins (60 to 70% of total protein). Higher levels of protein (1 gm/kg IBW) are provided if BUN levels remain within acceptable parameters (Zeman, 1991). Meats and milk products contribute significant amounts of protein and phosphorus; therefore, their intake needs to be monitored. A high-kilocalorie diet (30 to 40 kcal/kg dry weight or 2000 to 3000 kcal) prevents protein being used for energy rather than for tissue repair.

Electrolytes

What are recommendations for protein, kilocalories, sodium, and potassium in glomerulonephritis?

Sodium is restricted to 500 to 1000 mg if a client has hypertension or edema. For oliguria, fluids are limited to 500 to 700 ml/day plus the volume of urine output for the previous day. When a client is oliguric, potassium may be restricted to prevent hyperkalemia.

NURSING APPLICATIONS

Assessment

Physical—for height, weight, IBW, dry body weight, growth rates in children; edema, dehydration, skin turgor, hypertension; I&O.
Dietary—for appetite; food and fluid intake, especially adequacy of protein intake.
Laboratory—for albumin, transferrin, TLC, BUN, creatinine, GFR; sodium, potassium; WBCs, calcium, alkaline phosphatase (see Table 29–3); urinalysis for urine specific gravity and protein; creatinine clearance.

Interventions

1. When assessing BUN, also consider specific gravity of urine and serum electrolytes because dehydration can elevate BUN.
2. Carefully monitor hydration status and sodium levels, as diuresis may lead to sodium depletion.
3. Position client in an upright position for eating, and elevate head of bed fol-

lowing food intake to prevent nausea and vomiting, which could lead to anorexia.
4. Do not advocate protein restriction if the client is malnourished, i.e., low albumin, transferrin, and TLC levels.
5. If fluids are restricted, distribute throughout the day. Use tips presented in Chapter 8, Table 8–2.
6. Provide children with calcitriol (vitamin D) to promote growth, if ordered.

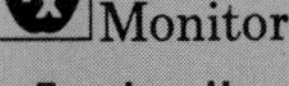Monitor potassium levels when diuretics are used.

Evaluation

* Client should follow dietary restrictions of sodium, fluids, and protein, and not develop renal failure.

Client Education

- Routine physical checkups are necessary to monitor renal functions to detect reoccurrence.
- Adequate fluid intake (at least 8 glasses a day) is important. Restriction of sodium intake is more effective in preventing fluid retention than restricting fluids.
- Smoky or coffee-colored urine indicates blood in the urine (Weaver, 1991).

NEPHROTIC SYNDROME (NEPHROSIS)

Physical Consequences

Nephrotic syndrome is characterized by heavy proteinuria, hypoalbuminemia, edema, and hypercholesterolemia, as discussed earlier under complications. Clients are extremely susceptible to infections and complain of weakness, anorexia, and headaches. Normal urinary protein is less than 0.15 gm protein in 24 hours; in nephrosis, between 3.5 and 30 gm protein may be lost.

Nephrotic syndrome, also called nephrosis, is characterized by degenerative lesions of renal tubules that result in increased permeability and loss of protein in the glomerular filtrate.

What are the symptoms of nephrosis?

Treatment

Along with use of diuretics, diet plays an important role in treatment of nephrotic syndrome. Diuretic medications inhibit tubular reabsorption of sodium and potassium, thus increasing diuresis. Diuretics do not alter the course of the disease, but increase the comfort of the client. If infection is present, antibiotics are prescribed.

Nutritional Care

Primary objectives of diet therapy are to control edema, replace protein losses, and prevent renal failure (see Table 29–4).

Protein and Kilocalories

Usually 0.8 to 1 gm protein/kg dry body weight is recommended. Increased proteinuria and protein catabolism occur when a high-protein diet is furnished (Al-Bander & Kaysen, 1991). Approximately 60 to 70% of the protein should be of high quality.

Replacement of protein losses must be balanced with a sufficient intake of nonprotein kilocalories. Increasing carbohydrate intake spares protein and prevents muscle catabolism. Depending on a client's current dry weight status, kilocaloric allowance may be between 40 and 60 kcal/kg/day.

Sodium

Edema is usually treated with a reduction in sodium intake. An appropriate level of sodium is 2000 to 3000 mg. Severe sodium restriction while ensuring adequate protein intake may be incompatible goals. When considering increased protein intake or further reduction in sodium, protein intake is more important because medications can be used to correct fluid retention. Compliance with sodium restriction usually alleviates the need for fluid restriction.

Fats

Although high serum lipid levels are known to increase risk of CHD, implementation of diet modifications has been controversial. A client's appetite and adequacy of food intake are important considerations when weighing the benefits of yet another dietary modification. If cholesterol and triglycerides are elevated, the Step-1 diet described in Chapter 24 has been suggested (Kean & Kasiske, 1990). A vegetarian soy diet with restricted proteins (0.7 gm/kg IBW) was effective in decreasing total serum cholesterol, HDL, and LDL, but triglyceride levels were unchanged (D'Amico et al, 1992).

Potassium

When diuretics are prescribed, caution must be exercised to prevent hypokalemia. High-potassium foods are suggested to replete potassium losses. Potassium supplements have an unpleasant taste and are gastric irritants and usually have a negative effect on food intake. To minimize these effects, provide the supplement with or after meals with a full glass of water or fruit juice (unless contraindicated).

Oral Intake

Providing appetizing meals is important to ensure that food is being eaten by these anorexic clients. If oral intake is poor, nutrition supplements or tube feeding may be necessary.

NURSING APPLICATIONS

Assessment

Physical—for height, weight/weight changes, IBW; BP, orthostatic hypotension, edema especially in ankles, I&O.

Dietary—for appetite, actual food intake, intake of sodium, protein, potassium, and fat.

Laboratory—for increased transferrin; increased cholesterol, triglycerides; SGOT (AST); elevated BUN, creatinine; sodium, alkaline phosphatase, decreased GFR; urine protein, urinalysis (see Table 29–3).

Interventions

1. Assist client in obtaining a salt substitute that improves palatability of food; avoid high-potassium substitutes if a potassium-sparing diuretic is prescribed (see Chapter 24, Table 24–9).
2. Monitor for vitamin D deficiency in clients with nephrotic syndrome since synthesis of the active form of vitamin D may be impaired.

3. If potassium-wasting diuretics are prescribed, monitor food intake for adequacy of potassium intake.
4. Since hyperlipidemia is a secondary effect and a high-fat intake may be necessary to provide adequate kilocalories, encourage the use of PUFA or monounsaturated fatty acids rather than saturated fats.
5. Help client plan appetizing meals.

Evaluation

* Desired outcomes include client consumes a diet that replaces lost protein, is low in sodium, and high in potassium-containing foods; does not develop infections; and has normal urine protein levels.

Client Education

- Frothy urine indicates protein in the urine (Weaver, 1991).

ACUTE RENAL FAILURE

Physical Consequences

In **acute renal failure,** kidneys suddenly cease to function normally because of circulatory, glomerular, or tubular deficiency. Generally renal function is restored when renal cells are regenerated. However, rapid accumulation of toxic substances may be fatal; mortality is around 50% for acute renal failure secondary to surgery or septicemia and 10 to 30% if secondary to dehydration or administration of nephrotoxins (Alvestrand & Bergström, 1988). Catabolism is a major contributing factor to the high mortality rate in clients following trauma or surgery.

Acute renal failure is characterized by an abrupt decline in renal function in clients with no previous history of renal disease and can be precipitated by infection, dehydration, burns, severe crushing injuries, transfusions, nephrotoxicity, anesthesia, shock, or sepsis.

Acute renal failure involves a rapid decrease in GFR with accumulation of nitrogenous waste products. The course of acute renal failure has 3 distinct phases. The first phase, or oliguria, is the hallmark characteristic of acute renal failure. To eliminate solute metabolic wastes, at least 600 ml/day must be excreted; urine excretion in these clients may be less than 400 to 500 ml. Hematuria, proteinuria, and abnormal fluid/electrolyte homeostasis occur. The second, or diuretic, phase is marked by increased urine output (up to several liters), but tubular **resorption** remains depressed. Therefore, uremia is present. During the recovery or third phase, renal function gradually improves, but it may take a year for total recovery. Some loss of function may be permanent.

Resorption—reabsorption.

Describe the 3 phases of acute renal failure.

Treatment

Dialysis may be used as a treatment during the oliguric or diuretic phase. An important therapy for acute renal failure is nutrition. However, diet is determined by a client's laboratory values and which medications are used to control metabolic and electrolyte imbalances: (1) Dietary phosphate may be restricted for clients with acute renal failure. However, this diet is poorly accepted, and phosphate-binding antacids are favored over dietary manipulations. (2) Normally medications are used to treat hyperuricemia and hypocalcemia rather than further dietary restrictions. (3) Because of the stressed condition and possible use of corticosteroid therapy to decrease inflammation, hyperglycemia is prevalent. Insulin is used to promote cellular uptake of glucose. (4) Diuretics also increase fluid excretion, but are usually used in diagnosing acute renal failure, not for treatment (Baer, 1990). (5) Aluminum or calcium hydroxide antacids may be used to counteract effects of excess HCl secretion.

Dialysis is removal of toxic substances from the blood and body fluids using a process of diffusion and filtration (osmosis) between solutions separated by a semipermeable membrane.

Antacids that contain sodium and magnesium (Maalox, Gelusil, Mylanta) may precipitate hypermagnesemia and should be avoided. (6) Protein requirements cannot be met from normal foods if the potassium restriction is less than 2000 mg (50 mEq). Therefore, other methods of reducing serum potassium levels may be used. **Cation** exchange resin drugs (such as Kayexalate) exchange sodium for potassium. However, these drugs are unpleasant and cause sodium retention, which could aggravate the edema already present. (7) To minimize edema, sorbitol may be given concurrently with cation exchange resins to eliminate sodium. Sorbitol increases fluid excretion through the GI tract. (8) IV glucose solutions and insulin may also be used to force potassium from serum into cells in an emergency situation.

Cation—positively charged ion.

Describe treatments for acute renal failure.

Nutritional Care

Optimal nutrition therapy is difficult to define. The following nutrients are of primary concern: energy, protein, sodium, potassium, and fluids (see Table 29–4). Nutritional requirements must be individualized, based on the different degrees of renal failure and catabolism. Objectives of nutritional management are to improve and maintain optimal nutritional status without inducing uremic symptoms or disturbing fluid and electrolyte balance. This can be a formidable task. Malnutrition and wasting often ensue or are worsened because of anorexia and poor food intake that adversely affect the healing process and recovery rate. Implementation of dialysis treatments allows the use of a more liberal diet. Nevertheless, some dietary restrictions are useful in decreasing frequency of dialysis.

What are goals of nutritional management in acute renal failure?

Protein

Even though by-products of protein metabolism are accumulating, enhancing onset of uremia, it is important that clients receive some protein to establish nitrogen balance. The optimal amount of protein given initially is controversial, but consensus is that it should be extremely low, unless dialysis treatments are used.

The amount of protein provided is individualized. When catabolism is not accelerated by an underlying condition, protein may be restricted to 0.55 to 0.60 gm/kg IBW/day, with 60 to 70% from high-quality protein to prevent uremic symptoms and avoid or reduce frequency of dialysis treatments. When a very low protein diet is ordered, EAA supplements (plus histidine) are recommended. As kidney function improves (reflected in GFR levels), protein intake is increased to at least the RDA of 0.8 gm/kg. (This is significantly below typical American intake).

In clients whose acute renal failure is secondary to burns, multiple trauma, or sepsis, protein requirements are elevated to prevent or diminish negative nitrogen balance resultant of catabolism. Dialysis is usually implemented as needed to permit adequate nutritional support in these clients.

What are the requirements for protein in acute renal failure?

Energy

Adequate kilocalories are furnished to prevent catabolism and weight loss. For most clients, 30 to 35 kcal/kg is adequate unless clients are severely catabolic because of their initial condition that precipitated the acute renal failure (Alvestrand & Bergström, 1988). Since protein intake is restricted, energy must be supplied from carbohydrates and fats. Even these must be low in electrolytes. When energy intake is limited, a weight loss of 0.2 to 0.3 kg/day may be expected; failure to lose 0.2 kg/day during the oliguric phase indicates fluid retention.

What is the recommended kcal/kg for acute renal failure?

Fluid and Electrolyte Balance

During both oliguric and diuretic phases of this disease, fluid intake is regulated according to fluid output. Dehydration and fluid overload are both potential

TABLE 29–5

CALCULATION OF MINIMAL FLUID REQUIREMENTS FOR RENAL FAILURE

Output		
24-hour urine output		− 500 ml
24-hour insensible water losses (variable, depending on room temperature, humidity and body temperature)		− 700 ml
Loss in vomitus		− 100 ml
Total Loss		− 1300 ml
Intake		
Metabolic water produced from oxidation of foods		+ 300 ml
Average fluid intake in solid foods*		+ 750 ml
Total Gain		1050 ml
Total Loss	− 1300	
Total Gain	+ 1050	
Additional Fluid Intake/24 hours	250	

* See Chapter 8, Table 8–1.

problems that should be guarded against by carefully monitoring a client's I&O, weight, serum sodium, and blood pressure. In some cases, I&O is monitored hourly.

During the oliguric phase, daily fluid allowance must not exceed losses. Fluids are initially restricted to the previous day's output plus a hypothetical allowance for insensible water losses (500 to 600 ml/day) and any losses from vomitus or diarrhea (Table 29–5). During this oliguric phase, a fluid challenge may be initiated. If urinary output does not increase, a potent diuretic (Mannitol and/or Lasix) may be prescribed (Baer, 1990).

When fluids are drastically restricted, certain foods with high fluid content such as soups, gelatin, popsicles, custard, fruit ices, and sherbets may be eliminated (see Chapter 8, Table 8–1).

Sodium is also dependent on the level of urinary excretion. During the oliguric phase, sodium restriction may be 500 to 1000 mg (20 to 40 mEq). The goal is to replace sodium losses. Weight and blood pressure are closely monitored because they reflect fluid balance. Any weight gain indicates fluid retention; to avoid congestive heart failure, fluid and sodium are decreased from the level a client was previously receiving.

During the oliguric phase, potassium levels are closely monitored, and intake is restricted accordingly. Hyperkalemia is a potential problem because potassium excretion is decreased when urine output is decreased, and tissue breakdown causes release of potassium from damaged cells. Because acute renal failure is usually sudden, hyperkalemia is a life-threatening situation and may be the main reason for initiating dialysis. Oral feedings may be restricted to 1000 to 1500 mg (25 to 50 mEq) potassium until urine output increases and serum potassium levels are normalized.

During the oliguric stage, what are suggestions for sodium and potassium intake? How are fluid requirements handled during the oliguric phase? What are suggestions for fluid, sodium, and potassium in the diuretic phase?

During the diuretic phase, fluid intake is increased to offset losses. Too much sodium and potassium may be lost. Sodium and fluid intake is liberalized, and potassium-containing foods that were previously restricted are encouraged. IV normal saline may be necessary.

Nutritional Requirements

Despite restriction of protein intake, kilocaloric requirements are relatively high. To meet these requirements, it may be necessary to use low-protein, high-energy, low-electrolyte commercial preparations. Kilocaloric-dense formulas or foods are needed because of fluid restrictions. Some of these are Sumacal (Sherwood Medical), Moducal (Mead Johnson), Polycose (Ross), and Microlipid (Sherwood Medical). Fruits, vegetables, and low-protein starches can be used to augment energy intake. Low-protein bread and cereal products and milk substitutes such as Alterna (Ross) are appropriate (Table 29–6).

TABLE 29–6

LOW-PROTEIN PRODUCTS AND THEIR SOURCES

Products

Breads/Crackers

LoPro Rice Starch Loaf[1,2]
LoPro Tapioca Bread[1,2]
dp Low Protein Bread[1,3]
Wel-Plan Low Protein Brown Bread[1,3]
Wel-Plan Low Protein Crackers[1,2,3]
Aproten Low Protein Rusks[1,2,3]
Low Protein Flat Bread[1]

Pastas/Rice

Aglutella Imitation Pasta (noodles, macaroni, spaghetti)[1,2]
Aproten Imitation Pasta (macaroni, noodles)[1,2,3]
Wel-Plan Imitation Pasta (macaroni, spaghetti)[1,2,3]
Aglutella Imitation Rice[1,2]

Baking Mixes

Unimix All Purpose Baking Mix[2]
dp Baking Mix[2,3]
Wel-Plan Baking mix[1,2,3]
dp Wheat Starch[2,3]
Kingsmill Cake and Cookie Base[1,2,3]
Egg Replacer (for cooking and baking only)[1,2]
Low Protein Bread Mix[1]

Cookies/Desserts

Lo-Pro Cookies (chocolate chip, spice, vanilla cream wafer)[1,2]
Kingsmill Cinnamon Cookies[1,2,3]
dp Cookies (chocolate chip, butterscotch chip)[2,3]
Wel-Plan Cookies (chocolate cream filled wafer, vanilla cream filled wafer, sweet cookie, chocolate cream filled)[1,2,3]
Doughnuts (banana, apple flavor, pumpkin)[1]
Belgian Style Waffles[1]
Ice Cream Cones[1]
Kingsmill Gelled Desserts (orange, cherry, strawberry, peach)[1,2,3]
Prono Gelled Desserts (orange, cherry, strawberry, lime, banana)[1,2,3]

Gravies/Sauces/Soups

Renal Meals Sauces (tomato flavored, creamy lemon herb, garlic herb)[1,3]
Med-Diet Gravies (rich brown, hearty mushroom, savory chicken)[2]
Med-Diet Sauces (zesty spaghetti, cheddar cheese)[2]
Med-Diet Broth/soup base (hearty beef, savory chicken, robust onion)[2]

Miscellaneous

Suplena—a high-kilocalorie (2 kcal/ml), low-protein nutritional supplement low in phosphorus, magnesium, and electrolytes; contains carnitine and taurine[2,4]
Nepro—high-kilocalorie, moderate-protein, low-electrolyte formula specially designed for renal clients[4]
Alterna—low-protein milk substitute[4]
Protein-Free Diet Powder Product 80056—powder that provides kilocalories (carbohydrate and fat) along with essential vitamins and minerals, but no protein[5]
Travasorb Renal—special amino acid formula contains both EAA and NEAA to promote better nitrogen utilization and balance for renal clients[6]
Aglutella Porridge[2]
Dietary Specialties Calorie Supplement[1,2]
Biocare Drink Mixes (orange, pineapple-apricot)[2]
Quench Gum[2]
Low Protein Potato Chips[1]

Sources

1. Ener-G Foods, Inc., 1526 Utah Ave., South, Seattle, WA 98134, (800)332–5222.
2. MedDiet, 3050 Ranchview Lane, Plymouth, MN 55447, (800)633–3438.
3. Dietary Specialties, Inc., P.O. Box 227, Rochester, NY 14601, (800)544–0099.
4. Ross Laboratories, Columbus, OH 43216.
5. Mead Johnson Laboratories, Evansville, IN 47721.
6. Clintec Nutrition Co, Affiliated with Baxter Healthcare Corporation and Nestle S.A., P.O. Box 760, Deerfield IL 60015–0760.

Critically ill clients usually are unable to take food orally, or the amounts needed to provide adequate nutrients for anabolism are not feasible. If the GI tract is functional, enteral feedings are implemented. When the GI tract is impaired, TPN must be used.

The appropriate form of nutrition support should be initiated as soon as it is evident that a client is unable to meet nutritional requirements with oral feedings. If nutrition support is to be implemented, dialysis is initiated before nutrition support so azotemia is not worsened by implementation of nutrition support. By using dialysis to lower waste products before providing nutrition support, these waste products are less likely to become toxic.

Supplementation of EAA may be required in severely uremic clients for a positive nitrogen balance. Travasorb Renal (Clintec), Amin-aid (Kendall McGaw), and Suplena (Ross) are available for oral intake as a nutrition supplement or enteral feeding. These products are frequently recommended not only because the total protein of the diet is limited, but also because the specific amino acid patterns are specially designed to meet a renal client's needs.

List foods and formulas used to provide adequate kilocalories, low-protein, and low-electrolyte diet. List formulas specially designed for uremic clients.

NURSING APPLICATIONS

Assessment

Physical—for height, weight/weight changes, dry body weight, IBW; BP; I&O, temperature, dehydration.
Dietary—for appetite, food/fluid intake, diet intake record.
Laboratory—for BUN over 30, creatinine; blood cultures; Hgb, Hct; TLC, transferrin, albumin, sodium, potassium, calcium, magnesium; cholesterol, triglyceride; glucose; alkaline phosphatase, carbon dioxide combining power, uric acid, creatinine clearance; urinalysis for osmolality and protein, urinary 3-methyl histidine.

Interventions

1. During the oliguric phase, implement strict I&Os. When calculating the amount of fluid to be given, err on the side of giving too little rather than too much. Monitor blood pressure and weights carefully to help determine whether a client is underhydrated or overhydrated.
2. Be careful with salt substitutes. Potassium-containing salt substitutes are not allowed during the oliguric phase.
3. During vomiting or diarrhea, liberalize sodium restriction.
4. Monitor weight daily because it accurately reflects fluid status.
5. Check any TPN feeding or enteral formula to be sure it contains carnitine, as the diseased kidney is unable to produce adequate quantities.
6. Use Table 29-3 to assess aberrant laboratory values and possible interventions.
7. Confer often with the dietitian regarding client status—intake, diet/changes, and other significant problems.

Evaluation

* The following should occur: (1) Fluid overload is averted; (2) fluid intake is appropriate; (3) metabolic acidosis does not occur; (4) fat and protein intake is limited; (5) low-sodium, low-potassium foods are ingested during oliguria phase, but sodium and potassium intake is increased during diuresis; and (6) infection is prevented.

Continued

Client Education

- Explain that TPN or enteral feedings can help prevent muscle wasting and shorten healing time.
- Discuss side effects of renal failure and relate them to the diet prescription.
- Excess protein leads to destruction of remaining glomeruli; therefore, protein intake must be closely regulated.

CHRONIC RENAL FAILURE

Describe the 4 phases of CRF.

Despite the kidney's recuperative powers from many types of renal insults, progressive loss of nephrons leads to CRF. Progression of CRF occurs in 4 stages (Table 29–7). These stages are not well-defined but are phases in a continuing degenerative process with increasing loss of functioning nephrons. Gradually kidney function diminishes, and the GFR may fall below 10 ml/min. At this point, uremic complications affect many organ systems (see Table 29–2). This stage is known as end-stage renal disease; dialysis or transplantation is inevitable.

Treatment

Treatment of CRF has been revolutionized by dialysis and renal transplants. However, these procedures are not implemented until kidney function is severely curtailed. Clients appear to feel well until the GFR has decreased to about 15 to 20 ml/min, when signs and symptoms of uremia appear. During the slow degenerative process, nutrient and fluid intakes are determined by functional capacity of the kidney to maintain homeostasis (see Table 29–4). With dietary manipulations, a client remains almost symptom free until the GFR decreases to approximately 10

TABLE 29–7

STAGES OF RENAL FAILURE

Stage of Renal Disease	Type of Renal Function Impairment	Loss of Renal Function	Glomerular Filtration Rate (ml/min)	Notes
Stage 1	Decreased renal reserve	55–66%	> 60	No symptoms
Stage 2	Renal insufficiency	80%	30–60	Mild azotemia (increased urea and creatinine); unable to adjust to wide variations in fluid, electrolyte, and protein intake, nocturia; mild anemia; hypertension
Stage 3	Renal failure	90%	12.5–30	Edema, azotemia, anemia, decreased concentrating ability, impaired ability to maintain electrolyte and acid–base balance, hypocalcemia, hyperphosphatemia; other neurologic, gastrointestinal, and cardiovascular complications
Stage 4	Uremia/uremic syndrome	90–100%	< 12.5	Oliguric, anemia, uremic symptoms involving many organ systems

ml/min. At this point, provision of adequate nutrition is impossible without development of severe uremic complications.

Nutritional Care

Objectives of the dietary regimen are to slow the rate of progression to end-stage renal disease, maintain optimal nutriture, prevent or minimize uremic toxicity, and provide for continuous growth in children. To meet these goals, nutritional management of CRF includes (Talbot, 1991) (1) restriction of protein to minimize azotemia and arrest progression of the disease, while providing adequate high-quality protein to prevent muscle wasting and maintain protein nutritional status; (2) adjustment of intake or absorption of minerals and electrolytes, such as sodium, potassium, and phosphorus; (3) provision of sufficient energy intake; (4) avoidance of potentially harmful intake of phosphorus, magnesium, aluminum, vitamins A and D, or citrate; and (5) replacement of deficient hormones, including erythropoietin and calcitriol. Optimal levels of these nutrients are individualized, depending on physiological factors and severity of renal failure.

In the first stage of CRF, the most frequently prescribed diet restriction is to control hypertension by limiting sodium and/or kilocalories (for weight loss), as needed. Adequate kilocalories are provided so protein is not used for energy.

What are the nutritional goals of CRF, and how are these met?

Effect of Nutrition on Progression of Renal Failure

Many research studies have been conducted to determine if dietary manipulations can slow progression of the disease. Several different factors have been examined in human studies—low-protein diets, very low protein diets supplemented with either EAA or **ketoacids** or **hydroxyacid analogues,** and protein and phosphorus restriction.

Ketoacids or hydroxyacid analogues are amino acids with the same structure as the original EAA except that an amino group is replaced by a keto group or hydroxy group with fewer nitrogen-containing amino groups. The body is able to change these groups to their respective EAAs. The overall effect is to decrease nitrogen load or waste products.

Very low protein diets relieve many of the uremic symptoms, and lower protein intake results in lower phosphorus intake, thereby helping to control hyperparathyroidism (Ihle et al, 1989; Rosman et al, 1984). Other investigators have reported altering progression of renal insufficiency by modifying a low-protein diet and/or using EAA supplements (Fouque et al, 1992; Alvestrand & Bergström, 1986). The overall results of either a very low protein diet or low-protein diet supplemented with EAA are similar. However, by using EAA supplements, the diet is somewhat liberalized, allowing more variety of protein-containing foods and resulting in better compliance.

Amino Acid:

```
    NH3
     |
R - C - COOH
     |
     H
```

Ketoacid:

```
     O
     ||
R - C - COOH
```

Hydroxyacid:

```
    OH
     |
R - C - COOH
     |
     H
```

Several groups studying the effects of ketoacid-supplemented, low-protein diets have almost universally reported slowed progression of renal degenerative changes (Mitch et al, 1984; Barsotti et al, 1983; Walser et al, 1983). Most studies investigating the role of protein and phosphorus restriction have used minimal protein levels and ketoacid analogue supplements. Results have indicated stabilization of GFR (Zeller et al, 1990; Walser, 1989; Viberti & Bending, 1988).

What are the findings of using a very low protein diet or a low protein diet with EAA supplements or ketoacid analogue–supplemented low-protein diets in CRF?

The National Institutes of Health (NIH) and Health Care Finance Administration are currently sponsoring a multicenter clinical trial to determine whether dietary protein and phosphorus restriction affect progression of chronic renal disease. Initial results have shown no evidence of overt malnutrition in clients who adhered to low-protein diets (Klahr, 1989).

Protein

For CRF, there is a fine line between avoiding uremic toxicity from excessive protein intake, while preventing malnutrition due to inadequate amounts of protein. Opinions differ as to when to initiate protein restriction and the level of protein to be provided. Most agree that protein restriction is recommended in clients with GFR values <20 to 25 ml/min to alleviate symptoms of uremia. Based on research already discussed, prudent protein restriction has been recommended (see Table 29–4; Table 29–8).

Low-protein diets are beneficial but may result in reduced quality of life because of unwelcome dietary changes (Table 29–9). Generally protein is restricted to 0.6 to 0.7 gm/kg IBW. Some clinicians use diets providing 0.3 gm protein/kg IBW supplemented with ketoacids or amino acids when GFR is less than 10 ml/min. A low-protein diet decreases nausea, vomiting, and fatigue. (For clients with protein losses, 0.8 to 1 gm protein/kg IBW is necessary to replenish losses.)

Dietary proportions of the individual EAA become especially important for uremic clients, in whom accumulation of nitrogenous products is critical. Each of the EAA must be present simultaneously in the intracellular pool. At least 60 to 70% of the protein should be of high quality for the diet to be effective in lowering BUN. Supplementation of EAA (discussed in the nutritional requirements section on acute renal failure) may be required in severely uremic clients for positive nitrogen balance. Since this low-protein diet is highly restrictive, client adherence is often unsuccessful. The use of EAA supplements with 20 gm unrestricted protein is a more popular regimen.

What are protein recommendations when GFR is <20 to 25 ml/min; when GFR is <10 ml/min?

Energy Intake

With severe protein restrictions, higher levels of carbohydrates (particularly those with little or no protein) and fats are provided to spare protein for growth and maintenance of tissues. Depending on a client's current nutritional status, 30 to 45 kcal/kg dry body weight is generally allowed, which can be calculated using guidelines in Table 29–4. Kilocaloric intake is frequently substantially below the desired level because of lack of appetite combined with protein restrictions.

Numerous commercially available carbohydrate and lipid supplements, dis-

TABLE 29–8

RECOMMENDED PROTEIN INTAKE AS DETERMINED BY GLOMERULAR FILTRATION RATE

Glomerular Filtration Rate (ml/min)	Amount of Protein Traditionally Recommended gm/kg (gm/day)	Potentially Beneficial* Protein Restriction gm/kg (gm/day)
20–50	1–1.2 (60–90)	0.6 (40)
15–20	0.7–0.8 (50–60)	0.6 (40)
10–15	0.6–0.7 (40–50)	0.6 (40)
<10	0.5–0.6 (35–40)	0.3 (20)+

* Data from Klahr S. Renal disease. *In* Brown ML, ed. *Present Knowledge in Nutrition.* 6th ed. Washington, D.C., International Life Sciences Institute, Nutrition Foundation, 1990: 377–384.

+ Supplemented with EAA or amino acid analogues.

TABLE 29–9

SAMPLE MENU FOR CHRONIC RENAL FAILURE

Food and Portion Size	Kilocalories	Protein (gm)	Phosphorus (mg)	Sodium (mg)	Potassium (mg)
Breakfast					
1 pear half	31	0.2	8	2.5	55
1 cup Rice Krispies	112	1.9	34.4	340	29.5
1 cup Ross Alterna	87	2.4	120	96	260
1 slice Lo Pro Rice Bread*	155	0.1	5	25	15
1 tsp margarine	34	0	1	51	1.8
1 package jelly	40	0	1	1.4	12
1 tbsp sugar	45	0	0	0.1	0
Lunch					
2 oz lean broiled pork chop	145	16	158	42.5	237
¼ cup MedDiet Brown Gravy*	15	0	NA	50	26
¼ cup imitation rice	263	0	NA	15	NA
½ cup boiled carrots with	35	0.9	24	52	177
1 tsp margarine	34	0	1	51	1.8
½ cup coleslaw with	8	0.4	8	6	86
2 tbsp mayonnaise	198	0.4	8	157	10
1 baked apple	91	0.5	13	1.7	150
4 oz cranberry juice	77	0	2.5	5	22.7
Dinner					
1½ oz beef cubes	86	13	104	28	172
½ cup Aglutella Noodles* with	150	0.2	25	8	4
2 tsp margarine	67	0	1.9	101	3.5
½ cup broccoli	26	2.9	50.5	22	166
1 sl Wel-Plan Brown Bread*	75	0.4	12	146	46
2 tsp margarine	67	0	1.9	101	3.5
½ cup blueberries	56	0.4	6.4	1.9	25.5
8 oz lemonade-flavor drink	102	0	34.3	6.1	32.8
Evening Snack					
8 oz orange soda	120	0	0	32	8
1 dp chocolate chip cookie*	70	0.1	4	22	15
Totals	2189	39.75	623.9	1364	1560

NA, Not available.
* Lo Pro, MedDiet, Aglutella, Wel-Plan, and dp are commercially available brand names of products specially designed for low-protein, low-electrolyte diets.
Nutrient data from Nutritionist III software, version 7.0; N-Squared Computing. Salem, OR.

cussed in the section on acute renal failure, are available to help in promoting energy intake. Complex carbohydrates, whether cereals, grains, or vegetables, contain some protein. Low-protein products can increase kilocaloric content and permit more high-quality protein (see Table 29–6).

Hard candies, gumdrops, jellies, honey, sugar, marshmallows, and popsicles can be used to increase kilocalories. However, even with urging, it is often impossible to motivate clients with renal disease to eat hard candy and other simple sugars because of their anorexia and altered taste perception.

Why is kilocalorie intake low in CRF clients? What is the kilocaloric requirement for CRF?

Fluid and Electrolyte Balance

For each 24 hours, a fluid intake level that totals 500 to 800 ml plus the previous 24-hour urine volume is recommended, as shown in Table 29–5. Fluids low in protein, sodium, and potassium are chosen. Water, cranberry juice, and sugar-sweetened, fruit-flavored drink mixes contain minimal amounts of these nutrients, so they are allowed liberally within the fluid volume limitation. Grape and apple juices are also permissible.

Clients with CRF who have no symptoms of fluid overload, hypertension, or heart failure are cautiously given increased amounts of sodium to determine their tolerance. A daily intake of 2000 to 3000 mg (40 to 130 mEq) sodium and 1500 to

3000 ml fluid maintains sodium and water balance in most clients with advanced renal failure. However, clients with excessive urinary sodium losses may require 6000 to 8000 mg/day of sodium to prevent hypotension and dehydration.

When end-stage renal disease occurs, clients may develop edema, hypertension, or congestive heart failure unless sodium and water are severely restricted. Sodium restriction may be below 1000 mg/day to decrease edema, lower blood pressure, and prevent fluid overload. (Reduced sodium diets are discussed in Chapter 24.)

When oliguria or anuria is present, a restriction of 0.5 mEq/kg/day of potassium (about 1500 mg or 35 to 40 mEq of potassium) is advised. A diet can easily contain 3 to 8 gm/day of potassium without careful selection of foods since fruits and vegetables (normally low in sodium and protein) contain appreciable amounts of potassium. An excess or depletion of potassium can cause cardiac arrhythmias. Hyperkalemia can occur quickly and without warning, causing cardiac depression, arrhythmias, and, eventually, cardiac arrest. Both potassium and sodium allowances are carefully planned by a dietitian.

What fluids are permissible with CRF clients? What are requirements for sodium; for potassium?

Acid-Base Balance

Diet modification to prevent acidosis is ineffective. Calcium carbonate (Os-Cal, Caltrate), sodium bicarbonate (Citrocarbonate), or sodium citrate (Bicitra) can be given. Sodium bicarbonate tablets cause excessive belching in some clients and are poorly tolerated.

Calcium and Phosphorus

Moderate dietary restriction of protein and control of serum calcium and phosphate should begin early in clients with renal failure to prevent or minimize secondary hyperparathyroidism and renal osteodystrophy from developing as well as to delay progression of CRF.

When serum creatinine exceeds 3 mg/dl, phosphate is retained, and intake should be restricted. To maintain a low to normal level of 2 to 3 mg/dl of serum phosphorus often requires reducing phosphorus intake to 700 mg/day (Table 29–10). Since protein intake is restricted, phosphorus is automatically limited to some extent because these nutrients occur in many of the same foods. A protein intake of 0.5 gm/kg IBW/day would supply about 800 mg of phosphorus if the types of animal products were not specified. Milk products significantly increase phosphorus content. By eliminating high phosphorus-containing foods (see Table 29–10), the daily phosphorus intake can be reduced to about 500 mg. Meat and fish may be boiled to remove phosphate further. Decreased phosphorus intake has proved effective in lowering phosphate levels, but difficulties arise when planning a workable food intake.

Because of unpalatability and lack of variety on an extremely low-phosphorus diet, phosphate-binding medications are frequently prescribed. Calcium and aluminum compounds are effective in controlling hyperphosphatemia (Mai et al, 1989). Use of an appropriate compound is based on physiological effect and client benefit and compliance (Schmitt, 1991). Medications can be effective in maintaining serum phosphorus levels below 6 mg/dl (Table 29–11).

Calcium compounds not only bind phosphorus, but also provide calcium. Frequently aluminum and calcium phosphate binders are coadministered to prevent hypercalcemia.

Calcium supplements (usually calcium carbonate, 1 gm/day) are started after a normal serum phosphorus level is achieved. If a client is on a low-phosphorus diet, small amounts of calcitriol (Rocaltrol), the active form of vitamin D, induce normal serum calcium levels with an adequate calcium intake. This leads to improved phosphorus metabolism and reduces osteodystrophy. Calcitriol is preferred because it has a shorter half-life than vitamin D. Vitamin D analogues may decrease daily calcium requirements by increasing intestinal calcium absorption.

Why is control of calcium and phosphorus started early in CRF? When should phosphorus be restricted? What are some ways to reduce phosphorus intake?

TABLE 29–10

PHOSPHORUS CONTENT OF SELECTED FOODS

Food Group and Food	Portion Size	Phosphorus (mg)
Meats and Substitutes		
Liver, beef	3 oz	392
Pink salmon	3 oz	280
Cottage cheese	½ cup	170
Cheddar cheese	1 oz	145
Hamburger patty	3 oz	134
Cod fish	3 oz	117
Chicken breast	3 oz	98
Whole egg	1 whole	89
Dairy Products		
Vanilla pudding	½ cup	188
Plain low-fat yogurt	½ cup	163
Baked custard	½ cup	155
Milk	½ cup	116
Half-and-half cream	½ cup	115
Frozen vanilla yogurt	½ cup	93
Vanilla ice cream	½ cup	67
Starches, Breads and Cereals		
Pinto beans	½ cup	137
Baked beans	½ cup	132
Cooked oatmeal	½ cup	89
Baked potato	1 medium	78
Lima beans	½ cup	77
Whole wheat bread	1 slice	73
Green peas	½ cup	66
Sweet potato	1 medium	62
Corn kernels	½ cup	39
White bread	1 slice	27
Corn flakes	½ cup	7
Miscellaneous		
Peanut butter	1 tbsp	52
Light cane molasses	¼ cup	36
Cola type soft drink	8 oz	29
Nondairy creamer (powder)	4 tbsp	0
Lemon lime soda	8 oz	0
Orange soda	8 oz	0

* Nutrient data from Nutritionist III software, version 7.0. N-Squared Computing, Salem, OR.

TABLE 29–11

NUTRITIONAL EFFECTS OF PHOSPHATE BINDERS

Binder*	Nutritional Effects
Aluminum compounds	
Aluminum hydroxide (AlternaGEL, Alu-Cap Capsules, Amphojel, Dialume, Nephrox)	May be constipating; source of aluminum (concentrates in CNS, especially the brain); may cause calcium (osteomalacia) and vitamin A deficiency; can cause dialysis dementia with long-term use
Calcium compounds	
Calcium carbonate (BioCal, Caltrate, Os-Cal, Tums)	Fewer side effects than aluminum compounds; source of calcium; may reduce iron absorption. Vitamin D must be present for calcium carbonate to be absorbed. Spinach or rhubarb may decrease calcium absorption
Calcium citrate (Citracal) Calcium acetate (Phos-Ex)	Source of calcium; may enhance aluminum compounds. Most effective of the calcium compounds for binding phosphorus; not as constipating as aluminum compounds

* To be effective as a binder, give with meals.

Data from Schmitt J. Selecting an appropriate phosphate binder. *J Renal Nutr* 1991 Jan; 1(1):38–40; Roe DA. *Handbook on Drug and Nutrient Interactions.* 4th ed. Chicago, American Dietetic Assoc, 1989; Allen AM. *Powers and Moore's Food Medication Interactions.* 7th ed. Tempe, AR, Ann Moore Allen, 1991.

Trace Elements

What drug has helped CRF clients return to a more active lifestyle? What is necessary to facilitate the effectiveness of this medicine?

The recent development of epoetin alfa (Epogen), a genetically engineered duplication of the protein, erythropoietin, has been effective in enabling clients with chronic uremia to produce their own RBCs and return to a more active lifestyle. However, adequate iron stores are necessary to facilitate effectiveness of Epogen. Oral ferrous sulfate supplements or intramuscular injections of iron may be needed. Zinc supplements (0.5 mg/kg of body weight) are often given for decreased taste perception.

Vitamins

What water-soluble vitamins are increased? For what problems is biotin given? Why are vitamin A supplements not given? Why are vitamin D supplements needed?

Myopathy—muscle disease, causing severe weakness.

Because of vitamin deficiencies observed in these clients, supplements are usually prescribed. Larger amounts of folate (1 mg), vitamin C (100 mg), and pyridoxine (5 mg) along with the RDA for other water-soluble vitamins are commonly used. Biotin supplements (10 mg/day) may be provided to treat neurological disorders related to uremia such as dementia, encephalopathy, and peripheral neuropathy.

Vitamin A intoxication has been observed. Supplements are avoided, as vitamin A increases PTH secretion, contributing to osteodystrophy. **Myopathy,** especially in the proximal muscles of the limbs, may result from vitamin D deficiency, which is associated with compromised renal function. Supplementation is usually in the form of calcitriol, the activated form of vitamin D.

Cholesterol and Fats

Physicians are beginning to address the problem of elevated serum cholesterol and triglycerides to lower the incidence of CHD. The Step-1 diet is being advocated to improve lipoprotein profiles. However, planning such diets adequate in kilocalories when protein levels are extremely low is difficult, and client compliance is poor. Use of monounsaturated fats rather than saturated fats is encouraged.

NURSING APPLICATIONS

Assessment

Physical—for height, dry weight, IBW, TSF, MAMC; overhydration/dehydration, BP, I&O, psychological state (denial, anxiety, anger, depression).

Dietary—for intake of protein, phosphorus, kilocalories, potassium, calcium, magnesium, vitamins A and D, iron, folate, vitamin C, and pyridoxine.

Laboratory—for transferrin, Hgb, Hct, uric acid, magnesium, creatinine, BUN, cholesterol, triglycerides, GFR; BUN/creatinine ratio; ABGs, sodium, chloride, glucose; urinary 3-methyl histidine; urinalysis for specific gravity and osmolality (see Table 29–3).

Interventions

1. For clients experiencing heavy proteinuria or receiving steroids, offer additional protein to replace losses.
2. If carbohydrate intolerance occurs, avoid offering concentrated sources of sugar.
3. Work closely with nutrition/food service to prevent serious errors in fluid and electrolyte balance among renal clients. Strict fluid limitations must allow enough water for medications. Try to schedule medications with meals to decrease the amount of fluid needed for this purpose.
4. Monitor for hypermagnesemia, as this may occur from antacids, laxatives, or enemas that contain large amounts of magnesium.
5. Encourage clients to eat; intake may be more important than discussing dietary limitations.

6. Monitor body weight daily along with serum sodium levels and blood pressure to estimate the most suitable sodium allowance. Rapid weight gain (with constant kilocalorie intake) and hypertension indicate that sodium and/or fluid intake is too high. Weight loss and decreased blood pressure imply too little sodium and/or fluid intake.
7. To help relieve thirst, suggest the following: Suck on hard candy, frozen juice, or ice cube (Carpenito, 1991). Use a spray bottle with mouthwash or water to relieve dry mouth.

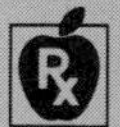 Hypercalcemia may result from supplementation of calcitriol; monitor calcium levels closely.

Evaluation

* Blood levels should return to near normal; required amounts of protein, carbohydrates, fats, kilocalories, fluids, electrolytes, trace elements, and vitamins are consumed by client; and reasons for these requirements are repeated by client/family.

Client Education

- Daily weights should be recorded.
- Helping a renal client understand the importance of controlling fluids cannot be overemphasized. If excessive fluids are removed by aggressive dialysis, severe muscle cramps, headache, nausea, vomiting, and a sudden drop in blood pressure may follow.
- Sodium content of all beverages (for example, water, coffee, tea, locally bottled carbonated and alcoholic beverages) is determined by sodium content of the water supply. Thus, if a community water supply is high in sodium, any beverages may contribute appreciably to sodium intake. Water softeners often add sodium to the water. Drinking water may have to be either restricted or distilled.

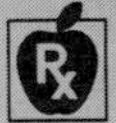 Large quantities of phosphate binders are needed. Since they are unpalatable, switching preparations may be useful; they may also be incorporated into recipes for cookies or breads.

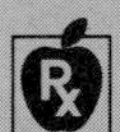 Most regular multivitamin pills are not advisable because they contain excessive vitamins A and D for a renal client.

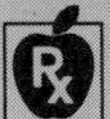 Ascorbic acid enhances GI absorption of aluminum; counsel clients who are taking aluminum compounds to avoid vitamin C supplements (Domingo et al, 1991).

PLANNING THE RENAL DIET

Creativity is necessary to avoid monotony and boredom in severely restricted renal diets. The more restrictions, the more difficult it is to please a client and maintain desired goals. Searching for variety, changing the diet daily, and avoiding the same meal on the same day of the week can improve compliance. Planning a renal diet is a difficult task, not only because of the number of nutrients to be considered, but also because of various metabolic problems associated with chronic renal disease. A diet may be calculated that is appropriate for a client's needs for protein, sodium, potassium, phosphorus, and fluid only to discover it is inadequate in kilocalories, calcium, trace minerals, or vitamins. Frequently priorities must be established, and supplements or medications may be used to meet nutritional requirements or decrease absorption of certain nutrients rather than further dietary restrictions. For example, when protein requirements are relatively high, it is difficult to meet optimal phosphorus level (which is low), and it may be necessary to use phosphorus binders.

The National Renal Diet has been developed to meet the varying needs of end-stage renal disease and hemodialysis and peritoneal dialysis clients (see Appendix D–3). The National Renal Diet Food Choices were modeled after the Exchange List for Meal Planning for diabetes mellitus, but in renal disease, more nutrients need to be controlled. Therefore, this planning tool was developed so varying levels of these nutrients could be modified easily.

Foods included in the exchange lists were altered (removed, portion sizes changed, or moved to a different exchange list), and additional lists were made. A few of the differences between the Exchange Lists for diabetes and Food Choices for renal disease are cited here. The National Renal Diet begins with milk and meat choices because quantity and quality of protein is top priority, and high-protein foods contain large quantities of phosphorus. Portion sizes of foods in the milk group are cut in half because of their high protein, phosphorus, and potassium content.

Because of large quantities of phosphorus, potassium, and NEAA present in dried beans and legumes, these foods are omitted from the starch/bread choices. Bran and whole grains are also limited because of their high phosphorus content; therefore fiber supplements may be recommended (Table 29–12). Because of omission of these items, protein content of the starch/bread food choices is 2 gm/serving rather than 3 gm/serving. Varying levels of potassium in fruits and vegetables necessitate 3 groups of each to control potassium intake. The fat food choices omit nuts and seeds because of low-quality protein, phosphorus, and potassium content.

An additional list is the milk substitute food choices. Because nondairy products are lower in phosphorus, potassium, and protein than regular dairy products, they can be included in the renal diet more easily. This group also includes nondairy frozen desserts and liquid nondairy creamers.

A high kilocalorie list can be used to provide additional kilocalories without adding protein. It includes concentrated sources of kilocalories for those with poor appetites or to meet high kilocaloric needs without exceeding optimal levels of protein or electrolytes. Since fluid limitations are frequently imposed, a beverage list is included to incorporate preferred beverages that may contain significant potassium or phosphorus.

What factors determine the diet prescription? Describe the milk group for renal diets. Describe the starch/bread group for the renal diet. Describe the fruit, vegetable, and fat list in the renal diet. Describe the milk substitute, high kilocalorie, and beverage list.

As previously discussed, some clients with renal insufficiency require specific amounts of sodium, which may not be consumed without the addition of some salt or salty foods. Salt choices include seasonings that provide 500 mg sodium, or the equivalent of ¼ tsp salt.

Approximately 33 to 50% of these clients have diabetes mellitus. Needs of a diabetic client vary from those of other renal clients. Carbohydrate must be quantified and modified to include more complex carbohydrate foods. Separate diet booklets are available for diabetic clients who have renal disease.

TABLE 29–12

COMMERCIAL FIBER SUPPLEMENTS

Production/Manufacturer	Amount	Fiber (gm)	Sodium (mg)	Potassium (mg)	Kilo-calories
Fibrad (Ross)	1 scoop	7	< 15	< 15	5
Fiberall (Rydell)	1 tsp (rounded)	3.4	1	60	6
Fibermed (Purdue Frederick)	2 wafers	10	Unknown	110	120
Metamucil (Procter & Gamble)	1 pkg	3.5	10	31	1–30
Unifiber (NuMed)	1 tbsp	3	0	0.8	0.4

NURSING APPLICATIONS

Assessment

Physical—for intellectual ability; type and severity of renal disease and treatment.
Dietary—for appetite, actual food intake, attitude about diet restrictions; knowledge of National Renal Diet.
Laboratory—see Table 29–3.

Interventions

1. Offer foods with sharp, distinct flavors, which may be more appealing because of taste changes.

Evaluation

* Client should be able to describe foods in each group.

Client Education

- Dietary adherence is the single most important factor in arresting progression of renal disease and in promoting overall well-being.
- Protein intake should be spread evenly throughout the day to minimize use of protein for energy, which results in more ammonia production.
- Meat produces more nitrogenous waste than milk and eggs; milk products contain more phosphorus.
- Clients with significant renal disease should be cautioned against eating large amounts of foods rich in potassium, such as dried fruits, oranges, bananas, and potatoes. Intake of potassium-containing foods should be distributed throughout the day because potassium is rapidly absorbed.

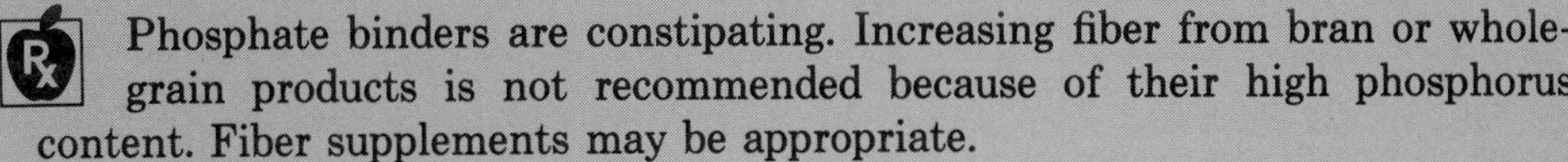

Phosphate binders are constipating. Increasing fiber from bran or whole-grain products is not recommended because of their high phosphorus content. Fiber supplements may be appropriate.

SPECIAL CONSIDERATIONS FOR DIALYSIS

When kidney function fails, dialysis must be employed. Dialysis can be used as a treatment for acute and chronic renal failure. Long-term prognosis for survival on maintenance dialysis is encouraging. Young adults without other systemic diseases and using outpatient dialysis face an annual mortality rate of less than 2%.

Even with dialysis and/or transplantation, nutritional care is still important. As many as one-third of dialysis clients have evidence of protein undernutrition (Marckmann, 1988). Hospitalized dialysis clients frequently are prescribed a diet restricted in protein, sodium, and potassium that is unpalatable to them (Sanders et al, 1991). Poor intake may also be related to seriousness of concurrent illness, anorexia, or depression. Even when clients are allowed a relatively liberal diet, nutritional status usually remains poor (Allman et al, 1990).

What causes poor intake in hospitalized dialysis clients?

Dietary Compliance

It is indeed naive when the physician, dietitian, and nurse assume that a client will accept a diet prescription even in the face of lethal consequences. Strict diet, fluid restrictions, and medication regimen facing a person dependent on dialysis top the list of psychological, social, and physical problems. About 50% of clients on dialysis adhere fairly well to dietary restrictions. Noncompliance can be obvious when elevated serum electrolytes, nitrogenous products, and weight are noted before dialysis treatments.

A thorough understanding of the causes of noncompliance has important prophylactic implications for nurses and clients. The psychological state of clients, their personality, attitudes, and beliefs can make the difference between rehabilitation and chronic invalidism.

Dependence on dialysis compounds the problem of diminished self-esteem associated with chronic disease. Apathy and helplessness may contribute to a client's feeling that deprivation is fruitless since eating may be his or her main enjoyable activity. The assault on a client's independence, self-esteem, body image, and physical sense of well-being is significant; all of these factors influence dietary compliance.

Dietary compliance can be more successful with a number of interventionist programs, e.g., client education, psychotherapy, behavioral strategies, and relaxation therapy. Behavioral therapy can have a significant impact by dealing with recurrent episodes of dietary abuse, sexual dysfunction, and marital conflicts as well as providing opportunities for developing new skills, eating habits, interests, and social roles. Most of all, clients gain satisfaction by being in control of their own affairs; this enhances compliance with the regimen and increases the pleasures of life.

What are some methods to increase dietary compliance with dialysis clients?

Praise and contingencies, such as tokens for preferred meals or access to early dialysis sessions, increase compliance. Immediate reinforcements are more beneficial than anticipation of completing long-range goals.

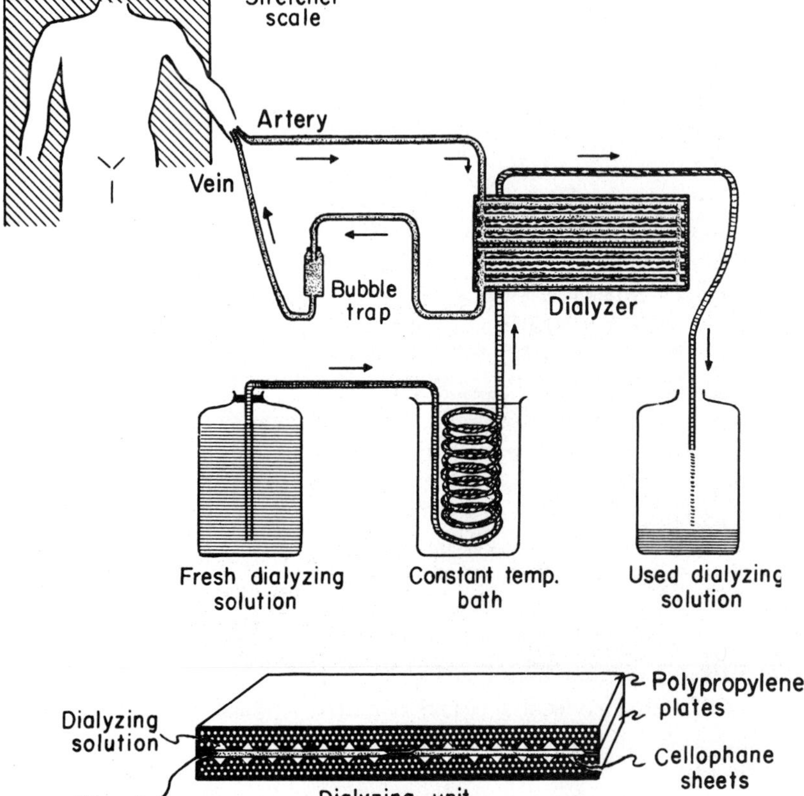

Figure 29–1 Diagram of the artificial kidney. (From Guyton AC. *Textbook of Medical Physiology*. 8th ed. Philadelphia, WB Saunders, 1991.)

Hemodialysis

A treatment for end-stage renal disease is **hemodialysis;** it is more efficient than peritoneal dialysis. A cannula is implanted in the arm or leg; blood passes through a thin membrane in an artificial kidney to the dialyzing fluid to remove unwanted substances (Fig. 29–1). An artificial kidney can function about twice as rapidly as 2 normal kidneys together. Length of time and frequency of intervals at which hemodialysis may be used are limited because of danger from excess heparin (added to prevent coagulation), hemolysis, and infection. Normally it is performed at a dialysis center for 4 to 6 hours, 2 to 3 times a week.

Hemodialysis is use of an artificial kidney machine to cleanse the blood of toxic materials via a synthetic semipermeable membrane.

Describe hemodialysis treatment.

Nutritional Care

Intermittent use of the "kidney" machine means toxic substances accumulate between treatments. Adherence to a moderately restricted diet affects frequency and effectiveness of treatment. However, the diet is liberalized as compared with that used in end-stage renal disease. Nutrient recommendations for hemodialysis clients are given in Table 29–4.

Protein requirement is affected by the fact that approximately 10 to 13 gm protein is lost in each dialysis session, which must be replaced. Although energy needs are relatively high, fat and cholesterol restriction is advisable to lower serum lipids. Because of accumulation of sodium and fluid between treatments, moderate restriction of sodium and fluid is the prudent approach. A specialized nutrition supplement, Nepro (Ross), is available that is high in kilocalories and protein but low in electrolytes; this is beneficial for many clients with poor intake.

Water-soluble vitamin supplements include the RDAs for each of the water-soluble vitamins except for increased amounts of pyridoxine, ascorbic acid, and folate, which are lost during dialysis (Makoff, 1991). Dialysis removes very little phosphorus; therefore, it should be limited somewhat, and a phosphorus-binding medication may be needed.

Why may a specialized nutrition supplement be needed? Explain why phosphorus is restricted.

NURSING APPLICATIONS

Assessment

Physical—for height, weight/dry weight/weight changes, IBW, TSF, MAMC, and blood pressure (in nonaccess arm); I&O, edema, temperature, psychosocial factors.

Dietary—for use of vitamin supplements; protein, phosphorus, sodium, and fat intake; attitude about diet restrictions.

Laboratory—for Hgb, Hct, iron, vitamin B_{12}, folate; creatinine, creatinine clearance, uric acid, urea, BUN, GFR; calcium, sodium, potassium, magnesium; albumin, alkaline phosphate; cholesterol, triglyceride.

Interventions

1. Offer foods high in vitamin C. The risk of infection is greatly increased during maintenance hemodialysis treatment. This impaired immune function may be reversed by improvement in nutritional status.
2. Consult with physician to supplement carnitine (2 gm/day) because carnitine deficiency contributes to hypertriglyceridemia in clients undergoing dialysis (Hellerstein et al, 1987).
3. Monitor for adequate protein intake; morbidity and mortality are high among clients with low-protein intake.
4. Excessive aluminum in the dialysate causes a progressive syndrome called

Continued

dialysis dementia and osteomalacia. Therefore, monitor dialysis clients for dementia (confusion) and osteomalacia (fragile bones).

Evaluation

* Client should comply with limited protein, potassium, sodium, and fluid intake. However, kilocalorie intake should be increased.

Client Education

- If nausea is experienced during dialysis, abstain from eating for 2 hours before treatment.
- Clients receiving maintenance hemodialysis should receive a calcium supplement.
- Weight gain between treatments should be less than 3 to 4 lbs.
- Discuss the role of sodium, potassium, and fluid intake between treatments. Appropriate limitations can be determined by checking a client's predialysis level of potassium and weight.
- Excesses of sodium and water between hemodialysis cause increases in weight and blood pressure; conversely, too little fluid intake or losses from nausea, vomiting, or diarrhea may lead to decreased GFR, hypotension, and dehydration.
- Protein intake is increased slightly to replace amounts lost during treatment, but high intakes may still cause azotemia. Meat contains large amounts of creatinine and phosphorus and should be moderate.
- Vitamin/mineral supplements should be used as prescribed by the physician/dietitian; excesses, especially of vitamin A and zinc, should be avoided.
- Cola beverages should be avoided because of their phosphate content.
- Counsel a client about the effects of high lipid levels and discuss the Step-1 diet.
- Discuss signs of uremia.

Peritoneal Dialysis

Peritoneal dialysis uses the peritoneal membrane as the semipermeable membrane. By inserting a catheter into the abdominal wall, dialysate is injected into the peritoneum. Dialysate, a hypertonic solution, causes fluid to flow into the peritoneal cavity.

IPD is usually performed 4 times a week for 10 hours. CAPD is the newest technical development in which the dialysate is left in the peritoneum and exchanged manually 3 to 5 times daily. In CCPD, a machine infuses 3 or 4 exchanges of dialysate at night. Approximately 2 L of dialysate remain in the peritoneal cavity during the daytime hours.

Some persons prefer **peritoneal dialysis.** Peritoneal dialysis can be **intermittent peritoneal dialysis (IPD), continuous ambulatory peritoneal dialysis (CAPD),** or **continuous cyclic peritoneal dialysis (CCPD).** Peritoneal dialysis may be administered at home or in centers; it can be initiated more quickly than hemodialysis because a dialyzing machine is not needed, anticoagulants are not necessary, and there is no need for vascular cannulization.

Nutritional Care

Protein losses in peritoneal dialysis may be extensive, as much as 5 to 20 gm/day, but clients are able to achieve positive nitrogen balance. The amount lost varies with the method used, volume of dialysate, and length of time the dialysate remains in the peritoneal cavity. As with clients receiving hemodialysis, clients frequently have low body weight and decreased fat, muscle, and serum protein levels.

Recommended energy intake is relatively normal, based on body size, activity, and concurrent illnesses (see Table 29–4). Clients on CAPD need to compensate their kilocaloric intake slightly because about 80% of the glucose from the dialysate is absorbed (Pemberton et al, 1988). (This is not true of IPD because of the shorter period of time the dialysate is in the peritoneal cavity.) Fat intake needs to be adjusted, as determined by lipoprotein levels.

As recommended for hemodialysis clients, the need for water-soluble vitamin supplementation is due to losses in dialysate. Sodium and fluid intake should be based on individual evaluation, but usually neither is severely restricted because this form of peritoneal dialysis is continuous or performed frequently. Clients performing dialysis at home maintain records of daily weight and blood pressure. Potassium restriction is usually unnecessary; however, potassium intake should be distributed throughout the day. Phosphate binders may be used since phosphorus restriction is inconsistent with the need to increase protein intake.

NURSING APPLICATIONS

Assessment

Same as for hemodialysis.

Interventions

1. Monitor for peritonitis (fever, abdominal pain, abdominal cramping, cloudy dialysis drainage, swelling and tenderness around catheter site, and elevated WBC), a major complication of long-term peritoneal dialysis. Peritonitis increases protein losses, and protein depletion increases chance of peritonitis.

Evaluation

* Client should consume a moderate increase in protein, not develop overhydration or dehydration or an infection, and have normal lipoprotein levels because of adjustments in fat intake.

Client Education

- Clients usually experience a feeling of fullness with the dialysis solution in the peritoneal cavity; this may cause anorexia.
- Anorexia in peritoneal dialysis may be due to fluid depletion and can be resolved with proper use of dialysis solutions.
- Large amounts of sodium removed with CAPD treatment may result in hypotension. Additional amounts of salt may be needed; this can be provided by putting salt into capsules.
- If phosphate binders cause constipation, suggest a fiber supplement.

SPECIAL CONSIDERATIONS FOR TRANSPLANTATION

The renal transplant diet should focus on optimal protein and kilocalorie intake to restore nitrogen balance (Edwards & Doster, 1990). Following a kidney transplant, protein intake should be increased to 1.2 to 2 gm/kg IBW, when BUN is less than 50 mg/dl and creatinine is less than 5 mg/dl, to promote healing (see Table 29–4).

Large amounts of immunosuppressive medications such as prednisone, azathioprine (Imuran), and cyclosporine prevent transplant rejection. These medications have many side effects on nutritional status (see Chapter 22, Table 22–4). Corticosteroids used for immunosuppression may cause increased catabolism of protein, negative nitrogen balance, decreased glucose tolerance, increased sodium and fluid retention, impaired calcium absorption, and increased serum lipids. Adverse effects of cyclosporine on plasma lipoprotein levels decrease when the medication is discontinued (Ballantyne et al, 1989).

To minimize hyperlipidemia, intake of cholesterol and saturated fat is restricted using the Step-1 diet. Increasingly lipid-lowering medications are being used. Nicotinic acid has been effective but is not well tolerated, unless it is initiated at a low level and gradually increased. Bile acid sequestrants, such as Questran, are avoided because they bind with immunosuppressive medications if taken together. HMG CoA reductase inhibitor, or lovastatin (Mevacor), has been used to lower serum cholesterol effectively (Melton, 1991). Lovastatin requires close monitoring for myopathy; increases in creatine kinase could lead to acute renal failure.

A diuretic or antihypertensive medication may be required for hypertension, but usually sodium is mildly restricted (2000 to 4000 mg). Potassium and phosphorus intake are individualized according to a client's serum values.

NURSING APPLICATIONS

Assessment

Physical—for height, dry weight, present weight, IBW, TSF, MAMC; anorexia, temperature, I&O, BP; anxiety level.

Dietary—for intake of fats, protein, calcium, and sodium.

Laboratory—for glucose, nitrogen balance, albumin, sodium, potassium, magnesium, chloride; Hgb, Hct, WBCs, TLC; GFR, BUN, creatinine, creatinine clearance; LDL, HDL, triglycerides.

Interventions

1. Consult the dietitian for individualization of diet.
2. Offer high-quality protein foods.
3. Monitor the following for increases, as these may indicate kidney rejection: BUN, creatinine, and weight (Cunningham & Smith, 1990).

Evaluation

* Client should consume 1.2 to 2 gm/kg IBW, increase kilocalorie intake to promote healing, and consume 2000 to 4000 mg sodium.
* Lipoprotein levels should be normal, and kidney rejection does not occur.

Client Education

- Intake of calcium-containing food should be 1 to 1.5 times the RDA to offset poor absorption.
- Discuss food safety issues (see section in Chapter 22 on depressed immune function).
- Drink 1 quart (1000 ml/day) fluid unless a limit is specifically prescribed by physician (Weaver, 1991).
- Refer to National Kidney Foundation, National Association of Patients on Hemodialysis and Transplantation, and American Kidney Foundation.

SPECIAL CONSIDERATIONS FOR CHILDREN WITH RENAL DISEASE

Achievement of normal growth in toddlers and catch-up growth in an older, growth-retarded uremic child is a true challenge. Catch-up growth is most difficult. Children whose CRF started at birth are especially small and have marked retardation in skeletal maturation. Children must be closely monitored because malnutrition and metabolic disturbances of uremia appear to be more severe in prepubertal children than in adults. Use of ketoacid analogue supplements may be effective in promoting more normal growth rates in these children (Jureidini et al, 1990). Energy intake should be close to 100% of the RDA for efficient use of dietary protein. Even with the RDA for the appropriate age group, potential growth in height is seldom achieved. This large amount of kilocalories is often difficult for these children to consume.

Protein usually is not restricted for children because of a history of growth retardation in children with renal failure; protein intake should be equal to or slightly exceed the RDA for the age group (Hanna et al, 1991). Emphasis is placed on providing high-quality proteins to ensure an adequate intake of EAA. In children with azotemia, dietary protein may be progressively reduced to minimal levels to maintain BUN concentration lower than 100 gm/dl (Foreman & Chan, 1988). Other energy sources in relation to the total diet are carbohydrates, 50%; and fat, 35 to 40% (Yang et al, 1988–89).

Few infants with renal failure need to be placed on fluid restrictions; sodium, potassium, and protein are usually the only problem nutrients. Breast milk is ideal because of its low solute load. The same principles apply for pureed foods (home or commercially prepared baby food) as for regular foods for adults, addressing individual needs for protein, sodium, potassium, and phosphorus.

As a child progresses to finger foods, the usual finger foods are often unacceptable. Thus, dry cereals, flavored gelatin cubes, fresh green beans or carrots, marshmallows, salt-free crackers with jelly or honey and margarine, julienne meat, and sticky rice are suitable.

Stressing allowances rather than restrictions is more optimistic, particularly for children. A child and his or her family should eat meals together with only slight modifications for the child. Preparation of fresh or frozen vegetables with no added sodium or potassium salt allows others to season their food at the table.

Therapeutic diets for children are composed of ordinary foods and low-protein products and/or nutrition supplements developed for renal disease. Portion sizes are modified and measured, particularly with exactness for total fluid intake. Children need to be involved in planning and implementing their diet. They should measure all fluids precisely rather than estimating intake. Youngsters usually become quite adept at taking medications with little fluid. Also, a child who carefully follows a sodium restriction experiences decreased thirst.

What are the recommended energy sources in relation to the total diet? Why is protein usually not restricted for children? If azotemia occurs, how is protein regulated? What is the ideal food for infants with CRF? What are appropriate finger foods for toddlers with CRF?

NURSING APPLICATIONS

Assessment

Physical—for age, weight, height, growth chart percentile; client/family psychosocial factors; BP; I&O.

Dietary—for adequate kilocalorie, carbohydrate, fat, protein intake; protein sources; where meals are taken; client/family's attitude about diet.

Laboratory—for BUN, creatinine, sodium, urine protein (see Table 29–3).

Interventions

1. Perform a complete clinical assessment. Particularly for children, an unusually high BUN value may not indicate an excessively high intake of protein but rather an inadequate dietary intake of nonprotein kilocalories. An unusually low BUN may denote poor nutritional intake, including inadequate protein and nonprotein kilocalories.
2. Offer glucose polymers since they are not as sweet and may help increase acceptance of products and thus increase energy intake. Uremic children have abnormally low preferences for sweet foods that can contribute to insufficient kilocaloric intake (Bellisle et al, 1990).

Evaluation

* Client should gain weight and consume 50% of total kilocalories from carbohydrate; 35 to 40% fat, and 10% protein. Eggs, milk, and meat are ingested.

Continued

Specific requirements are followed according to a client's age, and dietary management appropriate for the age is performed by the child.

Client Education

- Use of nondairy creamers and whipped toppings allows more variety.
- Recipes are available for preparing candies and cookies made with margarine and honey.
- Children must be taught adequate oral hygiene and dental care to prevent dental caries from the high-carbohydrate intake.
- Avoid all-you-can-eat situations to prevent overindulgence, but do not avoid special occasions entirely.
- Small, hard candies are surprisingly easy to aspirate and should not be offered to young children.

NEPHROLITHIASIS AND UROLITHIASIS

Nephrolithiasis is the occurrence of small gravel-like particles, composed of mineral salts, in any part of the kidney.

What dietary factors correlate with kidney stones?

Another serious problem occurring in the renal system is that of urinary calculi, or stone formation. **Nephrolithiasis** has an annual incidence of 7 to 21 cases per 10,000 Americans (Consensus Conference, 1988). This condition is more prevalent in men between 20 and 30 years of age. The only dietary factors that correlate consistently with stone occurrence are a high intake of animal protein, particularly meat, fish, and poultry, and sodium (Kok et al, 1990).

Physical Consequences

Supersaturated refers to concentration of a stone-forming salt to the point it exceeds its solubility in urine and precipitates.

Urolithiasis is a calculus or stone in any part of the urinary tract.

A stone may form when urine is **supersaturated** with respect to its constituent crystals. Progressive deposits of crystalline material form around a nucleus, causing **urolithiasis.** Approximately 70 to 80% of stones are principally calcium oxalate crystals; the rest are composed of calcium phosphate salts, uric acid, struvite (magnesium, ammonium, and phosphate), or the amino acid cystine. Small stones can be "passed," but some become trapped in the urinary tract.

Causes

Sarcoidosis—development of a tumor-like mass of reticuloendothelial cells frequently in the lymph nodes, liver, spleen, lungs, skin, eyes.

Certain conditions increase risk of hypercalciuria predisposing urolithiasis: hyperparathyroidism, renal tubular acidosis, **sarcoidosis,** vitamin D intoxication, and "idiopathic" hypercalciuria. Hereditary metabolic disorders or disorders caused by intestinal disease or diet may contribute to hyperoxaluria.

"Recumbency" stones develop within 14 to 21 days among 15 to 30% of all immobilized clients; these are caused by incomplete bladder emptying. In a horizontal position, urine stagnates because gravity is not aiding in urine drainage (Fig. 29–2). Tiny particles and crystals that ordinarily would be excreted stay in the renal pelvis and form nuclei for renal stones. Other factors that contribute to recumbency stones include (1) a slightly alkaline urine (common during bed rest), (2) UTIs (common with catheterization), (3) elevated urinary calcium concentrations (urinary calcium can triple after only 2 weeks of immobilization), and (4) elevated phosphorus.

What are the majority of stones composed of? What conditions cause hypercalciuria? What factors contribute to recumbency stones?

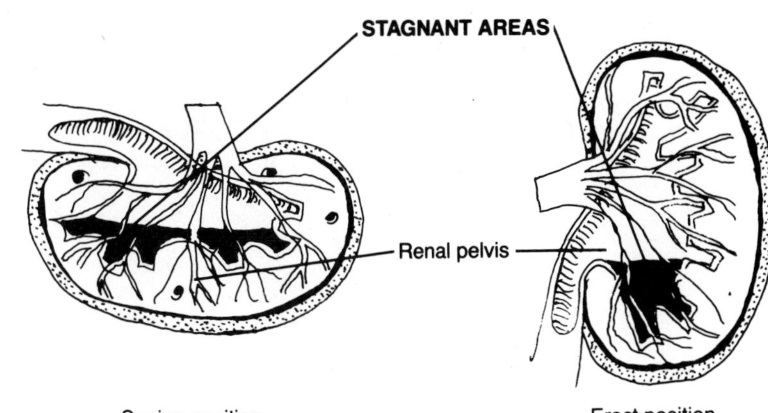

Figure 29–2 When the body is in a horizontal position, as when a client is confined to bed, urine stagnates in the renal pelvis, increasing risk of infections and stones.

Treatment

Fluid intake is important for any type of stone formation. Increased fluid intake lowers the concentration of substances involved in stone formation. A goal of doubling urine output or a 24-hour urinary output greater than 2 L is recommended to reduce new stone formation (Consensus Conference, 1988).

In the past, surgical procedures were necessary to remove these stones, but extracorporeal shock-wave lithotripsy is the current mode of therapy. With lithotripsy, stones are crushed small enough to be passed out of the body.

Chemical analysis identifies primary components of stones to prescribe dietary modifications. A diet history is useful in determining excesses of dietary components that may influence stone formation (calcium, oxalate, sodium, phosphorus, purine, cystine, acid-ash or alkaline-ash, and protein content). Recommendations for nutritional care are presented for each type of stone in which dietary changes are beneficial.

What measure can reduce new stone formation? Which dietary components can influence stone formation?

Calcium Oxalate Stones

Most calcium oxalate stones are of unknown cause and thus are called "idiopathic." The objective of treatment is to reduce abnormal urinary calcium and oxalate excretion. Hypercalciuria usually results from increased intestinal calcium absorption; absorptive hypercalciuria requires a calcium restriction. However, interactions of calcium and oxalate in the GI tract complicate therapy. Normally dietary calcium intake and intestinal oxalate absorption are inversely correlated. Less calcium is absorbed because it combines with oxalate in the intestine. Therefore, a very low calcium diet leads to increased oxalate absorption. Since oxalate cannot be metabolized, urinary excretion is increased. Small elevations in urinary oxalate concentration increase the risk of calcium oxalate stones; therefore, both calcium and oxalate intake are restricted.

Thiazide diuretics, which increase calcium reabsorption, are frequently prescribed to reduce renal calcium excretion. High salt intake decreases the effectiveness of thiazides and increases calcium excretion. Clients are advised to limit calcium intake to 800 to 1000 mg/day (RDA is 800 mg) and avoid high sodium intake.

Oxalate-containing foods should not be eaten in excessive amounts (Table 29–13). Alcohol consumption, particularly beer, is associated with higher urinary calcium and uric acid levels (Hughes & Norman, 1992). Oxalic acid is a metabolic byproduct of vitamin C, and large amounts from vitamin supplements should be avoided. Dietary fiber combines with dietary oxalate in the GI tract, significantly decreasing urinary calcium and oxalate (Firth & Norman, 1990).

Why is calcium intake lowered, and what effect does this have on oxalate? How do thiazide diuretics help? Why is a high sodium intake undesirable? Describe ways to decrease oxalate in diet. When are dietary restrictions contraindicated?

TABLE 29–13

NUTRITIONAL PRINCIPLES FOR CLIENTS WITH KIDNEY STONES
1. Drink plenty of water each day; 8 cups is recommended 2. Limit calcium intake by limiting dairy products to 2 to 3 servings/day 3. Avoid high sodium intake; limit intake of highly processed foods, especially canned soups, salted snacks, sauerkraut, ham, bacon, pickles, and olives; do not add salt at the table 4. Refrain from excessive amounts of meat products. Limit meat products to 6 oz/day and exclude organ meats 5. Limit intake of purine-containing foods: anchovies, sardines, meat extracts, gravy, broth and bouillon, organ meats (liver, heart, gizzards) 6. Limit intake of oxalate-containing foods: spinach, chard, parsley, other green leafy vegetables, beets, rhubarb, cocoa, chocolate, walnuts, almonds, peanuts, pecans, wheat germ, and tea 7. Increase fiber intake with whole-grain breads and cereals, fruits, and vegetables 8. Abstain from large amounts of vitamin C. Vitamin supplements should contain no more than the RDA

Dietary restrictions are contraindicated for calcium oxalate stones secondary to hyperparathyroidism, sarcoidosis, renal tubular acidosis, or primary hyperoxaluria. These conditions represent only 10% of all calcium oxalate renal stones.

Struvite or Triple Phosphate

Clients with chronic UTIs from bacterial organisms and alkaline urine tend to develop struvite stones. Paraplegics are the largest group at risk for this type of kidney stone since they often have a neurogenic bladder.

What clients are prone to struvite stones? List foods on an acid-ash diet. Describe treatment for struvite stones.

Ingestion of cranberry juice is sometimes recommended to acidify urine. However, commercially prepared cranberry juices contain only about 26% cranberry juice and are not thought to be consistently effective. Use of an acid-ash diet may be of some benefit. Cranberries, plums, prunes, meat, and bread are acid-ash foods. The most effective treatment is complete removal of the stones and appropriate antibacterial therapy.

Uric Acid

Uric acid stone disease (gout) accounts for approximately 10% of the renal stones in the US. Clients with persistently acid urine or increased urinary uric acid excretion are at risk. Allopurinol (Zyloprim) treatment is used for recalcitrant uric acid stones (Consensus Conference, 1988). Pharmacological agents such as bicarbonate or citrate are used to alkalinize urine. An alkaline-ash diet is recommended (see Appendix D–4): Milk, fruits (except cranberries, plums, and prunes), and vegetables (especially legumes and green vegetables).

Describe nutritional care for uric acid stones.

Reduction of purine or protein intake to normal levels is highly recommended. Meat, fish, and poultry intake should be limited to 6 to 7 oz/day. Alcohol inhibits uric acid excretion and should be eliminated or restricted.

NURSING APPLICATIONS

Assessment

Physical—for height, weight, IBW; excruciating flank pain; nausea, vomiting, burning and urinary frequency, paraplegia.
Dietary—for protein, calcium, oxalate, sodium, phosphorus, purine, acid or alkaline ash, and fluid intake.
Laboratory—for calcium, uric acid, serum oxalate levels, BUN, creatinine, phosphate; urinalysis for calcium and stone content.

Interventions

1. If client has calcium oxalate stones, offer high-fiber foods.
2. In clients with struvite stones, provide an acid-ash diet.
3. For clients with uric acid stones, offer an alkaline-ash diet and foods low in purine.
4. For immobilized clients, suggest an acid-ash diet to lower urine pH and prevent UTI.
5. Avoid catheterization if at all possible to prevent infection.
6. For bedfast clients, limit calcium intake to about 800 mg/day during the first 3 to 6 months, or until there is weight-bearing activity.
7. If nausea and vomiting are present, contact the physician. IV fluids may be needed to prevent stone formation.
8. Strain urine.

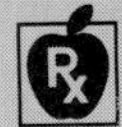
Monitor potassium levels when thiazide diuretics are used. Encourage high-potassium foods.

Evaluation

* Desired outcomes include client willingly complies/consumes diet to decrease incidence of stone formation and ingests 3000 ml/day of fluid with 1500 ml as water.

Client Education

- Bloody urine (hematuria), severe flank pain (renal colic), backache, nausea, and vomiting can result from renal stones.
- No matter what type of renal stone, fluid intake should be at least 3000 ml/day to dilute urine. Clients should drink 8 to 10 oz of water (or fluid) every hour during the day with 2 large glasses before bedtime. Nocturnal voiding should be followed with another glass of water. At least half the fluid ingested should be water.
- Encourage clients to become ambulatory as soon as possible.
- Frequently adults who have consumed excessive amounts of calcium (more than 3 servings per day) overreact when stones form. The admonition to consume less calcium does not mean to eliminate all milk products. Calcium should not be reduced to less than 600 mg/day. If it is, negative calcium balance and increased oxalate excretion may result.
- Since oxalic acid or oxalate results from metabolism of vitamin C, long-term, excessive intakes (about 4 gm or more over a long period of time) may precipitate oxalic acid stones. Acidic urine caused by high vitamin C intake promotes uric acid stone formation.
- Abstain from alcohol or use in moderation.

SUMMARY

When irreversible kidney disorders occur, dietary prescription is one of the most significant tools to delay the course of illness. Protein is restricted to decrease metabolic waste products and minimize uremic toxicity. Carbohydrates and fats are carefully selected to provide protein-sparing kilocalories for energy needs and controlling electrolyte intake. Metabolism and requirements for many nutrients may change frequently in renal failure. Maintaining electrolyte levels within normal limits, treating hypertension, preventing protein catabolism while restricting protein intake to lessen work of the kidneys, and avoiding dehydration and overhydration are goals of dietary intervention. Finally, maintenance of optimal nutritional status for as normal growth and health as possible is imperative.

Nephrolithiasis and urolithiasis, or kidney stones, may cause excruciating pain. Causes and composition of kidney stones vary, but fluid intake is a primary cause (inadequate) and treatment (increased). Immobilization is a strong conducive factor; bacterial infections may precipitate stones. Diet modifications and increased fluid intake are effective in both preventing and treating urolithiasis.

NURSING PROCESS IN ACTION

A client with CRF experiencing anorexia and altered taste sensations is admitted to the hospital. Dialysis is not required at present. Mild hypertension is present, but heart failure is absent. Current weight is 70 kg. Calcitriol is ordered.

Nutritional Assessment

- IBM, height, weight, TSF, MAMC.
- Food preferences, meal patterns.
- Intake of protein, fat, carbohydrate, salt, potassium, fluid, calcium, and phosphorus.
- Knowledge of dietary restrictions.
- Psychological status.
- Serum potassium, sodium, protein, albumin, BUN, creatinine; GFR.

Dietary Nursing Diagnosis

Altered nutrition: Less than body requirements RT anorexia and altered taste sensations.

Nutritional Goals

Client will eat 75 to 100% of ordered diet, verbalize understanding of dietary restrictions, and comply with nutritional regimen.

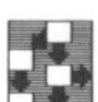

Nutritional Implementation 

Intervention: Discuss low-protein diet prescription (42 to 49 gm protein with 60 to 70% HBV protein) with client, and monitor foods provided on the tray and/or foods brought in by family and friends.

Rationale: Protein is restricted to 0.6 to 0.7 gm/kg IBW to decrease nausea, vomiting, and fatigue. At least 60 to 70% of the protein should be of high quality to provide EAA.

Intervention: Encourage food intake so client receives 2100 to 3150 kcal daily. Additional kilocalories may be added by using glucose polymers and salt-free margarine or oils.

Rationale: Generally 30 to 45 kcal/kg IBW is needed to prevent weight loss and spare protein.

Intervention: Offer favorite foods.

Rationale: Client is more likely to eat favorite foods, thus increasing energy intake.

Intervention: Monitor strict I&O.

Rationale: For each 24 hours, a fluid intake level that totals 500 to 800 ml plus the previous 24-hour urine volume is recommended.

Intervention: Offer water; cranberry juice; sugar-sweetened, fruit-flavored drinks; and grape and apple juice.

Rationale: These drinks contain minimal amounts of protein, sodium, and potassium; they also can be used to increase kilocaloric intake since they contain simple sugars.

Intervention: Provide 1000 to 2000 mg sodium.

Rationale: Since client is mildly hypertensive, mild sodium restriction is needed to maintain sodium and water balance.

Intervention: Avoid offering foods high in phosphorus; provide adequate calcium intake and prescribed amounts of calcitriol.

Rationale: Control of serum calcium and phosphate should begin early in clients with renal failure to prevent renal osteodystrophy from developing as well as delay the progression of CRF. Calcitriol induces normal serum calcium levels with an adequate calcium intake. Calcitriol may also prevent vitamin D deficiency.

Intervention: Emphasize not taking large doses of vitamin A.

Rationale: Vitamin A intoxication may occur.

Intervention: Refer to dietitian.

Rationale: With all the intricacies of the diet, expert knowledge is needed to manage this chronic disease.

Intervention: Allow client to vent feelings about dietary restrictions and offer support.

Rationale: Meeting self-esteem and self-actualization needs are necessary for compliance. Encouraging intake may be more important than discussing dietary limitations.

Intervention: Follow the National Renal Diet Food choices.

Rationale: These have been developed to meet varying needs of renal clients.

Evaluation

Client consumes 75 to 100% of ordered diet, talks about protein and phosphorus restrictions, and complies with these restrictions. Additionally, client should maintain "dry" weight, drink appropriate amounts of fluid, consume enough kilocalories to spare protein, and maintain normal blood pressure.

STUDENT READINESS

1. A renal client asks why a high-potency vitamin is undesirable. How would you respond?
2. What nutrients are usually supplemented in CRF?
3. How are diets modified for kidney disorders?
4. Plan a diet for 1 day for 40 gm of protein, 1500 mg of potassium, and 1000 mg of sodium.

CASE STUDY

Mr. G. M. awoke suddenly in the middle of the night with excruciating back pain just below his rib cage. After entering the hospital emergency room, a diagnosis of calcium renal stones was made.

1. What are the next steps in his medical care plan?
2. What can he do to prevent recurrences of kidney stones?
3. What types of food would you offer him?

CASE STUDY

Mr. G. J., a 57-year-old business executive, has been treated for hypertension and hypertensive renal disease for the past 23 years. He is now in end-stage renal failure and being treated with hemodialysis 3 times weekly. A 2000 kcal diet with 60 gm protein, 2000 mg sodium, 1500 mg potassium, and 800 ml fluid is ordered.

1. Why is protein intake not restricted to less than 40 gm to decrease BUN?
2. What is the desirable weight gain between dialysis treatments?
3. If protein intake were increased by 20 gm, why would the potassium intake have to be increased?
4. List 5 foods that have high potassium levels.
5. Write a sample menu plan for Mr. G. J.
6. If a 2000 kcal diet is prescribed, are vitamin supplements necessary?

REFERENCES

Al-Bander H, Kaysen GA. Ineffectiveness of dietary protein augmentation in the management of the nephrotic syndrome. *Pediatr Nephrol* 1991 July; 5(4):482–486.

Allman MA, et al. Energy supplementation and the nutritional status of hemodialysis patients. *Am J Clin Nutr* 1990 Apr; 51(4):558–562.

Alvestrand A, Bergström J. Renal diseases. *In* Kinney JM, et al. eds. *Nutrition and Metabolism in Patient Care.* Philadelphia, WB Saunders, 1988: 531–557.

Alvestrand A, Bergström J. Amino acid supplements and the course of chronic renal disease. *In* Mitch WE, ed. *The Progressive Nature of Renal Disease.* Vol 14. New York: Churchill Livingston, 1986: 219–229.

Baer CL. Acute renal failure: Recognizing and reversing its deadly course. *Nursing* 1990 June; 20(6):34–39.

Ballantyne CM, et al. Effects of cyclosporine therapy on plasma lipoprotein levels. *JAMA* 1989 July 7; 262(1):53–56.

Barsotti G, et al. Three years experience with a very low nitrogen diet supplemented with essential amino acids and keto analogues in the treatment of chronic uremia. *Proc Eur Dial Transplant Assoc* 1983; 19:773–778.

Bellisle F, et al. Perceptions of and preferences for sweet taste in uremic children. *J Am Diet Assoc* 1990 July; 90(7):951–954.

Carpenito LF. *Nursing Care Plans and Documentation: Nursing Diagnoses and Collaborative Problems.* Philadelphia, JB Lippincott, 1991.

Consensus Conference. Prevention and treatment of kidney stones. *JAMA* 1988 Aug 19; 260(7): 977–981.

Cunningham N, Smith SL. Postoperative care of the renal transplant patient. *Crit Care Nurse.* 1990 Oct; 10(9):74–80.

D'Amico G, et al. Effect of vegetarian soy diet on hyperlipidaemia in nephrotic syndrome. *Lancet* 1992 May; 339 (8802):1131–1134.

Domingo JL, et al. Effect of ascorbic acid on gastrointestinal aluminum absorption (Letter). *Lancet* 1991 Dec 7; 338(8780):1467.

Edwards MS, Doster S. Renal transplant diet recommendations: Results of survey of renal dietitians in the United States. *J Am Diet Assoc* 1990 June; 90(6):843–846.

Firth WA, Norman RW. The effects of modified diets on urinary risk factors for kidney stone disease. *J Can Diet Assoc* 1990 Fall; 51(4):404–408.

Foreman JW, Chan JCM. Chronic renal failure in infants and children. *J Pediatr* 1988 Nov; 133(5):793–800.

Fouque D, et al. Controlled low protein diets in chronic renal insufficiency: Meta-analysis. *Br Med J* 1992 Jan 25; 304(6821):216–220.

Hanna JD, et al. Chronic renal insufficiency in infants and children. *Clin Pediatr (Phila)* 1991 June; 30(6):365–384.

Hellerstein S, et al. Nutritional management of children with chronic renal failure. Summary of the task force on nutritional management of children with chronic renal failure. *Pediatr Nephrol* 1987 Apr; 1(2):195–211.

Hoppel CL, Ricanati ES. Carnitine requirements in renal disease. *In* Gussler J, Silverman E, eds. Renal Nutrition. Report of the Eleventh Ross Roundtable on Medical Issues. Columbus, OH, 1991: 68–71.

Hughes J, Norman RW. Diet and calcium stones. *Can Med Assoc J* 1992 Jan 15; 146(2):137–143.

Ihle BE, et al. The effect of protein restriction on the progression of renal insufficiency. *N Engl J Med* 1989 Dec 28; 321(26):1773–1777.

Joven J, et al. Abnormalities of lipoprotein metabolism in patients with the nephrotic syndrome. *N Engl J Med* 1990 Aug 30; 323(9):579–584.

Jureidini KJ, et al. Evaluation of long-term aggressive dietary management of chronic renal failure in children. *Pediatr Nephrol* 1990 Jan; 4(1):1–10.

Kean WJ, Kasiske B. Hyperlipidemia in the nephrotic syndrome. *N Engl J Med* 1990 Aug 30; 323 (9):603–604.

Klahr S. The modification of diet in renal disease study. *N Engl J Med* 1989 March 30; 320(13): 864–866.

Kok DJ, et al. The effects of dietary excesses in animal protein and in sodium on the composition and the crystallization kinetics of calcium oxalate monohydrate in urines of healthy men. *J Clin Endocrinol Metab* 1990 Oct; 71(4):861–867.

Mai ML, et al. Calcium acetate, an effective phosphorus binder in patients with renal failure. *Kidney Int* 1989 Oct; 36(4):690–695.

Makoff R. Water-soluble vitamin status in patients with renal disease treated with hemodialysis or peritoneal dialysis. *J Renal Nutr* 1991 Apr; 1(2):56–73.

Marckmann P. Nutritional status of patients on hemo-dialysis and peritoneal dialysis. *Clin Nephrol* 1988 Feb; 29(2):75–78.

Melton LB. Management of hyperlipidemia in renal disease (Abstract). *J Am Diet Assoc* 1991 Sept; 91(suppl 9):A141.

Mitch WE, et al. The effect of a keto acid-amino acid supplement diet to a restricted diet on the progression of chronic renal failure. *N Engl J Med* 1984 Sept 6; 311(10):623–629.

Nolan C, et al. Influence of calcium acetate or calcium citrate on intestinal aluminum absorption. *Kidney Int* 1990 Nov; 38(5):937–941.

Ofek I, et al. Anti-*escherichia coli* adhesin activity of cranberry and blueberry juices. *N Engl J Med* 1991 May 30; 324(22):1599.

Pemberton CM, et al. *Mayo Clinic Diet Manual.* 6th ed. Philadelphia, BC Decker, 1988.

Physician's Guide to Non-Insulin-Dependent (Type II) Diabetes: Diagnosis and Treatment. 2nd ed. Alexandria VA, American Diabetes Association, 1988.

Rosman JB, et al. Prospective randomized trial of early dietary protein restriction in chronic renal failure. *Lancet* 1984 Dec 8; 2(8415):1291–1296.

Sanders HN, et al. Hospitalized dialysis patients have lower nutrient intakes on renal diet than on regular diet. *J Am Diet Assoc* 1991 Oct; 91(10):1278–1280.

Schmitt J. Selecting an appropriate phosphate binder. *J Renal Nutr* 1991 Jan; 1(1):38–40.

Strauss J, et al. Less commonly recognized features of childhood nephrotic syndrome. *Pediatr Clin North Am* 1987 June; 34(3):591–607.

Talbot JM. Guidelines for the scientific review of enteral food products for special medical purposes. *JPEN* 1991 May-June; 15(3):1S–174S.

Viberti GC, Bending JJ. Preventive approach to diabetic kidney disease. *Contrib Nephrol* 1988; 61:91–100.

Walser M. Weighted least squares regression analysis of factors contributing to progression of chronic renal failure. *Contrib Nephrol* 1989; 75:127–133.

Walser M, et al. Supplements containing amino acids and keto acids in the treatment of chronic uremia. *Kidney Int* 1983 Dec; 16(suppl):S285–S289.

Weaver SH. Renal and urological care. *In* Shaw M, et al, eds. *Illustrated Manual of Nursing Practice.* Springhouse, PA, Springhouse, 1991: 603–680.

Yang W, et al. Chronic renal insufficiency—conservative management. *Child Nephrol Urol* 1988–89; 9(6):301–311.

Zeller DR, et al. The effect of dietary protein and phosphorus restriction on renal function in diabetic nephropathy—results of a 5 year study (Abstract). *Kidney Int* 1990 Jan; 37(1):246.

Zeman FJ. *Clinical Nutrition and Dietetics.* 2nd ed. New York, Macmillan, 1991.

APPENDICES

A. FOOD COMPOSITION TABLES
- A-1. Nutritive Values of Food
- A-2. Product Information for Medical Foods
- A-3. Nutritional Analysis of Fast Foods
- A-4. Caffeine Content of Foods

B. RECOMMENDED NUTRIENT INTAKES
- B-1. Recommended Daily Intake (see App. B-1)
- B-2. Recommended Nutrient Intakes (RNI), Canada, 1990, Based on Age, Energy, and Body Weight Expressed as Daily Rates

C. NUTRITIONAL ASSESSMENT CRITERIA
- C-1. 1983 Metropolitan Height and Weight Tables
- C-2. Body Mass Index
- C-3. Nomogram for Determining Abdominal/Gluteal Circumference Ratio (Waist/Hip Ratio)
- C-4. Determination of Body Frame Size from Wrist Circumference
- C-5. Arm Anthropometry Nomograms
  - C-5a. Adults
  - C-5b. Children
- C-6. Percentiles for Triceps Skinfold for Whites of the United States Health and Nutrition Examination Survey I of 1971 to 1974
- C-7. Percentiles for Upper Arm Circumference (mm) and Estimated Upper Arm Muscle Circumference (mm) for Whites of the United States Health and Nutrition Examination Survey I of 1971 to 1974
- C-8. Growth Charts
  - C-8a. Girls: Birth to 36 Months Physical Growth NCHS Percentiles
  - C-8b. Boys: Birth to 36 Months Physical Growth NCHS Percentiles
  - C-8c. Girls: 2 to 18 Years Physical Growth NCHS Percentiles
  - C-8d. Boys: 2 to 18 Years Physical Growth NCHS Percentiles
- C-9. Nutrients Detrimentally Affected by Drugs
- C-10. Timing of Drugs
- C-11. Drugs Requiring Increased Amounts of Fluids

D. SPECIALIZED TABLES FOR MODIFIED DIETS
- D-1. Diabetic Food Exchange Lists
- D-2. Diabetic Exchange Values for Fast Foods
- D-3. Exchange Lists for the National Renal Diet
- D-4. Acid–Base Ash Resulting from Metabolism of Foods

E. SOURCES FOR RELIABLE NUTRITION INFORMATION
- E-1. Nutrition Resources
- E-2. Recommended Journals and Newsletters

F. METRIC SYSTEM AND CONVERSIONS
- F-1. Commonly Used Equivalents
- F-2. Conversions to and from Metric Measures
- F-3. Conversions of Milligrams to Milliequivalents

G. ANSWERS TO NQ

Food Composition Tables

APPENDIX A

APPENDIX A–1 **NUTRITIVE VALUES OF FOOD**

	Approximate Measure	Weight (gm)	H_2O (gm)	Kcal	Protein (gm)	Carbohydrate (gm)	Dietary Fiber (gm)	Fat (gm)	MUFA (gm)	PUFA (gm)	Cholesterol (mg)	Calcium (mg)
Fats, Oils, and Related Products												
Butter												
Regular	1 tbsp	14	2	100	0	0	0	11	3.3	0.4	31	3
Regular, pat	1	5	0.8	36	<1	<1	0	4	1.2	0.2	11	1
Whipped	1 tbsp	9	1	65	<1	0	0	7	2.1	0.3	20	2
Whipped, pat	1	4	0.6	27	<1	0	0	3	0.9	0.1	8	1
Margarine												
Extra light	1 tbsp	14	—	50	0	0	0	6	—	2	0	—
Regular, hard	1 tbsp	14	2.2	101	<1	<1	0	11	5.0	3.6	0	4
Regular, hard, pat	1	5	0.8	36	<1	<1	0	4	1.8	1.3	0	2
Corn, soft	1 tbsp	14	2.4	101	0	0	0	11	4.5	4.5	0	4
Whipped	1 tbsp	9	1.4	70	0	0	0	8	2.5	3.1	0	2
Oil, cooking or salad												
Corn	1 tbsp	13.6	0	120	0	0	0	14	3.3	8.0	0	0
Olive	1 tbsp	13.5	0	119	0	0	0	14	9.9	1.1	0	0
Peanut	1 tbsp	13.5	0	119	0	0	0	14	6.2	4.3	0	0
Safflower	1 tbsp	13.6	0	120	0	0	0	14	1.6	10.1	0	0
Soybean	1 tbsp	13.6	0	120	0	0	0	14	5.9	5.1	0	0
Soybean/cottonseed	1 tbsp	13.6	0	120	0	0	0	14	4.0	6.6	0	0
Salad dressing, commercial												
French	1 tbsp	15.6	6	67	<1	3	0.1	6.4	1.2	3.4	2	2
French, low kcal	1 tbsp	16.3	11	22	<1	4	0.1	0.9	0.2	0.6	1	2
Italian	1 tbsp	15	6	69	0	2	0.1	7.1	1.7	4.1	0	1
Italian, low kcal	1 tbsp	15	12	16	0	1	0.1	1.5	0.3	0.9	1	0
Mayonnaise, soy	1 tbsp	14	2	99	<1	<1	0	11	3.1	5.7	8	2
Mayonnaise, reduced kcal	1 tbsp	14	—	40	0	1	—	4	—	2	0	—
Miracle Whip, Light	1 tbsp	14	—	45	0	2	0	4	—	—	5	—
Ranch style	1 tbsp	15	—	54	<1	1	0	6	—	—	—	—
Ranch, light	1 tbsp	14	—	30	0	1	—	3	—	—	0	—
Salad dressing, mayonnaise-type	1 tbsp	15	6	57	<1	5	0	5	1.3	2.7	3.8	2
Thousand Island	1 tbsp	16	7	59	<1	2	1	6	1.3	3.1	4.9	2
Thousand Island, low kcal	1 tbsp	15	11	24	<1	3	<1	2	0.4	1.0	2.0	2
Tartar sauce	1 tbsp	14	5	75	0	1	—	8	1.8	4.1	9.0	3
Fish and Shellfish Products												
Bluefish, baked with butter	3 oz	85	58	135	23	0	0	4	1	2.2	59	25
Clams												
Cooked, moist heat	3 oz	85	54	126	22	4	0	2	0.2	0.5	57	78
Canned, solid and liquid	3 oz	85	73	38	7	2	0	1	0	0	53	47
Cod, cooked, dry heat	3 oz	85	65	89	19	0	0	1	0.1	0.3	46	12
Crab meat, king, canned	3 oz	85	66	85	15	<1	0	2	0.4	1.3	85	38
Fish sticks, breaded, frozen, cooked	3 oz	85	40	231	13	20	2	10	4.3	2.7	95	17
Flounder/sole, baked	3 oz	85	62	99	21	0	0	1	0.3	0.4	58	15

Phosphate (mg)	Magnesium (mg)	Iron (mg)	Zinc (mg)	Sodium (mg)	Potassium (mg)	Vitamin A (RE)	Vitamin C (mg)	Thiamin (mg)	Riboflavin (mg)	Niacin (mg)	Vitamin B_6 (mg)	Folate (mcg)
3	<1	0.02	0.01	116	4	105	0	<0.01	<0.01	<0.01	0	<1
1	<1	0.01	<0.01	41	1	8	0	0	<0.01	<0.01	0	<1
2	<1	0.01	<0.01	74	2	68	0	0	<0.01	<0.01	0	<1
1	<1	0.01	<0.01	31	1	29	0	0	<0.01	<0.01	0	<1
—	—	—	—	55	5	—	—	—	—	—	—	—
3	<1	<0.01	0	132	6	139	<1	<0.01	<0.01	<0.01	<0.01	<1
1	<1	<0.01	0	47	2	15	<1	<0.01	<0.01	<0.01	0	<1
3	<1	0	0	152	5	141	<1	0	<0.01	<0.01	0	<1
2	<1	0	—	97	2	310	0	0	0	0	<0.01	<1
0	0	0	0	0	0	0	0	0	0	0	0	0
0	0	0.05	<0.01	<0.01	0	0	0	0	0	0	0	0
0	0	<0.01	<0.01	0.02	<1	—	0	0	0	0	0	0
0	0	0	0	0	0	0	0	0	0	0	0	0
0	0	0	0	0	0	0	0	0	0	0	0	0
0	0	0	0	0	0	0	0	0	0	0	0	0
2	0	0.10	0.01	214	12	3	0	<0.01	<0.01	0	<0.01	<1
2	0	0.10	0.03	128	13	0	0	0	0	0	0	0
1	<1	0	0.02	116	2	4	0	0	0	0	<0.01	<1
1	0	0	0.02	118	2	0	0	0	0	0	0	0
4	<1	0.10	0.02	78	5	12	0	0	0	0	0.08	1
0	—	—	—	110	0	—	—	—	—	—	—	—
—	—	—	—	95	—	—	—	—	—	—	—	—
—	—	—	—	97	—	—	—	—	—	—	—	—
—	—	—	—	130	—	—	—	—	—	—	—	—
4	<1	0.03	0.03	104	1	10	0	<0.01	<0.01	0	<0.01	<1
3	<1	0.10	0.02	109	18	15	0	0	0	0	<0.01	1
3	<1	0.10	0.02	153	17	15	0	0	0	0	<0.01	<1
4	—	0.10	—	98	11	3	0	0	0	0	—	—
244	24	0.60	—	88	—	13	—	0.09	0.09	1.59	—	—
287	16	23.81	2.32	95	534	145	19	0.13	0.36	2.9	0.09	—
116	—	3.50	1.04	44	119	—	—	<0.01	0.90	0.90	—	—
117	36	0.42	0.49	66	207	12	<1	0.08	0.07	2	0.24	7
155	18	0.69	3.67	425	94	—	—	0.07	0.07	1.64	—	—
154	21	0.63	0.56	494	222	26	0	0.11	0.15	1.79	0.05	15
246	50	0.29	0.54	89	292	10	—	0.07	0.10	1.86	0.20	—

Table continued on following page

APPENDIX A–1 **NUTRITIVE VALUES OF FOOD** *Continued*

	Approximate Measure	Weight (gm)	H_2O (gm)	Kcal	Protein (gm)	Carbohydrate (gm)	Dietary Fiber (gm)	Fat (gm)	MUFA (gm)	PUFA (gm)	Cholesterol (mg)	Calcium (mg)
Haddock, breaded, fried	3 oz	85	56	140	17	5	<1	5	2.2	1.2	42	34
Halibut, broiled, dry	3 oz	85	61	119	23	0	0	3	0.8	0.8	35	51
Herring, broiled	3 oz	85	54	173	20	0	0	10	4.1	2.3	66	63
Oysters												
Breaded, fried	3 oz	85	55	167	8	10	<1	11	4.0	2.8	69	53
Pacific, raw	3 oz	85	70	69	8	4	0	2	0.3	0.8	43	7
Salmon, chum, canned	3 oz	85	60	120	18	0	0	5	1.6	1.3	33	212
Sardines, canned in oil	3 oz	85	51	177	21	0	0	10	3.3	4.4	120	325
Scallops, breaded, fried	3 oz	85	50	183	15	9	<1	9	4.0	2.4	53	36
Shark, raw	3 oz	85	63	111	18	0	0	4	1.3	1.3	43	29
Shrimp, canned	3 oz	85	62	102	20	1	0	2	0.3	0.6	147	50
French fried	3 oz	85	45	206	18	10	1	10	3.2	4.3	150	57
Trout, rainbow, cooked, dry heat	3 oz	85	54	128	22	0	0	4	1.1	1.3	62	73
Tuna, canned in oil, drained	3 oz	85	51	168	25	0	0	7	2.5	2.5	15	11
Canned in water	3 oz	85	61	111	25	0	0	1	0.1	0.1	15	10
Salad	3 oz	85	60	145	13	3	<1	9	2.6	2.8	28	17
Fruits and Fruit Products												
Apple juice, canned/bottled	1 cup	248	218	116	<1	29	0.5	<1	<0.1	<0.1	0	17
Apples												
Fresh, unpeeled	1	138	116	81	<1	21	3.0	1	<0.1	0.2	0	10
Fresh, peeled	1	128	108	73	<1	19	2.4	<1	<0.1	0.1	0	5
Applesauce, canned												
Sweetened	1 cup	255	203	194	1	51	3.1	<1	<0.1	0.1	0	10
Unsweetened	1 cup	244	216	105	<1	28	3.7	<1	<0.1	<0.1	0	7
Apricot												
Canned, in juice	1 cup	248	215	119	2	31	2.8	<1	<0.1	<0.1	0	30
Dried, uncooked	1 cup	130	40	309	5	80	10.1	1	0.3	0.1	0	59
Fresh, without pit	1	35	31	17	1	4	0.7	<1	0.1	<0.1	0	5
Apricot nectar, canned	1 cup	251	213	141	1	36	1.5	<1	0.1	<0.1	0	18
Avocados, fresh, all varieties	1 cup	230	171	370	5	17	—	35	22	4.5	0	25
Banana flakes, dehydrated or powdered	1 tbsp	6.2	<1	22	<1	6	0.6	<1	<0.1	<0.1	0	1
Bananas, fresh, peeled	1	114	85	105	1	27	1.8	<1	<0.1	0.1	0	7
Blackberries, fresh	1 cup	144	123	75	1	18	8.9	1	0.2	0.3	0	46
Blueberries, fresh	1 cup	145	123	81	1	21	3.3	1	0.2	0.3	0	8
Cherries												
Sour, canned in water	1 cup	244	219	88	2	22	0.6	<1	<0.1	0.1	0	27
Sweet, canned, in juice	1 cup	250	212	135	2	35	0.6	<0.1	<0.1	<0.1	0	35
Cranberry juice												
Bottled	1 cup	253	215	144	0	36	0	0.3	0	0	0	8
Low kcal	8 fl oz	256	215	48	<1	38	0	0.1	0	0	0	8
Cranberry sauce, canned, sweetened	1 tbsp	17	11	26	<1	7	0.2	<0.1	<0.1	<0.1	0	1
Dates, natural, dried, whole	10 items	83	19	228	2	61	7.2	0.4	0	0	0	27
Fruit cocktail, canned in juice	1 cup	248	217	114	1	29	1.5	<0.1	<0.1	<0.1	0	20
Fruit roll up, cherry	1	14	—	50	0	12	—	1	—	—	0	—
Grapefruit juice												
Canned, sweetened	1 cup	250	218	115	2	28	0	0.2	<0.1	<0.1	0	20
Canned, unsweetened	1 cup	247	223	94	1	22	0.4	0.3	<0.1	<0.1	0	17
Grapefruit												
Canned in light syrup	1 cup	254	212	152	1	39	1.6	0.3	<0.1	<0.1	0	36
Fresh, pink and red	1	246	225	74	1	19	3.2	0.3	<0.1	<0.1	0	36
Fresh, white	1	236	214	78	2	20	2.5	0.2	<0.1	<0.1	0	28
Grapes, fresh, slip skin type	1 cup	92	75	58	<1	16	1.5	0.3	<0.1	<0.1	0	13
Grape juice												
Canned/bottled	1 cup	253	213	154	1	38	0	0.2	<0.1	<0.1	0	23
Frozen, diluted	1 cup	250	217	128	<1	32	0	0.2	<0.1	<0.1	0	10
Grape drink, canned	1 cup	253	213	154	1	38	0	0.2	<0.1	<0.1	0	23

Phosphate (mg)	Magnesium (mg)	Iron (mg)	Zinc (mg)	Sodium (mg)	Potassium (mg)	Vitamin A (RE)	Vitamin C (mg)	Thiamin (mg)	Riboflavin (mg)	Niacin (mg)	Vitamin B_6 (mg)	Folate (mcg)
210	—	1.00	—	150	296	—	2	0.03	0.06	2.70	—	—
242	91	0.91	0.45	59	490	46	0	0.06	0.08	6.06	0.34	12
258	35	1.20	1.08	98	356	26	<1	0.10	0.25	3.50	0.30	10
135	49	5.91	74.14	354	207	77	3	0.13	0.17	1.40	0.05	12
138	19	4.34	14.11	90	143	69	7	0.06	0.20	1.71	0.04	9
301	—	—	—	414	—	15	—	—	—	—	—	—
417	33	2.48	1.11	429	337	57	0	0.07	0.19	4.47	0.14	10
201	50	0.70	0.90	395	284	19	2	0.03	0.10	1.33	0.12	16
179	41	0.71	0.37	67	136	60	0	0.04	0.05	2.50	0.34	3
198	35	2.33	1.07	144	179	15	2	0.02	0.03	2.35	0.09	2
185	34	1.07	1.17	292	191	48	1	0.11	0.12	2.61	0.08	7
273	33	2.07	1.18	29	539	19	3	0.07	0.19	5.87	0.39	15
264	26	1.18	0.77	301	176	20	0	0.03	0.10	10.5	0.09	5
158	25	2.72	0.37	303	267	20	0	0.03	0.10	10.5	0.32	4
121	—	1.12	—	180	—	49	<1	0.03	0.10	4.27	—	—
18	8	0.92	0.07	7	296	<1	2	0.05	0.04	0.25	0.07	<1
10	6	0.25	0.05	1	159	7	8	0.02	0.02	0.11	0.07	4
9	4	0.09	0.05	0	144	6	5	0.02	0.01	0.12	0.06	<1
17	7	0.89	0.10	8	156	3	4	0.03	0.07	0.48	0.07	2
17	7	0.29	0.07	5	183	7	3	0.03	0.06	0.46	0.06	1
50	24	0.74	0.27	9	409	420	12	0.05	0.05	0.85	0.13	4
152	61	6.11	0.97	13	1791	941	3	0.01	0.20	3.90	0.20	13
7	3	0.19	0.09	<1	104	92	4	0.01	0.01	0.21	0.02	3
23	13	0.96	0.23	9	286	330	2	0.02	0.04	0.65	—	3
95	90	2.35	0.97	24	1378	141	18	0.25	0.28	4.42	0.64	142
5	7	0.07	0.04	<1	92	2	<1	0.01	0.02	0.17	—	—
22	33	0.35	0.18	1	451	9	10	0.05	0.11	0.62	0.66	22
30	29	0.82	0.39	0	282	24	30	0.04	0.06	0.58	0.08	49
15	7	0.25	0.16	9	129	15	19	0.07	0.07	0.52	0.05	9
24	15	3.34	0.17	17	239	184	5	0.04	0.10	0.43	0.11	20
55	30	1.45	0.25	8	328	31	6	0.05	0.06	1.02	0.08	11
5	5	0.38	0.18	10	46	0	90	0.02	0.02	0.09	0.05	<1
3	8	0.40	0.05	10	61	0	108	0.02	0.04	0.13	—	<1
1	1	0.04	0.01	5	5	<1	<1	<0.01	<0.01	0.02	<0.01	—
33	29	0.95	0.24	3	541	4	0	0.07	0.08	1.83	0.16	11
35	17	0.52	0.22	10	236	76	7	0.03	0.04	0.99	0.13	6
—	—	—	—	5	45	—	—	—	—	—	—	—
28	25	0.90	0.15	5	405	0	67	0.10	0.06	0.80	0.05	26
27	25	0.49	0.22	3	378	2	72	0.10	0.05	0.57	0.05	26
25	25	1.02	0.20	5	328	0	54	0.10	0.05	0.62	0.05	22
22	20	0.30	0.18	0	312	64	91	0.10	0.05	0.49	0.10	23
19	21	0.14	0.17	0	349	2	79	0.09	0.05	0.63	0.10	24
9	5	0.27	0.04	2	176	9	4	0.09	0.05	0.28	0.10	4
28	25	0.61	0.13	8	334	2	<1	0.07	0.09	0.66	0.16	7
10	10	0.25	0.10	5	53	2	60	0.04	0.07	0.31	0.11	3
28	25	0.61	0.13	8	334	2	<1	0.07	0.09	0.66	0.16	7

Table continued on following page

APPENDIX A–1 **NUTRITIVE VALUES OF FOOD** *Continued*

	Approximate Measure	Weight (gm)	H_2O (gm)	Kcal	Protein (gm)	Carbohydrate (gm)	Dietary Fiber (gm)	Fat (gm)	MUFA (gm)	PUFA (gm)	Cholesterol (mg)	Calcium (mg)
Lemonade, frozen, diluted	1 cup	248	221	105	0	28	0.6	0	0	0	0	2
Lemon juice												
Canned and bottled	1 cup	244	226	51	1	16	0.7	0.7	<0.1	0.2	0	27
Frozen	1 cup	244	225	54	1	16	0.7	0.8	<0.1	0.2	0	20
Lemons, fresh	1	108	94	22	1	12	1.0	0.3	<0.1	0.1	0	66
Limeade, frozen, diluted	1 cup	247	220	100	0	27	0.5	0	0	0	0	3
Lime juice, fresh	1 cup	246	222	66	1	22	0	0.3	<0.1	<0.1	0	22
Melons, cantaloupe, fresh	1 cup	160	144	56	1	13	1.2	0.5	0	0	0	18
Melons, honeydew, fresh	1 cup	170	152	60	1	16	1.5	0.2	0	0	0	10
Oranges, fresh												
All varieties	1	131	114	62	1	15	3.1	0.2	<0.1	<0.1	0	53
Fresh, sections	1 cup	180	156	85	2	21	3.6	0.2	<0.1	<0.1	0	72
Orange juice												
Fresh	1 cup	248	219	111	2	26	1.9	0.5	0.1	0.1	0	27
Canned	1 cup	249	222	104	2	25	0.3	0.4	<0.1	<0.1	0	20
Frozen, diluted	1 cup	249	219	112	2	27	0.5	0.2	<0.1	<0.1	0	22
Papayas, fresh	1 cup	140	124	55	1	14	1.3	0.2	<0.1	<0.1	0	34
Peaches, canned												
Juice pack	1 cup	248	217	109	2	29	—	0.1	<0.1	<0.1	0	15
Water pack	1 cup	244	227	59	1	15	1.1	0.2	<0.1	<0.1	0	5
Peaches, dried, uncooked	1 cup	160	51	382	6	98	14	1.2	<0.1	0.5	0	45
Peaches, fresh												
Sliced	1 cup	170	149	73	1	19	2.7	0.2	<0.1	<0.1	0	9
Whole	1	87	76	37	1	10	1.4	0.1	<0.1	<0.1	0	4
Peaches, frozen, sliced, sweetened	1 cup	250	187	235	2	60	5.9	0.3	0.1	0.2	0	8
Peach nectar, canned	1 cup	249	213	134	1	35	0.4	0.1	<0.1	<0.1	0	13
Pears, canned in juice	1 cup	248	214	124	1	32	4.7	0.2	<0.1	<0.1	0	22
Pears, fresh												
Bartlett, unpeeled	1	166	139	98	1	25	4.3	0.7	0.1	0.2	0	18
D'Anjou, unpeeled	1	200	168	118	1	30	5.2	0.8	0.2	0.2	0	22
Bosc, unpeeled	1	141	118	83	1	21	3.7	0.6	0.1	0.1	0	16
Pear nectar, canned	1 cup	250	210	150	<1	39	1.6	<0.1	<0.1	<0.1	0	13
Pineapple												
Canned in juice	1 cup	250	209	150	1	39	1.9	0.2	<0.1	<0.1	0	35
Fresh, diced	1 cup	155	134	76	<1	19	1.9	0.7	<0.1	0.2	0	11
Pineapple juice, canned	1 cup	250	214	140	<1	35	0.3	0.2	<0.1	<0.1	0	43
Plums												
Fresh, Japanese/hybrid	1	66	56	36	<1	8.6	1.4	0.4	0.3	<0.1	0	3
Purple, canned in juice	1 cup	252	212	146	1	38	0.9	<0.1	<0.1	<0.1	0	25
Prune juice, canned and bottled	1 cup	256	208	182	2	45	2.6	<0.1	<0.1	<0.1	0	31
Prunes, dehydrated, uncooked	1 cup	132	5	448	5	118	—	1.0	0.6	0.2	0	96
Raisins												
Seedless	1 cup	145	22	435	5	115	7.7	0.7	<0.1	0.2	0	71
Seedless, packet	1	14	2	42	<1	11	0.7	<0.1	<0.1	<0.1	0	7
Raspberries												
Fresh	1 cup	123	106	60	1	14	5.5	0.7	<0.1	0.4	0	27
Frozen, sweetened	1 cup	250	182	258	2	65	11	0.4	<0.1	0.2	0	38
Rhubarb												
Fresh, cooked with sugar	1 cup	270	170	380	1	97	5.4	0	0	0	0	211
Frozen, cooked with sugar	1 cup	240	163	278	1	75	4.8	0.1	0	0	0	348
Strawberries												
Fresh, whole	1 cup	149	136	45	1	11	3.9	0.6	<0.1	0.3	0	21
Frozen, sliced	1 cup	255	187	245	1	66	20	0.3	<0.1	0.2	0	28
Tangerine juice, canned, sweetened	1 cup	249	217	125	1	30	0.6	0.5	<0.1	<0.1	0	45

Phosphate (mg)	Magnesium (mg)	Iron (mg)	Zinc (mg)	Sodium (mg)	Potassium (mg)	Vitamin A (RE)	Vitamin C (mg)	Thiamin (mg)	Riboflavin (mg)	Niacin (mg)	Vitamin B_6 (mg)	Folate (mcg)
3	—	0.10	—	0	40	1	17	0.01	0.02	0.20	—	12
22	20	0.32	0.15	51	249	4	61	0.10	0.02	0.48	0.11	25
20	20	0.29	0.12	2	217	3	77	0.14	0.03	0.33	0.15	23
16	13	0.76	0.11	3	157	3	83	0.05	0.04	0.22	0.12	—
3	—	0	—	2	32	0	6	0	0	0	—	—
17	15	0.07	0.15	3	268	3	72	0.05	0.03	0.25	0.11	20
27	18	0.34	0.26	14	494	516	68	0.06	0.03	0.92	0.18	27
17	12	0.12	—	17	461	7	42	0.13	0.03	1.02	0.10	—
18	13	0.13	0.09	0	237	27	70	0.11	0.05	0.37	0.08	40
25	18	0.18	0.13	0	326	37	96	0.16	0.07	0.51	0.11	55
42	27	0.50	0.12	2	496	50	124	0.22	0.07	0.99	0.10	75
35	27	1.10	0.17	5	436	44	86	0.15	0.07	0.78	0.22	45
40	25	0.25	0.13	3	473	19	97	0.20	0.05	0.50	0.11	109
7	14	0.14	0.10	4	359	282	87	0.04	0.05	0.47	0.03	53
43	18	0.66	0.26	11	317	95	9	0.02	0.04	1.44	—	—
24	12	0.78	0.22	7	242	130	7	0.02	0.05	1.27	0.05	8
190	67	6.50	0.91	11	1594	346	8	<0.01	0	7.00	0.11	<1
21	12	0.19	0.24	0	335	91	11	0.03	0.07	1.68	0.03	6
10	6	0.10	0.12	0	171	47	6	0.02	0.04	0.86	0.02	3
28	13	0.93	0.13	15	325	71	236	0.03	0.09	1.63	0.05	8
15	10	0.47	0.20	17	100	64	13	<0.01	0.04	0.72	0.02	4
30	17	0.72	0.22	10	238	1	4	0.03	0.03	0.50	0.04	3
18	10	0.42	0.20	0	208	3	7	0.03	0.07	0.17	0.03	12
22	12	0.50	0.24	1	250	4	8	0.04	0.08	0.20	0.04	15
16	9	0.35	0.17	<1	176	3	6	0.03	0.06	0.14	0.03	10
8	8	0.65	0.18	10	33	<1	3	<0.01	0	0.32	0.04	3
15	35	0.70	0.25	4	305	10	24	0.24	0.05	0.71	0.19	12
11	22	0.57	0.12	2	175	4	24	0.14	0.06	0.65	0.14	16
20	33	0.65	0.28	3	335	1	27	0.14	0.06	0.64	0.24	58
7	5	0.07	0.07	0	114	21	6	0.03	0.06	0.33	0.05	2
38	<1	0.84	0.28	3	388	254	7	0.06	0.15	1.19	0.07	7
64	36	3.02	0.54	10	707	1	11	0.04	0.18	2.01	0.56	1
147	85	4.64	0.99	7	1397	233	0	0.16	0.22	3.95	0.98	3
141	48	3.02	0.39	17	1089	1	5	0.23	0.13	1.19	0.36	5
14	5	0.29	0.04	2	105	<1	<1	0.02	0.01	0.12	0.04	<1
15	22	0.70	0.57	0	187	16	31	0.04	0.11	1.11	0.07	32
43	33	1.63	0.45	3	285	15	41	0.05	0.11	0.58	0.09	65
41	32	1.60	0.22	5	548	22	16	0.05	0.14	0.80	0.05	14
19	29	0.50	0.19	2	230	17	8	0.04	0.06	0.48	0.05	13
28	15	0.57	0.19	2	247	4	85	0.03	0.10	0.34	0.09	26
33	18	1.50	0.15	8	250	6	106	0.04	0.13	1.02	0.08	38
35	20	0.50	0.08	3	443	105	55	0.15	0.05	0.25	0.08	12

Table continued on following page

APPENDIX A–1 **NUTRITIVE VALUES OF FOOD** *Continued*

	Approximate Measure	Weight (gm)	H_2O (gm)	Kcal	Protein (gm)	Carbohydrate (gm)	Dietary Fiber (gm)	Fat (gm)	MUFA (gm)	PUFA (gm)	Cholesterol (mg)	Calcium (mg)
Tangerines, fresh, peeled	1	84	74	37	<1	9	1.7	0.2	<0.1	<0.1	0	12
Watermelon, fresh	1 cup	160	146	51	1	12	0.6	0.7	—	—	0	13
Grain Products (Breads and Cereals)												
Bagel												
Egg	1	55	16	163	6	31	1.2	1	—	—	8	23
Water	1	55	16	163	6	31	1.2	1	0.4	0.6	0	23
Barley, pearled, light, cooked	1 cup	157	108	193	4	44	8.9	1	0.1	0.3	0	17
Biscuits												
Home recipe	1	28.4	8	105	2	13	0.4	5	2.0	1.2	0	34
Prepared/mix	1	28.4	8	104	2	13	0.5	5	1.3	0.2	1	34
Breadcrumbs, dry, grated	1 cup	100	7	390	13	73	3.7	5	1.6	1.4	0	122
Bread												
Boston brown, canned	1 slice	45	20	95	2	21	2.1	1	0.2	0.2	0	41
Corn	1 slice	45	23	108	2	16	1.2	4	—	—	0	49
Cracked wheat	1 slice	25	9	66	2	13	1.3	1	0.2	0.2	0	16
French, enriched	1 slice	35	12	98	3	18	0.8	1	0.4	0.4	0	39
Italian, enriched	1 slice	30	10	85	3	17	0.8	0	0	0	0	5
Mixed grain	1 slice	25	9	64	3	12	1.6	1	—	—	0	26
Oatmeal	1 slice	34	—	90	3	17	1	1	—	—	0	—
Pita	1	38	12	105	4	21	0.6	1	—	—	0	31
Pumpernickel	1 slice	32	12	82	3	15	1.9	1	—	—	0	23
Raisin, enriched	1 slice	25	8	70	2	13	0.6	1	0.3	0.2	0	26
Rye, American, light	1 slice	25	9	66	2	12	1.5	1	—	—	0	20
Vienna, enriched	1 slice	25	9	70	2	13	0.8	1	0.3	0.3	0	28
White, firm	1 slice	23	9	61	2	11	0.4	1	0.3	0.3	0	29
White, firm, toasted	1 slice	20	5	65	2	12	0.5	1	0.3	0.3	0	22
White, soft	1 slice	25	9	67	2	12	0.7	1	0.3	0.3	0	32
White soft, toasted	1 slice	22	6	67	2	12	0.6	1	0.3	0.3	0	32
Whole wheat, soft	1 slice	28.4	11	69	3	13	3.2	1	—	—	0	20
Whole wheat, firm	1 slice	25	10	61	2	11	2.8	1	0.2	0.3	0	18
Breakfast cereal, cooked												
Bulgur, cooked	1 cup	182	142	152	6	34	6.8	0.4	0.1	0.2	0	18
Corn grits, enriched	1 cup	242	206	145	3	32	0.6	<1	0.1	0.2	0	0
Corn grits, unenriched	1 cup	242	206	145	3	32	0.6	<1	0.1	0.2	0	0
Cream of wheat, regular	1 cup	251	219	133	4	28	1.9	<1	0	0	0	50
Farina, cooked, enriched	1 cup	233	205	117	3	25	3.3	<1	<0.1	<0.1	0	5
Malt O Meal, cooked	1 cup	240	210	122	4	26	0.6	<1	0	0	0	5
Oatmeal, cooked	1 cup	234	200	145	6	25	2.1	2	0.8	0.9	0	19
Wheat, rolled, cooked	1 cup	240	192	180	5	41	2.9	1	<0.1	0.5	0	19
Wheat, whole meal	1 cup	245	216	110	4	23	1.6	1	<0.1	0.5	0	17
Breakfast cereal, ready to eat												
All bran	1 cup	85	3	212	12	63	26	2	—	—	0	69
Bran flakes	1 cup	39	1	127	5	31	5.5	<1	0	0	0	19
Corn flakes	1 cup	22.7	<1	88	2	20	0.5	<1	0	0	0	1
Corn, shredded with added sugar	1 cup	25	<1	95	2	22	1.5	0	0	0	0	1
Frosted flakes	1 cup	38	<1	149	2	34	0.8	<1	0	0	0	4
Oats, puffed with added sugar	1 cup	25	<1	100	3	19	2.6	1	<0.1	0.5	0	44
Raisin Bran	1 cup	49	4	154	5	37	5.3	<1	—	—	0	17
Rice, puffed, plain	1 cup	14	<1	56	1	13	0.1	<1	0	0	0	<1
Rice, puffed, sugar	1 cup	28.4	<1	115	1	26	0.2	0	0	0	0	3
Wheat flakes, with added sugar	1 cup	30	1	105	3	24	2.7	0	0	0	0	12
Wheat germ, toasted	1 cup	113	6	432	33	56	14.6	12	1.7	7.5	0	51
Wheat, puffed, plain	1 cup	12	<1	44	2	10	0.4	0.1	0	0	0	3
Wheat, shredded, biscuit	1	23.6	2	83	3	19	2.2	0.3	0	0	0	10
Cornmeal, degermed, enriched, cooked	1 cup	240	28	878	20	186	1.9	4.0	1.0	1.7	0	12

Phosphate (mg)	Magnesium (mg)	Iron (mg)	Zinc (mg)	Sodium (mg)	Potassium (mg)	Vitamin A (RE)	Vitamin C (mg)	Thiamin (mg)	Riboflavin (mg)	Niacin (mg)	Vitamin B_6 (mg)	Folate (mcg)
8	10	0.08	0.20	<1	132	77	26	0.09	0.02	0.13	0.06	17
14	18	0.27	0.11	3	186	59	15	0.13	0.03	0.32	0.23	4
37	11	1.46	0.29	198	41	24	0	0.21	0.16	1.94	0.02	13
37	11	1.46	0.29	198	41	0	0	0.21	0.16	1.94	0.02	13
85	35	2.09	1.29	5	146	2	0	0.13	0.10	3.24	0.18	26
49	6	0.40	—	175	33	0	0	0.08	0.08	0.70	—	—
99	3	0.62	0.11	221	33	37	0	0.10	0.07	1.75	0.01	2
141	32	3.60	—	736	152	0	0	0.35	0.35	4.80	—	—
72	—	0.90	—	112	131	0	0	0.06	0.04	0.70	—	—
44	8	0.67	0.21	126	42	7	0	0.08	0.08	0.68	0.03	5
32	9	0.67	—	108	33	0	0	0.10	0.10	0.84	0.02	—
28	7	1.08	0.22	193	30	0	0	0.16	0.12	1.40	0.02	13
23	—	0.70	—	152	22	0	0	0.12	0.07	1.00	0.02	11
53	12	0.82	0.30	103	55	0	0	0.10	0.10	1.04	0.03	16
—	—	—	—	200	—	—	—	—	—	—	—	—
38	—	0.92	—	215	45	0	0	0.17	0.08	1.40	—	—
70	22	0.88	0.37	173	139	0	0	0.11	0.17	1.06	0.05	—
23	6	0.78	0.16	94	60	0	0	0.08	0.16	1.02	<0.01	9
36	6	0.68	0.32	174	51	0	0	0.10	0.08	0.83	0.02	10
20	5	0.77	0.16	138	22	0	0	0.12	0.09	1.00	0.02	9
25	5	0.65	0.14	118	26	0	0	0.11	0.07	0.86	<0.01	8
23	5	0.60	0.14	117	28	0	0	0.07	0.06	0.80	<0.01	8
27	5	0.71	0.16	129	28	0	0	0.12	0.08	0.94	<0.01	9
27	5	0.72	0.16	129	28	0	0	0.10	0.08	0.94	<0.01	9
73	26	0.96	0.47	178	49	0	0	0.10	0.06	1.07	0.05	15
65	23	0.86	0.42	159	44	0	0	0.09	0.05	0.96	0.05	14
73	59	1.75	1.04	9	124	0	0	0.10	0.05	1.82	0.15	33
29	10	1.55	0.17	0	53	—	—	0.24	0.15	1.96	0.06	2
29	10	1.55	0.17	0	53	—	—	0.24	0.15	1.96	0.06	2
42	10	10.3	0.33	2	43	0	0	0.25	0	1.51	0.04	10
28	5	1.17	0.16	0	30	—	—	0.19	0.12	1.28	0.02	5
24	5	9.60	0.17	2	31	0	0	0.48	0.24	5.76	0.02	5
178	56	1.59	1.15	2	131	5	—	0.26	0.05	0.30	0.05	9
182	53	1.70	1.15	535	202	0	0	0.17	0.07	2.20	—	26
127	54	1.20	1.18	535	118	0	0	0.15	0.05	1.50	—	27
794	318	13.50	11.20	961	1051	1125	45	1.11	1.28	15.00	1.53	301
192	71	24.80	5.15	303	248	516	0	0.51	0.59	6.86	0.70	138
14	3	1.43	0.06	232	21	300	12	0.30	0.34	4.00	0.41	80
10	4	0.60	0.09	247	—	0	13	0.33	0.05	4.40	0.45	88
10	3	0.95	0.82	247	24	503	20	0.49	0.57	6.69	0.68	3
102	28	4.00	0.69	294	—	275	13	0.33	0.38	4.40	0.45	6
183	64	22.30	5.02	359	256	500	0	0.49	0.59	6.69	0.69	133
14	4	0.15	0.14	<1	16	0	0	0.02	0.01	0.42	0.01	3
14	8	0.00	1.48	21	43	300	15	0	0	0	0.51	99
83	33	4.80	0.67	368	81	330	16	0.40	0.45	5.30	0.54	9
1295	362	10.30	18.80	5	1070	50	7	1.89	0.93	6.31	1.11	398
43	17	0.57	0.28	<1	42	0	0	0.02	0.03	1.30	0.02	4
86	40	0.74	0.59	<1	77	0	0	0.07	0.06	1.08	0.06	12
202	96	9.91	1.73	7	389	98	0	1.72	0.98	12.10	0.62	115

Table continued on following page

APPENDIX A–1 **NUTRITIVE VALUES OF FOOD** *Continued*

	Approximate Measure	Weight (gm)	H_2O (gm)	Kcal	Protein (gm)	Carbohydrate (gm)	Dietary Fiber (gm)	Fat (gm)	MUFA (gm)	PUFA (gm)	Cholesterol (mg)	Calcium (mg)
Crackers												
Cheese	4	4	<1	22	<1	2	0.1	1.3	0.4	0.1	—	4
Graham—plain	4	28	2	110	2	20	0.9	2	1	0.6	0	12
Rye wafers	4	26	2	90	4	20	4.2	0	0	0	0	14
Saltines	4	11	<1	50	1	8	0.3	1	0.4	0.2	3	2
Wheat Thins	4	7	—	36	<1	5	0.4	1.4	—	—	0	—
Croissant	1	26	6	109	2	11	0.6	6.1	—	—	—	12
Flour												
Buckwheat, whole	1 cup	120	13	402	15	85	16.9	3.7	1.1	1.1	0	49
Wheat, enriched, sifted	1 cup	115	14	419	12	88	3.1	1.1	0.1	0.5	0	17
Wheat, enriched, unsifted	1 cup	125	15	455	13	95	3.4	1.2	0.1	0.5	0	18
Wheat, white, self-rising	1 cup	125	13	443	12	93	3.4	1.2	0.1	0.5	0	423
French toast	1	65	34	153	5.7	17	2.0	6.7	—	—	—	72
Macaroni, cooked	1 cup	130	86	183	6.2	37	2.1	0.9	0.1	0.4	0	9
Muffins												
Blueberry	1	40	16	110	3	17	0.9	4.0	1.4	0.7	21	34
Bran	1	40	14	112	3	17	2.5	5.1	1.4	0.8	21	54
Corn	1	40	13	125	3	19	1.0	4	1.6	0.9	21	42
English, plain	1	56	24	133	4	26	1.3	1.1	—	—	0	91
Plain	1	40	15	120	3	17	0.9	4	1.7	1	21	42
Noodles, chow mein, enriched	1 cup	45	<1	237	4	26	1.8	14	3.5	7.8	0	9
Noodles, egg, enriched, cooked	1 cup	160	114	200	7	37	3.5	2	—	—	50	16
Pancakes												
Buttermilk mix, complete	1	53.4	—	180	5	38	—	1	—	0	5	150
Plain, from mix	1	27	15	59	1.9	8	0.4	2.2	0.7	0.3	20	36
Piecrust												
Home recipe—baked	1	180	27	900	11	79	4.7	60	26	15	0	25
Mix, prepared	1	160	30	743	10	71	4.2	47	20	12	0	66
Popcorn												
Cheese flavor	1 cup	11	<1	58	1	6	—	3.7	1.1	1.7	1	12
Popped, oil and salt	1 cup	9	<1	40	1	5	0.4	2	0.2	0.2	0	1
Popped, plain	1 cup	6	<1	25	1	5	0.4	0	0	0	0	1
Pretzels												
Dutch, twisted	1	16	<1	60	2	12	—	1	—	—	0	4
Thin, stick	10	3	1	12	<1	2	—	0.1	0	0	0	1
Rice, cooked												
Brown, long grain	1 cup	195	143	216	5	45	3.3	1.8	0.6	0.6	0	20
White, long grain	1 cup	205	141	264	6	57	2.1	0.6	0.2	0.2	0	23
White, parboil	1 cup	175	127	199	4	43	0.9	0.5	0.1	0.1	0	33
Wild	1 cup	164	121	166	7	35	2.6	0.6	0.1	0.4	0	5
Rolls												
Brown and serve, enriched	1	26	7	85	2	14	0.9	2	0.7	0.5	0	20
Cloverleaf, home recipe	1	35	9	120	3	20	1.3	3	1.1	0.7	0	16
Hamburger/hotdog buns	1	40	14	114	3	20	1.0	2.1	0.8	0.6	0	54
Hard, enriched	1	50	13	155	5	30	1.5	2	0.6	0.5	0	24
Submarine/hoagie, enriched	1	135	42	390	12	75	3.8	4	1.4	1.4	0	58
Spaghetti	1 cup	140	102	155	5	32	2.2	1	—	—	0	11
Stuffing mix, traditional herb	1 cup	57	—	220	8	44	—	2	—	—	—	40
Toaster pastries/Pop Tart	1	50	6	196	2	35	0.7	6	—	—	0	97
Tortilla												
Corn	1	30	14	67	2	13	1.6	1	—	—	0	42
Flour	1	30	—	95	3	17	0.8	2	—	—	0	46
Waffles												
Enriched, from mix with egg and milk	1	75	32	205	7	27	1.1	8	2.9	1.2	45	179

Phosphate (mg)	Magnesium (mg)	Iron (mg)	Zinc (mg)	Sodium (mg)	Potassium (mg)	Vitamin A (RE)	Vitamin C (mg)	Thiamin (mg)	Riboflavin (mg)	Niacin (mg)	Vitamin B_6 (mg)	Folate (mcg)
8	1	0.14	0.04	48	7	—	0	0.02	0.02	0.33	—	—
42	14	1.00	0.21	132	110	0	0	0.04	0.16	1	0.02	4
100	—	1.00	—	228	156	0	0	0.08	0.06	0.40	—	—
10	3	0.50	0.07	147	13	0	0	0.50	0.05	0.40	<0.01	2
—	—	—	—	—	—	—	—	—	—	—	—	—
32	7	1.04	—	140	40	8	0	0.28	0.10	1.20	—	—
404	301	4.87	3.74	13	692	0	0	0.50	0.23	7.4	0.70	64
124	25	5.34	0.81	2	123	0	0	0.90	0.57	6.79	0.05	30
135	27	5.80	0.88	2	134	—	0	0.98	0.62	7.38	0.06	33
744	24	5.84	0.78	1588	155	0	0	0.84	0.52	7.29	0.06	53
85	12	1.34	0.55	257	86	22	0	0.12	0.16	1.01	0.04	18
70	23	1.82	0.69	1	40	0	0	0.27	0.13	2.18	0.05	1
53	10	0.60	—	252	46	18	0	0.09	0.10	0.70	—	—
111	35	1.26	1.08	168	99	40	3	0.10	0.11	1.26	0.11	17
68	18	0.70	—	192	54	25	0	0.10	0.10	0.70	—	—
63	11	1.58	0.40	358	314	0	0	0.26	0.18	2.10	0.02	18
60	11	0.60	—	176	50	8	0	0.09	0.12	0.90	—	—
73	23	2.13	0.63	198	54	4	0	0.26	0.19	2.68	0.05	10
94	43	1.40	—	3	70	11	0	0.22	0.13	1.90	0.14	19
350	—	1.08	—	720	80	0	0	0.23	0.17	2	—	—
71	5	0.27	0.19	160	43	8	0	0.04	0.06	0.25	0.06	3
90	25	3.10	—	1099	89	0	0	0.47	0.40	5	—	—
136	—	3.05	—	1300	90	0	0	0.54	0.40	4.95	—	—
40	10	0.25	0.22	98	29	5	0.10	0.01	0.03	0.16	0.03	—
19	16	0.20	0.50	0	—	—	0	—	0.01	0.10	0.01	—
17	—	0.20	0.40	174	—	—	0	—	0.01	0.20	—	—
21	4	0.20	0.17	258	21	0	0	0.05	0.04	0.70	<0.01	3
3	1	0.06	0.03	48	3	0	0	0	0.01	0.13	0	<1
162	84	0.82	1.23	10	84	0	0	0.19	0.05	2.98	0.28	8
96	27	2.25	0.94	4	80	0	0	0.33	0.03	3.03	0.19	6
74	21	1.97	0.54	5	65	0	0	0.44	0.03	2.45	0.03	6
134	53	0.98	2.20	5	166	0	0	0.09	0.14	2.11	0.22	43
23	6	0.80	0.19	144	25	0	0	0.10	0.06	0.90	0.02	10
36	7	0.70	0.26	193	41	6	0	0.12	0.12	1.20	0.02	13
33	8	1.19	0.25	241	37	0	0	0.20	0.13	1.58	0.01	15
46	12	1.20	0.30	312	49	0	0	0.20	0.12	1.70	0.02	30
115	—	3.00	—	761	122	0	0	0.54	0.32	4.50	0.05	—
70	24	1.40	0.70	1	103	0	0	0.23	0.13	1.80	0.08	16
—	—	2.16	—	1100	140	0	0	0.30	0.20	2.40	—	—
97	9	2.00	0.29	230	85	96	0	0.16	0.17	2.10	0.19	40
55	20	0.57	0.43	53	52	—	0	0.05	0.03	0.38	0.09	6
25	7	1.10	—	—	—	<1	0	0.01	0.08	<1	—	—
257	—	1.00	—	514	146	34	0	0.14	0.22	0.90	—	—

Table continued on following page

APPENDIX A–1 **NUTRITIVE VALUES OF FOOD** *Continued*

	Approximate Measure	Weight (gm)	H_2O (gm)	Kcal	Protein (gm)	Carbohydrate (gm)	Dietary Fiber (gm)	Fat (gm)	MUFA (gm)	PUFA (gm)	Cholesterol (mg)	Calcium (mg)
Enriched, home recipe	1	75	28	245	7	26	1.1	13	2.8	1.4	45	154
Frozen	1	37	15	103	2	16	0.9	4	—	—	0	30
Legumes (dry), nuts, seeds, and related products												
Beans, dried												
Baked, home recipe	1 cup	253	165	382	14	54	19.5	13	5.4	1.9	13	154
Great northern, cooked	1 cup	180	124	210	14	38	9.7	1	—	—	0	90
Kidney, boiled, all types	1 cup	177	118	225	15	40	—	0.9	<0.1	0.5	0	50
Navy pea, cooked	1 cup	190	131	225	15	40	9	1	—	—	0	95
Pinto, boiled	1 cup	171	110	235	14	44	—	0.9	0.2	0.3	0	82
Pork and beans with frankfurters, canned	1 cup	257	178	365	17	40	12.8	17	7.3	2.2	15	123
Red kidney, canned	1 cup	255	194	230	15	42	12.5	1	—	—	0	74
Refried beans	1 cup	253	183	271	16	47	11.6	3	1.2	0.4	0	116
Small white, boiled	1 cup	179	113	254	16	46	7.9	1.2	0.1	0.5	0	131
Nuts												
Almonds, shelled, chopped	1 oz	28.4	1	167	6	6	2.6	15	9.6	3.1	0	75
Brazil, dried, shelled	1 oz	28.4	1	186	4	4	2.2	19	6.5	6.9	0	50
Cashews, dry roasted	1 oz	28.4	1	163	4	9	2.1	13	7.7	2.2	0	13
Coconut, dried, shredded	1 oz	28.4	4	142	1	14	1.2	10	0.4	0.1	0	4
Filbert/hazel, dried, chopped	1 oz	28.4	2	179	4	4	2.4	18	14	1.7	0	53
Peanut, roasted in oil, low sodium	1 cup	144	3	848	39	24	—	74	33	26	0	78
Pecans, dried, halves	1 oz	28.4	1	189	2	5	1.8	19	12	4.8	0	10
Walnut, black, dried, chopped	1 oz	28.4	1	172	7	3	2	16	3.6	10.6	0	16
Walnut, Persian/English	1 oz	28.4	1	182	4	5	1.4	18	4.0	11	0	27
Peanut butter												
Smooth type	1 tbsp	16	<1	94	4	3	1	8	3.8	2.3	0	5
Chunk style	1 tbsp	16	<1	95	4	4	1	8	3.8	2.3	0	7
Peas, dried, cooked												
Cowpeas/blackeye, boiled	1 cup	165	125	160	5	34	11	<1	0.1	0.3	0	212
Lentils, whole	1 cup	198	138	231	18	40	9.8	<1	0.1	0.4	0	37
Peas, split	1 cup	197	22	671	48	119	—	2	0.5	1.0	0	108
Seeds												
Pumpkin/squash, dried	1 oz	28.4	2	153	7	5	3	13	4.0	5.9	0	12
Pumpkin/squash, roasted	1 oz	28.4	1	126	5	15	13	6	1.7	2.5	0	16
Sesame, roasted, whole	1 oz	28.4	1	161	5	7	5.3	14	5.1	5.9	0	281
Sunflower, dried	1 oz	28.4	2	162	7	5	1.9	14	2.7	9.3	0	33
Meats (beef, lamb, pork)												
Beef, cooked												
Chuck blade, lean and fat, choice, braised	3 oz	85	40	296	23	0	0	22	9.5	0.8	88	11
Chuck blade, lean, all grades, braised	2.5 oz	71	39	179	22	0	0	9	4.1	0.3	75	9
Cuts, lean and fat, simmered/roasted	3 oz	85	40	297	21	0	0	23	10.2	0.9	78	9
Cuts, lean, simmered/roasted	2.5 oz	71	29	289	16	<1	0	25	11.4	0.9	65	6
Hamburger patty, extra lean	3 oz	85	49	218	22	0	0	14	6.1	0.5	71	6
Hamburger patty, lean	3 oz	85	48	231	21	0	0	16	6.9	0.6	74	9
Hamburger, baked	3 oz	85	47	244	20	0	0	18	7.8	0.7	74	9
Heart, cooked, simmered	3 oz	85	55	149	25	<1	0	5	1.1	1.2	164	5

Phosphate (mg)	Magnesium (mg)	Iron (mg)	Zinc (mg)	Sodium (mg)	Potassium (mg)	Vitamin A (RE)	Vitamin C (mg)	Thiamin (mg)	Riboflavin (mg)	Niacin (mg)	Vitamin B_6 (mg)	Folate (mcg)
135	17	1.48	0.65	445	129	28	0	0.18	0.24	1.46	0.05	14
141	8	1.80	0.30	256	78	95	0	0.17	0.20	1.93	0.10	<1
276	109	5.03	1.85	1068	906	<1	3	0.34	0.12	1.03	0.23	122
266	—	4.90	1.80	12	749	0	0	0.25	0.13	1.30	1.01	63
252	80	5.20	1.89	4	713	0	2	0.28	0.10	1.02	0.21	229
281	—	5.10	1.80	13	790	0	0	0.27	0.13	1.30	1.06	67
273	95	4.47	1.85	3	800	0	4	0.32	0.16	0.68	0.27	294
267	72	4.45	4.81	1105	604	39	6	0.15	0.14	2.32	0.12	77
278	10	4.60	1.91	833	673	1	8	0.13	0.10	1.50	1.12	36
213	99	4.48	3.47	1073	994	0	15	0.12	0.14	1.23	0.25	211
302	122	5.08	1.95	4	828	0	0	0.42	0.11	0.49	0.23	245
147	84	1.04	0.83	3	208	0	<1	0.06	0.22	0.95	0.03	17
170	64	0.96	1.30	<1	170	—	<1	0.28	0.04	0.46	0.07	1
139	74	1.70	1.59	5	160	0	0	0.06	0.06	0.40	0.07	20
30	14	0.55	0.52	74	95	0	<1	0.01	<0.01	0.13	0.08	2
89	81	0.93	0.68	<1	126	2	<1	0.14	0.03	0.32	0.17	20
460	230	2.38	4.43	9	881	0	0	0.13	0.22	20.60	0.35	181
82	36	0.60	1.55	<1	111	4	1	0.24	0.04	0.25	0.05	11
132	57	0.87	0.97	1	149	8	1	0.06	0.03	0.20	0.16	19
90	48	0.69	0.78	3	142	4	1	0.11	0.04	0.30	0.16	19
52	25	0.27	0.40	77	115	—	0	0.02	0.02	2.09	0.06	13
51	26	0.31	0.45	78	121	0	0	0.02	0.02	2.21	0.07	15
85	85	1.85	1.70	7	689	130	4	0.17	0.24	2.32	0.11	209
356	71	6.59	2.50	4	731	2	3	0.34	0.15	2.10	0.35	358
722	227	8.72	5.93	30	1932	29	4	1.43	0.42	5.69	0.34	539
333	152	4.25	2.12	5	229	11	<1	0.06	0.09	0.50	0.06	16
26	74	0.94	2.92	5	260	2	<1	0.01	0.02	0.08	0.01	3
181	101	4.18	2.03	3	135	<1	0	0.23	0.07	1.30	0.23	28
200	100	1.92	1.44	<1	195	1	<1	0.65	0.07	1.28	0.22	64
173	17	2.68	7.22	55	199	0	0	0.06	0.21	2.08	0.22	5
167	17	2.61	7.28	50	187	0	0	0.06	0.20	1.89	0.20	4
164	18	2.21	4.67	50	244	0	0	0.07	0.18	2.94	0.26	6
123	11	1.54	3.76	46	155	0	0	0.04	0.13	2.03	0.16	5
137	18	2.00	4.63	60	266	6	0	0.05	0.23	4.22	0.23	8
134	18	1.79	4.56	65	256	9	0	0.04	0.18	4.39	0.22	8
116	13	2.05	4.16	51	188	0	0	0.03	0.14	4.04	0.20	8
213	21	6.38	2.66	54	198	0	1	0.12	1.31	3.46	0.18	1

Table continued on following page

APPENDIX A–1 **NUTRITIVE VALUES OF FOOD** *Continued*

	Approximate Measure	Weight (gm)	H_2O (gm)	Kcal	Protein (gm)	Carbohydrate (gm)	Dietary Fiber (gm)	Fat (gm)	MUFA (gm)	PUFA (gm)	Cholesterol (mg)	Calcium (mg)
Liver, fried in margarine	3 oz	85	47	184	23	7	0	7	1.5	1.5	410	9
Roast, bottom, lean and fat	3 oz	85	46	222	25	0	0	13	5.7	0.5	81	5
Roast, bottom, lean	2.5 oz	70.9	41	157	22	0	0	7	3.1	0.3	68	4
Roast, rib, lean and fat	3 oz	85	40	308	18	0	0	26	11.4	0.9	73	9
Roast, rib, lean	2.5 oz	70.9	41	170	19	0	0	10	4.3	0.3	57	7
Steak, rib	3 oz	85	50	188	24	0	0	10	4.2	0.3	68	11
Steak, round, lean and fat	3 oz	85	50	179	26	0	0	8	3.1	0.3	72	5
Steak, round, lean, broiled	2.5 oz	70.9	43	135	22	0	0	4	1.7	0.2	60	4
Steak, sirloin, lean and fat	3 oz	85	45	238	23	0	0	15	6.9	0.6	77	9
Steak, sirloin, lean, broiled	2.5 oz	70.9	42	147	22	0	0	6	2.7	0.3	63	8
Beef, processed												
Corned beef, canned	3 oz	85	49	213	23	<1	0	13	5.1	0.5	73	17
Dried, cured, chipped	3 oz	85	48	140	25	1	0	3	1.4	0.2	78	5
Salami, beef	1 oz	28.4	17	74	4	1	0	6	2.7	0.3	19	3
Lamb, cooked												
Chop, lean and fat, broiled	3 oz	85	40	307	19	0	0	25	10.3	2.0	84	16
Chop, rib, lean, broiled	2.5 oz	70.9	42	167	20	0	0	9	3.7	0.8	65	11
Leg, lean and fat, roasted	3 oz	85	49	219	22	0	0	14	5.9	1.0	79	9
Leg, lean, roasted	2.5 oz	70.9	45	136	20	0	0	6	2.4	0.4	63	6
Loin, lean and fat, broiled	3 oz	85	44	268	21	0	0	20	8.3	1.4	85	17
Loin, lean, broiled	2.5 oz	70.9	43	153	21	0	0	7	3.0	0.5	67	13
Shoulder, arm, lean and fat, broiled	3 oz	85	47	239	21	0	0	17	6.8	1.3	82	16
Shoulder, arm, lean, braised	2.5 oz	70.9	35	198	25	0	0	10	4.4	0.7	86	18
Shoulder blade, lean and fat, broiled	3 oz	85	48	237	20	0	0	17	7.2	1.2	81	20
Shoulder blade, lean, broiled	2.5 oz	70.9	44	149	18	0	0	8	3.5	0.5	65	18
Pork, cured, cooked												
Bacon, broiled/fried	2 slices	12.6	2	73	4	<1	0	6	2.9	0.7	11	2
Bacon, simulated, all types	1 oz	28.4	14	88	3	2	—	8	2.0	4.4	0	7
Canadian bacon, grilled	1 oz	28.4	17	52	7	<1	0	2	1.1	0.2	16	3
Ham, canned, 13% fat	3 oz	85	52	192	17	<1	0	13	6.0	1.5	53	7
Ham, canned, extra lean, 4% fat	3 oz	85	59	115	18	<1	0	4	2.1	0.4	26	5
Ham, regular, roasted	3 oz	85	55	151	19	0	0	8	3.8	1.2	50	7
Pork, luncheon meats												
Bologna	1 oz	28.4	17	70	4	<1	0	6	2.8	0.6	17	3
Deviled ham, canned	1 oz	28.4	15	98	4	0	0	9	3.9	0.9	22	2
Frankfurter/hot dog	1	57	31	183	6	1	0	17	7.8	1.6	29	6
Ham and cheese loaf/roll	1 oz	28.4	16	74	5	<1	—	6	2.6	0.6	16	17
Ham, lunch meat, 11% fat	1 oz	28.4	18	52	5	<1	0	3	1.4	0.3	16	2
Pimento/pickle loaf	1 oz	28.4	17	74	3	2	—	6	2.7	0.7	10	27
Salami, dry or hard	1 oz	28.4	10	115	6	<1	0	10	4.5	1.1	22	4
Vienna sausage, canned, beef/pork	1 oz	28.4	17	79	3	<1	0	7	3.6	0.5	15	3
Pork, fresh, cooked												
Chop, lean and fat, broiled	3 oz	85	41	295	20	0	0	23	10.6	2.6	80	6
Loin, lean and fat, roast	3 oz	85	44	259	22	0	0	19	8.5	2.1	77	4
Loin, lean, roasted	2.5 oz	70.9	41	170	20	0	0	9	4.2	1.1	65	4

Phosphate (mg)	Magnesium (mg)	Iron (mg)	Zinc (mg)	Sodium (mg)	Potassium (mg)	Vitamin A (RE)	Vitamin C (mg)	Thiamin (mg)	Riboflavin (mg)	Niacin (mg)	Vitamin B_6 (mg)	Folate (mcg)
392	20	5.34	4.63	90	309	9221	20	0.18	3.52	12.30	1.22	187
217	20	2.76	4.36	43	248	0	0	0.06	0.21	3.29	0.29	9
193	18	2.45	3.88	36	218	0	0	0.05	0.18	2.89	0.26	8
140	17	1.77	4.28	52	257	0	0	0.07	0.15	2.65	0.25	5
151	18	1.85	4.92	52	267	0	0	0.06	0.15	2.92	0.21	6
177	23	2.19	5.95	59	335	0	0	0.09	0.18	4.08	0.34	7
203	26	2.39	4.59	51	365	0	0	0.10	0.22	4.98	0.46	10
174	22	2.04	3.95	43	314	0	0	0.08	0.19	4.28	0.40	9
185	24	2.56	4.89	54	306	15	0	0.10	0.22	3.29	0.34	8
173	23	2.38	4.62	47	286	4	0	0.09	0.21	3.04	0.32	7
95	12	1.77	3.03	856	116	0	<1	0.02	0.20	2.90	0.11	3
149	27	3.83	4.46	2952	377	—	0	0.06	0.28	3.23	—	—
32	4	0.62	0.61	333	64	0	5	0.03	0.05	0.92	0.06	<1
151	20	1.60	3.40	65	230	0	0	0.08	0.19	5.95	0.09	12
150	21	1.57	3.73	60	221	0	0	0.07	0.18	4.64	0.11	15
162	20	1.69	3.74	56	266	—	—	0.09	0.23	5.60	0.13	17
146	19	1.51	3.49	48	240	—	—	0.08	0.21	4.49	0.12	16
166	21	1.54	2.96	65	278	—	—	0.09	0.21	6.04	0.11	16
160	20	1.42	2.93	59	267	—	—	0.08	0.20	4.85	0.12	18
168	22	1.78	4.16	65	263	—	—	0.08	0.23	5.97	0.10	16
164	21	1.92	5.17	53	239	—	—	0.05	0.19	4.49	0.09	16
168	20	1.46	4.78	70	286	—	—	0.08	0.21	5.42	0.13	15
153	18	1.28	4.59	63	260	—	—	0.07	0.19	4.30	0.12	15
42	3	0.20	0.41	202	61	0	4	0.09	0.04	0.93	0.03	<1
20	5	0.68	0.12	415	48	3	0	1.25	0.14	2.15	0.14	12
84	6	0.23	0.48	438	110	0	6	0.23	0.06	1.96	0.13	1
207	15	1.17	2.13	800	304	0	12	0.70	0.22	4.51	0.26	4
178	18	0.78	1.90	965	296	0	23	0.88	0.21	4.16	0.38	4
239	19	1.14	2.10	1276	348	0	19	0.62	0.28	5.23	0.26	3
39	4	0.22	0.58	335	80	0	10	0.15	0.04	1.11	0.08	1
26	4	0.65	0.52	349	—	0	—	0.04	0.02	0.44	0.09	—
49	6	0.66	1.05	638	95	0	15	0.11	0.07	1.50	0.08	2
72	5	0.26	0.57	380	83	7	7	0.17	0.05	0.98	0.07	<1
70	5	0.28	0.61	373	94	0	8	0.25	0.07	1.49	0.10	<1
40	5	0.29	0.40	393	96	2	4	0.08	0.07	0.58	0.05	1
65	6	0.37	1.19	641	107	0	0	0.26	0.09	1.59	0.17	<1
14	2	0.25	0.46	269	28	0	0	0.03	0.03	0.46	0.04	1
200	21	0.69	2.09	56	299	2	<1	0.72	0.31	4.48	0.32	4
166	16	0.84	1.74	54	274	2	<1	0.70	0.20	4.29	0.34	<1
156	15	0.77	1.61	49	257	2	<1	0.64	0.19	3.87	0.32	<1

Table continued on following page

APPENDIX A–1 **NUTRITIVE VALUES OF FOOD** *Continued*

	Approximate Measure	Weight (gm)	H_2O (gm)	Kcal	Protein (gm)	Carbohy-drate (gm)	Dietary Fiber (gm)	Fat (gm)	MUFA (gm)	PUFA (gm)	Cholesterol (mg)	Calcium (mg)
Shoulder, lean, roasted	2.5 oz	70.9	42	173	18	0	0	11	4.8	1.3	69	6
Tenderloin, lean, roasted	2.5 oz	70.9	46	118	20	0	0	3	1.5	0.4	66	6
Pork, sausages, cooked												
Braunschweiger	1 oz	28.4	14	102	4	<1	0	9	4.2	1.1	44	3
Link	1	13	6	48	3	<1	0	4	1.8	0.5	11	4
Patty	1 oz	28.4	13	105	6	<1	0	.9	3.9	1.1	24	10
Veal, cooked												
All cuts, lean and fat	3 oz	85	49	197	26	0	0	10	3.7	0.7	97	19
All cuts, lean	2.5 oz	70.9	43	138	23	0	0	5	1.7	0.4	83	17
Shoulder blade, lean, roasted	2.5 oz	70.9	48	122	18	0	0	5	1.8	0.4	84	20
Milk products (cheese, cream, imitation cream, and related products)												
Cheese												
Blue	1 oz	28.4	12	100	6	1	0	8	2.2	0.2	20	150
Camembert	1 oz	28.4	15	85	6	<1	0	7	2.0	0.2	20	110
Cheddar, cut pieces	1 oz	28.4	10	114	7	<1	0	9	2.7	0.3	30	204
Cheddar, shredded	1 cup	113	42	455	28	2	0	38	10.6	1.1	119	815
Cheddar, low sodium, low fat	1 oz	28.4	—	80	8	1	—	5	—	0	20	—
Cottage, creamed (4% fat)	1 cup	225	178	232	28	6	0	10	2.9	0.3	34	135
Cottage, low fat (2% fat)	1 cup	226	179	203	31	8	0	4	1.2	0.1	19	155
Cottage, low fat (1% fat)	1 cup	226	186	164	28	6	0	2	0.7	0.1	10	138
Cottage, uncreamed	1 cup	145	116	123	25	3	0	1	0.2	<0.1	10	46
Cream	1 oz	28.4	15	100	2	1	0	10	2.8	0.4	31	23
Mozzarella, whole milk	1 oz	28.4	15	80	6	1	0	6	1.9	0.2	22	147
Mozzarella, skim milk	1 oz	28.4	15	72	7	1	0	5	1.3	0.1	16	183
Parmesan, grated	1 oz	28.4	5	129	12	1	0	9	2.5	0.2	23	390
Swiss	1 oz	28.4	12	95	7	1	0	7	2.0	0.2	24	219
Processed												
American	1 oz	28.4	11	106	6	1	0	9	2.6	0.3	27	174
Cheese food, American	1 oz	28.4	12	93	6	2	0	7	2.0	0.2	18	163
Cheese spread	1 oz	28.4	14	82	5	3	0	6	1.8	0.2	16	159
Provolone	1 oz	28.4	12	100	7	1	0	8	2.1	0.2	20	214
Ricotta, whole milk	1 oz	28.4	20	49	3	1	0	4	1.0	0.1	14	59
Ricotta, skim milk	1 oz	28.4	21	39	3	2	0	2	1.0	0.1	9	78
Romano	1 oz	28.4	9	110	9	1	0	8	2.2	0.1	29	301
Swiss	1 oz	28.4	11	107	8	1	0	8	2.1	0.3	26	272
Swiss, low sodium, low fat	1 oz	28.4	—	90	10	0	0	5	—	0	17	—
Cream, sour												
Cultured	1 tbsp	14.4	10	31	1	1	0	3	0.9	0.1	7	17
Imitation	1 oz	28.4	20	59	1	2	0	6	0.2	<0.1	0	1
Cream, sweet												
Half & Half	1 tbsp	15	12	20	1	1	0	2	0.5	0.1	6	16
Light, coffee	1 tbsp	15	11	29	<1	1	0	3	0.8	0.1	10	14
Cream, whipping												
Light	1 tbsp	15	10	44	<1	<1	0	5	1.4	0.1	17	10
Heavy	1 tbsp	15	9	51	<1	<1	0	6	1.6	0.2	20	10
Imitation, frozen liquid	1 tbsp	15	12	21	<1	2	0	2	1.2	<0.1	0	1
Imitation, frozen	1 tbsp	4.7	2	15	<1	1	0	1	0.1	<0.1	0	<1
Imitation, powdered	1 tbsp	5.9	<1	32	<1	3	0	2	0.1	<0.1	0	1
Mocha mix, nondairy	1 tbsp	15	—	20	1	1	1	2	0.8	0.8	0	—
Nondairy, light	1 tbsp	12	—	24	3	6	—	3	3	0	0	—
Whipped, imitation powdered	1 tbsp	5	3	9	<1	1	0	1	<0.1	<0.1	1	5
Whipped, imitation, pressurized	1 tbsp	5	3	12	<1	1	0	1	0.1	<0.1	0	<1
Whipped topping, pressurized	1 tbsp	4	2	10	<1	1	0	1	0.2	<0.1	3	4
Eggnog, commercial	1 cup	254	189	342	10	34	0	19	5.7	0.9	149	330

Phosphate (mg)	Magnesium (mg)	Iron (mg)	Zinc (mg)	Sodium (mg)	Potassium (mg)	Vitamin A (RE)	Vitamin C (mg)	Thiamin (mg)	Riboflavin (mg)	Niacin (mg)	Vitamin B_6 (mg)	Folate (mcg)
164	14	1.08	3.00	54	250	2	<1	0.41	0.26	3.05	0.28	4
204	18	1.09	2.13	47	382	2	<1	0.66	0.28	3.32	0.30	4
48	3	2.65	0.80	324	56	1195	3	0.07	0.43	2.38	0.09	12
24	2	0.16	0.33	168	47	0	<1	0.10	0.03	0.59	0.04	<1
53	5	0.36	0.71	366	102	0	0	0.21	0.07	1.28	0.09	<1
204	23	0.98	4.04	74	276	—	—	0.05	0.28	6.78	0.27	13
178	20	0.83	3.61	63	240	—	—	0.04	0.24	5.97	0.23	11
153	18	0.71	4.05	72	220	—	—	0.05	0.25	4.13	0.18	8
110	7	0.09	0.75	394	73	61	0	0.01	0.11	0.29	0.05	10
99	6	0.09	0.67	239	53	78	0	0.01	0.14	0.18	0.06	18
145	8	0.19	0.88	176	28	90	0	0.01	0.11	0.02	0.02	5
579	31	0.77	3.5	701	111	359	0	0.03	0.42	0.09	0.08	21
—	—	—	—	140	30	—	—	—	—	—	—	—
297	11	0.32	0.83	911	189	110	0	0.05	0.37	0.28	0.15	27
340	14	0.36	0.95	918	217	47	0	0.05	0.42	0.33	0.17	30
302	12	0.32	0.86	918	193	25	0	0.05	0.37	0.29	0.15	28
151	6	0.33	0.68	19	47	13	0	0.04	0.21	0.23	0.12	21
30	2	0.34	0.15	85	34	122	0	0.01	0.06	0.03	0.01	4
105	5	0.05	0.63	106	19	68	0	<0.01	0.07	0.02	0.02	2
131	7	0.06	0.78	132	24	50	0	<0.01	0.09	0.03	0.02	2
229	15	0.27	0.90	528	30	60	0	0.01	0.11	0.09	0.03	2
216	8	0.17	1.02	387	61	69	0	<0.01	0.08	0.01	0.01	2
211	6	0.11	0.85	405	46	103	0	<0.01	0.10	0.02	0.02	2
130	9	0.24	0.85	336	79	78	0	<0.01	0.13	0.04	0.04	2
202	8	0.09	0.73	380	69	67	0	0.01	0.12	0.04	0.03	2
141	8	0.15	0.92	248	39	69	0	<0.01	0.09	0.04	0.02	3
45	3	0.10	0.33	24	30	42	0	<0.01	0.06	0.03	0.01	4
52	4	0.12	0.38	35	36	37	0	<0.01	0.05	0.02	<0.01	4
215	12	0.22	0.73	339	25	49	0	0.01	0.11	0.02	0.02	2
171	10	0.05	1.11	74	31	72	0	<0.01	0.10	0.03	0.02	2
—	—	—	—	60	30	—	—	—	—	—	—	—
12	2	0.01	0.04	8	21	34	<1	<0.01	0.02	0.01	<0.01	2
13	2	0.11	0.33	29	46	0	0	0	0	0	0	0
14	2	0.01	0.08	6	20	20	<1	<0.01	0.02	0.01	<0.01	1
12	1	0.01	0.04	6	18	32	<1	<0.01	0.02	<0.01	<0.01	1
9	1	<0.01	0.04	5	14	51	<1	<0.01	0.02	<0.01	<0.01	<1
9	1	<0.01	0.03	6	11	66	<1	<0.01	0.02	<0.01	<0.01	<1
10	0	<0.01	<0.01	12	29	4	0	0	0	0	0	0
<1	<1	<0.01	<0.01	1	<1	12	0	0	0	0	0	0
25	<1	0.07	0.03	11	48	4	0	0	0.01	0	0	0
—	—	—	—	5	20	—	—	—	—	—	—	—
—	—	—	—	15	15	—	—	—	—	—	—	—
4	<1	<0.01	0.01	3	8	5	<1	<0.01	<0.01	<0.01	<0.01	<1
1	<1	<0.01	<0.01	3	1	6	0	0	0	0	0	0
3	<1	<0.01	0.01	5	6	10	0	<0.01	<0.01	<0.01	<0.01	<1
278	47	0.51	1.17	138	420	268	4	0.09	0.48	0.27	0.13	2

Table continued on following page

APPENDIX A–1 **NUTRITIVE VALUES OF FOOD** *Continued*

	Approximate Measure	Weight (gm)	H_2O (gm)	Kcal	Protein (gm)	Carbohydrate (gm)	Dietary Fiber (gm)	Fat (gm)	MUFA (gm)	PUFA (gm)	Cholesterol (mg)	Calcium (mg)
Milk												
Buttermilk	1 cup	245	221	99	8	12	0	2	0.6	0.1	9	285
Canned												
Evaporated, whole	1 cup	252	187	338	17	25	0	19	5.9	0.6	73	658
Evaporated, skim	1 cup	255	202	199	19	29	0	1	0.2	<0.1	10	740
Condensed, sweetened	1 cup	306	83	982	24	166	0	27	7.4	1.0	104	868
Chocolate												
Low fat (2% fat)	1 cup	250	209	179	8	26	<1	5	1.5	0.2	17	284
Low fat (1% fat)	1 cup	250	211	158	8	26	<1	3	0.8	0.1	7	287
Whole	1 cup	250	206	208	8	26	<1	9	2.5	0.3	30	280
Low fat (2% fat)	1 cup	244	218	121	8	12	0	5	1.4	0.2	18	297
Milk solids added	1 cup	245	218	125	9	12	0	5	1.4	0.2	18	313
Protein fortified	1 cup	246	216	137	10	14	0	5	1.4	0.2	19	352
Low fat (1% fat)	1 cup	244	220	102	8	12	0	3	0.8	0.1	10	300
Milk solids added	1 cup	245	220	104	9	12	0	2	0.7	0.1	10	313
Protein fortified	1 cup	246	218	119	10	14	0	3	0.8	0.1	10	349
Malted beverage, with 1 cup milk and ¾ oz powder												
Chocolate	1 cup	265	215	229	9	30	<1	9	2.6	0.4	34	304
Natural	1 cup	265	215	237	10	27	<1	10	2.8	0.6	37	354
Nondairy, tofu	1 cup	250	—	90	2	10	—	5	—	—	—	500
Nonfat, skim	1 cup	245	222	86	8	12	0	<1	0.1	<0.1	4	302
Solids added	1 cup	245	221	90	9	12	0	1	0.2	<0.1	5	316
Protein fortified	1 cup	246	220	100	10	14	0	1	0.2	<0.1	5	352
Whole (3.3% fat)	1 cup	244	215	150	8	11	0	8	2.4	0.3	33	291
Yogurt												
Fruit flavor, low fat	1 cup	227	169	231	10	43	1	3	0.7	0.1	10	345
Plain, low fat	1 cup	227	193	144	12	16	0	4	1.0	0.1	14	415
Plain, whole	1 cup	227	200	139	8	11	0	7	2.0	0.2	29	274
Mixed entrees and soups												
Beef and vegetable stew	1 cup	245	201	220	16	15	3	11	4.5	0.5	72	29
Beef potpie—home recipe	1 cup	245	135	601	25	46	5	35	15.0	8.6	51	34
Chicken chow mein—canned	1 cup	250	223	95	7	18	1	0	0	0	98	45
Chicken chow mein—home recipe	1 cup	250	195	255	31	10	1	10	3.4	3.1	98	58
Chicken/noodles, cooked—home recipe	1 cup	240	170	365	22	26	1	18	7.1	3.5	96	26
Chicken potpie, baked—home recipe	1 cup	245	139	576	25	44	4	33	14.2	5.8	76	74
Chili con carne/beans—canned	1 cup	255	184	340	19	31	5	16	7.2	1.0	38	82
Corned beef hash—canned	1 cup	220	147	400	19	24	—	25	10.9	0.5	50	29
Macaroni and cheese, enriched—canned	1 cup	240	192	230	9	26	1	10	3.1	1.4	42	199
Macaroni and cheese, enriched—home recipe	1 cup	200	116	430	17	40	1	22	8.8	2.9	42	362
Pizza, cheese	1 slice	63	30	140	8	21	2	3	1.0	0.5	9	116
Pizza, pepperoni	1 slice	71	33	181	10	20	2	7	3.1	1.2	14	65
Soups, canned, condensed												
Clam chowder, New England, chunky	1 serving	269	—	250	7	22	—	15	—	—	—	—
Cream of celery, prepared with water	1 cup	244	225	90	2	9	—	6	1.3	2.5	15	40
Cream of chicken, prepared with milk	1 cup	248	210	191	8	15	0.5	12	4.5	1.6	27	181
Cream of chicken, prepared with water	1 cup	244	221	117	3	9	0.5	7	3.3	1.5	9.8	34
Cream of mushroom, prepared with milk	1 cup	248	210	203	6	15	—	14	3.0	4.6	20	178

Phosphate (mg)	Magnesium (mg)	Iron (mg)	Zinc (mg)	Sodium (mg)	Potassium (mg)	Vitamin A (RE)	Vitamin C (mg)	Thiamin (mg)	Riboflavin (mg)	Niacin (mg)	Vitamin B_6 (mg)	Folate (mcg)
219	27	0.12	1.03	257	371	24	2	0.08	0.38	0.14	0.08	12
509	61	0.48	1.94	267	764	184	5	0.12	0.80	0.49	0.13	20
497	69	0.74	2.30	293	847	300	3	0.12	0.79	0.44	0.14	23
775	78	0.58	2.88	389	1136	302	8	0.28	1.27	0.64	0.16	34
254	33	0.60	1.02	150	422	150	2	0.09	0.41	0.32	0.10	12
256	33	0.60	1.02	152	426	150	2	0.1	0.42	0.32	0.10	12
251	33	0.60	1.02	149	417	91	2	0.09	0.41	0.31	0.10	12
232	33	0.12	0.95	122	377	150	2	0.10	0.40	0.21	0.11	12
245	35	0.12	0.98	128	397	150	3	0.10	0.42	0.22	0.11	13
276	40	0.15	1.11	145	447	150	3	0.11	0.48	0.25	0.13	15
235	34	0.12	0.95	123	381	150	2	0.10	0.41	0.21	0.11	12
245	35	0.12	0.98	128	397	150	3	0.10	0.42	0.22	0.11	13
273	39	0.15	1.11	143	444	150	3	0.11	0.47	0.25	0.12	15
265	47	0.50	1.09	172	499	80	3	0.13	0.44	0.63	0.14	16
303	52	0.29	1.13	223	529	94	3	0.20	0.59	1.31	0.19	22
—	—	0	—	120	10	50	6	0.15	0.43	2.0	0.20	40
247	28	0.10	0.98	126	406	150	2	0.09	0.34	0.22	0.10	13
255	36	0.12	1	130	418	150	3	0.10	0.43	0.22	0.11	13
275	40	0.15	1.11	144	446	150	3	0.11	0.48	0.25	0.12	15
228	33	0.12	0.93	120	370	92	2	0.09	0.40	0.2	0.1	12
271	33	0.16	1.68	133	442	31	1.5	0.08	0.40	0.22	0.09	21
326	40	0.18	2.02	159	531	45	1.8	0.1	0.5	0.26	0.11	25
215	26	0.11	1.3	105	351	84	1.2	0.07	0.32	0.17	0.07	17
184	—	2.90	—	1006	613	480	17	0.15	0.17	4.70	—	—
174	—	4.43	—	695	390	401	7	0.35	0.35	6.42	—	—
85	—	1.30	—	722	418	30	13	0.05	0.10	1.00	—	—
293	—	2.50	—	717	473	56	10	0.08	0.23	4.30	—	—
247	—	2.20	—	600	149	80	0	0.05	0.17	4.30	—	—
245	—	3.17	—	626	362	653	5	0.36	0.33	5.81	—	—
321	—	4.30	—	1354	594	30	—	0.08	0.18	3.30	0.26	—
147	—	4.40	—	1188	440	—	—	0.02	0.20	4.60	—	—
182	—	1.00	—	729	139	52	0	0.12	0.24	1.00	—	—
322	52	1.80	—	1086	240	172	0	0.20	0.40	1.80	—	—
113	16	0.58	0.82	336	110	74	1	0.18	0.16	2.48	0.04	59
75	8	0.94	0.52	267	153	54	2	0.14	0.23	3.05	0.05	53
—	—	—	—	1050	—	—	—	—	—	—	—	—
37	6	0.62	0.15	949	123	31	<1	0.03	0.05	0.33	0.01	2
151	17	0.68	0.68	1046	273	94	1	0.07	0.26	0.92	0.07	8
37	2	0.61	0.63	986	88	56	<1	0.03	0.06	0.82	0.02	2
156	20	0.59	0.64	1076	270	38	2	0.08	0.28	0.91	0.06	10

Table continued on following page

APPENDIX A–1 **NUTRITIVE VALUES OF FOOD** *Continued*

	Approximate Measure	Weight (gm)	H_2O (gm)	Kcal	Protein (gm)	Carbohydrate (gm)	Dietary Fiber (gm)	Fat (gm)	MUFA (gm)	PUFA (gm)	Cholesterol (mg)	Calcium (mg)
Cream of mushroom, prepared with water	1 cup	244	220	129	2	9	0.9	9	1.7	4.2	2.4	46
Bean with bacon, prepared with water	1 cup	253	213	173	8	23	3.2	6	2.2	1.8	2.5	81
Beef broth/bouillion, ready to serve	1 cup	240	234	17	3	0.1	0	<1	0.2	<0.1	0	14
Beef noodle, prepared with water	1 cup	244	224	84	5	9	—	3	1.2	0.5	4.9	15
Minestrone, prepared with water	1 cup	241	220	82	4	11	1.9	3	0.7	1.1	2.4	34
Pea, split, prepared with water	1 cup	253	207	189	10	28	—	4	1.8	0.6	7.6	23
Tomato, prepared with milk	1 cup	248	210	161	6	22	0.8	6	1.6	1.1	17.4	159
Tomato, prepared with water	1 cup	244	220	85	2	17	0.9	2	0.4	1.0	0	12
Vegetarian, prepared with water	1 cup	241	223	72	2	12	1.2	2	0.8	0.7	0	22
Soups, dehydrated												
Beef broth, cubed	1 item	3.6	<1	6	<1	<1	—	<1	<0.1	<0.1	0.1	2
Onion, prepared with water	1 cup	246	237	27	1	5	0.4	<1	0.3	<0.1	0	12
Spaghetti and tomato sauce with cheese—home recipe	1 cup	250	193	260	9	37	3	9	5.4	<1	4	80
Spaghetti and tomato sauce with cheese—canned	1 cup	250	200	190	6	39	3	2	0.3	0.4	4	40
Spaghetti with tomato sauce and meat—home recipe	1 cup	248	174	330	19	39	3	12	6.3	0.9	75	124
Spaghetti with tomato sauce and meat—canned	1 cup	250	195	260	12	29	3.0	10	3.3	3.9	39	53
Poultry and poultry products												
Chicken, cooked												
Boneless, canned	3 oz	85	58	140	18	0	0	7	2.7	1.5	53	12
Chicken frankfurter	1	45	26	116	6	3	0	9	3.8	1.8	46	43
Breast, fried in batter	3 oz	85	44	221	21	8	—	11	4.7	2.7	72	17
Breast, roasted	3 oz	85	53	167	25	0	0	7	2.6	1.4	72	12
Drumstick, meat only, fried	3 oz	85	53	166	24	0	0	7	2.5	1.7	81	10
Drumstick, meat and skin, battered and fried	3 oz	85	45	228	19	7	—	13	5.5	3.2	73	14
Drumstick, meat only, roasted	3 oz	85	57	147	24	0	0	5	1.6	1.2	79	10
Liver, simmered	3 oz	85	58	133	21	<1	0	5	1.1	0.8	536	12
Eggs, cooked, large (24 oz/doz)												
Fried	1	46	32	92	6	1	0	7	2.8	1.3	211	25
Hard boiled	1	50	37	77	6	1	0	5	2.0	0.7	213	25
Poached, whole	1	50	38	74	6	1	0	5	1.9	0.7	212	25
Scrambled	1	61	45	101	7	1	0	8	2.9	1.3	215	44
Egg substitute, frozen	¼ cup	60	44	96	7	2	0	7	1.5	3.8	1.2	44
Turkey												
All parts, roasted	3 oz	85	53	174	24	<1	—	8	2.6	2.1	81	22
Dark meat, no skin	3 oz	85	54	159	24	0	0	6	1.4	1.8	72	27
Light meat, no skin, roasted	3 oz	85	56	133	26	0	0	3	0.5	0.7	59	16
Light and dark meat, no skin	3 oz	85	55	145	25	0	0	4	0.9	1.2	65	21
Loaf, breast	3 oz	85	61	93	19	0	0	1	0.4	0.2	35	6
Pastrami	3 oz	85	60	120	16	1	0	5	1.7	1.4	46	8
Roll, light/dark meat	3 oz	85	60	127	15	2	0	6	1.9	1.5	47	27

Phosphate (mg)	Magnesium (mg)	Iron (mg)	Zinc (mg)	Sodium (mg)	Potassium (mg)	Vitamin A (RE)	Vitamin C (mg)	Thiamin (mg)	Riboflavin (mg)	Niacin (mg)	Vitamin B_6 (mg)	Folate (mcg)
49	5	0.51	0.59	1032	100	0	1	0.05	1	0.73	0.02	5
132	46	2.05	1.03	952	403	89	2	0.09	0.03	0.57	0.04	32
31	5	0.41	0	782	130	0	0	<0.01	0.05	1.87	0.02	5
46	6	1.10	1.54	952	99	63	<1	0.07	0.06	1.07	0.04	4
55	7	0.92	0.74	911	313	234	1	0.05	0.04	0.94	0.10	16
213	48	2.28	1.32	1008	399	44	2	0.15	0.08	1.48	0.07	3
149	22	1.81	0.29	932	449	108	68	0.13	0.25	1.52	0.16	21
34	8	1.76	0.24	871	263	69	66	0.09	0.05	1.42	0.11	15
35	7	1.08	0.46	822	209	300	2	0.05	0.05	0.92	0.06	11
8	2	0.08	0.01	864	15	<1	0	<0.01	<0.01	0.12	<0.01	1
30	5	0.15	0.06	849	64	0	<1	0.03	0.06	0.48	0	2
135	—	2.30	—	955	408	216	13	0.25	0.18	2.30	—	—
88	28	2.80	—	955	303	186	10	0.35	0.28	4.50	—	—
236	—	3.70	—	1009	665	—	22	0.25	0.30	4.00	—	—
113	28	3.30	—	1220	245	200	5	0.15	0.18	2.30	—	—

Phosphate (mg)	Magnesium (mg)	Iron (mg)	Zinc (mg)	Sodium (mg)	Potassium (mg)	Vitamin A (RE)	Vitamin C (mg)	Thiamin (mg)	Riboflavin (mg)	Niacin (mg)	Vitamin B_6 (mg)	Folate (mcg)
95	10	1.34	1.20	428	117	60	2	0.01	0.11	5.39	0.30	3
48	5	0.90	0.47	617	38	17	0	0.03	0.05	1.39	0.14	2
157	21	1.06	0.81	234	171	17	0	0.10	0.12	8.96	0.36	5
182	23	0.90	0.87	60	208	24	0	0.06	0.10	10.8	0.47	3
158	20	1.11	2.73	81	213	16	0	0.07	0.20	5.23	0.34	8
125	16	1.15	1.97	229	158	21	0	0.10	0.18	4.34	0.24	7
157	21	1.10	2.71	81	209	16	0	0.06	0.20	5.16	0.33	8
265	18	7.23	3.69	43	119	4183	14	0.13	1.49	3.79	0.50	654
89	5	0.72	0.55	162	61	114	0	0.03	0.24	0.04	0.07	18
86	5	0.60	0.52	62	63	84	0	0.03	0.26	0.03	0.06	22
89	5	0.72	0.55	140	60	95	0	0.03	0.22	0.03	0.06	18
104	7	0.73	0.61	171	84	119	0	<1	0.27	0.05	0.07	18
43	9	1.19	0.59	120	128	81	<1	0.07	0.23	0.08	0.08	10
170	21	1.71	2.69	57	231	58	<1	0.05	0.18	4.21	0.34	17
174	21	1.99	3.80	67	247	0	0	0.05	0.21	3.10	0.30	8
187	24	1.14	1.73	54	259	0	0	0.05	0.11	5.81	0.46	5
181	23	1.51	2.64	60	254	0	0	0.05	0.16	4.63	0.39	6
195	17	0.34	0.96	1216	237	0	0	0.03	0.09	7.07	0.31	3
170	12	1.41	1.84	889	221	0	0	0.05	0.21	3.00	0.23	4
143	15	1.15	1.70	497	230	0	0	0.08	0.24	4.07	0.23	4

Table continued on following page

APPENDIX A–1 **NUTRITIVE VALUES OF FOOD** *Continued*

	Approximate Measure	Weight (gm)	H_2O (gm)	Kcal	Protein (gm)	Carbohydrate (gm)	Dietary Fiber (gm)	Fat (gm)	MUFA (gm)	PUFA (gm)	Cholesterol (mg)	Calcium (mg)
Sugars, sweets, and desserts												
Apple butter	1 tbsp	20	10	37	<1	9	—	<1	—	—	—	3
Cake icing												
Chocolate, prepared from mix	1 cup	275	39	1035	9	185	—	38	11.7	1.0	0	165
Fudge, prepared from mix	1 cup	245	37	830	7	183	—	16	6.7	3.1	0	96
White, boiled	1 cup	94	17	295	1	75	0	0	0	0	0	2
White, uncooked	1 cup	319	35	1200	2	260	0	21	5.1	0.5	0	48
Cakes												
Angel food, prepared from mix	1 slice	53	17	142	4	32	<0.1	<1	—	—	0	5
Brownies, commercial	1 item	60	8	243	3	39	1.3	10	3.8	2.6	9	25
Cheese, New York, Jello	1 piece	43	—	175	4	33	0.3	3	—	—	1	95
Coffee, prepared from mix	1 slice	72	22	230	5	38	2.4	7	2.7	1.5	—	44
Cupcake, no icing	1 item	25	7	90	1	14	0.3	3	1.2	0.7	0	40
Cupcake with chocolate icing	1 item	36	8	130	2	21	0.4	5	1.7	0.7	15	47
Cupcake, devils food with icing	1 item	35	8	120	2	20	0.7	4	1.4	0.5	40	21
Fruit, dark—home recipe	1 slice	15	3	57	1	9	0.3	2	1.3	0.5	7	11
Gingerbread, prepared from mix	1 slice	63	23	175	2	32	1.8	4	1.8	1.1	1	57
Pound—home recipe	1 slice	33	5	160	2	16	0.1	10	3	0.6	68	6
Sheet, uncooked icing	1 slice	121	25	445	4	77	0	14	5.5	2.7	1	61
Sheet, no icing—home recipe	1 slice	86	22	315	4	48	0.9	12	4.9	2.6	1	55
Sponge—home recipe	1 slice	66	22	188	5	36	0	3	1.3	0.5	162	25
White, super moist, prepared from mix	1 serving	43	—	180	2	36	—	3	2	0	0	60
Candy												
Caramels, plain with chocolate	1 oz	28.4	2	115	1	22	0.8	2.9	1.1	0.1	0	42
Chocolate-coated peanuts	1 oz	28.4	<1	160	5	11	—	12	4.7	2.1	0	33
Fondant, uncoated	1 oz	28.4	2	105	0	25	0	0.9	0.3	0.1	0	4
Fudge, chocolate marshmallow	1 piece	20	2	84	<1	14	—	3.4	1.1	0.1	5	9
Gumdrops	1 oz	28.4	3	100	0	25	0	0	0	0	0	2
Hard	1 oz	28.4	<1	110	0	28	0	0	0	0	0	6
Life Savers	2 items	4	—	16	0	4	0	<0.1	0	0	0	1
Jelly beans	1 oz	28.4	2	67	0	27	0	0	0	0	0	3
Marshmallows	1 oz	28.4	5	90	1	23	0	0	0	0	0	5
Milk chocolate, plain	1 oz	28.4	<1	145	2	16	—	9	2.9	0.3	0	65
Chocolate beverage												
Powder with nonfat dry milk	1 oz	28.4	<1	100	5	20	—	1	0.3	0	2	167
Drink, no milk, dry	1 oz	28.4	<1	99	1	26	—	1	0.3	<0.1	0	11
Cookies												
Chocolate chip, home recipe	2 items	20	<1	93	1	13	0.5	5.4	2.3	1.6	11	7
Chocolate chip, from mix	2 items	21	<1	100	1	14	0.6	4.8	1.8	1.2	11	6
Fig bar	2 items	28	3	106	1	21	1.3	1.9	0.6	0.4	0	20
Gingersnap, home recipe	2 items	14	<1	69	<1	9	0.6	3.2	—	—	0	5
Macaroon	2 items	38	2	180	2	25	0.9	9	—	—	0	10
Oatmeal/raisin, from mix	2 items	26	1	123	1	18	0.7	5.2	1.7	1	0	9
Plain, mix	2 items	24	1	120	1	16	0.3	6	2.6	1.5	0	9
Sandwich, chocolate/vanilla	2 items	20	<1	100	1	14	0.3	4.5	1.9	1.1	0	5
Vanilla wafer	2 items	8	<1	37	<1	6	<0.1	1.2	0.4	0.2	5	3

Phosphate (mg)	Magnesium (mg)	Iron (mg)	Zinc (mg)	Sodium (mg)	Potassium (mg)	Vitamin A (RE)	Vitamin C (mg)	Thiamin (mg)	Riboflavin (mg)	Niacin (mg)	Vitamin B_6 (mg)	Folate (mcg)
4	—	0.10	—	0	50	0	—	—	—	—	—	—
305	—	3.30	—	882	536	174	1	0.06	0.28	0.60	—	—
218	—	2.70	—	568	238	0	0	0.05	0.20	0.70	—	—
2	—	0	—	134	17	0	0	0	0.03	0	—	—
38	—	0	—	156	57	258	0	0	0.06	0	—	—
63	6	0.45	0.11	142	52	0	0	0.06	0.12	0.59	<0.01	5
87	16	1.29	0.55	153	83	3	3	0.07	0.13	0.58	0.03	4
134	11	0.40	0	320	145	4	0	0.08	0.15	0.50	0.01	2
125	—	1.20	—	310	78	24	0	0.14	0.15	1.30	—	—
59	—	0.30	—	113	21	8	0	0.05	0.05	0.40	—	—
71	—	0.40	—	120	42	12	0	0.05	0.06	0.40	—	—
37	—	0.50	—	91	46	10	0	0.03	0.05	0.30	—	2
17	—	0.42	—	24	74	4	<1	0.02	0.02	0.17	—	—
63	14	0.90	0.28	90	173	0	0	0.09	0.11	0.80	0.05	5
24	—	0.50	—	58	20	16	0	0.05	0.06	0.40	—	2
91	—	0.80	—	274	74	48	0	0.14	0.16	1.10	—	7
88	12	0.90	0.30	382	68	30	0	0.13	0.15	1.10	0.02	6
65	7	1.11	0.80	164	59	25	0	0.09	0.13	0.73	0.04	15
—	—	0.72	—	260	25	0	0	0.09	0.07	0.80	—	—
35	1	0.40	—	74	54	0	0	0.01	0.05	0.10	—	—
84	—	0.40	—	16	143	0	0	0.10	0.05	2.10	—	—
2	—	0.30	—	60	1	0	0	0	0	0	—	—
13	7	0.19	0.11	21	28	16	0	<0.01	0.02	0.03	<0.01	0
0	—	0.10	—	10	1	0	0	0	0	0	—	—
2	—	0.50	—	9	1	0	0	0	0	0	—	—
<1	—	0.08	—	1	0	0	0	0	0	0	—	—
1	—	0.30	—	3	0	0	0	0	—	—	—	—
2	—	0.50	0.01	11	2	0	0	0	0	0	—	—
65	16	0.30	—	28	109	24	0	0.02	0.10	0.10	—	2
155	23	0.50	0.34	147	227	3	1	0.04	0.21	0.20	<0.01	—
36	28	0.89	0.44	60	168	<1	<1	0.01	0.04	0.14	<0.01	2
17	7	0.50	0.09	41	41	2	0	0.03	0.03	0.29	<0.01	2
15	5	0.46	0.11	76	27	12	0	0.03	0.04	0.39	<0.01	2
17	7	0.68	0.18	90	81	6	0	0.04	0.04	0.36	0.03	2
7	3	0.32	0.06	39	27	1	0	0.03	0.02	0.24	<0.01	1
32	—	0.30	—	12	176	0	0	0.02	0.06	0.20	—	—
29	7	0.57	0.17	74	45	4	0	0.04	0.04	0.48	0.01	3
18	2	0.30	0.07	131	12	15	0	0.05	0.04	0.45	0.01	2
48	10	0.35	0.17	126	8	0	0	0.03	0.05	0.35	<0.01	<1
5	1	0.12	—	20	6	2	0	0.02	0.02	0.16	—	—

Table continued on following page

APPENDIX A–1 **NUTRITIVE VALUES OF FOOD** *Continued*

	Approximate Measure	Weight (gm)	H_2O (gm)	Kcal	Protein (gm)	Carbohydrate (gm)	Dietary Fiber (gm)	Fat (gm)	MUFA (gm)	PUFA (gm)	Cholesterol (mg)	Calcium (mg)
Doughnuts												
Cake, plain	1 item	25	5	104	1	12	0.3	6	1.2	2	10	11
Yeast, glazed	1 item	50	13	205	3	22	1.1	11	5.8	3.3	13	16
Granola bar	1 item	24	<1	109	2	16	1.0	4	—	—	—	14
Jams/preserves												
Regular, packet	1 item	14	4	40	0	10	0.1	0	0	0	0	3
Regular	1 tbsp	20	6	55	0	14	0.2	0	0	0	0	4
Strawberry, low kcal	1 tsp	6	—	8	0	2	0.1	0	0	0	0	—
Milk desserts												
Custard, baked	1 cup	265	204	305	14	29	1	15	5.4	0.7	278	297
Ice cream												
Vanilla, hard (10% fat)	1 cup	133	81	269	5	32	0	14	4.1	0.5	59	176
Vanilla, soft serve	1 cup	173	103	377	7	38	0	23	5.9	0.7	153	236
Vanilla, hard (16% fat)	1 cup	148	87	349	4	32	0	24	6.8	0.9	88	151
Ice milk												
Vanilla, hard (4.3% fat)	1 cup	131	90	184	5	29	0	6	1.4	0.1	18	176
Vanilla, soft (2.6% fat)	1 cup	175	122	223	8	38	0	5	1.2	0.1	13	274
Milkshake												
Chocolate, thick	8 oz	227	164	269	7	48	1	6	1.8	0.2	24	299
Vanilla, thick	8 oz	227	169	254	9	40	<1	7	2.0	0.3	27	331
Pudding—home recipe												
Vanilla (Blanc-mange)	1 cup	255	194	285	9	41	0	10	2.5	0.2	36	298
Tapioca cream	1 cup	165	119	220	8	28	1	8	2.5	0.5	80	173
Pudding, mixed with milk												
Chocolate, cooked	1 cup	260	182	320	9	59	0	8	2.6	2.0	32	265
Chocolate, instant	1 cup	260	179	325	8	63	0	7	2.2	0.3	28	374
Sherbet, orange (2% fat)	1 cup	193	127	270	2	59	0	4	1.0	0.1	14	103
Yogurt, frozen, soft												
Chocolate	1 cup	144	92	230	6	36	—	9	2.5	0.3	6	212
Vanilla	1 cup	144	94	228	6	35	—	8	2.3	0.3	4	206
Molasses												
Cane, blackstrap	1 tbsp	20	5	45	0	11	0	—	—	—	0	137
Cane, light	1 tbsp	20	5	50	0	13	0	—	—	—	0	33
Pastry, danish												
Plain	1 item	65	17	250	4	29	0.6	14	6.1	3.2	0	69
Cheese	1 item	91	31	353	6	29	0.6	25	15.6	2.4	20	70
Pie												
Apple—home recipe	1 slice	135	69	323	3	49	2.2	14	6.4	3.6	0	12
Banana cream—home recipe	1 slice	130	70	285	6	40	1.4	12	4.7	2.3	40	86
Blueberry—home recipe	1 slice	135	69	325	3	47	1.7	15	6.2	3.6	0	15
Cherry—home recipe	1 slice	135	64	350	4	52	1.1	15	6.4	3.6	0	19
Custard—home recipe	1 slice	130	75	285	8	30	2.1	14	5.5	2.5	—	125
Lemon meringue—home recipe	1 slice	120	57	300	4	47	1.4	11	4.8	2.3	0	16
Mince—home recipe	1 slice	135	58	365	3	56	1.9	16	6.6	3.6	0	38
Peach—home recipe	1 slice	135	65	345	3	52	1.8	14	6.2	3.6	0	14
Pecan—home recipe	1 slice	118	24	495	6	61	4.1	27	14.4	6.3	0	55
Pumpkin—home recipe	1 slice	130	77	275	5	32	3.5	15	5.4	2.4	0	66
Popsicle	1	95	76	70	0	18	—	0	0	0	0	0
Sorghum	1 tbsp	21	5	55	0	14	0	—	—	—	0	35
Sugar												
Brown, pressed down	1 cup	220	4	820	0	212	0	0	0	0	0	187
White, granulated	1 cup	192	2	720	0	192	0	0	0	0	0	0
White, powdered, sifted	1 cup	100	1	385	0	100	0	0	0	0	0	0

Phosphate (mg)	Magnesium (mg)	Iron (mg)	Zinc (mg)	Sodium (mg)	Potassium (mg)	Vitamin A (RE)	Vitamin C (mg)	Thiamin (mg)	Riboflavin (mg)	Niacin (mg)	Vitamin B_6 (mg)	Folate (mcg)
55	6	0.37	0.13	139	27	2	0	0.06	0.05	0.43	<0.01	2
33	10	0.60	—	117	34	5	0	0.10	0.10	0.80	—	11
67	—	0.76	—	67	78	—	—	0.07	0.03	—	—	—
1	—	0.10	—	1	12	0	0	0	0	0	<0.01	1
2	—	0.20	—	2	18	0	0	0	0.01	0	<0.01	2
—	—	—	—	6	—	—	—	—	—	—	—	—
310	—	1.10	—	209	387	87	1	0.11	0.50	0.30	—	—
134	18	0.12	1.41	116	257	133	1	0.05	0.33	0.13	0.06	3
199	25	0.43	1.99	153	338	199	1	0.08	0.45	0.18	0.10	9
115	16	0.10	1.21	108	221	207	1	0.04	0.28	0.12	0.05	2
129	19	0.18	0.55	105	265	52	1	0.08	0.35	0.12	0.09	3
202	29	0.28	0.86	163	412	44	1	0.12	0.54	0.18	0.13	5
286	36	0.70	1.09	252	508	59	0	0.11	0.50	0.28	0.06	11
262	27	0.23	0.88	217	414	78	0	0.07	0.44	0.33	0.10	15
232	—	0	—	165	352	82	2	0.08	0.41	0.30	—	—
180	—	0.70	—	257	223	60	2	0.07	0.30	0.20	—	—
247	—	0.80	—	335	354	68	2	0.05	0.39	0.30	—	—
237	—	1.30	—	322	335	68	2	0.08	0.39	0.30	—	—
74	15	0.31	1.33	88	198	39	4	0.03	0.09	0.13	0.03	14
200	38	—	0.72	142	376	—	<1	0.05	0.30	0.44	0.11	16
186	20	0.44	0.62	126	304	82	1	0.05	0.32	0.41	0.12	8
17	—	3.20	—	18	585	—	—	0.02	0.04	0.40	0.04	—
9	—	0.90	—	3	183	—	—	0.01	0.01	0	0.04	—
66	10	1.20	0.55	249	61	11	0	0.16	0.15	1.47	—	—
80	16	1.85	0.63	320	116	43	3	0.27	0.21	2.55	0.06	15
31	11	1.22	0.23	207	115	5	2	0.15	0.11	1.24	0.04	7
107	—	1.00	—	252	264	66	1	0.11	0.22	1	—	—
31	10	1.40	—	361	88	8	4	0.15	0.11	1.40	—	—
34	10	0.90	—	410	142	118	0	0.16	0.12	1.40	—	—
147	—	1.20	—	373	178	60	0	0.11	0.27	0.80	—	—
48	7	0.90	0.34	223	53	33	4	0.10	0.12	0.72	0.03	11
51	24	1.90	—	604	240	0	1	0.14	0.12	1.40	—	—
39	10	1.20	—	361	21	198	4	0.15	0.14	2	—	—
122	—	3.70	—	260	145	40	0	0.26	0.14	1	—	—
90	17	1	—	278	208	320	0	0.11	0.18	1	—	—
—	—	0	—	0	—	0	0	0	0	0	—	—
5	—	2.60	—	2	—	—	—	—	0.02	0	—	—
42	—	7.50	—	66	757	0	0	0.02	0.07	0.40	—	—
0	—	0	0.10	2	0	0	0	0	0	0	—	—
0	—	0.10	—	1	3	0	0	0	0	0	—	—

Table continued on following page

APPENDIX A–1 **NUTRITIVE VALUES OF FOOD** *Continued*

	Approximate Measure	Weight (gm)	H_2O (gm)	Kcal	Protein (gm)	Carbohydrate (gm)	Dietary Fiber (gm)	Fat (gm)	MUFA (gm)	PUFA (gm)	Cholesterol (mg)	Calcium (mg)
Sugar substitutes												
Equal, packet	1 item	1	—	4	0	1	—	0	0	0	0	0
Sweet & Low, packet	1 item	1	—	4	—	1	—	—	—	—	0	—
Syrup												
Chocolate flavored, fudge	1 fl oz	38	10	125	2	20	—	5	1.6	0.1	0	48
Chocolate flavored, thin	1 fl oz	38	12	83	<1	22	0.1	<1	0.1	<0.1	0	6
Corn, table, light/dark	1 fl oz	42	10	120	0	30	0	0	0	0	0	18
Corn, high fructose	1 fl oz	39	9	109	0	30	—	0	0	0	0	0
Corn, table, light/dark	1 fl oz	42	10	120	0	30	0	0	0	0	0	18
Pancake, light, low kcal	1 fl oz	39	—	60	0	15	—	0	0	0	0	—
Pancake, low kcal	1 fl oz	28.4	16	46	0	13	—	0	0	0	0	0
Pancake with 2% maple	1 fl oz	39.4	12	104	0	27	—	<1	—	—	0	2
Vegetables and vegetable products												
Alfalfa seeds, sprouted, raw	1 cup	33	30	10	1	1	0.7	<1	<0.1	0.1	0	11
Asparagus												
Canned, spears	1 cup	242	227	48	5	6	3.5	2	0.1	0.7	0	46
Fresh spears, boiled	1 cup	180	166	44	5	8	2.2	1	<0.1	0.3	0	36
Fresh tips, boiled	1 cup	180	166	44	5	8	2.2	1	<0.1	0.3	0	36
Frozen spears, boiled	1 cup	180	164	50	5	9	2.2	1	<0.1	0.3	0	41
Frozen tips, boiled	1 cup	180	164	50	5	8	2.2	1	<0.1	0.3	0	41
Beans												
Green, canned, low sodium	1 cup	136	127	26	2	6	1.8	<1	<0.1	0.1	0	32
Green, frozen, french	1 cup	135	124	36	2	8	2.2	0.2	<0.1	0.1	0	61
Lima, canned	1 cup	248	198	186	11	34	10.4	1	<0.1	0.4	0	70
Lima, frozen, boiled, drained	1 cup	170	125	170	10	32	8.3	1	<0.1	0.3	0	38
Mung, fresh, sprouted	1 cup	104	94	32	3	6	1.6	0.2	<0.1	<0.1	0	14
Mung, sprouted, boiled	1 cup	125	116	26	3	5	2.7	0.1	<0.1	<0.1	0	15
Snap, green, boiled	1 cup	135	124	36	2	8	2.2	<1	<0.1	0.1	0	61
Beet greens, boiled, drained	1 cup	145	128	40	4	8	4.4	0.3	0.1	0.1	0	165
Beets												
Canned, whole	1 cup	246	225	71	2	17	2.0	0.2	<0.1	0.1	0	34
Whole, boiled, drained	1	50	46	16	1	3	1.1	<0.1	<0.1	<0.1	0	6
Broccoli												
Boiled, drained	1 cup	155	141	44	5	8	4	0.5	<0.1	0.3	0	72
Fresh	1 cup	88	78	24	3	5	3	0.3	<0.1	0.2	0	42
Frozen, boiled, drained	1 cup	185	167	51	6	10	7.3	0.2	<0.1	0.1	0	94
Brussels sprouts												
Fresh, boiled	1 cup	156	136	60	4	14	7	0.8	<0.1	0.4	0	56
Frozen, boiled	1 cup	155	134	65	6	13	5	0.6	<0.1	0.3	0	38
Cabbage												
Boiled, drained	1 cup	145	136	31	1	7	4	0.4	<0.1	0.2	0	48
Raw, shredded	1 cup	90	83	22	1	5	2	0.2	<0.1	0.1	0	42
Red, raw, shredded	1 cup	70	64	19	1	4	2	0.2	<0.1	0.1	0	36
Savoy, raw, shredded	1 cup	70	64	19	1	4	2	0.1	<0.1	<0.1	0	25
Carrot juice, canned	1 cup	246	219	98	2	23	6	0.4	<0.1	0.2	0	58
Carrots												
Boiled, drained, sliced	1 cup	156	136	70	2	16	6	0.3	<0.1	0.1	0	48
Canned, low sodium	1 cup	246	229	56	2	12	3	0.4	<0.1	0.2	0	62
Fresh, shredded, scraped	1 cup	110	97	48	1	11	4	0.2	<0.1	0.1	0	30
Fresh, whole, scraped	1	72	63	31	1	7	2	0.1	<0.1	0.1	0	19
Cauliflower												
Fresh, chopped	1 cup	100	92	24	2	5	2	0.2	0	0	0	29
Fresh, boiled, drained	1 cup	124	115	30	2	6	3	0.2	<0.1	0.1	0	34
Frozen, boiled	1 cup	180	169	34	3	7	3	0.4	<0.1	0.2	0	30

Phosphate (mg)	Magnesium (mg)	Iron (mg)	Zinc (mg)	Sodium (mg)	Potassium (mg)	Vitamin A (RE)	Vitamin C (mg)	Thiamin (mg)	Riboflavin (mg)	Niacin (mg)	Vitamin B$_6$ (mg)	Folate (mcg)
0	0	0	0	0	0	0	0	0	0	0	0	0
—	—	—	—	4	3	—	—	—	—	—	—	—
60	—	0.50	0.30	27	107	18	0	0.02	0.08	0.20	—	—
35	21	0.60	0.30	20	106	0	0	0.01	0.03	0.20	<0.01	2
6	<1	1.60	0.02	29	2	0	0	0	0	0	—	—
—	0	0.01	<0.01	<1	0	0	0	—	<0.01	0	0	0
6	<1	1.60	0.02	29	2	0	0	0	0	0	—	—
—	—	—	—	—	—	—	—	—	—	—	—	—
12	0	0	0.01	57	1	0	0	—	—	—	0	0
4	1	0.03	0.09	24	2	—	0	<0.01	<0.01	—	0	0
23	9	0.32	0.30	2	26	5	3	0.03	0.04	0.16	0.01	12
127	22	4.44	0.98	903	403	194	36	0.15	0.24	1.82	0.13	231
96	18	1.32	0.76	20	288	96	19	0.22	0.23	1.95	0.22	264
96	18	1.32	0.76	20	288	96	19	0.22	0.23	1.95	0.22	264
99	23	1.15	1	7	392	147	44	0.12	0.19	1.87	0.04	242
99	23	1.15	1	7	392	147	44	0.12	0.19	1.87	0.04	242
26	18	1.22	0.40	3	148	—	6	0.02	0.08	0.27	—	43
33	29	1.11	0.84	17	151	71	11	0.07	0.10	0.56	0.08	44
176	84	3.94	1.58	618	668	43	22	0.07	0.11	1.32	0.15	—
153	58	2.32	0.74	90	694	32	22	0.12	0.10	1.80	0.21	111
56	22	0.94	0.42	6	154	2	14	0.09	0.13	0.78	0.09	63
34	18	0.81	0.58	12	125	2	14	0.06	0.13	1.01	—	166
33	29	1.11	0.84	17	151	71	11	0.07	0.10	0.56	0.08	45
58	97	2.74	0.72	346	1308	734	36	0.17	0.42	0.72	0.19	—
39	39	1.65	0.56	648	349	3	10	0.03	0.09	0.37	0.14	71
12	19	0.31	0.13	25	156	<1	3	0.02	<0.01	0.14	0.02	27
92	38	1.30	0.60	40	456	216	116	0.09	0.18	0.90	0.22	78
58	22	0.78	0.36	24	286	136	82	0.06	0.10	0.56	0.14	62
101	37	1.13	0.56	44	332	348	74	0.10	0.15	0.84	0.24	104
88	32	1.88	0.50	34	494	112	97	0.17	0.12	0.95	0.28	94
84	37	1.15	0.55	36	504	91	71	0.16	0.18	0.83	0.45	157
36	22	0.57	0.23	28	297	13	35	0.08	0.08	0.33	0.09	29
21	14	0.50	0.16	16	221	11	43	0.05	0.03	0.27	0.09	51
29	11	0.35	0.15	7	144	3	40	0.04	0.02	0.21	0.15	15
29	20	0.28	—	20	161	70	22	0.05	0.02	0.21	0.13	—
102	34	1.14	0.44	72	720	6335	21	0.23	0.14	0.95	0.53	9
48	20	0.96	0.46	104	354	3830	4	0.05	0.09	0.79	0.38	22
50	22	1.50	0.70	96	426	3239	7	0.05	0.07	1.04	0.28	20
48	16	0.54	0.22	38	356	3094	10	0.11	0.06	1.02	0.16	15
32	11	0.36	0.14	25	233	2025	7	0.07	0.04	0.67	0.11	10
46	14	0.58	0.18	15	355	2	72	0.08	0.06	0.63	0.23	66
44	14	0.52	0.30	8	400	2	69	0.08	0.06	0.68	0.25	63
44	16	0.74	0.24	32	250	4	56	0.07	0.10	0.56	0.16	74

Table continued on following page

APPENDIX A–1 **NUTRITIVE VALUES OF FOOD** *Continued*

	Approximate Measure	Weight (gm)	H_2O (gm)	Kcal	Protein (gm)	Carbohydrate (gm)	Dietary Fiber (gm)	Fat (gm)	MUFA (gm)	PUFA (gm)	Cholesterol (mg)	Calcium (mg)
Celery												
Pascal, fresh, diced	1 cup	120	114	20	1	4	2	0.2	<0.1	0.1	0	48
Pascal, fresh, stalk	1	40	38	6	<1	2	1	0.1	<0.1	<0.1	0	16
Collards												
Fresh, boiled, drained	1 cup	128	118	34	2	8	2	0.2	—	—	0	30
Frozen, boiled, drained	1 cup	170	150	61	5	12	5	0.7	—	—	0	357
Corn												
Cream, canned, low sodium	1 cup	256	202	186	5	46	3	1.1	0.3	0.5	0	8
Frozen, boiled, kernels	1 cup	165	124	134	5	34	4	0.1	<0.1	0.1	0	4
Kernels from 1 ear	1	77	54	83	3	19	7	1.0	0.3	0.5	0	2
Sweet, canned, cream style	1 cup	256	202	186	5	46	3	1.1	0.3	0.5	0	8
Sweet, canned, vacuum pack	1 cup	210	161	166	5	41	10	1.1	0.3	0.5	0	10
Cucumber, raw, sliced	1 cup	104	100	14	1	3	1	0.1	<0.1	<0.1	0	14
Dandelion greens, boiled	1 cup	105	94	35	2	7	4	0.6	—	—	0	147
Endive, raw, chopped	1 cup	50	47	8	1	2	—	0.1	<0.1	<0.1	0	26
Kale, frozen, boiled, drained	1 cup	130	118	39	4	7	4	0.6	0.1	0.3	0	179
Kohlrabi, raw	1 cup	140	127	38	3	9	3	0.1	<0.1	<0.1	0	34
Lettuce												
Butterhead, leaves	1 slice	15	14	2	<1	<1	<1	<0.1	<0.1	<0.1	0	5
Iceberg, raw, chopped	1 cup	55	53	7	<1	1	1	0.1	<0.1	0.1	0	11
Iceberg, raw, leaves	1 piece	20	19	3	1	<1	<1	<0.1	<0.1	<0.1	0	4
Romaine, raw, shredded	1 cup	56	53	9	1	1	1	0.1	<0.1	0.1	0	20
Mushrooms												
Boiled, drained	1	12	11	3	<1	1	<1	0.1	<0.1	<0.1	0	1
Canned, drained	1	12	11	3	<1	1	<1	<0.1	<0.1	<0.1	0	1
Raw, chopped	1 cup	70	64	18	2	3	1	0.3	<0.1	0.1	0	4
Okra, raw, boiled, drained	1 cup	160	144	51	3	12	2	0.3	<0.1	0.1	0	101
Onion rings, frozen	1	10	3	41	1	4	<1	2.7	1.1	0.5	0	3
Onions												
Mature, boiled, drained	1 cup	210	185	93	3	21	2	0.4	0.1	0.2	0	46
Mature, raw, chopped	1 cup	160	144	61	2	14	3	0.3	<0.1	0.1	0	32
Young green	1	5	5	1	<1	<1	<1	<0.1	0	0	0	3
Parsley, raw, chopped	1 tbsp	4	4	1	<1	<1	<1	<0.1	<0.1	<0.1	0	5
Parsnips, sliced, boiled, drained	1 cup	156	121	126	2	31	8	0.5	0.2	0.1	0	58
Peas												
Green, canned, drained	1 cup	170	139	118	8	21	7	0.6	<0.1	0.3	0	34
Green, frozen, boiled, drained	1 cup	160	127	125	8	23	6	0.4	<0.1	0.2	0	38
Peppers												
Hot chili, canned	1 cup	136	126	34	1	8	2	0.1	<0.1	0.1	0	10
Sweet, boiled, drained	1	73	67	20	<1	5	1	0.2	<0.1	0.1	0	7
Sweet, raw	1	74	68	20	1	5	1	0.1	<0.1	0.1	0	7
Potato chips—salt added	10 items	20	1	105	1	10	<1	7.1	1	3.6	4	5
Potato												
Au gratin, from mix	1 cup	245	193	228	6	32	4	32	2.8	0.3	—	204
Baked, flesh and skin	1	202	144	220	5	51	5	0.2	<0.1	0.1	0	20
Boiled, peel after	1	136	105	118	3	27	2	0.1	<0.1	0.1	0	7
Boiled, peel before	1	135	105	116	2	27	2	0.1	<0.1	0.1	0	10
French fried, frozen	1	5	3	11	<1	2	<1	0.4	0.2	<0.1	0	1
Hash brown, home recipe	1 cup	156	96	239	4	12	3.1	22	9.7	2.5	—	13
Mashed, dehydrated	1 cup	210	171	166	4	28	1.2	4.6	1.4	1.3	4	65
Mashed, fresh, prepared with milk	1 cup	210	165	162	4	37	1.2	1.2	0.3	0.1	4	55

Phosphate (mg)	Magnesium (mg)	Iron (mg)	Zinc (mg)	Sodium (mg)	Potassium (mg)	Vitamin A (RE)	Vitamin C (mg)	Thiamin (mg)	Riboflavin (mg)	Niacin (mg)	Vitamin B_6 (mg)	Folate (mcg)
30	14	0.48	0.16	104	340	16	8	0.05	0.05	0.39	0.10	34
10	4	0.16	0.05	35	115	5	3	0.02	0.02	0.13	0.04	11
10	10	0.20	0.14	21	168	349	15	0.03	0.07	0.37	0.07	8
46	52	1.90	0.46	85	427	1017	45	0.08	0.20	1.08	0.19	129
130	44	0.98	1.36	8	344	25	12	0.06	0.14	2.46	0.16	115
78	30	0.50	0.56	8	228	41	4	0.11	0.12	2.10	0.16	33
79	24	0.47	0.37	13	192	17	5	0.17	0.06	1.24	0.05	36
130	44	0.98	1.36	730	344	25	12	0.06	0.14	2.46	0.16	115
134	48	0.88	0.96	572	390	51	17	0.09	0.15	2.45	0.12	104
18	12	0.28	0.24	2	156	5	5	0.03	0.02	0.31	0.05	14
44	—	1.89	—	46	244	1229	19	0.14	0.18	—	—	—
14	8	0.42	0.40	12	158	103	3	0.04	0.04	0.20	0.01	71
36	23	1.22	0.23	20	417	826	33	0.06	0.15	0.87	0.11	19
64	27	0.56	—	28	490	5	87	0.07	0.03	0.56	0.21	—
4	2	0.04	0.03	1	39	15	1	0.01	0.01	0.05	<0.01	11
11	5	0.28	0.12	5	87	18	2	0.03	0.02	0.10	0.02	31
4	2	0.10	0.04	2	32	7	<1	<0.01	<0.01	0.04	<0.01	11
25	3	0.62	0.14	5	162	146	13	0.06	0.06	0.28	0.03	76
10	1	0.21	0.10	<1	43	0	<1	<0.01	0.04	0.54	0.01	2
8	2	0.10	0.09	51	16	0	0	0.01	<0.01	0.19	<0.01	2
73	7	0.87	0.51	3	259	0	3	0.07	0.31	2.88	0.07	15
90	91	0.72	0.88	8	515	92	26	0.21	0.09	1.39	0.30	73
8	2	0.17	0.04	38	13	2	<1	0.14	0.01	0.36	<0.01	1
74	23	0.50	0.44	6	349	0	11	0.09	0.05	0.35	0.27	32
53	16	0.35	0.30	5	251	0	10	0.07	0.03	0.24	0.19	30
2	1	0.10	0.02	<1	13	25	2	<0.01	<0.01	<0.01	—	<1
2	2	0.25	0.03	2	21	21	4	<0.01	<0.01	0.05	<0.01	7
108	45	0.91	0.41	16	573	0	20	0.13	0.08	1.13	0.15	91
114	30	1.62	1.20	372	294	131	16	0.21	0.13	1.24	0.11	75
144	46	2.51	1.50	139	269	107	16	0.45	0.16	2.37	0.18	94
23	19	0.68	0.23	1595	254	1617	92	0.03	0.07	1.09	0.21	14
13	7	0.34	0.09	2	121	43	54	0.04	0.02	0.35	0.17	11
14	7	0.34	0.09	2	131	47	66	0.05	0.02	0.38	0.18	16
31	12	0.24	0.21	94	260	0	8	0.03	0	0.84	0.10	9
233	37	0.78	0.59	1078	537	76	81	0.05	0.20	2.30	0.10	16
115	55	2.75	0.65	16	844	—	26	0.22	0.07	3.32	0.70	22
60	30	0.42	0.41	5	515	—	18	0.14	0.03	1.96	0.41	14
54	26	0.42	0.37	7	443	—	10	0.13	0.03	1.77	0.36	12
4	1	0.07	0.02	2	23	0	<1	<0.01	<0.01	0.12	0.01	<1
66	31	1.26	0.47	37	501	0	9	0.12	0.03	3.12	0.43	12
92	34	1.26	0.53	491	704	27	6	0.06	0.11	1.68	0.42	15
101	38	0.57	0.61	636	628	40	14	0.19	0.08	2.35	0.49	17

Table continued on following page

APPENDIX A–1 **NUTRITIVE VALUES OF FOOD** *Continued*

	Approximate Measure	Weight (gm)	H_2O (gm)	Kcal	Protein (gm)	Carbohy-drate (gm)	Dietary Fiber (gm)	Fat (gm)	MUFA (gm)	PUFA (gm)	Cholesterol (mg)	Calcium (mg)
Salad	1 cup	250	190	358	6.7	28	5.3	21	6.2	9.3	170	48
Scalloped, prepared from mix	1 cup	245	198	228	5	31	4.7	11	3.0	0.5	—	88
Pumpkin, canned	1 cup	245	220	83	2.7	20	5.0	0.7	0.1	<0.1	0	64
Radishes, raw	1	4.5	4	1	<1	<1	<1	<0.1	<0.1	<0.1	0	1
Rutabagas, boiled, drained	1 cup	170	153	58	1.9	13	2.5	0.3	<0.1	0.1	0	71
Sauerkraut, canned	1 cup	236	218	45	2.2	10	6.1	0.3	<0.1	0.1	0	71
Spinach, canned, solids/liquids	1 cup	234	218	45	4.9	7	5.1	0.9	<0.1	0.4	0	194
Fresh, boiled, drained	1 cup	180	164	41	5.4	7	4.0	0.5	<0.1	0.2	0	245
Frozen, boiled, chopped	1 cup	205	184	57	6.4	11	4.5	0.4	<0.1	0.2	0	299
Raw, chopped	1 cup	56	51	12	1.6	2	1.5	0.2	<0.1	<0.1	0	55
Squash												
Acorn, baked	1 cup	205	170	115	2.3	30	4.3	0.3	<0.1	0.1	0	90
Butternut, baked	1 cup	205	180	82	1.8	22	3.5	0.2	<0.1	<0.1	0	84
Summer, boiled, sliced	1 cup	180	169	36	1.6	8	2.5	0.6	<0.1	0.2	0	49
Zucchini, frozen, boiled	1 cup	223	211	38	2.6	8	3.2	0.3	<0.1	0.1	0	38
Succotash, boiled, drained	1 cup	192	131	222	9.7	47	14	1.5	0.3	0.7	0	32
Sweet potato												
Baked, peeled	1	114	83	118	2.0	28	3.4	0.1	<0.1	<0.1	0	32
Candied	1 piece	105	70	144	0.9	29	1.1	3.4	0.7	0.2	0	27
Canned, vacuum	1 cup	200	152	183	3.3	42	4.8	0.4	<0.1	0.2	0	44
Tomato juice, canned	1 cup	244	228	42	1.9	10	2.9	0.1	<0.1	0.1	0	20
Tomato												
Raw, red, ripe	1	123	115	26	1.0	6	1.6	0.4	0.1	0.2	0	6
Red, canned, stewed	1 cup	225	233	68	2.4	17	2.0	0.4	0.1	0.2	0	84
Turnip greens												
Frozen, boiled	1 cup	164	149	50	6	8	5.1	0.7	0.1	0.3	0	251
Raw, boiled	1 cup	144	134	29	2	6	2.9	0.3	<0.1	0.1	0	198
Turnips, boiled, drained, diced	1 cup	156	146	28	1	8	3.1	0.1	<0.1	<0.1	0	34
V-8 vegetable juice	1 cup	243	—	49	0	10	2.4	0	0	0	0	29
Water chestnuts, Chinese, canned	1 cup	140	121	70	1	17	—	0.1	<0.1	<0.1	0	6
Miscellaneous items												
Baking chocolate												
Unsweetened/liquid	1 oz	28.4	<1	134	4	10	—	14	3	3	0	15
Chocolate chips, real, semisweet	1 oz	28.4	—	132	1	19	—	8	—	—	0	8
Baking powder for home use, sodium aluminum sulfate with:												
Monocalcium phosphate monohydrate	1 tsp	3	<0.1	4	<1	1	—	0	0	0	0	58
Monocalcium phosphate monohydrate and calcium sulfate	1 tsp	3.8	<0.1	5	<1	1	—	0	0	0	0	239
Low sodium	1 tsp	4.3	<0.1	7	<1	2	—	0	0	0	0	207
Beer												
Regular	12 fl oz	356	329	146	1	13	0.8	0	0	0	0	18
Light	12 fl oz	354	337	99	<1	5	0	0	0	0	0	18
Carbonated beverages												
Club soda	8 fl oz	237	237	0	0	0	0	0	0	0	0	12
Cola-type soft drink	12 fl oz	370	330	151	0	38	0	0	0	0	0	11
Diet cola soft drink with Nutrasweet	12 fl oz	355	354	4	<1	<1	0	0	0	0	0	14
Cream soda	12 fl oz	371	322	190	0	49	0	0	0	0	0	19
Orange soda	12 fl oz	372	326	180	0	46	—	0	0	0	0	24
Root beer	12 fl oz	370	330	151	0	39	0	0	0	0	0	19
Tonic water, quinine soda	8 fl oz	244	222	83	0	21	0	0	0	0	0	2

Phosphate (mg)	Magnesium (mg)	Iron (mg)	Zinc (mg)	Sodium (mg)	Potassium (mg)	Vitamin A (RE)	Vitamin C (mg)	Thiamin (mg)	Riboflavin (mg)	Niacin (mg)	Vitamin B_6 (mg)	Folate (mcg)
130	38	1.63	0.78	1323	635	83	25	0.19	0.15	2.23	0.35	17
137	34	0.93	0.61	835	498	51	81	0.04	0.14	2.59	0.10	23
86	56	3.41	0.42	12	505	5404	10	0.06	0.13	0.90	0.14	30
<1	<1	0.01	0.01	1	10	<1	1	0	<0.01	0.01	<0.01	1
83	36	0.80	0.51	31	488	0	37	0.12	0.06	1.07	0.15	26
47	31	3.47	0.45	1560	401	5	35	0.05	0.05	0.34	0.31	56
75	131	3.70	0.98	746	538	1505	32	0.04	0.25	0.63	0.19	136
101	157	6.43	1.37	126	839	1474	18	0.17	0.43	0.88	0.44	262
98	141	3.12	1.44	176	611	1595	25	0.12	0.34	0.86	0.30	220
27	44	1.52	0.30	44	312	376	16	0.04	0.11	0.41	0.11	108
92	88	1.91	0.35	8	896	88	22	0.34	0.03	1.81	0.40	38
55	60	1.23	0.27	8	582	1435	31	0.15	0.04	1.99	0.25	39
69	44	0.65	0.71	2	346	52	10	0.08	0.07	0.92	0.12	36
56	29	1.07	0.45	5	433	96	8	0.09	0.09	0.86	0.10	17
224	102	2.93	1.22	32	787	56	16	0.32	0.18	2.55	0.22	—
62	23	0.52	0.33	12	397	2488	28	0.08	0.15	0.69	0.28	26
27	12	1.19	0.16	73	198	440	7	0.02	0.04	0.41	0.04	12
98	45	1.77	0.36	107	625	1597	53	0.07	0.11	1.48	0.38	33
46	28	1.42	0.36	882	536	136	45	0.11	0.08	1.64	0.27	48
30	13	0.55	0.11	11	273	77	24	0.07	0.06	0.77	0.10	18
51	29	1.86	0.42	647	611	142	34	0.12	0.09	1.82	—	7
56	42	3.18	0.68	25	368	1308	36	0.09	0.12	0.77	0.11	65
41	32	1.15	0.20	41	293	792	40	0.07	0.10	0.59	0.26	171
30	13	0.34	—	78	211	0	18	0.04	0.04	0.47	0.11	14
—	—	1.46	—	819	513	342	49	0.05	0.05	1.70	—	—
28	6	1.22	0.54	12	164	<1	2	0.02	0.03	0.50	—	—
96	75	1.18	1.04	3	330	—	—	0.01	—	0.59	—	—
43	31	0.73	0.67	<1	89	6	0	<0.01	0.03	0.13	<0.01	<1
87	—	0	—	329	5	0	0	0	0	0	—	—
359	—	0	—	312	7	0	0	0	0	0	—	—
314	—	0	—	<1	471	0	0	0	0	0	—	—
43	21	0.11	0.07	18	89	0	0	0.02	0.09	1.62	0.18	21
43	18	0.14	0.11	11	64	0	0	0.04	0.11	1.39	0.12	14
0	2	0.02	0.24	50	5	0	0	0	0	0	0	0
44	4	0.11	0.04	15	4	0	0	0	0	0	0	0
32	4	0.11	0.29	21	0	0	0	0.01	0.08	0	0	0
0	4	0.18	0.26	45	4	0	0	0	0	0	0	0
0	0	0.24	0.36	48	12	0	0	0	0	0	0	0
0	4	0.18	0.26	48	4	0	0	0	0	0	0	0
0	0	0.02	0.25	10	0	0	0	0	0	0	0	0

Table continued on following page

APPENDIX A–1 **NUTRITIVE VALUES OF FOOD** *Continued*

	Approximate Measure	Weight (gm)	H_2O (gm)	Kcal	Protein (gm)	Carbohydrate (gm)	Dietary Fiber (gm)	Fat (gm)	MUFA (gm)	PUFA (gm)	Cholesterol (mg)	Calcium (mg)
Coffee												
Brewed	8 fl oz	235	237	<1	<1	1	0	0	0	0	0	5
Instant	8 fl oz	239	237	5	<1	<1	0	0	0	<0.1	0	7
Gatorade	8 fl oz	241	225	60	0	15	0	0	0	0	0	0
Gelatin, dry, envelope	1 item	7	1	25	6	0	0	0	0	0	0	0
Gelatin dessert, prepared	1 cup	240	202	140	4	34	0	0	0	0	0	—
Mineral water	8 fl oz	237	237	0	0	0	0	0	0	0	0	33
Mustard, yellow, prepared	1 tsp	5	4	5	<1	<1	<0.1	<1	0	0	0	4
Olives												
Green, pickled, canned	4	16	13	15	<1	<1	0.4	2	1	0.1	0	8
Mission, ripe, canned	4	12	9	20	<1	<1	0.4	3	2	0.1	0	12
Pickles												
Pickle/hot dog relish	1 oz	28.4	18	35	0	8	—	0	0	0	0	6
Dill, cucumber, medium	4	260	242	20	0	4	3.1	0	0	0	0	68
Sweet/gherkin, small	4	60	37	80	0	20	0.7	0	0	0	0	8
Sauces												
Barbecue	1 tbsp	15.6	13	12	<1	2	0.1	<1	0.1	0.1	0	3
White, medium, enriched	1 cup	250	183	405	10	22	—	31	8	0.8	33	288
Tea												
Brewed	8 fl oz	237	236	2	0	<1	0	0	0	<0.1	0	0
Instant, sweetened	8 fl oz	259	236	88	<1	22	0	0	<0.1	<0.1	0	5
Tomato catsup	1 tbsp	15	10	15	0	4	—	0	0	0	0	3
Vinegar, cider	1 tbsp	15	14	0	0	1	0	0	0	0	0	1
Whiskey/gin/rum/vodka												
80 proof	1 fl oz	27.8	19	64	0	0	0	0	0	0	0	0
86 proof	1 fl oz	27.8	18	70	0	0	0	0	0	0	0	0
90 proof	1 fl oz	27.7	17	73	0	0	0	0	0	0	0	0
Yeast												
Bakers, dry, packet	1 serving	7	<1	20	3	3	2.2	0	0	0	0	3
Brewers, dry	1 tbsp	8	<1	25	3	3	—	0	0	0	0	17

Nutrient data from *Nutritionist III*, version 7.0 software. Salem, OR.

Phosphate (mg)	Magnesium (mg)	Iron (mg)	Zinc (mg)	Sodium (mg)	Potassium (mg)	Vitamin A (RE)	Vitamin C (mg)	Thiamin (mg)	Riboflavin (mg)	Niacin (mg)	Vitamin B_6 (mg)	Folate (mcg)
2	12	0.12	0.05	5	128	0	0	0	0	0.53	0	<1
7	10	0.12	0.07	7	86	0	0	0	<0.1	0.67	0	0
22	2	0.12	0.05	96	27	0	0	0.02	0	0	0	0
0	—	0.40	—	8	180	—	4	0	0	0	0	—
—	—	—	—	0	—	—	—	—	—	—	—	—
0	0	0	0	2	0	0	0	0	0	0	0	0
4	2	0.10	—	65	7	—	—	—	—	—	—	—
2	—	0.20	—	323	7	4	—	—	—	—	—	<1
1	—	0.13	0.04	77	3	4	—	0	0	—	0	<1
4	—	0.19	—	200	—	—	—	—	—	—	—	—
56	31	2.80	0.70	3712	520	28	16	0	0.04	0	0.02	3
8	<1	0.80	0.08	512	—	4	4	0	0	0	<0.01	<1
3	3	0.14	0.03	127	27	14	1	<0.01	<0.01	0.14	0.01	<1
233	38	0.50	0.52	796	348	115	2	0.12	0.43	0.70	0.06	—
2	7	0.05	0.05	7	88	0	0	0	<0.01	0	0	12
3	5	0.05	0.08	8	49	0	0	0	0.05	0.09	<1	10
8	4	0.10	0.03	156	54	21	2	0.01	0.01	0.20	0.02	<1
1	—	0.10	0.02	<1	15	—	—	—	—	—	0	—
1	0	0.03	0.02	<1	<1	0	0	<0.01	0	0	0	0
1	0	0.01	0.01	<1	<1	0	0	<0.01	0	0.01	0	0
0	0	0	0	<1	0	0	0	0	0	0	0	0
90	4	1.10	—	1	140	0	0	0.16	0.38	2.60	0.14	286
140	18	1.40	—	9	152	0	0	1.25	0.34	3.00	0.20	313

APPENDIX A–2 **PRODUCT INFORMATION FOR MEDICAL FOODS***

Product (Manufacturer)	Kcal/ml	mOsm/kg	CHO, gm (% kcal)	Protein, gm (% kcal)	Fat, gm (% kcal)	Fiber, gm	Volume (ml) for 100% RDA	Comments
Milk-Based Products for Nutritional Supplements								
Carnation Instant Breakfast† (Clintec)	1.0	671–758**	126 (53)	53 (21)	30 (26)	None	1060‡	Powder; flavored; contains lactose
Delmark Instant Breakfast† (Delmark)	1.0	500	137 (53)	48 (19)	32 (29)	None	1000	Contains lactose; available in powdered or liquid form
Forta Shake† (Ross)	1.0		148 (51)	68 (24)	32 (25)	None	1000	Contains lactose
Meritene Powder† (Sandoz)	1.06	690	120 (45)	69 (26)	34 (29)	None	1040	Powder; contains lactose; flavored
Sustacal Powder† (Mead Johnson)	1.35	1000	180 (54)	77 (23)	35 (23)	None	810	Contains lactose
1.0 kcal/ml Polymeric Formulas for Tube Feeding or Nutrition Supplements§								
Ensure with Fiber (Ross)	1.1	480	162 (55)	40 (15)	37 (31)	14	1400	Flavored
Ensure (Ross)	1.06	470	145 (55)	37 (14)	37 (32)	None	1887	Flavored
Ensure HN (Ross)	1.06	470	141 (53)	44 (17)	36 (30)	None	1321	Flavored; nutrient dense, high nitrogen
Nutrilan, flavors (Elan Pharma)	1.06	450	143 (54)	38 (14)	37 (31)	None	1900	Flavored
Nutren 1.0 (Clintec)	1.00	300–390**	127 (51)	40 (16)	38 (33)	None	1500	Available in flavors and with fiber (14 gm/1000 ml)
Promote (Ross)	1.0	350	130 (52)	62 (25)	26 (23)	None	1250	Flavored; high nitrogen, nutrient-dense, fat blend recommended by American Heart Association, contains omega-3 fatty acids, fortified with ultratrace minerals,§ carnitine and taurine
Resource (Sandoz)	1.06	430	140 (54)	37 (14)	37 (32)	None	1890	Flavored
Sustacal Liquid (Mead Johnson)	1.0	650	140 (55)	61 (24)	23 (21)	None	1080	High nitrogen, flavored
Sustacal with Fiber (Mead Johnson)	1.06	480	140 (53)	46 (17)	35 (30)	6	1420	Flavored
Sustacal 8.8 (Mead Johnson)	1.06	500	148 (56)	37 (14)	35 (30)	None	1890	Nutrient dense, flavored
1.0 kcal/ml Polymeric Formulas Primarily for Tube Feedings								
Attain (Sherwood)	1.0	300	135 (54)	40 (16)	35 (30)	None	1250	50% of fats from MCT
Compleat Modified (Sandoz)	1.07	300	140 (53)	43 (16)	37 (31)	4.2	1500	Blenderized from natural foods; contains ultratrace minerals‖
Compleat Regular (Sandoz)	1.07	450	130 (48)	43 (16)	43 (36)	4.2	1500	Blenderized from natural foods; contains lactose and ultratrace minerals‖
Entralife (Corpak)	1.0	300	137 (55)	35 (14)	35 (31)	None	1285	50% of fat from MCT
Entralife HN (Corpak)	1.0	300	133 (53)	42 (17)	34 (30)	None	1250	Available with fiber (14 gm/1000 ml); 50% of fat from MCT

APPENDIX A–2 **PRODUCT INFORMATION FOR MEDICAL FOODS**[*] *Continued*

Product (Manufacturer)	Kcal/ml	mOsm/kg	CHO, gm (% kcal)	Protein, gm (% kcal)	Fat, gm (% kcal)	Fiber, gm	Volume (ml) for 100% RDA	Comments
Entralife HN-II (Corpak)	1.25	300	153 (49)	61 (20)	44 (31)	None	1250	Fortified with ultratrace minerals;[ǁ] 50% of fat from MCT
Entrition (Clintec)	1.0	300	136 (55)	35 (14)	35 (32)	None	2000	
Entrition, half strength (Clintec)	0.5	120	68 (55)	18 (14)	18 (32)	None	N/A	Diluted strength for transitional feedings or intolerance
Entrition, HN (Clintec)	1.0	300	114 (46)	44 (18)	41 (37)	None	1300	High nitrogen
Entrition RDA (Clintec)	1.0	300	135 (54)	36 (14)	35 (32)	None	1500	For volume-sensitive clients or with fluid restriction
Entrition with Fiber (Clintec)	1.0	300	127 (51)	40 (16)	38 (33)	14	1500	Contains ultratrace minerals[ǁ]
Fibersource (Sandoz)	1.2	390	170 (56)	43 (14)	41 (30)	10	1500	Contains ultratrace minerals[ǁ] and 50% of fat from MCT
Fibersource HN (Sandoz)	1.2	390	160 (52)	53 (18)	41 (30)	6.8	1500	High nitrogen; contains ultratrace minerals,[ǁ] 50% of fat from MCTs
Introlite (Ross)	0.53	250	71 (54)	22 (17)	18 (30)	None	700	Diluted strength for transitional feedings or intolerance; fortified with ultratrace minerals[ǁ]
Isocal (Mead Johnson)	1.06	270	135 (50)	34 (13)	44 (37)	None	1890	General isotonic formula for tube feeding
Isocal HN (Mead Johnson)	1.06	270	123 (46)	44 (17)	45 (37)	None	1250	Nutrient dense, high nitrogen
Isosource (Sandoz)	1.2	360	170 (56)	43 (14)	41 (30)	None	1500	Contains ultratrace minerals,[ǁ] 50% of fat from MCT
Isosource HN (Sandoz)	1.2	330	160 (52)	53 (18)	41 (30)	None	1500	High nitrogen; contains ultratrace minerals,[ǁ] taurine and carnitine; 50% of fat from MCT
Isotein HN (Sandoz)	1.2	300	160 (52)	68 (23)	34 (25)	None	1770	Powder; high nitrogen; contains ultratrace minerals[ǁ]
Jevity (Ross)	1.06	310	152 (53)	44 (17)	37 (30)	14	1320	Fortified with ultratrace minerals,[ǁ] taurine and carnitine; 50% fat from MCTs
Introlan (Elan Pharma)	0.53	150	70 (53)	23 (17)	18 (30)	None	2000	Fortified with ultratrace minerals;[ǁ] 50% fat from MCTs
Nitrolan (Elan Pharma)	1.24	310	160 (52)	60 (19)	40 (29)	None	1250	Fortified with ultratrace minerals;[ǁ] 50% fat from MCTs

Table continued on following page

Product (Manufacturer)	Kcal/ml	mOsm/kg	CHO, gm (% kcal)	Protein, gm (% kcal)	Fat, gm (% kcal)	Fiber, gm	Volume (ml) for 100% RDA	Comments
Isolan (Elan Pharma)	1.06	300	144 (54)	40 (15)	36 (31)	None	1250	Fortified with ultratrace minerals;‖ 50% fat from MCTs
Fiberlan (Elan Pharma)	1.2	310	160 (52)	50 (17)	40 (30)	14	1250	Fortified with ultratrace minerals;‖ 50% fat from MCTs
Osmolite (Ross)	1.06	300	145 (55)	37 (14)	39 (31)	None	1887	50% of fats from MCTs; fortified with ultratrace minerals‖
Osmolite HN (Ross)	1.06	300	141 (53)	44 (17)	37 (30)	None	1321	50% of fats from MCTs; fortified with ultratrace minerals‖
Preattain (Sherwood)	0.5	150	120 (48)	40 (16)	40 (36)	None	1600	Diluted strength for transitional feeding or intolerance
Profiber (Sherwood)	1.0	300	132 (48)	40 (16)	40 (36)	12	1500	Fortified with ultratrace minerals‖
Replete (Clintec)	1.0	350	113 (45)	63 (25)	33 (30)	None	1500	Flavored; high nitrogen; available with fiber
Ultracal (Mead Johnson)	1.06	310	123 (46)	44 (17)	45 (37)	14	1180	High nitrogen; nutrient dense; 60% canola oil, 40% MCT; flavored
Vitaneed (Sherwood)	1.0	300	128 (48)	40 (16)	40 (36)	8	1500	Blenderized using natural foods
> 1.5 kcal/ml Polymeric Formulas for Tube Feedings or Nutrition Supplement								
Comply (Sherwood)	1.5	410	180 (48)	60 (16)	60 (36)	None	1000	Unflavored and flavored available
Ensure Plus (Ross)	1.5	690	200 (53)	55 (15)	53 (32)	None	1420	High kilocalorie, flavored
Ensure Plus HN (Ross)	1.5	690	200 (53)	63 (17)	50 (30)	None	947	High kilocalorie; high nitrogen; flavored
Entrition (Clintec)	1.5	420	170 (45)	60 (16)	68 (39)	None	1000	Contains MCT and ultratrace minerals‖
Isocal HCN (Mead Johnson)	2.0	640	200 (40)	75 (15)	102 (45)	None	1000	High kilocalorie; high nitrogen; fortified with ultratrace minerals‖
Magnacal (Sherwood)	2.0	590	250 (50)	70 (14)	80 (36)	None	1000	Flavored
Ultra (Elan Pharma)	1.5	610	202 (54)	60 (16)	50 (30)	None	1000	Fortified with ultratrace minerals,‖ 50% fat from MCTs
Nutren 1.5 (Clintec)	1.5	410–590**	170 (45)	60 (16)	68 (39)	None	1000	Flavored available; less sweet taste; 50% of fat from MCTs
Nutren 2.0 (Clintec)	2.0	710	196 (39)	80 (16)	106 (45)	None	750	Flavored; less sweet taste
Resource Plus (Sandoz)	1.5	600	200 (53)	55 (15)	53 (32)	None	1600	Flavored
Sustacal HC (Mead Johnson)	1.5	670	190 (50)	61 (16)	58 (34)	None	1180	Flavored
Two Cal HN (Ross)	2	690	217 (43)	84 (17)	91 (40)	None	947	High nitrogen, fortified with ultratrace minerals;‖

Product (Manufacturer)	Kcal/ml	mOsm/kg	CHO, gm (% kcal)	Protein, gm (% kcal)	Fat, gm (% kcal)	Fiber, gm	Volume (ml) for 100% RDA	Comments
								designed for stressed clients
Formulas for Specific Conditions								
METABOLICALLY STRESSED								
Criticare HN (Mead Johnson)	1.06	650	220 (82)	38 (14)	5 (5)	None	1890	Equal percentage of free amino acids and small peptides; fortified with additional amounts of vitamin C and B-complex vitamins
Impact (Sandoz)	1.0	375	132 (53)	56 (22)	28 (25)	None	1500	High protein (intact), enriched with arginine, RNA, and omega-3 fatty acids; contains ultratrace minerals;[‖] available with fiber (10 gm/1000 ml)
Perative (Ross)	1.3	425	177 (55)	67 (21)	37 (25)	None	1155	Small peptides (elemental); enriched with arginine, carnitine, taurine, and ultratrace minerals[‖]
Reabilan HN (O'Brien)	1.33	490	158 (48)	58 (18)	52 (35)	None	1875	High nitrogen; small peptides
Replete (Clintec)	1.0	290–350	113 (45)	63 (25)	33 (30)	None	1000	Available flavored and unflavored without or with fiber (10 gm fiber/1000 ml); foritifed with vitamins A and C, zinc, and glutamine to promote healing
Stresstein (Sandoz)	1.2	910	170 (57)	70 (23)	28 (20)	None	2000	Powder; BCAA enriched; contains MCTs and ultratrace minerals[‖]
Traumacal (Mead Johnson)	1.5	490	145 (38)	83 (22)	68 (40)	None	3000	High kilocalorie; high nitrogen; moderate CHO; increased amounts of nutrients needed for wound healing
Traum-Aid (McGaw)	1.0	760	166 (66)	56 (22)	5 (4)	None	3000	Powder; amino acids, BCAA-enriched; 40% MCT
IMPAIRED GI FUNCTION								
Accupep HPF (Sherwood)	1.0	490	188 (76)	40 (16)	10 (9)	None	1600	Powder, hydrolyzed protein (elemental), 50% of fat from MCTs

Table continued on following page

APPENDIX A–2 **PRODUCT INFORMATION FOR MEDICAL FOODS*** *Continued*

Product (Manufacturer)	Kcal/ml	mOsm/kg	CHO, gm (% kcal)	Protein, gm (% kcal)	Fat, gm (% kcal)	Fiber, gm	Volume (ml) for 100% RDA	Comments
Alitraq (Ross)	1.0	575	165 (66)	53 (21)	16 (13)	None	1500	Powdered; flavored; peptides and free amino acids (elemental), supplemented with glutamine and arginine; fortified with ultratrace minerals,‖ taurine and carnitine; designed for metabolically stressed clients with impaired GI function
Lipisorb (Mead Johnson)	1.0	320	116 (46)	35 (14)	48 (40)	None	1970	Powder; flavored; unique MCT formulation for fat malabsorption
Peptamen (Clintec)	1.0	270	127 (51)	40 (16)	39 (33)	None	1500	Flavored; peptides and free amino acids (elemental); supplemented with glutamine, arginine, ultratrace minerals,‖ taurine and carnitine; 70% of fat from MCT; designed for metabolically stressed client with impaired GI function
Reabilan (Elan Pharma)	1	350	131 (53)	31 (13)	39 (35)	None	2250	Short-chain peptides
Travasorb HN (Clintec)	1.0	560	175 (70)	45 (18)	14 (12)	None	2000	Powder; peptide (elemental); 60% of fat from MCT
Tolerex (Sandoz)	1.0	550	230 (91)	21 (8)	2 (1)	None	3160	Powder; free amino acids (elemental)
Vital HN (Ross)	1.0	500	185 (74)	42 (17)	11 (9)	None	1500	Powder; free amino acids (elemental); high nitrogen; enriched with ultratrace minerals‖
Vivonex TEN (Sandoz)	1.0	630	206 (82)	38 (15)	3 (3)	None	2000	Powder; free amino acids; BCAA-enriched with glutamine and arginine
GLUCOSE INTOLERANCE								
Glucerna (Ross)	1.0	375	94 (33)	42 (17)	56 (50)	None	1422	Oral or tube feeding use; fat blend emphasizing monounsaturated fatty acids; fortified with ultratrace minerals,‖ carnitine and taurine

APPENDIX A–2 **PRODUCT INFORMATION FOR MEDICAL FOODS*** *Continued*

Product (Manufacturer)	Kcal/ml	mOsm/kg	CHO, gm (% kcal)	Protein, gm (% kcal)	Fat, gm (% kcal)	Fiber, gm	Volume (ml) for 100% RDA	Comments
RENAL DISORDERS								
Amin-aid (Kendall McGaw)	1.9	700	366 (75)	19 (4)	46 (21)	None	N/A	Nutritionally incomplete; powder; EAA plus histamine
Nepro (Ross)	2	635	215 (43)	70 (14)	96 (43)	None	950¶	Flavored; high kilocalorie, moderate protein, low electrolytes, low fluid; designed for clients with chronic or acute renal failure on dialysis
Suplena (Ross)	2	600	255 (51)	30 (6)	96 (43)	None	950¶	High kilocalorie, low protein, low electrolyte, low fluid; contains carnitine and taurine; designed for nondialyzed renal clients; flavored
Travasorb Renal (Clintec)	1.35	590	270 (81)	23 (7)	18 (12)	None	N/A	Nutritionally incomplete (only water-soluble vitamins present); EAA, contains histidine and arginine; 70% fat from MCT
HEPATIC CONDITIONS								
Hepatic-Aid II (Kendall McGaw)	1.17	560	168 (57)	44 (15)	36 (28)	None	N/A	Nutritionally incomplete; powder; amino acids; BCAA-enriched; low aromatic amino acids and methionine; contains arginine
Travasorb Hepatic (Clintec)	1.1	600	215 (77)	29 (11)	15 (12)	None	2268	Powder; flavors available; high in BCAA, low in aromatic amino acids; 70% of fat from MCT
PULMONARY CONDITIONS								
Nutrivent (Clintec)	1.5	450	100 (27)	68 (18)	94 (55)	None	1000	High fat with MCT
Pulmocare (Ross)	1.5	520	106 (28)	63 (17)	92 (55)	None	950	Flavored; high fat, low CHO; fortified with ultratrace minerals‖

* Medical foods have been defined by FDA to be foods that are formulated to be consumed or administered enterally under the supervision of a physician and intended for the specific dietary management of a disease or condition for which distinctive nutritional requirements based on recognized scientific principles are established by medical evaluation. These foods are exempt from current food labeling laws. Unless otherwise indicated, all formulas are liquid, ready to use, lactose free, and nutritionally adequate when the amount indicated is provided.

† Made with 8 oz whole milk.

‡ Except biotin.

§ Formulas are frequently flavored, making them suitable for oral or tube feedings.

‖ Ultratrace minerals include selenium, chromium, and molybdenum.

¶ Except phosphorus, magnesium, and vitamins A and D, which are limited on renal diets.

** Variations due to added flavors.

Clintec Nutrition Co., Deerfield IL 60015-0760; Delmark Foods, a division of Sandoz Nutrition Food Service, Minneapolis, MN 55440; Ross Laboratories, Columbus, OH 43216; Mead Johnson Enteral Nutritionals, Evansville, IN 47721; Sandoz Nutrition Corporation, Minneapolis, MN 55440; Corpak, Inc., Wheeling, IL 60090; Elan Pharma, Cambridge, MA 02141; Sherwood Medical Company, St. Louis, MO 63103; Kendall McGaw Inc., Irvine, CA 92714-5895.

(CHO, carbohydrate; MCT, medium chain triglycerides; BcAA, branched chain amino acids; EAA, essential amino acids; ROA, recommended dietary allowances; N/A, not available.)

Nutrient data from *Nutritionist III,* Version 7.0 software. Salem, OR.

APPENDIX A–3 **NUTRITIONAL ANALYSIS OF FAST FOODS**

	Approximate Measure	Weight (mg)	Kcal	Protein (gm)	Carbohydrate (gm)	Fat (gm)	MUFA (mg)	PUFA (mg)	Cholesterol (mg)
Arby's									
Beef and Cheese Sandwich	1 item	176	402	32	27	18	3.7	3.5	77
Chicken Breast Sandwich	1 item	184	493	23	48	25	9.6	10.3	91
Club Sandwich	1 item	252	560	30	43	30	—	—	100
Ham and Cheese Sandwich	1 item	146	353	21	33	16	6.7	1.4	58
Roast Beef Sandwich	1 item	139	346	22	34	14	6.8	1.7	52
Boston Clam Chowder	1 serving	227	207	10	18	11	5	2	28
Tomato Florentine Soup	1 serving	227	84	3	15	2	1	1	2
Wisconsin Cheese Soup	1 serving	227	287	9	19	19	8	3	31
Super Roast Beef	1 item	234	501	25	50	22	8.2	5.4	40
Turkey Deluxe	1 item	236	510	28	46	24	—	—	70
Burger King									
Bacon Double Cheeseburger Deluxe	1 serving	195	592	33	28	39	14	6	111
Barbecue Bacon Double Cheese	1 item	174	536	32	31	31	13	2	105
Broiler	1 item	168	379	24	31	18	—	—	53
Broiler Sauce	1 serving	14	90	0	0	10	2	5	7
Chicken Tender	1 piece	90	39	3	2	2	<1	0.5	8
Croissant with Egg and Cheese	1 item	127	369	13	24	25	7.5	1.4	216
Croissant with Egg, Cheese, Ham	1 item	152	475	19	24	34	11	2.4	213
Double Cheeseburger	1 item	172	483	30	29	27	11	2	100
Fish Tenders	1 serving	99	267	12	18	16	7	4	28
Mushroom, Swiss, Double Cheese Burger	1 item	176	473	31	27	27	11	2	95
Ranch Dip Sauce	1 serving	28	171	0	2	18	4	10	0
Sweet/Sour Sauce	1 serving	28	45	0	11	0	0	0	0
Tartar Dip Sauce	1 serving	28	174	0	3	18	4	11	16
Tater Tenders	1 serving	71	213	2	25	12	6	3	3
Whopper Hamburger	1 item	261	630	26	50	36	14	2.2	104
Dairy Queen									
Banana Split	1 item	383	540	10	91	15	—	—	30
Dip Cone—regular	1 item	156	300	7	40	13	—	—	20
Float	1 item	397	330	6	59	8	—	—	20
Cone—regular	1 item	142	226	5	33	8	2.5	0.5	38
Malt—regular	1 item	418	600	15	89	20	—	—	50
Sundae—regular	1 item	177	319	6	53	10	2.6	0.9	23
Hardees									
Bacon and Egg Biscuit	1 serving	124	410	15	35	24	14	5	155
Bacon, Egg, and Cheese Biscuit	1 serving	137	460	17	35	28	15	5	165
Big Country Breakfast with Bacon	1 serving	217	660	24	51	40	22	8	305
Big Country Breakfast with Country Ham	1 serving	254	670	29	52	38	21	8	345
Big Country Breakfast with Ham	1 serving	251	620	28	51	33	19	8	325
Big Country Breakfast with Sausage	1 serving	274	850	33	51	57	31	11	340
Big Roast Beef	1 serving	134	300	18	32	11	5	2	45
Big Twin	1 serving	173	450	23	34	25	9	5	55
Biscuit n' Gravy	1 serving	221	440	9	45	24	14	5	15
Chick n' Pasta Salad	1 serving	414	230	27	23	3	1	1	55
Crispy Curls	1 serving	85	300	4	36	16	8	5	0
Grilled Chicken Sandwich	1 serving	192	310	24	34	9	3	5	60
Ham and Egg Biscuit	1 serving	138	370	15	35	19	12	4	160
Ham, Egg, and Cheese Biscuit	1 serving	151	420	18	35	23	13	4	170
Mushroom n' Swiss Burger	1 serving	186	490	30	33	27	12	2	70
Regular Roast Beef	1 serving	114	260	15	31	9	4	2	35
The Lean One	1 item	220	420	27	37	18	8	2	85
Three Pancakes	1 serving	137	280	8	56	2	1	1	15
Jack in the Box									
Breakfast Jack Sandwich	1 item	121	301	18	28	13	—	—	182
Jumbo Jack Hamburger	1 item	246	551	28	45	29	12.6	2.4	80
Jumbo Jack with Cheese	1 item	272	628	32	45	35	12.6	2.0	110
Moby Jack	1 item	141	455	17	38	26	—	—	56
Onion Rings—bag	1 item	83	275	4	31	16	6.7	0.7	14

Calcium (mg)	Iron (mg)	Sodium (mg)	Potassium (mg)	Vitamin A (RE)	Vitamin C (mg)	Thiamin (mg)	Riboflavin (mg)	Niacin (mg)	Vitamin B_6 (mg)	Folate (mcg)
183	5.05	1634	345	58	0	0.38	0.46	5.90	0.34	41
—	—	1019	330	—	—	—	—	—	—	—
200	3.60	1610	—	—	—	0.68	0.43	7.00	—	—
130	3.25	772	290	96	3	0.31	0.49	2.69	0.20	71
54	4.23	792	316	63	2	0.38	0.31	5.86	0.27	40
—	—	1157	319	100	4	—	—	—	—	—
—	—	910	221	100	12	—	—	—	—	—
—	—	1129	441	90	2	—	—	—	—	—
—	—	798	503	—	—	—	—	—	—	—
80	2.7	1220	—	—	—	0.45	0.34	8	—	—
—	—	804	—	—	—	—	—	—	—	—
—	4.0	795	—	—	—	—	—	—	—	—
—	—	764	—	—	—	—	—	—	—	—
—	—	95	—	—	—	—	—	—	—	—
—	—	90	—	—	—	—	—	—	—	—
244	2.2	551	174	300	<1	0.19	0.38	1.51	0.10	36
144	2.13	1080	272	135	11	0.52	0.30	3.19	0.23	36
—	—	851	—	—	—	—	—	—	—	—
—	—	870	—	—	—	—	—	—	—	—
—	4.14	746	—	—	—	—	—	—	—	—
—	—	208	—	—	—	—	—	—	—	—
—	—	52	—	—	—	—	—	—	—	—
—	—	302	—	—	—	—	—	—	—	—
—	—	318	—	—	—	—	—	—	—	—
104	6	990	520	192	13	0.02	0.03	5.20	0.31	31
350	1.8	—	—	225	18	0.60	0.6	0.8	—	—
200	0.40	—	—	90	0	0.09	0.34	0	—	—
200	0	—	—	30	0	0.12	0.17	0	—	—
212	0.21	126	233	87	2	0.07	0.36	0.42	0.09	7
500	3.60	—	—	225	4	0.12	0.60	0.80	—	—
232	0.66	204	443	75	3	0.07	0.34	1.20	0.14	11
—	—	990	180	—	—	—	—	—	—	—
—	—	1220	200	—	—	—	—	—	—	—
—	—	1540	530	—	—	—	—	—	—	—
—	—	2870	710	—	—	—	—	—	—	—
—	—	1780	620	—	—	—	—	—	—	—
—	—	1980	670	—	—	—	—	—	—	—
—	—	880	320	—	—	—	—	—	—	—
—	4	580	280	—	—	—	—	—	—	—
—	—	1250	210	—	—	—	—	—	—	—
—	9	380	620	—	—	—	—	—	—	—
—	—	840	370	—	—	—	—	—	—	—
—	3	890	410	—	—	—	—	—	—	—
—	—	1050	210	—	—	—	—	—	—	—
—	—	1270	230	—	—	—	—	—	—	—
—	—	940	370	—	—	—	—	—	—	—
—	—	730	260	—	—	—	—	—	—	—
—	—	760	510	—	—	—	—	—	—	—
—	—	890	240	—	—	—	—	—	—	—
177	2.5	1037	190	133	3	0.41	0.47	5.1	0.14	—
134	4.5	1134	492	74	4	0.47	0.34	11.6	0.30	—
273	4.6	1666	499	220	5	0.52	0.38	11.3	0.31	—
167	1.7	837	246	72	1	0.30	0.21	4.5	0.12	—
73	0.9	430	129	2	<1	0.09	0.10	0.92	0.06	11

Table continued on following page

APPENDIX A–3 **NUTRITIONAL ANALYSIS OF FAST FOODS** *Continued*

	Approximate Measure	Weight (mg)	Kcal	Protein (gm)	Carbohydrate (gm)	Fat (gm)	MUFA (mg)	PUFA (mg)	Cholesterol (mg)
Kentucky Fried Chicken									
Chicken Hot Wings	1 piece	119	63	4	3	4	—	0.7	25
Chicken Sandwich	1 serving	166	482	21	39	27	—	9	47
Crispy Chicken, Breast	1 piece	135	342	33	12	20	—	2	114
Crispy Chicken, Drumstick	1 piece	69	204	14	6	14	—	2	71
Crispy Chicken, Thigh	1 piece	119	406	20	14	30	—	4	129
Cripsy Chicken, Wing	1 piece	65	254	12	9	19	—	3	67
Long John Silver's									
Breaded Shrimp Feast	1 piece	420	51	1	6	2	1.6	0.3	6
Catfish Fillet Dinner	1 serving	373	860	28	90	42	26	6	65
Chicken, Light Herb	1 serving	498	630	35	85	17	5	7	85
Clam Chowder with Cod	1 serving	198	140	11	10	6	3	2	20
Clam Dinner	1 serving	363	980	21	122	45	30	6	15
Cole Slaw	1 serving	98	140	1	20	6	2	4	15
Fish and Chicken Entree	1 serving	398	870	35	91	40	26	5	70
Fish and More	1 serving	381	800	31	88	37	23	5	70
Chicken Plank Dinner	1 serving	415	940	39	94	44	29	5	70
Fries	1 serving	85	220	3	30	10	7	1	5
Garden Salad	1 serving	246	170	9	13	9	—	—	5
Gumbo with Cod and Shrimp	1 serving	198	120	9	4	8	3	3	25
Homestyle Fish Sandwich	1 serving	196	510	22	58	22	13	3	45
Homestyle Fish Sandwich Platter	1 serving	379	870	26	108	38	22	7	55
Hushpuppy	1 piece	24	70	2	10	2	1	1	5
Light Portion Fish with Paprika	1 serving	284	300	24	45	2	1	1	70
Light Portion Fish with Lemon Crumb	1 serving	291	320	24	49	4	1	1	75
Mixed Vegetables	1 serving	113	60	2	9	2	1	1	0
9 Piece Batter Shrimp	1 piece	357	95	3	10	5	3	1	14
Ocean Chef Salad	1 serving	321	250	24	19	9	2	2	80
Rice Pilaf	1 serving	142	210	5	43	2	1	1	0
Seafood Plate	1 serving	400	970	30	109	46	30	6	70
Seafood Salad	1 serving	337	270	16	36	7	2	3	90
Seafood Salad—Scoop Size	1 serving	142	210	14	26	5	2	3	90
Shrimp and Fish Dinner	1 serving	348	770	25	85	37	23	5	80
Shrimp, Fish, and Chicken Dinner	1 serving	380	840	31	89	40	26	5	80
Shrimp Scampi, Baked	1 serving	529	610	25	87	18	6	7	220
Homestyle Fish	1 piece	513	1260	49	124	64	43	6	130
Fish—3 Piece	1 serving	456	960	43	97	44	29	5	100
Fish and Fryes, 3-Piece Dinner	1 serving	358	810	42	77	38	27	2	85
McDonald's									
Apple Bran Muffin	1 serving	85	190	5	46	0	0	0	0
Apple Pie	1 serving	83	260	2	30	15	9.1	0.9	0
Barbecue Sauce	1 serving	32	50	<1	12	<1	0.2	0.2	0
Big Mac Hamburger	1 item	215	560	25	43	32	20.1	1.5	103
Bacon and Egg Biscuit	1 serving	156	440	18	33	26	16.1	2	253
Egg and Sausage Biscuit	1 item	180	520	20	33	35	20	2.5	275
Sausage Biscuit	1 item	123	440	13	32	29	17.2	2.5	49
Biscuit with Spread	1 serving	75	260	5	32	13	8.6	0.6	1
Cheeseburger	1 item	116	310	15	31	14	7.7	0.9	53
Chef Salad	1 serving	283	230	21	8	13	6.5	0.9	128
Chicken McNuggets	1 serving	113	290	19	17	16	10.4	1.8	65
Chocolate Shake	1 serving	293	320	12	66	2	0.9	<0.1	10
Chunky Chicken Salad	1 serving	250	140	23	5	3	2	0.5	78
Cookie, Chocolaty	1 serving	56	330	4	42	16	10.2	0.4	4
Cookie, McDonaldland	1 serving	56	290	4	47	9	6.8	0.5	0
Croutons	1 serving	11	50	1	7	2	1.3	0.1	0
Apple Danish	1 slice	115	390	6	51	18	10.8	2.0	26
Cinnamon Raisin Danish	1 item	110	440	6	58	21	13	1.6	35
Raspberry Danish	1 item	117	410	6	62	16	10.2	1.1	26
Egg McMuffin	1 item	138	290	18	28	11	6.1	1.3	226
English Muffin	1 serving	59	170	5	27	5	1.7	0.5	9
Filet O Fish	1 item	142	440	14	38	26	10.2	10.8	50

Calcium (mg)	Iron (mg)	Sodium (mg)	Potassium (mg)	Vitamin A (RE)	Vitamin C (mg)	Thiamin (mg)	Riboflavin (mg)	Niacin (mg)	Vitamin B_6 (mg)	Folate (mcg)
—	—	113	—	—	—	—	—	—	—	—
—	—	1060	—	—	—	—	—	—	—	—
—	—	790	—	—	—	—	—	—	—	—
—	—	324	—	—	—	—	—	—	—	—
—	—	688	—	—	—	—	—	—	—	—
—	—	422	—	—	—	—	—	—	—	—
—	—	85	41	—	—	—	—	—	—	—
—	—	990	1180	—	—	—	—	—	—	—
—	—	2170	790	—	—	—	—	—	—	—
—	—	590	380	—	—	—	—	—	—	—
—	—	1200	870	—	—	—	—	—	—	—
—	—	260	190	—	—	—	—	—	—	—
—	—	1520	1290	—	—	—	—	—	—	—
—	—	1390	1260	—	—	—	—	—	—	—
—	—	1660	1320	—	—	—	—	—	—	—
—	—	60	390	—	—	—	—	—	—	—
—	—	380	20	—	—	—	—	—	—	—
100	—	740	310	300	—	—	—	—	—	—
—	18	780	470	—	—	—	—	—	—	—
—	—	1110	1050	—	—	—	—	—	—	—
—	—	25	65	—	—	—	—	—	—	—
—	—	650	460	—	—	—	—	—	—	—
—	—	900	470	—	—	—	—	—	—	—
—	—	330	120	75	—	—	—	—	—	—
—	—	163	94	—	—	—	—	—	—	—
—	—	1340	160	—	—	—	—	—	—	—
—	—	570	140	—	—	—	—	—	—	—
—	—	1540	1100	—	—	—	—	—	—	—
—	—	670	100	—	—	—	—	—	—	—
—	—	570	100	250	—	—	—	—	—	—
—	—	1250	1030	—	—	—	—	—	—	—
—	—	1450	1170	—	—	—	—	—	—	—
—	—	2120	560	—	—	—	—	—	—	—
—	—	1590	1660	—	—	—	—	—	—	—
—	—	1890	1540	—	—	—	—	—	—	—
—	—	1630	1340	—	—	—	—	—	—	—
31	0.6	230	—	1	<1	0.02	0.08	0.4	—	—
11	0.7	240	—	0	11	0.06	0.02	0.3	—	—
13	0.3	340	—	30	2	0.01	0.01	0.17	—	—
256	4	950	237	106	2	0.48	0.41	6.81	0.27	21
185	2.56	1230	—	160	0	0.36	0.33	2.47	—	—
116	3.16	1250	319	88	<1	0.53	0.35	3.99	0.20	40
83	1.98	1080	—	0	0	0.49	0.21	3.96	—	—
75	1.31	730	—	0	0	0.23	0.11	1.65	—	—
199	2.30	750	223	118	2	0.29	0.21	3.86	0.12	18
256	1.51	490	—	411	14	0.31	0.29	3.60	—	—
13	1	520	—	0	0	0.11	0.12	8.97	—	—
332	0.84	240	—	92	0	0.13	0.50	0.40	—	—
34	1.02	230	—	366	20	0.22	0.17	8.5	—	—
24	2.18	280	—	0	0	0.18	0.21	2.47	—	—
9	2.07	300	—	0	0	0.25	0.18	2.54	—	—
7	0.35	140	—	0	<1	0.05	0.03	0.42	—	—
14	1.37	370	—	35	16	0.28	0.20	2.2	—	—
35	1.81	430	—	33	3	0.32	0.24	2.8	—	—
14	1.47	310	—	35	3	0.33	0.21	2.1	—	—
256	2.77	740	213	150	1	0.47	0.33	3.71	0.16	44
151	1.61	270	—	37	0	0.33	0.14	2.47	—	—
165	1.83	1030	150	44	<1	0.3	0.15	2.68	0.10	20

Table continued on following page

APPENDIX A–3 **NUTRITIONAL ANALYSIS OF FAST FOODS** *Continued*

	Approximate Measure	Weight (mg)	Kcal	Protein (gm)	Carbohydrate (gm)	Fat (gm)	MUFA (mg)	PUFA (mg)	Cholesterol (mg)
French Fries, Large	1 serving	122	400	6	46	22	11.6	0.9	16
French Fries, Medium	1 serving	97	320	4	36.	17	9.2	0.7	12
French Fries, Small	1 serving	68	220	3	26	12	6.5	0.5	9
Garden Salad	1 serving	213	110	7	6	7	3.2	0.5	83
Hamburger	1 item	102	260	12	31	10	5.1	0.8	37
Hashbrown Potato	1 serving	55	130	1	15	7	3.7	0.4	9
Honey Sauce	1 serving	14	45	0	12	0	0	0	0
Hot Cakes with Syrup	1 serving	176	410	8	74	9	3.1	2.5	21
Hot Caramel Sundae	1 serving	174	270	7	59	3	1.2	0.1	13
Hot Fudge Sundae	1 serving	169	240	7	51	3	0.8	0.1	6
Hot Mustard Sauce	1 serving	30	70	<1	8	4	1.2	1.9	5
Iced Cheese Danish	1 serving	110	390	7	42	22	12.1	1.8	47
McChicken	1 serving	190	490	19	40	29	11.5	11.6	43
McDLT Hamburger	1 item	234	580	26	36	37	16.7	8.5	109
McLean, Deluxe	1 serving	206	320	22	35	10	5	1	60
Milk Shake, Low Fat	1 serving	293	320	12	66	2	1	0	10
Pork Sausage	1 serving	48	180	8	0	16	8.5	1.9	48
Quarter Pounder Hamburger	1 item	166	410	23	34	21	11.4	1.2	86
Quarter Pounder Hamburger with Cheese	1 item	194	520	29	35	29	16.5	1.5	118
Sausage McMuffin	1 item	117	370	17	27	22	11.1	2.4	64
Sausage and Egg McMuffin	1 item	167	440	23	28	27	14.2	3.2	263
Scrambled Eggs	1 serving	98	140	12	1	10	5.0	1.4	399
Side Salad	1 serving	115	60	4	3	3	1.6	0.3	41
Strawberry Sundae	1 serving	171	210	6	49	1	0.4	<0.1	5
Sweet and Sour Sauce	1 serving	32	60	<1	14	<1	0.1	0.1	0
Vanilla Frozen Yogurt	1 serving	80	100	4	22	1	0.3	0.1	3
Vanilla Shake, Low Fat	1 serving	293	290	11	60	1	0.7	0.1	10
Subway									
Buttermilk Ranch Salad Dressing	1 serving	56.7	348	1	2	37	7	24	6
Lite Italian Salad Dressing	1 serving	56.7	23	1	4	1	—	—	—
BMT Sub, Honey Wheat	1 item	220	1011	45	88	57	25	7	133
BMT Sub, Italian Roll	1 item	213	982	44	83	55	24	7	133
Cold Cut Combo, Wheat	1 item	191	883	48	88	41	15	10	166
Cold Cut Combo, Italian	1 item	184	853	46	83	40	15	10	166
Ham and Cheese, Honey Wheat	1 item	194	673	39	86	22	8	4	73
Ham and Cheese, Italian Roll	1 item	184	643	38	81	18	8	4	73
Meatball, Honey Wheat	1 item	224	947	44	101	45	18	4	88
Meatball, Italian Roll	1 item	215	918	42	96	44	17	4	88
Roast Beef, Wheat Roll	1 item	189	717	41	89	24	9	4	75
Roast Beef, Italian Roll	1 item	184	689	42	84	23	9	4	—
Seafood and Crab, Wheat	1 item	219	1015	31	100	58	16	28	56
Seafood and Crab, Italian	1 item	210	986	29	94	57	15	28	56
Spicy Italian, Italian	1 item	213	1043	42	83	63	28	7	137
Steak and Cheese, Italian	1 item	213	765	43	83	32	12	4	82
Club Sub, Honey Wheat	1 item	220	722	47	89	23	9	4	84
Club Sub, Italian Roll	1 item	213	693	46	83	22	8	4	84
Turkey Breast, Wheat	1 item	192	674	42	88	20	7	7	67
Taco Bell									
Bean Burrito	1 item	168	332	17	43	12	4	0.6	79
Beef Burrito	1 item	110	262	13	29	10	4	0.4	33
Beefy Tostada	1 item	225	334	16	30	17	4	0.5	75
Burrito Supreme	1 item	225	457	21	43	22	7	1.7	126
Beef Burrito Supreme	1 item	255	457	24	42	22	—	2.1	57
Enchirito	1 item	213	382	20	31	20	—	1.5	54
Mexican Pizza	1 serving	223	575	21	40	37	—	9.7	52
Nachos Bellgrande	1 serving	287	649	22	61	35	—	2.6	36
Nachos	1 serving	106	346	8	38	19	—	1.6	9
Pintos and Cheese	1 serving	128	190	9	19	9	—	0.8	16
Soft Taco	1 item	92	228	12	18	12	—	1.2	32
Taco Bellgrande	1 item	163	355	18	18	23	—	1.3	56

Calcium (mg)	Iron (mg)	Sodium (mg)	Potassium (mg)	Vitamin A (RE)	Vitamin C (mg)	Thiamin (mg)	Riboflavin (mg)	Niacin (mg)	Vitamin B_6 (mg)	Folate (mcg)
18	0.93	200	866	0	15	0.24	0	3.29	0.32	40
14	0.73	150	692	0	12	0.19	0	2.60	0.25	32
10	0.52	110	484	0	8	0.14	0	1.84	0.18	22
149	1.26	160	—	391	14	0.10	0.16	0.59	—	—
122	2.29	500	215	46	2	0.28	0.16	3.84	0.12	17
6	0.27	330	—	0	2	0.06	0.02	0.85	—	—
—	0.07	0	—	0	<1	0	0.01	0.04	—	—
114	2.08	640	187	52	5	0.32	0.33	2.82	0.12	9
222	0.08	180	—	87	0	0.08	0.35	0.26	—	—
235	0.48	170	—	64	0	0.08	0.35	0.30	—	—
15	0.22	250	—	2	<1	0.01	0.01	0.15	—	—
33	1.42	420	—	38	1	0.29	0.23	2.10	—	—
143	2.61	780	—	31	2	0.96	0.21	8.92	—	—
225	3.91	990	—	226	7	0.39	0.36	6.87	—	—
—	—	670	290	—	—	—	—	—	—	—
332	—	240	—	—	—	—	—	—	—	—
8	0.67	350	—	0	0	0.27	0.10	2.31	—	—
142	3.68	660	322	67	3	0.36	0.29	6.70	0.27	23
295	3.72	1150	341	211	3	0.37	0.39	6.73	0.23	23
235	2.3	830	—	72	1	0.60	0.29	4.8	—	—
263	3.34	980	—	150	0	0.64	0.42	4.82	—	—
57	2.08	290	—	156	1	0.07	0.26	0.05	—	—
76	0.67	85	—	217	7	0.05	0.08	0.32	—	—
190	0.16	95	—	64	1	0.07	0.29	0.25	—	—
11	0.17	190	—	65	<1	0	0.01	0.08	—	—
112	0.23	80	—	38	0	0.04	0.18	0.37	—	—
327	0.10	170	—	92	0	0.13	0.48	0.31	—	—
—	—	492	17	—	—	—	—	—	—	—
—	—	952	13	—	—	—	—	—	—	—
—	—	3199	1002	—	—	—	—	—	—	—
—	—	3139	917	—	—	—	—	—	—	—
—	—	2278	1010	—	—	—	—	—	—	—
—	—	2218	876	—	—	—	—	—	—	—
—	—	2508	918	—	—	—	—	—	—	—
—	—	1710	834	—	—	—	—	—	—	—
—	—	2082	1498	—	—	—	—	—	—	—
—	—	2022	1210	—	—	—	—	—	—	—
—	—	2348	994	—	—	—	—	—	—	—
—	—	2288	910	—	—	—	—	—	—	—
—	—	2027	641	—	—	—	—	—	—	—
—	—	1967	557	—	—	—	—	—	—	—
—	—	2282	880	—	—	—	—	—	—	—
—	—	1556	909	—	—	—	—	—	—	—
—	—	2777	1055	—	—	—	—	—	—	—
—	—	2717	971	—	—	—	—	—	—	—
—	—	2520	605	—	—	—	—	—	—	—
144	3.84	1030	405	240	3	0.28	0.6	3.86	0.21	73
42	3.05	746	370	42	1	0.12	0.5	3.23	0.16	20
190	2.45	870	490	383	4	0.09	0.5	2.85	0.26	<1
146	3.80	367	350	216	8	0.45	0.9	6.17	0.27	43
145	3.95	1053	431	286	9	0.43	2.19	3.7	—	—
269	2.84	1243	—	290	28	0.26	0.42	2.3	—	—
257	3.74	1031	408	295	31	0.32	0.33	3.0	—	—
297	3.48	997	674	341	58	0.10	0.34	2.2	—	—
191	0.93	399	159	169	2	<0.1	0.16	0.7	—	—
156	1.42	642	—	132	51	0.05	0.15	0.4	—	—
116	2.27	516	178	64	1	0.39	0.22	2.7	—	—
182	1.92	472	334	254	6	0.11	0.29	2.0	—	—

Table continued on following page

APPENDIX A–3 **NUTRITIONAL ANALYSIS OF FAST FOODS** *Continued*

	Approximate Measure	Weight (mg)	Kcal	Protein (gm)	Carbohydrate (gm)	Fat (gm)	MUFA (mg)	PUFA (mg)	Cholesterol (mg)
Taco, Regular	1 item	171	370	21	27	21	7	1.0	57
Taco, Light	1 item	170	410	19	18	29	—	5.4	56
Salad, No Shell, No Salsa	1 serving	530	502	30	26	31	—	1.7	80
Taco Salad with Salsa and Shell	1 serving	595	941	36	63	61	—	12.1	80
Taco Salad with Salsa, No Shell	1 serving	530	520	31	30	31	—	1.7	80
Tostada, Regular	1 item	144	223	10	27	10	3	0.8	30
Wendy's									
Bacon and Cheese Potato	1 serving	347	450	15	57	18	—	—	10
Big Classic, Quarter Pound Hamburger	1 serving	277	570	27	46	33	—	—	85
Broccoli and Cheese Potato	1 serving	377	400	9	59	16	—	—	0
Cheese Potato	1 serving	348	470	13	57	21	—	—	0
Cheese Sauce	1 serving	56	40	1	5	2	—	—	0
Cheese Tortellini in Spaghetti Sauce	1 serving	112	120	4	24	1	—	—	5
Chicken Club Sandwich	1 serving	231	500	30	42	24	—	—	75
Chicken Salad	1 serving	56	120	7	4	8	—	3	0
Chili	1 serving	255	220	21	23	7	—	—	45
Double Hamburger	1 item	226	540	34	40	27	10	3	122
French Fries, Regular	1 serving	134	440	5	53	23	—	—	25
Kid Meal Hamburger	1 serving	104	260	14	30	9	—	—	35
Refried Beans	1 serving	56	70	4	10	3	—	1	0
Seafood Salad	1 serving	56	110	4	7	7	—	4	0
Single Cheeseburger with Everything	1 serving	252	490	29	35	27	—	—	90
Single Hamburger	1 item	218	511	26	40	27	11.4	2.2	86
Single Hamburger with Everything	1 serving	234	420	25	35	21	—	—	70
Spanish Rice	1 serving	56	70	2	13	1	—	1	0
Taco Salad with Taco Chips	1 serving	791	660	40	46	37	—	—	35
Triple Hamburger	1 item	259	693	50	29	42	18.2	2.7	142
Tuna Salad	1 serving	56	100	8	4	6	—	3	0

Nutrient data from *Nutritionist III*, version 7.0 software, Salem, OR.

Calcium (mg)	Iron (mg)	Sodium (mg)	Potassium (mg)	Vitamin A (RE)	Vitamin C (mg)	Thiamin (mg)	Riboflavin (mg)	Niacin (mg)	Vitamin B_6 (mg)	Folate (mcg)
221	2.42	802	473	257	2	0.15	0.45	3.2	0.24	23
155	2.44	594	316	199	5	0.20	0.33	2.5	—	—
331	4.54	1056	988	572	74	0.25	0.50	3.2	—	—
398	7.10	1662	1212	888	77	0.51	0.75	4.8	—	—
367	5.14	1431	1151	908	76	0.26	0.64	3.2	—	—
211	1.88	543	403	187	1	0.10	0.33	1.3	0.17	75
—	—	1125	1580	—	—	—	—	—	—	—
—	—	1075	590	—	—	—	—	—	—	—
—	—	470	1555	—	—	—	—	—	—	—
—	—	580	1435	—	—	—	—	—	—	—
—	—	300	70	—	—	—	—	—	—	—
—	—	280	110	—	—	—	—	—	—	—
—	14.4	950	515	—	—	—	—	16	—	—
—	—	215	60	—	—	—	—	—	—	—
—	6.3	750	495	—	—	—	—	—	—	—
102	6.0	791	569	31	1	0.36	0.39	7.6	0.54	27
—	—	265	855	—	—	—	—	—	—	—
—	—	545	205	—	—	—	—	—	—	—
—	—	215	210	—	—	—	—	—	—	—
—	—	455	40	—	—	—	—	—	—	—
—	—	1155	495	—	—	—	—	—	—	—
96	4.92	825	479	93	3	0.42	0.38	7.28	0.33	36
—	—	865	495	—	—	—	—	—	—	—
—	—	440	130	—	—	—	—	—	—	—
—	—	1110	1330	—	—	—	—	—	—	—
65	8.33	713	785	47	1	0.31	0.56	11	0.62	31
—	—	290	90	—	—	—	—	—	—	—

APPENDIX A–4 **CAFFEINE CONTENT OF FOODS**

Product	Amount (oz)	Caffeine Content	
		Average (mg)	***Range (mg)***
Coffee*			
Brewed, drip method	5	115	60–180
Brewed, percolator	5	80	40–170
Instant	5	65	30–120
Brewed decaffeinated	5	3	2–5
Instant decaffeinated	5	2	1–5
Tea*			
Brewed, major U.S. brands	5	40	20–90
Brewed, imported brands	5	60	25–110
Instant	5	30	25–50
Iced	12	70	67–76
Cocoa beverage*	5	4	2–20
Chocolate milk beverage*	8	5	2–7
Milk chocolate*	1	6	1–15
Dark chocolate, semisweet*	1	20	5–35
Baker's chocolate*	1	26	26
Chocolate-flavored syrup*	1	4	4
Soft drinks†			
Regular colas	12	—	30–46
Decaffeinated colas	12	—	trace
Diet colas	12	—	0–59
Decaffeinated diet colas	12	—	0–trace
Orange, lemon-lime, root beer, tonic, ginger ale, club soda	12	—	0
Other regular	12	—	0–93

* From Lecos C. The latest caffeine scorecard. *FDA Consumer* March 1984. (Data from FDA, Food Additive Chemistry Evaluation Branch, based on evaluations of existing literature on caffeine levels.)

† Data from *What's in Soft Drinks.* Washington, D.C., National Soft Drink Association, July 1985.

Recommended Nutrient Intakes

APPENDIX B

APPENDIX B–1 **RECOMMENDED DAILY INTAKE***

	Adults and Children Over 4 yrs.†	Children Under 4 yrs.	Infants Under 13 months	Pregnant or Lactating Women
Protein	65 gm‡	28 gm‡	25 gm‡	**
Vitamin A	5,000 IU	2,500 IU	1,500 IU	8,000 IU
Vitamin C	60 mg	40 mg	35 mg	60 mg
Thiamin	1.5 mg	0.7 mg	0.5 mg	1.7 mg
Riboflavin	1.7 mg	0.8 mg	0.6 mg	2.0 mg
Niacin	20 mg	9.0 mg	8.0 mg	20 mg
Calcium	1.0 gm	0.8 gm	0.6 gm	1.3 gm
Iron	18 mg	10 mg	15 mg	18 mg
Vitamin D	400 IU	400 IU	400 IU	400 IU
Vitamin E	30 IU	10 IU	5.0 IU	30 IU
Vitamin B_6	2.0 mg	0.7 mg	0.4 mg	2.5 mg
Folacin	0.4 mg	0.2 mg	0.1 mg	0.8 mg
Vitamin B_{12}	6 mcg	3 mcg	2 mcg	8 mcg
Phosphorus	1.0 gm	0.8 gm	0.5 gm	1.3 gm
Iodine	150 mcg	70 mcg	45 mcg	150 mcg
Magnesium	400 mg	200 mg	70 mg	450 mg
Zinc	15 mg	8 mg	5 mg	15 mg
Copper	2 mg	1 mg	0.6 mg	2 mg
Biotin	0.3 mg	0.15 mg	0.5 mg	0.3 mg
Pantothenic acid	10 mg	5 mg	3 mg	10 mg

* For use in nutrition labeling of foods, including foods that are vitamin and mineral supplements.

** Not specified because this RDI is used only in vitamin and mineral supplements for pregnant or lactating women.

† These values are on most nutrition labels.

‡ If protein efficiency ratio of protein is equal to or better than that of casein U.S. RDA is 45 gm for adults and pregnant or lactating women, 20 gm for children under 4 years of age and 18 gm for infants.

From U.S. Dept. of Health and Human Services, Food and Drug Administration, Office of Public Affairs, Rockville, MD 20857. HHS Publication (FDA) 81–2146; revised March 1981.

APPENDIX B–2 RECOMMENDED NUTRIENT INTAKES (RNI), CANADA, 1990, BASED ON AGE, ENERGY, AND BODY WEIGHT EXPRESSED AS DAILY RATES*

Age	Sex	Energy (kcal)	Weight (kg)	Thiamin (mg)	Riboflavin (mg)	Niacin (NE)†	n-3 PUFA‡ (g)	n-6 PUFA (g)	Protein (g)
Months									
0–4	Both	600	6.0	0.3	0.3	4	0.5	3	12‖
5–12	Both	900	9.0	0.4	0.5	7	0.5	3	12
Years									
1	Both	1100	11	0.5	0.6	8	0.6	4	19
2–3	Both	1300	14	0.6	0.7	9	0.7	4	22
4–6	Both	1800	18	0.7	0.9	13	1.0	6	26
7–9	Male	2200	25	0.9	1.1	16	1.2	7	30
	Female	1900	25	0.8	1.0	14	1.0	6	30
10–12	Male	2500	34	1.0	1.3	18	1.4	8	38
	Female	2200	36	0.9	1.1	16	1.1	7	40
13–15	Male	2800	50	1.1	1.4	20	1.4	9	50
	Female	2200	48	0.9	1.1	16	1.2	7	42
16–18	Male	3200	62	1.3	1.6	23	1.8	11	55
	Female	2100	53	0.8	1.1	15	1.2	7	43
19–24	Male	3000	71	1.2	1.5	22	1.6	10	58
	Female	2100	58	0.8	1.1	15	1.2	7	43
25–49	Male	2700	74	1.1	1.4	19	1.5	9	61
	Female	2000	59	0.8	1.0	14	1.1	7	44
50–74	Male	2300	73	0.9	1.3	16	1.3	8	60
	Female	1800	63	0.8‡‡	1.0‡‡	14‡‡	1.1‡‡	7‡‡	47
75+	Male	2000	69	0.8	1.0	14	1.0	7	57
	Female§§	1700	64	0.8‡‡	1.0‡‡	14‡‡	1.1‡‡	7‡‡	47
Pregnancy (additional)									
1st Trimester		100		0.1	0.1	0.1	0.05	0.3	5
2nd Trimester		300		0.1	0.3	0.2	0.16	0.9	20
3rd Trimester		300		0.1	0.3	0.2	0.16	0.9	24
Lactation (additional)		450		0.2	0.4	0.3	0.25	1.5	20

* From Recommended Nutrient Intakes for Canadians. Bureau of Nutritional Sciences, Ottawa, 1990.
† NE = niacin equivalents.
‡ PUFA = polyunsaturated fatty acids.
§ RE = retinol equivalents.
‖ Protein is assumed to be from breast milk and must be adjusted for infant formula.
¶ Infant formula with high phosphorus should contain 375 mg calcium.
** Breast milk is assumed to be the source of the mineral.
†† Smokers should increase vitamin C by 50%.
‡‡ Level below which intake should not fall.
§§ Assumes moderate physical activity.

Vitamin A (RE)§	Vitamin D (μg)	Vitamin E (mg)	Vitamin C (mg)	Folate (μg)	Vitamin B_{12} (μg)	Calcium (mg)	Phosphorus (mg)	Magnesium (mg)	Iron (mg)	Iodine (μg)	Zinc (mg)
400	10	3	20	50	0.3	250¶	150	20	0.3**	30	2**
400	10	3	20	50	0.3	400	200	32	7	40	3
400	10	3	20	65	0.3	500	300	40	6	55	4
400	5	4	20	80	0.4	550	350	50	6	65	4
500	5	5	25	90	0.5	600	400	65	8	85	5
700	2.5	7	25	125	0.8	700	500	100	8	110	7
700	2.5	6	25	125	0.8	700	500	100	8	95	7
800	2.5	8	25	170	1.0	900	700	130	8	125	9
800	5	7	25	180	1.0	1100	800	135	8	110	9
900	5	9	30	150	1.5	1100	900	185	10	160	12
800	5	7	30	145	1.5	1000	850	180	13	160	9
1000	5	10	40††	185	1.9	900	1000	230	10	160	12
800	2.5	7	30††	160	1.9	700	850	200	12	160	9
1000	2.5	10	40††	210	2.0	800	1000	240	9	160	12
800	2.5	7	30††	175	2.0	700	850	200	13	160	9
1000	2.5	9	40††	220	2.0	800	1000	250	9	160	12
800	2.5	6	30††	175	2.0	700	850	200	13	160	9
1000	5	7	40††	220	2.0	800	1000	250	9	160	12
800	5	6	30††	190	2.0	800	850	210	8	160	9
1000	5	6	40‡‡	205	2.0	800	1000	230	9	160	12
800	5	5	30††	190	2.0	800	850	210	8	160	9
100	2.5	2	0	300	1.0	500	200	15	0	25	6
100	2.5	2	10	300	1.0	500	200	45	5	25	6
100	2.5	2	10	300	1.0	500	200	45	10	25	6
400	2.5	3	25	100	0.5	500	200	65	0	50	6

Nutritional Assessment Criteria

APPENDIX C

APPENDIX C–1 **1983 METROPOLITAN HEIGHT AND WEIGHT TABLES***

Men					Women				
Height					Height				
FEET	INCHES	Small Frame	Medium Frame	Large Frame	FEET	INCHES	Small Frame	Medium Frame	Large Frame
5	2	128–134	131–141	138–150	4	10	102–111	109–121	118–131
5	3	130–136	133–143	140–153	4	11	103–113	111–123	120–134
5	4	132–138	135–145	142–156	5	0	104–115	113–126	122–137
5	5	134–140	137–148	144–160	5	1	106–118	115–129	125–140
5	6	136–142	139–151	146–164	5	2	108–121	118–132	128–143
5	7	138–145	142–154	149–168	5	3	111–124	121–135	131–147
5	8	140–148	145–157	152–172	5	4	114–127	124–138	134–151
5	9	142–151	148–160	155–176	5	5	117–130	127–141	137–155
5	10	144–154	151–163	158–180	5	6	120–133	130–144	140–159
5	11	146–157	154–166	161–184	5	7	123–136	133–147	143–163
6	0	149–160	157–170	164–188	5	8	126–139	136–150	146–167
6	1	152–164	160–174	168–192	5	9	129–142	139–153	149–170
6	2	155–168	164–178	172–197	5	10	132–145	142–156	152–173
6	3	158–172	167–182	176–202	5	11	135–148	145–159	155–176
6	4	162–176	171–187	181–207	6	0	138–151	148–162	158–179

* Weights for adults age 25 to 59 years based on lowest mortality. For determination of frame size, see Appendix C–4. Weight in pounds according to frame in indoor clothing (5 pounds for men and 3 pounds for women) wearing shoes with 1-inch heels.

Source of basic data *1979 Build Study,* Society of Actuaries and Association of Life Insurance Medical Directors of America. Courtesy of the Metropolitan Life Insurance Company, 1983.

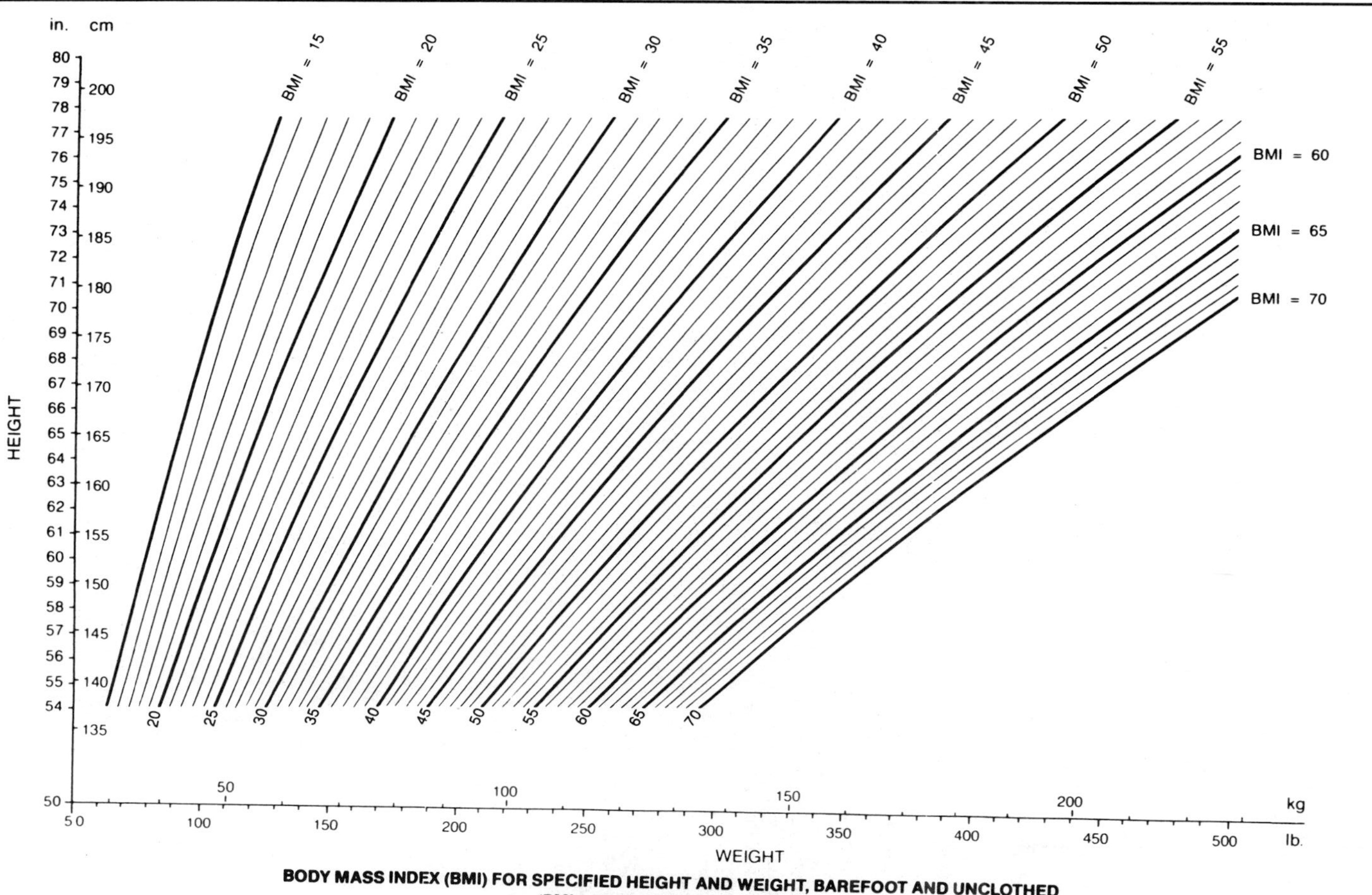

BODY MASS INDEX (BMI) FOR SPECIFIED HEIGHT AND WEIGHT, BAREFOOT AND UNCLOTHED
(BMI = Weight (kg) / [Height (m)]²)

Appendix C–2. To determine a client's BMI: (1) Locate the client's height (without shoes) on the left side of the chart. (2) Using a pencil and index card, draw a line across the graph. (3) Locate the client's weight without clothes on the grid at the bottom of the chart. Draw a line up from the mark to cross the horizontal line already drawn. (4) The lines will cross at, or very near, the curved line, which shows the client's body mass index. (Copyright Portland Health Institute, Inc. The Portland Health Institute Body Mass Index Graph is reproduced with permission from Herman M. Frankel, M.D., Portland Health Institute, Inc, 9045 S.W. Barbur Boulevard, Portland, OR 97219. Single copies on 8 1/2 × 11 in. stock, and instructions for use, will be sent at no charge to interested health professionals and others on receipt of a stamped, self-addressed envelope. (See Frankel HM. Determination of body mass index. *JAMA* 1986;255:1292.))

APPENDIX C–3 **NOMOGRAM FOR DETERMINING ABDOMINAL/GLUTEAL CIRCUMFERENCE RATIO (WAIST/HIP RATIO)**

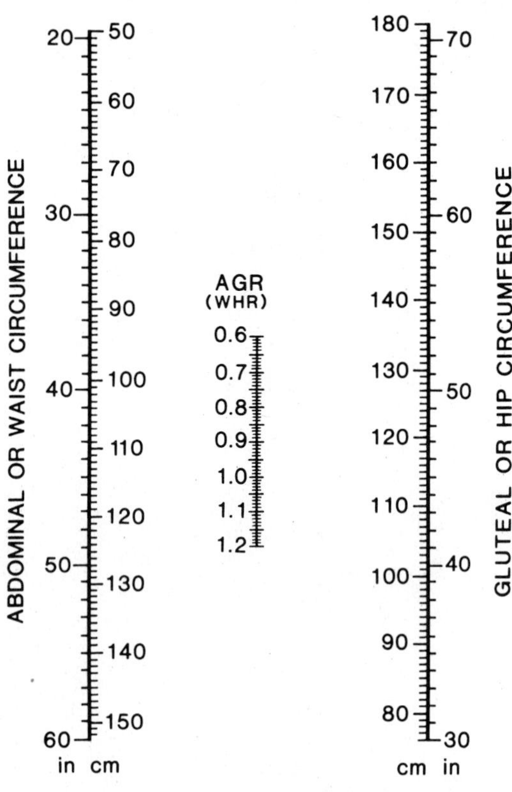

Appendix C–3. Nomogram for determining the ratio of abdominal (waist) circumference to gluteal (hips) circumference. Place a straight edge between the column for waist circumference and the column for hip circumference and read the ratio from the point where this straight edge crosses the AGR or WHR line. The waist or abdominal circumference is the smallest circumference below the rib cage and above the umbilicus, and the hips or gluteal circumference is taken as the largest circumference at the posterior extension of the buttocks. (From Bray GA. Overweight is risking fate. Definition, classification, prevalence and risks. *Ann NY Acad Sci* 1987;249:14. [Copyright 1988, George A. Bray, M.D. Used with permission].)

APPENDIX C–4 DETERMINATION OF BODY FRAME SIZE FROM WRIST CIRCUMFERENCE

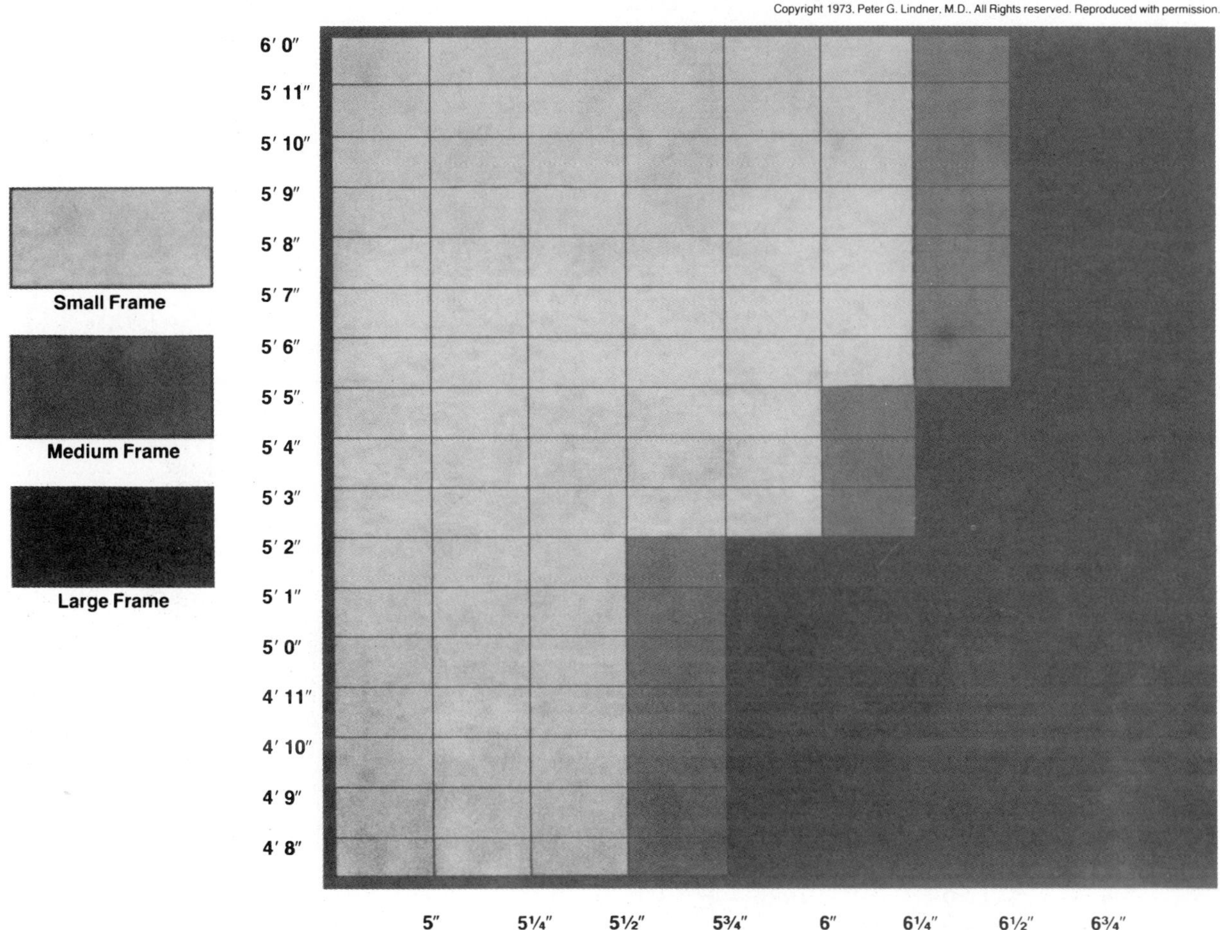

Appendix C–4. The wrist is measured distal to styloid process of radius and ulna at smallest circumference. Use height without shoes and inches for wrist size to determine frame type from this chart. (Copyright 1973. Peter G. Lindner, M.D. All rights reserved.)

APPENDIX C–5a **ARM ANTHROPOMETRY NOMOGRAM FOR ADULTS**

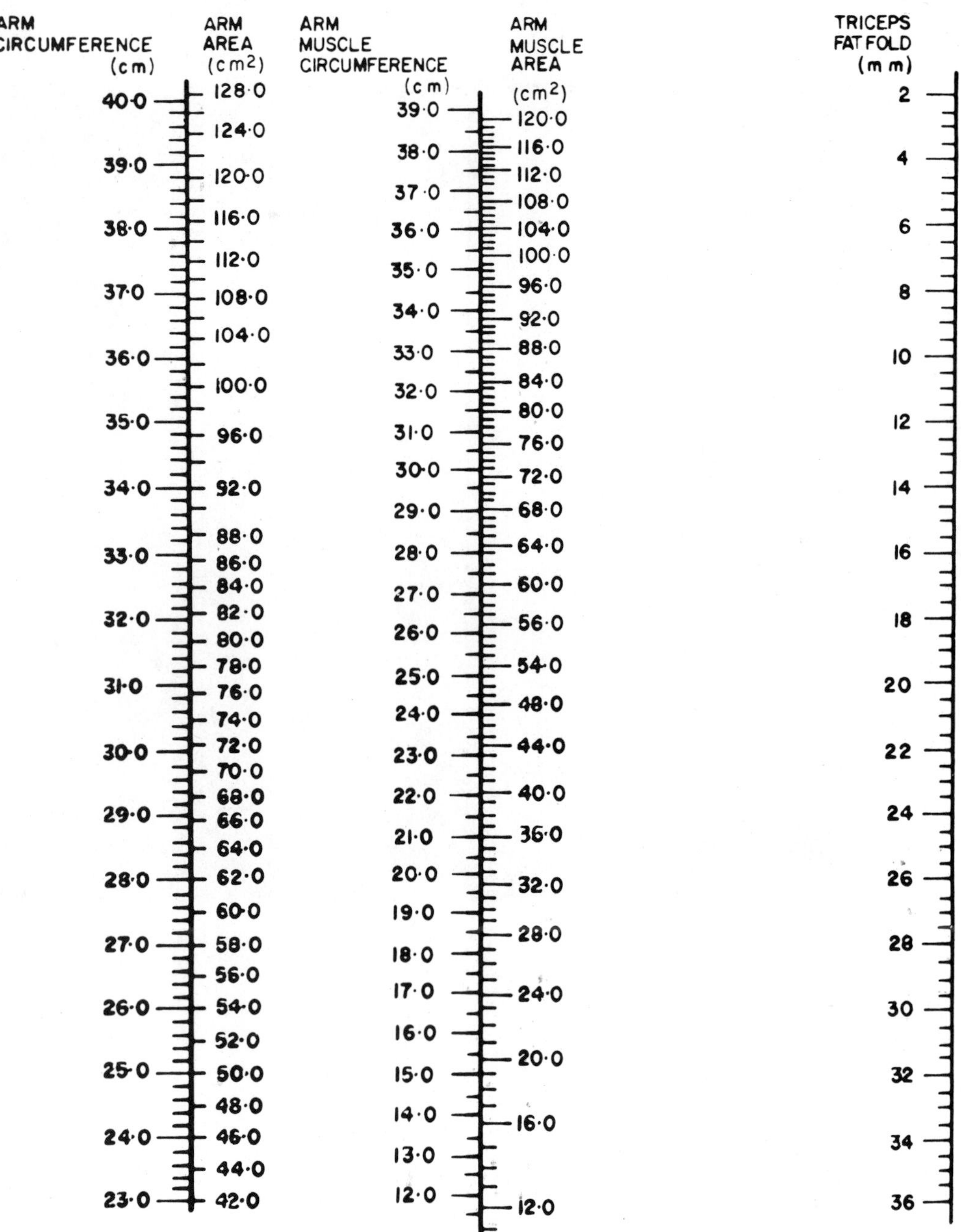

Appendix C–5a. To obtain muscle circumference: (1) Lay ruler between values of arm circumference and fatfold. (2) Read off muscle circumference on middle line. To obtain tissue areas: (1) The arm areas and muscle areas are alongside their respective circumferences. (2) Fat area = arm area − muscle area. (From Gurney JM, Jelliffe DB. Arm anthropometry in nutritional assessment: Nomogram for rapid calculation of muscle circumference and cross-sectional muscle fat areas. *Am J Clin Nutr* 1973;26(9):912. © American Society for Clinical Nutrition.)

APPENDIX C–5b **ARM ANTHROPOMETRY NOMOGRAM FOR CHILDREN**

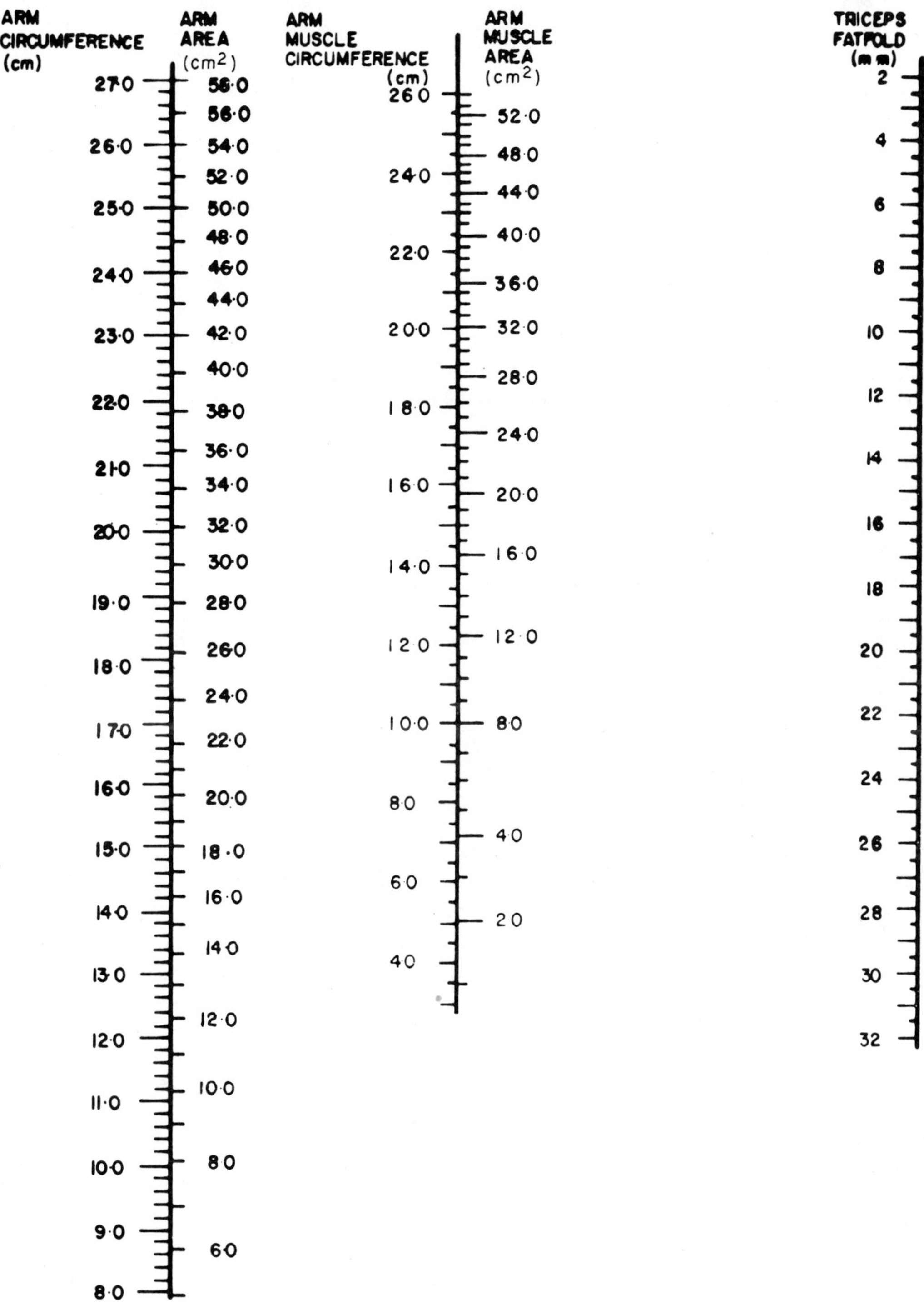

Appendix C–5b. To obtain muscle circumference: (1) Lay ruler between values of arm circumference and fatfold. (2) Read off muscle circumference on middle line. To obtain tissue areas: (1) The arm areas and muscle areas are alongside their respective circumferences. (2) Fat area = arm area − muscle area. (From Gurney JM, Jelliffe DB. Arm anthropometry in nutritional assessment: Nomogram for rapid calculation of muscle circumference and cross-sectional muscle fat areas. *Am J Clin Nutr* 1973;26(9):912. © American Society for Clinical Nutrition.)

APPENDIX C–6 **PERCENTILES FOR TRICEPS SKINFOLD FOR WHITES OF THE UNITED STATES HEALTH AND NUTRITION EXAMINATION SURVEY I OF 1971 TO 1974**

	Triceps Skinfold Percentiles (mm²)															
	n	***5***	***10***	***25***	***50***	***75***	***90***	***95***	***n***	***5***	***10***	***25***	***50***	***75***	***90***	***95***
Age Group	**MALES**								**FEMALES**							
1–1.9	228	6	7	8	10	12	14	16	204	6	7	8	10	12	14	16
2–2.9	223	6	7	8	10	12	14	15	208	6	8	9	10	12	15	16
3–3.9	220	6	7	8	10	11	14	15	208	7	8	9	11	12	14	15
4–4.9	230	6	6	8	9	11	12	14	208	7	8	8	10	12	14	16
5–5.9	214	6	6	8	9	11	14	15	219	6	7	8	10	12	15	18
6–6.9	117	5	6	7	8	10	13	16	118	6	6	8	10	12	14	16
7–7.9	122	5	6	7	9	12	15	17	126	6	7	9	11	13	16	18
8–8.9	117	5	6	7	8	10	13	16	118	6	8	9	12	15	18	24
9–9.9	121	6	6	7	10	13	17	18	125	8	8	10	13	16	20	22
10–10.9	146	6	6	8	10	14	18	21	152	7	8	10	12	17	23	27
11–11.9	122	6	6	8	11	16	20	24	117	7	8	10	13	18	24	28
12–12.9	153	6	6	8	11	14	22	28	129	8	9	11	14	18	23	27
13–13.9	134	5	5	7	10	14	22	26	151	8	8	12	15	21	26	30
14–14.9	131	4	5	7	9	14	21	24	141	9	10	13	16	21	26	28
15–15.9	128	4	5	6	8	11	18	24	117	8	10	12	17	21	25	32
16–16.9	131	4	5	6	8	12	16	22	142	10	12	15	18	22	26	31
17–17.9	133	5	5	6	8	12	16	19	114	10	12	13	19	24	30	37
18–18.9	91	4	5	6	9	13	20	24	109	10	12	15	18	22	26	30
19–24.9	531	4	5	7	10	15	20	22	1060	10	11	14	18	24	30	34
25–34.9	971	5	6	8	12	16	20	24	1987	10	12	16	21	27	34	37
35–44.9	806	5	6	8	12	16	20	23	1614	12	14	18	23	29	35	38
45–54.9	898	6	6	8	12	15	20	25	1047	12	16	20	25	30	36	40
55–64.9	734	5	6	8	11	14	19	22	809	12	16	20	25	31	36	38
65–74.9	1503	4	6	8	11	15	19	22	1670	12	14	18	24	29	34	36

From Frisancho AR. New norms of upper limb fat and muscle areas for assessment of nutritional status. *Am J Clin Nutr* 1981;34(11):2530. © American Society for Clinical Nutrition.

APPENDIX C–7 **PERCENTILES FOR UPPER ARM CIRCUMFERENCE (mm) AND ESTIMATED UPPER ARM MUSCLE CIRCUMFERENCE (mm) FOR WHITES OF THE UNITED STATES HEALTH AND NUTRITION EXAMINATION SURVEY I OF 1971 TO 1974**

	Arm Circumference (mm)							Arm Muscle Circumference (mm)						
	5	10	25	50	75	90	95	5	10	25	50	75	90	95
Age Group							**MALES**							
1–1.9	142	146	150	159	170	176	183	110	113	119	127	135	144	147
2–2.9	141	145	153	162	170	178	185	111	114	122	130	140	146	150
3–3.9	150	153	160	167	175	184	190	117	123	131	137	143	148	153
4–4.9	149	154	162	171	180	186	192	123	126	133	141	148	156	159
5–5.9	153	160	167	175	185	195	204	128	133	140	147	154	162	169
6–6.9	155	159	167	179	188	209	228	131	135	142	151	161	170	177
7–7.9	162	167	177	187	201	223	230	137	139	151	160	168	177	190
8–8.9	162	170	177	190	202	220	245	140	145	154	162	170	182	187
9–9.9	175	178	187	200	217	249	257	151	154	161	170	183	196	202
10–10.9	181	184	196	210	231	262	274	156	160	166	180	191	209	221
11–11.9	186	190	202	223	244	261	280	159	165	173	183	195	205	230
12–12.9	193	200	214	232	254	282	303	167	171	182	195	210	223	241
13–13.9	194	211	228	247	263	286	301	172	179	196	211	226	238	245
14–14.9	220	226	237	253	283	303	322	189	199	212	223	240	260	264
15–15.9	222	229	244	264	284	311	320	199	204	218	237	254	266	272
16–16.9	244	248	262	278	303	324	343	213	225	234	249	269	287	296
17–17.9	246	253	267	285	308	336	347	224	231	245	258	273	294	312
18–18.9	245	260	276	297	321	353	379	226	237	252	264	283	298	324
19–24.9	262	272	288	308	331	355	372	238	245	257	273	289	309	321
25–34.9	271	282	300	319	342	362	375	243	250	264	279	298	314	326
35–44.9	278	287	305	326	345	363	374	247	255	269	286	302	318	327
45–54.9	267	281	301	322	342	362	376	239	249	265	281	300	315	326
55–64.9	258	273	296	317	336	355	369	236	245	260	278	295	310	320
65–74.9	248	263	285	307	325	344	355	223	235	251	268	284	298	306
							FEMALES							
1–1.9	138	142	148	156	164	172	177	105	111	117	124	132	139	143
2–2.9	142	145	152	160	167	176	184	111	114	119	126	133	142	147
3–3.9	143	150	158	167	175	183	189	113	119	124	132	140	146	152
4–4.9	149	154	160	169	177	184	191	115	121	128	136	144	152	157
5–5.9	153	157	165	175	185	203	211	125	128	134	142	151	159	165
6–6.9	156	162	170	176	187	204	211	130	133	138	145	154	166	171
7–7.9	164	167	174	183	199	216	231	129	135	142	151	160	171	176
8–8.9	168	172	183	195	214	247	261	138	140	151	160	171	183	194
9–9.9	178	182	194	211	224	251	260	147	150	158	167	180	194	198
10–10.9	174	182	193	210	228	251	265	148	150	159	170	180	190	197
11–11.9	185	194	208	224	248	276	303	150	158	171	181	196	217	223
12–12.9	194	203	216	237	256	282	294	162	166	180	191	201	214	220
13–13.9	202	211	223	243	271	301	338	169	175	183	198	211	226	240
14–14.9	214	223	237	252	272	304	322	174	179	190	201	216	232	247
15–15.9	208	221	239	254	279	300	322	175	178	189	202	215	228	244
16–16.9	218	224	241	258	283	318	334	170	180	190	202	216	234	249
17–17.9	220	227	241	264	295	324	350	175	183	194	205	221	239	257
18–18.9	222	227	241	258	281	312	325	174	179	191	202	215	237	245
19–24.9	221	230	247	265	290	319	345	179	185	195	207	221	236	249
25–34.9	233	240	256	277	304	342	368	183	188	199	212	228	246	264
35–44.9	241	251	267	290	317	356	378	186	192	205	218	236	257	272
45–54.9	242	256	274	299	328	362	384	187	193	206	220	238	260	274
55–64.9	243	257	280	303	335	367	385	187	196	209	225	244	266	280
65–74.9	240	252	274	299	326	356	373	185	195	208	225	244	264	279

From Frisancho AR. New norms of upper limb fat and muscle areas for assessment of nutritional status. *Am J Clin Nutr* 1981;34(11):2530.

APPENDIX C–8a **GIRLS: BIRTH TO 36 MONTHS PHYSICAL GROWTH NCHS PERCENTILES**

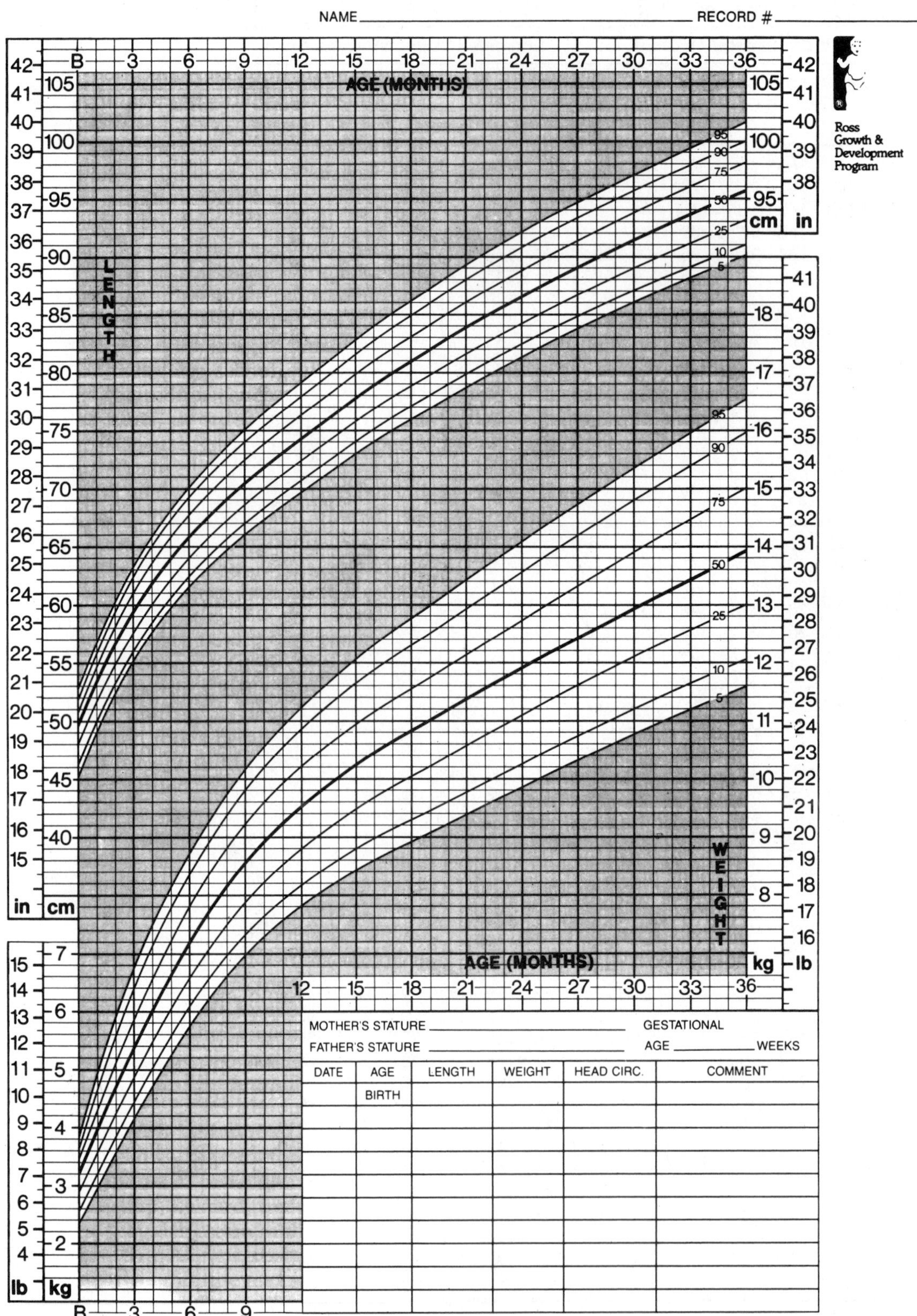

Appendix C–8a. Physical growth of girls: Birth to 36 months. (Adapted from Hamill PW, et al. Physical growth: National Center for Health Statistics percentiles. *Am J Clin Nutr* 1979;32:607–629. Data from the Fels Longitudinal Study, Wright State University School of Medicine, Yellow Springs, Ohio. © 1982 Ross Laboratories.)

APPENDIX C–8b **BOYS: BIRTH TO 36 MONTHS PHYSICAL GROWTH NCHS PERCENTILES**

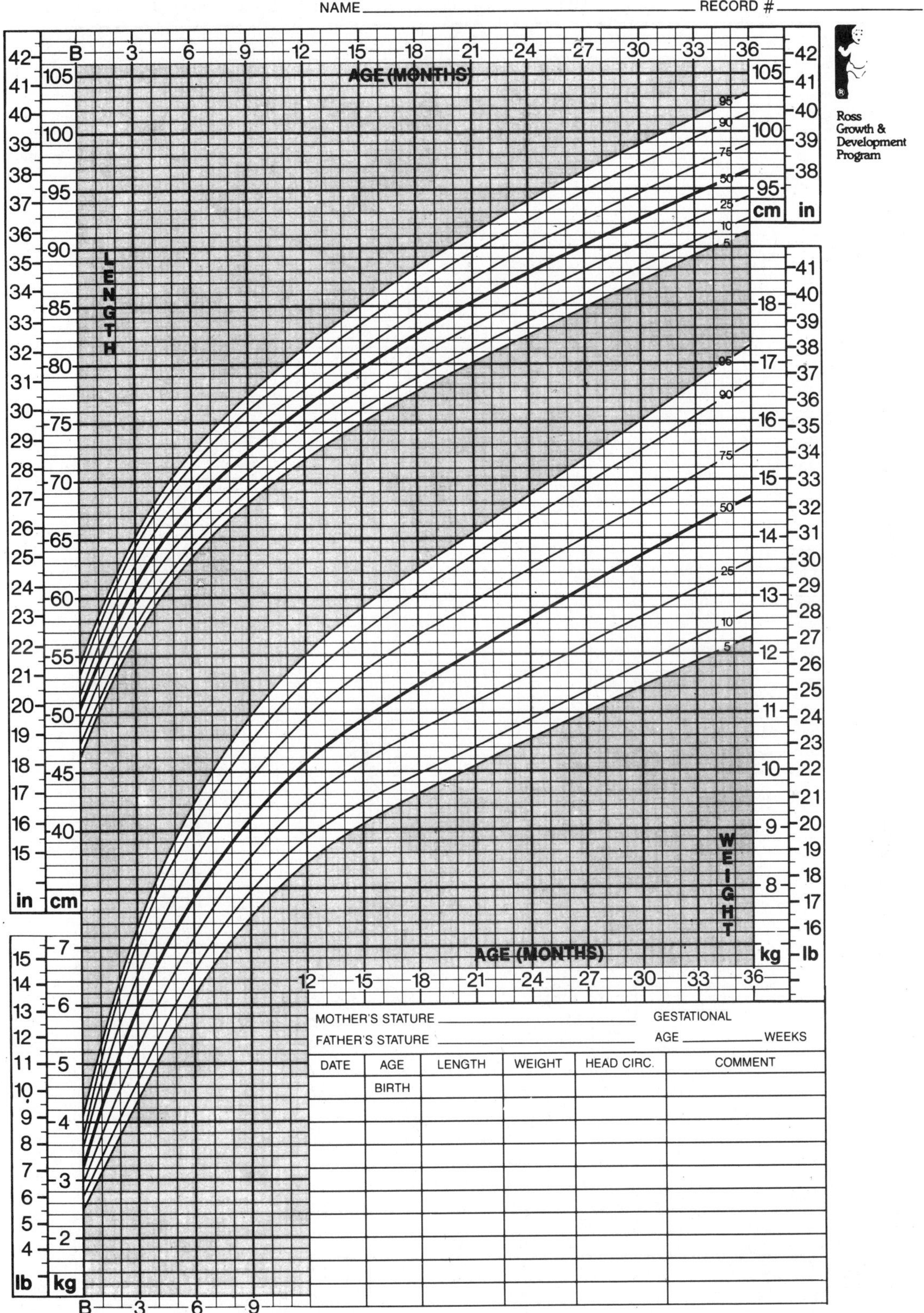

Appendix C–8b. Physical growth of boys: Birth to 36 months. (Adapted from Hamill PW, et al. Physical growth: National Center for Health Statistics percentiles. *Am J Clin Nutr* 1979;32:607–629. Data from the Fels Longitudinal Study, Wright State University School of Medicine, Yellow Springs, Ohio. © 1982 Ross Laboratories.)

APPENDIX C–8c **GIRLS: 2 TO 18 YEARS PHYSICAL GROWTH NCHS PERCENTILES**

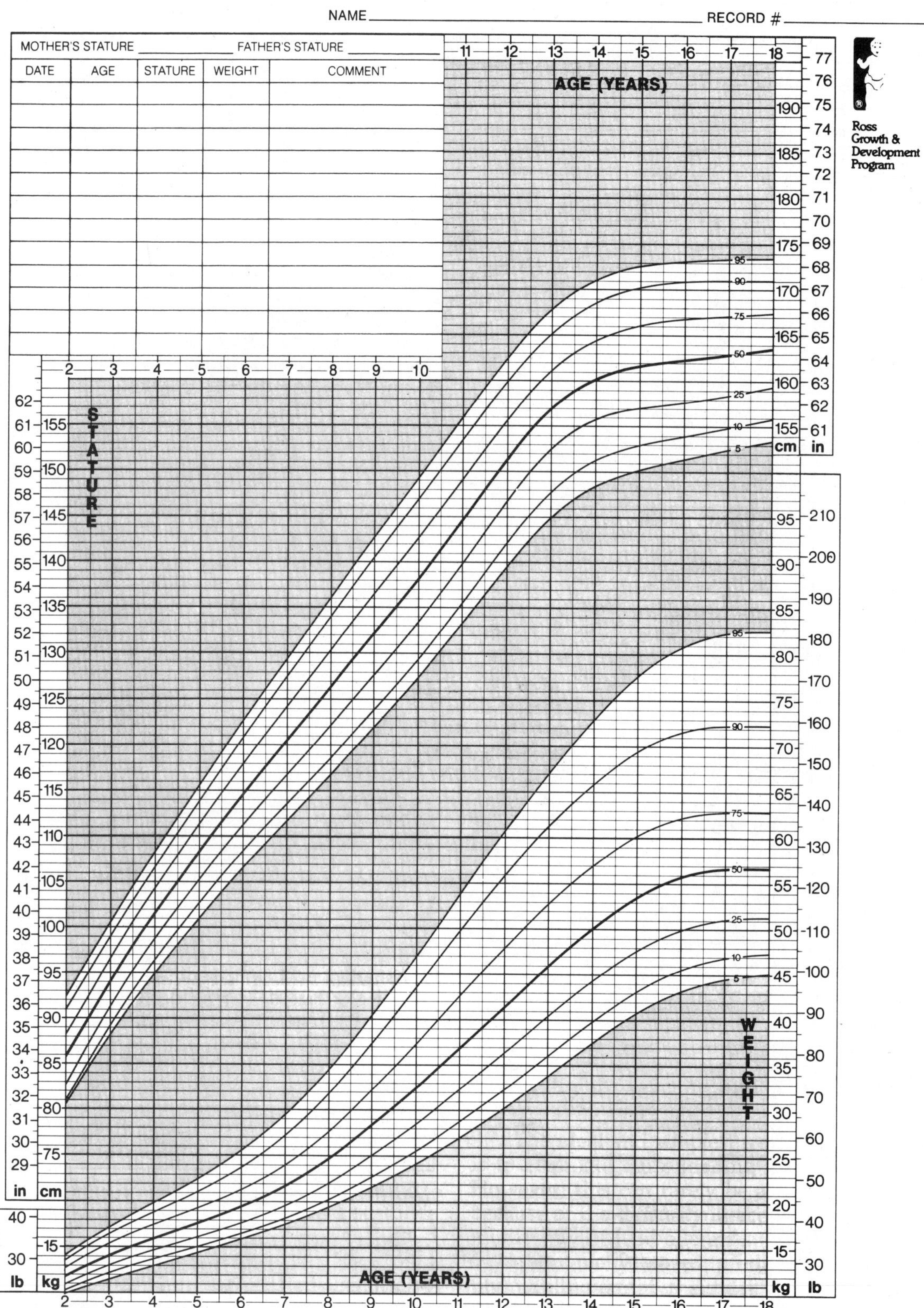

Appendix C–8c. Physical growth of girls: 2 to 18 years old. (Adapted from Hamill PW, et al. Physical growth: National Center for Health Statistics percentiles. *Am J Clin Nutr* 1979;32:607–629. Data from the National Center for Health Statistics (NCHS), Hyattsville, Maryland. © 1982 Ross Laboratories.)

APPENDIX C–8d **BOYS: 2 TO 18 YEARS PHYSICAL GROWTH NCHS PERCENTILES**

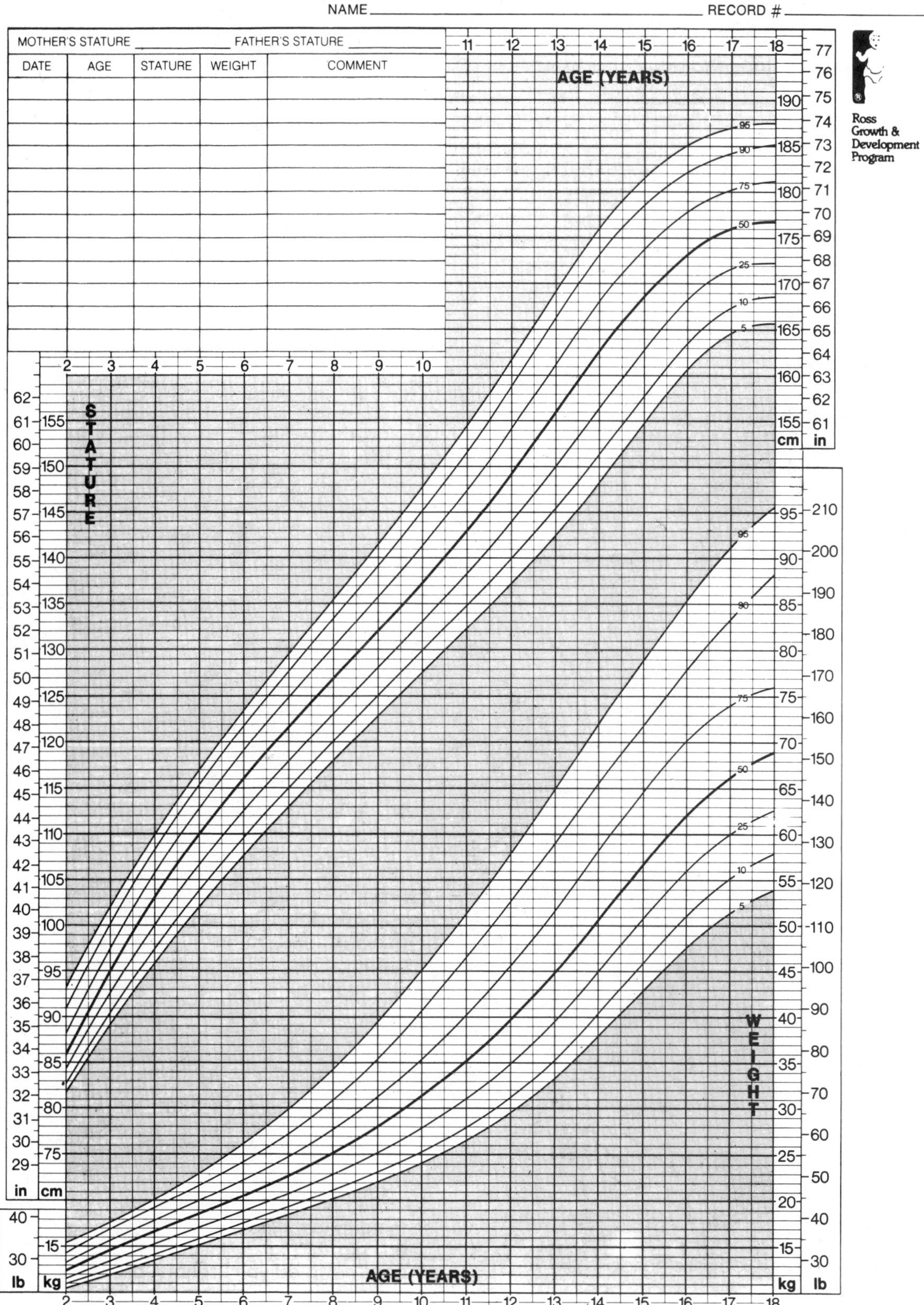

Appendix C–8d. Physical growth of boys: 2 to 18 years old. (Adapted from Hamill PW, et al. Physical growth: National Center for Health Statistics percentiles. *Am J Clin Nutr* 1979;32:607–629. Data from the National Center for Health Statistics (NCHS), Hyattsville, Maryland. © 1982 Ross Laboratories.)

APPENDIX C–9 **NUTRIENTS DETRIMENTALLY AFFECTED BY DRUGS***

Drugs by Classification	GI Disturbances	Anorexia	Protein Metabolism	Carbohydrate Metabolism	Fat Metabolism	Vitamin A	Vitamin D	Vitamin K	Thiamin	Riboflavin	Niacin	Vitamin B_{12}	Vitamin B_6	Folate	Vitamin C	Calcium	Phosphorus	Iron	Sodium	Potassium	Magnesium	Zinc	Remarks
Analgesics																							
Alcohol									X			X		X							X	X	
Aspirin			X					X							X					X			
Antacids																							
Aluminum hydroxide									X								X						
Magnesium hydroxide (and others)									X									X					
Sodium bicarbonate																							Can cause alkalosis if taken with milk
Anticoagulants																							
Coumarin derivatives								X															Antagonized by high levels of vitamins K and E
Anticonvulsants																							
Phenobarbital							X					X	X	X		X					X		
Phenytoin							X					X	X	X		X					X		Supplement with less than 5 mg/day folic acid
Primidone		X					X					X	X	X		X							
Antidepressants																							
Lithium carbonate	X			X												X					X		Force fluids
MAO inhibitors																							Avoid foods high in tyramine
Antigout																							
Colchicine			X	X	X	X						X							X	X			Decreased serum cholesterol
Antimicrobials																							
Chloramphenicol										X		X	X	X				X					
Penicillin																				X			Do not take with acidic beverages
Tetracycline	X	X	X	X				X							X	X		X			X	X	Do not take with milk products, iron, or antacids
Neomycin		X	X	X	X	X	X	X				X				X		X	X	X			Can lead to deficiency of fat-soluble vitamins

Erythromycin	X																						Do not take with acidic beverages
Sulfonamides	X	X												X				X		X			
Griseofulvin	X	X																					Optimal absorption with high-fat meal
Antineoplastic																							Force fluids; avoid alcohol
Methotrexate	X	X		X	X							X		X									
5-Fluorouracil	X	X	X																				
Antiparkinsonian	X	X	X										X		X				X	X			Antagonized by high-protein, B_6-rich foods
Levodopa																							
Antitubercular																							
Para-aminosalicylic acid				X	X							X		X				X					Force fluids
Isonicotinic acid hydrazide											X		X	X									Avoid foods high in tyramine
Cycloserine			X									X	X	X		X					X		
Cathartics																							Alkaline foods will dissolve coating, causing GI irritation
Bisacodyl				X																X			
Mineral oil						X	X	X								X	X						
Phenolphthalein							X									X							
Chelating agents																							
Penicillamine	X	X											X									X	Force fluids (16 oz at bedtime)
Corticosteroids	X		X	X	X		X						X	X	X	X	X			X		X	Food may protect stomach against ulceration
Diuretics									X				X			X				X	X	X	Encourage foods high in potassium and calcium
Furosemide				X												X				X	X		
Thiazides				X						X						X				X	X	X	Avoid imported licorice; encourage high-potassium foods
Triamterene														X		X							Avoid high-potassium foods
Spironolactone																X					X		
Hypocholesterolemics																							
Cholestyramine resin				X	X	X	X	X				X		X		X		X					
Clofibrate	X			X		X						X						X	X	X			

Table continued on following page

APPENDIX C–9 **NUTRIENTS DETRIMENTALLY AFFECTED BY DRUGS** *Continued*

Drugs by Classification	***GI Disturbances***	***Anorexia***	***Protein Metabolism***	***Carbohydrate Metabolism***	***Fat Metabolism***	***Vitamin A***	***Vitamin D***	***Vitamin K***	***Thiamin***	***Riboflavin***	***Niacin***	***Vitamin B_{12}***	***Vitamin B_6***	***Folate***	***Vitamin C***	***Calcium***	***Phosphorus***	***Iron***	***Sodium***	***Potassium***	***Magnesium***	***Zinc***	**Remarks**
Hypotensive agents																							Take with food to increase bio-availability
Hydralazine	X	X											X										
Methyldopa													X										
Oral contraceptives	X		X							X		X	X	X	X						X	X	
Sedatives/hypnotics																							
Glutethimide							X									X							
Barbiturates							X		X			X		X	X								
Uricosuric																							
Allopurinol										X							X		X	X	X		Force fluids
Probenecid										X							X		X	X	X		Force fluids

* Adapted from Roe DA. *Handbook: Interaction of Selected Drugs and Nutrients in Patients.* Chicago, American Dietetic Association, 1982.

APPENDIX C-10 **TIMING OF DRUGS**

Drugs to be Given on an Empty Stomach

Classification and Drug	*Effect of Food on Drug Absorption* DECREASES	DELAYS	*Comments*
Analgesics			
Acetaminophen (Datril, Phenaphen, Tylenol)		X	
Enteric-coated acetylsalicylic acid		X	
Antacids			
Aluminum hydroxide, calcium carbonate, magnesium hydroxide			1–3 hr after each meal and at bedtime
Antiarthritic			
Penicillamine (Cuprimine, Depen)	X		
Nonsteroidal anti-inflammatory drugs (NSAIDs)		X	
Anticonvulsants			
Phenobarbital	X		
Antihypertensives			
Atenolol (Tenoretic, Tenormin)	X		
Captopril (Capoten, Capozide)	X		Maximum effectiveness if given on empty stomach 1 hr before meals
Anti-infectives			
Amoxicillin (Amoxil, Polymox, Trimox, Wymox)		X	Give with 8 oz water
Ampicillin (Omnipen, Polycillin)	X		Give with 8 oz water
Cephalexin (Biocef, Keflex)		X	
Clindamycin (Cleocin)	X		
Cloxacillin (Tegopen)	X		Give with 8 oz water
Didanosine (ddI)	X		
Erythromycin/erythromycin salts (Erythromycin Base, E.E.S., Pediazole, others)	X		Give with 8 oz water. Enteric-coated erythromycin base and erythromycin ethylsuccinate may be given with food
Metronidazole (Flagyl)		X	May give with fruit juice/fruit to decrease epigastric distress
Nafcillin Na (Nafcil, Unipen)	X		
Penicillin G potassium (Pentids)	X		Give with 8 oz water
Penicillin-VK (Pen-Vee K, Veetids)	X		
Sulfdisoxazole (Gantrisin, others)		X	
Tetracycline (Achromycin V, Sumycin)	X		Do not give with iron or calcium supplements, antacids, or milk products
Anti-parkinsonism agents			
Isoniazid (INH; Rifamate); rifampin (Rifadin, Rimactane)	X		

Table continued on following page

APPENDIX C–10 **TIMING OF DRUGS** *Continued*

Drugs to be Given on an Empty Stomach

Classification and Drug	*Effect of Food on Drug Absorption* DECREASES	DELAYS	*Comments*
Cardiac drugs			
Digoxin (Lanoxin)		X	High fiber or calcium decreases absorption. Maintain high potassium intake
Quinidine (Duraquin, Quinaglute)	X		Give with 8 oz water. Avoid excessive consumption of citrus juices (orange, grapefruit, and pineapple)
Diuretics			
Furosemide (Lasix)		X	
Hydrochlorothiazide (Aldactazide, Aldoril, Dyazide, Esidrix, HydroDIURIL, Maxzide, Oretic)	X		
Laxatives			
Bisacodyl (Dulcolax)		X	Interferes with absorption of nutrients. Give with at least 8 oz water 1 hr after a meal
Docusate (Colace, Senokot, Surfak)		X	Oral solution has a bitter taste; mix with milk
Mineral oil		X	Interferes with absorption of nutrients
Respiratory			
Theophylline (Bronkodyl, Quibron, Slo-phyllin, Theostat)		X	Take with 8 oz water

Drugs to be Given Prior to Meals (30 min Before Meals)

Classification and Drug	*Rationale*
Anorexiants	
Phentermine (Ionamin) and phenmetrazine (Preludin)	For maximum psychological and pharmacological effectiveness
Anticholinergic agents	
Atropine sulfate and scopolamine (Donnagel, Donnatal, Lomotil, Ru-Tuss); clidinium bromide (Librax), belladonna and its alkaloids (Bellergal-S, Cafergot); glycopyrrolate (Robinul); and propantheline (Pro-Banthine)	Anticholinergic drugs inhibit vagal effects on gastric glands and gastric secretion when the gastric acid is reaching a maximum. They are more effective against basal secretion when taken after gastric secretions are stimulated
Antidepressants	
Monomine oxidase inhibitors (Nardil, Parnate) and methylphenidate (Ritalin)	Give 30 min before meals to avoid interference with absorption
Antidiabetic	
Glyburide (DiaBeta, Micronase)	Should be in blood stream before breakfast for maximum activity
Antiulcer	
Sucralfate (Carafate)	Food interferes with disaccharide that coats stomach ulcers
Promotility agent	
Metoclopramide (Reglan)	Presence of food decreases effectiveness

APPENDIX C–10 **TIMING OF DRUGS** *Continued*

Drugs not to be Given with Antacids

Drugs	*Rationale*
Bisacodyl (Dulcolax)	Enteric coating dissolves in antacids, releasing the irritant drug in the stomach
Ciprofloxacin (Cipro)	Magnesium and aluminum antacids complex, decreasing absorption
Iron preparations	Complexes with antacids, decreasing absorption
Tetracycline (Achromycin) and its derivatives, such as demeclocycline (Declomycin) and doxycycline (Vibramycin)	Complexes with antacids, decreasing absorption

Drugs not to be Given with Milk or Milk Products

Drugs	*Rationale*
Bisacodyl (Dulcolax)	Enteric coating dissolves in basic medium such as milk
Enteric-coated aspirin (Ecotrin)	Enteric coating dissolves in basic medium such as milk
Enteric-coated erythromycin (E-Mycin, Erythrocin)	Milk enhances dissolution of the protective coating, which protects the acid-labile drug from degradation in the stomach
Methotrexate	Complexes with the alkaline medium, decreasing absorption
Potassium chloride or iodide	Complexes with alkaline medium, decreasing absorption
Tetracycline and its derivatives (Vibramycin, Sumycin, and Achromycin)	Complexes with the alkaline medium, decreasing absorption

Drugs to be Given with Food*

Classification and Drug	*Rationale*
Analgesics	
Aspirin (A.S.A., Ecotrin, Empirin); aspirin with codeine; ibuprofen (Motrin, Nuprin); indomethacin (Indocin); phenylbutazone (Butazolidin)	Food delays and reduces absorption but prevents nausea, vomiting, and GI irritation
Propoxyphene (Darvon, Wygesic)	Food increases absorption
Antineoplastic agents	
Busulfan (Myleran), cyclophosphamide (Cytoxan), hydroxyurea (Hydrea), melphalan (Alkeran), mercaptopurine (Purinethol), methotrexate, procarbazine (Matulane), and thiaguanine (Lanvis)	Generally given on a full stomach. Food may be withheld if the nausea and vomiting associated with these drugs occurs. Force fluids
Sedatives and hynotics	
Chloral hydrate (Noctec)	Food minimizes nausea and vomiting. Give with 8 oz of liquid
Psychotropic	
Phenothiazines (Thorazine, Chlorpromazine, Mellaril, others)	Food minimizes GI side effects
Diazepam (Valium)	Food increases solubilization; increases absorption
Lithium (Lithane, Eskalith)	Take after meal or snack to reduce stomach upset, tremors or weakness and to prevent laxative effect

Table continued on following page

APPENDIX C–10 **TIMING OF DRUGS** *Continued*

Drugs to be Given with Food*

Classification and Drug	***Rationale***
Antidiabetic agents	
Chlorpropamide (Diabinese), tolbutamide (Orinase)	Food delays absorption but minimizes GI upsets
Steroids	
Cortisone (Cortone), methylprednisolone (Medrol), prednisone (Deltasone), and dexamethazone (Decadron)	Absorption is delayed by food, but more consistent blood levels are established when given with food
Antilipemic agents	
Cholestyramine (Questran)	Take immediately before meals for clinical effect
Clofibrate (Atromid-S)	Food decreases absorption but minimizes GI side effects
Anticoagulants	
Dicumarol (Coumadin)	Food enhances absorption; limit foods with vitamin K
Anticonvulsants	
Phenytoin (Dilantin), carbamazepine (Tegretol)	Food enhances absorption and minimizes gastric irritation
Anti-infective drugs	
Doxycycline (Vibramycin)	In contrast to many tetracyclines, better tolerated with food
Griseofulvin (Fulvicin, Grifulvin, Grisactin)	High-fat meals enhance absorption
Isoniazid (INH)	Food decreases absorption but minimizes gastric irritation
Ketoconazole (Nizoral)	Food minimizes gastric irritation
Metronidazole (Flagyl)	Food delays absorption but minimizes gastric irritation
Minocycline (Minocin)	In contrast to many tetracyclines, better tolerated with food
Nitrofurantoin (Furadantin, Macrodantin)	Food increases absorption
Antihypertensive drugs	
Hydralazine (Apresoline)	Food enhances absorption
Hydrochlorothiazide (Dyazide, Esidrix, HydroDIURIL, Oretic, others)	Food increases absorption; prevents nausea and vomiting
Propranolol (Inderal)	Food, especially high-protein foods, enhances absorption
Reserpine (Diupres, Serpasil)	Food minimizes gastric irritation
Diuretics	
Chlorthalidone (Hygroton); triamterene (Dyazide, Dyrenium, Maxzide); chlorothiazide (Diuril); and furosemide (Lasix)	Food minimizes stomach upset and delays absorption, but bioavailability is not affected
Spironolactone (Aldactone) and hydrochlorothiazide (Dyazide, Esidrix, HydroDIURIL, Oretic, others)	Food increases absorption; prevents nausea and vomiting
Antisecretory drugs	
Cimetidine (Tagamet)	Food delays absorption, but bioavailability is not affected. Do not give concurrently with antacids
Antiarthritic and antigout	
Allopurinol (Zyloprim), phenylbutazone (Butazolidin), trihexyphenidyl (Artane)	Food delays absorption and prevents nausea and vomiting, but bioavailability is not significantly affected
Replacement supplements	
Potassium products	Food delays absorption, but minimizes GI irritation
Iron preparations	Food minimizes GI side effects

APPENDIX C-10 **TIMING OF DRUGS** *Continued*

Drugs to be Given with Food*	
Classification and Drug	***Rationale***
Antilipid agents	
Clofibrate (Atromid-S), lovastatin (Mevacor), nicotinic acid, probucol (Lorelco)	Food minimizes GI side effects

* These drugs are *too irritating* to be taken on an empty stomach, or their absorption is enhanced when taken immediately before, during, or after meals or with milk.

APPENDIX C-11 **DRUGS REQUIRING INCREASED AMOUNTS OF FLUIDS***

Drugs	**Rationale**
Aspirin, iron preparation, methotrexate, tetracycline	Full glass of water (8 oz) promotes dispersion and dissolution of the drug and reduces the risk of esophageal or peptic ulceration or minimizes acid degradation in the stomach and enhances bioavailability
Liquid potassium chloride (K-LOR, Kaon CL, Kay Ciel, K-Lyte, others)	Liquid potassium preparations must be diluted with water to avoid GI injury. (Doses of 78 mg of potassium should be taken with at least 3 or 4 oz of water, fruit juice, or a carbonated beverage)
Ampicillin (Omnipen, Polycillin); cloxacillin (Tegopen); erythromycin stearate (Erythrocin, Wyamycin); and penicillin G (Bicillin, Pentids, Wycillin)	A full glass of water (8 oz) enhances gastric emptying and dilutes the gastric contents of these acid-labile drugs
Sulfamethoxazole/trimethoprim (Bactrim, Septra)	Enhances absorption. Reduces gastric irritation. Helps flush kidneys
Allopurinol (Zyloprim), probenecid (Benemid), and sulfonamides (Gantrisin, Thiosulfil, Gantanol)	At least 8 oz of water should be taken with these drugs; 8–10 glasses a day prevents crystalluria or formation of urinary calculi
Methylcellulose and psyllium hydrophilic mucilloid (Metamucil)	To be taken with at least 8 oz of water; a generous quantity of fluid is necessary to the bulk-forming effect of these laxatives and to prevent obstruction
Penicillamine (Cuprimine)	When prescribed for cysteinuria, about 1 pint of water should be consumed at bedtime and again during the night, when the urine is more acid
Cyclophosphamide (Cytoxan, Neosar)	To ensure prompt excretion of toxic active metabolites, drug administration should be followed by 2000–3000 ml of fluid
Cholestyramine (Questran)	High fluid intake (minimum of 6 cups) needed to prevent constipation
Activated charcoal	Mix with at least 8 oz water. Do not mix with milk or ice cream, as this will decrease effectiveness of charcoal.

* These drugs should be administered with at least 8 oz of fluid.

Specialized Tables for Modified Diets

APPENDIX D

APPENDIX D–1 **EXCHANGE LISTS FOR MEAL PLANNING**

STARCH/BREAD LIST

Each item in this list contains approximately 15 gm of carbohydrate, 3 gm of protein, a trace of fat, and 80 kcal. Whole-grain products average about 2 gm of fiber per serving. Starch exchanges can be chosen from any of the items on this list. The general rule is that:

½ cup of cereal, grain, or pasta is 1 serving.
1 oz of a bread product is 1 serving.

Cereals/Grains/Pasta

🌾 Bran cereals, concentrated	⅓ cup
🌾 Bran cereals, flaked (such as Bran Buds, All Bran)	½ cup
Bulgur (cooked)	½ cup
Cooked cereals	½ cup
Cornmeal (dry)	2½ tbsp
Grapenuts	3 tbsp
Grits (cooked)	½ cup
Other ready-to-eat unsweetened cereals	¾ cup
Pasta (cooked)	½ cup
Puffed cereal	1½ cup
Rice, white or brown (cooked)	⅓ cup
Shredded wheat	½ cup
🌾 Wheat germ	3 tbsp

Dried Beans Peas/Lentils

🌾 Beans and peas (cooked) (such as kidney, white, split, blackeye)	⅓ cup
🌾 Lentils (cooked)	⅓ cup
🌾 Baked beans	¼ cup

Starchy Vegetables

🌾 Corn	½ cup
🌾 Corn on cob, 6 in. long	1
🌾 Lima beans	½ cup
🌾 Peas, green (canned or frozen)	½ cup
🌾 Plantain	½ cup
Potato, baked	1 small (3 oz)
Potato, mashed	½ cup
🌾 Squash, winter (acorn, butternut)	¾ cup
Yam, sweet potato, plain	⅓ cup

Bread

Bagel	½ (1 oz)
Bread sticks, crisp, 4 in. long × ½ in.	2 (⅔ oz)
Croutons, low fat	1 cup
English muffin	½
Frankfurter or hamburger bun	½ (1 oz)
Pita, 6 in. across	½
Plain roll, small	1 (1 oz)
Raisin, unfrosted	1 slice (1 oz)
Rye, pumpernickel	1 slice (1 oz)
Tortilla, 6 in. across	1
White (including French, Italian)	1 slice (1 oz)
Whole wheat	1 slice (1 oz)

Crackers/Snacks

Animal crackers	8
Graham crackers, 2½ in. square	3
Matzoth	¾ oz
Melba toast	5 slices
Oyster crackers	24
Popcorn (popped, no fat added)	3 cups
Pretzels	¾ oz
Rye crisp, 2 in. × 3½ in.	4
🌾 Saltine-type crackers	6
🌾 Whole-wheat crackers, no fat added (crisp breads, such as Finn, Kavli, Wasa)	2–4 slices (¾ oz)

Starch Foods Prepared with Fat
(Count as 1 starch/bread serving, plus 1 fat serving.)

Biscuit, 2½ in. across	1
Chow mein noodles	½ cup
Corn bread, 2 in. cube	1 (2 oz)
Cracker, round butter type	6
French Fried potatoes, 2 in. to 3½ in. long	10 (1½ oz)
Muffin, plain, small	1
Pancake, 4 in. across	2
Stuffing, bread (prepared)	¼ cup
Taco shell, 6 in. across	2
Waffle, 4½ in. square	1
🌾 Whole wheat crackers, fat added (such as Triscuits)	4–6 (1 oz)

🌾 3 gm or more of fiber per serving

MEAT LIST

Each serving of meat and substitutes on this list contains about 7 gm of protein. The amount of fat and number of kilocalories vary, depending on what kind of meat or substitute is chosen. The list is divided into 3 parts based on the amount of fat and kilocalories: lean meat, medium-fat meat, and high-fat meat. One ounce (meat exchange) of each of these included:

	Carbohydrate (gm)	Protein (gm)	Fat (gm)	Kilocalories
Lean	0	7	3	55
Medim-Fat	0	7	5	75
High-Fat	0	7	8	100

Lean Meat and Substitutes *(One exchange is equal to any one of the following items.)*		
Beef	USDA Good or Choice grades of lean beef, such as round, sirloin, and flank steak; tenderloin; and chipped beef	1 oz
Pork	Lean pork, such as fresh ham; canned, cured, or boiled ham ; Canadian bacon , tenderloin	1 oz
Veal	All cuts are lean except for veal cutlets (ground or cubed). Examples of lean veal are chops and roasts	1 oz
Poultry	Chicken, turkey, Cornish hen (without skin)	1 oz
Fish	All fresh and frozen fish	1 oz
	Crab, lobster, scallops, shrimp, clams (fresh or canned in water)	2 oz
	Oysters	6 medium
	Tuna (canned in water)	¼ cup
	Herring (uncreamed or smoked)	1 oz
	Sardines (caned)	2 medium
Wild Game	Venison, rabbit, squirrel	1 oz
	Pheasant, duck, goose (without skin)	1 oz
Cheese	Any cottage cheese	¼ cup
	Grated parmesan	2 tbsp
	Diet cheeses (with less than 55 kcal per ounce)	1 oz
Other	95% fat-free luncheon meat	1 oz
	Egg whites	3 whites
	Egg substitutes with less than 55 kcal per ½ cup	¼ cup

Medium-Fat Meat and Substitutes *(One exchange is equal to any one of the following items.)*		
Beef	Most beef products fall into this category: Examples are all ground beef, roast (rib, chuck, rump), steak (cubed, Porterhouse, T-bone), and meatloaf	1 oz
Pork	Most pork products fall into this category. Examples are chops, loin roast, Boston butt, cutlets	1 oz
Lamb	Most lamb products fall into this category. Examples are chops, leg, and roast	1 oz
Veal	Cutlet (ground or cubed, unbreaded)	1 oz
Poultry	Chicken (with skin), domestic duck or goose (well-drained of fat), ground turkey	1 oz
Fish	Tuna (canned in oil and drained)	¼ cup
	Salmon (canned)	¼ cup
Cheese	Skim or part-skim milk cheeses, such as:	
	Ricotta	¼ cup
	Mozzarella	1 oz
	Diet cheeses (with 56–80 kcal per ounce)	1 oz
Other	86% fat-free luncheon meat	1 oz
	Egg (high in cholesterol, limit to 3 per week)	1
	Egg substitutes with 56–80 kcal per ¼ cup	¼ cup
	Tofu (2½ in. × 2¾ in. × 1 in.)	4 oz
	Liver, heart, kidney, sweetbreads (high in cholesterol)	1 oz

Table continued on following page

High-Fat Meat and Substitutes

(One exchange is equal to any one of the following items.)

Remember, these items are high in saturated fat, cholesterol, and kilocalories, and should be used only 3 times per week.

Beef	Most USDA Prime cuts of beef, such as ribs, corned beef	1 oz
Pork	Spareribs, ground pork, pork sausage (patty or link)	1 oz
Lamb	Patties (ground lamb)	1 oz
Fish	Any fried fish product	1 oz
Cheese	All regular cheeses, such as American, Blue, Cheddar, Monterey, Swiss	1 oz
Other	Luncheon meat, such as bologna, salami, pimento loaf	1 oz
	Sausage, such as Polish, Italian	1 oz
	Knockwurst, smoked	1 oz
	Bratwurst	1 oz
	Frankfurter (turkey or chicken)	1 frank (10/lb)
	Peanut butter (contains unsaturated fat)	1 tbsp
	Count as 1 high-fat meat plus 1 fat exchange:	
	Frankfurter (beef, pork, or combination)	1 frank (10/lb)

VEGETABLE LIST

Each vegetable serving on this list contains about 5 gm of carbohydrate, 2 gm of protein, and 25 kcal. Vegetables contain 2–3 gm of dietary fiber.

Vegetables are a good source of vitamins and minerals. Fresh and frozen vegetables have more vitamins and less added salt. Rinsing canned vegetables removes much of the salt.

Unless otherwise noted, the serving size for vegetables (1 vegetable exchange) is:

½ cup of cooked vegetables or vegetable juice
1 cup of raw vegetables

Artichoke (½ medium)
Asparagus
Beans (green, wax, Italian)
Bean sprouts
Beets
Broccoli
Brussels sprouts
Cabbage, cooked
Carrots
Cauliflower
Eggplant
Greens (collard, mustard, turnip)
Kohlrabi
Leeks
Mushrooms, cooked
Okra
Onions
Pea pods
Peppers (green)
Rutabaga
Sauerkraut
Spinach, cooked
Summer squash (crookneck)
Tomato (one large)
Tomato/vegetable juice
Turnips
Water chestnuts
Zucchini, cooked

Starchy vegetables such as corn, peas, and potatoes are found on the Starch/Bread list.

For free vegetables, see Free Food List.

400 mg or more of sodium per exchange

Continued

FRUIT LIST

Each item on this list contains about 15 gm of carbohydrate, and 60 kcal. Fresh, frozen, and dry fruits have about 2 gm of fiber per serving. Fruit juices contain very little dietary fiber. The carbohydrate and kilocalorie content for a fruit serving is based on the usual serving of the most commonly eaten fruits. Use fresh fruits or fruits frozen or canned without sugar added. Whole fruit is more filling than fruit juice and may be a better choice for those who are trying to lose weight. Unless otherwise noted, the serving size for 1 fruit serving is:

½ cup of fresh fruit or fruit juice
¼ cup of dried fruit

Fresh, Frozen, and Unsweetened Canned Fruit

Apple (raw, 2 in. across)	1 apple
Applesauce (unsweetened)	½ cup
Apricots (medium, raw) or	4 apricots
Apricots (canned)	½ cup, or 4 halves
Banana (9 in. long)	½ banana
Blackberries (raw)	¾ cup
Blueberries (raw)	¾ cup
Cantaloupe (5 in. across)	⅓ melon
(cubes)	1 cup
Cherries (large, raw)	12 cherries
Cherries (canned)	½ cup
Figs (raw, 2 in. across)	2 figs
Fruit cocktail (canned)	½ cup
Grapefruit (medium)	½ grapefruit
Grapefruit (segments)	¾ cup
Grapes (small)	15 grapes
Honeydew melon (medium)	⅛ melon
cubes	1 cup
Kiwi (large)	1 kiwi
Mandarin oranges	¾ cup
Mango (small)	½ mango
Nectarine (1½ in. across)	1 nectarine
Orange (2½ in. across)	1 orange
Papaya	1 cup
Peach (2¾ in. across)	1 peach, or ¾ cup
Peaches (canned)	½ cup, or 2 halves
Pear	½ large, or 1 small
Pears (canned)	½ cup or 2 halves
Persimmon (medium, native)	2 persimmons
Pineapple (raw)	¾ cup
Pineapple (canned)	⅓ cup
Plum (raw, 2 in. across)	2 plums
Pomegranate	½ pomegranate
Raspberries (raw)	1 cup
Strawberries (raw, whole)	1¼ cup
Tangerine (2½ in. across)	2 tangerines
Watermelon (cubes)	1¼ cup

Dried Fruit

Apples	4 rings
Apricots	7 halves
Dates	2½ medium
Figs	1½
Prunes	3 medium
Raisins	2 tbsp

Fruit Juice

Apple juice/cider	½ cup
Cranberry juice cocktail (regular)	⅓ cup
Grapefruit juice	½ cup
Grape juice	⅓ cup
Orange juice	½ cup
Pineapple juice	½ cup
Prune juice	⅓ cup

MILK LIST

Each serving of milk or milk products on this list contains about 12 gm of carbohydrate and 8 gm of protein. The amount of fat in milk is measured in percent of butterfat. The kilocalories vary, depending on what kind of milk is chosen. The list is divided into 3 parts based on the amount of fat and kilocalories: skim/very low-fat milk, low-fat milk, and whole milk. 1 serving (1 milk exchange) of each of these includes:

	Carbohydrate (gm)	Protein (gm)	Fat (gm)	Kilocalories
Skim/very low-fat	12	8	trace	90
Low-fat	12	8	5	120
Whole	12	8	8	150

3 gm or more of fiber per serving

Table continued on following page

Skim and very Low-Fat Milk

Skim milk	1 cup
½% milk	1 cup
1% milk	1 cup
Low-fat buttermilk	1 cup
Evaporated skim milk	½ cup
Dry nonfat milk	⅓ cup
Plain nonfat yogurt	8 oz

Low-Fat Milk

2% milk	1 cup fluid
Plain low-fat yogurt (with added nonfat milk solids)	8 oz

Whole Milk

The whole milk group has much more fat per serving than the skim and lowfat groups. Whole milk has more than 3¼% butterfat. Limit choices from the whole milk group as much as possible.

Whole milk	1 cup
Evaporated whole milk	½ cup
Whole plain yogurt	8 oz

FAT LIST

Each serving on the fat list contains 5 gm of fat and 45 kcal. The foods on the fat list contain mostly fat, although some items may also contain a small amount of protein. All fats are high in kilocalories and should be carefully measured. Everyone should modify fat intake by eating unsaturated fats instead of saturated fats. The sodium content of these foods varies widely. Check the label for sodium information.

Unsaturated Fats

Avocado	⅛ medium
Margarine	1 tsp
Margarine, diet*	1 tbsp
Mayonnaise	1 tsp
Mayonnaise, reduced-calorie*	1 tbsp
Nuts and seeds:	
Almonds, dry roasted	6 whole
Cashews, dry roasted	1 tbsp
Pecans	2 whole
Peanuts	20 small or 10 large
Walnuts	2 whole
Other nuts	1 tbsp
Seeds, pine nuts, sunflower (without shells)	1 tbsp
Pumpkin seeds	2 tsp
Oil (corn, cottonseed, safflower, soybean, sunflower, olive, peanut)	1 tsp
Olives*	10 small or 5 large
Salad dressing, mayonnaise-type	2 tsp
Salad dressing, mayonnaise-type, reduced-calorie	1 tbsp
Salad dressing (oil varieties)*	1 tbsp
* Salad dressing, reduced-calorie	2 tbsp

(Two tablespoons of low-calorie salad dressing is a free food.)

Saturated Fats

Butter	1 tsp
Bacon*	1 slice
Chitterlings	½ oz
Coconut, shredded	2 tbsp
Coffee whitener, liquid	2 tbsp
Coffee whitener, powder	4 tsp
Cream (light, coffee, table)	2 tbsp
Cream, sour	2 tbsp
Cream (heavy, whipping)	1 tbsp
Cream cheese	1 tbsp
Salt pork*	¼ oz

FREE FOODS

A *free food* is any food or drink that contains less than 20 kcal per serving. You can eat as much as you want of those items that have no serving size specified. You may eat 2 or 3 servings per day of those items that have a specific serving size. Be sure to spread them out through the day.

Drinks
Bouillon or broth without fat
Bouillon, low-sodium
Carbonated drinks, sugar-free
Carbonated water
Club soda
Cocoa powder, unsweetened (1 tbsp)
Coffee/tea
Drink mixes, sugar-free
Tonic water, sugar-free

Nonstick pan spray

Fruit
Cranberries, unsweetened (½ cup)
Rhubarb, unsweetened (½ cup)

Vegetables (raw, 1 cup)
Cabbage
Celery
Chinese cabbage
Cucumber
Green onion
Hot peppers
Mushrooms
Radishes
Zucchini

Salad greens
Endive
Escarole
Lettuce
Romaine
Spinach

Sweet substitutes
Candy, hard, sugar-free
Gelatin, sugar-free
Gum, sugar-free
Jam/jelly, sugar-free (2 tsp)
Pancake syrup, sugar-free (1–2 tbsp)
Sugar substitutes (saccharin, aspartame)
Whipped topping (2 tbsp)

Condiments
Catsup (1 tbsp)
Horseradish
Mustard
Pickles, dill, unsweetened
Salad dressing, low-calorie (2 tbsp)
Taco sauce (1 tbsp)
Vinegar

Seasonings can be very helpful in making food taste better. Be careful of how much sodium you use. Read the label, and choose those seasonings that do not contain sodium or salt.

Basil (fresh)
Celery seeds
Cinnamon
Chili powder
Chives
Curry
Dill
Flavoring extracts (vanilla, almond, walnut, peppermint, butter, lemon)
Garlic
Garlic powder
Herbs
Hot pepper sauce
Lemon
Lemon juice
Lemon pepper
Lime
Lime juice
Mint
Onion powder
Oregano
Paprika
Pepper
Pimento
Spices
Soy sauce
Soy sauce, low sodium ("lite")
Wine, used in cooking (¼ cup)
Worcestershire sauce

COMBINATION FOODS

Much of the food we eat is mixed together in various combinations. These combination foods do not fit into only 1 exchange list.

Food	Amount	Exchanges
Casseroles, homemade	1 cup (8 oz)	2 starch, 2 medium-fat meat, 1 fat
Cheese pizza, thin crust	¼ of 15 oz or ¼ of 10 in	2 starch, 1 medium-fat meat, 1 fat
Chili with beans, (commercial)	1 cup (8 oz)	2 starch, 2 medium-fat meat, 2 fat
Chow mein, (without noodles or rice)	2 cups (16 oz)	1 starch, 2 vegetable, 2 lean meat
Marcaroni and cheese	1 cup (8 oz)	2 starch, 1 medium-fat meat, 2 fat
Soup		
Bean	1 cup (8 oz)	1 starch, 1 vegetable, 1 lean meat
Chunky, all varieties	10¾ oz can	1 starch, 1 vegetable, 1 medium-fat meat
Cream (made with water)	1 cup (8 oz)	1 starch, 1 fat
Vegetable or broth	1 cup (8 oz)	1 starch

Table continued on following page

Food	Amount	Exchanges
Spaghetti and meatballs (canned)	1 cup (8 oz)	2 starch, 1 medium-fat meat, 1 fat
Sugar-free pudding (made with skim milk)	½ cup	1 starch
If beans are used as a meat substitute		
Dried beans, peas, lentils	1 cup (cooked)	2 starch, 1 lean meat

FOODS FOR OCCASIONAL USE

Moderate amounts of some foods can be used in your meal plan, despite their sugar or fat content, as long as blood-glucose control is maintained. The following list includes average exchange values for some of these foods. Because they are concentrated sources of carbohydrate, portion sizes are very small.

Food	Amount	Exchanges
Angel food cake	1/12 cake	2 starch
Cake, no icing	1/12 cake, or a 3 in. square	2 starch, 2 fat
Cookies	2 small (1¾ in. across)	1 starch, 1 fat
Frozen fruit yogurt	⅓ cup	1 starch
Gingersnaps	3	1 starch
Granola	¼ cup	1 starch, 1 fat
Granola bars	1 small	1 starch, 1 fat
Ice cream, any flavor	½ cup	1 starch, 2 fat
Ice milk, any flavor	½ cup	1 starch, 1 fat
Sherbert, any flavor	¼ cup	1 starch
Snack chips, all varieties	1 oz	1 starch, 2 fat
Vanilla wafers	6 small	1 starch, 1 fat

3 gm or more of fiber per serving.

400 mg or more of sodium per exchange.

* If more than one or two servings are eaten, these foods have 400 mg or more of sodium.

This material has been modified from *Exchange Lists for Meal Planning,* which is the basis of a meal planning system designed by a committee of the American Diabetes Association and the American Dietetic Association. Although designed primarily for people with diabetes and others who must follow special diets, the Exchange Lists are based on principles of good nutrition that apply to everyone.

APPENDIX D–2 **DIABETIC EXCHANGE VALUES FOR FAST FOODS**

Products	Serving Size	Starch/ Bread	Lean Meat	Medium-Fat Meat	Vegetables	Fruit	Fat
Arby's							
Beef and Cheddar Sandwich	1 (7 oz)	2		3			2
Chicken Breast Sandwich	1 (6.9 oz)	2½		3			2

APPENDIX D–2 **DIABETIC EXCHANGE VALUES FOR FAST FOODS** *Continued*

Products	Serving Size	Starch/ Bread	Lean Meat	Medium-Fat Meat	Vegetables	Fruit	Fat
Chicken Club Sandwich	1 (7 oz)	4		2			4
Ham and Cheese Sandwich	1 (5.5 oz)	1		3			
Roast Beef Sandwich, Regular	1 (5.2 oz)	2		2			1
Roast Beef Sandwich, King	1 (6.7 oz)	3		3			
Roast Beef Sandwich, Super	1 (8.3 oz)	3		3			1
Turkey Deluxe	1 (7 oz)	2		3			
Burger King							
Bacon Double Cheeseburger	1	2		4			2
Bagel with Bacon, Egg, Cheese	1	3		2			1
Breakfast Croissan'wich	1	1½		1			3
Cheeseburger	1	2		2			1
Chicken Bundles	1	2		1			4
Chicken Salad without Salad Dressing	1		2		1		
Chicken Specialty Sandwich	1	4		2			5
Chicken Tenders	6 pieces	1		2			
Croissant with Egg, Cheese, Ham	1	1½		2			2
Ham and Cheese Specialty Sandwich	1	3		3			1
Shrimp and Pasta Salad	1	1	1				1
Whaler Fish Sandwich	1	3		2			3
Whopper Sandwich	1	3		3			4
Whopper with Cheese	1	3		4			4
Dairy Queen							
Chicken Breast Fillet	1 (202 gm)	3		3			3
Chicken Sandwich	1 (220 gm)	3		3			5
Cone, Regular	1	2½					1
Dip Cone, Small	1	1½					2
Double Hamburger	1 (239 gm)	2		5			3
Double with Cheese	1 (210 gm)	2		4			2
Fish Sandwich	1 (170 gm)	3		2			1
French Fries, Regular	1	1½					2
Hot Dog with Chili	1 (128 gm)	1½		1			2
Hot Dog with Cheese	1 (114 gm)	1½		1			3
Single Hamburger	1 (148 gm)	2		2			1
Single with Cheese	1 (162 gm)	2		3			1
Super Hot Dog	1 (175 gm)	3		1			4
Super Hot Dog with Cheese	1 (196 gm)	3		2			4
Super Hot Dog with Chili	1 (218 gm)	3		2			4
Triple Hamburger	1 (272 gm)	2		6			3
Triple with Cheese	1 (301 gm)	2		7			3
Hardees							
Bacon and Egg Biscuit	1 (124 gm)	2		1			4
Bacon, Egg, and Cheese Biscuit	1 (137 gm)	2		2			4
Big Country Breakfast with Bacon	1 (217 gm)	3½		3			4
Big Country Breakfast with Ham	1 (284 gm)	3½		3			4
Big Country Breakfast with Sausage	1 (274 gm)	3½		4			6
Big Deluxe	1 (216 gm)	2		3			3
Biscuit 'n Gravy	1 (210 gm)	3					4
Chicken Fillet	1 (173 gm)	3		2			
Chick 'n Pasta Salad	1 (414 gm)	1½	3				
French Fries, Regular	1 (2.5 oz)	2					2

Table continued on following page

APPENDIX D–2 **DIABETIC EXCHANGE VALUES FOR FAST FOODS** *Continued*

Products	Serving Size	Starch/ Bread	Lean Meat	Medium-Fat Meat	Vege-tables	Fruit	Fat
Ham 'n Cheese	1 (149 gm)	2		2½			
Ham and Egg Biscuit	1 (138 gm)	2		1½			2
Ham, Egg, and Cheese Biscuit	1 (171 gm)	2		2			3
Mushroom 'n Swiss Burger	1 (186 gm)	2		3½			2
Roast Beef Sandwich, Big	1 (134 gm)	2		2			
Roast Beef Sandwich, Regular	1 (114 gm)	2		1			1
Jack In the Box							
Bacon Cheeseburger	1 (230 gm)	3		3			4
Breakfast Jack Sandwich	1 (126 gm)	2		2			1
Cheeseburger	1 (113 gm)	2		1½			2
Cheese Nachos	1 (170 gm)	3		1			6
Club Pita without Sauces	1 (179 gm)	2	2				
Hamburger	1 (103 gm)	2		1			1
Hot Club Supreme	1 (213 gm)	2½		3			3
Jumbo Jack Hamburger	1 (222 gm)	3		3			3
Jumbo Jack with Cheese	1 (242 gm)	3		3½			4
Moby Jack	1 (137 gm)	2½		1½			3
Onion Rings—Bag	1 (108 gm)	2½					4
Swiss and Bacon Burger	1 (187 gm)	2		3½			6
Kentucky Fried Chicken							
Buttermilk Biscuits	1 (75 gm)	2					3
Center Breast Chicken, Original Recipe	1 (107 gm)	½		3			
Center Breast, Extra Crispy	1 (135 gm)	1		3			1
Chicken Gravy	1 (78 gm)						1
Chicken Wing, Original Recipe	1 (56 gm)	½		1½			1
Chicken Wing, Extra Crispy	1 (65 gm)	½		1½			2
Drumstick, Original Recipe	1 (58 gm)		2				
Drumstick, Extra Crispy	1 (69 gm)	½		2			
Side Breast, Original Recipe	1 (95 gm)	½		3			
Side Breast, Extra Crispy	1 (98 gm)	1		2			3
Thigh, Original Recipe	1 (96 gm)	½		2			2
Thigh, Extra Crispy	1 (119 gm)	1		2			4
Long John Silver's							
Baked Fish with Sauce	1 (5.5 oz)		4				
Battered Shrimp Dinner	9 pieces	5		2			7
Breaded Shrimp Platter	21 pieces	8		1			8
Catfish Fillet Dinner	2 fillets	6		3			4
Chicken Plank (a la Carte)	1 (2.2 oz)	1		1			
Clam Chowder with Cod	1 (6.6 oz)	1		1			
Clam Dinner	1	8		2			5
Cole Slaw	1	1					1
Fish and Chicken Entree	1	6		3			4
Fish and Fryes, 3-piece Dinner	3 pieces fish	6		4			4
Fish and More	2 pieces fish	6		3			5
Fryes	1 (3 oz)	2					2
Garden Salad with Crackers	1	1		1			1
Gumbo with Cod and Shrimp	1		1		1		1
Homestyle Fish Sandwich	1	4		2			1
Homestyle Fish Sandwich Dinner	6 pieces	8		4			7
Hushpuppy	1 piece	½					½
Mixed Vegetables	1 (4 oz)				2		
Ocean Chef Salad with Crackers	1	1	3				

APPENDIX D–2 **DIABETIC EXCHANGE VALUES FOR FAST FOODS** *Continued*

Products	Serving Size	Starch/ Bread	Lean Meat	Medium-Fat Meat	Vegetables	Fruit	Fat
Seafood Platter	1	7		2			6
Seafood Salad	1 scoop	1½	2				
Seafood Salad with Crackers	1	2	2				
Shrimp and Fish Dinner	1	5		2			5
Shrimp, Fish, and Chicken Dinner	1	5		3			5
McDonald's							
Apple Pie	1 (83 gm)	2					3
Barbecue Sauce	1 (32 gm)					1	
Big Mac Hamburger	1 (215 gm)	3		3			3
Biscuit with Eggs and Sausage	1 (180 gm)	2		2			5
Biscuit with Sausage	1 (123 gm)	2		1			5
Biscuit with Spread	1 (75 gm)	2					2½
Cheeseburger	1 (114 gm)	2		1½			1
Chef Salad	1 (283 gm)			3	1		
Chicken McNuggets	1 (113 gm)	1		2			1
Chunky Chicken Salad	1 (250 gm)		3		1		
Egg McMuffin	1 (138 gm)	2		2			
English Muffin with Butter	1 (59 gm)	2					1
Filet O Fish	1 (142 gm)	2½		1			4
French Fries, Large	1 (122 gm)	3					4
French Fries, Medium	1 (97 gm)	2½					3
French Fries, Small	1 (68 gm)	2					2
Garden Salad	1 (213 gm)			1	1		
Hamburger	1 (102 gm)	2		1			1
Hashbrown Potato	1 (53 gm)	1					1½
Hot Mustard Sauce	1 (30 gm)					1	
McChicken	1	2½		2			2
McDLT Hamburger	1 (234 gm)	2½		3			4
McLean, Deluxe	1	2		3			
Pork Sausage	1 (48 gm)			1			3
Quarter Pounder Hamburger	1 (166 gm)	2		3			1
Quarter Pounder Hamburger with Cheese	1 (194 gm)	2		3½			2
Sausage McMuffin	1 (117 gm)	2		2			2
Sausage and Egg McMuffin	1 (167 gm)	2		3			2
Scrambled Eggs	1 (100 gm)		2				
Side Salad	1 (115 gm)				1		½
Sweet and Sour Sauce	1 (32 gm)					1	
Vanilla Frozen Yogurt	1 (86 gm)	1½					
Taco Bell							
Bean Burrito	1 (191 gm)	3½		1			1
Beef Burrito	1 (191 gm)	2½		2			1
Beefy Tostada	1 (196 gm)	1½		1½			2
Burrito Supreme	1 (248 gm)	3		1½			2
Enchirito	1 (213 gm)	2		2			2
Mexican Pizza	1 (269 gm)	3		3			6
Nachos	1 (106 gm)	2½					4
Nachos Bellgrande	1 (287 gm)	4		2			6
Pintos and Cheese	1 (127 gm)	1		1			1
Soft Taco	1 (92 gm)	1		1½			1
Taco Bellgrande	1 (170 gm)	1		2			3
Taco, Regular	1 (78 gm)	1	2				
Taco Light Platter	1 (488 gm)	6		3			8
Taco Salad without Salsa	1 (510 gm)	4		3½			8
Taco Salad with Salsa	1 (601 gm)	4		4			8
Taco Salad without Beans	1 (516 gm)	3		3			8
Tostada, Regular	1 (156 gm)	2		1			1

Table continued on following page

APPENDIX D–2 **DIABETIC EXCHANGE VALUES FOR FAST FOODS** *Continued*

Products	Serving Size	Starch/ Bread	Lean Meat	Medium-Fat Meat	Vege-tables	Fruit	Fat
Taco Salad with Salsa	1 (601 gm)	4		4			8
Taco Salad without Beans	1 (516 gm)	3		3			8
Tostada, Regular	1 (156 gm)	2		1			1
Wendy's							
Bacon and Cheese Potato	1 (350 gm)	3½		1			5
Bacon Cheeseburger	1 (151 gm)	2		3			2
Big Classic Hamburger on Kaiser Bun	1 (241 gm)	2		3			2
Broccoli and Cheese Potato	1 (365 gm)	3½					5
Cheese Potato	1 (350 gm)	3½		1			5
Cheese Sauce	1 (2 oz)			1			2
Chili	9 oz (256 gm)	1	3				
Chili and Cheese Potato	1 (400 gm)	4		1½			2
Double Hamburger	1 (203 gm)	2		6			
French Fries, Regular	1 serving	2					3
Kid Meal Hamburger	1 (72 gm)	1		2			
Single Hamburger Patty on White Bun	1 (127 gm)	2		3			
Double Hamburger Patty on White Bun	1 (203 gm)	2		6			
Double Hamburger Patty with Cheese	1 (221 gm)	2		6			1
Taco Salad with Taco Chips	1 (791 gm)	3		5			1

Data from Franz MJ. *Fast Food Facts.* Wayzata, MN, DCI Publishing, 1990.

APPENDIX D–3 **EXCHANGE LISTS FOR THE NATIONAL RENAL DIET**

AVERAGE CALCULATION FIGURES FOR PLANNING CHRONIC RENAL INSUFFICIENCY DIET*

Food Choices	kcal	Protein (gm)	Sodium (mg)	Phosphate (mg)
Milk	120	4.0	80	110
Milk substitutes†	140	0.5	40	30
Meat	65	7.0	25	65
Starches	90	2.0	80	35
Vegetables‡	25	1.0	15	20
Fruits	70	0.5	Trace	15
Fats	45	Trace	55	5
High-kcal choices§	100	Trace	15	5
Salt choices	—	—	250	—

* Serving sizes for each food choice are shown in the food lists in table.
† Milk substitute choices are nondairy products, which can be used in lieu of milk and milk products.
‡ Average sodium level values do not include canned vegetables. Add 250 mg sodium for canned vegetables with added salt.
§ High-kilocalorie choices are foods high in carbohydrates that contain only a trace of protein and minimal electrolytes. These should be used to raise kilocalorie intake to the desired level.

FOOD LISTS FOR CHRONIC RENAL INSUFFICIENCY DIET

Milk Choices	
Average per choice: 4 gm protein, 120 kcal, 80 mg sodium, 110 mg phosphorus	
Milk (nonfat, low-fat, whole)	½ cup
Alterna	1 cup

FOOD LISTS FOR CHRONIC RENAL INSUFFICIENCY DIET *Continued*

Buttermilk, cultured	½ cup
Chocolate milk	½ cup
Light cream or half-and-half	½ cup
Ice milk or ice cream	½ cup
Yogurt, plain or fruit flavored	½ cup
Evaporated milk	¼ cup
Cream cheese	3 tbsp
Sour cream	4 tbsp
Sherbet	1 cup
Sweetened condensed milk	¼ cup
Nondairy Milk Substitutes	
Average per choice: 0.5 gm protein, 140 kcal, 40 mg sodium, 30 mg phosphorus	
Dessert, nondairy frozen	½ cup
Dessert topping, nondairy frozen	½ cup
Liquid nondairy creamer, polyunsaturated	½ cup
Meat Choices	
Average per ounce: 7 gm protein, 65 kcal, 25 mg sodium, 65 mg phosphorus	
Prepared without Added Salt	
Beef	
Round, sirloin, flank, cubed, T-bone, and porterhouse steak; tenderloin, rib, chuck, and rump roast; ground beef and ground chuck	1 oz
Pork	
Fresh ham, tenderloin, chop, loin roast, cutlet	1 oz
Lamb	
Chop, leg, roast	1 oz
Veal	
Chop, roast, cutlet	1 oz
Poultry	
Chicken, turkey, Cornish hen, domestic duck and goose	1 oz
Fish	
All fresh and frozen fish	1 oz
Lobster, scallops, shrimp, clams	1 oz
Crab, oysters	1½ oz
Canned tuna, canned salmon (unsalted)	1 oz
Sardines* (unsalted)	1 oz
Wild game	
Venison, rabbit, squirrel, pheasant, duck, goose	1 oz
Egg	
Whole	1 large
Egg white or yolk	2 large
Low-cholesterol egg product	¼ cup
Chitterlings	2 oz
Organ meats*	1 oz
Prepared with Added Salt	
Beef	
Deli-style roast beef†	1 oz
Pork	
Boiled or deli-style ham†	1 oz
Poultry	
Deli-style chicken or turkey†	1 oz
Fish	
Canned tuna, canned salmon†	1 oz
Sardines*†	
Cheese	
Cottage†	¼ cup
High in Sodium, Phosphorus, and/or Saturated Fat (should be used in limited quantities)	
Bacon	
Frankfurters, bratwurst, Polish sausage	
Lunch meats including bologna, braunschweiger, liverwurst, picnic loaf, salami, summer sausage	
All cheeses except cottage cheese	

Table continued on following page

FOOD LISTS FOR CHRONIC RENAL INSUFFICIENCY DIET *Continued*

Starch Choices

Average per choice: 2 gm protein, 90 kcal, 80 mg sodium, 35 mg phosphorus

Breads and Rolls	
Bread (French, Italian, raisin, light rye, sourdough white)	1 slice (1 oz)
Bagel	½ small (1 oz)
Bun, hamburger or hot dog type	½
Danish pastry or sweet roll, no nuts	½ small
Dinner roll or hard roll	1 small
Doughnut	1 small
English muffin	½
Muffin, no nuts, bran or whole wheat	1 small (1 oz)
Pancake‡§	1 small
Pita or pocket bread	½ 6-in.
Tortilla, corn or	2 6-in.
flour	1 6-in.
Waffle‡§	1 small (1 oz)
Cereals and Grains	
Cereals, ready to eat, most brands§	¾ cup
Puffed rice	2 cups
Puffed wheat	1 cup
Cooked cereal	
Cream of rice or wheat, farina, Malt-O-Meal	½ cup
Oat bran or oatmeal, Ralston	⅓ cup
Corn meal, cooked	¾ cup
Grits, cooked	½ cup
Flour, all-purpose	2½ tbsp
Pasta (noodles, macaroni, spaghetti), cooked	½ cup
Pasta made with egg (egg noodles), cooked	⅓ cup
Rice, white or brown, cooked	½ cup
Starchy Vegetables	
Corn	⅓ cup or ½ ear
Green peas	¼ cup
Potatoes, boiled, mashed	½ cup
Potatoes, baked, white or sweet	1 small (3 oz)
Potatoes, french fried	½ cup or 10 small
Potatoes, hashed brown	½ cup
Squash, butternut, mashed	½ cup
Squash, winter, baked (all other varieties), cubed	1 cup
Crackers and Snacks	
Crackers (saltines, round butter)	4
Graham crackers	3 squares
Melba toast	3 oblong
RyKrisp§	3
Popcorn, plain	1½ cups popped
Potato chips	1 oz (14 chips)
Tortilla chips	¾ oz (9 chips)
Pretzels,§ sticks or rings	¾ oz (10 sticks)
Desserts	
Cake, angelfood	1/20 cake or 1 oz
Cake	2 × 2-in square or 1½ oz
Sandwich cookies†§	4
Shortbread cookies	4
Sugar cookies	4
Sugar wafers	4
Vanilla wafers	10
Fruit pie (apple, berry, cherry, peach)	⅛ pie
Sweetened gelatin	½ cup

High in Poor-Quality Protein and Phosphorus (should be used rarely and in limited quantities)

Bran cereal or muffins, Grape-Nuts, granola cereal or bars
Boxed, frozen, or canned meals, entrees, or side dishes
Pumpernickel, dark rye, whole-wheat, or oatmeal breads
Whole-wheat crackers
Whole-wheat cereals

FOOD LISTS FOR CHRONIC RENAL INSUFFICIENCY DIET *Continued*

Vegetable Choices

Average per choice: 1 gm protein, 25 kcal, 15 mg sodium, 20 mg phosphorus. See Starch List for other vegetables. Prepared or canned without added salt||

1 Cup Serving

Alfalfa sprouts
Cabbage
Celery
Cucumber (or ½ whole)
Eggplant
Endive
Escarole
Lettuce, all varieties
Pepper, green, sweet
Radishes, sliced (or 15 small)
Turnips
Watercress

½ Cup Serving

Artichoke
Bamboo shoots
Bean sprouts
Beans, green or wax
Beets
Carrots (or 1 small)
Cauliflower
Chard
Chinese cabbage
Collard greens
Kale
Kohlrabi
Mushrooms, fresh (or 4 medium)
Onions
Parsnips¶
Pumpkin
Rutabagas¶
Squash, summer
Tomato (or 1 medium)
Tomato juice, unsalted
Tomato juice, regular#
Tomato puree
Turnip greens
Vegetable juice cocktail, unsalted
Vegetable juice cocktail, regular#

¼ Cup Serving

Asparagus (or 2 spears)
Avocado (¼ whole)
Beet greens
Broccoli
Brussels sprouts
Chili pepper
Mushrooms, cooked
Mustard greens
Okra
Snow peas
Spinach
Tomato sauce

Fruit Choices

Average per choice: 0.5 gm protein, 70 kcal, 15 mg phosphorus

1 Cup Serving

Apple (1 medium)
Apple juice
Applesauce
Cranberries
Cranberry juice cocktail
Papaya nectar
Peach nectar
Pear nectar
Pear, canned or fresh (1 medium)
Tangerine (1 medium)

½ Cup Serving

Apricot nectar
Banana (½ small)
Blueberries
Figs, canned
Fruit cocktail
Grapes (15 small)
Grape juice
Grapefruit (½ medium)
Grapefruit juice
Gooseberries
Kiwifruit (½ medium)
Lemon (½ medium)
Lemon juice
Mango (½ medium)
Nectarine (½ medium)
Orange (½ medium)
Peach, canned or fresh (½ medium)
Pineapple
Plums, canned or fresh (1 medium)
Rhubarb
Strawberries
Watermelon

¼ Cup Serving

Apricots (2 halves)
Apricots, dried (2)
Blackberries
Cantaloupe (⅛ small)
Cherries
Dates (2 tbsp)
Figs, dried (1 whole)
Honeydew melon (⅛ small)
Orange juice
Papaya (¼ medium)

Table continued on following page

FOOD LISTS FOR CHRONIC RENAL INSUFFICIENCY DIET *Continued*

Prune juice	Raisins (2 tbsp)
Prunes, cooked (5)	Raspberries
Fat Choices	
Average per choice: trace protein, 45 kcal, 55 mg sodium, 5 mg phosphorus	
Unsaturated Fats	
Margarine	1 tsp
Reduced-kilocalorie margarine	1 tbsp
Mayonnaise	1 tsp
Low-kilocalorie mayonnaise	1 tbsp
Oil	
Safflower, sunflower, corn, soybean, olive, peanut, canola	1 tsp
Salad dressing, mayonnaise-type	2 tsp
Salad dressing, oil-type	1 tbsp
Low-kilocalorie salad dressing (mayonnaise-type)**	2 tbsp
Low-kilocalorie salad dressing (oil-type)**	2 tbsp
Tartar sauce	1½ tsp
Saturated Fats	
Butter	1 tsp
Coconut	2 tbsp
Powdered coffee whitener	1 tbsp
Solid shortening	1 tsp
High-Kilocalorie Choices	
Average per choice: trace protein, 100 kcal, 15 mg sodium, 20 mg potassium, 5 mg phosphorus	
Beverages (Count within fluid allowance)	
Carbonated beverages	1 cup
Fruit flavors, root beer, colas†† or pepper type	
Cranberry juice cocktail	1 cup
Fruit-flavored drink	1 cup
Kool-Aid	1 cup
Limeade	1 cup
Lemonade	1 cup
Tang	1 cup
Wine‡‡	½ cup
Frozen Desserts (Count within fluid allowance)	
Fruit ice	½ cup
Juice bar (3 oz)	1 bar
Popsicle (3 oz)	1 bar
Sorbet	½ cup
Candy and Sweets	
Candy corn	20 or 1 oz
Gumdrops	15 small
Hard candy	4 pieces
Jellybeans	10
LifeSavers or cough drops	12
Marshmallows	5 large
Honey	2 tbsp
Sugar, brown or white	2 tbsp
Jam or jelly	2 tbsp
Sugar, powdered	3 tbsp
Marmalade	2 tbsp
Syrup	2 tbsp
Butter mints	14
Fruit chews	4
Chewy fruit snacks	1 pouch
Fruit Roll-Ups	2
Cranberry sauce or relish	¼ cup
Special Low-Protein Products	
Low-protein gelled dessert	½ cup
Low-protein bread	1 slice
Low-protein cookies	2
Low-protein pasta	½ cup
Low-protein rusk	2 slices

FOOD LISTS FOR CHRONIC RENAL INSUFFICIENCY DIET *Continued*

Salt Choices	
Average per choice: 250 mg sodium	
Salt	1/8 tsp
Seasoned salts (onion, garlic)	1/8 tsp
Accent	1/4 tsp
Barbecue sauce	2 tbsp
Bouillon	1/3 cup
Catsup	1½ tbsp
Chili sauce	1½ tbsp
Dill pickle	1/6 large or ½ oz
Mustard	4 tsp
Olives, green	2 medium or 1/3 oz
Olives, black	3 large or 1 oz
Soy sauce	¾ tsp
Steak sauce	2½ tsp
Sweet pickle relish	2½ tbsp
Taco sauce	2 tbsp
Tamari sauce	¾ tsp
Teriyaki sauce	1¼ tsp
Worcestershire sauce	1 tbsp

* High phosphorus—≥100 mg/serving.
† High sodium—each serving counts as 1 meat choice and 1 salt choice.
‡ High phosphorus—≥70 mg/serving.
§ High sodium—each serving counts as 1 starch choice and 1 salt choice.
‖ For vegetables canned with salt, add 250 mg sodium and count as 1 vegetable choice and 1 salt choice.
¶ High phosphorus—≥40 mg/serving.
# Very high sodium—each serving counts as 1 vegetable choice and 2 salt choices.
** High sodium—each serving counts as 1 fat choice and 1 salt choice.
†† High phosphorus—≥20 mg/serving.
‡‡ Check with physician for recommendation regarding alcohol.
Alterna, Ross Laboratories, Columbus, OH 43216; Malt-O-Meal, Malt-O-Meal Co, Minneapolis, MN 55402; Ralston, RyKrisp, Ralston Purina Co, St Louis, MO 63164; Grape-Nuts, Kool-Aid, Tang, General Foods Corp, White Plains, NY 10625; Popsicle, Popsicle Industries Inc, Englewood, NJ 07631; LifeSavers, Nabisco Brands, Inc, East Hanover, NJ 07936; Fruit Roll-Ups, General Mills, Inc, Minneapolis, MN 55440; Accent, Pet, Inc, St Louis, MO 63102.

APPENDIX D–4 ACID–BASE ASH RESULTING FROM METABOLISM OF FOODS

Acid Ash		**Alkaline Ash**	**Neutral**
Meats	Walnuts	Milk products	Butter and margarine
Beef	Fruit	Milk	Sugars and syrups
Fish	Cranberries	Cream	Fats and oils
Fowl	Plums	Buttermilk	Beverages
Shellfish	Prunes	Nuts	Coffee
Eggs	Bread	Almonds	Tea
Cheese	Bread (all types)	Chestnuts	Starches
Peanut butter	Crackers	Coconut	
Vegetables	Macaroni	Vegetables	
Corn	Spaghetti	All types	
Lentils	Noodles	Fruit	
Fat	Dessert	Citrus	
Bacon	Cakes	All others	
Nuts	Cookies	Jams and jellies	
Brazil		Honey	
Filberts			
Peanuts			

Sources for Reliable Nutrition Information

APPENDIX E

APPENDIX E–1 **NUTRITION RESOURCES**

AGING

AARP Fulfillment
American Association of Retired Persons
Box 22738
Long Beach, CA 90801

Administration on Aging
Information Specialist
Division of Technical Information and Dissemination
Dept. of Health and Human Services
330 Independence Ave., S.W., Rm 4746
Washington, DC 20201

Alzheimer's Association
70 E. Lake St., Ste. 600
Chicago, IL 60601

National Institute on Aging
Public Affairs Officer
DHHS
Bldg. 31, Rm. 5C-35
Bethesda, MD 20892

National Osteoporosis Foundation
1625 Eye Street, N.W., Ste. 822
Washington, DC 20006

National Screening Initiative
2626 Pennsylvania Ave., N.W.
Washington, DC 20037

AIDS

Centers for Disease Control
Center for Infectious Diseases
AIDS Program
Atlanta, GA 30333

National AIDS Information Clearinghouse (NAIC)
National A-I-C
P.O. Box 6003
Rockville, MD 20850
(800) 458-5231

Task Force on Nutrition Support in AIDS
Wang Associates, Inc.
19 W. 21st St.
New York, NY 10010

U.S. Public Health Service
Hubert H. Humphrey Bldg., Rm. 725-H
Washington, DC 20201

ALLERGIES

Asthma and Allergy Foundation of America
1717 Massachusetts, Ste. 305
Washington, DC 20036

Food Allergy Center
Box 654
Greenwich, CT 06836
(800) 937-7354

Food Allergy Network
4744 Holly Ave.
Fairfax, VA 22030

National Institute of Allergy and Infectious Diseases
Office of Research Reporting and Public Response
9000 Rockville Pike
Bethesda, MD 20205

ANOREXIA

American Anorexia and Bulimia Association
418 E. 76th St.
New York, NY 10021

Anorexia Nervosa and Related Eating Disorders
P.O. Box 5102
Eugene, OR 97405

Bulimia Anorexia Self Help (BASH)
522 North New Ballas Rd., Ste. 206
St. Louis, MO 63141

Center for the Study of Anorexia and Bulimia
Resource Center
1 W. 91st St.
New York, NY 10024

National Association of Anorexia Nervosa and
Associated Disorders
P.O. Box 7
Highland Park, IL 60035

CANCER

American Cancer Society
1599 Clifton Road, N.E.
Atlanta, GA 30329-4251
(800) ACS-2345

American Institute for Cancer Research
1759 R St., N.W.
Washington, DC 20069-2012
(800) 843-8114

Leukemia Society of America, Inc.
National Headquarters
600 Third Ave.
New York, NY 10016

National Cancer Institute
Cancer Information Service
Health Promotion Sciences Branch
Division of Cancer Prevention and Control
DHHS
Blair Bldg., Rm. 414
9000 Rockville Pike
Bethesda, MD 20892-4200
(800) 4-CANCER

CARDIOVASCULAR DISEASE (CHOLESTEROL, HYPERTENSION, HEART DISEASE)

American Heart Association
National Center
7320 Greenville Ave.
Dallas, TX 75231

Cholesterol/Smoking Information
National Institutes of Health
Director, Information Services
Bldg. 31-A, Rm. 4A-21
Bethesda, MD 20892

High Blood Pressure Information Center
Information Specialist
120/80 National Institutes of Health
Bethesda, MD 20892

Information Center
NHLBI Education Programs
4733 Bethesda Ave., Ste 530
Bethesda, MD 20814

National Cholesterol Education Program
National Heart, Lung, and Blood Institute C-200
National Institutes of Health
Bethesda, MD 20892

National High Blood Pressure Education Program
Information Center
4733 Bethesda Ave., Ste. 530
Bethesda, MD 20814

DIABETES

American Diabetes Association
National Center
1660 Duke St.
P.O. Box 25757
Alexandria, VA 22314
(800) 232-3472

HCF Diabetes Foundation
P.O. Box 22124
Lexington, KY 40522

Juvenile Diabetes Foundation International
432 Park Ave., South
New York, NY 10016

National Diabetes Information Clearinghouse
National Institutes of Health
Box NDIC
Bethesda, MD 20892

Sugarfree Center
P.O. Box 114
Van Nuys, CA 91408

GASTROINTESTINAL DISEASES

American Celiac Society
45 Gifford Ave.
Jersey City, NJ 07304

American Liver Foundation
998 Pompton Ave.
Cedar Grove, NJ 07009

Celiac Sprue Association
P.O. Box 31700
Omaha, NE 68131-0700

Center for Ulcer Research and Education Foundation
11661 San Vincente Blvd., Ste. 304
Los Angeles, CA 90049

Crohn's and Colitis Foundation of America
144 Park Ave. S.
New York, NY 10016-7374

Gluten Intolerance Group
P.O. Box 23053
Seattle, WA 98102-0353

National Digestive Disease Information Clearinghouse
Box NDDIC
Bethesda, MD 30892

National Foundation for Ileitis & Colitis
444 Park Ave., South
New York, NY 10016-7374

The Community (newsletter for people with Crohn's disease and ulcerative colitis)
P.O. Box 264
Concord, MA 01742

United Ostomy Association
36 Executive Park, Ste. 120
Irvine, CA 92714

KIDNEY

American Association of Kidney Patients
1 Davis Blvd.
Suite LL1
Tampa, FL 33606

American Council on Transplantation
700 North Fairfax St., Ste. 505
Alexandria, VA 22314

National Kidney and Urologic Disease Information Clearinghouse
Box NKUDIC
Bethesda, MD 20892

National Kidney Foundation, Inc.
30 East 33rd St.
New York, NY 10016

PEDIATRICS

American Cleft Palate–Craniofacial Association
1218 Grandview Ave.
Pittsburgh, PA 15211

Beech-Nut Nutrition Corporation
P.O. Box 127
Fort Washington, PA 19034

Children's Foundation
1420 New York Ave. N.W., Ste. 800
Washington, DC 20005

Gerber Products Company
445 State St.
Fremont, MI 49412

Mead Johnson
Nutrition Division
2400 W. Pennsylvania St.
Evansville, IN 47721

USDHHS
Office of Child Development
200 Independence Ave., S.W.
Washington, DC 20201

PREGNANCY AND LACTATION

Healthy Mother Coalition
Directory of Educational Materials
U.S. Department of Health and Human Services
200 Independence Ave., S.W.
Room 740-G
Washington, DC 20201

La Leche League International
9615 Minneapolis Ave.
Franklin Park, IL 60131-8209

Maternal and Child Health
National Center for Education
Program Director
38th and R Sts. N.W.
Washington, DC 20057

National Foundation/March of Dimes
1275 Mamaroneck Ave.
White Plains, NY 10605

WIC Supplemental Food Section
Dept. of Health Services
WIC Warehouse
1103 N B St., Ste. E
Sacramento, CA 94814

PULMONARY DISEASE

American Lung Association
1740 Broadway
New York, NY 10019

Cystic Fibrosis Foundation
6931 Arlington Road
Bethesda, MD 20814

National Heart, Lung, and Blood Institute
Information Center/Publications
4733 Bethesda Ave., Ste. 530
Bethesda, MD 20814

OTHER

American Council on Science and Health
1995 Broadway, 18th floor
New York, NY 10023

American Dietetic Association
216 West Jackson Blvd., Ste. 800
Chicago, IL 60606-6995
(800) 366-1655 (National Center for Nutrition and Dietetics consumer hotline)

American Medical Association
Department of Foods and Nutrition
515 North State St.
Chicago, IL 60610

American National Red Cross
Food and Nutrition Consultant
17th and D N.W.
National Headquarters
Washington, DC 20006

American Public Health Association
1015 Fifteenth St., N.W.
Washington, DC 20005

Arthritis Foundation National Office
3400 Peachtree Road, N.E.
Atlanta, GA 30326

Center for Science in the Public Interest (CSPI)
1755 S St., N.W.
Washington, DC 20009

Community Nutrition Institute
1146 19th St., N.W.
Washington, DC 20036

Consumer Health Information Research Institute (CHIRI)
National Patient Education Library
3521 Broadway
Kansas City, MO 64111

Food and Drug Administration
Public Information Office
Park Office Center 3101
Park Center Drive
Alexandria, VA 22302

Food and Nutrition Information Center
National Agricultural Library Bldg., Rm. 304
10301 Baltimore Blvd.
Beltsville, MD 20705

Food Research and Action Center (FRAC)
2011 I St., N.W.
Washington, DC 20006

International Food Information Council
1331 Pennsylvania Ave., N.E., Ste. 707
Washington, DC 20004

Metropolitan Life Insurance Company
Health and Welfare Division
One Madison Ave.
New York, NY 10010

National Association for Sickle Cell Disease
3345 Wilshire Blvd, Ste. 1106
Los Angeles, CA 90010-1880

National Council Against Health Fraud
P.O. Box 1276
Loma Linda, CA 92354

National Dairy Council
11 North Canal St.
Chicago, IL 60606

National Live Stock and Meat Board
Nutrition Research Department
444 North Michigan Ave.
Chicago, IL 60611

National Nutritional Consortium
1635 I St., Ste. 1
Washington, DC 20036

Nutrition Foundation, Inc.
Office of Education and Public Affairs
888 Seventeenth St., N.W.
Washington, DC 20006

President's Council on Physical Fitness and Sports
Director of Information
DHHS
405 Fifth St., N.W., Ste. 7103
Washington, DC 20001

Society for Nutrition Education
2001 Killebrew Dr., Ste. 340
Minneapolis, MN 55425-1882

U.S. Department of Agriculture
Washington, DC 202050
Agricultural Research Service
Extension Service
Food and Nutrition Service
Office of Information

SUBSTANCE ABUSE

Alateen (for members 12–20 years of age whose lives have been adversely affected by someone else's drinking problem)
c/o Al-Anon Family Group Headquarters
P.O. Box 862
Midtown Station
New York, NY 10018

Al-Anon Family Group Headquarters
P.O. Box 862
Midtown Station
New York, NY 10018

Cocaine Anonymous World Service
3740 Overland Ave., Ste. G
Los Angeles, CA 90036

Narcotics Anonymous
P.O. Box 9999
Van Nuys, CA 91409

National Clearinghouse for Alcohol Information
Box 2345
Rockville, MD 20850

National Council on Alcoholism
733 Third Ave.
New York, NY 10017

Women for Sobriety
P.O. Box 618
Quakertown, PA 18951

World Services, Inc.
(Alcoholics Anonymous)
P.O. Box 459
Grand Central Station
New York, NY 10163

Recommended Journals and Newsletters

APPENDIX E–2 RECOMMENDED JOURNALS AND NEWSLETTERS

American Journal of Clinical Nutrition
American Journal of Nursing
American Journal of Public Health
Contemporary Nutrition (General Mills)
Dietetic Currents (Ross Laboratories)
Dairy Council Digest (National Dairy Council)
Diabetes
Diabetes Care
Diabetes Forecast
Diabetes Talk
FDA Consumer
Journal of the American College of Nutrition
Journal of the American Dietetic Association
Journal of the American Medical Association
Journal of Nutrition Education
Journal of Parenteral and Enteral Nutrition
Nutrition and the MD
Nutrition Reviews
Nutrition Today
RD (Norwich Eaton)
RN

Metric System and Conversions

APPENDIX F

APPENDIX F–1 **COMMONLY USED EQUIVALENTS**

Measure	Equivalent
60 drops	1 tsp, 5 ml, 5 gm
1 gm	1 ml
1 tsp	5 gm
3 tsp	1 tbsp
1 tbsp	15 gm
1 tbsp	1 oz
1 oz (fluid)	30 gm
4 oz	120 gm
8 oz	240 gm
16 tbsp	1 cup
1 qt	960 gm
1 lb	454 gm
1.06 qt	1 L
1 L	1000 ml

APPENDIX F–2 **CONVERSIONS TO AND FROM METRIC MEASURES**

Known	Multiply by	To Know
Length		
inches	25.4	millimeters
inches	2.54	centimeters
feet	30.48	centimeters
meters	3.281	feet
Weight		
grains	64.7999	milligrams
ounces	28.35	grams
pounds	454.0	grams
pounds	0.454	kilograms
kilograms	2.205	pounds
Capacity (Liquid)		
teaspoons	4.7	milliliters
tablespoons	14.1	milliliters
fluid ounces	29.573	milliliters
cups (8 oz)	238.0	milliliters
pints	0.473	liters
quarts	0.946	liters
Energy Units		
kilocalories	4.184	kilojoules
kilojoules	0.239	kilocalories

Temperature

To convert Celsius degrees into Fahrenheit, multiply by 9⁄5 and add 32:

$$25°C = \left(25 \times \frac{9}{5}\right) + 32° = (45 + 32) = 77°F$$

Table continued on following page

APPENDIX F–2 **CONVERSIONS TO AND FROM METRIC MEASURES** *Continued*

To convert Fahrenheit degrees into Celsius, subtract 32 and multiply by 5/9:

$$95°F = (95 - 32) \times \frac{5}{9} = 63 \times \frac{5}{9} = 35°C$$

Frequently used temperatures:

Boiling point of water	100°C	212°F
Body temperature	37°C	98.6°F
Freezing point of water	0°C	32°F

Weight

To convert pounds to kilograms, divide the pounds by 2.2:

$$\frac{160\ \text{lb}}{2.2} = 72.72\ \text{kg}$$

Height

To convert feet and inches to centimeters, multiply the inches by 2.54:

$$6\ \text{feet} = 72\ \text{inches}$$
$$72 \times 2.54 = 182.8\ \text{cm}$$

APPENDIX F–3 **CONVERSIONS OF MILLIGRAMS TO MILLIEQUIVALENTS***

To convert milligrams (mg) to milliequivalents (mEq):

$$\frac{\text{Milligrams}}{\text{Atomic weight}} \times \text{Valence} = \text{Milliequivalents}$$

Mineral Element	**Chemical Symbol**	**Atomic Weight**	**Valence**
Chlorine	Cl	35.4	1
Potassium	K	39	1
Sodium	Na	23	1
Calcium	Ca	40	2
Magnesium	Mg	24.3	2
Sulfur	S	32	
Sulfate	SO_4	96	2

Sodium (mg)	**Sodium (mEq)**
500	21.8
1000	43.5
1500	75.3
2000	87.0

APPENDIX G

Answers to NQ

■ ANSWERS TO NQ (CHAPTER 1)

1. False—No single food contains all the essential nutrients in the amounts needed for optimal health.
2. False—Food fads are characterized by exaggerated beliefs about the value of nutrition in health and disease and do not possess healing qualities.
3. True.
4. False—RDAs are based on healthy clients' nutrient needs and stand for recommended dietary allowances.
5. True.
6. False—Three to 5 servings are recommended for vegetables and 2 to 4 servings for fruit.
7. True.
8. False—Organic food just means food has been grown without synthetic pesticides or fertilizers. It does not mean it is more nutritious.
9. True.
10. True.

■ ANSWERS TO NQ (CHAPTER 2)

1. True.
2. False—This is the hydrolysis of lipids or fat. Carbohydrate yields monosaccharides.
3. False—Absorption occurs primarily in the small intestine.
4. False—Long-chain triglycerides enter the lymphatic system; short-chain and medium-chain triglycerides enter the portal circulation.
5. False—Laxatives increase the rate of transit time, thereby decreasing nutrient absorption.
6. False—Most enzymes end in "ase" (e.g., lactase).
7. True.
8. False—Villi are located in the small intestine.
9. True.
10. True.

■ ANSWERS TO NQ (CHAPTER 3)

1. False—These foods are digested to constituent amino acids before absorption just like any other protein and have no specific effect on aging.

2. False—The breed of hen determines the color of eggshell, and color is not related to its nutritional value.
3. False—Gelatin does not contain all the EAAs.
4. False—The protein requirement is at least equal to that of the young adult or may be increased.
5. True.
6. True.
7. True.
8. False—It is both a protein and kilocalorie deficiency disorder.
9. False—In addition to foods from plants, dairy products are consumed. Eggs are excluded.
10. True.

ANSWERS TO NQ (CHAPTER 4)

1. False—The FDA has labeled raw sugar as unfit for direct use as a food or a food ingredient because of the impurities it contains.
2. True.
3. True.
4. False—A blood glucose level below 70 mg/dl is called hypoglycemia; 110 mg/dl is hyperglycemia.
5. True.
6. True.
7. True.
8. False—Sucrose is table sugar.
9. True.
10. True.

ANSWERS TO NQ (CHAPTER 5)

1. False—All foods are digested by the body; it just takes a longer time to digest fats, and they are retained in the stomach longer than carbohydrate or proteins.
2. False—Many manufacturers have responded by eliminating tropical oils from processed foods. Americans currently consume less than 2% of kilocalories from tropical oils.
3. True.
4. True.
5. False—Bananas contain a trace of fat; avocados are 88% fat. However, they are both plant products, so they do not contain any cholesterol.
6. False—All fats produce 9 kcal/gm.
7. True.
8. False—Label reading is essential because some products are high in fats or saturated fats even though they do not contain cholesterol.
9. True.
10. True.

■ ANSWERS TO NQ (CHAPTER 6)

1. True.
2. True.
3. True.
4. True.
5. False—Retinol is the principal dietary source of vitamin A from animals. Beta-carotene is the principal vitamin A present in plants.
6. True.
7. True.
8. False—A deficiency of vitamin D causes rickets.
9. True.
10. False—Vitamin K is the antidote for warfarin overdose. Protamine sulfate is the antidote for heparin.

■ ANSWERS TO NQ (CHAPTER 7)

1. False—All substances are potentially toxic if the dose is large enough.
2. True.
3. True.
4. False—Vitamin D is called the sunshine vitamin because the sun facilitates the body's production of vitamin D; vitamin B_6 can be called pyridoxine, pyridoxal, or pyridoxamine.
5. False—Beriberi is caused from a thiamin deficiency; niacin deficiency causes pellagra.
6. True.
7. False—They should take niacin only under a physician's supervision because of adverse side effects, including liver damage and toxicity.
8. True.
9. False—Liver, leafy vegetables, legumes, grapefruit, and oranges are rich sources of folate. Carrots are high in vitamin A.
10. True.

■ ANSWERS TO NQ (CHAPTER 8)

1. True.
2. True.
3. True.
4. False—Both liquid and solid foods provide water.
5. False—Normal sodium levels are 135 to 145 mEq/L. Potassium levels are 3.5 to 5 mEq/L.
6. True.
7. False—Potassium is principally within the cells (intracellular). Sodium is found in extracellular fluid.
8. True.
9. False—Potassium is present in most foods; thus, dietary deficiency is rare.
10. True.

■ ANSWERS TO NQ (CHAPTER 9)

1. True.
2. False—Supplements are not recommended without laboratory testing to indicate a deficiency.
3. False—Dolomite is produced from animal bone that has accumulated lead, possibly causing lead poisoning with prolonged use.
4. False—No evidence exists to support these allegations.
5. True.
6. True.
7. False—Calcium supplements by themselves probably are not beneficial to women over 30 years of age.
8. True.
9. True.
10. True.

■ ANSWERS TO NQ (CHAPTER 10)

1. True.
2. True.
3. False—BMR stands for basal metabolic rate, the amount of energy needed to maintain involuntary physiological functions.
4. True.
5. True.
6. False—Hunger is the physiological drive to eat, whereas appetite implies a desire for specific types of food.
7. False—Salt lost in sweat can be provided from a normal diet.
8. False—Their use is warranted only for heavy exercise and/or when the temperature-humidity index is high.
9. False—A steak is undesirable because of the slow digestive process. A light meal with a high level of carbohydrate is better.
10. False—Only fats, carbohydrate, protein, and alcohol provide energy.

■ ANSWERS TO NQ (CHAPTER 11)

1. False—Assessment is gathering data, whereas interventions are actions nurses do for clients.
2. True.
3. True.
4. False—The first step is assessment. Analysis is the second step.
5. True.
6. False—This is an example of an intervention or implementation.
7. True.
8. True.
9. False—A diet history involves gathering data from an interview with the client/family concerning several aspects of diet.
10. True.

■ ANSWERS TO NQ (CHAPTER 12)

1. False—This diet is inadequate in all nutrients and should only be used for 24 to 48 hours.
2. True.
3. False—Prune and tomato juice are not allowed.
4. False—Dysphagia problems usually require a texture modification (from pureed to chopped) and possibly liquid consistency or NPO status. A soft diet addresses possible GI problems and does not relate to texture.
5. True.
6. True.
7. True.
8. True.
9. False—These are not advisable because of possible *Salmonella* contamination.
10. True.

■ ANSWERS TO NQ (CHAPTER 13)

1. True.
2. False—They are not considered nutrition support; a liter of D_5W provides only 170 kcal. IV feedings are primarily for hydration.
3. True.
4. False—These are usually better accepted if served cold.
5. False—A formulary is a list of interchangeable products that can be substituted when the one specified is not available.
6. True.
7. True.
8. False—When oral intake reaches 500 kcal or more, tube feedings can be gradually decreased.
9. True.
10. False—The head of the bed should be elevated at least 30 degrees.

■ ANSWERS TO NQ (CHAPTER 14)

1. False—These do not reflect natural instincts for required nutrients and may cause harm.
2. True.
3. True.
4. False—Although she is "eating for 2," normal energy requirements are not doubled. An additional 300 kcal are recommended during the second and third trimester.
5. False—Weight gain is individualized for each woman.
6. True.
7. True.
8. False—Breast milk is normally thin and is nutritionally adequate.
9. False—The more often an infant nurses, the more milk is produced. Milk production is most active during infant sucking.
10. True.

■ ANSWERS TO NQ (CHAPTER 15)

1. True.
2. False—Goat's milk is inadequate in folate and vitamin B_{12}; additionally, the solute load is high because of its sodium, potassium, and protein content.
3. False—Solid foods are introduced between 4 and 6 months of age, not 6 weeks.
4. False—It is one of the last because of the high frequency of allergies.
5. False—Infants benefit nutritionally from continued feedings.
6. True.
7. True.
8. True.
9. False—Breakfast is the meal skipped most frequently.
10. True.

■ ANSWERS TO NQ (CHAPTER 16)

1. False—Denture wearers need to learn to swallow liquids, then chew soft foods, and, last, bite and pulverize regular foods.
2. True.
3. False—Intake is lower as a result of menopause.
4. True.
5. False—Toxicity may occur.
6. True.
7. False—Fat-soluble vitamins are not absorbed when mineral oil is taken regularly.
8. False—Lethal amounts of cyanide are found in oils extracted from American apricot kernels.
9. False—Scientific evidence does not substantiate this theory.
10. True.

■ ANSWERS TO NQ (CHAPTER 17)

1. True.
2. True.
3. False—They believe in the "hot" and "cold" theory of food balance.
4. False—Dried beans are eaten at every meal, not tacos.
5. True.
6. True.
7. False—Normally, breakfast is light.
8. True.
9. False—Kimchi is a popular staple for Koreans, not the Japanese.
10. True.

■ ANSWERS TO NQ (CHAPTER 18)

1. False—It is one-fifth, not one-third.
2. True.
3. True.

4. False—Kwashiorkor is mainly a protein deficiency, whereas marasmus is an energy deficiency.
5. False—A deficiency of iron causes iron deficiency anemia.
6. True.
7. True.
8. False—Calcium losses are increased not decreased.
9. True.
10. False—Weight loss is especially effective.

■ ANSWERS TO NQ (CHAPTER 19)

1. False—Overweight is 10 to 20% above DBW, whereas obesity is 20% above DBW.
2. False—Appestat is a theory that proposes a set-point (appestat) that dictates how much fat a client will have.
3. True.
4. True.
5. True.
6. False—In general, although drugs may be used for weight loss, they are not the sole answer to management of obseity.
7. False—Not enough fat can be removed to affect obesity significantly.
8. False—Strict kilocaloric restriction is not advisable; high kilocaloric foods may be curtailed while providing adequate kilocalories for growth and energy.
9. True.
10. True.

■ ANSWERS TO NQ (CHAPTER 20)

1. True.
2. True.
3. False—Clients with anorexia nervosa are prone to hypokalemia.
4. False—Folate levels are low in clients with bulimia.
5. True.
6. True.
7. False—Cough mixtures could cause a disulfiram reaction and are not advocated.
8. False—This reinforces the delusion.
9. True.
10. True.

■ ANSWERS TO NQ (CHAPTER 21)

1. True.
2. False—Vitamin C excretion is increased during stressful periods.
3. False—Hypermetabolism is an increase in resting energy requirements, whereas hypercatabolism is a marked loss of protein and fat.
4. True.

5. False—A weekly weight gain at a rate of more than 2 lbs per week reflects fluid retention.
6. True.
7. False—Sepsis is bacteria in the blood; fever usually accompanies sepsis.
8. True.
9. True.
10. True.

■ ANSWERS TO NQ (CHAPTER 22)

1. False—Adequate intake is needed to prevent the tumor from "stealing" nutrients from the body.
2. True.
3. False—Straws should be used rather than wide-angle cups.
4. False—Avoid favorite foods to prevent learned aversions.
5. True.
6. True.
7. False—Severe dementia can significantly affect nutritional status.
8. False—TLC is affected by the disease and an invalid parameter for nutrition status in AIDS clients. Serial measurements of TLC can be used to measure the effectiveness of nutrition support.
9. False—Acidic beverages are irritating to oral lesions.
10. False—There is no scientific proof that it can control this condition.

■ ANSWERS TO NQ (CHAPTER 23)

1. False—Only 1 to 2% of Americans suffer from food allergies.
2. False—Cow milk allergy is attributed to protein, whereas lactose intolerance is attributed to sugar.
3. True.
4. False—Tofu contains soy and should be avoided.
5. True.
6. True.
7. True.
8. True.
9. False—Asthmatics occasionally are adversely affected by sulfites.
10. True.

■ ANSWERS TO NQ (CHAPTER 24)

1. False—Compliance is hard to achieve, and the antihypertensive and potassium-sparing effects are limited.
2. True.
3. True.
4. False—Cholesterol intake has the least effect on serum cholesterol.
5. True.
6. True.

7. True.
8. False—Fat intake should be limited to 30% of kilocalories; saturated fats should be limited to 10%.
9. False—The overall balance of harm and benefit does not favor a recommendation to drink alcohol to prevent CHD.
10. True.

■ ANSWERS TO NQ (CHAPTER 25)

1. False—Tilting the head forward during swallowing facilitates glottis closure.
2. False—Heartburn is not caused by inadequate digestion; therefore, additional enzymes are not appropriate.
3. False—The diet is dictated by client food intolerances; a bland diet may be used as a transitional diet.
4. True.
5. True.
6. True.
7. False—Malnutrition is common in clients with Crohn's disease as a result of inadequate intake and malabsorption.
8. False—A low-fiber diet is needed to allow bowel rest and prevent fiber from accumulating in the pouches.
9. False—This syndrome may occur 20 minutes to 3 hours after meals in clients who have had gastric surgery; diarrhea rather than vomiting (emesis) occurs.
10. True.

■ ANSWERS TO NQ (CHAPTER 26)

1. False—Steatosis is a result of injury to the liver, i.e., infections, nutritional deficiencies, or toxins. The most common nutritional deficiency is protein.
2. True.
3. False—These are usually well tolerated by hepatitis clients.
4. False—Laennec's cirrhosis is a result of alcoholism and malnutrition.
5. False—This vein carries nutrients from the GI tract to the liver.
6. False—Dietary composition plays only a small role in the cause of gallstones.
7. True.
8. False—Hypocalcemia can result.
9. True.
10. True.

■ ANSWERS TO NQ (CHAPTER 27)

1. True.
2. True.
3. False—Some form of carbohydrate is needed, preferably milk or carbohydrate food that contains some protein to help maintain the blood glucose until the next meal; insulin would make hypoglycemia worse.
4. True.

5. True.
6. True.
7. False—The diabetic diet is based on regular foods; dietetic foods are unnecessary.
8. False—These clients produce little or no insulin; oral hypoglycemics would not work.
9. True.
10. True.

■ ANSWERS TO NQ (CHAPTER 28)

1. True.
2. False—A high-protein, moderate-carbohydrate diet is used to prevent hypoglycemia associated with Addison's disease.
3. True.
4. False—A high-kilocalorie diet (> 3000 kcal) is required because of the elevated BMR.
5. True.
6. False—Calcium intake is needed to improve the low calcium levels.
7. True.
8. True.
9. True.
10. False—Organ meats contain large amounts of purines and should be avoided by clients with gout.

■ ANSWERS TO NQ (CHAPTER 29)

1. False—Cranberry is indicated to acidify urine and prevent *E. coli* from adhering to mucosa cells of the bladder.
2. True.
3. False—Usually 0.8 to 1 gm protein/kg is recommended; this is decreased from the normal American diet but slightly more than the RDA.
4. True.
5. False—Low-protein breads are beneficial to make the low-protein diet more palatable and increase kilocaloric intake.
6. False—Diet modification to prevent acidosis is ineffective.
7. False—Phosphorus is restricted because it is not excreted.
8. True.
9. True.
10. False—These foods need to be restricted.

Index

Note: Page numbers in *italics* refer to illustrations; page numbers followed by t refer to tables.

Hyperlipidemia *(Continued)*
secondary, 774
type and quantity of dietary fat and, 779–780
Hyperlipoproteinemia: Specific high levels of various plasma lipoproteins (very low density, low density, high density), 777, 778t
Hypermetabolism: Elevated metabolic rate, 267
in AIDS, 707
in stress, 655
Hypernatremia: Elevated serum sodium levels, 211
Hyperosmolar hyperglycemic nonketosis syndrome, 893–894
Hyperparathyroidism, 956
vs. hypoparathyroidism, 955t
Hyperphagia, 268
Hyperphosphatemia, 230
Hyperplasty: Increased numbers of fat cells.
Hypertension: A persistent elevation of systolic blood pressure above 140 mmHg and of diastolic pressure above 90 mmHg in clients less than 45 years of age, 761–773
causes of, 762
in Black Americans, 524
in elderly, 489
management of, 764–766
alcohol in, 772
calcium in, 771–772
nonpharmacologic therapies in, 764–765, 767t
pharmacologic therapies in, 765t–766t, 765–766
potassium in, 769, 771, 771t
sodium in, 767–768, 768t–771t
weight control in, 767
nutrition care in, 766–773
nutrition resources for, 1105
nutritional risk factors in, 762–764
pregnancy-induced, 415
prevalence of, 762, *762*
salt intake and, 17
Hyperthyroidism, 951–953
vs. hypothyroidism, 952t
Hypertonic solutions: Solutions that have a greater osmolality than plasma, 202
Hypertrophy: Increase in size due to increased number of body cells, 587–588
Hyperuricemia: Elevated serum uric acid.
fasting and, 594
fat oxidation and, 132
Hypoalbuminemia, diarrhea due to, in enteral nutrition, 365
Hypocalcemia, 227–228
Hypochlorhydria: Decreased amount of hydrochloric acid in the stomach.
Hypochromic: Abnormally pale (said of erythrocytes lacking hemoglobin).
Hypodipsia: Diminished thirst, 207
Hypogeusia: Loss of taste, 42
due to cancer, 703
in elderly, 489
Hypoglycemia: Lowered glucose levels, 101, 939–943
alimentary. See *Dumping syndrome.*
diagnosis of, 941
due to diabetes mellitus, 895
fasting/organic, 940
testing for, *942*
functional, 939–940
nutritional care in, 942–943
oral glucose tolerance curves in, *940*
premenstrual syndrome and, 431t
reactive, 939–940
testing for, *941*
sample menu for, *943*
total parenteral nutrition and, 385
treatment of, 942
warning signs, causes, and treatment of, 896t
Hypoglycemic agents, oral, in diabetes mellitus, 919–920, 919t
Hypokalemia: Lowered potassium levels, 215
in infants, diabetes mellitus and, 926
in uremia, 977
Hyponatremia: Lowered serum sodium levels, 212–213
diagnostic tree for, *212*
Hypoparathyroidism, *954*, 954–955
vs. hyperparathyroidism, 955t
Hypophosphatemia, 230
Hypoproteinemia, in stress, 657
Hyposmia: Abnormally decreased sensitivity to odors.
due to cancer, 702
Hypothalamic–anterior pituitary–gonadal axis, in anorexia nervosa, 619
Hypothalamus, 268
hunger control and, 268–269
in lactation, 418–419
Hypothyroidism, 949–950
obesity and, 589
vs. hyperthyroidism, 952t
Hypotonia: Decreased strength, 186
Hypotonic solutions: Solutions that have a lesser osmolality than plasma, 202
Hypotony: Decreased tone or strength in the GI tract that deters transit time.
gastric, in diabetes mellitus, 907
Hypovolemia: Decreased circulating plasma.
in diabetes mellitus, 889
in renal disorders, 976
Hypoxemic: Lacking adequate oxygen in the blood.
Hypoxia: Reduction in oxygen supply to the tissues; in anemia, this is due to reduced oxygen-carrying capacity of the blood.

Iatrogenic illness: Adverse condition inadvertently induced by a physician or a prescribed treatment.
Ice cream, nutritive values of, 1040t–1041t
ICF. See *Intracellular fluid (ICF).*
Ideal body weight (IBW), deviations from, weight classification based on, 292t
IgE. See *Gamma E immunoglobulin (IGE).*
Ileostomy, 844–846, 845t
Ileus: Failure of the gastrointestinal tract to function properly in propelling intestinal contents to be expelled.
Illness, appetite and, 321
children during, nutritional needs of, 478
effect of, on nutrient requirements, 321
psychosocial needs and, 320–321, *322*
Immobilization, nutritional effects of, 681
Immune function, depressed, in AIDS, 713
in cancer, 705–706
in elderly, 492
Immune response, nutrient deficiency and, 667
Immunocompetence: The ability to produce an immune response after exposure to an allergen.
in cancer, 698
Immunologic system, food allergies and, 728
Immunopolysaccharides, function of, 102t
Immunosuppression: Diminished ability to fight infection, 347
in transplants, 716–717, 717t
Immunotherapy: Treatment with preformed antibodies administered to enhance the host's response to harmful substances or conditions, e.g., tumors.
Impact, product information for, 1053t
Impaction: Hardened feces that may block the intestinal tract, 41, 490, 604
Implementation: Actual carrying out of interventions, 304–309
client education in, 305t, 305–307, *306*
referrals in, 307t, 307–309, 308t
Imuran, side effects of, 717t
Infant(s). See also *Children; Newborn(s); Toddler(s).*
Canadian recommended nutrient intakes for, 1066t–1067t
choline deficiency in, 193
developmental milestones in, 453t–454t
fat-soluble vitamin requirements for, 152t
feeding progression of, 452–457
food allergy diagnosis in, 731
food allergy risk in, 743–744, 744t
full-term, nutritional requirements for, 445
hypercalcemia and, 227
hypokalemia in, diabetes mellitus and, 926
introduction of foods to, 454–456
low birth weight, nutritional requirements for, 446
macrosomia in, diabetes mellitus and, 925
NCHS growth percentiles in, 1076–1077
neuromuscular maturation of, 452, 454
nutrition resource referral chart for, 308t
nutritional requirements for, 445–446
nutritional status of, effect of breast milk on, 423–424
nutrition-related problems of, 457–465
baby bottle tooth decay in, 460–461, *461*

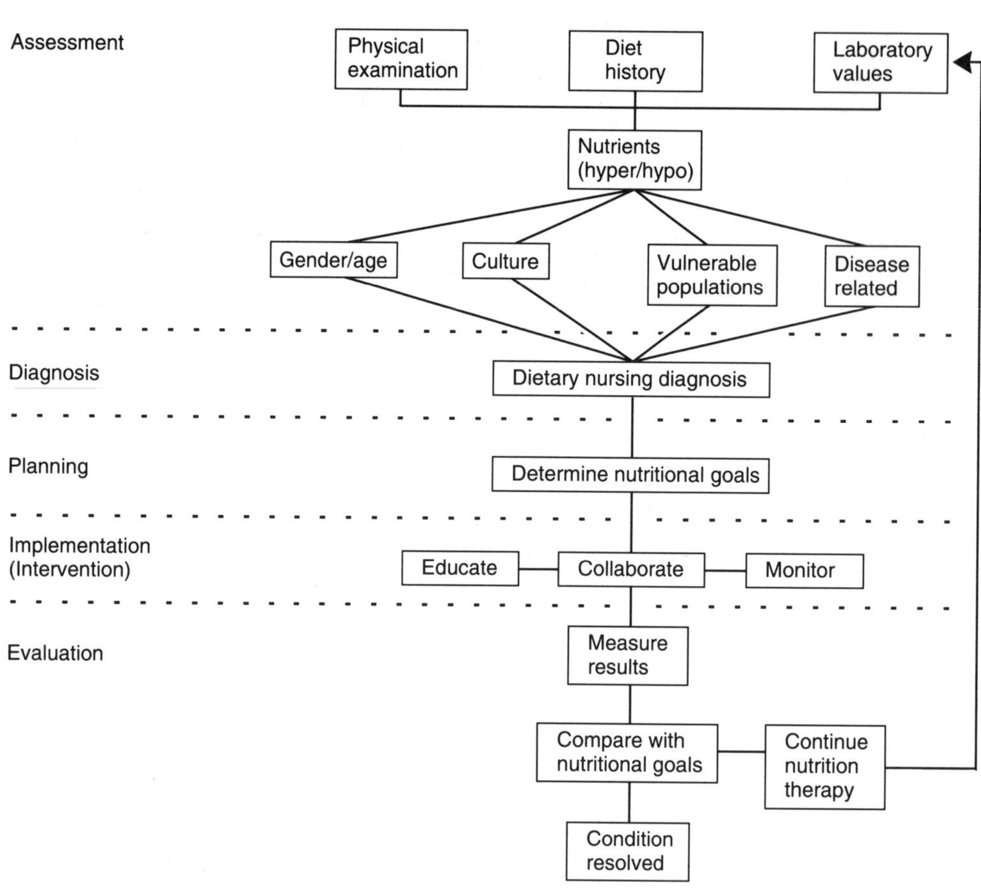

Nursing process
Nutritional care
Assessment
Physical examination
Diet history
Laboratory values
Nutrients (hyper/hypo)
Gender/age
Culture
Vulnerable populations
Disease related
Diagnosis
Dietary nursing diagnosis
Planning
Determine nutritional goals
Implementation (Intervention)
Educate
Collaborate
Monitor
Evaluation
Measure results
Compare with nutritional goals
Continue nutrition therapy
Condition resolved

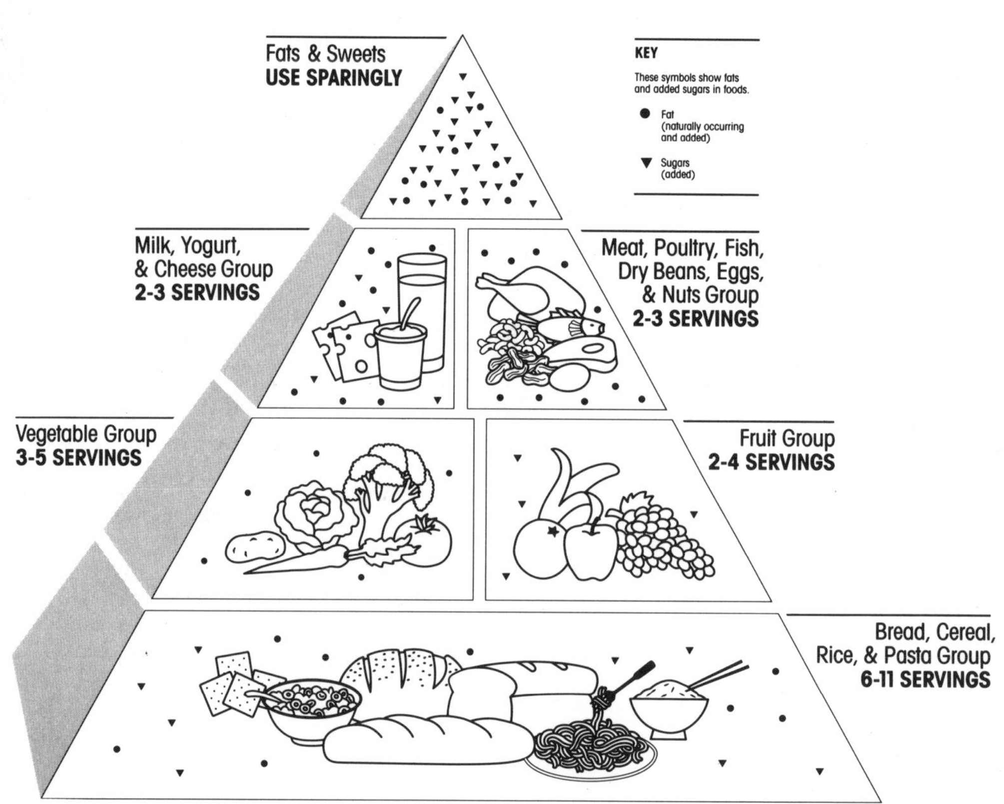

Fats & Sweets
USE SPARINGLY
KEY
These symbols show fats and added sugars in foods.
Fat (naturally occurring and added)
Sugars (added)
Milk, Yogurt, & Cheese Group
2-3 SERVINGS
Meat, Poultry, Fish, Dry Beans, Eggs, & Nuts Group
2-3 SERVINGS
Vegetable Group
3-5 SERVINGS
Fruit Group
2-4 SERVINGS
Bread, Cereal, Rice, & Pasta Group
6-11 SERVINGS